Yamada's Atlas of Gastroenterology

Yamada's Atlas of Gastroenterology

Fifth Edition

Edited by

Editor-in-Chief
Daniel K. Podolsky MD
President
University of Texas Southwestern Medical Center
Professor of Internal Medicine
Department of Internal Medicine
University of Texas Southwestern Medical School
Dallas, TX, USA

Associate Editors
Michael Camilleri MD
Executive Dean for Development
Atherton and Winifred W. Bean Professor
Professor of Medicine, Physiology and Pharmacology
Distinguished Investigator, Mayo Clinic
Rochester, MN, USA

J. Gregory Fitz MD FAASLD
Executive Vice President for Academic Affairs and Provost
University of Texas Southwestern Medical Center
Dean
Professor of Internal Medicine
Department of Internal Medicine
University of Texas Southwestern Medical School
Dallas, TX, USA

Anthony N. Kalloo MD
Professor of Medicine
Johns Hopkins University School of Medicine
Director, Division of Gastroenterology & Hepatology
Johns Hopkins Hospital
Baltimore, MD, USA

Fergus Shanahan MD
Professor and Chair
Department of Medicine
Director, Alimentary Pharmabiotic Centre
University College Cork, National University of Ireland
Cork, Ireland

Timothy C. Wang MD
Chief, Division of Digestive and Liver Diseases
Silberberg Professor of Medicine
Department of Medicine and Irving Cancer Research Center
Columbia University Medical Center
New York, NY, USA

WILEY Blackwell

This edition first published 2016 © 2016 by John Wiley and Sons Ltd.
Fourth Edition © 2009, Blackwell Publishing Ltd.

Registered office: John Wiley & Sons, Ltd, The Atrium, Southern Gate, Chichester, West Sussex, PO19 8SQ, UK

Editorial offices: 9600 Garsington Road, Oxford, OX4 2DQ, UK
The Atrium, Southern Gate, Chichester, West Sussex, PO19 8SQ, UK
111 River Street, Hoboken, NJ 07030-5774, USA

For details of our global editorial offices, for customer services and for information about how to apply for permission to reuse the copyright material in this book please see our website at www.wiley.com/wiley-blackwell

The right of the author to be identified as the author of this work has been asserted in accordance with the UK Copyright, Designs and Patents Act 1988.

Library of Congress Cataloging-in-Publication Data are available

ISBN: 9781118496435

A catalogue record for this book is available from the British Library.

Wiley also publishes its books in a variety of electronic formats. Some content that appears in print may not be available in electronic books.

Cover images: Reproduced from figures within the book. See the captions for (from left to right on the front cover) figures 16.13, 32.10c, 59.13, 77.15d, 68.12, 76.6a, and 76.6b for more details.

Cover design by John Wiley & Sons Ltd.

Set in 9.5/12pt MinionPro-Regular by Toppan Best-set Premedia Limited
Printed and bound in Malaysia by Vivar Printing Sdn Bhd

1   2016

Contents

List of contributors, ix

Preface, xix

About the companion website, xxi

PART 1 Anatomy and development

1 Esophagus: anatomy and structural anomalies, 3
 Ikuo Hirano

2 Stomach and duodenum: anatomy and structural
 anomalies, 13
 Eric Goldberg and Jean-Pierre Raufman

3 Small intestine: anatomy and structural anomalies, 19
 Deborah C. Rubin and Jacob C. Langer

4 Colon: anatomy and structural anomalies, 24
 Konstantin Umanskiy and Jeffrey B. Matthews

5 Pancreas: anatomy and structural anomalies, 30
 David G. Heidt, Michael W. Mulholland,
 and Diane M. Simeone

6 Abdominal cavity: anatomy, structural anomalies,
 and hernias, 36
 Kevin P. Murphy, Michael M. Maher,
 and Owen J. O'Connor

7 Gallbladder and biliary tract: anatomy and structural
 anomalies, 43
 Theodore H. Welling

8 Liver: anatomy, microscopic structure, and cell types, 50
 Gary C. Kanel

PART 2 Gastrointestinal diseases

A Esophagus

9 Motility disorders of the esophagus, 61
 Joan W. Chen, John E. Pandolfino, and Peter J. Kahrilas

10 Gastroesophageal reflux disease, 72
 Kumar Krishnan, John E. Pandolfino, and Peter J. Kahrilas

11 Eosinophilic esophagitis, 82
 Yael Haberman Ziv, Margaret H. Collins,
 and Marc E. Rothenberg

12 Esophageal infections and disorders associated with
 acquired immunodeficiency syndrome, 85
 C. Mel Wilcox

13 Esophageal neoplasms, 93
 Adam J. Bass and Anil K. Rustgi

14 Miscellaneous diseases of the esophagus: foreign
 bodies, physical injury, and systemic and dermatological
 diseases, 102
 Seth D. Crockett, Evan S. Dellon, and Nicholas J. Shaheen

B Stomach

15 Disorders of gastric emptying, 115
 Henry P. Parkman

16 Peptic ulcer disease, 124
 Jonathan R. White, Krish Ragunath, and John C. Atherton

17 Zollinger–Ellison syndrome, 135
 Robert T. Jensen

18 Gastritis and gastropathy, 140
 David Y. Graham and Robert M. Genta

19 Tumors of the stomach, 149
 Emad M. El-Omar and Chun-Ying Wu

20 Miscellaneous diseases of the stomach, 153
 Tamas A. Gonda and Yanghee Woo

C Small intestine

21 Dysmotility of the small intestine and colon, 157
 Michael Camilleri, Silvia Delgado-Aros,
 and Lawrence Szarka

22 Bacterial, viral, and toxic causes of diarrhea,
 gastroenteritis, and anorectal infections, 170
 Gail A. Hecht, Jerrold R. Turner, and Phillip I. Tarr

23 Chronic infections of the small intestine, 177
 George T. Fantry, Lori E. Fantry, Stephen P. James,
 and David H. Alpers

24 Disorders of epithelial transport, metabolism,
 and digestion in the small intestine, 184
 Richard J. Grand

25 Short bowel syndrome, 189
 Richard N. Fedorak, Leah M. Gramlich, and Lana Bistritz

26 Tumors of the small intestine, 202
    Barbara H. Jung and Maria Rosario Ferreira

27 Miscellaneous diseases of the small intestine, 208
    Marc S. Levin

D Inflammatory Bowel Disease

28 Ulcerative colitis: clinical manifestations
    and management, 216
    *William F. Stenson, William J. Tremaine,
    and Russell D. Cohen*

29 Crohn's disease: clinical manifestations
    and management, 225
    Gil Y. Melmed and Stephan R. Targan

E Colon

30 Polyps of the colon and rectum, 234
    Daniel C. Chung and John J. Garber III

31 Malignant tumors of the colon, 238
    Jay Luther and Andrew T. Chan

32 Polyposis syndromes, 246
    Randall W. Burt, Mary P. Bronner, and Kory W. Jasperson

33 Colorectal cancer screening, 266
    Uri Ladabaum

34 Anorectal diseases, 270
    Adil E. Bharucha and Arnold Wald

F Pancreas

35 Acute pancreatitis, 287
    Hana Algül and Roland M. Schmid II

36 Chronic pancreatitis, 307
    Joachim Mössner, Albrecht Hoffmeister, and Julia Mayerle

37 Hereditary diseases of the pancreas, 317
    Carlos G. Micames and Jonathan A. Cohn

38 Cystic lesions of the pancreas, 324
    James J. Farrell

39 Neuroendocrine tumors of the pancreas, 329
    Peter J. Carolan and Daniel C. Chung

G Gallbladder and biliary tract

40 Gallstones, 335
    Piero Portincasa and David Q. H. Wang

41 Primary sclerosing cholangitis and
    other cholangiopathies, 354
    Russell H. Wiesner and Kymberly D.S. Watt

42 Cystic diseases of the liver and biliary tract, 361
    James L. Buxbaum and Shelly C. Lu

43 Tumors of the biliary tract, 368
    Tushar Patel

H Liver

44 Acute viral hepatitis, 374
    Marc G. Ghany and T. Jake Liang

45 Chronic hepatitis B viral infection, 387
    Robert G. Gish

46 Hepatitis C virus infection, 392
    Raymond T. Chung and Andrew Tai

47 Drug-induced liver disease, 397
    Frank V. Schiødt and William M. Lee

48 Autoimmune hepatitis, 405
    Richard Taubert and Michael P. Manns

49 Primary biliary cirrhosis, 409
    Marlyn J. Mayo and Dwain L. Thiele

50 Hemochromatosis, 415
    Paul C. Adams

51 Metabolic diseases of the liver, 419
    Ronald J. Sokol and Mark A. Lovell

52 Alcoholic liver disease, 423
    Jose Altamirano, Eric S. Orman, and Ramon Bataller

53 Nonalcoholic fatty liver disease, 428
    M. Shadab Siddiqui and Arun J. Sanyal

54 Hepatic fibrosis, 436
    Don C. Rockey

55 Approach to the patient with ascites
    and its complications, 447
    Guadalupe Garcia-Tsao

56 Liver transplantation, 459
    Alyson N. Fox and Robert S. Brown, Jr.

57 Hepatocellular carcinoma, 465
    Jorge A. Marrero and Amit Singal

58 Liver abscess, 469
    Roman E. Perri and David S. Raiford

59 Vascular diseases of the liver, 472
    Susana Seijo and Laurie D. DeLeve

I Miscellaneous

60 Intraabdominal abscesses and fistulae, 477
    Peter Irving and Nyree Griffin

61 Diseases of the peritoneum, retroperitoneum, mesentery,
    and omentum, 484
    Jennifer W. Harris, Scott D. Stevens, and B. Mark Evers

62 Obesity: treatment and complications, 491
Louis A. Chaptini and Steven Peikin

63 Bariatric surgery and complications, 495
Obos Ekhaese, Danny O. Jacobs, and Russell LaForte

64 Complications of AIDS and other immunodeficiency
states, 501
*Phillip D. Smith, Nirag C. Jhala, C. Mel Wilcox,
and Edward N. Janoff*

65 Gastrointestinal manifestations of immunological
disorders, 509
Paula O'Leary and Fergus Shanahan

66 Parasitic diseases: protozoa, 515
Ellen Li and Samuel L. Stanley Jr.

67 Helminthic infections of the gastrointestinal tract
and liver, 524
Thormika Keo, John Leung, and Joel V. Weinstock

68 Gastrointestinal manifestations of systemic
diseases, 544
Eran Israeli and Charles N. Bernstein

69 Skin lesions associated with gastrointestinal and liver
diseases, 554
Kim B. Yancey and Travis W. Vandergriff

70 Oral manifestation of gastrointestinal diseases, 574
Vidyasagar Ramappa and Yashwant R. Mahida

71 Intestinal ischemia and vasculitides, 582
Juan-Ramón Malagelada and Carolina Malagelada

72 Radiation injury in the gastrointestinal tract, 597
Steven M. Cohn and Stephen J. Bickston

PART 3 Diagnostic and therapeutic modalities in gastroenterology

A Endoscopic

73 Upper gastrointestinal endoscopy, 605
*Ebubekir S. Daglilar, Abdurrahman Kadayifci,
and William R. Brugge*

74 Capsule and small bowel endoscopy, 621
Jonathan A. Leighton and Shabana F. Pasha

75 Colonoscopy and flexible sigmoidoscopy, 626
*Peter H. Rubin, Steven Naymagon, Christopher B. Williams,
and Jerome D. Waye*

76 Endoscopic retrograde cholangiopancreatography:
diagnostic and therapeutic, 634
Mustafa A. Arain and Martin L. Freeman

77 Gastrointestinal dilation and stent placement, 643
Shayan Irani and Richard A. Kozarek

78 Management of upper gastrointestinal hemorrhage related
to portal hypertension, 664
Tinsay A. Woreta and Zhiping Li

79 Endoscopic diagnosis and treatment of nonvariceal upper
gastrointestinal hemorrhage, 675
David J. Bjorkman

80 Endoscopic therapy for polyps and tumors, 680
Mouen A. Khashab, Sergey V. Kantsevoy, and Heiko Pohl

81 Laparoscopy and laparotomy, 698
Ricardo Zorron and Gustavo Carvalho

82 Natural orifice translumenal endoscopic
surgery (NOTES), 702
Vivek Kumbhari and Anthony N. Kalloo

B Imaging

83 Plain and contrast radiology, 722
Marc S. Levine and Stephen E. Rubesin

84 Transabdominal sonography, 732
Stephanie F. Coquia, Linda C. Chu, and Ulrike M. Hamper

85 Endoscopic ultrasonography, 741
Marcia Irene Canto and Mouen A. Khashab

86 Computed tomography of the gastrointestinal tract, 756
*Siva P. Raman, Karen M. Horton, Pamela T. Johnson,
and Elliot K. Fishman*

87 Magnetic resonance imaging, 768
Diane Bergin

88 Positron emission tomography in the
gastrointestinal tract, 782
*Manuela Matesan, Jonathan Sham, James Park,
and Satoshi Minoshima*

89 Radionuclide imaging of the gastrointestinal tract, 804
Harvey A. Ziessman

90 Abdominal angiography, 820
Kyung Jae Cho

91 Interventional radiology, 842
*Todd R. Schlachter, Julius Chapiro, Rafael Duran,
Vania Tacher, Camila Zamboni, Luke Higgins, and
Jean-Francois Henri Geschwind*

C Pathology

92 Liver biopsy and histopathological diagnosis, 860
Sugantha Govindarajan

93 Endoscopic mucosal biopsy: histopathological
interpretation, 878
Elizabeth Montgomery and Anthony N. Kalloo

Index, 931

List of contributors

Paul C. Adams MD
Professor of Medicine
Chief of Gastroenterology
Western University
London, ON, Canada

Hana Algül MD MPH
Professor
Head, Outpatient Clinic for Pancreatic Diseases
Technical University of Munich
Munich, Germany

Jose Altamirano MD MMSc
Research Scientist
Institut d'Investigacions Biomèdiques August Pi i Sunyer (IDIBAPS)
Barcelona, Spain

David H. Alpers MD
William B Kountz Professor of Medicine and Geriatrics
Department of Internal Medicine
Center for Human Nutrition
Washington University School of Medicine
St Louis, MO, USA

Mustafa A. Arain MD
Assistant Professor of Medicine
Division of Gastroenterology
University of Minnesota
Minneapolis, MN, USA

John C. Atherton MD FRCP
Professor of Gastroenterology
Nottingham Digestive Diseases Centre
National Institute of Health Research Biomedical Research Unit in
Gastrointestinal and Liver Diseases at
Nottingham University Hospitals NHS Trust
School of Medicine, University of Nottingham
Nottingham, UK

Adam J. Bass MD
Assistant Professor of Medicine
Dana-Farber Cancer Institute and Harvard Medical School
Boston, MA, USA

Ramon Bataller MD
Associate Professor
Departments of Medicine and Nutrition
The University of North Carolina at Chapel Hill
Chapel Hill, NC, USA

Diane Bergin MD
Consultant Radiologist
Department of Radiology
University Hospital Galway
Galway, Ireland

Charles N. Bernstein MD
Distinguished Professor of Medicine
Head, Section of Gastroenterology
Director University of Manitoba IBD Clinical and Research Centre
Bingham Chair in Gastroenterology
College of Medicine
Faculty of Health Science
University of Manitoba
Winnipeg, MB, Canada

Adil E. Bharucha MD MBBS
Professor of Medicine
Department of Gastroenterology and Hepatology
Mayo Clinic College of Medicine
Rochester, MN, USA

Lana Bistritz MD
Associate Professor
Division of Gastroenterology
University of Alberta
Edmonton, AB, Canada

Stephen J. Bickston MD AGAF
Professor of Internal Medicine
Associate Chair for Gastroenterology
Virginia Commonwealth University
Richmond, VA, USA

David J. Bjorkman MD MSPH
Dean and Executive Director of Medical Affairs
Charles E. Schmidt College of Medicine
Florida Atlantic University
Boca Raton, FL, USA

Mary P. Bronner MD
HCI Senior Leader
Division Chief of Anatomic Pathology and Molecular Oncology
University of Utah
Salt Lake City, CT, USA

Robert S. Brown Jr. MD MPH
Vice Chair, Transitions of Care, Department of Medicine
Interim Chief, Division of Gastroenterology and Hepatology
Weill Cornell Medical College
Director, Center for Liver Disease and Transplantation
New York Presbyterian Hospital
New York, NY, USA

William R. Brugge MD
Professor of Medicine
Harvard Medical School
Director, Pancreas Biliary Center
Massachusetts General Hospital
Boston, MA, USA

Randall W. Burt MD
Barnes Professor of Medicine
University of Utah
Director of High Risk Clinics
Huntsman Cancer Institute
Salt Lake City, UT, USA

James L. Buxbaum MD
Assistant Professor of Clinical Medicine
Director of Endoscopy
Los Angeles County Medical Center
Department of Medicine
Division of Gastroenterology and Liver Diseases
Keck School of Medicine
University of Southern California
Los Angeles, CA, USA

Michael Camilleri MD
Executive Dean for Development
Atherton and Winifred W. Bean Professor
Professor of Medicine, Physiology and Pharmacology
Distinguished Investigator, Mayo Clinic
Rochester, MN, USA

Marcia Irene Canto MD MHS
Professor of Medicine and Oncology
Johns Hopkins University
Baltimore, MD, USA

Peter J. Carolan MD
Instructor in Medicine
Gastrointestinal Unit
Massachusetts General Hospital
Boston, MA, USA

Gustavo Carvalho MD PhD
Associate Professor
Department of General Surgery
Universidade Federal de Pernambuco
Recife, Brazil

Andrew T. Chan MD MPH
Vice-Chief, Gastroenterology
Chief, Clinical and Translational Epidemiology Unit
Massachusetts General Hospital;
Associate Professor of Medicine
Harvard Medical School
Boston, MA, USA

Julius Chapiro MD
Post-Doctoral Research Fellow
Johns Hopkins University School of Medicine
Baltimore, MD, USA

Louis A. Chaptini MD
Assistant Professor of Medicine
Section of Digestive Diseases
Yale University School of Medicine
New Haven, CT, USA

Joan W. Chen MD
Clinical Lecturer, Internal Medicine
University of Michigan
Ann Arbor, MI, USA

Kyung Jae Cho MD FSIR
William Martel Emeritus Professor of Radiology
Department of Radiology
Vascular and Interventional Radiology
University of Michigan Cardiovascular Center
Ann Arbor, MI, USA

Linda C. Chu MD
Assistant Professor of Radiology
Russell H. Morgan Department of Radiology and Radiological Science
Johns Hopkins University School of Medicine
Baltimore, MD, USA

Daniel C. Chung MD
Clinical Chief, Gastrointestinal Unit
Director, GI Cancer Genetics Program
Massachusetts General Hospital
Associate Professor of Medicine
Harvard Medical School
Boston, MA, USA

Raymond T. Chung MD
Director of Hepatology and Liver Center
Vice-Chief, Gastroenterology
Massachusetts General Hospital
Boston, MA, USA

Russell D. Cohen MD
Professor of Medicine, Pritzker School of Medicine
Director, Inflammatory Bowel Disease Center
Co-Director, Advanced IBD Fellowship Program
University of Chicago Medical Center
Chicago, IL, USA

Jonathan A. Cohn MD
Professor of Medicine
Associate Professor of Cell Biology
Professor of Pediatrics
Department of Medicine
Duke University School of Medicine
Durham, NC, USA

Steven M. Cohn MD PhD
Paul Janssen Professor of Medicine and Immunology
Division of Gastroenterology and Hepatology
University of Virginia School of Medicine
Charlottesville, VA, USA

Margaret H. Collins MD
Professor
Division of Gastroenterology, Hepatology, and Nutrition
Cincinnati Children's Hospital Medical Center
Cincinnati, OH, USA

Stephanie F. Coquia MD
Assistant Professor of Radiology
Russell H. Morgan Department of Radiology and Radiological Science
Johns Hopkins University School of Medicine
Baltimore, MD, USA

Seth D. Crockett MD MPH
Assistant Professor
Division of Gastroenterology and Hepatology
University of North Carolina School of Medicine
Chapel Hill, NC, USA

Ebubekir S. Daglilar MD
Division of Gastroenterology
Massachusetts General Hospital
Boston, MA, USA

Laurie D. DeLeve MD PhD FAASLD
Professor of Medicine
Senior Associate Chair for Scientific Affairs
Division of Gastrointestinal and Liver Diseases
Keck School of Medicine of USC
Los Angeles, CA, USA

Silvia Delgado-Aros MD MSc
Metge Adjunt Servei Digestiu
Hospital del Mar (IMAS)
Barcelona, Spain

Evan S. Dellon MD MPH
Associate Professor
Center for Esophageal Diseases and Swallowing
Division of Gastroenterology and Hepatology
University of North Carolina School of Medicine
Chapel Hill, NC, USA

Rafael Duran MD
Radiologist
Johns Hopkins Radiology
Johns Hopkins University School of Medicine
Baltimore, MD, USA

Obos Ekhaese DO
Assistant Professor
Department of Surgery
University of Texas Medical Branch
Galveston, TX, USA

Emad M. El-Omar BSc(Hons) MB ChB MD (Hons) FRCP(Edin) FRSE
Professor of Gastroenterology/Honorary Consultant Physician
Institute of Medical Sciences
School of Medicine & Dentistry
Aberdeen University
Aberdeen, UK

B. Mark Evers MD
Professor and Vice-Chair for Research
Department of Surgery
Director, Lucille P. Markey Cancer Center
University of Kentucky
Lexington, KY, USA

George T. Fantry MD
Associate Professor of Medicine
Assistant Dean for Student Research and Education
University of Maryland School of Medicine
Baltimore, MD, USA

Lori E. Fantry MD MPH
Associate Professor of Medicine
Institute of Human Virology
Department of Medicine
University of Maryland School of Medicine
Baltimore, MD, USA

James J. Farrell MD
Director, Yale Center for Pancreatic Disease
Associate Professor of Medicine
Yale University
New Haven, CT, USA

Richard N. Fedorak MD FRCPC
Professor
Division of Gastroenterology
University of Alberta
Edmonton, AB, Canada

Maria Rosario Ferreira MD
Assistant Professor of Medicine
Division of Gastroenterology and Hepatology
Northwestern University, Feinberg School of Medicine
Evanston, IL, USA

Elliot K. Fishman MD
Professor of Radiology and Radiological Science
Johns Hopkins University
Baltimore, MD, USA

Alyson N. Fox MD MSCE
Center for Liver Disease and Transplantation
Columbia University College of Physicians and Surgeons
New York Presbyterian Hospital
New York, NY, USA

Martin L. Freeman MD FACG FASGE
Professor of Medicine
President, American Pancreatic Association 2012–2013
Director, Division of Gastroenterology
Hepatology and Nutrition Medical Director
Total Pancreatectomy and Islet Autotransplantation Director
Advanced Endoscopy and Pancreaticobiliary Endoscopy Fellowship
University of Minnesota
Minneapolis, MN, USA

John J. Garber III MD
Assistant in Medicine
Gastrointestinal Unit
Massachusetts General Hospital
Instructor, Harvard Medical School
Boston, MA, USA

Guadalupe Garcia-Tsao MD
Professor of Medicine
Yale University School of Medicine;
New Haven, CT;
Chief, Digestive Diseases
VA-CT Healthcare System
West Haven, CT, USA

Robert M. Genta MD
Clinical Professor
Miraca Life Sciences Research Institute
Irving, TX;
Pathology, Internal Medicine
University of Texas Southwestern Medical Center
Dallas, TX, USA

Jean-Francois Henri Geschwind MD
Professor of Radiology, Surgery and Oncology
Director, Vascular and Interventional Radiology
Director, Interventional Radiology Center
Johns Hopkins University School of Medicine
Baltimore, MD, USA

Marc G. Ghany MD MHSc
Investigator
Liver Diseases Branch
National Institute of Diabetes and Digestive and Kidney Diseases
National Institutes of Health
Bethesda, MD, USA

Robert G. Gish MD
Clinical Professor of Medicine (Consultant)
Stanford University, Palo Alto, CA;
Hepatitis B Foundation, Doylestown, PA, USA

Eric Goldberg MD
Associate Professor of Medicine
Division of Gastroenterology and Hepatology
University of Maryland, School of Medicine
Baltimore, MD, USA

Tamas A. Gonda MD
Assistant Professor of Medicine
Department of Medicine
Columbia University Medical Center
New York, NY, USA

Sugantha Govindarajan MD
Professor
Department of Pathology
USC Keck School of Medicine
Downey, CA, USA

David Y. Graham MD MACG
Professor
Medicine-Gastroenterology
Baylor College of Medicine
Houston, TX. USA

Leah M. Gramlich MD FRCP
Professor of Medicine
Division of Gastroenterology
University of Alberta
Edmonton, AB, Canada

Richard J. Grand MD
Director Emeritus, Inflammatory Bowel Disease Center;
Director Emeritus, Clinical and Translational Study Unit
Professor of Pediatrics, Harvard Medical School
Boston Children's Hospital
Boston, MA, USA

Nyree Griffin MD FRCR
Consultant Radiologist
Guys and St Thomas' Hospital NHS Foundation Trust
London, UK

Yael Haberman Ziv MD PhD
Assistant Professor
Division of Gastroenterology, Hepatology and Nutrition
Cincinnati Children's Hospital Medical Center
Cincinnati, OH, USA

Ulrike M. Hamper MD MBA FACR
Professor of Radiology, Urology and Pathology
Director, Division of Ultrasound
Russell H. Morgan Department of Radiology and Radiological Science
Johns Hopkins University School of Medicine
Baltimore, MD, USA

Jennifer W. Harris MD
Department of Surgery
University of Kentucky
Lexington, KY, USA

Gail A. Hecht MD
Professor
Division Director, Gastroenterology and Nutrition
Department of Medicine
Loyola University Medical Centre
Maywood, IL, USA

David G. Heidt MD
Clinical Lecturer/Fellow
Department of Surgery, Section of General Surgery
University of Michigan
Ann Arbor, MI, USA

Luke Higgins MD PhD
Medical Resident
Department of Radiology
Johns Hopkins University School of Medicine
Baltimore, MD, USA

Ikuo Hirano MD
Professor of Medicine
Department of Gastroenterology and Hepatology
Northwestern University School of Medicine
Chicago, IL, USA

Albrecht Hoffmeister MD
Division of Gastroenterology and Rheumatology
Department of Medicine, Neurology, and Dermatology
University Hospital of Leipzig
Leipzig, Germany

Karen M. Horton MD
Executive Vice Chair of Radiology
Professor of Radiology and Radiological Science
Johns Hopkins University
Baltimore, MD, USA

Shayan Irani MBBS MD
Head of Pancreatic Center of Excellence
Digestive Disease Institute
Virginia Mason Medical Center
Seattle, WA, USA

Peter Irving MA MD FRCP
Consultant Gastroenterologist
Guy's and St Thomas' Hospital NHS Foundation Trust
London, UK

Eran Israeli MD
Head, IBD Unit
Institute of Gastroenterology and Liver Disease
Hadassah-Hebrew University Medical Centre
Jerusalem, Israel

Danny O. Jacobs MD MPH FACS
Executive Vice President and Provost
Dean, School of Medicine
Thomas N. and Gleaves T. James Distinguished Chair
Provost Administration
University of Texas Medical Branch
Galveston, TX, USA

Stephen P. James MD
Director, Division of Digestive Diseases and Nutrition
National Institute of Diabetes and Digestive and Kidney Disease
Bethesda, MD, USA

Edward N. Janoff MD
Professor of Medicine, Immunology and Microbiology
Director, Mucosal and Vaccine Research Center (MAVRC)
University of Colorado Denver;
Denver Veterans Affairs Medical Center
Denver, CO, USA

Kory W. Jasperson MS CGC
Certified Genetic Counselor
Department of Medical Affairs
Ambry Genetics
Aliso Viejo, CA, USA

Robert T. Jensen MD
Digestive Diseases Branch
National Institute of Diabetes and Digestive and Kidney Diseases
National Institutes of Health
Bethesda, MD, USA

Nirag C. Jhala MD
Professor, Pathology and Laboratory Medicine
Director, Anatomic Pathology/Cytology
Temple University
Philadelphia, PA, USA

Pamela T. Johnson MD
Associate Professor
Department of Radiology and Radiological Science
Johns Hopkins University
Baltimore, MD, USA

Barbara H. Jung MD
Associate Professor of Medicine
University of Illinois at Chicago
Chicago, IL, USA

Abdurrahman Kadayifci MD
Research Fellow
Division of Gastroenterology
Massachusetts General Hospital
Boston, MA, USA,
Division of Gastroenterology
Faculty of Medicine
University of Gaziantep, Turkey

Peter J. Kahrilas MD
Gilbert H. Marquardt Professor in Medicine
Division of Gastroenterology and Hepatology
Northwestern University Feinberg School of Medicine
Chicago, IL, USA

Anthony N. Kalloo MD
Professor of Medicine
Johns Hopkins University School of Medicine
Director, Division of Gastroenterology & Hepatology
Johns Hopkins Hospital
Baltimore, MD, USA

Gary C. Kanel MD
Professor of Clinical Pathology
Department of Pathology
University of Southern California Keck School of Medicine
Los Angeles, CA, USA

Sergey V. Kantsevoy MD
Assistant Professor of Medicine
Johns Hopkins University School of Medicine
Baltimore, MD, USA

Thormika Keo MD PhD
Clinical Fellow Division of Gastroenterology-Hepatology
Tufts Medical Center
Boston, MA, USA

Mouen A. Khashab MD
Associate Professor of Medicine
Department of Gastroenterology
Johns Hopkins University
Baltimore, MD, USA

Richard A. Kozarek MD
Clinical Professor of Medicine
University of Washington;
Executive Director
Digestive Disease Institute
Virginia Mason Medical Center
Seattle, WA, USA

Kumar Krishnan MD
Assistant Professor of Medicine
Division of Gastroenterology
Houston Methodist Hospital
Weill Cornell Medical College
Houston, TX, USA

Vivek Kumbhari MD
Fellow in Advanced Endoscopy
Johns Hopkins University School of Medicine
Baltimore, MD, USA

Uri Ladabaum MD MS
Professor of Medicine
Division of Gastroenterology and Hepatology
Stanford University School of Medicine
Stanford, CA, USA

Russell LaForte MD
Assistant Professor
Division of General Internal Medicine
University of Texas Medical Branch
Galveston, TX, USA

Jacob C. Langer MD
Professor of Surgery
University of Toronto
Chief of General Surgery
Hospital for Sick Children
Toronto, ON, Canada

William M. Lee MD
Professor
Department of Internal Medicine and Biomedical Engineering
University of Texas Southwestern Medical Center
Dallas, TX, USA

Jonathan A. Leighton MD
Professor of Medicine
Division of Gastroenterology and Hepatology
Mayo Clinic
Scottsdale, AZ, USA

John Leung MD
Assistant Professor of Medicine
Director, Food Allergy Center
Division of Gastroenterology-Hepatology
Tufts Medical Center
Boston, MA, USA

Marc S. Levin MD AGAF
Professor of Medicine
Division of Gastroenterology and VA Medicine
Washington University in St. Louis
School of Medicine and Staff Physician, Gastroenterology
VA St. Louis Health Care System
St. Louis, MO, USA

Marc S. Levine MD
Chief, Gastrointestinal Radiology
University of Pennsylvania Medical Center;
Professor of Radiology and Advisory Dean
Hospital of the University of Pennsylvania
Philadelphia, PA, USA

Ellen Li MD PhD
Chief, Division of Gastroenterology and Hepatology
Professor of Medicine
Director of GI Translational Research
Stony Brook University Hospital
Stony Brook, NY, USA

Zhiping Li MD
Associate Professor of Medicine
Director of Hepatology
Johns Hopkins University
Baltimore, MD, USA

T. Jake Liang MD
Chief, Liver Diseases Branch
Deputy Director of Translational Research
National Institute of Diabetes and Digestive and Kidney Diseases
National Institutes of Health
Bethesda, MD, USA

Mark A. Lovell MD
Professor, Vice-Chair for Pediatric Pathology at UCD
Chair of the Department of Pathology at TCH
University of Colorado School of Medicine and Children's Hospital Colorado
Aurora, CO, USA

Shelly C. Lu MD
Professor of Medicine
Director, Division of Gastroenterology
Cedars-Sinai Medical Center
Los Angeles, CA, USA

Jay Luther MD
Clinical and Research Instructor
Department of Gastroenterology
Massachusetts General Hospital;
Harvard Medical School
Boston, MA, USA

Michael M. Maher MD
Professor of Radiology
Department of Radiology
University College Cork
Cork, Ireland

Yashwant R. Mahida
Professor of Medicine
Faculty of Medicine & Health Sciences
University of Nottingham and Nottingham
University Hospitals NHS Trust
Nottingham, UK

Carolina Malagelada MD PhD
Attending Gastroenterologist
Hospital Universitari Vall d'Hebron
Autonomous University of Barcelona
Barcelona, Spain

Juan-Ramón Malagelada MD
Associate Professor of Medicine
Hospital Universitari Vall d'Hebron
Autonomous University of Barcelona
Barcelona, Spain

Michael P. Manns MD
Professor and Chairman
Director of Gastroenterology, Hepatology and Endocrinology
Hannover Medical School
Hannover, Germany

Jorge A. Marrero MD MS
Professor of Medicine
Chief of Clinical Hepatology
Medical Director of Liver Transplantation
University of Texas Southwestern Medical Center
Dallas, TX, USA

Manuela Matesan MD PhD
Assistant Professor
Department of Radiology
University of Washington
Seattle, WA, USA

Jeffrey B. Matthews MD
Surgeon-in-Chief and Chairman, Department of Surgery
Dallas B. Phemister Professor of Surgery
The University of Chicago Medicine and Biological Sciences
Chicago, IL, USA

Julia Mayerle MD
Professor of Medicine
Division of Internal Medicine A
University Hospital of Ernst-Moritz-Arndt-University of Greifswald
Greifswald, Germany

Marlyn J. Mayo MD
Associate Professor of Internal Medicine
University of Texas Southwestern Medical Center
Dallas, TX, USA

Gil Y. Melmed MD MS
Director, Clinical Inflammatory Bowel Disease
Inflammatory Bowel & Immunobiology Research Institute
Cedars-Sinai Medical Center
Los Angeles, CA, USA

Carlos G. Micames MD
Adjunct Professor of Medicine
Division of Gastroenterology
University of Puerto Rico
Rio Piedras, Puerto Rico

Satoshi Minoshima MD PhD
Professor and Chair of Radiology
Department of Radiology
University of Utah
Salt Lake City, UT, USA

Elizabeth Montgomery MD
Professor of Pathology, Oncology, and Orthopedic Surgery
Department of Pathology
Johns Hopkins University
Baltimore, MD, USA

Joachim Mössner MD (FACP hon)
Professor of Medicine
Director, Division of Gastroenterology and Rheumatology
Department of Medicine, Neurology and Dermatology
University Hospital of Leipzig
Leipzig, Germany

Michael W. Mulholland MD PhD
Frederick A. Coller Distinguished Professor Surgery
Chair, Department of Surgery
University of Michigan
Ann Arbor, MI, USA

Kevin P. Murphy MB MRCS FFRRCSI
Lecturer in Radiology
Cork University Hospital and University College Cork
Cork, Ireland

Steven Naymagon MD
Assistant Professor of Medicine and Gastroenterology
Icahn School of Medicine at Mount Sinai
New York, NY, USA

Owen J. O'Connor MD MRCSI FFRRCSI
Consultant Radiologist and Senior Lecturer
Cork University Hospital, Mercy University Hospital
and University College Cork
Cork, Ireland

Paula O'Leary MD FRCPI FRCPath(imm)
Senior Lecturer in Medicine and Consultant Physician
Department of Medicine
University College Cork
Cork, Ireland

Eric S. Orman MSCR
Assistant Professor of Medicine
Department of Medicine
Indiana University School of Medicine
Indianapolis, IN, USA

John E. Pandolfino MD MSCI
Hans Popper Professor of Medicine
Division Chief, Gastroenterology and Hepatology
Northwestern University Feinberg School of Medicine
Chicago, IL, USA

James Park MD
Associate Professor
Department of Surgery
University of Washington
Seattle, WA, USA

Henry P. Parkman MD
Professor of Medicine
Department of Medicine
Section of Gastroenterology
Temple University School of Medicine
Philadelphia, PA, USA

Shabana F. Pasha MD
Associate Professor of Medicine
Division of Gastroenterology and Hepatology
Mayo Clinic
Scottsdale, AZ, USA

Tushar Patel MB ChB
James C. and Sarah K. Kennedy Dean for Research
Professor of Medicine
Mayo Clinic
Jacksonville, FL, USA

Steven R. Peikin MD
Professor of Medicine
Head, Division of Gastroenterology and Liver Diseases
Cooper Medical School of Rowan University
Cooper University Hospital
Camden, NJ, USA

Roman E. Perri MD
Assistant Professor of Medicine
Division of Hepatobiliary Surgery and Liver Transplantation
Vanderbilt University Medical Center
Nashville, TN, USA

Heiko Pohl MD
Department of Gastroenterology
Dartmouth-Hitchcock Medical Center
VA White River Junctio
White River Junction, VT, USA

Piero Portincasa MD PhD
Professor of Internal Medicine
Department of Biomedical Sciences and Human Oncology
University of Bari Medical School
Bari, Italy

Krish Ragunath MD FRCP FASGE
Professor of Gastrointestinal Endoscopy
Nottingham Digestive Diseases Centre
National Institute of Health Research Biomedical Research Unit in
Gastrointestinal and Liver Diseases at Nottingham University Hospitals
NHS Trust
School of Medicine, University of Nottingham
Nottingham, UK

David S. Raiford MD
Professor of Medicine
Vanderbilt University Medical Center
Nashville, TN, USA

Siva P. Raman MD
Assistant Professor of Radiology
Department of Radiology
Johns Hopkins University
Baltimore, MD, USA

Vidyasagar Ramappa MBBS MD
Specialist Registrar in Gastroenterology
University of Nottingham and Nottingham University Hospitals NHS Trust
Nottingham, UK

Jean-Pierre Raufman MD
Professor of Medicine
Division of Gastroenterology and Hepatology
University of Maryland, School of Medicine
Baltimore, MD, USA

Don C. Rockey MD
Chairman, Department of Internal Medicine
Medical University of South Carolina
Charleston, SC, USA

Marc E. Rothenberg MD PhD
Professor of Pediatrics
Director, Division of Allergy and Immunology
Director, Cincinnati Center for Eosinophilic Disorders
Cincinnati Children's Hospital Medical Center;
University of Cincinnati College of Medicine
Cincinnati, OH, USA

Stephen E. Rubesin MD
Professor of Radiology
Hospital of the University of Pennsylvania
Philadelphia, PA, USA

Deborah C. Rubin MD AGAF
Professor of Medicine and Developmental Biology
Division of Gastroenterology/Department of Medicine
Washington University School of Medicine
Saint Louis, MO, USA

Peter H. Rubin MD
Associate Clinical Professor of Medicine and Gastroenterology
Icahn School of Medicine at Mount Sinai
New York, NY, USA

Anil K. Rustgi MD
T. Grier Miller Professor of Medicine and Genetics
Chief of Gastroenterology
American Cancer Society Professor
University of Pennsylvania Perelman School of Medicine
Philadelphia, PA, USA

Arun J. Sanyal MD MBBS ISc
Charles M. Caravati Professor in Gastroenterology
Virginia Commonwealth University
Richmond, VA, USA

Frank V. Schiødt MD
Chief of Gastroenterology and Hepatology, Dr.Sci.
Abdominalcenter K
Bispebjerg Hospital
Copenhagen
Denmark

Roland M. Schmid II MD
Professor and Direcor II. Medizinische Klinik
Specialist in Gastroenterology and Endocrinology
Technical University of Munich
Munich, Germany

Todd R. Schlachter MD
Clinical Instructor of Vascular and Interventional Oncology
Department of Radiology
Johns Hopkins University School of Medicine
Baltimore, MD, USA

Susana Seijo MD PhDtaub
Hepatic Hemodynamic Laboratory
Liver Unit, Institut de Malalties Digestives i Metaboliques
Hospital Clínic-Institut de Investigacions Biomèdiques August Pi I Sunyer
(IDIBAPS)
Barcelona, Spain

Nicholas J. Shaheen MD MPH
Professor, Center for Esophageal Diseases and Swallowing
Chief, Division of Gastroenterology and Hepatology
University of North Carolina School of Medicine
Chapel Hill, NC, USA

Jonathan Sham MD
Physician
Department of Surgery
University of Washington
Seattle, WA, USA

Fergus Shanahan MD

Professor and Chair
Department of Medicine
Director, Alimentary Pharmabiotic Centre
University College Cork, National University of Ireland
Cork, Ireland

M. Shadab Siddiqui MD

Assistant Professor of Medicine
Division of Gastroenterology, Hepatology and Nutrition
Virginia Commonwealth University
Richmond, VA, USA

Diane M. Simeone MD

Lazar J. Greenfield Professor of Surgery and Professor of Molecular and
Integrative Physiology
Director, Translational Oncology Program
Director, Pancreatic Cancer Center
Department of Surgery, Section of General Surgery
University of Michigan
Ann Arbor, MI, USA

Amit Singal MD

Associate Professor of Internal Medicine
Department of Clinical Science
University of Texas Southwestern Medical Center
Dallas, TX, USA

Phillip D. Smith MD

Mary J. Bradford Professor in Gastroenterology
Professor of Medicine and Microbiology
University of Alabama at Birmingham
Birmingham Veterans Affairs Medical Center
Birmingham, AL, USA

Ronald J. Sokol MD

Arnold Silverman MD Endowed Chair in Digestive Health
Professor and Vice Chair of Pediatrics
Chief of Pediatric Gastroenterology, Hepatology and Nutrition
University of Colorado School of Medicine
Children's Hospital Colorado
Aurora, CO, USA

Samuel L. Stanley Jr. MD

Professor Medicine
President, Stony Brook University
Stony Brook, NY, USA

William F. Stenson MD

Dr. Nicholas V. Costrini Professor of Gastroenterology
and Inflammatory Bowel Disease
Washington University School of Medicine
St Louis, MO, USA

Scott D. Stevens MD

Chief, Division of Abdominal Radiology
Associate Professor of Radiology
University of Kentucky
Lexington, KY, USA

Lawrence Szarka MD

Assistant Professor of Medicine
Department of Gastroenterology and Hepatology
Mayo Clinic
Rochester, MN, USA

Vania Tacher MD

Post-doctoral Research Fellow
John Hopkins Radiology
Johns Hopkins University School of Medicine
Baltimore, MD, USA

Andrew W. Tai MD PhD

Assistant Professor of Internal Medicine and Microbiology & Immunology
University of Michigan;
Staff Physician
VA Ann Arbor Healthcare System
Ann Arbor, MI, USA

Stephan R. Targan MD

Director, F. Widjaja Foundation Inflammatory Bowel and Immunobiology
Research Institute
Cedars Sinai Medical Center
Los Angeles, CA, USA

Phillip I. Tarr MD

Co-Leader, Pathobiology Research Unit, Department of Pediatrics
Director, Division of Pediatric Gastroenterology and Nutrition
Melvin E. Carnahan Professor of Pediatrics
Professor of Molecular Microbiology
Washington University
St. Louis, MO, USA

Richard Taubert MD

Department of Gastroenterology, Hepatology and Endocrinology
Hannover Medical School
Hannover, Germany

Dwain L. Thiele MD

Senior Associate Dean for Strategic Development
Jan and Henri Bromberg Chair in Internal Medicine
Professor of Internal Medicine
University of Texas Southwestern Medical School
Dallas, TX, USA

William J. Tremaine MD

Professor of Medicine
Department of Gastroenterology and Hepatology
Mayo Clinic College of Medicine
Rochester, MN, USA

Jerrold R. Turner MD PhD

Sara and Harold Lincoln Thompson Professor
Associate Chair, Department of Pathology
University of Chicago
Chicago, IL, USA

Konstantin Umanskiy MD FACS FASCRS

Associate Professor of Surgery
The University of Chicago Pritzker School of Medicine
Chicago, IL, USA

Travis W. Vandergriff MD

Assistant Professor of Dermatology
University of Texas Southwestern Medical Center
Dallas, TX, USA

Arnold Wald MD
Section of Gastroenterology and Hepatology
University of Wisconsin
School of Medicine and Public Health
Madison, WI, USA

David Q.-H. Wang MD PhD
Associate Professor of Medicine, Biochemistry and Molecular Biology
Division of Gastroenterology and Hepatology
Department of Internal Medicine
Saint Louis University School of Medicine
St. Louis, MO, USA

Kymberly D.S. Watt MD
Associate Professor of Medicine
Department of Gastroenterology and Hepatology
Mayo Clinic
Rochester, MN, USA

Jerome D. Waye MD
Professor of Medicine
Icahn School of Medicine at Mount Sinai
Director, Center for Advanced Colonoscopy and Polypectomy
New York, NY, USA

Joel V. Weinstock MD
Professor of Medicine
Chief of the Division of Gastroenterology-Hepatology
Tufts Medical Center
Boston, MA, USA

Theodore H. Welling MD
Associate Professor of Surgery
Co-Director, Multidisciplinary Liver Tumor Program
Section of Transplantation
University of Michigan Health System
Ann Arbor, MI, USA

Jonathan R. White MBChB MRCP
Clinical Research Fellow in Gastroenterology
Nottingham Digestive Diseases Centre, School of Medicine, University of Nottingham;
Centre for Biomolecular Sciences
University of Nottingham;
NIHR Biomedical Research Unit in Gastrointestinal and Liver Diseases at Nottingham University Hospitals NHS Trust
Nottingham, UK

Russell H. Wiesner MD
Professor of Medicine
Department of Gastroenterology and Hepatology
Mayo Clinic
Rochester, MN, USA

C. Mel Wilcox MD MSPH
Professor of Medicine
Division of Gastroenterology and Hepatology
University of Alabama at Birmingham
Birmingham, AL, USA

Christopher B. Williams
Retired

Yanghee Woo MD FACS
Associate Clinical Professor
Director, Gastrointestinal Minimally Invasive Therapy
Division of Surgical Oncology
Department of Surgery
City of Hope Medical Center
Duarte, CA, USA

Tinsay A. Woreta MD MPH
Assistant Professor of Medicine
Division of Gastroenterology and Hepatology
Johns Hopkins University
Baltimore, MD, USA

Chun-Ying Wu MD PhD MPH LL.M LL.B
Professor of Medicine, National Yang-Ming University
Professor of Law, Tunghai University
Taichung Veterans General Hospital
Taipei, Taiwan

Kim B. Yancey MD
Professor and Chair
Department of Dermatology
University of Texas Southwestern Medical Center
Dallas, TX, USA

Camila Zamboni MD
Graduate Student
Johns Hopkins University School of Medicine
Baltimore, MD, USA

Harvey A. Ziessman MD
Professor of Radiology
Russell H. Morgan Department of Radiology
Division of Nuclear Medicine
Johns Hopkins University
Baltimore, MD, USA

Ricardo Zorron MD PhD
Professor of Surgery
Director, Innovative Surgery Division
Bariatric Center
Klinikum Bremerhaven Reinkenheide
Bremerhaven, Germany

Preface

As the field of gastroenterology has evolved, a rich variety of modalities have contributed to progress in the practice of its art and science. This fifth edition of *Yamada's Atlas of Gastroenterology* endeavors to provide illustrative examples that collectively provide a pictorial survey of the field. It accompanies the publication of the sixth edition of *Yamada's Textbook of Gastroenterology*.

With these newest editions of the original *Textbook* and companion *Atlas*, editorial responsibility has transitioned to a new set of editors; however, the goals of the books remain the same. The *Textbook* continues to provide comprehensive coverage of the field, incorporating significant advances since the last edition. It is global in scope, both literally and figuratively. Figuratively in the sense that it covers all facets of gastroenterology as well as key ancillary relevant disciplines, and literally in considering the challenges encountered in the practice of gastroenterology as they may vary in different regions of the world.

This newest edition of the *Atlas* is a companion intended to fulfill those same expectations. It is a compendium of supplementary images to the varied aspects of gastroenterology covered in the *Textbook*, spanning the many technologies and related fields important to the clinical practice of gastroenterology. These include gross and microscopic anatomy, and the full range of imaging modalities and endoscopies that inform the practice of gastroenterology. In addition, the *Atlas* includes graphics that supplement those of the *Textbook* to highlight key insights into many of the topics covered in the latter.

The organization of this *Atlas* follows that of the newest edition of the *Textbook*, which itself has been refreshed in some notable ways. Most significantly, the *Textbook* now encompasses a section comprising chapters that provide the clinician with a practical approach to the most common symptoms prompting a patient to seek a gastroenterologist's expertise. These and other changes reflected in both the *Textbook* and *Atlas* are intended to make them even more useful to our readers, including students, specialty and subspecialty trainees, practicing clinicians, and academicians. The student of gastroenterology, whether entirely new to the field or seeking continued learning after many decades, will find collectively a comprehensive source to guide the intellectual and practical grasp of gastroenterology. The *Atlas* provides visual images to bring to life the substance of the *Textbook*.

Neither the *Textbook* nor the *Atlas* would be possible without the benefit of legions of mentors, colleagues, and patients who have taught the editors over the years and provided the knowledge which serves as the foundation for these newest editions. The new group of editors is deeply appreciative of the enormous efforts made by contributing authors to provide the supplementary contents of this *Atlas* as a resource to readers. We also thank the many individuals at the publisher, Wiley, who worked with us on this project to bring it to a state of completion. I am especially grateful to Ms. Julia Kanellos whose outstanding editorial support was invaluable throughout.

On behalf of all the editors, it is our hope that this *Atlas* will truly be a resource to all those interested in a deeper understanding of gastroenterology.

Daniel K. Podolsky, MD

About the companion website

Companion website

This book is accompanied by a companion website:

www.yamadagastro.com/atlas

The website includes:
- Videos from the following chapters:
  - Chapter 56, Liver transplantation
  - Chapter 58, Liver abscess
  - Chapter 63, Bariatric surgery and complications
  - Chapter 74, Capsule and small bowel endoscopy
  - Chapter 75, Colonoscopy and flexible sigmoidoscopy
  - Chapter 77, Gastrointestinal dilation and stent placement
  - Chapter 78, Management of upper gastrointestinal hemorrhage related to portal hypertension
  - Chapter 80, Endoscopic therapy for polyps and tumors
  - Chapter 81, Laparoscopy and laparotomy
  - Chapter 91, Interventional radiology
- Figures from the book, to download as PowerPoint slides

PART 1

Anatomy and development

CHAPTER 1

Esophagus: anatomy and structural anomalies

Ikuo Hirano

Northwestern University School of Medicine, Chicago, IL, USA

An understanding of the normal and abnormal histology and structure is essential to the clinical care of patients with esophageal disorders. Esophageal biopsies obtained during endoscopy sample the squamous mucosa and less commonly the lamina propria of the esophageal wall. The histologic evaluation of submucosal glands, Meissner's and Myenteric ganglia, and the muscularis propria depicted in Figure 1.1 typically requires surgical biopsy. Methods of endoscopic mucosal resection have allowed sampling of the esophageal submucosa and muscularis mucosa. Per oral esophageal myotomy may allow for histologic evaluation of deeper mural structures. Endoscopic ultrasonography can evaluate the structural integrity and anomalies of deeper structures including the muscularis propria. Extrinsic compression of the esophagus by adjacent mediastinal structures as shown in Figure 1.2 is better appreciated on radiographic barium examination, or cross sectional imaging than endoscopy. Feline esophagus, so-called eosinophilic esophagitis, is depicted in Figure 1.3 and can be mistaken for esophageal rings. The feline pattern is a transient phenomenon visualized with retching and esophageal shortening and may represent contraction of the muscularis mucosa. Upon relaxation of the esophageal musculature and distension with air insufflation, the plications disappear.

Esophageal developmental anomalies include vascular lesions, duplications and heterotopic gastric mucosa. Kartagener's syndrome leads to right-sided rather than left-sided aortic arch esophageal compression (Figure 1.4). Patients with dysphagia lusoria present with swallowing difficulties arising from extrinsic compression of the thoracic esophagus by congenital anomalies of the aortic arch, most commonly by an aberrant take-off of the right subclavian artery from the left side of the aortic arch (Figure 1.5). Congenital venous malformations illustrated in Figure 1.6 represent another vascular anomaly and are distinct from esophageal varices as vascular obstruction or portal hypertension is not present in the former. Congenital esophageal duplications assume both tubular

(Figure 1.7) and cystic (Figure 1.8 and 1.9) forms. While most are apparent before the age of 1 year, 25% can present in adults with symptoms of dysphagia. Heterotopic gastric mucosa (inlet patch) shown in Figure 1.10 is a common congenital anomaly, with a prevalence of 4% based on an autopsy series. Infrequently, this anomaly is associated with cervical esophageal stricture (Figure 1.11) and web formation (Figure 1.12). Other uncommon developmental anomalies include esophageal atresia, congenital esophageal stenosis, and bronchopulmonary foregut malformations.

Structural esophageal anomalies include esophageal rings and webs, cricopharyngeal bar, pharyngoesophageal diverticula and diffuse idiopathic skeletal hyperostosis of the cervical spine. The most widely recognized structural anomaly is the lower esophageal mucosal or Schatzki ring that is found in about 10% of adults. It is one of the most common causes of dysphagia and food impaction, although the majority of Schatzki rings are asymptomatic. The inner diameter of the ring is a critical determinant for dysphagia and can be assessed on endoscopic retroflexed view (Figure 1.13), or ingestion of a barium tablet of known diameter. A cricopharyngeal bar is found in 5%–19% of radiographic studies of the pharynx. The majority are not associated with dysphagia. Pathologic and physiologic studies support shared features between symptomatic cricopharyngeal bars and Zenker's diverticula. The patient in Figure 1.14 has both a cricopharyngeal bar and small diverticulum. Therapeutic options of symptomatic cricopharyngeal bars and Zenker's diverticula include both endoscopic and surgical approaches. Epiphrenic diverticula arise from the distal esophagus and are often associated with an underlying spastic esophageal motility disorder (Figure 1.15a and b). With time, the diverticula can increase in size resulting in food retention, bezoar formation and symptoms of regurgitation (Figure 1.16). Treatment for large or symptomatic epiphrenic diverticula is most commonly surgical and includes not only a diverticulectomy but also treatment of the underlying motility disorder. Intramural

Yamada's Atlas of Gastroenterology, Fifth Edition. Edited by Daniel K. Podolsky, Michael Camilleri, J. Gregory Fitz, Anthony N. Kalloo, Fergus Shanahan, and Timothy C. Wang.
© 2016 John Wiley & Sons, Ltd. Published 2016 by John Wiley & Sons, Ltd.
Companion website: www.yamadagastro.com/atlas

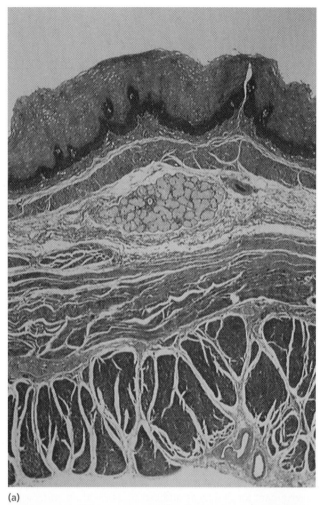

(a)

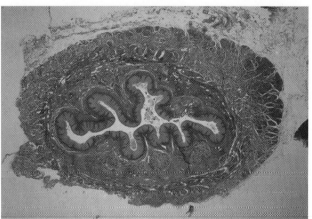

(b)

Figure 1.1 (a) This cross section (×2.5) from the middle third of the esophagus has a mixture of skeletal and predominantly smooth muscle in the muscularis propria. The submucosal glands are clearly shown. An esophageal cardiac gland in which a small focus of glandular epithelium interrupts the squamous mucosa is a normal finding, seen in at least 1% of all esophagi. (b) Longitudinal section of esophageal wall (×10). Source: Courtesy of Rodger C. Haggitt, M.D., Seattle, WA.

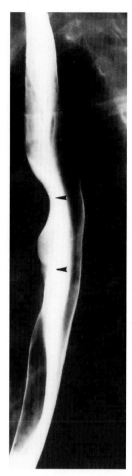

Figure 1.2 Barium esophagram shows normal indentation of the esophageal lumen but the aorta (top arrowhead) and left mainstem bronchus (bottom arrowhead).

pseudodiverticulosis is a rare finding best appreciated on barium esophagram rather than upper endoscopy. The disorder results from dilation on excretory ducts of submucosal esophageal glands and is associated with proximal esophageal strictures and esophageal candidiasis. Diffuse idiopathic skeletal hyperostosis (DISH) of the cervical spine leads to ossification of the anterolateral ligaments and enthuses. Dysphagia may result from extrinsic compression of the cervical esophagus (Figure 1.17).

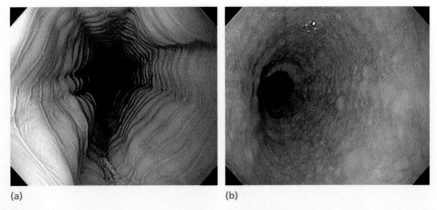

(a)   (b)

Figure 1.3 (a) Feline esophagus demonstrating rippling or plications of the esophageal mucosa. This is a transient occurrence and disappears with continued observation. **(b)** Eosinophilic esophagitis can present with a similar appearance but the rings persist with air insufflation and less tightly spaced apart.

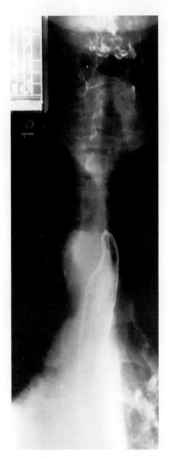

Figure 1.4 Barium esophagram of a patient with Kartagener's syndrome showing esophageal compression by the right sided aortic arch and dextrocardia.

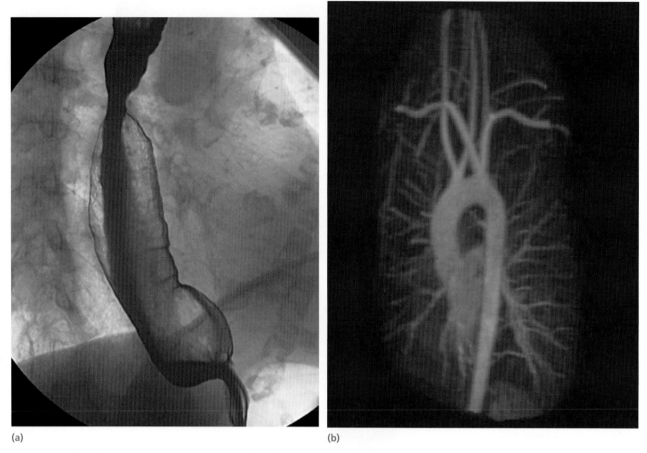

(a) (b)

Figure 1.5 Dysphagia lusoria represents symptomatic esophageal compression by a vascular anomaly of the aortic arch, most commonly by an aberrant right subclavian artery. **(a)** Barium esophagram in a patient reveals thoracic esophageal compression by an aberrant right subclavian artery posterior to the esophagus. **(b)** Magnetic resonance angiography reveals an aberrant right subclavian artery arising from the aortic arch.

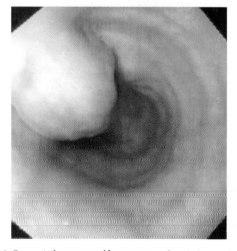

Figure 1.6 Congenital venous malformations as depicted may also be referred to as primary esophageal varices when no secondary cause such as portal hypertension can be identified. These venous structures rarely bleed spontaneously. Endosonography confirmed a conglomerate of venous channels in this case.

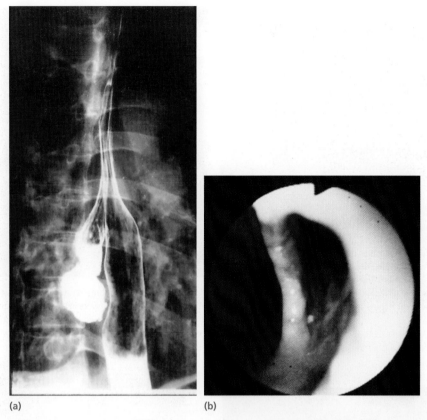

(a)   (b)

Figure 1.7 (a) Radiograph showing a large, congenital, tubular duplication of the esophagus. **(b)** Endoscopic view showing the opening to the tubular duplication (right) and esophageal lumen (left). Congenital esophageal duplications may be tubular or cystic.

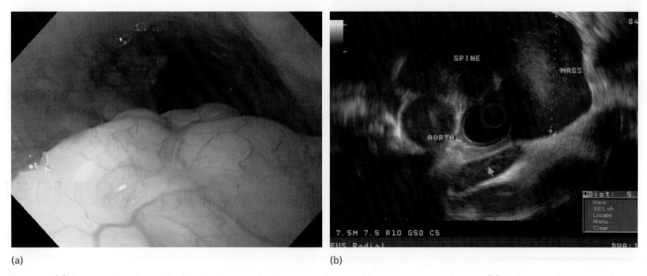

(a)   (b)

Figure 1.8 (a) Congenital esophageal duplication cysts may be present as submucosal lesions on upper endoscopy. **(b)** Endoscopic ultrasonographic image of a large duplication cyst. Duplication cysts are the second most common benign esophageal submucosal lesion with stromal tumors being more common. Source: Images courtesy of Sri Komanduri, MD.

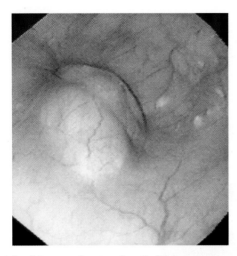

Figure 1.9 Small intramural cysts such as the bilobate type shown here are not symptomatic and are typically identified on barium esophagram or endoscopy for another indication. The cystic nature of the lesion can be confirmed using endoscopic ultrasonography. The differential diagnosis includes submucosal esophageal lesions and esophageal varices.

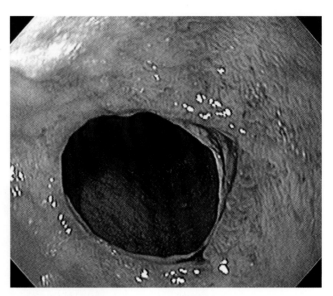

Figure 1.11 A large, circumferential focus of heterotopic gastric mucosa in the cervical esophagus associated with a circumferential mucosal web immediately distally. The web in this case likely represents a form of peptic stricture related to acid secretion from parietal cells within the inlet patch.

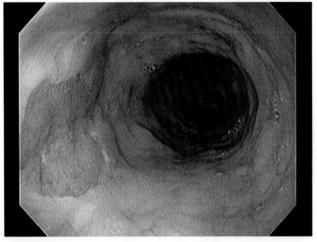

Figure 1.10 Heterotopic gastric mucosa (inlet patch) in the cervical esophagus. The reported prevalence approximates 4%. The lesions can be unifocal as in the case illustrated, multifocal or circumferential.

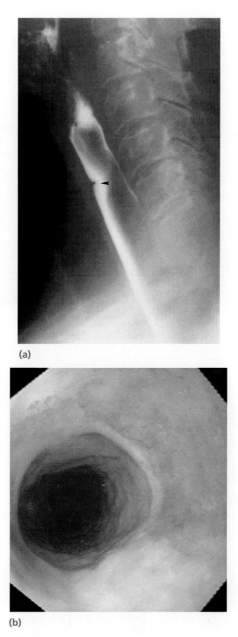

(a)

(b)

Figure 1.12 (a) Barium contrast radiograph showing a mucosal web in the cervical esophagus, often an incidental finding. **(b)** Corresponding endoscopic view of the cervical web from A demonstrates a proximal gastric inlet patch with web creating a shelf or lip at the distal aspect of the heterotopic gastric mucosa.

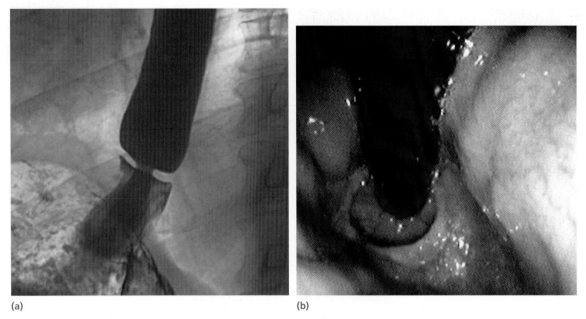

(a)   **(b)**

Figure 1.13 **(a)** A high grade stenosis from a Schatzki ring located at the esophagogastric junction on a barium esophagram. **(b)** Retroflexed endoscopic view of a Schatzki ring. Schatzki's rings are almost invariably seen in association with hiatal hernia as is the cases here. The inner ring diameter of a Schatzki ring is an important determinant of whether the ring is associated with dysphagia.

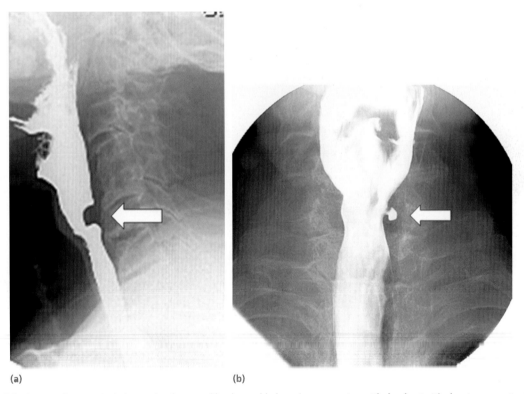

(a)   **(b)**

Figure 1.14 **(a)** Barium esophagram depicting a cricopharyngeal bar in an elderly patient presenting with dysphagia. The bar is a posterior indentation (arrow) arising from the cricopharyngeus muscle. **(b)** A small Zenker's diverticulum (arrow) is seen in the same patient originating from the left lateral aspect of the posterior pharynx in this anterior-posterior view. Physiologic data links the pathogenesis of Zenker's diverticula with increased intraluminal pressure that develops as a result of limited opening of the upper esophageal sphincter.

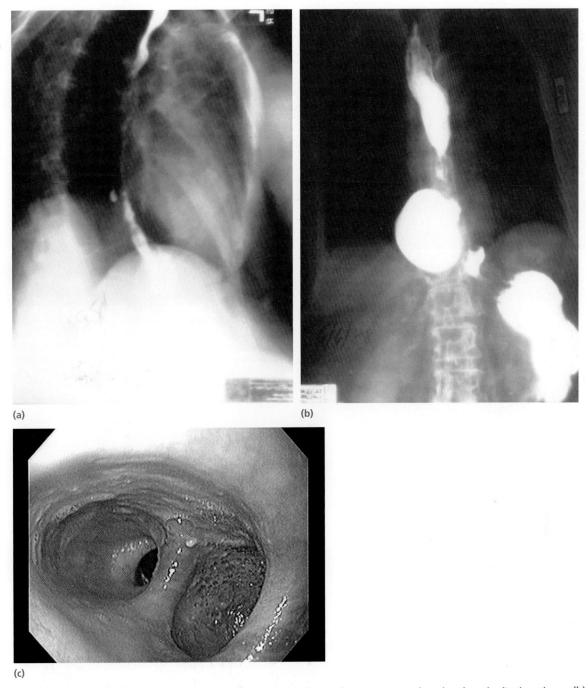

Figure 1.15 **(a)** Esophagram of a 75 year old woman shows a tiny epiphrenic diverticulum projecting to the right side in the distal esophagus. **(b)** Eight years later, there was a marked increase in the size of the diverticulum and the patient developed symptoms of dysphagia and chest pain. **(c)** In another patient, a moderate sized, wide mouthed diverticulum originates to the right of the esophageal lumen.

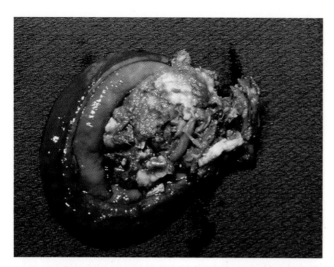

Figure 1.16 Surgical specimen of a resected esophageal diverticulum which contained a large bezoar. Source: Courtesy of Thomas W. Rice, MD.

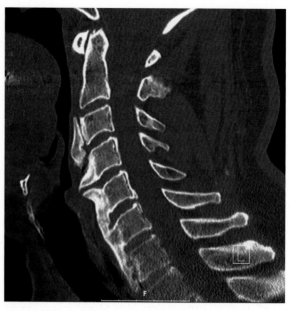

Figure 1.17 Sagittal computed tomography view of the cervical spine of a 62 year old man with diffuse idiopathic skeletal hyperostosis and moderate dysphagia. Anterior ossification of C3–C7 produces extrinsic compression of the esophageal inlet and cervical esophagus. Source: Verlaan J-J, Boswijk PFE, de Ru JA, Dhert WJA, Oner FC. The Spine Journal 2011(11);1058–1067. Reproduced with permission from Elsevier.

CHAPTER 2

Stomach and duodenum: anatomy and structural anomalies

Eric Goldberg and Jean-Pierre Raufman
University of Maryland School of Medicine, Baltimore, MD, USA

The gross and microscopic anatomy of the stomach and duodenum are intrinsically aligned with their functions. A thorough understanding of the regional anatomy facilitates understanding normal function as well as the pathophysiological mechanisms underlying disease. As an example, a dense anastomotic network of arteries supplies oxygen to the stomach (Figure 2.1). Therefore, it is uncommon to have gastric ischemia unless there are severe systemic perturbations in blood flow. In addition, the stomach and duodenum are in close proximity to other vital abdominal organs such as the pancreas, liver, and biliary system. Cross-sectional imaging such as computed tomography (CT) scan or magnetic resonance imaging (MRI) (Figures 2.2, 2.3, 2.4, and 2.5) demonstrate these anatomic relationships. Diseases of these adjacent organs may affect the stomach and duodenum but their close proximity also allows the stomach and duodenum to be exploited as portals to access these structures for diagnostic and therapeutic procedures. Endoscopic ultrasonography (EUS) can be used to diagnose and treat gastric disorders (Figures 2.6 and 2.7). EUS can also be used to drain pancreatic cysts that impinge on the stomach and to biopsy lesions in the pancreas and neighboring lymph nodes. Recognizing the normal histology and embryology of the stomach and duodenum facilitates an understanding of certain disease processes. Figure 2.8 is an endoscopic image showing ectopically located gastric epithelium in the proximal esophagus called a gastric inlet patch. These patches are probably embryologic remnants and have been associated with dysphagia and even esophageal adenocarcinoma. Another example of ectopic gastric tissue is a Meckel's diverticulum (Figure 2.9). Pyloric stenosis is a narrowing of the gastric outlet that causes nausea, vomiting, and dehydration (Figures 2.10 and 2.11). It can be congenital or acquired. Treatment is endoscopic dilation or surgery.

Esophagogastroduodenoscopy (EGD) has emerged as the "gold standard" for evaluation of upper gastrointestinal disorders. It allows direct viewing of the mucosal surface of the upper gastrointestinal tract, thereby facilitating diagnosis and treatment of inflammation, peptic ulcer disease, neoplasia, and other conditions (Figures 2.12, 2.13, 2.14, and 2.15). Directed endoscopic biopsies permit histological confirmation of gastric and duodenal diseases. Undoubtedly, further advances in imaging, such as real-time histological assessment using confocal microscopy, will improve both our diagnostic and therapeutic capabilities. While fluoroscopic examinations such as UGI series have largely been supplanted by direct endoscopy, they still have a role in the diagnosis of gastrointestinal disorders such as intestinal malrotation (Figure 2.16).

Yamada's Atlas of Gastroenterology, Fifth Edition. Edited by Daniel K. Podolsky, Michael Camilleri, J. Gregory Fitz, Anthony N. Kalloo, Fergus Shanahan, and Timothy C. Wang.
© 2016 John Wiley & Sons, Ltd. Published 2016 by John Wiley & Sons, Ltd.
Companion website: www.yamadagastro.com/atlas

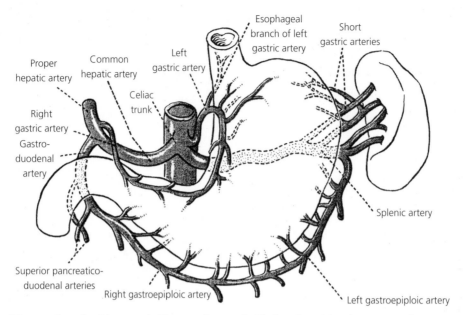

Figure 2.1 Illustration of the arterial supply of the stomach. The stomach is supplied by branches of the celiac artery. A dense anastomotic network of arteries encircle the stomach. Source: Hollinshead WH, Rosse C. Textbook of Anatomy, Lippincott–Williams and Wilkens, 1985. Reproduced with permission from Wolters Kluwer Health.

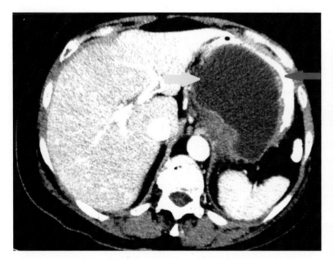

Figure 2.2 Pancreatic pseudocyst (yellow arrow) abutting and compressing the contrast-filled stomach (red arrow). This image demonstrates the close location of the pancreas posterior to the stomach

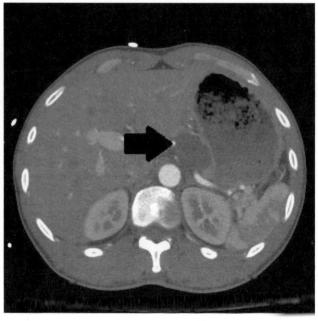

Figure 2.3 Computed tomography (CT) scan of the abdomen demonstrating a gastric duplication cyst (arrow). Source: Courtesy of Barry Daly, MD, University of Maryland School of Medicine.

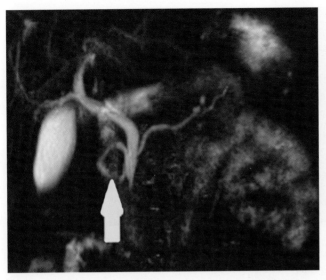

Figure 2.4 Magnetic resonance cholangiopancreatography (MRCP) image demonstrating annular pancreas. The pancreatic duct (yellow arrow) can be seen encircling the second portion of the duodenum. Source: Courtesy of Barry Daly, MD, University of Maryland School of Medicine.

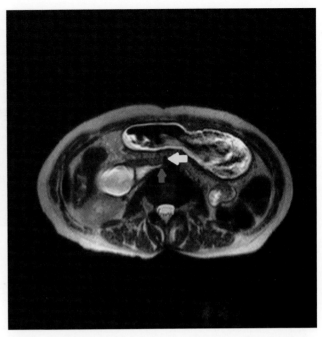

Figure 2.5 Magnetic resonance imaging of the abdomen demonstrating superior mesenteric artery syndrome. The contrast-filled duodenum (blue arrow) is compressed and partially obstructed by the superior mesenteric artery (yellow arrow). Source: Courtesy of Barry Daly, MD, University of Maryland School of Medicine.

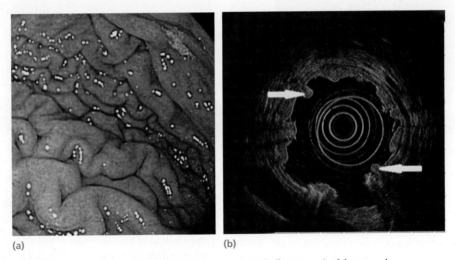

(a)   (b)

Figure 2.6 **(a)** Endoscopic and **(b)** endoscopic ultrasonographic image of the rugae (yellow arrows) of the stomach.

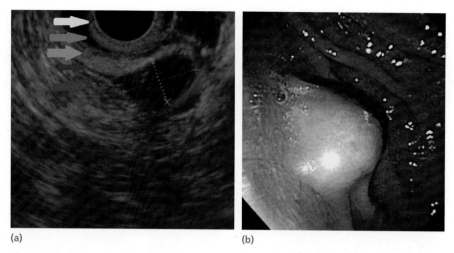

Figure 2.7 (a) Endoscopic ultrasonographic image of the stomach demonstrating the five layers of the stomach: mucosa (yellow arrow); muscularis mucosa (orange arrow); submucosa (green arrow); muscularis (red arrow); and serosa (blue arrow). A gastrointestinal stromal tumor (GIST) can be seen arising from the fourth layer (crossed dashed lines). (b) Endoscopic image of the gastrointestinal stromal tumor in the antrum of the stomach. Source: Courtesy of Lance Uradomo, MD, University of Maryland School of Medicine.

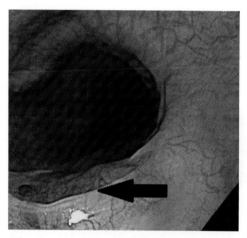

Figure 2.8 Gastric inlet patch, an example of ectopic gastric mucosa, in the proximal esophagus (black arrow).

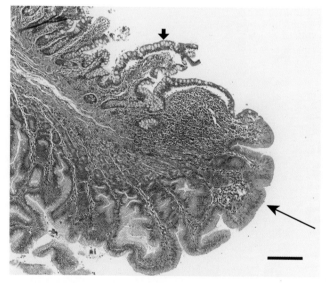

Figure 2.9 Pathological specimen of a Meckel diverticulum. The short thick arrow shows small intestinal mucosa and the longer thin arrow shows ectopic gastric mucosa. The solid bar is 200 μm in length. Source: Courtesy of William Twaddell, MD, University of Maryland School of Medicine.

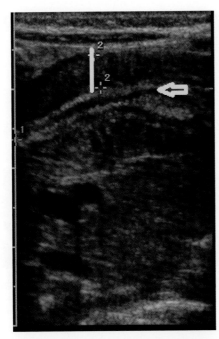

Figure 2.10 Ultrasonographic image demonstrating congenital hypertrophic pyloric stenosis. The vertical line indicates the hypertrophic pyloric muscle and the arrow indicates the narrowed pyloric lumen. Source: Courtesy of Barry Daly, MD, University of Maryland School of Medicine.

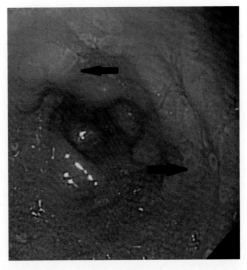

Figure 2.12 Endoscopic image showing Brunner's gland hyperplasia of the duodenum. The black arrows indicate a few of the many visible Brunner's glands.

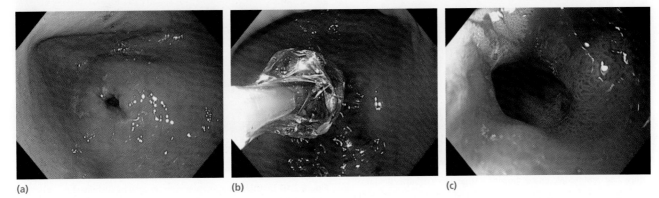

(a)   (b)   (c)

Figure 2.11 Acquired pyloric stenosis secondary to peptic ulcer disease. (a) Endoscopic image demonstrating narrow lumen. (b) Endoscopic balloon dilation of the stenotic pylorus. (c) Postdilation image of the pylorus. Source: Courtesy of Bruce Greenwald, MD, University of Maryland School of Medicine.

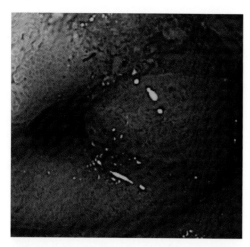

Figure 2.13 Endoscopic image showing an inflammatory stricture in the duodenal bulb.

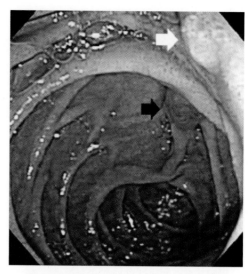

Figure 2.15 Second portion of the duodenum demonstrating the major papilla (black arrow) and the minor papilla (white arrow). The minor papilla is typically located a few centimeters proximal to the major papilla.

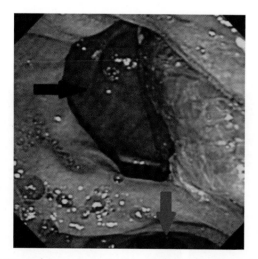

Figure 2.14 Endoscopic image showing a large duodenal diverticulum (black arrow) in the second portion of the duodenum. The diverticulum contains food and bile debris. The duodenal lumen can be seen at the bottom of the image (red arrow).

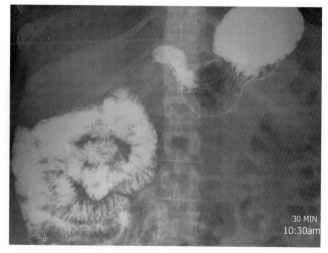

Figure 2.16 Intestinal malrotation seen on upper gastrointestinal series with small bowel follow through. The duodenum and the jejunum are seen right of the midline in this image. Source: Courtesy of Barry Daly, MD, University of Maryland School of Medicine.

CHAPTER 3
Small intestine: anatomy and structural anomalies

Deborah C. Rubin[1] and Jacob C. Langer[2]
[1] Washington University School of Medicine, Saint Louis, MO, USA
[2] University of Toronto and Hospital for Sick Children, Toronto, ON, Canada

Embryology of the small intestine

The primitive human gut forms when the dorsal part of the yolk sac is incorporated into the embryo at 4 weeks' development, giving rise to the foregut, midgut, and hindgut. The foregut is the progenitor of the esophagus, stomach, duodenum up to the biliary duct ampulla, pharynx, respiratory tract, liver, pancreas, and biliary tract. The midgut gives rise to the duodenum distal to the common bile duct, jejunum, ileum, cecum, appendix, ascending colon, and one-half to two-thirds of the transverse colon. The rest of the colon and superior anal canal are derived from the hindgut.

The gut endoderm is the precursor of the gastrointestinal tract epithelium. Its endothelium arises from the ectoderm of the stomodeum and proctodeum as well as the endoderm. The splanchnic mesenchyme supplies the muscular and connective tissue components of the gastrointestinal tract. The midgut first freely communicates with the yolk sac and then narrows to be connected by the omphalomesenteric or vitelline duct. The primitive gut forms a U-shaped loop that grows so rapidly compared with the embryo that it herniates into the umbilical cord at the sixth week of gestation (Figure 3.1). The proximal limb of the loop elongates into multiple intestinal loops, whereas the distal limb simply develops into the cecal diverticulum. The first stage of rotation is 90° counterclockwise around the superior mesenteric artery axis. At 10 weeks, the intestines return into the abdominal cavity and rotate a further 180° counterclockwise in the second stage. Finally, the cecum and appendix descend from the right upper quadrant to the right lower quadrant, and the proximal part of the colon elongates to form the hepatic flexure and ascending colon (third stage of rotation). Fixation occurs as the ascending colonic mesentery fuses with the parietal peritoneum and becomes fixed retroperitoneally. The mesentery of the small intestine attains a broad-based attachment to the posterior abdominal wall and extends from the duodenojejunal junction to the ileocecal region. The end result of this process is the normal location of the small and large intestines.

Congenital anomalies

A brief review of the main features of the common congenital anomalies is presented and illustrated with pictures of surgical specimens.

Meckel diverticulum

Meckel diverticulum is the most common congenital anomaly of the gastrointestinal tract. It results from failure of the vitelline duct to be completely resorbed (Figure 3.2). Large autopsy series indicate a 2%–3% prevalence of Meckel diverticulum in the general population. Meckel diverticula are true diverticula, containing all layers of the bowel from serosa to mucosa. Heterotopic tissue is present approximately 50% of the time and includes gastric mucosa, pancreatic tissue, and, less commonly, colonic mucosa, Brunner glands, and jejunal or hepatobiliary tissue. The presence of heterotopic mucosa correlates with increased risk for symptomatic, complicated Meckel diverticulum.

The complications of Meckel diverticulum include bleeding, intestinal obstruction, diverticulitis, perforation, and carcinoma. The frequency of specific complications varies between adult and pediatric patients. Among children, the most common complications are gastrointestinal bleeding and obstruction. For adults, intestinal obstruction is by far the most frequent complication and gastrointestinal bleeding is rare.

The diagnosis of Meckel diverticulum remains a challenge. Sodium pertechnetate technetium-99m radionuclide scanning is particularly useful in the care of children. This isotope is taken up into gastric mucosal cells and can help detect Meckel diverticula that contain ectopic gastric mucosa.

Management of complicated Meckel diverticulum is surgical. The management of asymptomatic Meckel diverticulum that is

Yamada's Atlas of Gastroenterology, Fifth Edition. Edited by Daniel K. Podolsky, Michael Camilleri, J. Gregory Fitz, Anthony N. Kalloo, Fergus Shanahan, and Timothy C. Wang.
© 2016 John Wiley & Sons, Ltd. Published 2016 by John Wiley & Sons, Ltd.
Companion website: www.yamadagastro.com/atlas

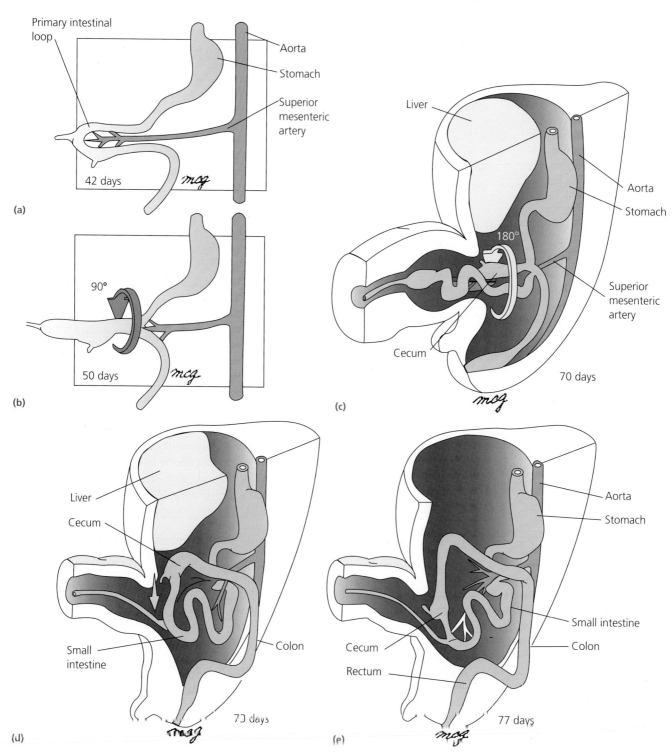

Figure 3.1 Herniation and rotation of the intestine. (a, b) At the end of the sixth week, the primary intestinal loop herniates into the umbilicus, rotating through 90° counterclockwise (in frontal view). (c) The small intestine elongates to form jejunoileal loops, the cecum and appendix grow, and at the end of the 10th week, the primary intestinal loop retracts into the abdominal cavity rotating an additional 180° counterclockwise. (d, e) During the 11th week, the retracting midgut completes this rotation as the cecum is positioned just inferior to the liver. The cecum is then displaced inferiorly, pulling down the proximal hindgut to form the ascending colon. The descending colon is simultaneously fixed on the left side of the posterior abdominal wall. The jejunum, ileum, and transverse and sigmoid colons remain suspended by mesentery. Source: Larsen WJ (ed.). Human Embryology, 2nd edn; 1997. Reproduced with permission of Elsevier.

an incidental finding remains controversial, although prophylactic removal seems to be safe and produces low morbidity and mortality rates.

Duplications

Duplications of the gastrointestinal tract are rare congenital cystic anomalies attached to the intestinal mesenteric border (Figure 3.3). Duplications may occur anywhere along the gastrointestinal tract, although those of small bowel origin are usually found in the ileum. Most duplications are diagnosed during infancy and early childhood, but duplications are occasionally newly discovered in adults. Symptoms in childhood include abdominal pain, obstructive symptoms, and hemorrhage. Adults frequently have no symptoms or have mild abdominal symptoms. Intussusception, gastrointestinal hemorrhage, or carcinoma occasionally develops in adults. Detection may be difficult. Small bowel

follow-through shows a duplication only if the lumen of the normal intestine communicates with the duplication. Ultrasonography or computed tomographic scanning is valuable for detecting a cystic mass. Duplications are managed surgically.

Intestinal atresia and stenosis

Intestinal atresia is a condition in which segments of the lumen contain areas of total occlusion (Figures 3.4 and 3.5). Atresia is one of the common causes of intestinal obstruction among neonates. Atresia may be single or multiple and is found from the esophagus through to the rectum. The prevalence is from 1

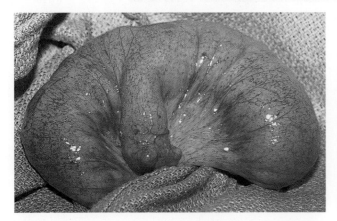

Figure 3.2 Meckel diverticulum. These true diverticula contain all layers of the intestinal wall. Ectopic gastric mucosa may appear as small, red nodules.

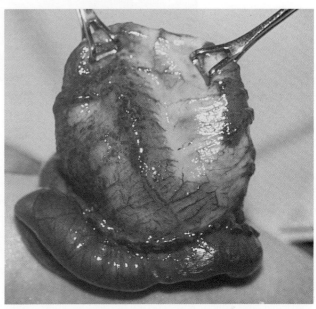

Figure 3.3 Jejunal duplication. Duplications are present on the mesenteric border and share a common blood supply with the adjacent bowel.

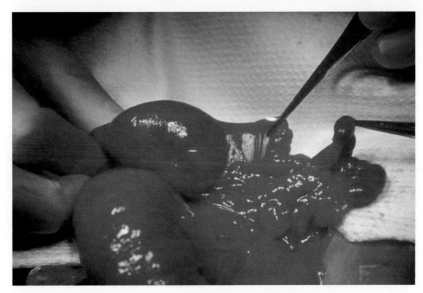

Figure 3.4 Jejunal atresia, type II. A cord-like fibrous segment connects the two ends of intestine.

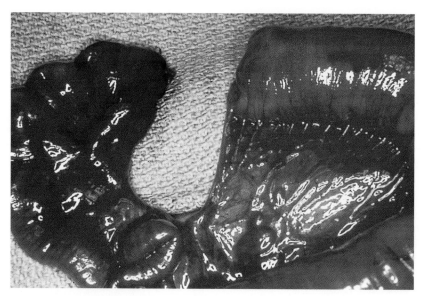

Figure 3.5 Atresia of the small intestine, type IIIa. There is complete separation of the blind ends of the small bowel and a mesenteric gap.

in 3000 to 5000 live births. In type I atresia, a membranous septum or diaphragm of mucosa and submucosa obstructs the lumen, but the intestinal wall and mesentery are intact. Type II is characterized by two blind bowel ends connected by a fibrous cord, with intact mesentery in between (see Figure 3.4). In type IIIa lesions (see Figure 3.5), two blind bowel ends are separated by a mesenteric gap. Type IIIb is "apple peel" atresia, in which there is proximal atresia in the small intestine and absence of the distal superior mesenteric artery (less than 5% of all instances of atresia). In this case, the bowel distal to the atresia is foreshortened and coiled, and receives retrograde blood supply from the ileocolic, right colic, or inferior mesenteric artery. Type IV denotes multiple areas of atresia throughout the small bowel, which have the appearance of a string of sausages; the atresia may be type I, II, or IIIa.

Polyhydramnios is frequently detected in proximal gastrointestinal atresia, but amniotic fluid may be normal in distal atresia. Bilious vomiting soon after birth is a characteristic symptom of proximal atresia, whereas abdominal distention, later vomiting, and failure to pass meconium are found in distal atresia. Diagnosis may be made by means of prenatal ultrasonography followed by plain radiography, and cautious contrast radiography after birth and before surgical intervention.

Gastroschisis and omphalocele

Gastroschisis occurs when there is a small defect in the abdominal wall to the right of the umbilicus through which there is massive evisceration of the intestines (Figure 3.6). The bowel has no membranous covering, has been exposed to amniotic fluid in utero, is thickened, and is covered with adhesions. Omphalocele occurs when the abdominal viscera herniate through the umbilical ring and persist outside the body covered by a membranous sac but not by skin (Figure 3.7). Omphalocele

may be associated with a variety of other structural or chromosomal anomalies. The diagnosis of an abdominal wall defect is suggested by the presence of a high maternal serum α-fetoprotein level. Prenatal ultrasonography also is a sensitive method of prenatal diagnosis. Prenatal detection allows for obstetric planning so that the patient can be at a tertiary care facility for delivery. Treatment is surgical by means of primary closure, or use of a surgical silo or polymeric silicone sac.

Volvulus

Volvulus is abnormal twisting of the intestine around the axis of its own mesentery, resulting in obstruction of the more proximal bowel (Figure 3.8). The twisting of the mesentery may involve the mesenteric vessels and make the involved loop particularly susceptible to strangulation and gangrene. Midgut volvulus is usually caused by a preexisting defect such as malrotation, which results in a narrow-based mesentery. Patients have symptoms of obstruction of the small intestine and an acute abdomen. The severity of pain may be out of proportion to the physical findings, which include abdominal distention, rebound tenderness, guarding and rigidity, and a palpable abdominal mass. Plain abdominal radiographs may demonstrate distended bowel with air–fluid levels consistent with obstruction, free air from a perforation, or a relatively gasless abdomen. Barium studies can be useful in depicting disorders of rotation by showing an abnormal position of the duodenojejunal junction. A typical corkscrew-like appearance of barium in the distorted duodenum and jejunum also is diagnostic. Ultrasound may show abnormal orientation of the superior mesenteric vessels, or a "whirlpool" sign if midgut volvulus has occurred. Rapid recognition of volvulus and prompt surgical intervention are the keys to decreasing the fatality rate associated with this condition.

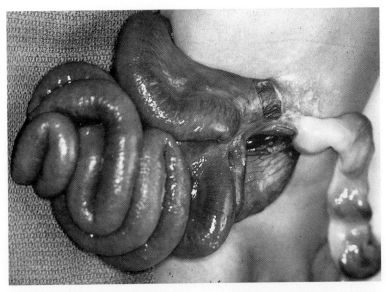

Figure 3.6 Gastroschisis. Multiple loops of exteriorized small intestine are depicted. The bowel is often dilated, edematous, and thickened, presumably because of direct exposure to amniotic fluid.

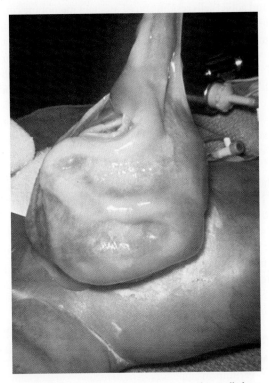

Figure 3.7 Omphalocele. Loops of intestine sit in a thin-walled sac composed of umbilical cord coverings. Source: Langer JC. Gastroschisis and omphalocele. Semin Pediatr Surg 1996;5:124. Reproduced with permission of Elsevier.

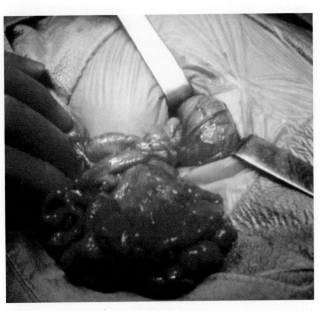

Figure 3.8 Volvulus. There is complete twisting of the small bowel around the axis of its mesentery. Although in this case the loops of the small intestine appear normal, ischemia or frank necrosis of the intestine may be present.

CHAPTER 4

Colon: anatomy and structural anomalies

Konstantin Umanskiy and Jeffrey B. Matthews

Pritzker School of Medicine, University of Chicago, Chicago, IL, USA

The colon is a tubular structure of approximately 150 cm in length that courses through the abdomen beginning at the right lower quadrant with the cecum followed by the ascending colon, which becomes the transverse colon at the hepatic flexure (Figure 4.1). The transverse colon crosses the upper abdomen towards the spleen, where it becomes the descending colon at the splenic flexure and terminates as the sigmoid colon in the left lower quadrant. The sigmoid colon makes a sweeping turn in the pelvis, joining the rectum at the sacral promontory.

The rectum is a tubular organ that is straight in its course towards the anus and measures 12–15 cm in size (Figure 4.2). The distal rectum continues inferiorly to become the anal canal. The anal canal measures 3.2–5.3 cm in men and 3–5 cm in women. It opens externally as the anus, an anterior–posterior slit that remains virtually closed at rest. Approximately in the middle of the anal canal, the distal rectal mucosa of endodermal origin transitions into lower (cutaneous) lining derived from ectoderm. This transition occurs at the dentate line, an area notable for tooth-like mucosal protrusions pointing cephalad. The folds of the distal rectal mucosa form the columns of Morgagni, which in turn form pits known as anal sinus crypts. Within these crypts are located the openings of the anal glands, which secrete mucus for lubrication of the anal canal to allow easier passage of stool. Internal hemorrhoids are the venous cushions located submucosally on the left lateral, right posterior, and right anterior aspect of the anal canal and are covered by a rather thin layer of anoderm.

The anal sphincter complex is formed by the muscles of the pelvic floor and the muscles located along the pelvic sidewall (Figure 4.3). The major muscle that contributes fibers to the external sphincter is the levator ani. The midline of the pelvic floor has several openings through which pass the lower rectum, urethra, and either the dorsal vein of the penis in the male or the vagina in the female. The levator ani is supplied by the roots of the sacral nerves S2–S4 as well as the perineal branch of the pudendal nerve.

The histological section in Figure 4.4 represents all layers of the colonic wall. At the top of the section is the colonic mucosa, with lymphoid aggregate extending into the submucosa. The muscularis propria consists of a circular smooth muscle layer and longitudinal layer. The exterior surface is covered by serosa.

Simple columnar surface epithelium (shown at the top of Figure 4.5) forms mucosal crypts arranged in parallel "row of test tubes." The lamina propria consists of the stromal elements investing the crypts and extending from the surface epithelium to the smooth muscle cells of the muscularis mucosa. Prominent vascular structures (arterioles, venules, and lymphatics) are noted within the submucosa. The colonic surface epithelium is a simple columnar cuboidal epithelium composed of absorptive and goblet cells residing on a basement membrane complex. Absorptive surface cells do not contain mucin within their cytoplasm and under normal hematoxylin and eosin (H&E) staining their cytoplasm appears eosinophilic. The nuclei of absorptive cells are oval and located towards the basement membrane. Nuclei of absorptive cells are uniform in their location and size and oriented in parallel with the long axis of the cells. Goblet cells synthesize and store mucous, and secrete mucous granules by exocytosis. Because the cytoplasm of goblet cells is almost entirely filled with mucin, which does not stain with standard H&E stain, it appears to be vacant.

The anal transition zone (ATZ) (Figure 4.6) epithelium consists of four to nine cell layers, with the surface cells arranged as a columnar, cuboidal, or polygonal layer, while the basal cells are small with their nuclei arranged perpendicular to the basement membrane. Within the ATZ small areas of mature squamous epithelium may be present, especially at the upper border of the anal canal. At the distal aspect of the ATZ, approximately at the level of the dentate line, squamous epithelium becomes more uniform, indicating the beginning of the squamous zone. Squamous epithelium in this zone is unkeratinized with short or no papillae.

Figure 4.7 shows a low-magnification view of a cross-section of the vermiform appendix. The irregular (stellate) lumen is lined by a single layer of surface epithelium. Note the characteristic lymphoid follicles within the lamina propria that also

Yamada's Atlas of Gastroenterology, Fifth Edition. Edited by Daniel K. Podolsky, Michael Camilleri, J. Gregory Fitz, Anthony N. Kalloo, Fergus Shanahan, and Timothy C. Wang.
Companion website: www.yamadagastro.com/atlas

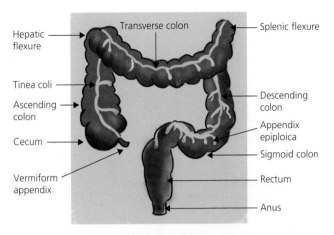

Figure 4.1 Schematic depiction of the colon and rectum and its anatomical segments.

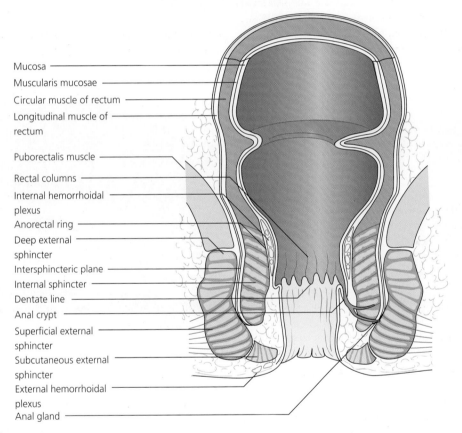

Figure 4.2 Anorectal anatomy.

extended to submucosa. The histology of the appendix varies slightly from that of colon. In contrast to the colon where crypts line up evenly like test tubes in a rack, appendiceal crypts are more irregular in shape, length, and distribution. In areas containing lymphoid tissue, crypts are typically absent. Appendiceal lymphoid aggregates can extend beneath the muscularis mucosa into the underlying submucosa. These aggregates are confluent and appear similar in composition and function to Peyer's patches of the small bowel.

The majority of patients with anorectal malformations also have an abnormal communication between the rectum and other pelvic organs or structures (vagina, bladder, or urethra) or perineum. In patients with cloaca, rectum, vagina, and urinary tract are fused together, forming a common channel (Figure 4.8). This single channel opens at a location where the urethra would be typically found in normal females.

The blood supply to the colon and rectum is derived from superior and inferior mesenteric arteries (Figure 4.9). The

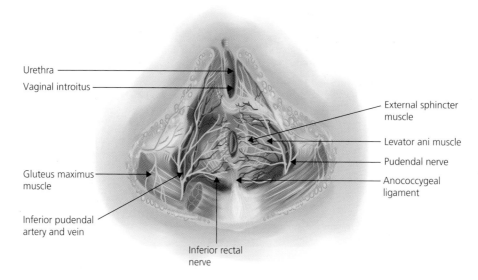

Figure 4.3 Pelvic floor (female) anatomy and anal sphincter innervation.

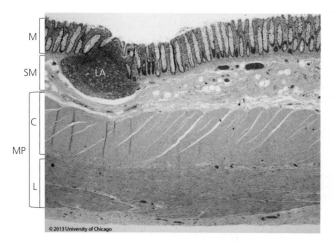

Figure 4.4 Anatomy of the colonic wall. C, circular muscle; L, longitudinal muscle; LA, lymphoid aggregate; M, colonic mucosa; MP, muscularis propria; SM, submucosa. Courtesy of Dr. Shu-Yuan Xiao, Department of Pathology, University of Chicago.

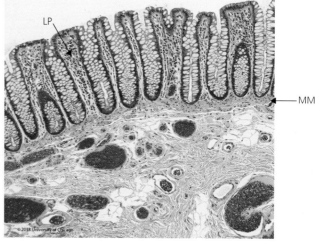

Figure 4.5 Normal colonic mucosa. H&E stain. LP, lamina propria; MM, muscularis mucosa. Courtesy of Dr. Shu-Yuan Xiao, Department of Pathology, University of Chicago.

superior mesenteric artery originates from the aorta posterior to the pancreas at the level of L1. It courses anteriorly to the third portion of the duodenum and continues in caudal fashion and slightly to the right, traveling within the mesentery of the small bowel as it gives off 12 to 20 jejunal and ileal branches and continues as the ileocolic artery towards the cecum. On the right side, the superior mesenteric artery gives off the middle and right colic arteries. The ileocolic artery bifurcates into an ascending branch, coursing superiorly and anastomosing with right colic artery and a posterior branch, which supplies the cecum and appendix. The middle colic artery bifurcates into left and right branches. The left branch supplies the distal half of the transverse colon and splenic flexure, while the right branch supplies the hepatic flexure and provides collateral circulation through anastomosis with branches of the ileocolic and right colic arteries.

The inferior mesenteric artery originates from the aorta about 3–4 cm cephalad to its bifurcation at the level of L2–L3 and courses caudally and to the left towards the pelvis. It gives off the left colic artery, which bifurcates into an ascending branch, contributing to the arc of Riolan, and a descending branch that runs caudally and supplies the descending colon. As the inferior mesenteric artery continues its course into the pelvis it gives off two to six sigmoidal arteries and becomes called the superior hemorrhoidal artery (superior rectal artery). The central

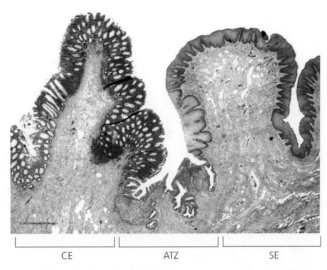

Figure 4.6 Anal canal. Transition between the colonic epithelium (CE) on the left, anal transition zone (ATZ), and squamous epithelium (SE) of the anal canal on the right. Courtesy of Dr. Shu-Yuan Xiao, Department of Pathology, University of Chicago.

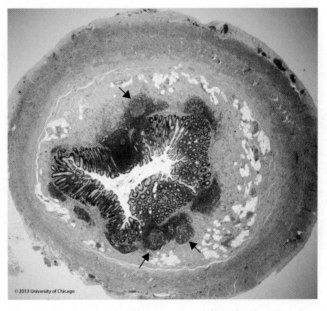

Figure 4.7 Appendix. Arrows, lymphoid follicles within the lamina propria. Courtesy of Dr. Shu-Yuan Xiao, Department of Pathology, University of Chicago.

anastomotic artery connecting the colonic mesenteric vascular beds is the marginal artery of Drummond. It provides collateral circulation between the superior and inferior mesenteric arterial systems as it runs along the mesenteric border of the entire colon. A potential watershed area between the inferior and superior mesenteric arterial systems is located at the splenic flexure and is called Griffiths' critical point. Another area of potentially diminished blood supply is Sudeck's point, located at the watershed area between the inferior mesenteric artery and the internal iliac artery. This point is located near the rectosigmoid junction. In addition to the artery of Drummond, a communicating arc between inferior and superior mesenteric systems is the arc of Riolan, a thick torturous vessel that often referred to as the meandering artery. It tends to become more pronounced as it plays a critical role in establishing collateral circulation between the middle colic artery and the ascending branch of the left colic artery in advanced atherosclerotic disease when either the superior or inferior mesenteric artery is occluded. Correspondingly, the presence of a meandering artery with antegrade flow indicates stenosis or occlusion of the inferior mesenteric artery, while retrograde flow indicates occlusion of the superior mesenteric artery.

Lymphatic drainage from upper and middle parts of the rectum proceeds along the superior hemorrhoidal artery through the inferior mesenteric lymph nodes (Figure 4.10). The caudal part of the rectum drains cephalad through superior rectal lymphatics into inferior mesenteric nodes and laterally into middle rectal lymphatics to the internal iliac nodes.

Lymphatic drainage from the anal canal above the dentate line proceeds cephalad via superior rectal lymphatics through inferior mesenteric nodes and laterally along both the middle rectal vessels and inferior rectal vessels through the ischioanal fossa towards the internal iliac lymph nodes. Lymph from the anal canal below the dentate line usually drains to the inguinal nodes.

In Figure 4.11 a massively dilated cecum occupies most of the abdomen. Gas-filled intestinal loops result in a "coffee bean" sign. The dilated cecum is displaced medially and superiorly across the mid-abdomen, extending into the left upper quadrant. Several loops of small bowel are also dilated.

Figure 4.12 shows a markedly dilated, gas-filled sigmoid colon with a "bent inner tube" sign. The sigmoid colon can undergo volvulus in either direction, clockwise or counterclockwise, and upon completion of the 360° turn a closed loop obstruction occurs within the affected segment. The hyperperistalsis and fluid secretion that follows further contribute to colonic distention and increased tension within the colonic wall, which in turn results in hypoperfusion, ischemia, and, eventually, colonic wall necrosis.

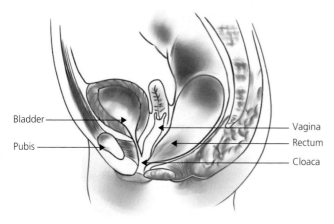

Figure 4.8 Cloacal abnormality.

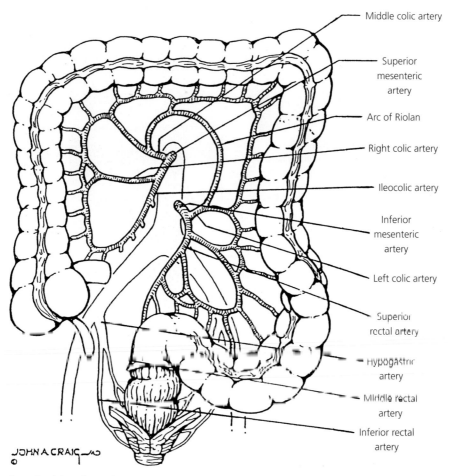

Figure 4.9 Arterial blood supply of the colon and rectum. Source: Kodner IJ, Fry RD, Fleshman JW, Birnbaum EH. Colon, rectum and anus. In: Schwartz SI (ed.). Principles of Surgery, 6th edn (1993). Reproduced with permission from the McGraw-Hill Companies.

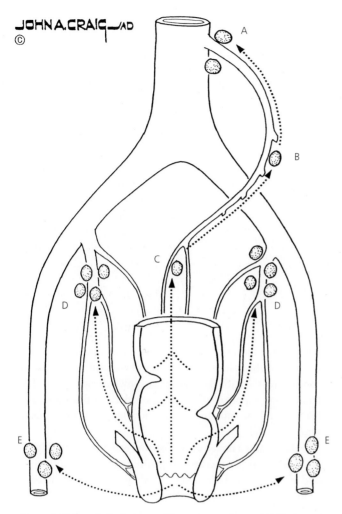

Figure 4.10 Lymphatic drainage of the rectum and anus. (A) Nodes at the origin of inferior mesenteric artery; (B) nodes at the origin of sigmoid branches; (C) sacral nodes; (D) internal iliac nodes; (E) inguinal nodes. Source: Kodner IJ, Fleshman JW, Fry RD. Anal and rectal cancer: principles of management. In: Schwartz SI, Ellis H (eds). Maingot's Abdominal Operations, 9th edn. Norwalk, CT: Appleton & Lange, 1989. Reproduced with permission from the McGraw- Hill Companies.

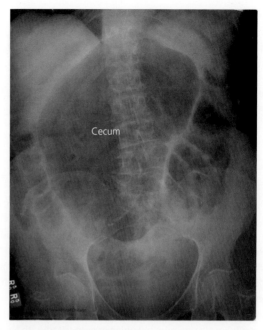

Figure 4.11 Radiograph of cecal volvulus.

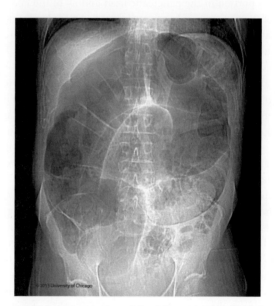

Figure 4.12 Computer tomogram of the abdomen (scout image) of a patient with sigmoid volvulus.

CHAPTER 5

Pancreas: anatomy and structural anomalies

David G. Heidt, Michael W. Mulholland, and Diane M. Simeone
University of Michigan Health System, Ann Arbor, MI, USA

Knowledge of the anatomic and structural relations of the pancreas has become increasingly important with the advent of cross-sectional imaging, innovations in endoscopy, and the introduction of methods for percutaneous biopsy of the gland. The central location of the gland in the upper retroperitoneum complicates the medical and surgical management of pancreatic disease.

Pancreatic development begins during the fourth week of gestation from two primordial anlagen associated with the duodenum (Figure 5.1). The dorsal pancreatic bud, destined to form a portion of the pancreatic head and all of the body and tail of the pancreas, enlarges more rapidly and extends into the dorsal mesentery. The ventral pancreatic bud, the source of the uncinate process and a portion of the pancreatic head, develops in association with the hepatic rudiment and biliary ductal structures. Rotation of the ventral pancreatic bud to the left of the duodenum brings it below the dorsal bud. Fusion occurs in the seventh week of gestation. In most instances, fusion of the ventral duct with the dorsal duct results in formation of a single pancreatic duct that empties through the ventral ductal segment (Figure 5.2). Failure of ductal fusion results in formation of the congenital anomaly pancreas divisum (Figures 5.3 and 5.4).

The pancreas is an elongated organ (12–20 cm in length in adults) that lies transversely in the upper retroperitoneum. The gland may be divided arbitrarily into head, uncinate process, neck, body, and tail (Figure 5.5). The head of the pancreas lies on the right in the concavity of the duodenal sweep. The head of the gland also is related to the gastroepiploic foramen, the right kidney, the inferior vena cava, and the right portion of the transverse mesocolon (Figures 5.6 and 5.7). The distal common bile duct traverses the head of the pancreas before entering the duodenum.

The neck of the pancreas is bordered inferiorly by both the transverse mesocolon and the root of the mesentery of the small intestine. Posteriorly, the neck of the pancreas is associated with the confluence of the superior mesenteric and splenic veins, which, together, form the portal vein (Figure 5.8). The body and tail of the pancreas are related, along the superior border, to the splenic artery and vein (Figure 5.9). The transverse mesocolon is attached to the inferior border of the tail of the gland; the stomach contacts the anterior surface. The tail of the pancreas extends to the left in the leaves of the splenorenal ligament to the hilum of the spleen. Some of these anatomic relations, as seen with cross-sectional imaging, are shown in Figure 5.10. The arterial blood supply of the pancreas is derived from both the celiac axis and the superior mesenteric artery. Venous drainage is entirely portal.

The pancreas is a mixed endocrine and exocrine gland (Figure 5.11). The exocrine pancreas is organized in lobular units composed of ductules and acini. Acinar cells are pyramidal and have a highly basophilic cytoplasm. Numerous zymogen granules are visualized by means of electron microscopic examination of the cellular apex. Centroacinar cells (which express the surface marker Hes-1, a Notch pathway signaling molecule) and ductal cells (which express cytokeratin-19) are more columnar. The acini rest on a thin basal lamina penetrated by numerous blood vessels and nerve fibers. Centroacinar cells have been recently implicated as a possible cell of origin in pancreatic ductal carcinoma.

The endocrine pancreas is composed of approximately 1 million islets of Langerhans. The islets contain endocrine cells that stain positively for insulin (75%–80%), glucagon (10%–20%), and somatostatin (5%). Pancreatic polypeptide and several other enteric peptides are also expressed within cells of the pancreatic islets.

Yamada's Atlas of Gastroenterology, Fifth Edition. Edited by Daniel K. Podolsky, Michael Camilleri, J. Gregory Fitz, Anthony N. Kalloo, Fergus Shanahan, and Timothy C. Wang.
© 2016 John Wiley & Sons, Ltd. Published 2016 by John Wiley & Sons, Ltd.
Companion website: www.yamadagastro.com/atlas

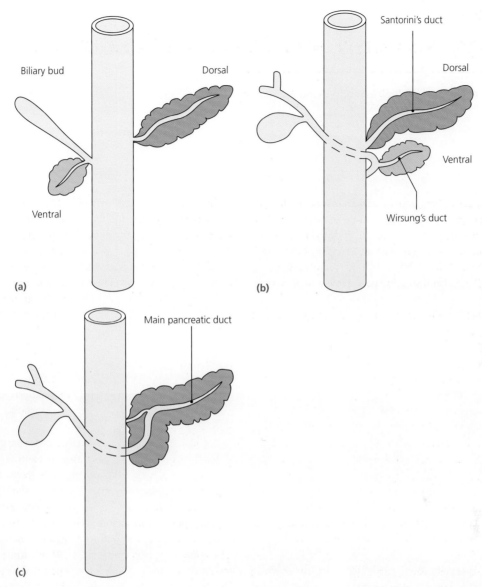

Figure 5.1 (a–c) Developmental anatomy of the pancreas. Source: Misiewicz JJ, Forbes A, Price A, et al. Atlas of Clinical Gastroenterology, 2nd edn. London: Wolfe, 1994. Copyright ©1994 Elsevier.

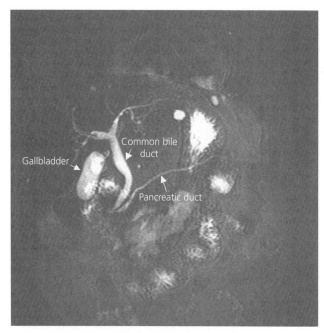

Figure 5.2 Magnetic resonance cholangiopancreatography demonstrates standard pancreatic ductal anatomy, with a single main pancreatic duct emptying through the ventral segment.

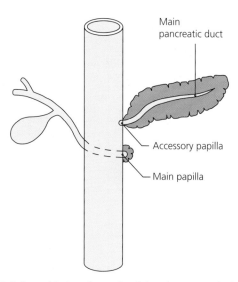

Figure 5.3 Failure of fusion of ventral and dorsal pancreatic buds results in pancreas divisum. Source: Misiewicz JJ, Forbes A, Price A, et al. Atlas of Clinical Gastroenterology, 2nd edn. London: Wolfe, 1994. Copyright ©1994 Elsevier.

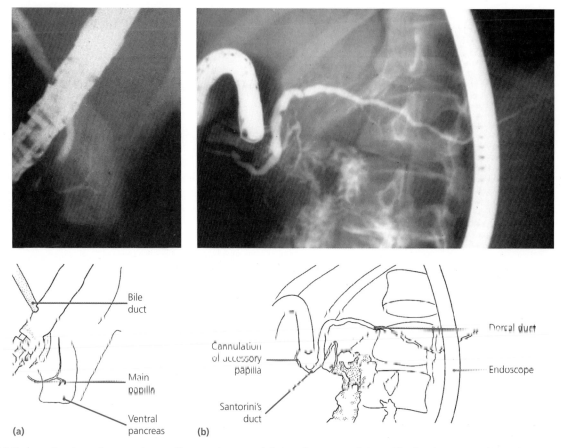

Figure 5.4 Endoscopic retrograde pancreatogram illustrates the congenital anomaly pancreas divisum. The dorsal pancreatic duct is filled through the accessory pancreatic duct **(a)**. The ventral pancreatic duct **(b)** fills through the major papilla. The two ductal systems do not communicate. Source: Misiewicz JJ, Forbes A, Price A, et al. Atlas of Clinical Gastroenterology, 2nd edn. London: Wolfe, 1994. Copyright ©1994 Elsevier.

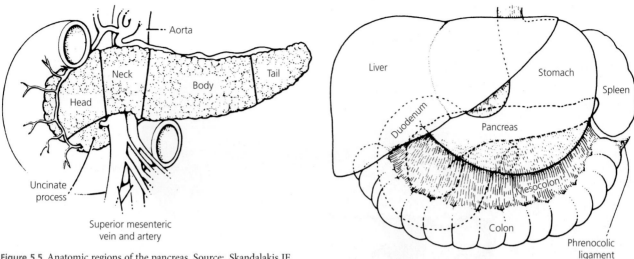

Figure 5.5 Anatomic regions of the pancreas. Source: Skandalakis JE, Gray SW, Rowe JS. Anatomical Complications in General Surgery. New York: McGraw-Hill, 1983. Reproduced with permission of Dr. Skandalakis.

Figure 5.6 Anterior relations of the pancreas. Source: Skandalakis JE, Gray SW, Rowe JS Jr., et al. Anatomical complications of pancreatic surgery. Contemp Surg 1979;15:17.

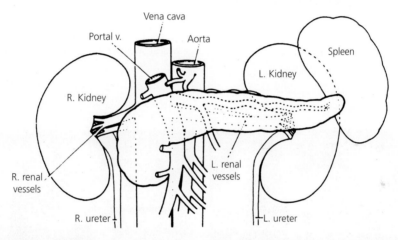

Figure 5.7 Anatomic relations posterior to the pancreas. L., left; R., right; v., vein. Source: Skandalakis JE, Gray SW, Rowe JS Jr., et al. Anatomical complications of pancreatic surgery. Contemp Surg 1979; 15:17.

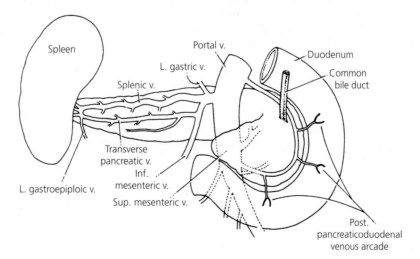

Figure 5.8 Posterior view of the pancreas demonstrates relations to portal venous tributaries. Inf., inferior; L., left; Post, posterior; Sup., superior; v., vein. Source: Skandalakis JE, Gray SW, Rowe JS Jr., et al. Anatomical complications of pancreatic surgery. Contemp Surg 1979;15:17.

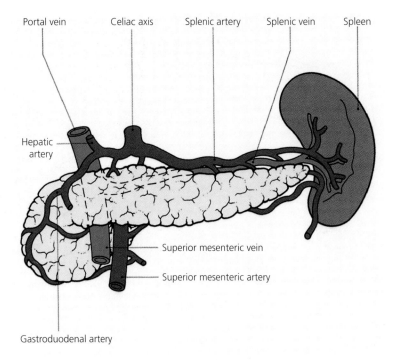

Portal vein   Celiac axis   Splenic artery   Splenic vein   Spleen

Hepatic artery

Superior mesenteric vein

Superior mesenteric artery

Gastroduodenal artery

Figure 5.9 Arterial supply to the pancreas. Source: Misiewicz JJ, Forbes A, Price A, et al. Atlas of Clinical Gastroenterology, 2nd edn. London: Wolfe, 1994. Copyright ©1994 Elsevier.

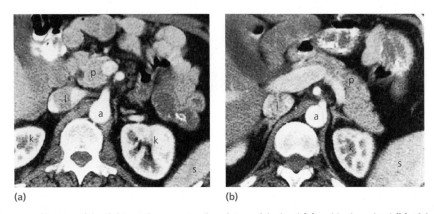

(a)   (b)

Figure 5.10 Computed tomographic scan of the abdomen demonstrates the relation of the head (a) and body and tail (b) of the pancreas to surrounding structures. a, aorta; l, inferior vena cava; k, kidney; p, pancreas; s, spleen.

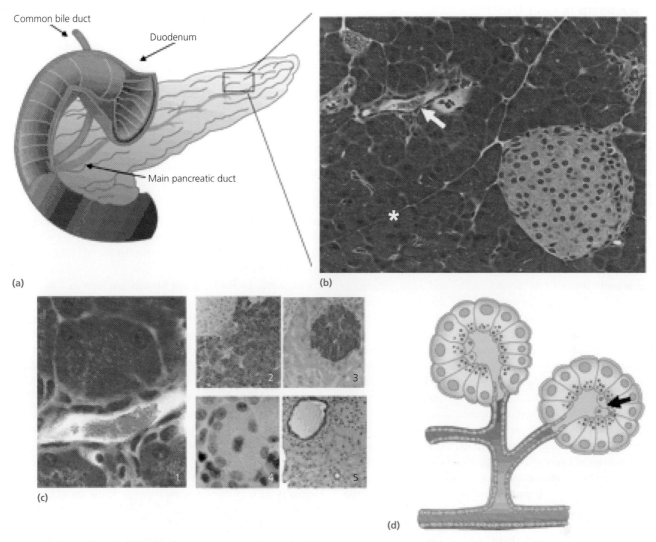

Figure 5.11 Anatomy of the pancreas. **(a)** Gross anatomy of the pancreas demonstrating its close anatomical relationship with the duodenum and common bile duct. **(b)** The major components of the pancreatic parenchyma on a histological level. At the lower right is an islet of Langerhans, the endocrine portion of the pancreas, which is principally involved in regulating glucose homeostasis. The asterisk is placed among acini, which are involved in secreting various digestive enzymes (zymogens) into the ducts (indicated by the solid arrow). **(c)** Photomicrographs of hematoxylin and eosin- and immunohistochemical-stained sections of pancreatic tissue, demonstrating the various cell types. (Panel 1) An acinar unit in relationship to the duct. (Panel 2) Acinar units visualized with an antibody to amylase are seen as brown owing to diaminobenzidine staining. (Panel 3) Islet of Langerhans shown stained with an antibody to insulin. (Panel 4) A centroacinar cell showing robust Hes1 staining. (Panel 5) Ductal cells (seen in cross-section) are stained with an antibody to cytokeratin-19. **(d)** Representation of an acinar unit showing the relationship to the pancreatic ducts. Also depicted are centroacinar cells (arrow), which sit at the junction of the ducts and acini. Source: Hezel AF, Kimmelman AC, Stanger BZ, et al. Genetics and biology of pancreatic ductal adenocarcinoma. Genes Dev 2006;20:1218. Reproduced with permission of Cold Spring Harbor Laboratory Press.

CHAPTER 6

Abdominal cavity: anatomy, structural anomalies, and hernias

Kevin P. Murphy, Michael M. Maher, and Owen J. O'Connor
Cork University Hospital and University College Cork, Cork, Ireland

Abdominal cavity anatomy

This Atlas provides a pictorial guide depicting anatomical structural anomalies encountered in the abdominal cavity. These may be broadly divided into developmental and adult patterns of anatomical variation. The boundaries of the abdominal cavity, intra- and retroperitoneal divisions, and the peritoneal cavity subdivisions determine the location and appearances of the various structural anomalies encountered since these are benign processes which tend to respect intact anatomy. The abdominopelvic cavity is bounded superiorly by the diaphragm, inferiorly by the pelvic floor, and circumferentially by the abdominal wall. The abdominopelvic cavity is divided into intraperitoneal and retroperitoneal components by the peritoneum. The peritoneal cavity is subdivided into several spaces and recesses via peritoneal reflections. They in turn are subdivided into ligaments, omenta, and mesenteries. Most notably, the peritoneal cavity is partitioned into supra and infra mesocolic compartments by the transverse mesocolon.

Developmental and childhood structural anomalies of the abdominal cavity

Any disorder of the physiological developmental rotation of the small bowel is termed malrotation. The key concern is the propensity for midgut volvulus with resultant obstruction and bowel ischaemia. Imaging confirmation is performed using an upper gastrointestinal fluoroscopic contrast study (Figure 6.1). Surgical management of symptomatic malrotation involves release of abnormal adhesions (Ladd's Bands), which sometimes also necessitates bowel resection.

Congenital intraabdominal cystic lesions include lymphangiomata, mesenteric cysts, enteric cysts, and enteric duplication cysts. Many are detected antenatally and are asymptomatic (Figure 6.2).

Exomphalos (omphalocoele) is a persistence of the physiological umbilical small bowel herniation and has coverings of amnion and peritoneum. Unlike gastroschisis, it is associated with other congenital anomalies in 54%. Gastroschisis involves an anterior abdominal wall hernia that lies lateral to the umbilicus and lacks coverings.

Congenital paediatric groin hernias are seen in 3%–5% of births and up to 30% of premature (male) infants. The vast majority are indirect inguinal hernias as a result of incomplete closure of the processus vaginalis (Canal of Nuck in females).

A Morgagni-type congenital diaphragmatic hernia is an anteromedial parasternal defect that is frequently right-sided (90%) (Figure 6.3). A Bochdalek hernia (Figure 6.4) is a left-side predominant (80%) congenital defect in the posterolateral diaphragm that is more common than Morgagni with higher mortality and morbidity. Pulmonary hypoplasia and pulmonary hypertension are key concerns.

Adult abdominal hernias

Hernia is: *"The protrusion of an organ or tissue out of the body cavity in which it normally lies."*

The key elements of a hernia are the hernia sac, neck, and contents. Any cause of increased intraabdominal pressure predisposes to abdominal wall hernia along with conditions that lead to weakening of the abdominal wall. Clinical evaluation is sufficient to diagnose an abdominal wall hernia in most cases. Irreducible (incarcerated) hernias may be associated with bowel obstruction, or bowel ischemia due to strangulation.

The inguinal canal is an oblique channel, approximately 4 cm long, through the inferomedial anterior abdominal wall, and a site of potential weakness. The adjacent femoral canal represents the medial compartment of the femoral sheath. Inguinal hernias account for over 70% of abdominal wall hernias with femoral hernias responsible for 5%–15% of cases. Direct inguinal hernia occurs due to protrusion of contents through the posterior canal wall medial to the epigastric vessels while the indirect type leads to extension of contents through the deep ring (Figures 6.5, 6.6, 6.7, 6.8, and 6.9).

Yamada's Atlas of Gastroenterology, Fifth Edition. Edited by Daniel K. Podolsky, Michael Camilleri, J. Gregory Fitz, Anthony N. Kalloo, Fergus Shanahan, and Timothy C. Wang.
© 2016 John Wiley & Sons, Ltd. Published 2016 by John Wiley & Sons, Ltd.
Companion website: www.yamadagastro.com/atlas

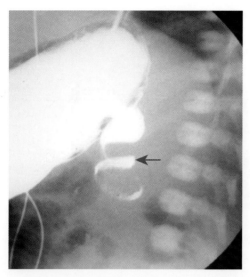

Figure 6.1 Upper GI study in a neonate with vomiting due to malrotation. Lateral view shows a "corkscrew" appearance of the duodenum (arrow) that has torted around itself in a neonate with malrotation.

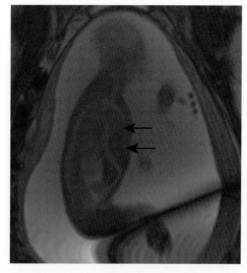

Figure 6.3 Fetal magnetic resonance image shows protrusion of part of the liver (arrows) through a right-sided Morgagni hernia.

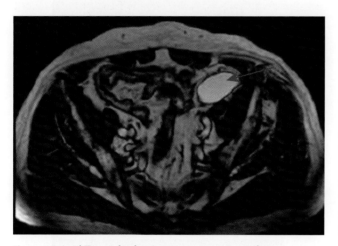

Figure 6.2 Axial T2-weighted magnetic resonance image that demonstrates an incidental simple left iliac fossa lymphangioma (arrow).

A wide variety of hernias occur in the abdominal cavity. These are described based on location, appearances, or sometimes eponymously:

- Pantaloon hernia occurs when direct and indirect ipsilateral inguinal hernias simultaneously exist.
- Littre's hernia contains a Meckels diverticulum.
- Amyand's hernia contains an incarcerated appendix (Figure 6.10).
- Richter Hernia contains a single wall, usually antimesenteric, of bowel; hence this type can strangulate without bowel obstruction.

- Maydl Hernia contains more than one loop of bowel meaning that this can result in closed loop obstruction.
- Femoral hernia leads to herniation of contents into the femoral canal through the femoral ring (Figure 6.11).

Surgical repair is the only definitive therapy for management of groin hernias and is recommended for the majority of these (Figure 6.12). Complications related to groin hernia repair such as recurrence, infection and postoperative collections occur in up to 20% (Figure 6.13).

An umbilical hernia is the most common nongroin abdominal wall hernia (Figure 6.14). Spigelian hernias pass through the anterior abdominal wall immediately lateral to the rectus abdominus muscles (Figure 6.15). Lumbar hernias are classified into superior or inferior types according to the divisions of the lumbar triangles (Figure 6.16). Incisional or parastomal hernias occur following 9.9% of laparotomies, and 0.7% of laparoscopies (Figure 6.17 and 6.18). Paraduodenal hernias represent approximately 53% of internal hernias; left-sided hernias are more common. Internal hernias are difficult to diagnose clinically and therefore CT is important for assessment (Figure 6.19). Intermittent abdominal pain or acute bowel obstruction (often closed-loop and strangulated) are the most commonly observed symptoms.

Noninternal pelvic hernias are frequently seen in elderly females with acquired pelvic floor weakness, with obturator hernias being the commonest (Figure 6.20). These are often associated with an obturator neuropathy (Howship-Romberg sign). Adult diaphragmatic hernias are most commonly post-traumatic in origin with the left hemidiaphragm being more frequently affected. Approximately 11% of congenital diaphragmatic hernias present during adulthood.

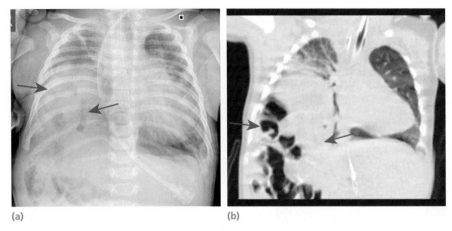

(a) (b)

Figure 6.4 (a and b) Chest radiograph and coronal CT in a neonate showing a Bochdalek-type defect in the right hemidiaphragm (inferior arrow) with bowel loops extending into the chest superiorly (superior arrows).

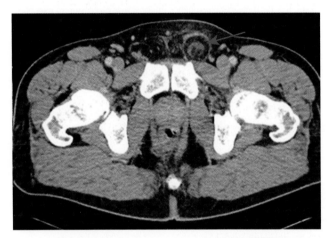

Figure 6.5 Axial intravenous contrast-enhanced CT image shows strangulated fat contained within an indirect left inguinal hernia (arrow).

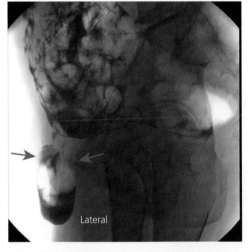

Figure 6.7 Lateral image from a herniogram. This demonstrated a large right inguinal hernia (arrows).

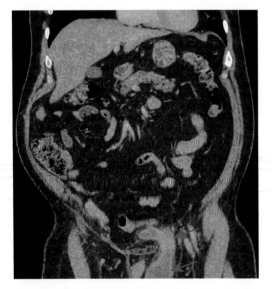

Figure 6.6 Coronal CT shows part of the bladder contained within a direct left inguino-scrotal hernia (arrows).

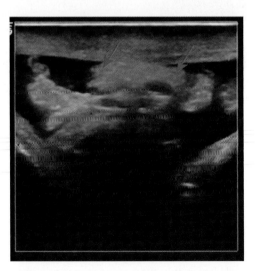

Figure 6.8 Ultrasound image demonstrating a right inguino-scrotal hernia, which contains fat and small bowel (arrows).

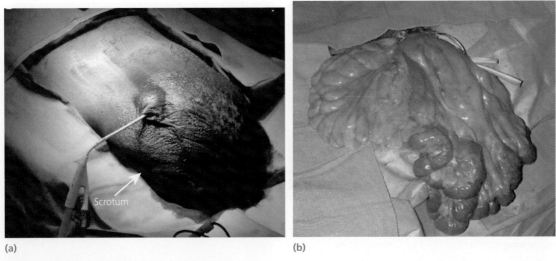

(a)   (b)

Figure 6.9 Giant inguinal hernia. **(a)** Large bilateral inguinal hernia. **(b)** The operation revealed that most of the small and large intestinal contents were present in the hernia sac in the scrotum.

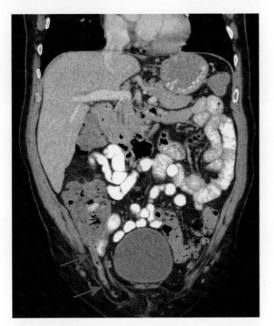

Figure 6.10 Coronal CT shows the appendix (arrows) extending into a right inguinal hernia (Amyand's hernia).

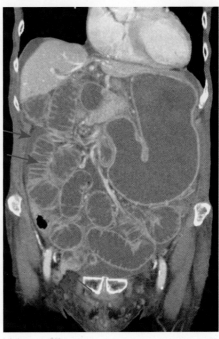

Figure 6.11 Coronal CT demonstrates an incarcerated right femoral hernia (inferior arrows) with resultant small bowel obstruction and ascites (superior arrows).

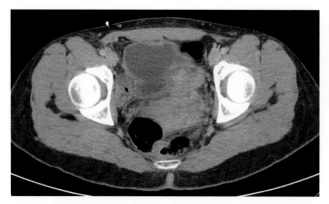

Figure 6.12 Axial CT image with normal appearances following a mesh plug repair (arrow) of a right femoral hernia, which was palpable in this case.

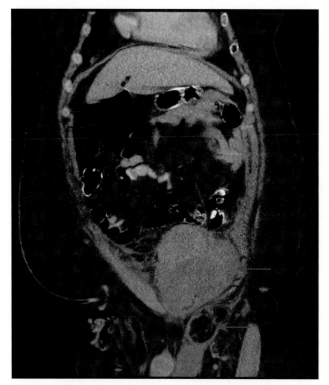

Figure 6.13 Coronal CT displays a recurrent left inguinal hernia (inferior arrow) with associated postoperative haematoma (superior arrow).

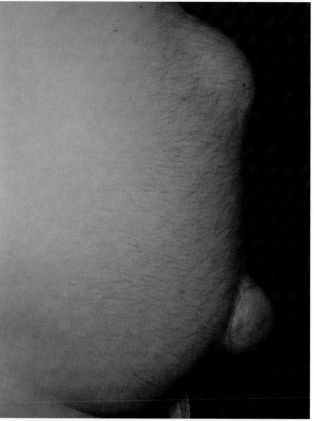

(a)

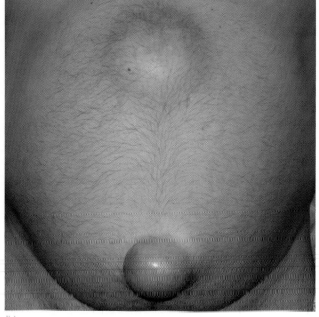

(b)

Figure 6.14 (a) Subxiphoid hernia (superior) and (b) umbilical hernia (inferior) in the same patient.

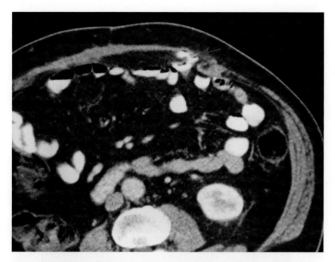

Figure 6.15 Axial CT image with a small left spigelian hernia (arrow).

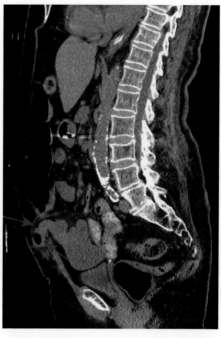

Figure 6.17 Sagittal CT reformat in a patient with a small bowel containing incisional hernia (arrows) from a prior laparotomy.

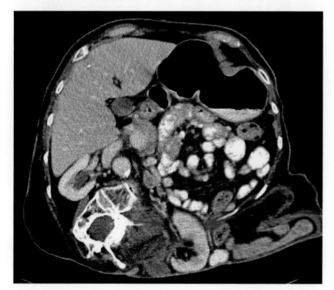

Figure 6.16 Axial CT image shows a defect in the left superior lumbar triangle (arrows). Part of the left kidney and bowel are contained within the sac.

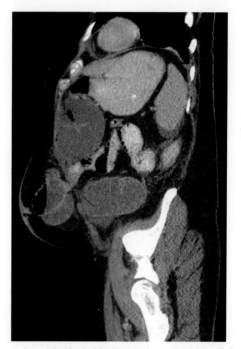

Figure 6.18 Sagittal CT image shows a small bowel containing parastomal hernia (arrow) with resultant dilated proximal small bowel loops as a result of bowel obstruction.

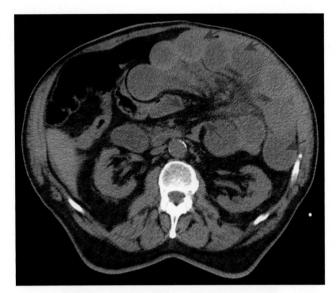

Figure 6.19 Axial CT image showing an internal hernia. Loops of small bowel have passed through a defect in the transverse mesocolon (posteromedial arrows) leading to small bowel obstruction (anterolateral arrows).

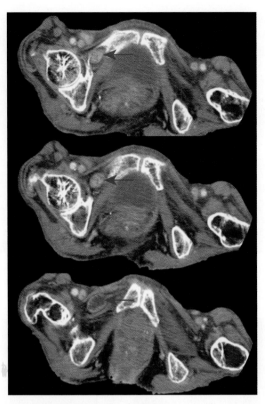

Figure 6.20 Right-sided obturator hernia demonstrated on CT. This contains a loop of small bowel (arrows) on axial intravenous contrast medium-enhanced CT.

CHAPTER 7

Gallbladder and biliary tract: anatomy and structural anomalies

Theodore H. Welling
University of Michigan Health System, Ann Arbor, MI, USA

Anatomy

The gallbladder lies in a depression along the inferior surface of the liver in a plane dividing the liver into its anatomic right and left lobes. The gallbladder is intimately attached to the liver by loose connective tissue that contains small veins and lymphatic vessels. The rest of the gallbladder, which is not in direct contact with the liver, is covered with peritoneum reflected from the liver and is in contact with the duodenum and hepatic flexure of the colon (Figure 7.1). The gallbladder is divided into four anatomic areas: fundus, body, infundibulum, and neck. The neck tapers into the cystic duct, which joins the common hepatic duct to become the common bile duct. Although the cystic duct typically joins the common hepatic duct directly, it may join the extrahepatic biliary tract anywhere from the right hepatic duct down to the level of the ampulla (Figures 7.2 and 7.3). The blood supply to the gallbladder and cystic duct is usually from a single artery arising from the right hepatic artery, although variations in this configuration are common (Figure 7.4). The gallbladder is innervated by branches of both the sympathetic and parasympathetic nervous systems (Figure 7.5), which play a role in modulating gallbladder contractility. The gallbladder has five layers: epithelium, lamina propria, muscularis, perimuscular connective tissue, and serosa. The gallbladder mucosa is lined with columnar epithelial cells that are covered with abundant microvilli and joined by tight junctions.

Bile drains from the liver into the right and left hepatic ducts, which usually join outside the liver to form the common hepatic duct. The cystic duct then joins the common hepatic duct to become the common bile duct. The common bile duct lies anterior to the portal vein and to the right of the hepatic artery. The common bile duct is divided into four segments: supraduodenal, retroduodenal, pancreatic, and intraduodenal.

The intraduodenal common bile duct joins the main pancreatic duct to form the ampulla of Vater, which empties into the lumen of the duodenum. The intraduodenal common bile duct and ampulla of Vater are surrounded by a sheath of smooth muscle fibers referred to as the sphincter of Oddi (Figure 7.6). Regulation of bile flow is controlled primarily by the sphincter of Oddi.

Embryology

The biliary tract is first apparent during the fifth week of gestation and develops as a ventral sacculation in the distal foregut (Figure 7.7). This sacculation grows into the ventral mesentery, which divides into two buds: the cranial bud develops into the liver and intrahepatic bile ducts, and the caudal bud develops into the gallbladder and cystic duct (Figure 7.8). Another small bud arises from the inferior aspect of the caudal bud and ultimately develops into the ventral pancreas (Figure 7.9). The ventral pancreatic bud rotates 180° from right to left, fusing with the dorsal pancreatic bud to form the complete pancreas. Because the lower end of the common bile duct is attached to the ventral pancreatic bud, it also rotates and fuses with the duodenum along its posteromedial wall (Figure 7.10). Variations in this developmental process give rise to structural anomalies in the biliary tract (Figure 7.11). In addition, viral etiologies along with host response may result in various forms of atresia (Figure 7.12). Type II and type III choledochal cysts are likely secondary to variations in development (Figure 7.13), whereas type I choledochal cysts are related to an aberrant junction of the pancreatic and biliary ducts such that a common channel of greater than a 20 mm (normal < 10 mm) exists, resulting in reflux of pancreatic juice into the biliary epithelium, leading to gradual inflammation and ectasia.

Yamada's Atlas of Gastroenterology, Fifth Edition. Edited by Daniel K. Podolsky, Michael Camilleri, J. Gregory Fitz, Anthony N. Kalloo, Fergus Shanahan, and Timothy C. Wang.
© 2016 John Wiley & Sons, Ltd. Published 2016 by John Wiley & Sons, Ltd.
Companion website: www.yamadagastro.com/atlas

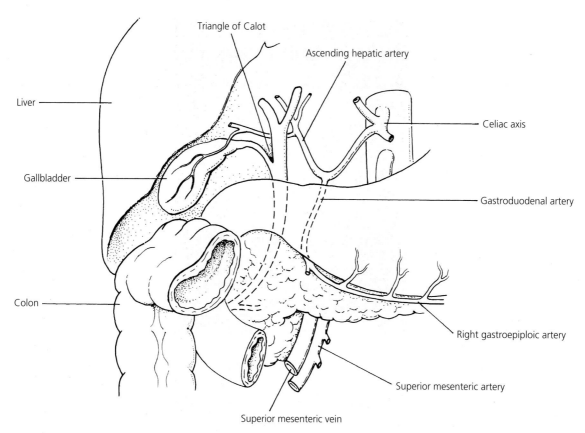

Figure 7.1 Relation of the gallbladder and extrahepatic biliary tract to the liver, duodenum, colon, and pancreas.

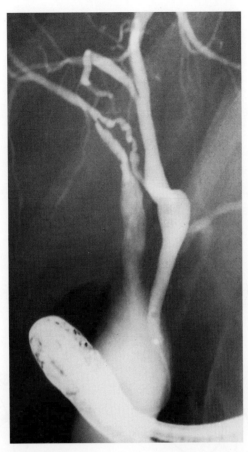

Figure 7.2 Endoscopic retrograde cholangiopancreatogram demonstrates an anomalous junction of the cystic duct with an accessory right hepatic duct.

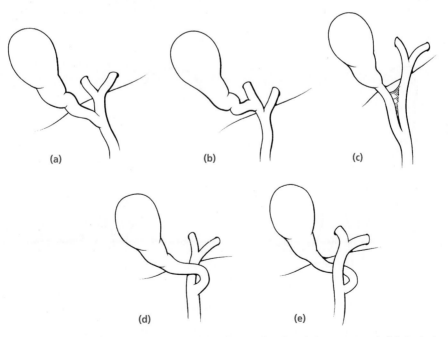

Figure 7.3 Variations in cystic duct anatomy. **(a)** Cystic duct joins common hepatic duct directly (most common). **(b)** Cystic duct joins the right hepatic duct. **(c)** Low junction of cystic duct with common hepatic duct. **(d)** Anterior spiral of cystic duct before joining common hepatic duct. **(e)** Posterior spiral of cystic duct before joining common hepatic duct.

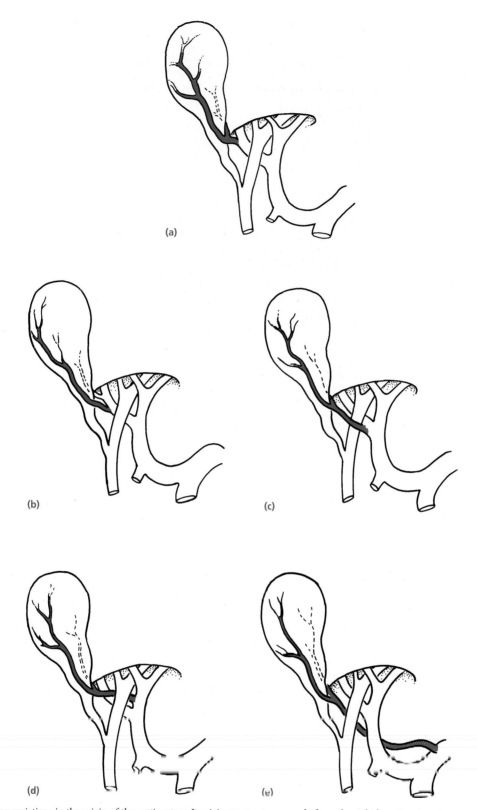

Figure 7.4 Common variations in the origin of the cystic artery. It originates most commonly from the right hepatic artery, traverses the triangle of Calot, and on reaching the gallbladder divides into two main branches **(a)**. Occasionally, the two branches come off the right hepatic artery independently **(b)**. The cystic artery may cross the hepatic duct anteriorly **(c)**, come off the left hepatic artery **(d)**, or, more rarely, come directly from the celiac axis **(e)**.

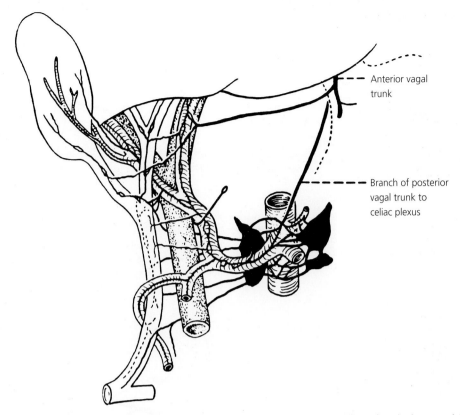

--- Anterior vagal trunk

--- Branch of posterior vagal trunk to celiac plexus

Figure 7.5 Schematic of the innervation of the gallbladder and extrahepatic biliary tract. The nerves originate from both vagi and from the celiac axis. They reach the biliary tract traveling along the walls of the hepatic artery, except for direct branches of the anterior vagus that cross through the gastrohepatic ligament.

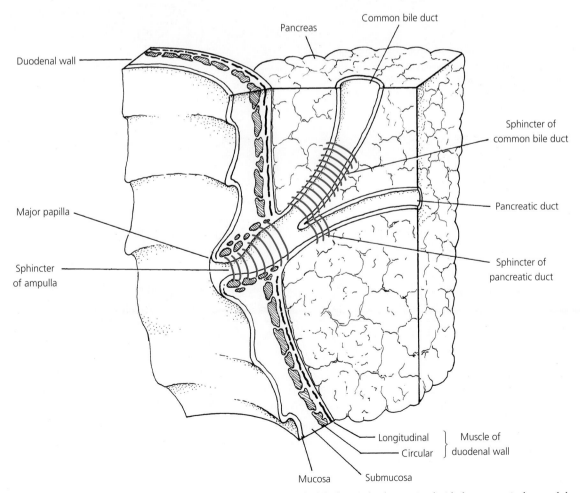

Pancreas

Common bile duct

Duodenal wall —

Sphincter of common bile duct

Major papilla

Pancreatic duct

Sphincter of ampulla

Sphincter of pancreatic duct

— Longitudinal
— Circular

Muscle of duodenal wall

Mucosa   Submucosa

Figure 7.6 Muscular apparatus at the terminal end of the common bile duct. The bile duct is closely associated with the pancreatic duct, and they both enter the medial wall of the duodenum tangentially. Each duct has its own sphincter, which is poorly developed in the pancreatic duct.

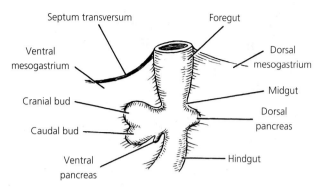

Figure 7.7 At the 3-mm stage of the embryo, the ventral bud enters the mesogastrium and soon divides into a cranial and a caudal bud. A smaller caudal bud represents the origin of the ventral pancreas.

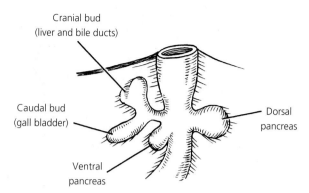

Figure 7.8 As the embryo reaches 5 mm, the cranial bud (which will form the liver and intrahepatic biliary tract) moves toward the septum transversum, pulling the caudal bud (gallbladder and extrahepatic bile ducts).

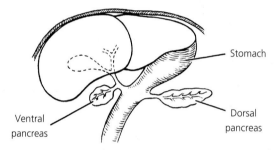

Figure 7.9 When the embryo reaches 7 mm, the right and left lobes of the liver occupy the position under the septum transversum. The ventral pancreas and the extrahepatic biliary tract are visible. As the ventral pancreas rotates to reach the dorsal pancreas, it pulls the lower end of the common bile duct with it.

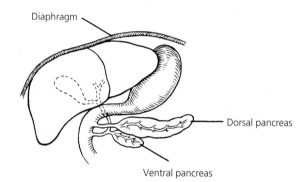

Figure 7.10 At the 12-mm stage, the ventral pancreas has rotated and the normal anatomic relations of the bile ducts and gastrointestinal tract have taken place.

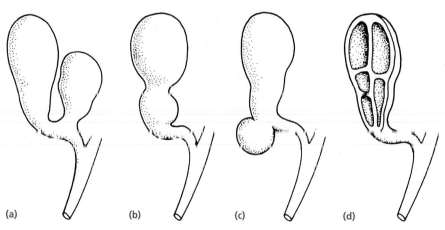

Figure 7.11 (a) Two gallbladders. **(b)** Bilobed gallbladder. **(c)** Diverticulum at the neck. **(d)** Septated gallbladder. All are anatomic variations that relate to the embryological development of the biliary tract.

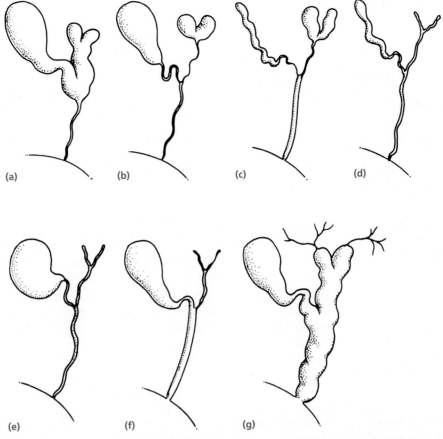

Figure 7.12 (a–g) Different forms of biliary atresia. Biliary atresia may be partial, affecting the intrahepatic or extrahepatic portions of the biliary tract, or may be a complete process.

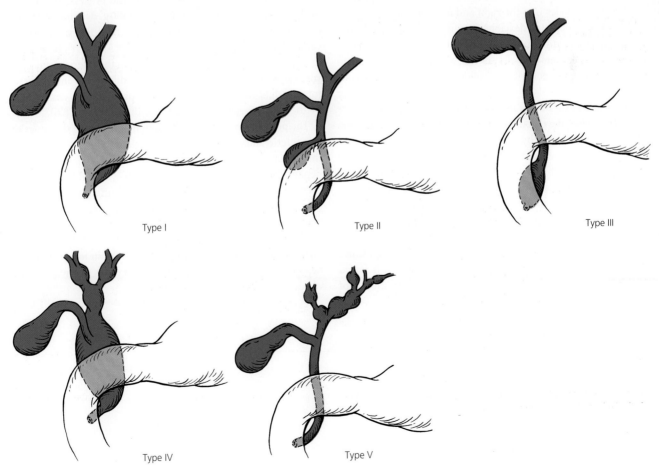

Type I

Type II

Type III

Type IV

Type V

Figure 7.13 Classification of choledochal cysts.

CHAPTER 8

Liver: anatomy, microscopic structure, and cell types

Gary C. Kanel

University of Southern California, Los Angeles, CA, USA

Embryology

The hepatic primordium anlage first appears towards the end of the third week of gestation and is seen as a hollow midline outgrowth stalk (*hepatic diverticulum*). By the fourth week the diverticulum enlarges by proliferation of the endodermal cell strands (*hepatoblasts*) and projects cranially into the mesoderm of the septum transversum, eventually giving rise to the hepatic parenchyma and intrahepatic duct structures.

The vascular network is originally derived from the development of both the vitelline and umbilical veins. The hepatic cords and vessels anastomose, forming the hepatic sinusoids. By week five most of the major vessels are identified, including the right and left umbilical veins, the transverse portal sinus, and the ductus venosus. The portal vein develops from the vitelline vein and then subdivides into the right and left branches.

The biliary apparatus develops from membranous infoldings occurring between the junctional complexes of adjacent hepatoblasts and appears initially as intercellular spaces with no distinct wall. A ductal plate develops from the hepatoblasts immediately adjacent to the portal mesenchyme, eventually forming an anastomosing network of portal duct structures.

During fetal development, the red blood cell precursors abound in the parenchyma (Figure 8.1), while myeloid and megakaryocytic precursors are more evident within the portal tracts. The hepatoblasts immediately adjacent to the mesenchyme of the portal tracts form the ductal plate, which is two-layered; by 3 months a lumen is seen within the ductal plate, with formation of double-layered tubular structures (Figure 8.2).

Individual cell functions become apparent at different times in embryological development. α-Fetoprotein, which is found in high amounts at birth, initially is present by 1 month of gestation, and continues throughout fetal development (Figure 8.3). Glycogen may be seen by 2 months, with glycogen synthesis becoming most apparent by 3 months, although at birth the amount of glycogen rapidly diminishes due to rapid and active glycogenolysis. Steatosis within the hepatocyte parallels that of glycogenesis. Hemosiderin is usually visible in early stages, becomes most marked as intrahepatic hematopoiesis decreases, and then gradually decreases but may still be seen at birth in the periportal hepatocytes.

Gross anatomy

The liver extends from the right lateral aspect of the abdomen 15–20 cm transversely towards the xiphoid process. The weight of the adult liver varies from 1200 to 1800 g, depending on the overall body size. Anatomically it has four lobes: right, left, caudate, and quadrate (Figures 8.4 and 8.5). The right and left lobes are divided by a line extending from the inferior vena cava superiorly to the middle of the gallbladder fossa inferiorly. A total of eight functional segments are present, each demarcated by their own vascular and biliary drainage (Figure 8.6).

The portal vein is formed through the merger of the superior mesenteric and splenic veins. The hepatic vein is composed of three major tributaries (right, middle, and left), while the hepatic artery ascends along the hepatoduodenal ligament and eventually divides into the right and left main branches. The biliary drainage of the right lobe is derived from anterior and posterior segmental branches that merge to form the right hepatic duct. Lateral and medial segmental branches merge to form the left hepatic duct, which drains the left lobe. The intrahepatic components of these vessels and ducts follow along the various hepatic segments (Figure 8.7)

Yamada's Atlas of Gastroenterology, Fifth Edition. Edited by Daniel K. Podolsky, Michael Camilleri, J. Gregory Fitz, Anthony N. Kalloo, Fergus Shanahan, and Timothy C. Wang.
© 2016 John Wiley & Sons, Ltd. Published 2016 by John Wiley & Sons, Ltd.
Companion website: www.yamadagastro.com/atlas

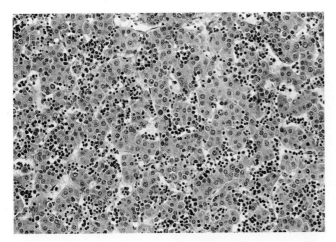

Figure 8.1 Embryonic development of the hepatic lobule. Extramedullary hematopoiesis is prominent in the hepatic lobules, begins at approximately 6 weeks, and is most active during the sixth and seventh months of gestation.

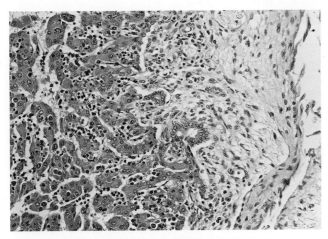

Figure 8.2 Embryonic development of the duct plate. Ductal plates form by invasion of hepatoblasts into the portal mesenchyme.

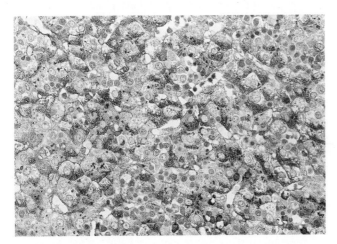

Figure 8.3 α-Fetoprotein during embryonic development. This protein, which is present at high concentration at birth, is initially identified in the liver at 1 month of gestation.

Microanatomy

The basic microanatomical structure of the liver can best be seen on a three-dimensional drawing of the portal tracts, parenchyma, and vascular flow (Figure 8.8). The portal tract (Figure 8.9) contains one to two interlobular bile ducts that are usually seen adjacent to the hepatic arterioles, the latter responsible for their blood supply. The portal venule is a single vascular structure. The fibrous tissue, which supports the major portal components, varies in amount depending on the distance of the portal tract from the hepatic hilum. The hepatic lobules (Figure 8.10) are composed predominantly of liver cell trabecular cords one cell thick. The adjacent sinusoids are lined by both endothelial and Kupffer cells, whereas the perisinusoidal space, located between the endothelial cells and hepatocytes, contains stellate cells and collagen fibers.

The hepatocytes average from 25 to 40 μm in diameter and are polyhedral and multifaceted. The cells have three distinct cell boundaries: sinusoidal, lateral (intercellular), and canalicular membranes. The liver cell nucleus is centrally located within the hepatocyte and measures approximately 10 μm in diameter.

The liver cell cytoplasm (Figures 8.11 and 8.12) contains numerous functionally important organelles. The superstructure is maintained by the cytoskeleton of the hepatocyte, which includes three major subdivisions: microfilaments, microtubules, and intermediate filaments. The numerous mitochondria maintain critical functions such as oxidative phosphorylation and fatty acid oxidation and also contain components that are essential for the urea and citric acid cycles. The endoplasmic reticulum (ER) is composed of a convoluted network of cisternae, saccules, tubules, and vesicles and is divided into two components, the rough ER and the smooth ER. The Golgi apparatus is composed of highly polarized parallel flattened dilated saccules or vesicles. Lysosomes appear as electron-dense pleomorphic single membrane-bound vesicles containing various enzymes such as acid phosphatase, esterases, proteases, and lipases.

The Kupffer cells are sinusoidal lining cells that function as tissue macrophages. The endothelial cells are flattened elongated sinusoidal cells. Numerous cytoplasmic projections and clustered fenestrae or gaps that range in size from 0.1 to 0.2 μm are present. The stellate cells are located within the perisinusoidal liver cell recesses along the space of Disse and often contain variably sized lipid droplets that carry a high concentration of vitamin A (retinol palmitate). The space of Disse lies between the hepatocytes and the endothelial cells.

The stroma overall supports the basic hepatic architectural arrangement and is composed of five basic types of collagen, with types I and III representing more than 95% of the total collagen. Type I represents mature collagen fibers and is seen predominantly within the portal tracts but also around the outflow veins, whereas type III collagen represents new collagen fibers which, along with the type IV collagen fibers, comprises the sinusoidal reticulin framework.

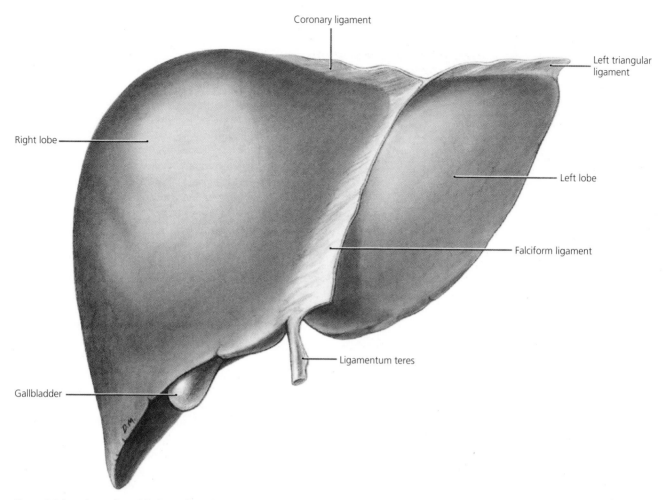

Coronary ligament

Left triangular ligament

Right lobe

Left lobe

Falciform ligament

Ligamentum teres

Gallbladder

Figure 8.4 Anterior surface of the liver. The right and left lobes are divided by the falciform ligament, with the ligamentum teres lying along its free edge. Source: Agur AMR, Lee MJ. Grant's Atlas of Anatomy, 10th edn; 1999. Reproduced with permission of Wolters Kluwer Health.

The biliary tract can be divided into its structural components, the smallest of which are the biliary canaliculi (Figure 8.13) which are located along the intercellular spaces between hepatocytes and are lined by microvilli. The canaliculi that enter the portal tracts, labeled the terminal ductules or ducts of Hering, are derived from hepatocytes located at the limiting plate and communicate with the interlobular bile ducts. The interlobular bile ducts within the smaller portal structures are lined by a single layer of cuboidal cells, whereas the larger interlobar and septal ducts have a fibrous wall and are lined by a single layer of cuboidal to columnar epithelium. These lead into the segmental ducts, eventually forming the major hilar ducts that ultimately branch into the main right and left hepatic ducts.

The major blood vessels that supply the liver are the portal vein and the hepatic artery. The portal vein sequentially develops interlobar, segmental, and interlobular veins, and preterminal branches. The terminal portal venules are seen in the smaller triangular portal tracts. The hepatic artery branches accompany the portal vein and divide within the smaller portal tracts into the periportal plexus and the peribiliary plexus, which supply blood to the accompanying interlobular bile ducts through small capillaries that are layered around the ducts.

The hepatic acinus can be divided into three segments: simple (Figure 8.14), complex, and acinar agglomerate. The simple acinus is the smallest functional parenchymal unit and centers on a portal tract. The acinus is divided into three zones (zones of Rappaport): periportal (zone 1), which includes the limiting plate; midzone (zone 2); and perivenular (zone 3), with the terminal hepatic venule at its outer lateral margin. The complex acinus is derived from three adjacent simple acini fed by a preterminal portal vein and arterial branch. The acinar agglomerate is composed of approximately four complex acini and is fed by a portal venous branch. In addition, the hepatocytes within these various zones have many different specialized physiological functions that are manifestations of nutrient and hormonal gradients, oxygen concentration gradients, and availability of numerous substrates and enzyme activities.

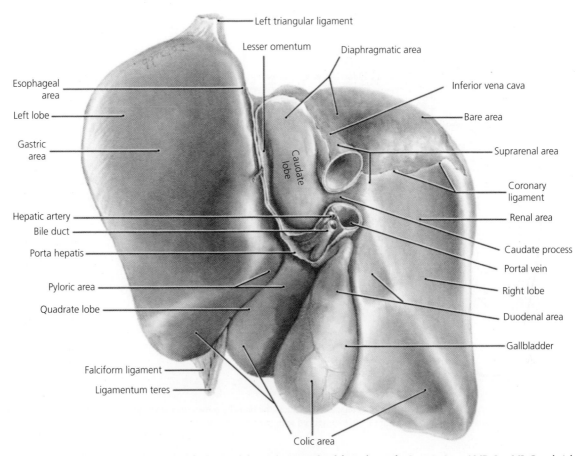

Figure 8.5 Inferior and posterior hepatic surfaces. The hepatic hilum is best visualized from this angle. Source: Agur AMR, Lee MJ. Grant's Atlas of Anatomy, 10th edn; 1999. Reproduced with permission of Wolters Kluwer Health.

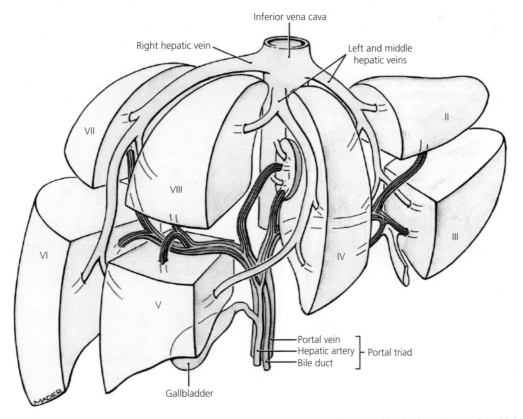

Figure 8.6 Segmental and vascular hepatic components. The eight functional components are demarcated by their vascular supply and biliary drainage. Source: Agur AMR, Lee MJ. Grant's Atlas of Anatomy, 10th edn; 1999. Reproduced with permission of Wolters Kluwer Health.

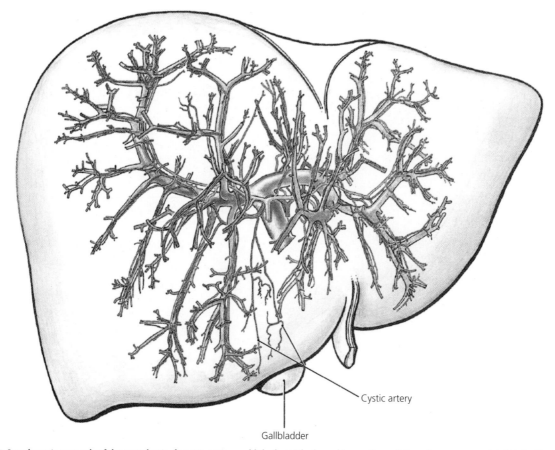

Cystic artery

Gallbladder

Figure 8.7 Intrahepatic network of the portal vein, hepatic artery, and bile duct. The branching patterns follow along a segmental distribution. Source: Agur AMR, Lee MJ. Grant's Atlas of Anatomy, 10th edn; 1999. Reproduced with permission of Wolters Kluwer Health.

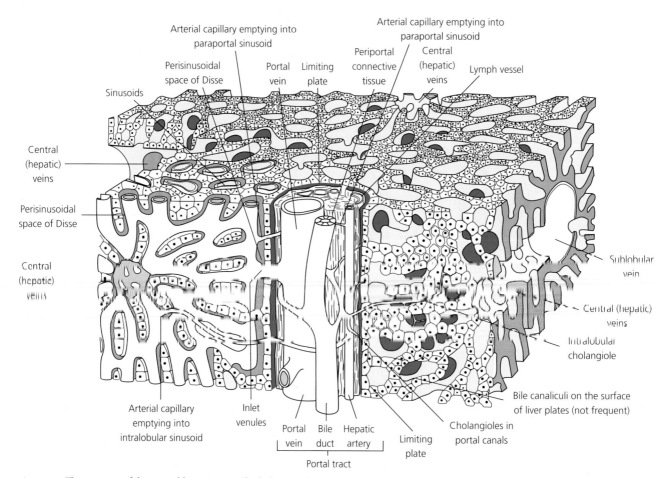

Figure 8.8 The structure of the normal liver. Source: Sherlock S, Dooley J. Diseases of the Liver and Biliary System, 11th edn; 2002. Reproduced with permission of John Wiley & Sons.

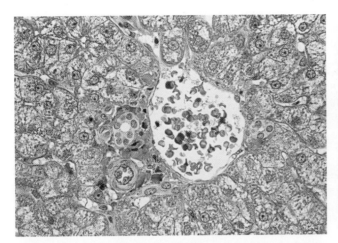

Figure 8.9 Portal tract (Masson trichrome stain). The major components include the hepatic arteriole, portal venule (large vessel), and bile ductule (cuboidal epithelium). There is a normal amount of collagen seen in this portal tract.

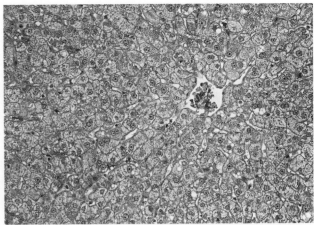

Figure 8.10 Parenchyma (Masson trichrome stain). The liver cell plates are one cell thick and are divided by sinusoids lined by Kupffer and endothelial cells, with vascular outflow via the terminal hepatic venule. No sinusoidal collagen deposition is appreciated on light microscopy in the normal liver.

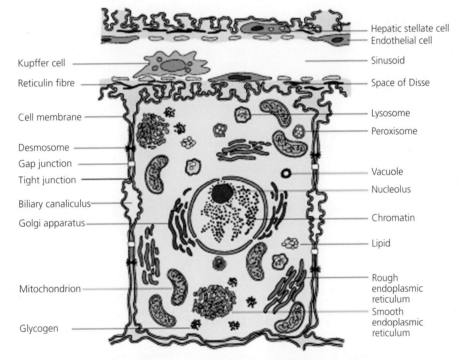

Figure 8.11 Drawing of a liver cell with organelles. This drawing illustrates the various components within the hepatocytes. Source: Sherlock S, Dooley J. Diseases of the Liver and Biliary System, 11th edn; 2002. Reproduced with permission of John Wiley & Sons.

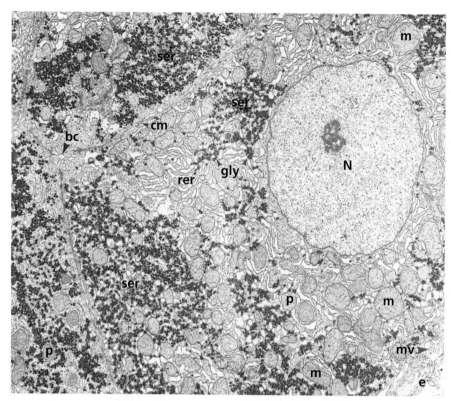

Figure 8.12 Hepatocyte (electron microscopic image). The hepatocyte is composed of a single nucleus (N). The cytoplasm demonstrates many mitochondria (m), rough (rer) and smooth (ser) endoplasmic reticulum, glycogen (gly), and peroxisomes (p). Also seen are the cell membrane (cm), a bile canaliculus (bc), endothelium (e), and microvilli (mv). Source: Phillips MJ, Poucell S, Patterson J, et al. The Liver: an Atlas and Text of Ultrastructural Pathology; 1987. Reproduced with permission of Wolters Kluwer Health.

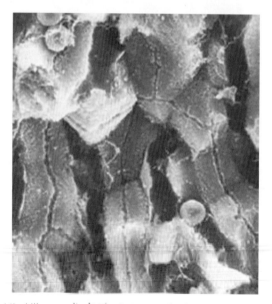

Figure 8.13 Scanning electron micrograph of the biliary canaliculi. The distinct canaliculi are seen in the center of the liver plates. Source: Sherlock S, Dooley J. Diseases of the Liver and Biliary System, 11th edn; 2002. Reproduced with permission of John Wiley & Sons.

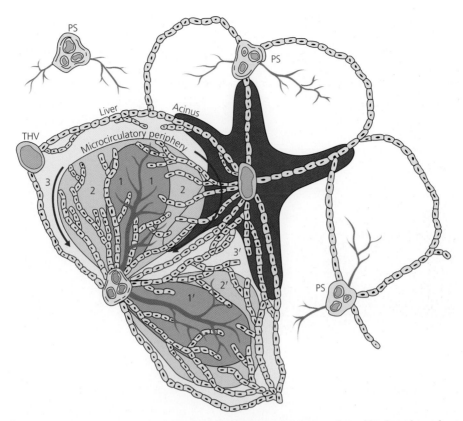

Figure 8.14 The simple liver acinus. The three hepatic zones and their relationship to the microcirculatory blood supply are demonstrated. PS, portal structures; THV, terminal hepatic venule. Source: Sherlock S, Dooley J. Diseases of the Liver and Biliary System, 11th edn; 2002. Reproduced with permission of John Wiley & Sons.

PART 2

Gastrointestinal diseases

CHAPTER 9

Motility disorders of the esophagus

Joan W. Chen,[1] John E. Pandolfino,[2] and Peter J. Kahrilas[2]

[1] University of Michigan, Ann Arbor, MI, USA
[2] Northwestern University, Feinberg School of Medicine, Chicago, IL, USA

The diagnosis and management of motility disorders of the esophagus has undergone a dramatic evolution over the last 5 years due to new technologies that have moved from the investigational realm into clinical practice. High-resolution manometry and intraluminal impedance (Figures 9.1, 9.2, and 9.3) are two exciting developments that have enhanced our ability to visualize esophageal motor patterns and the dynamics of bolus transit through the esophagus. These techniques have improved our accuracy to assess esophageal motor function and have also allowed us to better define clinical phenotypes with important prognostic function. These tools have also expanded our ability to develop treatment paradigms focused on these important motor abnormalities and have also provided greater confidence in diagnosis. The role of contrast studies and endoscopy (Figures 9.4, 9.5, 9.6, and 9.7) still remain crucial to the evaluation of esophageal motor disorders, however, and they remain an important complementary diagnostic option in the evaluation of dysphagia, chest pain, and gastroesophageal reflux disease.

With this background, the current chapter will focus on describing esophageal motility disorders and their complications using a complement of radiographic studies and advanced motility techniques that utilize esophageal pressure topography (Figures 9.8–9.17).

Acknowledgment

This work was supported by R01 DK079902 (JEP) and R01 DK56033 (PJK) from the Public Health Service.

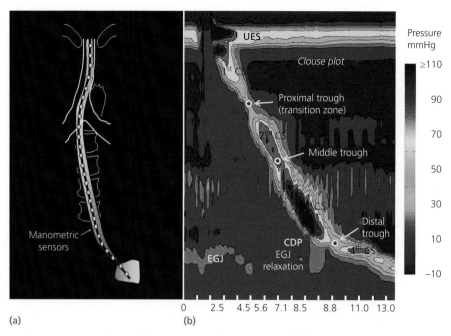

Figure 9.1 Representation of a normal swallow illustrated with high-resolution manometry (HRM) plotted in esophageal pressure topography (EPT). **(a)** placement of a HRM catheter with closely spaced circumferential pressure sensors along the length of the esophagus. **(b)** HRM data can be displayed as pressure topography, also known as a "Clouse plot," where pressure values between the closely spaced sensors are interpolated and the pressure magnitude indicated by color. Sterotypic features of the topographic architecture of the peristaltic contraction is evident in **(b)**. The four contraction segments (CS) and troughs between contractions, including the transition zone, are labeled on the EPT. UES, upper esophageal sphincter; EGJ, esophagogastric junction; CDP, contractile deceleration point. Source: Courtesy of the Esophageal Center at Northwestern.

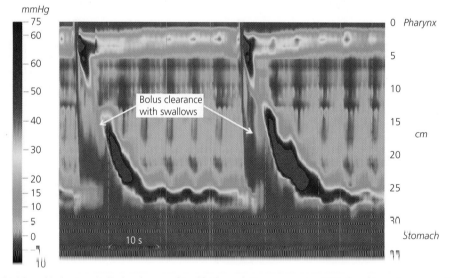

Figure 9.2 Normal peristalsis and bolus transit displayed on combined high-resolution manometry (HRM) and impedance recording. The combined HRM-Impedance catheter and recording system provides bolus transit information in addition to esophageal contraction pattern. Impedance data, indicated by pink overlying the esophageal pressure topography plot, indicate the disposition of the swallowed bolus and demonstrate complete clearance in this example. Source: Courtesy of the Esophageal Center at Northwestern.

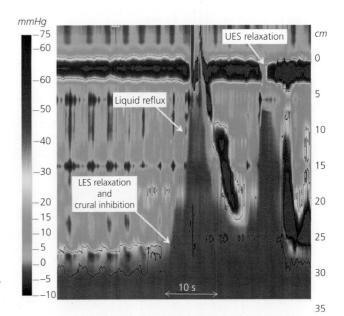

Figure 9.3 Reflux event seen on combined high-resolution manometry–impedance tracing. In this example, a transient lower esophageal sphincter (LES) relaxation is associated with liquid reflux from the stomach. This was followed by a swallow and repeated reflux with a microburp. The bolus is then cleared by secondary peristalsis. UES, upper esophageal sphincter. Source: Courtesy of the Esophageal Center at Northwestern.

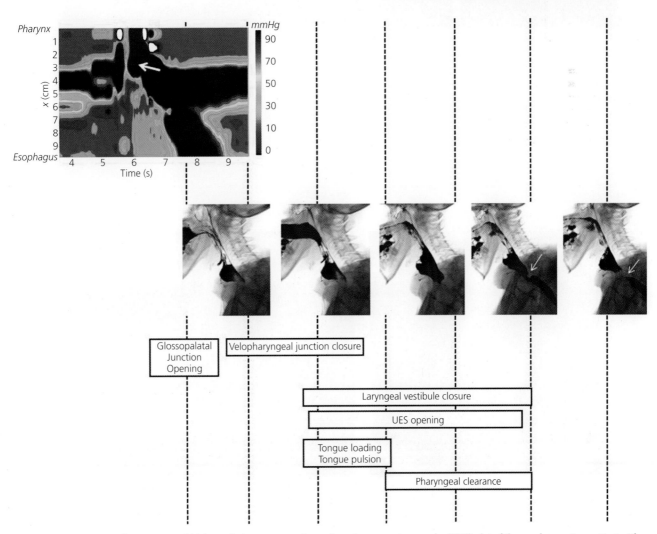

Figure 9.4 Concomitant fluoroscopy and high-resolution manometric esophageal pressure topography (EPT) plot of the oropharynx in a patient with a cricopharyngeal (CP) bar. The white arrow on the EPT plot indicates the high-pressure zone at the noncompliant CP muscle. The fluoroscopic images are presented in sequence during a barium swallow. As in a typical swallow, glossopalatal junction opening occurs in synchrony with upper esophageal sphincter (UES) relaxation. This is followed by velopharyngeal junction closure, sealing off the nasopharynx to prevent regurgitation. Laryngeal vestibule closure and UES opening occurs as the epiglottis is inverted, and the bolus is rapidly pushed through the UES. Bolus transit continues with pharyngeal stripping and clearance and concludes with laryngeal vestibule closure. The latter two fluoroscopic images in this patient demonstrate a prominent CP (white arrows) at the level of C5-6. Source: Courtesy of the Esophageal Center at Northwestern.

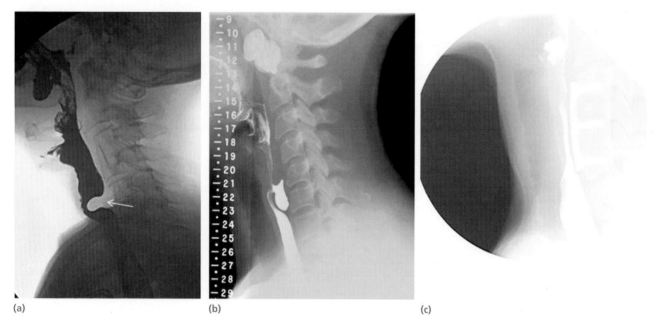

(a) (b) (c)

Figure 9.5 **(a)** Cricopharyngeal (CP) bar found on barium esophagram of a patient with oropharyngeal dysphagia. The posterior indentation of the barium column is caused by a noncompliant cricopharyngeus muscle (white arrow). **(b)** Zenker's diverticulum originating above the cricopharyngeus muscle. **(c)** Large cervical spine fixation plates located at C5-C6 level with associated esophageal luminal narrowing in a patient with dysphagia. Source: Courtesy of the Esophageal Center at Northwestern.

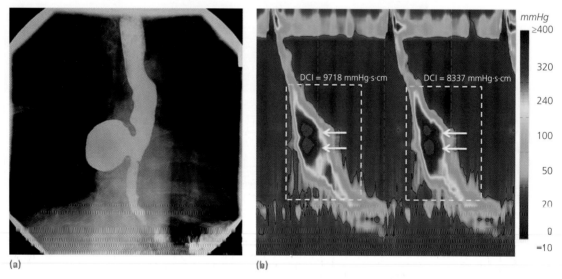

(a) (b)

Figure 9.6 Midesophageal diverticulum. **(a)** Barium x-ray of a large diverticulum in the midesophagus in a patient with dysphagia and regurgitation. **(b)** High-resolution manometry (HRM) study showed a jackhammer pattern. White arrows on the HRM–esophageal pressure topography plot point to two high-pressure zones during distal esophageal contraction, which correlate with contractions above and below the diverticulum. DCI, distal contractile integral. Source: Courtesy of the Esophageal Center at Northwestern.

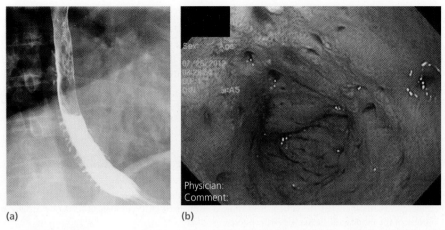

Figure 9.7 Esophageal intramural pseudodiverticulosis. **(a)** Barium x-ray and **(b)** endoscopic image of small outpouches in the wall of the esophagus, consistent with pseudodiverticula, believed to represent dilated excretory ducts of esophageal submucosal glands. Source: Courtesy of the Esophageal Center at Northwestern.

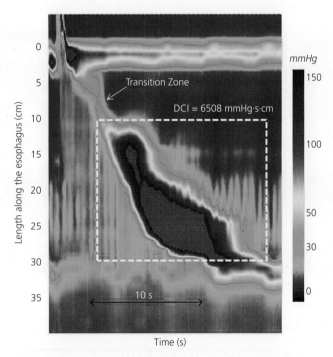

Figure 9.8 Hypertensive peristalsis defined in the Chicago Classification using the distal contractile integral (DCI). DCI is the metric used to assess contractile vigor of the esophagus distal to the transition zone. Normal DCI is less than 5000 mmHg·s·cm. A hypertensive swallow has a DCI greater than 5000 mmHg·s·cm but less than 8000 mmHg·s·cm. Source: Courtesy of the Esophageal Center at Northwestern.

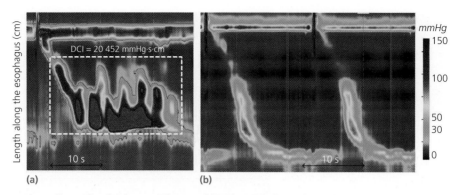

Figure 9.9 **(a)** Illustration of a swallow with a distal contractile integral (DCI) greater than 8000 mmHg·s·cm, consistent with a "Jackhammer" contraction, based on the Chicago Classification. **(b)** The same patient showed normalized DCI on sildenafil 25 mg twice daily and symptomatic improvement. Source: Courtesy of the Esophageal Center at Northwestern.

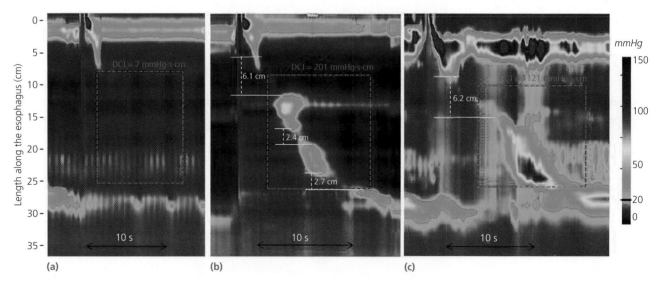

Figure 9.10 High-resolution manometric recordings of three types of weak peristalsis. **(a)** Absent peristalsis. **(b)** Weak peristalsis – ineffective esophageal motility (IEM), associated with breaks in the 20-mmHg isobaric contour at each pressure trough and a distal contractile integral (DCI) <450 mmHg·s·cm. **(c)** Weak peristalsis with a large transition zone (TZ) defect. Source: Courtesy of the Esophageal Center at Northwestern.

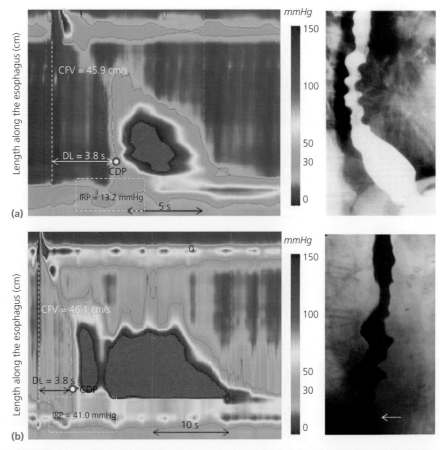

Figure 9.11 The definition of distal esophageal spasm (DES) in high-resolution manometry is based on the latency of the distal contraction and requires identification of the contractile deceleration point (CDP). The CDP is the inflection point in velocity of the contractile wavefront defined by the 30-mmHg isobaric contour. The contractile front velocity (CFV) is defined as the slope of the tangent approximating the 30-mmHg isobaric contour between the proximal pressure trough and the CDP. The timing of the distal contraction is assessed using the distal latency (DL), defined as the interval between upper esophageal relaxation and the CDP. **(a)** Rapid and premature distal esophageal contractions defined by elevated CFV and shortened DL are consistent with DES. To the right is a corresponding corkscrew esophagus on barium x-ray in a patient with symptomatic DES. **(b)** An example of spastic achalasia with a premature distal contraction and elevated integrated relaxation pressure (IRP). A corkscrew esophagus is again seen on barium x-ray (right panel). However, the GEJ in this patient shows a characteristic bird beak pattern (white arrow). Source: Courtesy of the Esophageal Center at Northwestern.

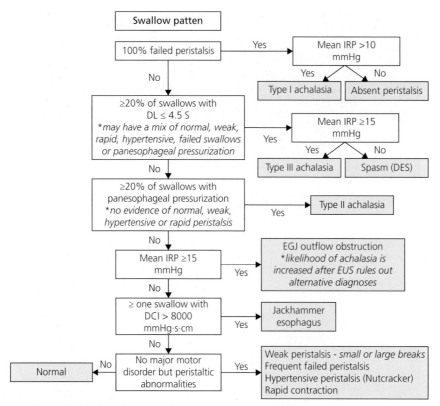

Figure 9.12 Algorithm for applying the Chicago Classification to the diagnosis of esophageal motor disorders associated with dysphagia and chest pain. Esophagogastric junction (EGJ) relaxation is characterized by the integrated relaxation pressure (IRP) to define the degree of EGJ outflow obstruction. If the IRP is abnormal, the patients are defined into subtypes of achalasia based on the dominant esophageal body contractile and pressurization patterns. Note that the IRP cutoff to define type I achalasia is lower than in other contractile patterns. If the patients have premature contractions (distal latency <4.5 s) in ≥20% of swallows and the mean IRP of 15 mmHg or greater, they are classified as type III or spastic achalasia. Patients with panesophageal pressurization in ≥20% swallows, they are defined as type II achalasia. Patients with an elevated IRP and evidence of intact or weak peristalsis without premature contractions, are classified as EGJ outflow obstruction. EGJ outflow obstruction may be an early form or variant presentation of achalasia, or related to a structural or infiltrative process. Advanced imaging, for example endoscopic ultrasound, should be used to clarify this diagnosis. One or more swallows with distal contractile integral (DCI) greater than 8000 mmHg·s·cm defines Jackhammer esophagus. If none of the above abnormalities are found, patients may have minor motor disorders (weak peristalsis, frequently failed peristalsis, hypertensive peristalsis, or rapid contraction) or normal contractility. DL, distal latency; DES, diffuse esophageal spasm. Source: Courtesy of the Esophageal Center at Northwestern.

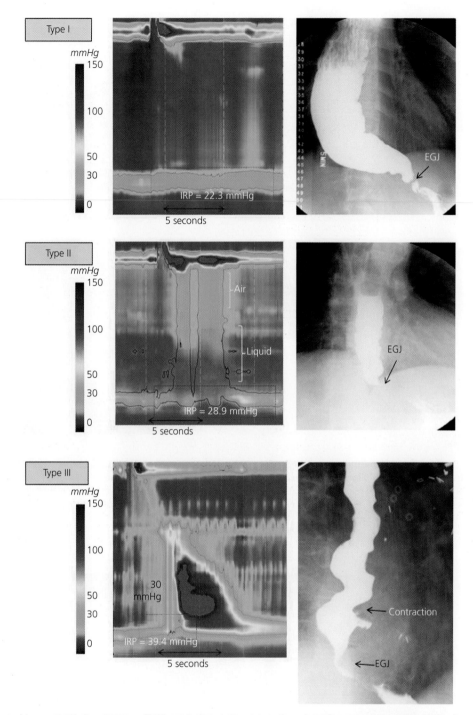

Figure 9.13 Achalasia subtypes. With the adoption of high-resolution manometry and esophageal pressure topography (EPT), three distinct subtypes of achalasia were defined using EPT metrics. All have impaired esophagogastric junction (EGJ) relaxation and absent peristalsis but the differentiating features are in the patterns of esophageal pressurization: type I has 100% failed swallows (aperistalsis); type II exhibits panesophageal pressurization in ≥20% swallows; and type III exhibits two or more premature (spastic) contractions. The panels to the right display examples of barium x-rays in patients with each achalasia subtype. Note how the impedance data in the type II patient corresponds to the level of barium retention in the x-ray. Several recent publications have shown differences in prognosis of these achalasia subtypes, supporting the classification scheme. IRP, integrated relaxation pressure. Source: Courtesy of the Esophageal Center at Northwestern.

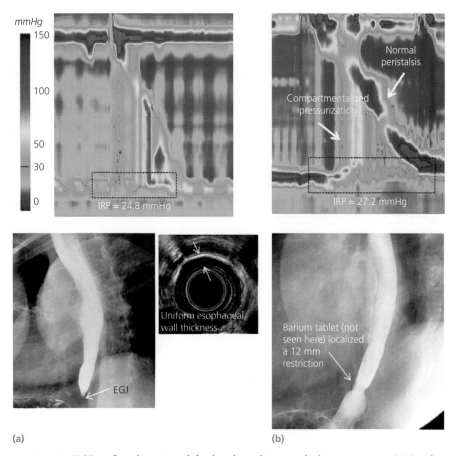

Figure 9.14 Esophagogastric junction (EGJ) outflow obstruction, defined as elevated integrated relaxation pressure (IRP) with intact or weak peristalsis and no premature contractions. EGJ outflow obstruction may represent an early form or variant presentation of achalasia. Alternatively, it may be related to a structural or infiltrative process at the EGJ. Two examples of outflow obstruction are shown here. **(a)** The high-resolution manometry (HRM) recording (upper panel) shows elevated IRP and distal pressurization. The patient was thought to have achalasia after barium esophagram (lower panel) and endoscopic ultrasound (lower central panel) ruled out an obstructive or infiltrative process. In the second example **(b)**, elevated IRP was seen in the setting of compartmentalized pressurization with normal distal peristalsis on HRM (upper panel). This patient was found to have a distal stricture that did not allow passage of a barium tablet on x-ray (lower panel). Source: Courtesy of the Esophageal Center at Northwestern.

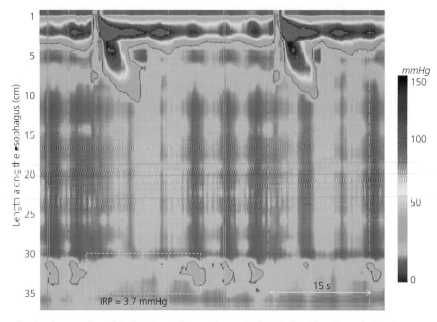

Figure 9.15 Scleroderma often involves esophageal dysfunction with smooth muscle fibrosis. Manifestations of scleroderma esophagus are typically dysphagia and heartburn. Manometric abnormalities include a hypotensive or absent lower esophageal sphincter pressure, hypotensive to absent distal esophageal peristalsis, and normal proximal esophageal peristalsis. IRP, integrated relaxation pressure. Source: Courtesy of the Esophageal Center at Northwestern.

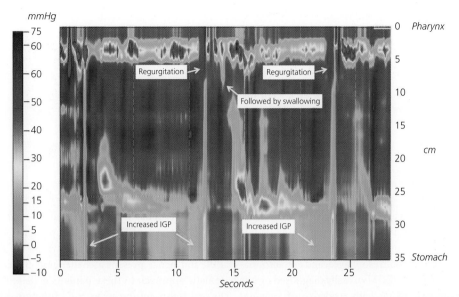

Figure 9.16 High-resolution manometry recording of rumination in a patient with recurrent postprandial regurgitation causing weight loss. The manometic tracing shows abrupt increases in intragastric pressure (IGP) followed by regurgitation consistent with rumination syndrome. Source: Courtesy of the Esophageal Center at Northwestern.

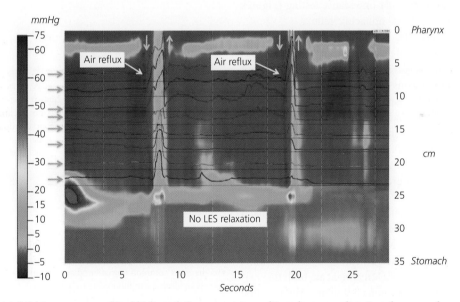

Figure 9.17 Supragastric belching seen on combined high-resolution manometry and impedance recording. Impedance waveforms (indicated by orange arrows to the left) demonstrate air transit in the esophagus, seen as abrupt increase in impedance. The lower esophageal sphincter (LES) remains contracted. The direction of air movement is indicated by the blue arrows. This is consistent with supragastric belching. Source: Courtesy of the Esophageal Center at Northwestern.

CHAPTER 10

Gastroesophageal reflux disease

Kumar Krishnan,[1] John E. Pandolfino,[2] and Peter J. Kahrilas[2]
[1] Houston Methodist Hospital, Weill Cornell Medical College, Houston, TX, USA
[2] Northwestern University Feinberg School of Medicine, Chicago, IL, USA

Gastroesophageal reflux disease (GERD) accounts for a large number of referrals to gastroenterologists (Figure 10.1). While typically presenting as heartburn, the spectrum of symptoms attributable to GERD includes both esophageal and extraesophageal symptoms (Figure 10.2). GERD is usually diagnosed on the basis of typical symptoms along with evidence of mucosal injury. This mucosal injury often results in the endoscopic appearance of esophagitis, esophageal stricture, or a metaplastic reaction from chronic reflux-related injury (Figures 10.3, 10.4, and 10.5). In some patients, formal testing for pathological reflux is required for diagnosis. This can include both acid reflux testing (Figure 10.6) as well as pH-impedance testing (Figures 10.7 and 10.8), which may reveal nonacidic reflux.

In healthy individuals, the most common physiological mechanism of gastroesophageal reflux is transient lower esophageal sphincter relaxation (Figure 10.9). Distinct anatomic and other physiological mechanisms result in more profound reflux in some patients. These mechanisms augment the refluxate/mucosa contact time. While manometric features are not diagnostic of GERD, a typical motility pattern is ineffective esophageal motility (Figure 10.10). Anatomically, the esophagogastric junction (EGJ) is the primary barrier to pathological reflux. The Hill classification grades variable incompetence of the EGJ (Figure 10.11). Perhaps the most significant anatomic abnormality predisposing to reflux is the presence of a hiatal hernia. Here, the stomach is displaced proximally into the chest. This results in separation of the lower esophageal sphincter from the crural diaphragm (Figure 10.12).

The primary objectives of GERD treatment are both the alleviation of symptoms and healing mucosal injury. The first-line for treatment of GERD is the use of oral proton pump inhibitors (PPI). While PPI have demonstrated excellent efficacy in healing of erosive esophagitis, they have variable efficacy for the alleviation of some GERD-related symptoms (Figure 10.13). Some patients with typical heartburn symptoms do not respond to PPI, and hence present a challenging clinical dilemma. A systematic approach to these patients is helpful and must include formal reflux testing to exclude functional heartburn (Figure 10.14). Surgical therapies for GERD have been shown to be as effective as medical therapy for relieving heartburn and healing esophagitis in patients with GERD. However, while relatively safe in expert centers, surgical complications do occur (Figure 10.15).

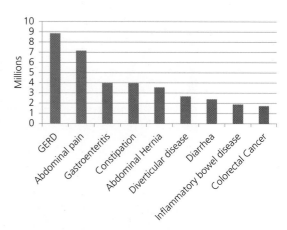

Figure 10.1 The burden of gastroesophageal reflux disease (GERD) in an ambulatory setting. Data of insurance claim records reveal that GERD was the most common outpatient diagnosis among gastroenterologist in 2009 with almost 9 million visits coded with GERD. There were roughly 2 million outpatient visits prompted by GERD. Source: Adapted from Peery AF, Dellon ES, Lund J, et al. Burden of gastrointestinal disease in the United States: 2012 update. Gastroenterology 2012;143:1179.

Yamada's Atlas of Gastroenterology, Fifth Edition. Edited by Daniel K. Podolsky, Michael Camilleri, J. Gregory Fitz, Anthony N. Kalloo, Fergus Shanahan, and Timothy C. Wang.
© 2016 John Wiley & Sons, Ltd. Published 2016 by John Wiley & Sons, Ltd.
Companion website: www.yamadagastro.com/atlas

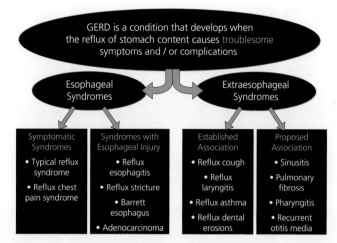

Figure 10.2 The Montreal definition of reflux disease. The clinical manifestations of gastroesophageal reflux disease (GERD) can be subdivided into esophageal and extraesophageal syndromes. The esophageal syndromes can be defined by any combination of reflux-related symptoms and/or reflux-related pathology. There are also multiple extraesophageal syndromes that have been attributed to reflux, some with strong pathophysiological associations and others are more speculative. Source: Modified from Vakil N, van Zanten SV, Kahrilas P, et al. The Montreal definition and classification of gastroesophageal reflux disease: a global evidence-based consensus. Am J Gastroenterol 2006;101:1900. Reproduced with permission of Nature Publishing Group.

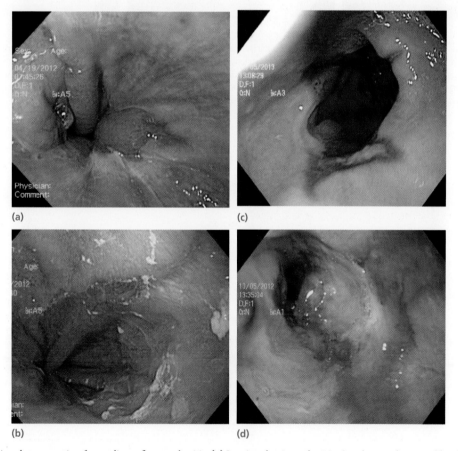

Figure 10.3 The Los Angeles convention for grading reflux esophagitis. **(a)** Los Angeles A esophagitis. One (or more) mucosal break on the top of mucosal folds less than 5 mm in length. Of note, this is present in 5% of asymptomatic patients. **(b)** At least one mucosal break >5 mm, but not bridging adjacent mucosal folds. **(c)** Mucosal break bridging mucosal folds, but <75% circumferential. **(d)** Mucosal breaks involving at least 75% of the luminal circumference. Source: Esophageal Center at Northwestern. Reproduced with permission.

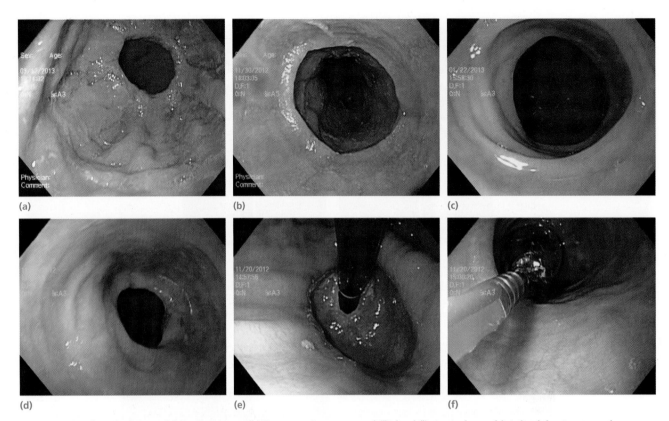

Figure 10.4 Esophageal strictures. **(a)** Peptic stricture. **(b)** For comparison, a mucosal ("Schatzki") ring is shown. **(c)** A distal dominant complex stricture in eosinophilic esophagitis. **(d)** Estimating the diameter of a stricture is essential when planning dilation therapy; this can be challenging in the forward view. **(e)** A useful technique is to evaluate the stricture on retroflexion in relation to the endoscope diameter. **(f)** Here, the stricture can be estimated to be 1.5× the diameter of the gastroscope, or roughly 15 mm, which guided selection of an 18-mm balloon dilator. Source: Esophageal Center at Northwestern. Reproduced with permission.

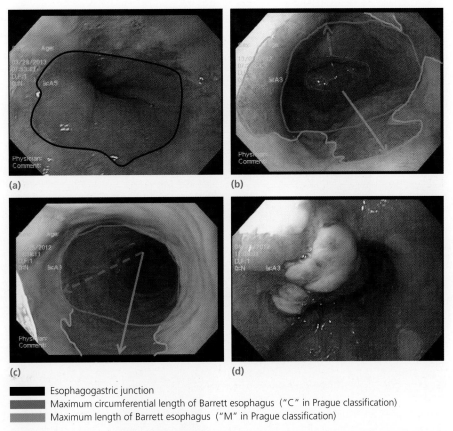

Esophagogastric junction
Maximum circumferential length of Barrett esophagus ("C" in Prague classification)
Maximum length of Barrett esophagus ("M" in Prague classification)

Figure 10.5 The Prague convention for measuring the extent of Barrett metaplasia. Intestinal metaplasia is graded based on circumferential and total length. **(a)** Irregular Z-line. **(b)** Short-segment Barrett esophagus (Prague classification C2M3). **(c)** Long-segment Barrett (Prague classification C5M7). **(d)** Esophageal adenocarcinoma. Source: Esophageal Center at Northwestern. Reproduced with permission.

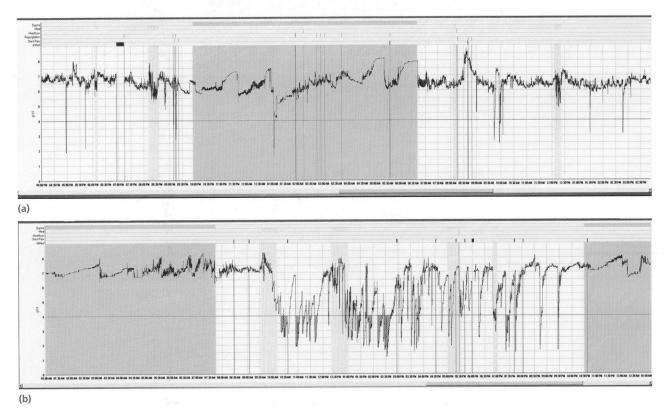

Figure 10.6 Wireless ambulatory pH testing. **(a)** Normal percent esophageal acid exposure time (0.5%). Yellow shading highlights meals and green highlights periods of sleep. **(b)** Abnormal ambulatory pH study in a patient with very abnormal daytime (postprandial) reflux but no nocturnal reflux.

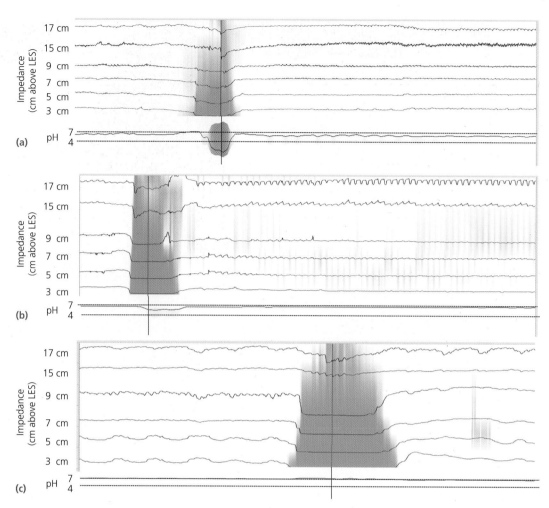

Figure 10.7 pH-impedance reflux testing. **(a)** Acidic reflux event. The sequential drop in impedance propagating from the distal sensor to more proximal sensors indicates a retrograde flow of acidic liquid (pH < 4). **(b)** Weakly acidic reflux (pH > 4 and <7). **(c)** Weakly acidic reflux not detected on the pH recording. LES, lower esophageal sphincter. Source: Krishnan K., Pandolfino J.E., Kahrilas P.J., et al. Increased risk for persistent intestinal metaplasia in patients with Barrett's esophagus and uncontrolled reflux exposure before radiofrequency ablation. Gastroenterology 2012;143:576. Reproduced with permission of Elsevier.

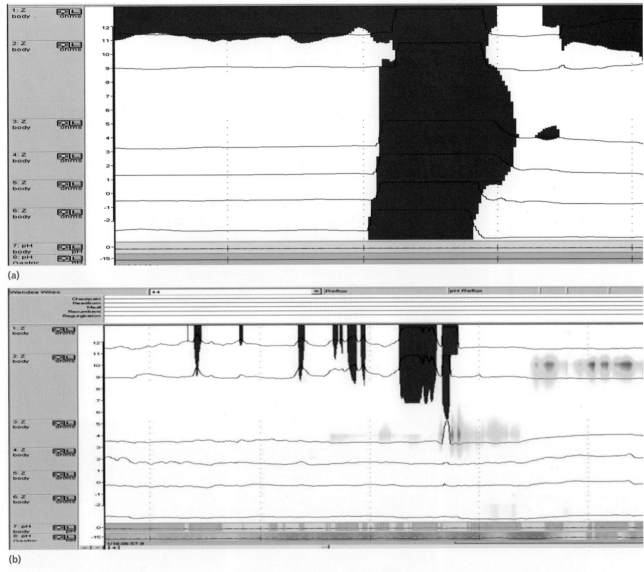

Figure 10.8 Belching seen with pH-impedance. (a) Gastric belch. Note the increase in impedance that propagates from the distal sensor to the most proximal sensor. (b) Supragastric belching can be confused with reflux. The rise in pH originates above the lower esophageal sphincter.

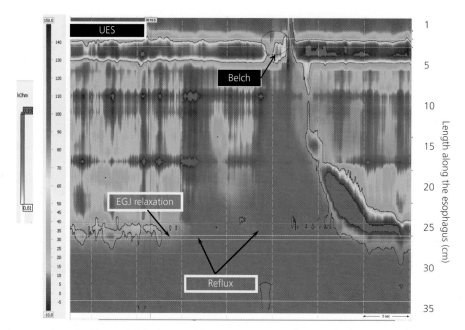

Figure 10.9 Transient lower esophageal sphincter (LES) relaxation. The most common mechanism of reflux. Transient esophagogastric junction (EGJ) relaxation is a vagovagal reflex triggered by proximal gastric distention and effecting LES relaxation, crural diaphragm inhibition, and esophageal shortening. UES, upper esophageal sphincter. It is the physiological mechanism of belching. Source: Esophageal Center at Northwestern. Reproduced with permission.

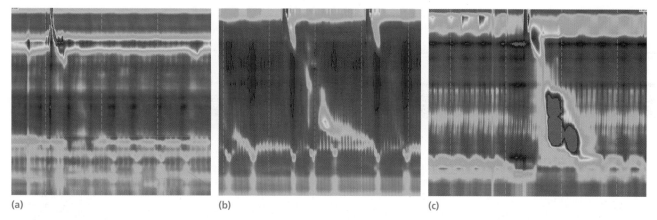

Figure 10.10 High-resolution esophageal manometric findings in patients with gastroesophageal reflux disease. **(a)** Failed swallow with hiatal hernia and hypotensive lower esophageal sphincter (LES). The combination of weak LES along with poor peristalsis causes prolonged esophageal acid exposure. **(b)** Weak peristalsis. Note the faint pressure signal at the LES. **(c)** Hypertensive peristalsis. This is a common finding in patients with reflux-related hypersensitivity. Source: Esophageal Center at Northwestern. Reproduced with permission.

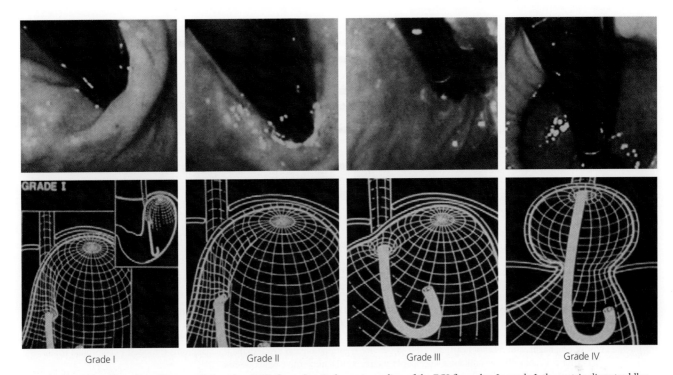

Grade I   Grade II   Grade III   Grade IV

Figure 10.11 Hill grade and esophagogastric junction (EGJ) flap valve. Endoscopic grading of the EGJ flap valve. In grade I, the gastric sling straddles the EGJ. In grade II, the ridge of mucosa adjacent to the EGJ is less prominent, and opens with respiration. In grade III, the hiatus is patulous. In grade IV, the hiatus is grossly patulous, and the Z-line is displaced proximally. Source: Hill LD, Kozarek RA, Kraemer SJ, et al. The gastroesophageal flap valve: in vitro and in vivo observations. Gastrointest Endosc 1996;44:541. Reproduced with permission of Elsevier.

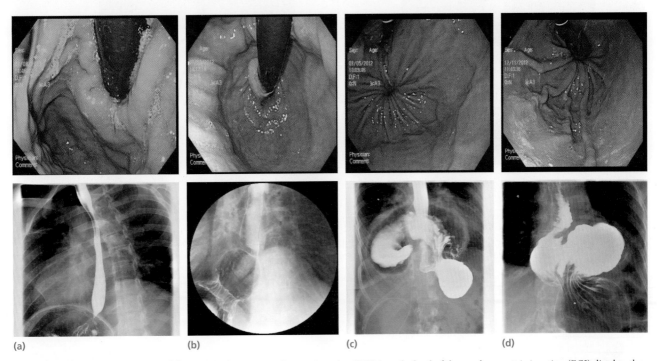

(a)   (b)   (c)   (d)

Figure 10.12 Types of hiatus hernia. **(a)** Normal. The squamocolumnar junction (SCJ) is at the level of the esophagogastric junction (EGJ) distal to the hiatus. **(b)** Type 1 (sliding) hiatus hernia. The EGJ is displaced proximally thus leaving a portion of gastric cardia above the diaphragm. **(c)** Type 2 paraesophageal hernia. A portion of gastric fundus herniates through the hiatal canal without proximal displacement of the EGJ. In the radiographic study, a substantial portion of the proximal stomach has herniated into the chest and subsequently has resulted in a mesenteric–axial volvulus. **(d)** Type 3 mixed hernia. There is herniation of the gastric cardia through the hiatal canal, along with a portion of the gastric fundus. Type 4 hiatus hernia (not shown) involves herniation of abdominal organs other than the stomach above the diaphragm. Source: Esophageal Center at Northwestern. Reproduced with permission.

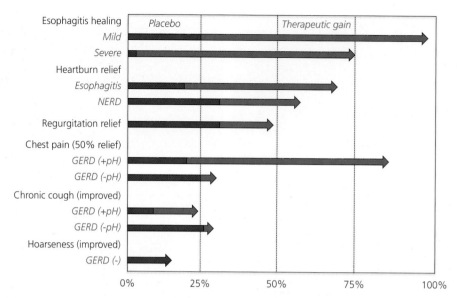

Figure 10.13 Efficacy of proton pump inhibitors (PPIs) for the treatment of gastroesophageal reflux disease (GERD). Summary of available randomized controlled trial data on PPI treatment for various potential manifestations of GERD. The length of the blue bars is the typically observed placebo response, while the green arrow extension is the therapeutic gain of the PPI beyond that observed with placebo. PPIs have excellent efficacy for the treatment of erosive esophagitis and relief of heartburn. The efficacy for regurgitation and extraesophageal symptoms is modest in controlled trials; however, it is better for patients with concomitant abnormal pH-metry. NERD, nonerosive reflux disease.

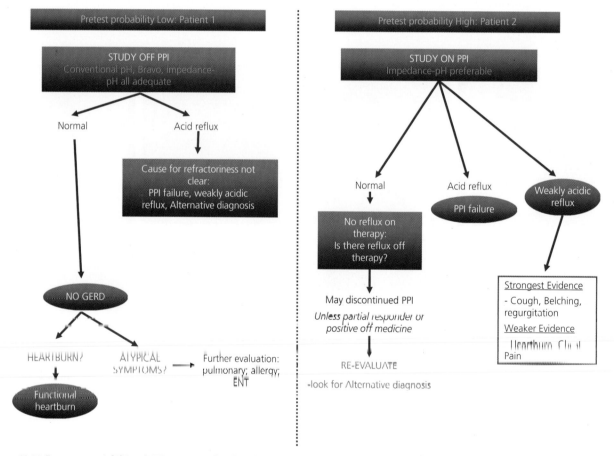

Figure 10.14 Proton pump inhibitor (PPI) nonresponder algorithm – algorithm for patients who fail empiric trials of PPI and have negative upper endoscopy. Formal reflux testing is often helpful. The patient's clinical symptoms can guide the ideal reflux testing approach (i.e., typical heartburn vs atypical symptoms). Patients with high pretest probability can be tested with pH-impedance while continuing PPI therapy. Those with low pretest probability should be studied after withholding PPI therapy for 1 week. Most importantly, PPIs should be discontinued in patients who do not exhibit objective evidence of reflux during the study. GERD, gastroesophageal reflux disease. Source: Pandolfino JE, Vela MF Esophageal-reflux monitoring. Gastrointest Endosc 2009;69:917. Reproduced with permission of Elsevier.

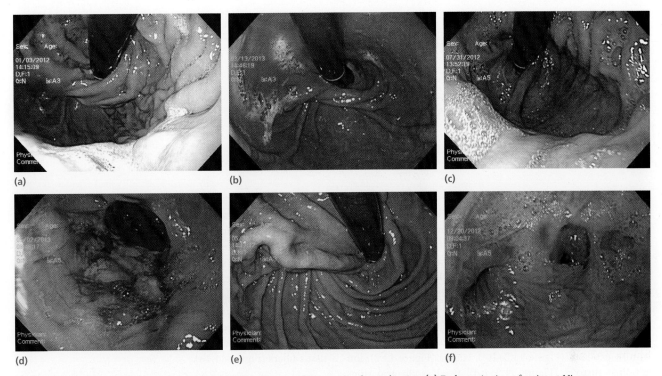

Figure 10.15 Surgical therapy for gastroesophageal reflux disease and its associated complication. **(a)** Endoscopic view of an intact Nissen fundoplication. **(b)** Partially disrupted fundoplication. **(c)** Completely disrupted fundoplication. **(d)** "Slipped" Nissen fundoplication. On retroflexed view, an intact fundoplication can be seen. **(e)** Paraesophageal hernia postfundoplication. **(f)** Fistula within the fundoplication. Source: Esophageal Center at Northwestern. Reproduced with permission.

CHAPTER 11
Eosinophilic esophagitis

Yael Haberman Ziv, Margaret H. Collins, and Marc E. Rothenberg
Cincinnati Children's Hospital Medical Center and University of Cincinnati College of Medicine, Cincinnati, OH, USA

Eosinophilic esophagitis (EoE) represents a chronic, immune/antigen-mediated esophageal disease characterized clinically by symptoms related to esophageal dysfunction, a distinctive spectrum of endoscopic findings, and histologically by eosinophil-predominant inflammation. Figure 11.1 represent normal esophageal endoscopic finding of the proximal (Figure 11.1a) and distal (Figure 11.1b) esophagus without thickening, furrowing, exudate, erythema, or erosion. Esophageal endoscopic abnormalities in patients with EoE include whitish exudates (Figure 11.2a,b,e), edema (Figure 11.2), longitudinal furrows (Figure 11.2a,c,d), fixed esophageal rings/trachealization (Figure 11.2d), and narrow-caliber esophagus or stricture (Figure 11.2e–g).

Typical histological findings of esophageal biopsy from a patient with EoE include a basal layer hyperplasia, numerous intraepithelial eosinophils (>15 eosinophils/high power field), dilated intercellular spaces, and thick and rope-like connective tissue fibers in the lamina propria (Figure 11.3a). This is different from an esophageal biopsy taken from uninflamed esophageal tissue, where the basal layer occupies a small portion of the epithelial thickness, intraepithelial eosinophils are not seen, and the lamina propria contains thin delicate connective tissue fibers (Figure 11.3b).

Yamada's Atlas of Gastroenterology, Fifth Edition. Edited by Daniel K. Podolsky, Michael Camilleri, J. Gregory Fitz, Anthony N. Kalloo, Fergus Shanahan, and Timothy C. Wang.
© 2016 John Wiley & Sons, Ltd. Published 2016 by John Wiley & Sons, Ltd.
Companion website: www.yamadagastro.com/atlas

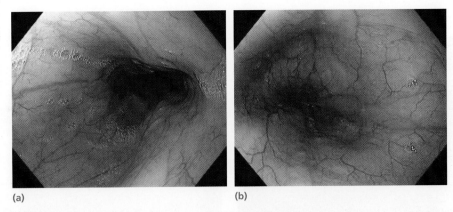

Figure 11.1 Normal esophagus endoscopy. Normal proximal **(a)** and distal **(b)** esophagus.

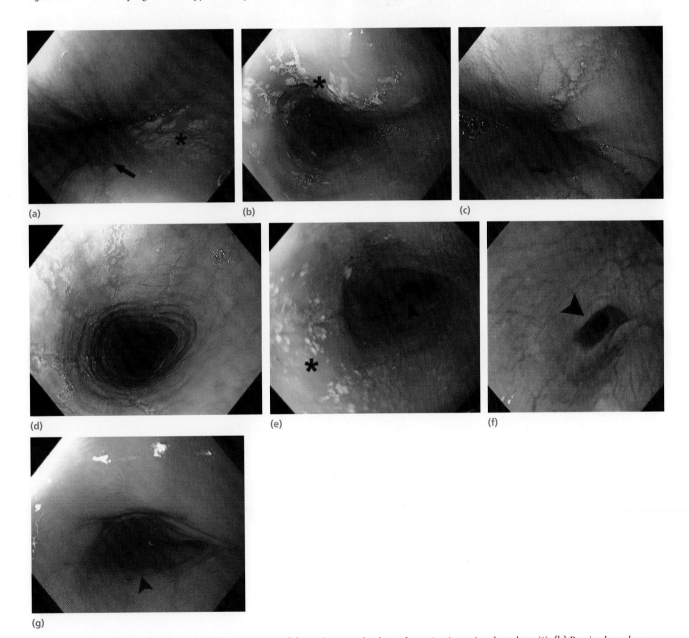

Figure 11.2 Endoscopic findings in eosinophilic esophagitis. **(a)** Esophagus with edema, furrowing (arrow) and exudates (*). **(b)** Proximal esophagus with edema and exudates (*). **(c)** Esophagus with edema and furrowing (arrow). **(d)** Esophagus with fixed esophageal rings/ trachealization and furrowing. **(e)** Esophagus with edema, exudate (*), and narrowing (arrow head). **(f)** Esophageal narrowing (arrow head). **(g)** Esophageal narrowing with mucosal fragility (arrow head).

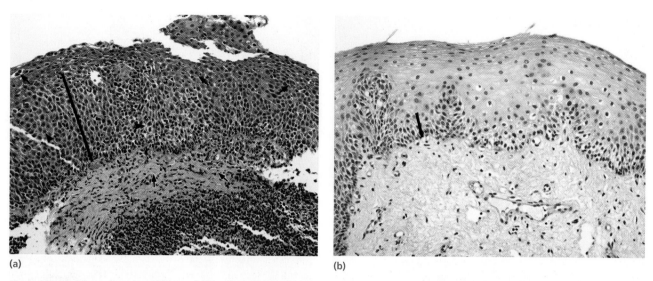

(a)   (b)

Figure 11.3 Histology of esophageal biopsy. **(a)** Esophageal biopsy from a patient with eosinophilic esophagitis showing a basal layer that occupies a significant portion of the epithelium (bar), numerous intraepithelial eosinophils, intercellular spaces are dilated (arrowheads), and the connective tissue fibers in the lamina propria are thick and ropey (outlined arrows). H&E, 200×. **(b)** Esophageal biopsy taken from uninflamed esophageal tissue, where the basal layer (bar) occupies a small portion of the epithelial thickness, intraepithelial eosinophils are not seen, and the lamina propria contains thin delicate connective tissue fibers. H&E 200×.

CHAPTER 12

Esophageal infections and disorders associated with acquired immunodeficiency syndrome

C. Mel Wilcox

University of Alabama-Birmingham, Birmingham, AL, USA

While the acquired immunodeficiency syndrome (AIDS) epidemic was the major contributor to the witnessed upsurge in esophageal infections observed in the 1980s and 1990s, more recently, with the widespread availability of highly active antiretroviral therapy, these infections are becoming much less common. In addition, the adoption of antimicrobial prophylaxis for high-risk immunocompromised patients and the development of more targeted immunomodulators, such as those post organ transplantation, has also led to an overall fall in the incidence of infections, including those involving the esophagus. Despite these advancements, however, esophageal infections will remain important complications of immunodeficiency states.

Esophageal infections can be categorized by the infecting organism. *Candida* spp. are the most common fungal pathogens with aspergillosis, histoplasmosis, and blastomycosis being very rare. Following fungi, viruses (herpes simplex virus [HSV] and cytomegalovirus [CMV]) are the most common cause of infection. Rare additional causes of esophagitis include bacteria, mycobacteria, and parasites. Odynophagia is the most common symptom of esophageal infection with dysphagia being reported less frequently. Although barium esophagography is helpful in suggesting the presence of infectious esophagitis, these studies are not definitive. Endoscopy provides the highest diagnostic accuracy.

Candida albicans is the most common pathogen causing esophageal infection. Classically, barium radiographs of esophageal candidiasis reveal a "shaggy" appearance resulting from diffuse plaque material that coats the esophageal mucosa, mimicking ulceration (Figure 12.1). The endoscopic appearance of *Candida* is well recognized and is essentially pathognomonic (Figures 12.2 and 12.3).

Candida rarely causes true ulceration; thus, the presence of esophageal ulcer associated with *Candida* esophagitis suggests an additional esophageal process (Figures 12.4 and 12.5). Esophageal brushings have the highest diagnostic yield for candidal infection. Mucosal biopsies will be diagnostic when more severe disease is present, and should be performed in the presence of ulceration. Fungal cultures are not widely available and provide no additional information over the endoscopic and histological findings unless fungi other than *Candida* are suspected.

Other fungi rarely cause esophageal disease. *Histoplasma* is the most frequent fungal pathogen reported to involve the esophagus, usually from mediastinal involvement (Figure 12.6).

In contrast to *Candida* esophagitis, barium radiographs of viral esophagitis demonstrate ulceration. The ulcers are usually well circumscribed but may coalesce to form a superficial esophagitis. Ulcers associated with HSV infection typically are small and well circumscribed, whereas those associated with CMV have a greater propensity to form larger well-circumscribed longitudinal or linear lesions. A diffuse viral esophagitis may result in a cobblestone or shaggy mucosal appearance, similar to that observed in esophageal candidiasis (Figure 12.7). Endoscopically, HSV ulcers correspond to the radiographic features appearing as well-circumscribed small volcano-like lesions, likely the site of a vesicle (Figure 12.8) or shallow ulcers (Figure 12.9); occasionally when multiple and small, the lesions may mimic esophageal candidiasis (Figure 12.10). Although esophageal ulcers caused by CMV may resemble HSV (Figure 12.11), in general, CMV causes larger or more extensive lesions, which are often very deep in patients with AIDS (Figures 12.12, 12.13, and 12.14), leading to bleeding, stricture, or rarely perforation. Multiple biopsies of the ulcer edge (for HSV) and ulcer base (for CMV) with careful histological examination of biopsy material should reveal the intranuclear (Cowdry type A) or cytoplasmic inclusions characteristic of HSV (Figure 12.15) or CMV infection (Figure 12.16), respectively.

Yamada's Atlas of Gastroenterology, Fifth Edition. Edited by Daniel K. Podolsky, Michael Camilleri, J. Gregory Fitz, Anthony N. Kalloo, Fergus Shanahan, and Timothy C. Wang.
© 2016 John Wiley & Sons, Ltd. Published 2016 by John Wiley & Sons, Ltd.

Companion website: www.yamadagastro.com/atlas

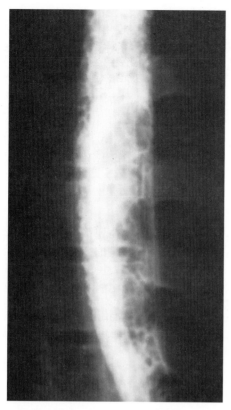

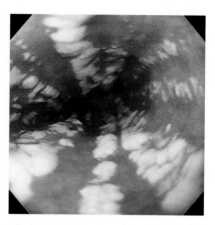

Figure 12.2 Multiple raised white plaques involving the esophagus with normal intervening mucosa. This would be classified as Grade II *Candida* esophagitis.

Figure 12.1 Barium esophagram shows multiple filling defects with irregularity of the mucosal surface resulting in a "shaggy" appearance due to esophageal candidiasis.

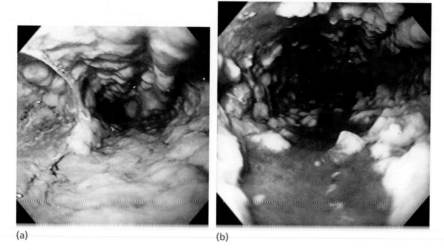

(a)   (b)

Figure 12.3 (a) Exuberant yellow plaque material encroaching on the esophageal lumen typical for severe *Candida* esophagitis (Grade IV). **(b)** The plaque material has been removed with the endoscope revealing relatively normal underlying mucosa without ulceration.

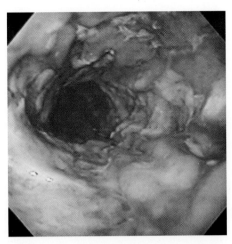

Figure 12.4 Diffuse ulceration with a surpigenious appearance with overlying candidal debris. This AIDS patient has cytomegalovirus esophagitis and *Candida* coinfection.

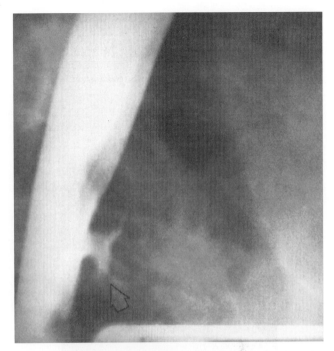

Figure 12.6 Ulcer seen in the mid-esophagus near the bronchus (arrow) caused by an infected lymph node from *Histoplasma capsulatum*. Courtesy of Robert Koehler, MD.

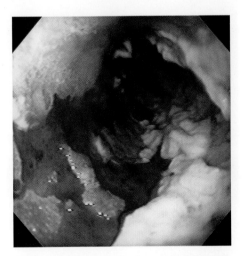

Figure 12.5 Diffuse candidal plaque has been removed with the endoscope revealing a shallow serpiginous ulceration, which on biopsy confirmed cytomegalovirus.

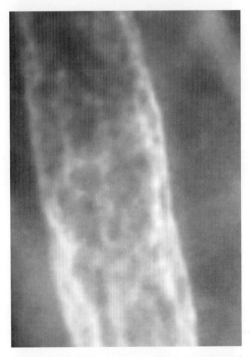

Figure 12.7 Barium esophagram showing diffuse mucosal irregularity resembling *Candida* esophagitis. This AIDS patient had diffuse erosive esophagitis due to herpes simplex virus.

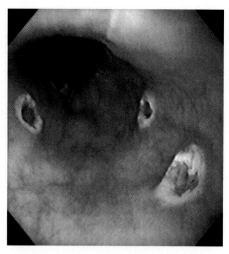

Figure 12.8 Small volcano-like ulcers due to herpes simplex virus.

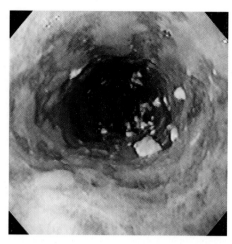

Figure 12.11 Shallow irregular ulceration with intervening areas of preserved but edematous squamous mucosa due to cytomegalovirus. Note also the candidal plaques in the distal esophagus. This endoscopic appearance is also compatible with herpes simplex virus esophagitis.

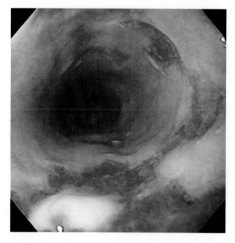

Figure 12.9 Multiple well-circumscribed, shallow esophageal ulcers due to herpes simplex virus esophagitis.

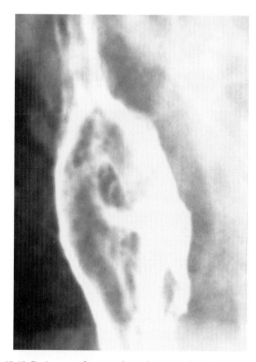

Figure 12.12 Barium esophagram shows large esophageal ulceration due to cytomegalovirus esophagitis in a patient with AIDS.

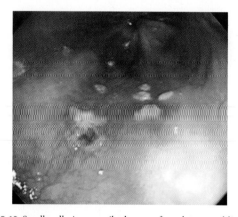

Figure 12.10 Small well-circumscribed areas of exudate resembling *Candida*. This is a classic appearance of mild herpes simplex virus esophagitis. This patient had neutropenia.

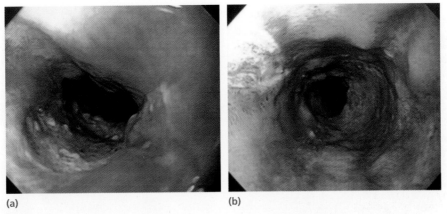

(a)   (b)

Figure 12.13 **(a)** Large deep ulceration in the proximal esophagus due to cytomegalovirus in a patient with AIDS. **(b)** Ulcerations in the distal esophagus are smaller, more linear, and not as deep. Ulceration may not be uniform in the same patient.

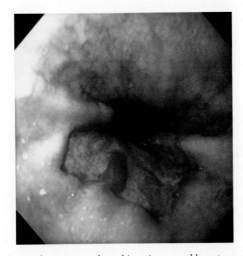

Figure 12.14 Solitary deep well-circumscribed ulcer at the gastroesophageal junction caused by cytomegalovirus.

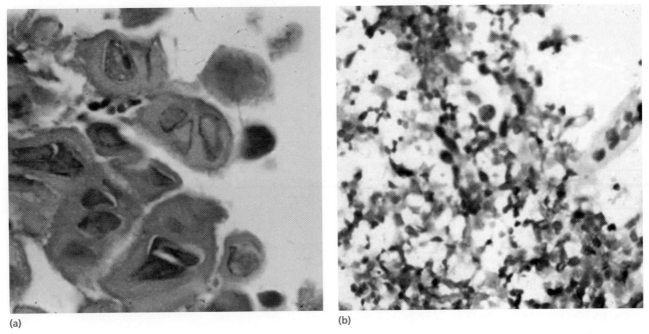

(a)   (b)

Figure 12.15 **(a)** Multinucleated giant cells in squamous mucosa characteristic of herpes simplex virus infection. **(b)** Immunohistochemical staining shows herpes simplex virus antigens, confirming infection.

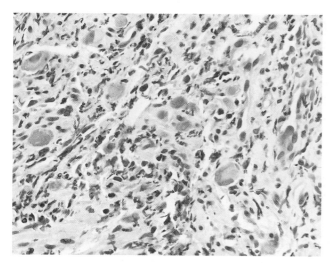

Figure 12.16 Multiple large cells with both intranuclear and intracytoplasmic inclusions typical for cytomegalovirus viral cytopathic effect.

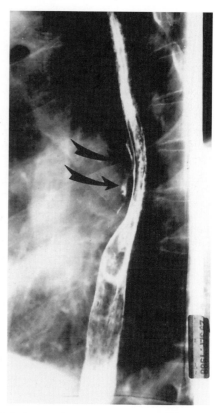

Figure 12.17 Barium esophagram reveals diffuse mucosal irregularity and a fistulous tract (arrows) to mediastinal lymph nodes in a patient with AIDS. This patient has tuberculosis. Endoscopy showed candidiasis and an ulcer at the opening of the fistulous tract. Courtesy of Dr. R. DeSilva.

Radiographic findings in esophageal tuberculosis are nonspecific but may show ulceration, stricture, or fistulas extending from the esophagus to the trachea, bronchi, or mediastinal lymph nodes (Figures 12.17 and 12.18).

An interesting disorder whose pathogenesis is not well defined is the HIV-associated idiopathic esophageal ulcer. Characteristically, these lesions become manifest when immunodeficiency is severe (CD4 lymphocyte count < 100/mm^3). The clinical, radiographic, and endoscopic manifestations are indistinguishable from CMV (Figures 12.19–12.21). These ulcers may be deep and result in esophagoesophageal fistula. Other esophageal diseases seen in AIDS patients include parasites and, rarely, neoplasms such as Kaposi sarcoma or non-Hodgkin lymphoma (Figure 12.22).

In summary, in most cases of infectious esophagitis, determination of the specific infection and institution of appropriate therapy will result in mucosal healing and relief of symptoms. Endoscopy is the most sensitive and specific technique for establishing the etiology of esophageal infections.

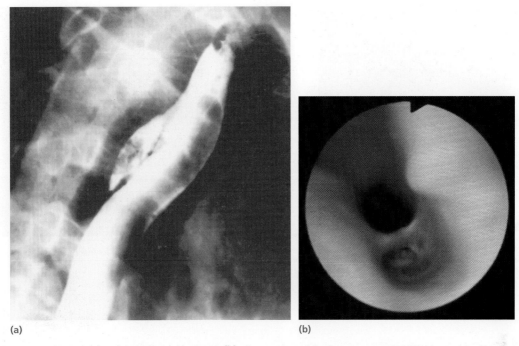

(a)
(b)

Figure 12.18 Barium esophagram **(a)** and endoscopic photograph **(b)** of an esophageal fistula in a man with AIDS, due to *Mycobacterium tuberculosis*. Courtesy of Dr. J. P. Raufman.

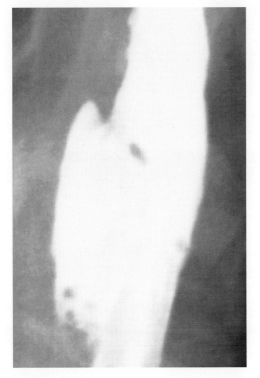

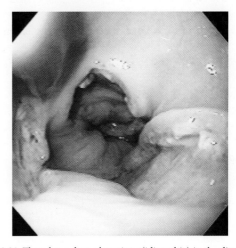

Figure 12.20 Three large deep ulcerations (idiopathic) in the distal esophagus in a patient with AIDS.

Figure 12.19 Barium esophagram showing large solitary ulceration in the mid-esophagus that was idiopathic in a patient with AIDS.

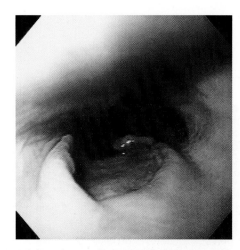

Figure 12.21 Solitary, large, well-circumscribed ulceration with a heaped-up appearance typical for the idiopathic esophageal ulceration of AIDS.

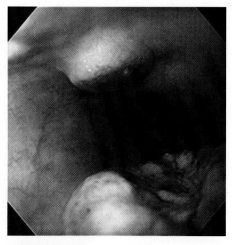

Figure 12.22 Heaped up ulcerated lesions in the mid-esophagus typical for non-Hodgkin lymphoma.

CHAPTER 13

Esophageal neoplasms

Adam J. Bass[1] and Anil K. Rustgi[2]
[1] Harvard Medical School Center, Boston, MA, USA
[2] University of Pennsylvania Perelman School of Medicine, Philadelphia, PA, USA

The most common malignant esophageal neoplasms are squamous cell carcinoma and adenocarcinoma, the latter typically arising in Barrett epithelium. Although esophageal squamous cell carcinoma is the more common of the two worldwide, adenocarcinoma is more frequent in the United States. Frequent symptoms resulting from lumenal masses include dysphagia, odynophagia, and weight loss, which require diagnosis by means of fiberoptic endoscopy with biopsy and cytology. On establishment of diagnosis, preoperative staging is needed before selection of therapy.

Esophageal squamous cell carcinoma occurs predominantly in lower socioeconomic groups within the United States, with predilection for African American males. Risk factors include tobacco and alcohol use, although in high-incidence areas of the world (northern China, India, Iran, southern Russia, South Africa, and some parts of South America) other factors appear more critical, such as exposure to nitrosamines and concomitant nutritional (minerals and vitamins) deficiencies. Clinical suspicion of squamous cell carcinoma merits performance of a barium esophagography. This may reveal an early cancer that manifests as a plaque-like lesion (Figure 13.1) or, alternatively, advanced cancer with an ulcerated polypoid lesion (Figure 13.2) or a circumferential annular lesion (Figures 13.3 and 13.4). Endoscopy with biopsies may demonstrate various stages: dysplasia, carcinoma in situ, or carcinoma (Figure 13.5). Preoperative staging is necessary, with endoscopic ultrasound to determine esophageal wall invasion and lymph node involvement (Figure 13.6). A computed tomography (CT) scan will exclude regional and distant metastases. Although surgical resection with esophagectomy and gastric interposition is preferred for cure of patients who are appropriate candidates, neoadjuvant therapy with chemotherapy and radiation therapy followed by surgery has shown promise. Palliation is needed for patients who cannot undergo potentially curative therapy (Figure 13.7).

Esophageal adenocarcinoma invariably develops in the setting of Barrett esophagus (Figure 13.8). An important factor in the development of Barrett esophagus is gastroesophageal reflux, although other unidentified factors may be important. Because Barrett esophagus may progress from metaplasia to low- and high-grade dysplasia with eventual adenocarcinoma, endoscopic surveillance with a systematic protocol for biopsies is warranted. Initial suspicion and diagnosis of Barrett dysplasia and esophageal adenocarcinoma require barium esophagography (Figure 13.9) and fiberoptic endoscopy (Figure 13.10). Pathology may reveal Barrett esophagus with varying degrees of dysplasia (Figure 13.11a,b) and adenocarcinoma (Figure 13.11c). As with squamous cell carcinoma, preoperative staging entails endoscopic ultrasound (Figure 13.12) and CT scanning. Therapy may be surgical or multimodal (neoadjuvant chemotherapy and radiation therapy followed by surgery) if the patient is an appropriate candidate. Otherwise, palliative therapy is provided. It should be noted that both esophageal neoplasms could have associated complications, such as fistula formation (Figure 13.13).

There are many other epithelial and nonepithelial esophageal neoplasms, both benign and malignant, but they are generally quite rare. An example of a benign nonepithelial tumor is leiomyoma, which is typically silent and patients are generally asymptomatic (Figure 13.14). Rare malignant esophageal neoplasms include carcinosarcoma, metastatic cancer (melanoma, breast cancer), neuroendocrine tumors, and various sarcomas (Figure 13.15).

Yamada's Atlas of Gastroenterology, Fifth Edition. Edited by Daniel K. Podolsky, Michael Camilleri, J. Gregory Fitz, Anthony N. Kalloo, Fergus Shanahan, and Timothy C. Wang.
© 2016 John Wiley & Sons, Ltd. Published 2016 by John Wiley & Sons, Ltd.
Companion website: www.yamadagastro.com/atlas

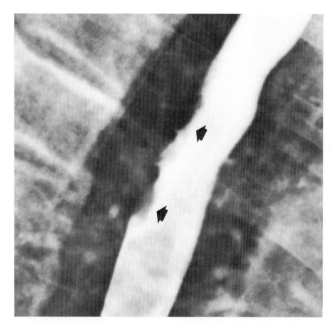

Figure 13.1 Early squamous cell carcinoma of the esophagus presenting as a plaque-like lesion (arrows) on the posterior wall. Source: Eisenberg RL. Gastrointestinal Radiology: A Pattern Approach, 4th edn. Philadelphia: Lippincott Williams & Wilkins, 2003. Reproduced with permission of Wolters Kluwer Health.

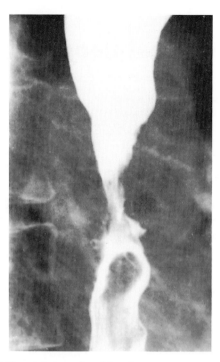

Figure 13.2 Ulcerated circumferential apple core-type squamous cell carcinoma. Source: Eisenberg RL. Gastrointestinal Radiology: A Pattern Approach, 4th edn. Philadelphia: Lippincott Williams & Wilkins, 2003. Reproduced with permission of Wolters Kluwer Health.

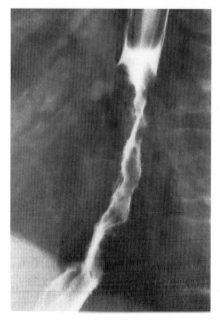

Figure 13.3 Esophagram shows extensive infiltrative lesion of the distal esophagus. Source: Eisenberg RL. Gastrointestinal Radiology: A Pattern Approach, 4th edn. Philadelphia: Lippincott Williams & Wilkins, 2003. Reproduced with permission of Wolters Kluwer Health.

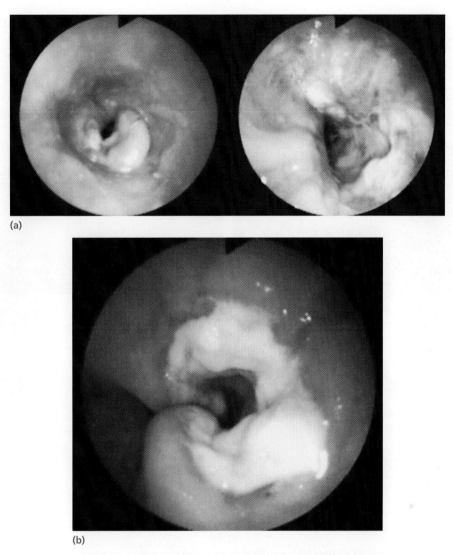

(a)

(b)

Figure 13.4 Endoscopic appearance of infiltrating squamous cell carcinoma. These three carcinomas have variously occluded the lumen and would present as dysphagia. Source: Silverstein FE, Tytgat GNJ. Gastrointestinal Endoscopy, 3rd edn. London: Mosby-Wolfe,1997. Reproduced with permission of Elsevier.

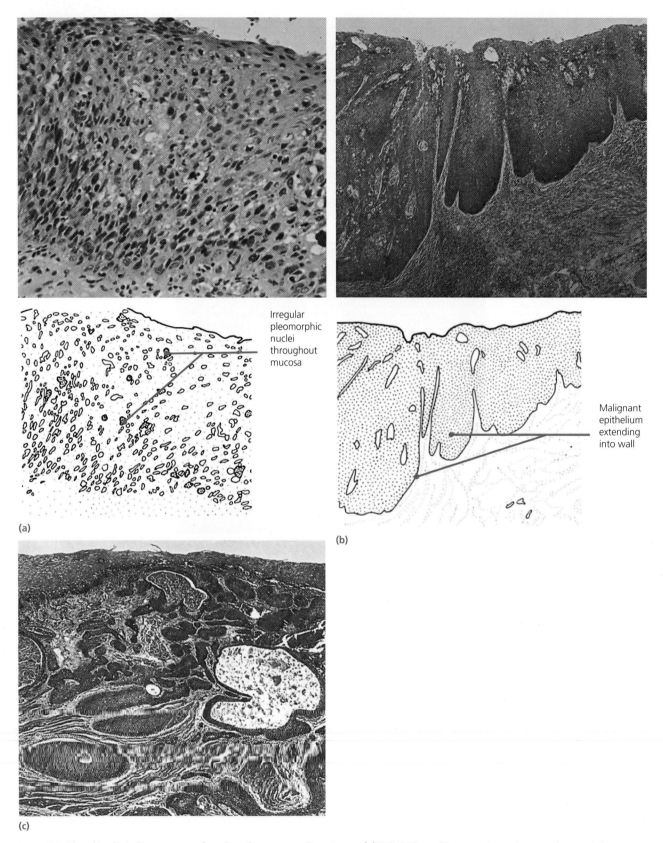

Irregular
pleomorphic
nuclei
throughout
mucosa

(a)

Malignant
epithelium
extending
into wall

(b)

(c)

Figure 13.5 Three histological appearances of esophageal squamous cell carcinoma. **(a)** Full-thickness biopsy specimen shows nuclear atypia but no invasion. This is carcinoma in situ. **(b)** Specimen shows early invasive squamous cell carcinoma with downward extension of the tumor into the submucosa. **(c)** Established infiltrating, well-differentiated carcinoma. There are islands of malignant tissue under essentially normal squamous epithelium. Source: Misiewicz JJ, Bartram CI, Cotton PB, et al. Atlas of Clinical Gastroenterology. London: Gower, 1988. Reproduced with permission of Elsevier.

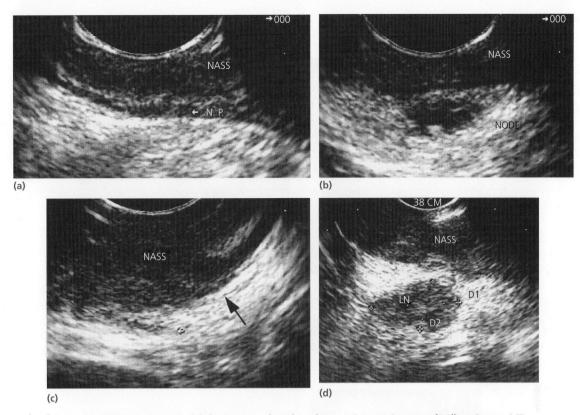

Figure 13.6 (a–d) Endoscopic ultrasound images of different stages of esophageal cancer. Source: Courtesy of William Brugge, MD.

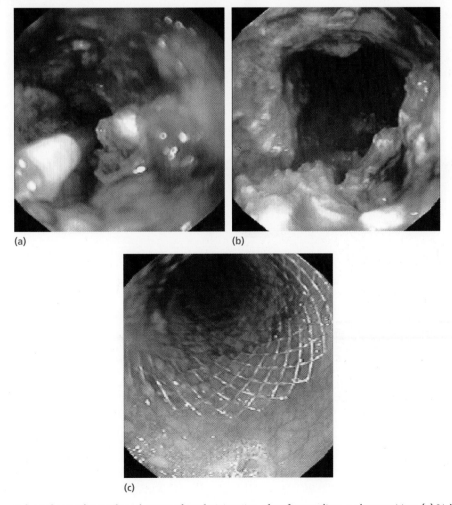

Figure 13.7 Photodynamic laser therapy for esophageal cancer after administration of porfimer sodium, a photosensitizer. **(a)** Light of 630 nm wavelength from a laser acts on cells that accumulate the photosensitizer. **(b)** After 6 days, there is some decrease in mass size. **(c)** After 12 days, the mass is markedly diminished in size, and a metallic endoprosthesis is inserted endoscopically. Source: Courtesy of Norman Nishioka.

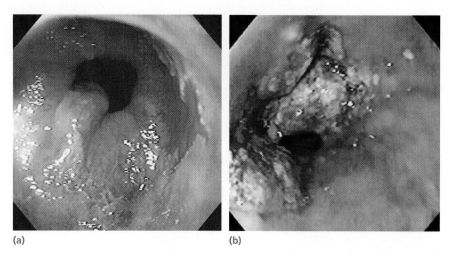

(a)   (b)

Figure 13.8 Barrett esophagus. **(a)** Upper endoscopy reveals short-segment Barrett esophagus. **(b)** Upper endoscopy reveals long-segment Barrett esophagus with inflammation and possible early cancer. Source: Courtesy of David Katzka, MD.

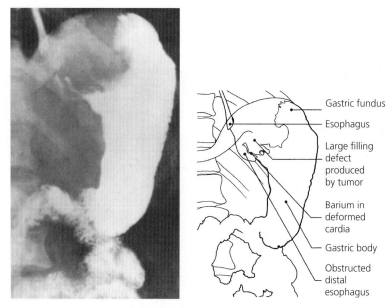

Figure 13.9 Adenocarcinoma of the distal esophagus may be difficult to differentiate from squamous cell carcinoma on the basis of radiographic appearance. However, as shown here, when the tumor extensively involves the fundus of the stomach, the diagnosis is more certain. Source: Misiewicz JJ, Bartram CI, Cotton PB, et al. Atlas of Clinical Gastroenterology. London: Gower, 1988. Reproduced with permission of Elsevier.

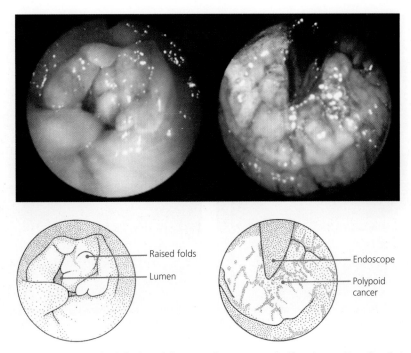

Figure 13.10 At endoscopy, adenocarcinoma may be difficult to differentiate from squamous cell carcinoma. Retroflexed views of the tumor from the stomach may help. Source: Silverstein FE, Tygat GNJ. Gastrointestinal Endoscopy, 3rd edn. London: Mosby-Wolfe,1997. Reproduced with permission of Elsevier.

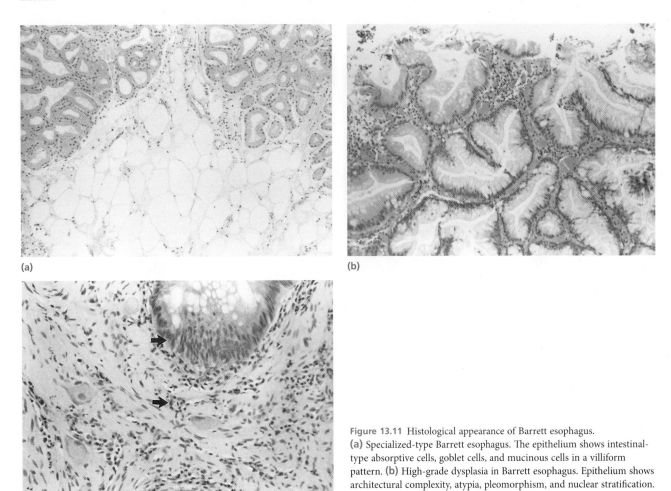

Figure 13.11 Histological appearance of Barrett esophagus.
(a) Specialized-type Barrett esophagus. The epithelium shows intestinal-type absorptive cells, goblet cells, and mucinous cells in a villiform pattern. **(b)** High-grade dysplasia in Barrett esophagus. Epithelium shows architectural complexity, atypia, pleomorphism, and nuclear stratification. **(c)** Intramucosal adenocarcinoma in Barrett esophagus. Tumor invasion beyond the basement membrane is present in the form of single cells, small glands, or sheets of cells. Source: Courtesy of Robert Odze, MD.

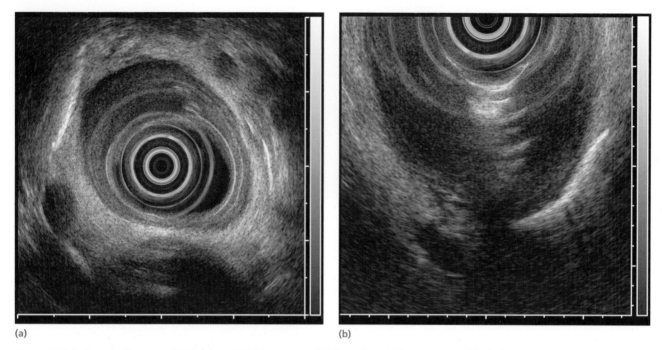

(a)　(b)

Figure 13.12 Endoscopic ultrasound (EUS). **(a)** An EUS demonstrates a T2N1 esophageal adenocarcinoma. **(b)** The lesion is invading the right pleura. Source: Courtesy of Michael Kochman, MD.

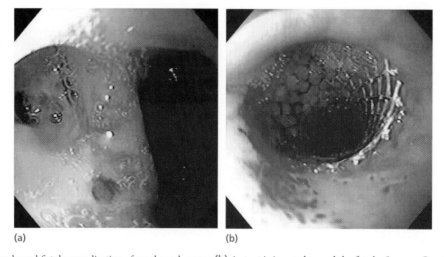

(a)　(b)

Figure 13.13 (a) An esophageal fistula complication of esophageal cancer. **(b)** A stent is inserted to seal the fistula. Source: Courtesy of Michael Kochman, MD.

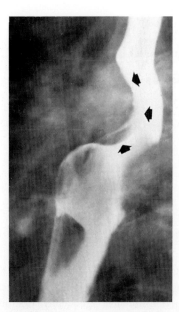

Figure 13.14 Leiomyoma usually presents itself as a smooth, rounded intramural defect (arrows) that encroaches on the barium column.
Source: Eisenberg RL. Gastrointestinal Radiology: A Pattern Approach, 4th edn. Philadelphia: Lippincott Williams & Wilkins, 2003. Reproduced with permission of Wolters Kluwer Health.

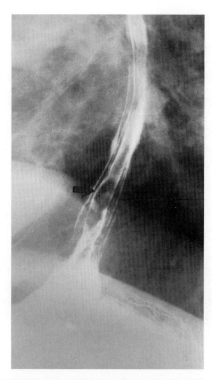

Figure 13.15 Kaposi sarcoma of the esophagus represented by a dumbbell-shaped submucosal mass (arrow) with superficial ulceration.
Source: Courtesy of Deborah Hall, MD.

CHAPTER 14

Miscellaneous diseases of the esophagus: foreign bodies, physical injury, and systemic and dermatological diseases

Seth D. Crockett, Evan S. Dellon, and Nicholas J. Shaheen
University of North Carolina School of Medicine, Chapel Hill, NC, USA

This chapter presents images from a selection of diseases of the esophagus not covered elsewhere in the textbook, including trauma, foreign body impaction, corrosive and pill esophagitis, lymphocytic esophagitis, acute esophageal necrosis, and rare manifestations of systemic and dermatological diseases.

Mallory–Weiss tears, mucosal lacerations at the gastroesophageal junction (GEJ) caused by a sudden rise in intraabdominal pressure during vomiting or retching, are common causes of upper GI hemorrhage. If either active bleeding or stigmata of recent bleeding is seen at endoscopy, hemostatic treatment is recommended (Figure 14.1). These tears can be subtle and, when suspected, careful antegrade and retroflexed examination of the GEJ is mandatory (Figure 14.2).

Perforation of the esophagus following pneumatic dilation of the lower esophageal sphincter in achalasia or after bougie dilation of an esophageal stricture should be suspected with chest pain, fever, or the presence of subcutaneous air after dilation (Figure 14.3). An esophagram with a water-soluble agent prior to the use of barium is recommended for initial diagnostic testing. Spontaneous rupture of the esophagus, Boerhaave syndrome (Figure 14.4), is life-threatening, requiring immediate management.

Esophageal intramural hematomas represent another type of trauma to the esophagus, usually due to a mechanical insult. On endoscopic evaluation, a bluish or violet mass protruding into the esophageal lumen is seen, sometimes in association with superficial ulceration (Figure 14.5). These often resolve spontaneously.

As the portal to the GI tract, the esophagus is the most common site of foreign body impaction. Accordingly, it is possible for a wide variety of objects to become lodged there. This may be due to qualities of the object, such as sharp edges or a large size, or to underlying structural or motility abnormalities

of the esophagus. When food bolus impaction is encountered, the bolus can often be gently advanced under endoscopic guidance into the stomach. Frequently, examination of the cleared esophagus reveals a Schatzki ring or peptic stricture (Figure 14.6).

Sharp bone fragments can also pierce the esophageal wall, causing localized trauma (Figure 14.7). Underlying strictures, in contrast, predispose solid objects, like fruit pits, to become stuck if ingested (Figure 14.8). Patients with psychiatric disease may swallow a panoply of unusual objects, including so-called "sporks," which are challenging to remove and can cause local ulceration (Figure 14.9). Coins, most commonly swallowed inadvertently by pediatric patients, may also become lodged in the esophagus. Because they are radiopaque, impacted coins can be detected and monitored with a plain radiograph, but if a coin does not spontaneously pass from the distal esophagus within 24 h, endoscopic removal is warranted (Figure 14.10).

Pill esophagitis is also caused by a chemical irritant to the esophagus, specifically a medication tablet. Some medications may become stuck in the esophagus and cause local inflammation or erosions without any underlying esophageal structural or motility disorder. In other cases, however, an area of esophageal narrowing may be the underlying cause of pill esophagitis (Figure 14.11).

Purposeful or accidental ingestion of corrosive substances, particularly strong alkali solutions found in some cleaning products, can lead to caustic esophagitis with long-term sequelae of persistent esophageal strictures and increased risk of esophageal squamous cell carcinoma. Endoscopy can be useful in grading the injury, which ranges from mucosal erythema, to sloughing and ulceration of the mucosa, to frank esophageal necrosis (Figure 14.12).

Yamada's Atlas of Gastroenterology, Fifth Edition. Edited by Daniel K. Podolsky, Michael Camilleri, J. Gregory Fitz, Anthony N. Kalloo, Fergus Shanahan, and Timothy C. Wang.
© 2016 John Wiley & Sons, Ltd. Published 2016 by John Wiley & Sons, Ltd.
Companion website: www.yamadagastro.com/atlas

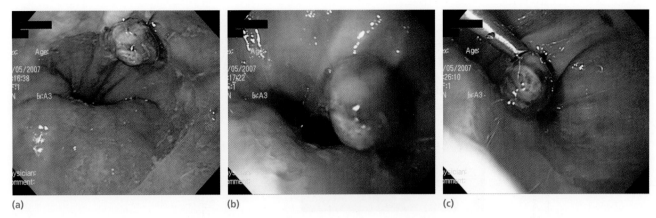

(a)   (b)   (c)

Figure 14.1 A Mallory–Weiss tear located at the gastroesophageal junction (a) with an overlying clot seen in close-up view (b). Treatment with application of a clip at the base of the lesion achieved hemostasis (c).

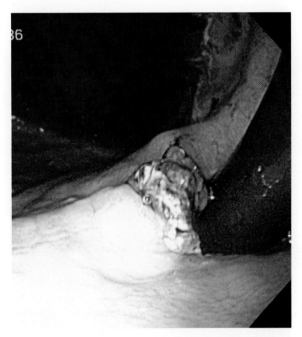

Figure 14.2 Mallory–Weiss tear seen in retroflexed view near the gastroesophageal junction.

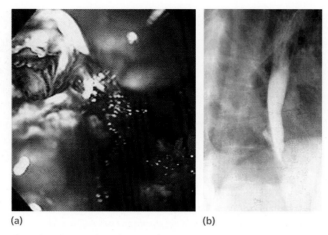

(a)   (b)

Figure 14.3 Endoscopic view of an esophageal perforation (seen between the 10 and 11 o'clock positions) after bougie dilation of the esophagus 2 days earlier **(a)**. A contained perforation was first demonstrated on barium swallow **(b)**. Source: Courtesy of Douglas O. Faigel.

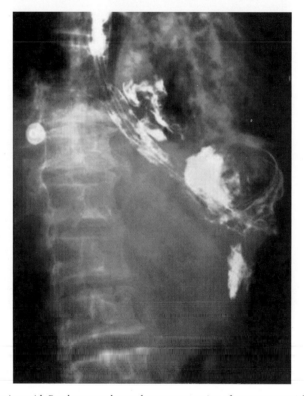

Figure 14.4 A barium swallow from a patient with Boerhaave syndrome shows extravasation of contrast material from the distal esophagus into the mediastinum. Source: Courtesy of Douglas O. Faigel.

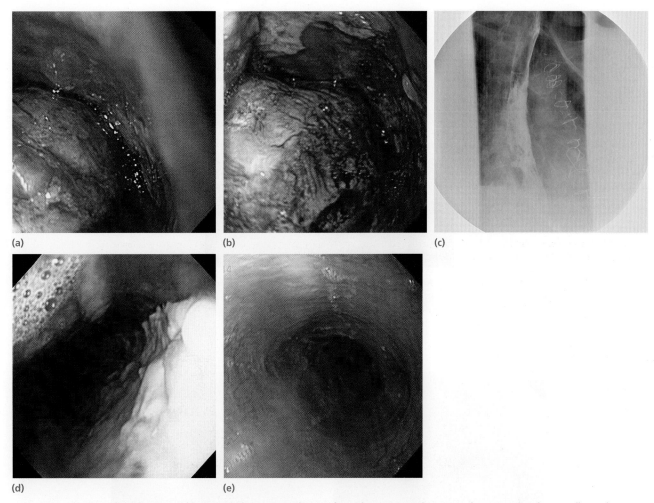

Figure 14.5 A large esophageal intramural hematoma due to a complication from placing a central venous catheter is seen endoscopically nearly obstructing the lumen (a) with an overlying area of ulceration (b). Barium swallow shows mucosal irregularity, a possible distal filling defect, and contrast that is slow to leave the esophagus (c). On endoscopies over the subsequent 2 months (d, e), the ulcerated area sloughs, the hematoma resorbs, and the mucosa heals with a mild stricture formed just above the gastroesophageal junction.

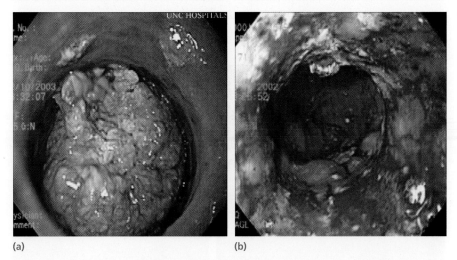

Figure 14.6 An example of food impaction in the distal esophagus (a) caused by a peptic stricture with overlying erosive esophagitis (b).

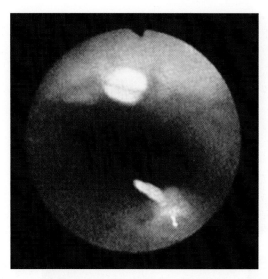

Figure 14.7 An endoscopic view of a fish bone lodged in the proximal esophagus. A contralateral ulcer is present in the 12 o'clock position. The patient sought treatment with severe neck pain after swallowing the bone. Source: Courtesy of Douglas O. Faigel.

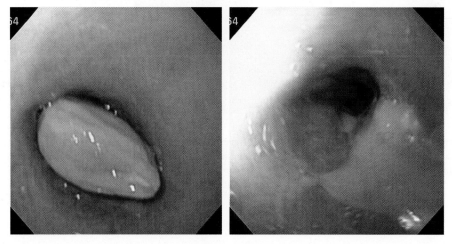

Figure 14.8 A fruit pit stuck in the esophagus (a) due to an underlying stricture (b).

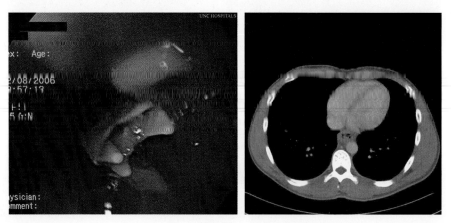

Figure 14.9 An endoscopic view of an impacted and folded plastic "spork" in the distal esophagus of a psychiatric patient (a). On a CT scan of the chest prior to the procedure, the foreign body can be seen in the distal esophagus, which is also thickened and mildly dilated (b).

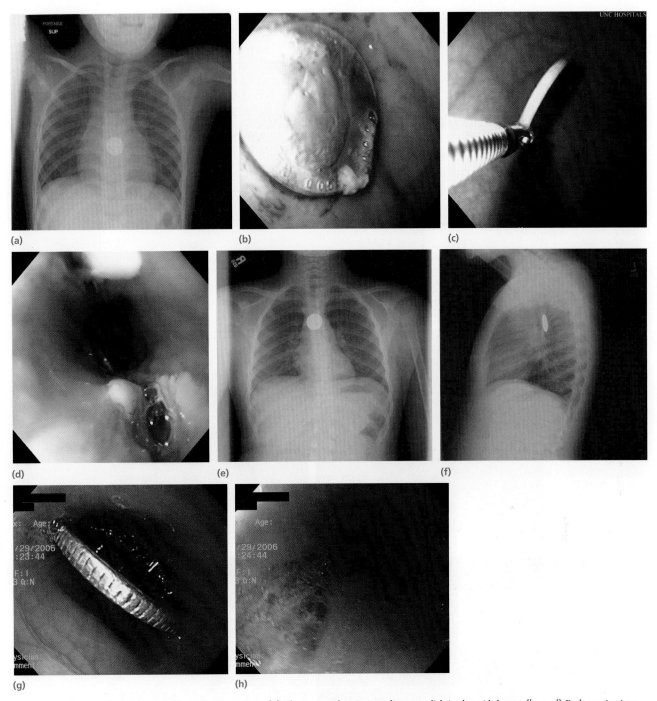

Figure 14.10 Images of coins impacted in pediatric patients. **(a)** Chest x-ray showing a radiopaque disk in the mid thorax. **(b, c, d)** Endoscopic views of the same patient, showing a penny in the esophagus with surrounding erosions, being removed by a pair of forceps, and the residual ulcerations left. **(e, f)** PA and lateral chest films showing a similar radiopaque disk, likely localizing to the esophagus and not passing after 24 hours. **(g, h)** A dime is found lodged in the esophagus, with residual esophageal erosions after foreign body removal.

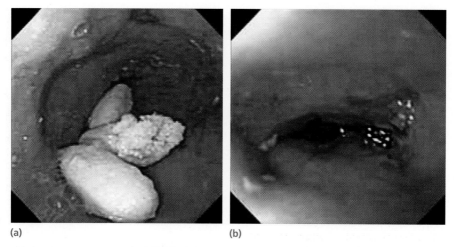

Figure 14.11 Three pill tablets (one partially dissolved) lodged in the midesophagus with nearby erosions **(a)**. After removal of the tablets, pill esophagitis and an underlying esophageal stricture are evident **(b)**.

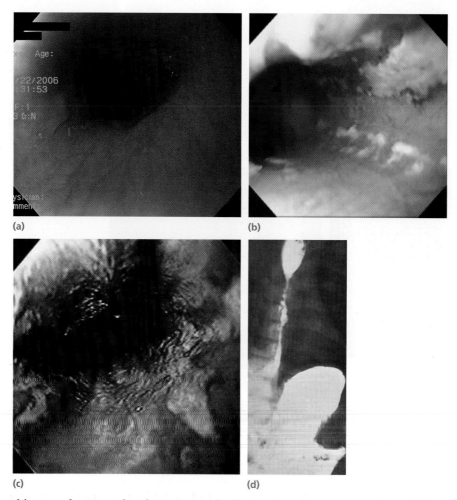

Figure 14.12 Examples of the range of caustic esophageal injury in several pediatric patients after ingestion of a household alkali cleaning agent. Grade 1 injury is manifest by mucosal erythema **(a)**, grade 2 injury results in sloughing of the mucosa with ulceration **(b)**, and grade 3 injury results in mucosal necrosis **(c)**. A long-term complication from severe injury is esophageal stricturing disease, seen here on a barium esophagram **(d)**.
Source: **(c, d)** Courtesy of Douglas O. Faigel.

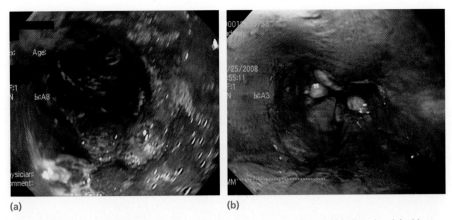

(a)　　　　　　　　　　(b)

Figure 14.13 Endoscopic appearance of acute esophageal necrosis, with characteristic circumferential blackened and friable mucosa involving the distal esophagus **(a)**, stopping abruptly at the gastroesophageal junction **(b)**.

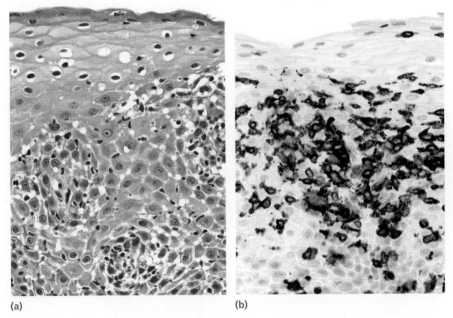

(a)　　　　　　　　　　(b)

Figure 14.14 Histopathology images from an esophageal mucosal biopsy from a patient with lymphocytic esophagitis showing dense inflammatory infiltrate consisting primary of lymphocytes **(a)**, and positive immunohistochemical staining for CD3, a T-cell marker **(b)**. Source: Haque S, Genta RM. Lymphocytic oesophagitis: clinicopathological aspects of an emerging condition. Gut 2012;61:1108. Reproduced with permission of BMJ Publishing Group Ltd.

Acute esophageal necrosis (AEN) or "black esophagus" is a condition typically characterized by circumferential necrosis of the esophagus. Endoscopically, the esophageal mucosa appears blackened, and involvement typically stops abruptly at the gastroesophageal junction (Figure 14.13). The necrotic esophageal epithelium is friable, with underlying hemorrhagic tissue. This condition can be reversible, but carries a high mortality risk likely owing to the fact that patients with AEN tend to have a substantial burden of comorbid illness.

Lymphocytic esophagitis (LyE) is an emerging condition characterized clinically by esophageal symptoms such as dys-phagia, heartburn, or chest pain, and histologically by an intense, lymphocyte-predominant inflammatory infiltrate in the esophageal mucosa in the absence of granulocytes (Figure 14.14). A range of endoscopic findings can be seen in LyE, including esophageal rings, strictures, furrows, plaques, erosive esophagitis, erythema, and nodularity (Figure 14.15).

A number of systemic diseases can affect the esophagus in rare instances. Sarcoidosis can cause extrinsic compression from enlarged lymph nodes, infiltration of the esophageal wall resulting in an achalasia-like syndrome, and esophageal strictures or mucosal nodularity (Figures 14.16). In the case of

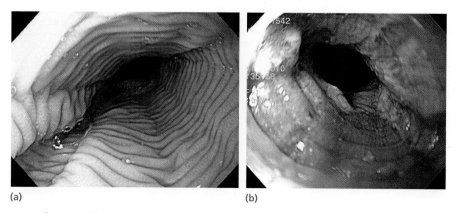

(a)   (b)

Figure 14.15 Endoscopic view of patient with lymphocytic esophagitis and dysphagia showing esophageal rings **(a)** and furrows, white plaques, and nodularity **(b)**. Source: Haque S, Genta RM. Lymphocytic oesophagitis: clinicopathological aspects of an emerging condition. Gut 2012;61:1108. Reproduced with permission of BMJ Publishing Group Ltd.

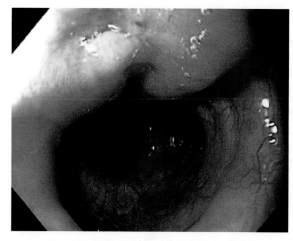

Figure 14.16 Extrinsic compression of the esophagus caused by sarcoidosis. Endoscopic view of lesion in midesophagus with normal overlying mucosa. Cross-sectional imaging in this case revealed adjacent lymphadenopathy, and endoscopic ultrasound-guided biopsy confirmed granulomatous inflammation consistent with sarcoidosis.
Source: Samarasena JB, Chu E, Muthusamy VR. An African American man with dysphagia: a unique initial presentation of sarcoidosis. Endoscopy 2012;44 (S02):E63. Reproduced with permission of Thieme Publishing Group.

Crohn's disease, the impact of esophageal involvement can be substantial. Due to chronic transmural inflammation, the esophagus can be narrowed with sinus tracts forming from deep ulcerations. In some instances, esophagotracheal or esophagobronchial fistulae may develop, causing recurrent pneumonitis, pneumonia, or empyema, and requiring surgical management (Figure 14.17).

While graft-versus-host disease (GVHD) more commonly affects the lower GI tract and the liver, it can affect the esophagus. Diagnosis is mostly made on biopsy, which also excludes opportunistic infections in the immunosuppressed bone marrow transplant patient. Esophageal erythema or friability, as well as webs or strictures, can be seen on endoscopic examination and barium studies can also show strictures (Figures 14.18 and 14.19). Behçet syndrome, characterized by oral and genital aphthous ulceration and ocular inflammation, is another systemic disease that rarely affects the esophagus (Figure 14.20). Additionally, primary or secondary amyloidosis may cause dysphagia due to amyloid deposition in the esophageal muscle or nerves (Figure 14.21).

Finally, blistering dermatological diseases can rarely have esophageal involvement. Pemphigus vulgaris, due to autoantibodies against desmoglein-3 in keratinocytes, can cause esophageal blistering (Figure 14.22). Bullous pemphigoid is caused by IgG autoantibodies directed against the basement membrane of the squamous epithelium. Esophageal involvement by bullous pemphigoid is also rare, but it can result in esophageal mucosal sloughing and upper GI bleeding (Figure 14.23). Benign mucous membrane pemphigoid (BMMP) is due to deposition of autoantibodies in the basement membrane of the esophageal mucosa, leading to tense blisters, with subsequent scarring and stricturing (Figures 14.24 and 14.25). Epidermolysis bullosa dystrophica (EPD), a heritable disease caused by a mutation in the collagen type VII gene, results in a cycle of recurrent blistering and scarring due to mild trauma (Figure 14.26). In the esophagus, the routine act of swallowing is enough to prompt this cycle, which leads to strictures, esophageal shortening, and dysmotility. Because endoscopy also induces trauma, it is reserved for therapeutic dilation, making a barium esophagram the preferred diagnostic test in this condition (Figure 14.27).

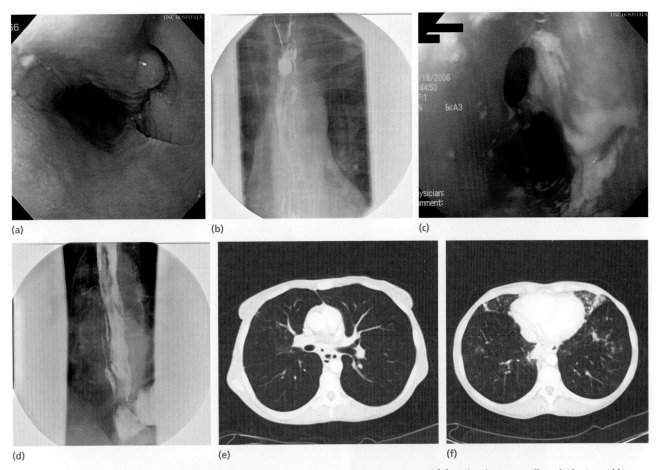

Figure 14.17 Examples of Crohn's esophagitis. Esophageal narrowing and deep sinus tracts are noted **(a)**, and on barium swallow, the barium tablet becomes lodged in the proximal esophagus **(b)**. Several fistulae with white exudate and possible candida are seen opening from the esophagus **(c)**, and barium swallow confirms a thin fistulous tract from the area of the gastroesophageal junction extending caudally to the right main-stem bronchus **(d)**. On computed tomography scan, a thickened esophagus with multiple sinus tracts is readily apparent **(e)**, and just above the gastroesophageal junction a fistulous tract is seen entering the lung **(f)**.

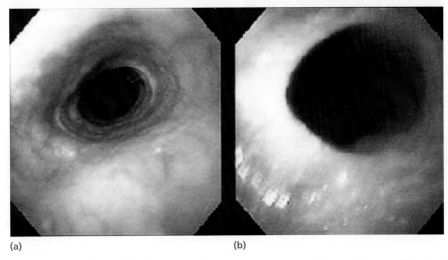

Figure 14.18 Graft-versus-host disease of the esophagus with multiple fine mucosal webs present. Source: Courtesy of Douglas O. Faigel.

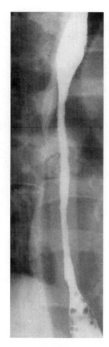

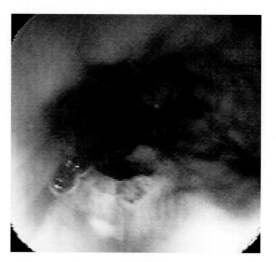

Figure 14.20 Endoscopic view of esophageal ulceration in a patient with Behçet disease. Source: Courtesy of Douglas O. Faigel.

Figure 14.19 A long, tight stricture of the middistal esophagus in a patient with graft-versus-host disease involving the esophagus. Source: Courtesy of Douglas O. Faigel.

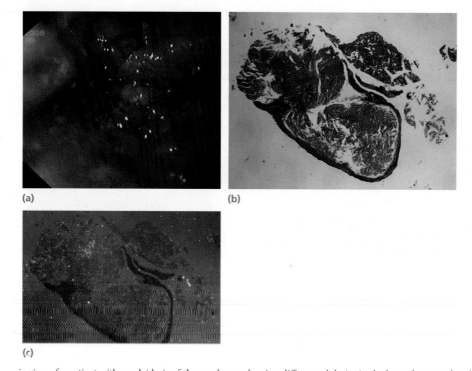

Figure 14.21 Endoscopic view of a patient with amyloidosis of the esophagus showing diffuse nodularity in the hypopharyngeal and postcricoid region **(a)** and corresponding histopathology, showing extracellular pink hyaline material deposition **(b)**, which was strongly positive with Congo red stain **(c)**. Source: Bhavani RSS, Lakhtakia S, Sekaran A, et al. Amyloidosis presenting as postcricoid esophageal stricture. Gastrointestinal Endoscopy 2010;71:180. Reproduced with permission of Elsevier.

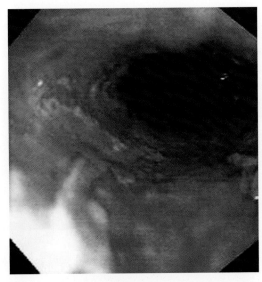

Figure 14.22 Desquamated esophageal mucosa in a patient with pemphigus vulgaris. Source: Courtesy of Douglas O. Faigel.

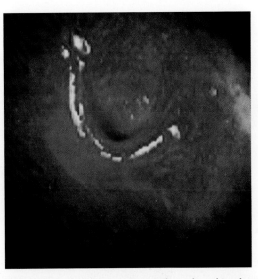

Figure 14.24 Endoscopic view of a patient with esophageal involvement of benign mucous membrane pemphigoid, showing a tight esophageal stricture. Source: Courtesy of Douglas O. Faigel.

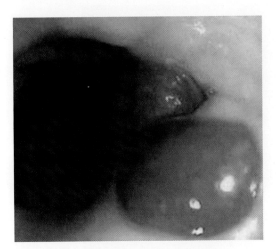

Figure 14.23 Endoscopic image from patient with bullous pemphigoid, showing hemorrhagic vesicles in the upper third of the esophagus. The affected patient presented with characteristic skin lesions and upper GI bleeding. Source: Maharshak N, Sagi M, Santos E, et al. Oesophageal involvement in bullous pemphigoid. Clin Exp Dermatol 2013;38:274. Reproduced with permission of John Wiley & Sons.

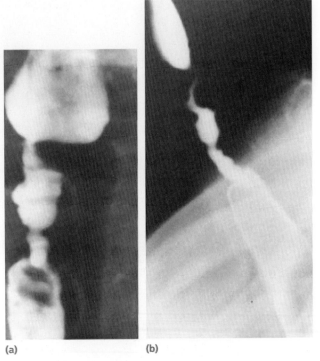

(a) (b)

Figure 14.25 Benign mucous membrane pemphigoid. Postinflammatory scarring caused a long, irregular area of narrowing suggestive of a malignant process on a barium swallow **(a, b)**. Source: Eisenberg RL. Gastrointestinal radiology: a pattern approach, 4th edn, 2003. Reproduced with permission of Wolters Kluwer Health.

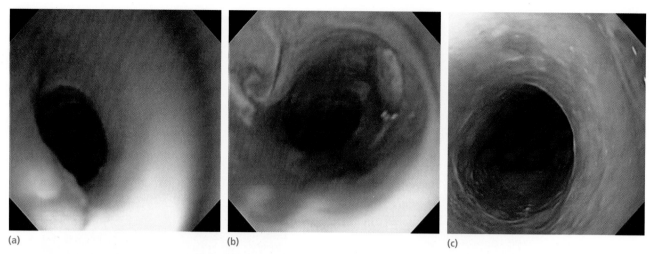

(a)   (b)   (c)

Figure 14.26 An endoscopic view of a tight esophageal stricture due to epidermolysis bullosa dystrophica before **(a)** and after **(b)** initial dilation. After multiple sessions of serial dilation, the stricture zone is much improved **(c)**.

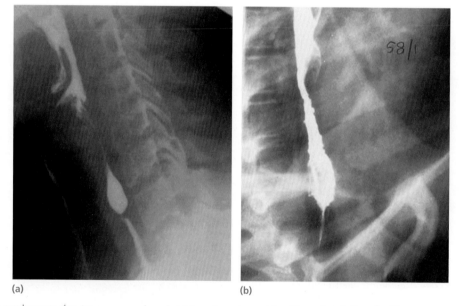

(a)   (b)

Figure 14.27 Barium esophagrams showing severe esophageal strictures in patients with epidermolysis bullosa **(a, b)**. Source. Courtesy of Douglas O. Faigel.

CHAPTER 15

Disorders of gastric emptying

Henry P. Parkman
Temple University School of Medicine, Philadelphia, PA, USA

Introduction

Gastric motility disorders include delayed gastric emptying (gastroparesis), rapid gastric emptying (as seen in dumping syndrome), and disorders with motor and sensory abnormalities (e.g., functional dyspepsia). Management of these patients requires an understanding of the pathophysiology, clinical tests, and treatment options.

Gastric motility

Gastric motility delivers ingested food into the duodenum at a rate that maximizes digestion and absorption. The motor activity of the stomach is generated by three different anatomic regions of the stomach: the proximal fundus, the distal antrum, and the pyloric sphincter. Each region has its own unique motility pattern. The proximal stomach accommodates to store the ingested meal; the distal stomach grinds down or triturates solid particles; and the pylorus allows emptying the meal in a regulated fashion into the duodenum. Thus, gastric emptying is a highly regulated process reflecting coordination between the propulsive forces of proximal fundic tone and distal antral contractions, and relaxation of the pylorus.

Gastroparesis

Gastroparesis is a disorder characterized by symptoms and evidence of gastric retention in the absence of mechanical obstruction. Gastroparesis has significant impact on quality of life and typically affects women. Although the true prevalence of gastroparesis is not known, it has been estimated that up to 4% of the population experiences symptomatic manifestations of this condition. Diabetes mellitus is the most common systemic disease associated with gastroparesis. A similar number

of patients present with idiopathic gastroparesis. Of patients with idiopathic gastroparesis, a previous viral infection antecedent to gastroparesis symptoms may be present in up to 23% of cases. Postsurgical gastroparesis, often with vagotomy or inadvertent damage to the vagus nerve, represents the third most common etiology of gastroparesis.

Symptoms of gastroparesis

The most frequently reported symptoms associated with gastroparesis include nausea, vomiting, early satiety, and postprandial fullness. Abdominal pain is also noted by many patients and represents a challenging symptom to treat. Weight loss, malnutrition, and dehydration may be prominent in severe cases. In diabetics, gastroparesis may adversely affect glycemic control. Although it has been a common assumption that gastrointestinal symptoms can be attributed to delayed gastric emptying, most investigations have observed only weak correlation between symptom severity and the degree of gastric stasis. Symptoms that suggest delayed gastric emptying in patients with dyspeptic symptoms are primarily postprandial fullness, nausea, and vomiting. In patients with diabetes, symptoms that have been associated with delayed gastric emptying are abdominal bloating/ fullness. A symptom questionnaire, the Gastroparesis Cardinal Symptom Index (GCSI), has been developed and validated for quantifying symptoms in patients with gastroparesis (Table 15.1). The GCSI is based on three subscales (postprandial fullness/ early satiety, nausea/ vomiting, and bloating) and represents a subset of the longer patient assessment of upper gastrointestinal disorders-symptoms (PAGI-SYM). The GCSI has also been validated for use as a daily diary.

Evaluation of gastroparesis

The diagnosis of gastroparesis is made when a documented delay in gastric emptying is present and endoscopic or radiographic testing exclude a mechanical blockage. The best accepted technique for measurement of gastric emptying is scintigraphy,

Yamada's Atlas of Gastroenterology, Fifth Edition. Edited by Daniel K. Podolsky, Michael Camilleri, J. Gregory Fitz, Anthony N. Kalloo, Fergus Shanahan, and Timothy C. Wang.
© 2016 John Wiley & Sons, Ltd. Published 2016 by John Wiley & Sons, Ltd.
Companion website: www.yamadagastro.com/atlas

Table 15.1 Gastroparesis Cardinal Symptom Index (GCSI). The GCSI is a nine-symptom questionnaire that has been developed for quantifying symptoms in patients with gastroparesis. Source: Revicki DA, Rentz AM, Dubois D, et al. Development and validation of a patient-assessed gastroparesis symptom severity measure: the Gastroparesis Cardinal Symptom Index. Aliment Pharmacol Ther 2003;18:141. Reproduced with permission of John Wiley & Sons.

	None	Very mild	Mild	Moderate	Severe	Very severe
1. Nausea (feeling sick to your stomach as though you might vomit)	0	1	2	3	4	5
2. Retching (heaving, as if to vomit, but nothing comes up)	0	1	2	3	4	5
3. Vomiting	0	1	2	3	4	5
4. Stomach fullness	0	1	2	3	4	5
5. Not able to finish a normal-sized meal	0	1	2	3	4	5
6. Feeling excessively full after meals	0	1	2	3	4	5
7. Loss of appetite	0	1	2	3	4	5
8. Bloating (feeling as though you need to loosen your clothes)	0	1	2	3	4	5
9. Stomach is visibly larger	0	1	2	3	4	5

using an egg meal cooked with a technetium radiolabel (^{99m}Tc). The gastric emptying test determines the percent gastric retention at both 2 and 4 h postprandially. Physicians from the American Neurogastroenterology and Motility Society with the Society of Nuclear Medicine have adopted the low-fat, egg-white sandwich with jelly as a test meal and imaging at 0, 1, 2, and 4 h postprandially (Figure 15.1). Imaging for gastric emptying up to 4 h, rather than 2 h, has been shown to increase the diagnosis of delayed gastric emptying and is now suggested as the standard in gastric emptying tests to obtain reliable results for the detection of gastroparesis (Figure 15.2). When gastric scintigraphy is performed for shorter durations, the test is less reliable because of the wide range in normal gastric emptying prior to the 4-h time.

Gastric emptying scintigraphy measures the net output of solids or liquids from the stomach but does not define the pathophysiological mechanisms that may impair gastric emptying. Technical advances in scintigraphy may provide more information on fundic and antral abnormalities. Regional gastric emptying can be used to assess intragastric meal distribution and transit from the proximal to distal portion of the stomach (Figure 15.3). Proximal retention has been described in gastroesophageal reflux disease (GERD), distal retention in functional dyspepsia, and global retention in gastroparesis. Dynamic antral contraction scintigraphy (DACS) with frequent imaging can visualize antral contractions (Figure 15.4). Gastric mucosal labeling with single photon emission computed tomography (SPECT), which measures gastric volume as an index of accommodation, can be combined with a scintigraphic test that measures gastric emptying using two different radionuclides (Figure 15.5). In this test, intravenous technetium 99m pertechnetate is used to image the gastric mucosa and an indium-111 radiolabeled solid meal is employed to measure gastric emptying.

Two other methods are available to measure gastric emptying. First, the wireless motility capsule, a Food and Drug Administration (FDA)-approved pH and pressure sensing capsule (SmartPill™), can assess gastric emptying by recording the duration of acidity from capsule ingestion to the change in pH, from the acidic stomach to the alkaline duodenum (Figure 15.6). This capsule can also record pressures as it passes through the gastrointestinal tract. Second, a stable isotope (e.g., ^{13}C-octanoate, ^{13}C-spirulina [the latter is now approved by FDA for diagnosis of gastric emptying delay]) breath test can be used for measuring gastric emptying, and has been shown to correlate significantly with gastric emptying for solids measured by scintigraphy. These breath tests are convenient, sensitive, and specific to detect delayed gastric emptying. Both of these tests can be performed as an outpatient or as an inpatient in a hospital room.

Electrogastrography is the cutaneous recording of myoelectric activity of the gastric smooth muscle by means of electrodes placed on the abdominal-wall skin overlying the stomach. The recorded signal is called an electrogastrogram (EGG) and usually consists of three cycles per minute (cpm) signal, reflecting gastric slow-wave (pacemaker) activity and the subsequent gastric contractions (Figure 15.7). Abnormalities in the EGG signal have been demonstrated in patients with gastroparesis and functional dyspepsia (Figure 15.8). A significant percentage of these patients may have very rapid, slow-wave frequencies (tachygastria) or slow-wave frequencies that are very slow (bradygastria). Multichannel EGG recording has been suggested as a way to assess gastric electrical slow-wave propagation velocity and to detect electromechanical uncoupling (Figure 15.9). In this technique, the EGG is recorded using electrodes placed at different positions overlying the stomach. Multichannel electrogastrography may enhance the diagnostic utility of the test compared with traditional one-channel recording in detecting abnormalities, such as ectopic gastric pacemaker and abnormal coupling of the electrical slow waves. Gastric dysrhythmias (tachygastria, bradygastria) and decreased postprandial amplitude (or power) of the EGG have been described in idiopathic and diabetic gastroparesis. Studies have suggested a good correlation between delayed gastric emptying measured

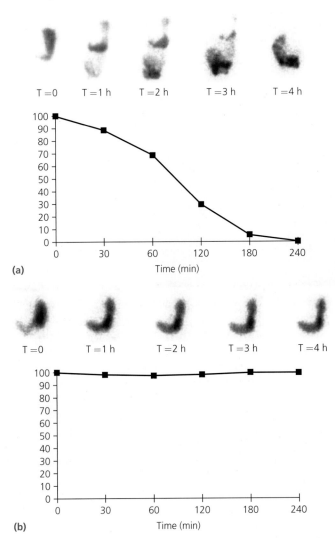

(a)

(b)

Figure 15.1 Gastric emptying scintigraphy. Gastric emptying scintigraphy using a technetium-99m-labeled egg sandwich. The percentages of gastric retention are shown for 0, 30, 60, 120, 180, and 240 min after meal ingestion. **(a)** Normal gastric emptying with only 30% retention at 2 h after meal ingestion (normal < 50%) and complete emptying at 4 h (normal < 10%). **(b)** Markedly delayed gastric emptying with little emptying at 4 h.

by scintigraphy and an abnormal EGG, particularly postprandial rhythm and amplitude abnormalities. An abnormal EGG is present in about 75% of patients with gastroparesis compared with only 25% of symptomatic patients with normal gastric emptying. Gastric dysrhythmias have been suggested to be better predictors of symptoms than delayed gastric emptying. In diabetic patients, hyperglycemia may itself provoke dysrhythmias, primarily tachygastrias. EGG is used to demonstrate gastric myoelectric abnormalities in patients with unexplained nausea and vomiting with abdominal discomfort or functional dyspepsia. The EGG is generally used as an adjunct to gastric emptying scintigraphy, as part of a comprehensive evaluation of patients with refractory symptoms suggestive of an upper GI motility disorder.

Diabetic gastroparesis

Gastroparesis is a well-recognized complication of diabetes mellitus. Diabetic gastroparesis is clinically important because it causes gastrointestinal symptoms, alterations in glycemic control, and changes in oral drug absorption. It is associated with long-standing, insulin-dependent (type 1) diabetes mellitus (IDDM) with the complications of retinopathy, nephropathy, and peripheral neuropathy. Longitudinal studies suggest that delayed gastric emptying of solid or nutrient liquid meals is common, not only in the 25%–40% of patients with long-standing type 1 diabetes, but also in the 10%–20% of patients with type 2 diabetes, a more common condition.

Hyperglycemia itself may reversibly impair gastric motility by decreasing antral contractility, reducing antral phase III migrating motor complex activity, increasing pyloric contractions, stimulating gastric dysrhythmias (primarily tachygastria), and thus delaying gastric emptying. The typical level of blood glucose associated with impaired gastric motor function is >230 mg/dL (or 13 mmol/L). Normalization of serum glucose in hyperglycemic patients has been shown to improve gastric myoelectric activity, accelerate gastric emptying, and restore antral phase III activity in some patients. In addition, hyperglycemia reduces the effect of prokinetic agents.

Changes of gastric motility may also significantly affect postprandial blood glucose concentrations. In some diabetic patients, delayed gastric emptying may contribute to poor glucose control because of unpredictable delivery of food into the duodenum. Impaired gastric emptying with continued administration of exogenous insulin may also produce hypoglycemia. Conversely, acceleration of emptying has been reported to cause hyperglycemia. Problems with blood sugar control may be the first indication that a diabetic patient is developing a gastric motility disorder. Interestingly, in some of these patients, gastroparetic symptoms may be mild or absent.

In addition to abnormalities in gastric emptying, subjects with IDDM have an increased perception of gastric distention produced with a gastric barostat, perhaps resulting in exaggerated nausea, bloating, and upper abdominal pain. Increased sensitivity of the proximal stomach may be responsible for dyspeptic symptoms in the postprandial period during which the proximal stomach is distended by a meal. Thus, in some patients with diabetic gastroparesis, there is visceral hypersensitivity similar to that described in functional dyspepsia. There is also an overlap between idiopathic gastroparesis and functional dyspepsia, in that delayed gastric emptying has been described in approximately 35% of patients with functional dyspepsia.

Treatment of gastroparesis

The goals of gastroparesis therapy include relief of symptoms, normalization of nutrition and hydration status, improvement of glycemic control in diabetics, and improvement of gastric

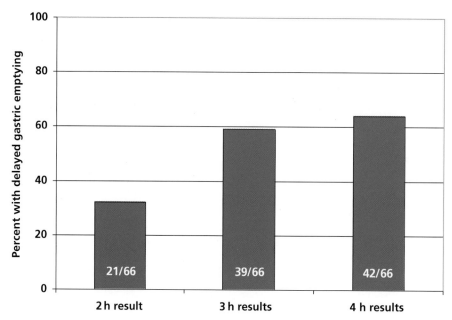

Figure 15.2 Gastric emptying scintigraphy with imaging up to 4 h. Imaging for gastric emptying up to 4 h increases the detection of delayed gastric emptying (see Chapter 23). Imaging up to 4 h increased the diagnostic yield for delayed gastric emptying from 31% of patients at 2 h to 63% at 4 h. Source: Guo JP, Maurer AH, Fisher RS, Parkman HP. Extending gastric emptying scintigraphy from two to four hours detects more patients with gastroparesis. Dig Dis Sci 2001;46:24–9. Reproduced with permission of Springer Science + Business Media.

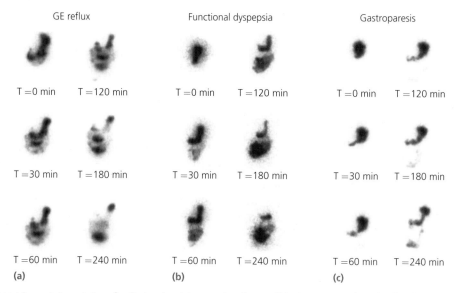

Figure 15.3 Regional gastric emptying scintigraphy. Regional gastric emptying abnormalities in gastroesophageal reflux disease, functional dyspepsia, and gastroparesis. (a) In patients with gastroesophageal reflux disease, there is retention of the radioactivity in the proximal portion of the stomach. (b) In patients with functional dyspepsia, there is retention of radioactivity in the distal portion of the stomach. (c) In patients with gastroparesis, there is a global retention throughout the whole stomach. Source: Gonlachanvit S, Maurer AH, Fisher RS, Parkman HP. Regional gastric emptying abnormalities in functional dyspepsia and gastro-oesophageal reflux disease. Neurogastroenterol Motil 2006;18:894–904. Reproduced with permission of John Wiley & Sons.

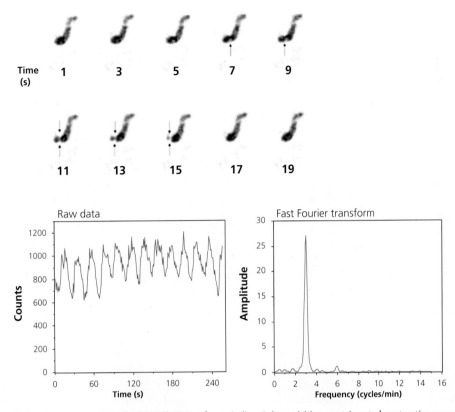

Figure 15.4 Dynamic antral contraction scintigraphy (DACS). Using dynamic (i.e., 1 s) acquisition, gastric antral contractions can be characterized noninvasively with scintigraphy; both the frequency and an estimate of the contractions can be obtained. An example of DACS with analysis is shown. With a region of interest drawn around the mid antrum, the time activity curves show the counts oscillate at about three contractions per minute. The amplitude of the fast Fourier transform (FFT) analysis gives an approximation of the ejection fraction (contraction strength). Source: Knight LC, Parkman HP, Brown KL, et al. Delayed gastric emptying and decreased antral contractility in normal premenopausal women compared with men. Am J Gastroenterol 1997;92:968–75. Reproduced with permission of John Wiley & Sons.

emptying when appropriate. Treatment of gastroparesis includes dietary modifications, prokinetic and antiemetic medications, measures to control pain and address psychological issues, and endoscopic or surgical options in selected instances. The different therapeutic modalities may be offered alone or in different combinations as dictated by the needs of the individual patient.

Prokinetic agents enhance the motility of the upper gastrointestinal tract and accelerate the aboral movement of the intralumenal contents. In general, prokinetic agents increase gastric antral contractility, correct gastric dysrhythmias, and improve antroduodenal coordination. Current prokinetic agents for treatment include oral agents metoclopramide and erythromycin. Cisapride (Propulsid) and Tegaserod (Zelnorm) have been removed from the market because of cardiac or vascular side effects. Domperidone is not available in the United States, although it is available through the FDA Investigative New Drug (IND) program. Intravenous agents currently used to treat hospitalized patients include metoclopramide and erythromycin. New medications in development are more selective 5-HT4 receptor agonists as well as motilin and ghrelin agonists.

Gastric electrical stimulation with an implanted neurostimulator is an emerging therapy for treatment of refractory gastroparesis. It has been intensely investigated over the last two decades. Only in the last 10 years, however, have promising results been reported. There are several ways to electrically stimulate the stomach. First is gastric electrical pacing. Here, the goal is to entrain and pace the gastric slow waves at a higher rate than the patient's normal 3.0 cpm. Pacing at 10% higher than the basal rate has been shown to accelerate gastric emptying and improve dyspeptic symptoms. Second is neuromodulation using high-frequency stimulation at four times the basal rate (12 cpm). With these stimulation parameters, there may be improvement in symptoms with little change in gastric emptying. It has been suggested that this type of stimulation activates sensory afferent nerves to suppress symptoms. Finally, early studies have used sequential circumferential direct muscle stimulation, employing bursts of very high frequency stimulation to sequentially induce direct muscle stimulation in a peristaltic fashion and accelerate gastric emptying.

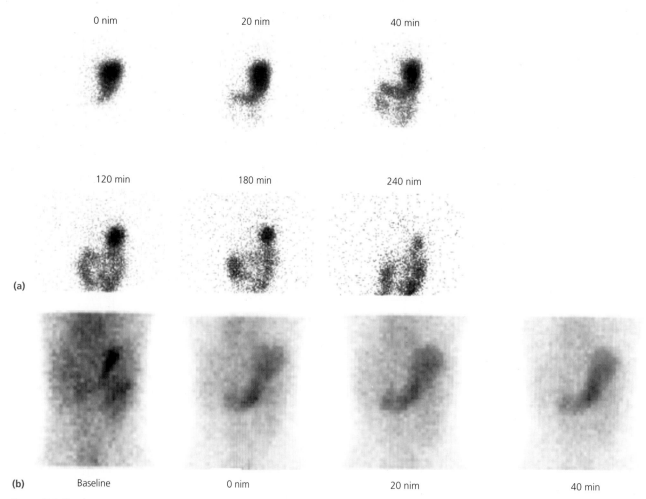

0 nim | 20 nim | 40 min

120 min | 180 min | 240 nim

(a)

(b) Baseline | 0 nim | 20 nim | 40 min

Figure 15.5 Simultaneous gastric emptying and gastric volume. Gastric mucosal labeling with single photon emission computed tomography (SPECT) imaging, which measures gastric volume as an index of accommodation, can be combined with a scintigraphic test that measures gastric emptying using two different radionuclides. In this test, intravenous technetium-99m pertechnetate is used to image the gastric mucosa and an indium-111 radiolabeled solid meal is employed to measure gastric emptying. **(a)** Gastric emptying of orally administered indium-111-labeled egg sandwich. **(b)** Gastric volume after intravenous technetium and orally administered egg sandwich. Source: Simonian HP, Kantor S, Knight LC, et al. Simultaneous assessment of gastric accommodation and emptying: Studies with liquid and solid meals. J Nuclear Med 2004;45:1155. Reproduced with permission.

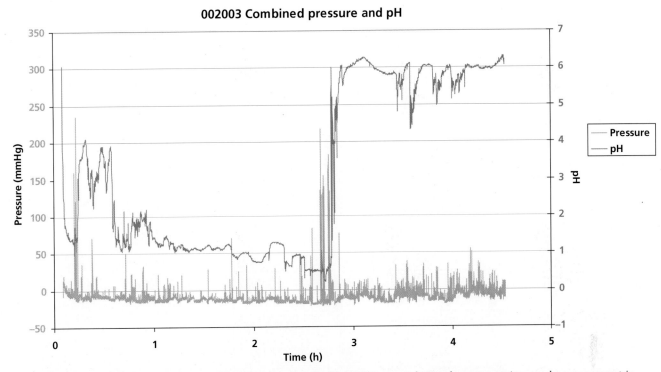

Figure 15.6 Wireless motility capsule recording. The wireless motility capsule, an FDA-approved pH and pressure-sensing capsule, can assess gastric emptying by recording the duration of acidity from capsule ingestion to the change in pH from the acidic stomach to the alkaline duodenum. This capsule can also record pressures as it passes through the gastrointestinal tract. High-amplitude contractions precede the gastric emptying of the SmartPill at 2.75 h, as indicated by the marked increase in pH.

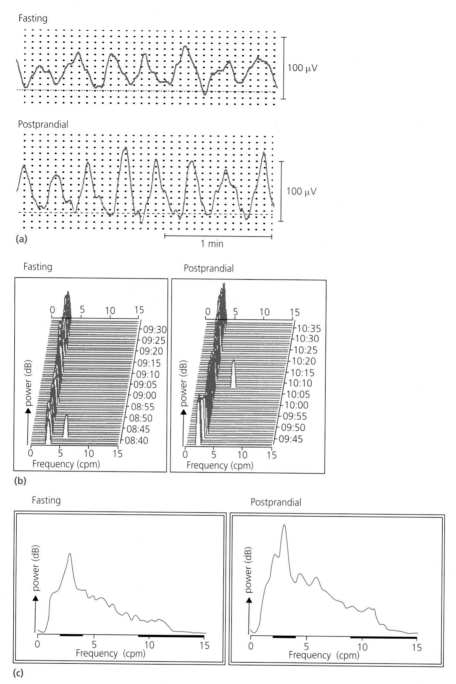

Figure 15.7 Single-channel electrogastrography. This figure shows the EGG tracings and computer analyses from a normal volunteer. The raw tracing (a) demonstrates a sinusoidal oscillation with a frequency of 3 cpm during both the fasting and postprandial periods. Signal amplitude increases with meal ingestion. Running spectral analysis (b) displays the dominant EGG frequencies as a function of time. Throughout the recording, the dominant frequency is in the frequency band 2–4 cpm. The power frequency spectrum (c) displays the dominant frequency for the entire fasting and postprandial periods (3 cpm). The increase in power with meal ingestion can be quantified using this analysis. Small peaks at harmonics of the dominant frequency are seen at 6 and 9 cpm. Source: Parkman HP, Hasler WL, Barnett JL, Eaker EY. American Motility Society Clinical GI Motility Testing Task Force. Electrogastrography. Neurogastroenterol Motil 2003;15:89–102. Reproduced with permission of John Wiley & Sons.

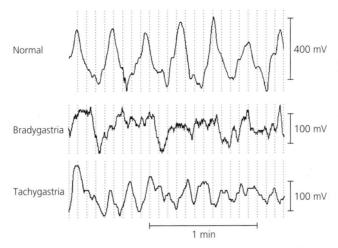

Figure 15.8 Gastric dysrhythmias recorded with electrogastrography (EGG). Representative EGG tracings showing examples of normal 3 cpm rhythm, bradygastria, and tachygastria. Source: Parkman HP, Hasler WL, Barnett JL, Eaker EY; American Motility Society Clinical GI Motility Testing Task Force. Electrogastrography. Neurogastroenterol Motil 2003;15:89–102. Reproduced with permission of John Wiley & Sons.

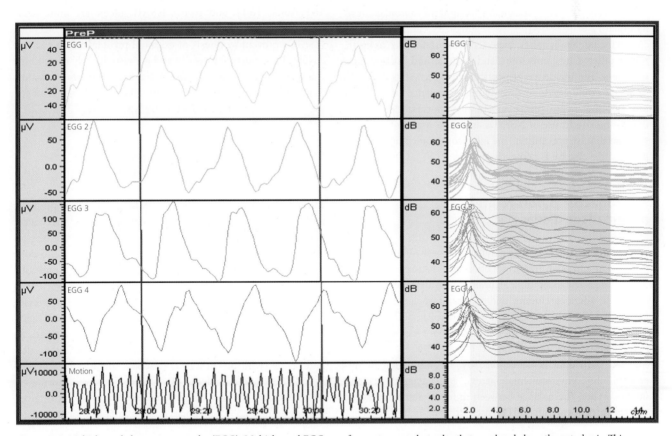

Figure 15.9 Multichannel electrogastrography (EGG). Multichannel EGG uses four cutaneous electrodes that are placed along the antral axis. This technique, as developed by Chen et al., can assess myoelectrical coupling between different leads. Coupling is defined as similar frequency in adjacent EGG leads. Multichannel EGG was used to assess electrical slow-wave coupling in addition to the dominant frequency, power, and percent normal rhythm in normal subjects to define the normal parameters. Similar multichannel EGG values were observed among different genders and ages. Body mass and ethnicity may impact on some of the EGG values. The motion tracing shows normal 3 cpm activity among the four different EGG leads placed along the antral axis. Source: Simonian HP, Panganamamula K, Parkman HP, Xu X, Chen JZ, Lindberg G, et al. Multichannel electrogastrography (EGG) in normal subjects: a multicenter study. Dig Dis Sci 2004;49:594–601. Reproduced with permission of Springer Science + Business Media.

CHAPTER 16

Peptic ulcer disease

Jonathan R. White, Krish Ragunath, and John C. Atherton
University of Nottingham, Nottingham, UK

Introduction

Peptic ulcer disease remains a common cause of morbidity and mortality in the 21st century. Through the endoscope (Figure 16.1), a peptic ulcer is identified as a mucosal break in the stomach or duodenum with depth. The arbitrary criterion (used in most clinical trials) is that an ulcer has a diameter of 5 mm or larger, and lesions smaller than 5 mm are designated erosions. The leading causes of peptic ulcer disease are *Helicobacter pylori* infection (Figures 16.2, 16.3, and 16.4) and nonsteroidal antiinflammatory drug (NSAID) use (Figures 16.5 and 16.6). Rarer causes include malignancy, hypersecretory states such as gastrinoma, other drugs, infections, and vascular and inflammatory disorders. The incidence of peptic ulcer disease has decreased in many countries following falling prevalence of *H. pylori* infection, but peptic ulcers remain an important clinical issue due to the rise in use of NSAIDs as well as aspirin for cardiovascular disease prevention. The most common complication of peptic ulcer disease is hemorrhage.

Helicobacter pylori-related peptic ulcer disease

H. pylori colonizes the gastric mucosa of over 50% the world's population and is an important etiological factor in both duodenal and gastric ulceration. *H. pylori* is also an important cause of gastric adenocarcinoma and mucosa-associated lymphoid tissue (MALT) lymphoma. *H. pylori* provokes both local and systemic inflammatory responses, which are essential in the pathogenesis of *H. pylori*-induced disease. Disease risk in an infected individual is determined by a combination of host susceptibility, environmental factors, and bacterial virulence factors. When the balance between mucosal damaging agents and the integrity of mucosal defenses is disturbed, peptic ulceration may occur (Figure 16.7). Eradication of *H. pylori* cures related ulcers and prevents their recurrence.

Nonsteroidal antiinflammatory drug-related peptic ulcer disease

Increasing NSAID and aspirin use has led to an increase in the relative proportion of gastric to duodenal ulcers (Figures 16.8, 16.9, 16.10, 16.11, and 16.12). NSAID ulcers are more likely than *H. pylori* ulcers to develop complications such as bleeding. NSAIDs prevent synthesis of essential prostaglandins that are required for mucosal integrity and are also directly toxic to the mucosa. The type of agent, dose, patient age, and other cofactors may influence who develops ulcers. The overall risk of peptic ulcer disease is increased 20-fold by NSAID use.

Management of acute upper gastrointestinal hemorrhage

Initial treatment is to resuscitate with fluids and blood products and to reverse or stop offending drugs. Widely used ulcer classification systems exist to predict risk of recurrent hemorrhage and associated mortality. Esophagogastroduodenoscopy (EGD) is often carried out for both diagnostic and therapeutic purposes. Endoscopic hemostasis is achieved by a variety of techniques, which include injection therapy around the vessel, thermal therapy with a heat probe leading to coagulation, delivery of hemostatic clips, or forming a physical barrier with an inorganic material. The use of proton pump inhibitors after endoscopy (with or without endoscopic therapy) is beneficial in individuals with evidence of acute hemorrhage. Alternatives to endoscopic therapy, depending on clinical circumstances, include angiography with endovascular embolization or surgery

Yamada's Atlas of Gastroenterology, Fifth Edition. Edited by Daniel K. Podolsky, Michael Camilleri, J. Gregory Fitz, Anthony N. Kalloo, Fergus Shanahan, and Timothy C. Wang.
© 2016 John Wiley & Sons, Ltd. Published 2016 by John Wiley & Sons, Ltd.
Companion website: www.yamadagastro.com/atlas

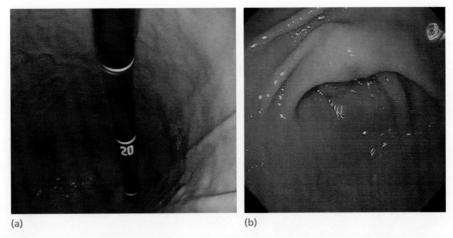

Figure 16.1 (a) The image with an endoscope shows a normal stomach with the endoscope in retroflection. The gastric lining is seen to consist of a regular array of folds, called rugae. **(b)** The endoscopic view of the gastric antrum shows a single nonsteroidal antiinflammatory drug-induced gastric erosion. Note that the antrum has a smooth surface.

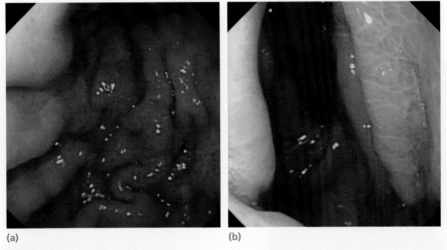

Figure 16.2 (a, b) *Helicobacter pylori*-associated gastritis. Although the stomach demonstrates edema and erythema in this case, these macroscopic changes correlate poorly with histological gastritis. Magnification endoscopy is more accurate, but ultimately "gastritis" is a histological diagnosis.

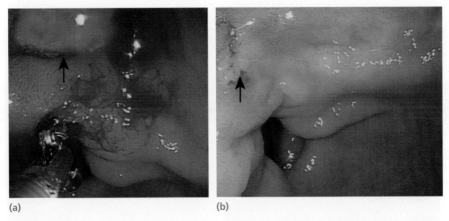

Figure 16.3 (a) Single ulcer in the gastric antrum (arrow): histology showed moderate numbers of *Helicobacter pylori* organisms. **(b)** After *H. pylori* eradication and proton pump inhibitor treatment the ulcer has almost completely healed but has left some scarring and deformity (arrow).

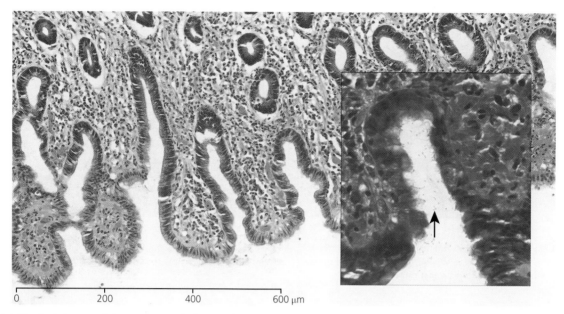

Figure 16.4 Histological image of chronic active *Helicobacter pylori*-associated gastritis in the antral mucosa in a patient with duodenal ulceration and prepyloric gastric erosions (20× hematoxylin and eosin staining). Inset shows a large number of *H. pylori* organisms (arrow), with the characteristic histological appearances of spiral bacilli demonstrated using toludine blue staining in the same biopsy (40×). Source: Courtesy of Dr R. Ingram and Dr A. Zaitoun, Nottingham University Hospital, UK.

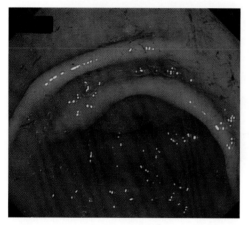

Figure 16.5 Gastric antrum showing petechial hemorrhages, seen as brown dots, which are a typical finding in nonsteroidal antiinflammatory drug or aspirin users.

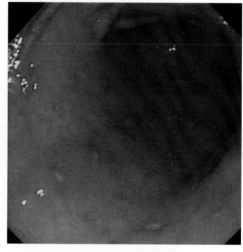

Figure 16.6 Drug-induced erosive gastritis.

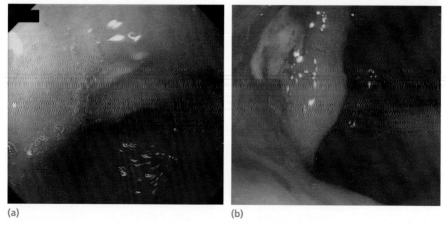

Figure 16.7 *Helicobacter pylori*-associated **(a)** erosive gastritis and **(b)** an ulcer in the gastric antrum.

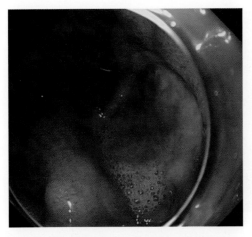

Figure 16.8 Endoscopic view of a clean-based gastric ulcer.

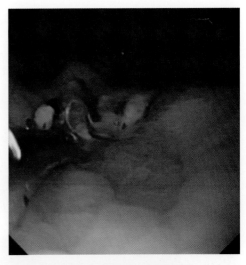

Figure 16.9 Nonsteroidal antiinflammatory drug-induced ulcer seen on the lesser curvature of the stomach.

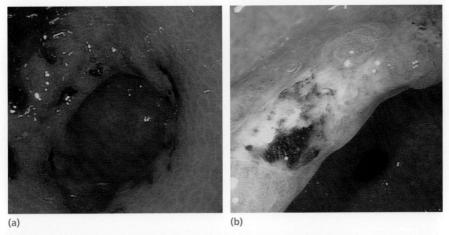

(a)   (b)

Figure 16.10 (a, b) Typical nonsteroidal antiinflammatory drug-induced superficial gastric antral ulcers.

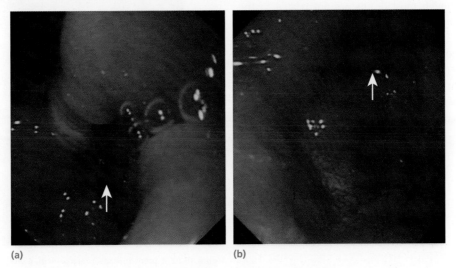

(a)   (b)

Figure 16.11 (a, b) Deep benign prepyloric antral ulcers with deformation of the surrounding area.

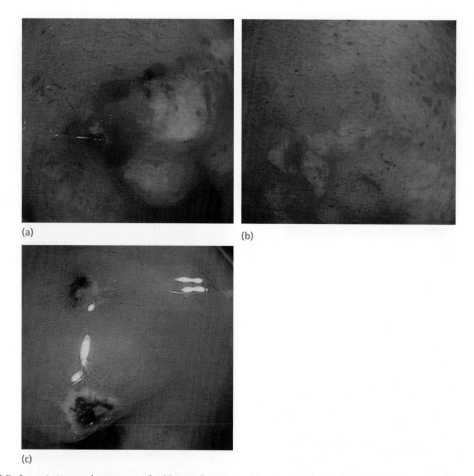

(a)

(b)

(c)

Figure 16.12 **(a, b)** Endoscopic images showing superficial hemorrhages caused by nonsteroidal antiinflammatory drugs (NSAIDs) in the first part of duodenum. The mucosal surface appears inflamed and the duodenal bulb is greatly shortened. **(c)** Endoscopic image showing superficial erosions throughout the stomach. This patient was taking NSAIDs and also had *Helicobacter pylori* infection.

(Figures 16.13–16.29). Despite these interventions mortality is still significant, although most deaths are not related to the hemorrhage itself but to cardiopulmonary complications or multiorgan failure.

Other complications of peptic ulcer disease include perforation, which carries a significant mortality, and gastric outlet obstruction, which occurs when the edematous, inflamed gastric mucosa or scarring obstructs the distal stomach. Ulcers can also penetrate adjacent organs and form fistulas.

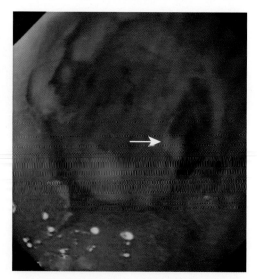

Figure 16.13 A prepyloric ulcer (arrow) with a visible vessel seen in a patient admitted with an acute upper gastrointestinal hemorrhage.

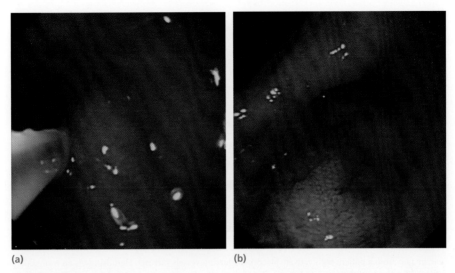

(a)   (b)

Figure 16.14 (a) Injection needle injecting 1 in 10 000 adrenaline to a nonbleeding vessel. **(b)** This provides volume tamponade and local vasoconstriction to stop further bleeding.

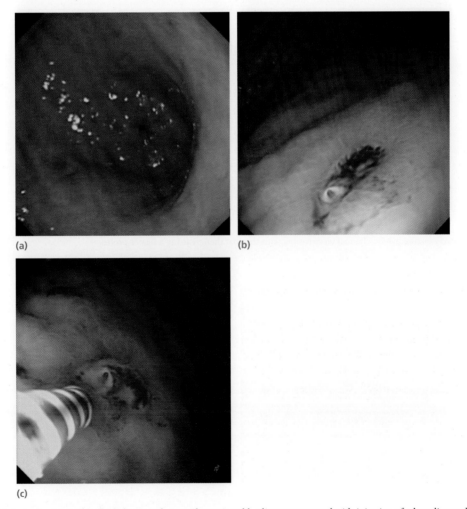

(a)   (b)

(c)

Figure 16.15 (a–c) Endoscopic views of multiple benign ulcers with previous bleeding areas treated with injection of adrenaline and coagulation with a bipolar gold probe.

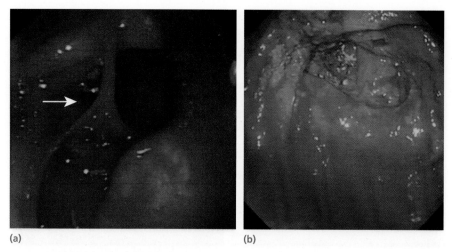

(a)   (b)

Figure 16.16 **(a)** Endoscopic images from a patient with actively bleeding, spurting vessels (arrow). Hemospray is an inorganic powder that can be applied in active ulcer bleeding. This is one of the novel endoscopy-based therapies that forms a physical barrier, halting the hemorrhage and encouraging the formation of clots. **(b)** Hemospray successfully arrested the bleeding in this patient.

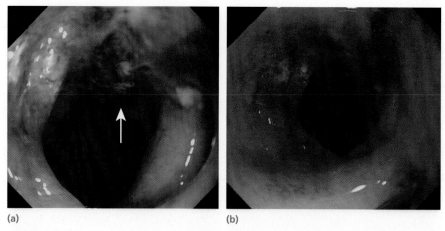

(a)   (b)

Figure 16.17 **(a, b)** Actively oozing pyloric channel ulcer treated with thermal therapy using a heater probe.

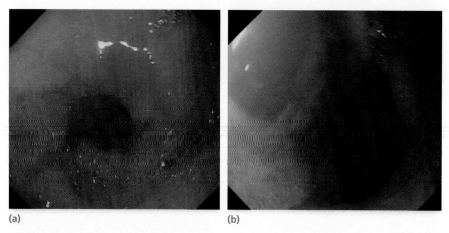

(a)   (b)

Figure 16.18 **(a)** Endoscopic images of a pyloric channel ulcer with severe stenosis. **(b)** The narrowing was widened by repeated endoscopic balloon dilatation.

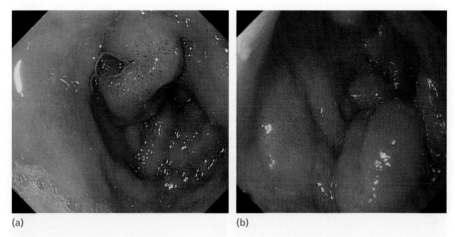

(a)   (b)

Figure 16.19 Duodenitis in the **(a)** first and **(b)** second parts of the duodenum. This is usually caused by *Helicobacter pylori* infection but can also commonly be caused by aspirin or nonsteroidal antiinflammatory drug use.

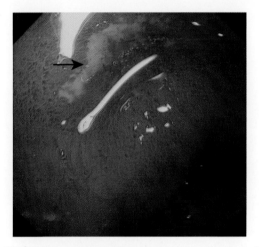

Figure 16.20 Endoscopic images of a superficial linear ulcer (arrow) located in the first part of the duodenum.

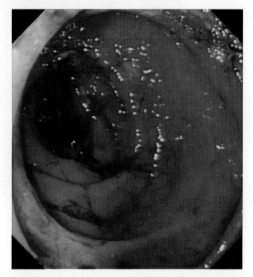

Figure 16.22 Blood in the duodenum from an actively bleeding proximal duodenal ulcer.

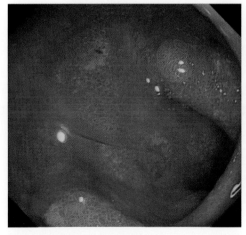

Figure 16.21 Moderate erosive duodenitis.

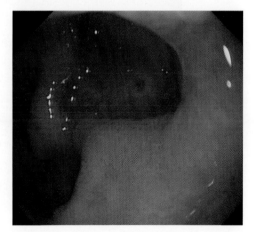

Figure 16.23 Endoscopic view of a duodenal ulcer with a clean base and an exposed vessel.

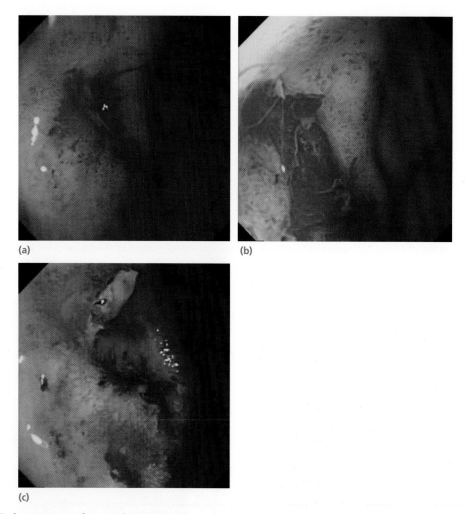

Figure 16.24 (a–c) Endoscopic views of an actively oozing D1 ulcer, treated with adrenaline injection and heater probe application. The duodenal bulb is inflamed, shorter and often deformed in patients with peptic ulcer disease.

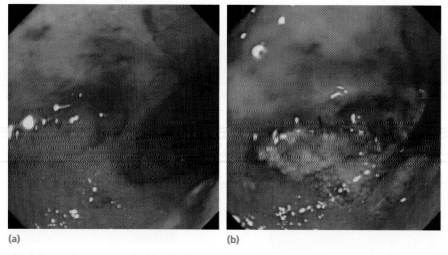

Figure 16.25 (a) A superficial ulcer in the anterior wall of the duodenum with a visible vessel was the cause of significant bleeding in this elderly patient. **(b)** The ulcer was treated with dual therapy consisting of adrenaline injection and heater probe application.

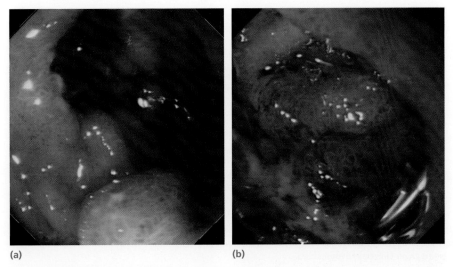

Figure 16.26 (a, b) Severe nonsteroidal antiinflammatory drug-induced ulcer with a visible clot at the D1/D2 junction. The deep ulcerations extend throughout the duodenum leading to deformity.

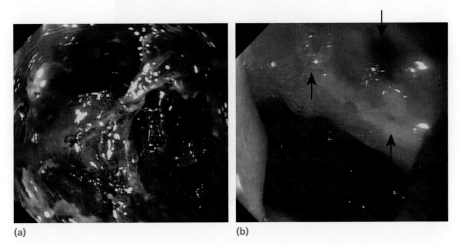

Figure 16.27 (a) A very large clot covering an ulcer in the first part of the duodenum. **(b)** The clot was washed away and revealed a linear ulcer with multiple bleeding points (arrows).

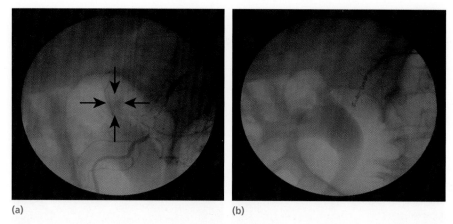

(a)   (b)

Figure 16.28 Radiological images of a patient undergoing endovascular embolization of the gastroduodenal artery. **(a)** Image showing a blush of contrast in the duodenal bulb (arrows). **(b)** Image showing successful insertion of a hemostatic coil to arrest the bleeding. Source: Courtesy of Professor K. Ragunath, Nottingham University Hospital, UK.

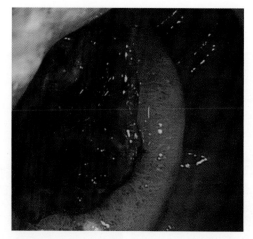

Figure 16.29 Rare malignant duodenal ulcer at the junction of the first and second part of the duodenum.

CHAPTER 17

Zollinger–Ellison syndrome

Robert T. Jensen
National Institutes of Health, Bethesda, MD, USA

Zollinger–Ellison syndrome (ZES) is a clinical syndrome characterized by symptoms due to excess gastric acid secretion (severe peptic ulcer disease [PUD], diarrhea, gastroesophageal reflux disease [GERD]) caused by the autonomous release of gastrin from a neuroendocrine tumor (NET; also called a gastrinoma, islet cell tumor, non-β cell islet cell tumor). Patients with ZES have two important therapeutic considerations: treatment of the acid hypersecretion and treatment of the gastrinoma per se. These are both required because the gastric acid hypersecretion, if untreated, leads to increased morbidity and mortality due to complications of refractory PUD/GERD. Treatment of the gastrinoma is needed because 60%–90% are malignant. ZES can occur either sporadically (not inherited) (75%) or as part of the multiple endocrine neoplasia type 1 syndrome (MEN1)(25%), an autosomal dominant disorder. These two forms need to be distinguished because they differ in many treatment options.

ZES is much less frequent than idiopathic PUD but can be suspected by the presence of severe PUD, family history of endocrinopathies with PUD, PUD with diarrhea or the presence of prominent gastric folds on upper gastrointestinal endoscopy (UGI) (Figure 17.1c,d) (due to trophic action of gastrin). This finding differs from small or lack of gastric folds on upper gastrointestinal endoscopy, characteristically seen in patients with atrophic gastritis (Figure 17.1b) (a frequent cause of hypergastrinemia, like ZES) compared to normal gastric folds (Figure 17.1a). The trophic action of gastrin on the gastric endocrine cells can lead to the development of gastric carcinoids in patients with ZES with MEN1 (MEN1/ZES) (arrows Figure 17.1d). ZES in MEN1/ZES patients characteristically occurs at an earlier age than in patients with sporadic ZES (Figure 17.1e).

Once the diagnosis is suspected, a fasting serum gastrin level (FSG) is usually the initial study because 99%–100% of ZES patients have an elevated level. However, the most common cause of hypergastrinemia is not ZES, but is due to physiological hypergastrinemia secondary to achlor /hypochlorhydria seen in atrophic gastritis, pernicious anemia, or due to use the of potent acid suppressants such as proton pump inhibitors (PPIs; e.g.,

omeprazole). To distinguish ZES, measurement of gastric pH is required because ZES patients have gastric acid hypersecretion both in their basal acid output and maximal acid outputs (Figure 17.2b), and have inappropriately elevated FSG levels because in normal subjects acid physiologically suppresses gastrin release. An elevated FSG in the presence of a gastric pH <2 is strongly suggestive of ZES; however, in patients with FSG <10-fold elevated, additional studies for diagnosis are required, including performing a secretin provocative test and assessing FSG levels (positive >120 pg/mL increase in FSG) (Figure 17.2a). In the past, a calcium infusion test (positive >395 pg/mL increase in FSG) (Figure 17.2a) or no/minimal increase in FSG with meal testing (Figure 17.2a) were used, but these two are rarely used at present.

After establishing the diagnosis, controlling the gastric acid hypersecretion (usually with PPIs), assessment for the presence of MEN1, and tumor localization studies to determine the location of the primary and extent of disease (cross-sectional imaging [computed tomography, magnetic resonance imaging], somatosatin receptor scintigraphy [Octreoscan or ^{68}Ga-labeled somatostatin analogs with computed tomography/positron emission tomography scanning]) are recommended. For patients with sporadic disease, surgical exploration by a surgeon familiar with pancreatic neuroendocrine tumors (pNETs) should be undertaken in those patients with resectable disease and no medical contraindications to surgery. This is recommended because 50%–60% of patients with sporadic ZES can be cured immediately postoperatively and 30%–40% at >10 years (Figure 17.3a). In contrast, patients with MEN1/ZES are rarely cured (Figure 17.3a) without aggressive resections such as a Whipple procedure, which are not recommended, and thus routinely do not undergo surgery for resection of abdominal pNETs unless it is >1.5–2 cm in diameter on imaging studies. In sporadic ZES, 70%–85% of gastrinomas occur in the duodenum not the pancreas, and in MEN1/ZES 85%–100% are found in the duodenum. Duodenal gastrinomas can be small (2–10 mm) and thus it is important to perform a duodenotomy with careful search of the duodenum at surgery, to achieve an

Yamada's Atlas of Gastroenterology, Fifth Edition. Edited by Daniel K. Podolsky, Michael Camilleri, J. Gregory Fitz, Anthony N. Kalloo, Fergus Shanahan, and Timothy C. Wang.
© 2016 John Wiley & Sons, Ltd. Published 2016 by John Wiley & Sons, Ltd.
Companion website: www.yamadagastro.com/atlas

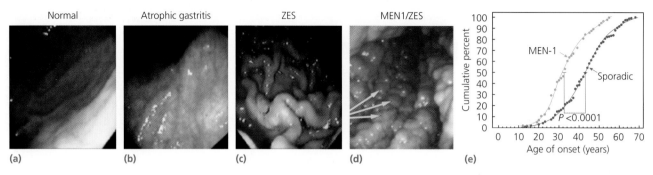

Figure 17.1 Endoscopic findings important in suspecting/diagnosing Zollinger–Ellison syndrome (ZES). **(a–c)** Show typical endoscopic findings of the gastric folds in normal patients, patients with atrophic gastritis (loss of folds, thin mucosa), or ZES (prominent folds, present in >94%). **(d)** Shows multiple gastric carcinoids (type 2) (arrows) that frequently occur in patients with multiple endocrine neoplasia type 1 syndrome (MEN1)/ZES (23%). **(e)** Shows the onset of ZES in patients with MEN1/ZES ($n = 58$) is 10 years earlier than in patients without MEN1 (sporadic ZES) ($n = 203$). Source: Data from Roy PK, Venzon DJ, Shojamanesh H, et al. Zollinger-Ellison syndrome: clinical presentation in 261 patients. Medicine (Baltimore) 2000;79:379 and Gibril F, Schumann M, Pace A, et al. Multiple endocrine neoplasia type 1 and Zollinger-Ellison syndrome. A prospective study of 107 cases and comparison with 1009 patients from the literature. Medicine (Baltimore) 2004;83:43.

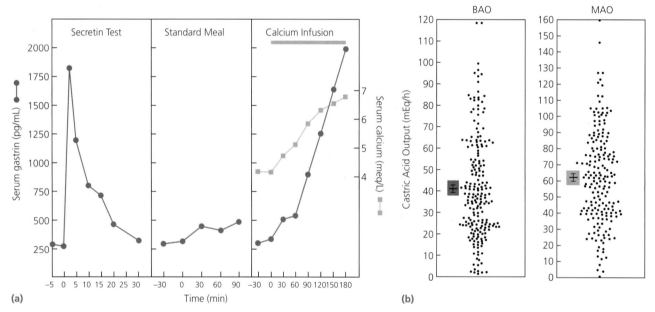

Figure 17.2 Provocative test results and acid secretory findings important in suspecting/diagnosing Zollinger–Ellison syndrome (ZES). **(a)** Shows the typical response in serum gastrin concentrations in patients with ZES with injection of secretin (positive >120 pg/mL increase) (secretin test), calcium infusion (≥395 pg/mL increase) (positive ≥395 pg/mL increase), and standard meal test (<100% basal increase). Only the secretin test is widely used today. Source: Data from Berna M.J., Hoffmann K.M., Long S.H., et al. Serum gastrin in Zollinger-Ellison syndrome: II. Prospective study of gastrin provocative testing in 293 patients from the National Institutes of Health and comparison with 537 cases from the literature. evaluation of diagnostic criteria, proposal of new criteria, and correlations with clinical and tumoral features. Medicine (Baltimore) 2006;85:331. **(b)** Shows the markedly elevated gastric basal acid secretion (BAO) (upper limit of normal [ULN] <15 mEq/h) and maximal acid secretion (MAO) (ULN 48 mEq/h) in 235 patients with ZES. Source: Data from Roy PK, Venzon DJ, Feigenbaum KM, et al. Gastric secretion in Zollinger-Ellison syndrome. Correlation with clinical expression, tumor extent and role in diagnosis — a prospective NIH study of 235 patients and a review of 984 cases in the literature. Medicine (Baltimore) 2001;80:189.

optimal cure rate (Figure 17.3b). Some patients have negative imaging and in these, in the past, some experts recommended observation without surgery. However, a recent study shows these patients also benefit from surgical exploration and have a similar benefit from surgery as sporadic cases (Figure 17.4a,b).

Important prognostic factors for patients with ZES include: adequate control of the gastric acid hypersecretory state; the primary location of the gastrinoma (Figure 17.5b), with pancreatic gastrinomas being more aggressive and associated with a decreased survival compared to a primary in the duodenum or lymph node; the extent of the disease (Figure 17.5a), with any extent of liver metastases associated with decreased survival. Increasing extent of liver metastases is associated with progressive worse survival (Figure 17.5a). Additional factors associated

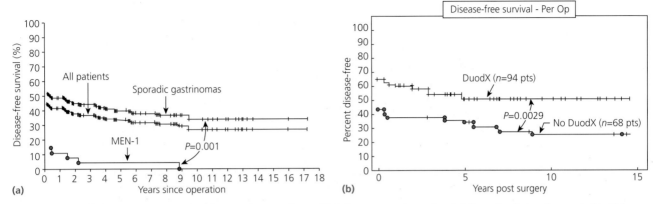

Figure 17.3 Surgical results in patients with Zollinger–Ellison syndrome (ZES) from prospective studies. **(a)** Shows the disease-free survival in 151 patients with ZES (sporadic = 123 patients with multiple endocrine neoplasia type 1 syndrome [MEN1]; ZES = 28 patients) after attempted surgical cure (without Whipple resection). Data show that 34% of sporadic ZES patients have a long-term cure (10 years), but none of the MEN1/ZES patients do. Source: Data from Norton JA, Fraker DL, Alexander HR, et al. Surgery to cure the Zollinger-Ellison syndrome. N Engl J Med 1999;341:635. **(b)** Shows the importance of performing a duodenotomy in 162 ZES patients. Duodenotomy results in more duodenal gastrinomas being found, in a higher cure rate, and a better ZES-related survival. Source: Data from Norton JA, Alexander HR, Fraker DL, et al. Does the use of routine duodenotomy (DUODX) affect rate of cure, development of liver metastases or survival in patients with Zollinger–Ellison syndrome (ZES). Ann Surg 2004;239:617.

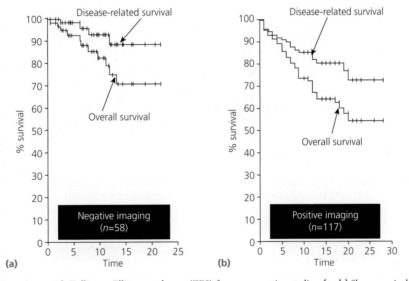

Figure 17.4 Surgical results in patients with Zollinger–Ellison syndrome (ZES) from prospective studies. **(a, b)** Show survival (disease-related and total survival) in patients with negative preoperative imaging (*n* = 58) or positive preoperative imaging (*n* = 117). These results demonstrate that the survival rates are as good in patients with negative preoperative imaging as those with positive imaging, and thus the lack of positive preoperative imaging should not be used to postpone surgery in patients with sporadic ZES. Source: Data from Norton JA, Fraker DL, Alexander HR, et al. Value of surgery in patients with negative imaging and sporadic Zollinger–Ellison syndrome. Ann Surg 2012;256:509.

with a poor prognosis include: the development of ectopic Cushing's syndrome (Figure 17.6); the presence of the sporadic form of ZES (Figure 17.7a); increasing size of the primary gastrinoma; increasing rate of growth of the gastrinoma; high proliferative rate of the gastrinoma; and high serum levels of tumor markers such as FSG levels or chromogranin A levels.

Patients with MEN1/ZES, if the acid hypersecretion is controlled, generally have a more benign course than those with sporadic disease (Figure 17.7a,b). However, their overall

survival is still shortened compared to the general population (mean age death 55 years) and their death is primarily related to a MEN1 cause (Figure 17.7b), with malignant pNETs or thymus carcinoids being the principal cause of early death. However, MEN1/ZES patients present at an age approximately 10 years earlier than sporadic ZES (Figure 17.1b), and they almost invariably have multiple gastrinomas as well as pancreatic pNETs (usually small microadenomas of the pancreas that do not produce a functional syndrome [nonfunctional pNETs,

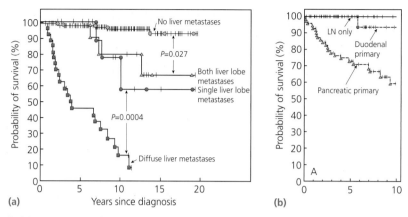

Figure 17.5 Effect on survival of disease extent and primary location in Zollinger–Ellison syndrome (ZES) patients. **(a)** Shows the effect of increasing the extent of liver metastases on survival in 212 ZES patients. Source: Data from Yu F, Venzon DJ, Serrano J, et al. Prospective study of the clinical course, prognostic factors and survival in patients with longstanding Zollinger-Ellison syndrome. J Clin Oncol 1999;17:615. **(b)** Shows the difference in survival for ZES patients with a pancreatic primary ($n = 20$), duodenal primary gastrinoma ($n = 42$), or gastrinoma only in the lymph nodes (LN) ($n = 24$). Source: Data from Weber HC, Venzon DJ, Lin JT, et al. Determinants of metastatic rate and survival in patients with Zollinger–Ellison syndrome: a prospective long-term study. Gastroenterology 1995;108:1637.

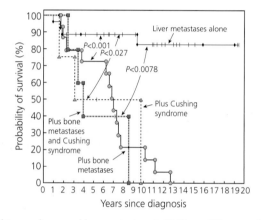

Figure 17.6 Effect on survival of ectopic Cushing syndrome and bone metastases in Zollinger–Ellison syndrome (ZES) patients. The results show the poor prognosis in ZES patients ($n = 27$) with liver metastases who develop Cushing syndrome ($n = 4$), bone metastases ($n = 15$), or both ($n = 5$). Source: Data from Yu F, Venzon DJ, Serrano J, et al. Prospective study of the clinical course, prognostic factors and survival in patients with longstanding Zollinger–Ellison syndrome. J Clin Oncol 1999;17:615.

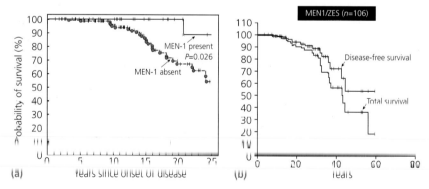

Figure 17.7 Effect on survival of the presence of multiple endocrine neoplasia type 1 syndrome (MEN1) in Zollinger–Ellison syndrome (ZES) patients. **(a)** Shows the difference in survival for ZES patients with ($n = 34$) or without MEN1 ($n = 151$). Source: Data from Weber HC, Venzon DJ, Lin JT, et al. Determinants of metastatic rate and survival in patients with Zollinger-Ellison syndrome: a prospective long-term study. Gastroenterology 1995;108:1637. **(b)** Shows the long-term survival in 106 MEN1/ZES patients followed at the National Institutes of Health (NIH). This survival is much better than reported in 182 MEN1/ZES patients in the literature. Source: Data from Ito T, Igarashi H, Uehara H, et al. Causes of death and prognostic factors in multiple endocrine neoplasia type 1: a prospective study: comparison of 106 MEN1/Zollinger-Ellison syndrome patients with 1613 literature MEN1 patients with or without pancreatic endocrine tumors. Medicine (Baltimore) 2013;92:135.

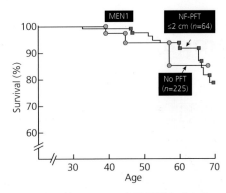

Figure 17.8 Effect on survival of a nonfunctional pancreatic endocrine tumor (NF-PET) in the presence of multiple endocrine neoplasia type 1 syndrome (MEN1) in Zollinger–Ellison syndrome (ZES) patients. The results show the effect on survival of a nonfunctional pancreatic endocrine tumor (NF-PET) ≤ 2 cm ($n = 64$) in patients with MEN1 compared to MEN1 patients ($n = 225$) with no pancreatic neuroendocrine tumor (No-pNET). This result, in addition to other studies showing very low cure rate and excellent long-term survival, lead to the North American Neuroendocrine Tumor Society (NANETS)/European Neuroendocrine Tumor Society (ENETS) recommendations not to routinely operate on MEN1 patients with or without ZES with small pNETs ≤ 2 cm. Source: Data from Triponez F, Goudet P, Dosseh D, et al. Is surgery beneficial for MEN1 patients with small (< or = 2 cm), nonfunctioning pancreaticoduodenal endocrine tumor? An analysis of 65 patients from the GTE. World J Surg 2006;30:654.

NF-pNETs]) and which cannot be cured without a total pancreatectomy. Long-term studies show that if NF-pNETs are <2 cm in diameter in MEN1 patients their survival is similar to patients with no pNETs imaged (Figure 17.8); also, patients with MEN1/ZES with imaged pNETs <2 cm have a 15-year survival of 100%. This has led both the European Neuroendocrine Tumor Society guidelines (ENETs) and the North American Neuroendocrine Tumor Society guidelines (NANETs) to recommend that these patients not routinely undergo surgical exploration.

CHAPTER 18

Gastritis and gastropathy

David Y. Graham[1] and Robert M. Genta[2]
[1] Michael E. DeBakey Veterans Affairs Medical Center, Baylor College of Medicine, Houston, TX, USA
[2] Miraca Life Sciences Research Institute, Irving, TX, and University of Texas Southwestern Medical Center, Dallas, TX, USA

Autoimmune gastritis

Autoimmune gastritis is a corpus-restricted chronic atrophic gastritis. It is usually associated with serum antiparietal cell and antiintrinsic factor antibodies and with intrinsic factor deficiency, with or without pernicious anemia. Most clinical manifestations of autoimmune gastritis result from the loss of parietal and chief cells of the oxyntic mucosa, and only become apparent in the florid or end-stage phases of the disease. Major effects include achlorhydria, hypergastrinemia, loss of pepsin and pepsinogens, iron deficiency with macrocytic anemia, vitamin B-12 deficiency with megaloblastic anemia, and increased risk of gastric neoplasms, particularly carcinoids.

Endoscopic appearance

In the corpus, the mucosa is usually thinner than normal (Figure 18.1); this explains why few folds are left and fine submucosal vessels are easily recognized at endoscopic examination, especially in advanced stages of disease (Figure 18.2). Figure 18.3 shows the appearance of an atrophic antrum.

Histopathological aspects

The main histopathological features of advanced autoimmune gastritis are the diffuse involvement of the oxyntic mucosa by chronic atrophic gastritis with moderate intestinal metaplasia and a gastric antrum that may be either normal or show reactive gastropathy (Figure 18.4).

Enterochromaffin-like cell hyperplasia (linear and micronodular) (Figure 18.5), and multiple carcinoids are commonly found in the advanced stages of the disease. Hyperplasia of gastrin cells, secondary to achlorhydria, is often seen.

Intestinal metaplasia

Intestinal metaplasia is the replacement of the mucous cells that line the normal gastric mucosa with an epithelium similar to that of the small intestine. Intestinal metaplasia is found most frequently in patients with either current or past *Helicobacter pylori* infection. The clinical significance of intestinal metaplasia is related to its association with dysplasia and adenocarcinoma in *H. pylori* gastritis. Recent studies suggest that the cell linage of intestinal metaplasia differs from that of gastric carcinoma and that it is either a likely dead end histologically and possibly transdifferentiation processes from pseudopyloric metaplasia (spasmolytic peptide-expressing metaplasia).

Endoscopic appearance

The endoscopic feature most commonly associated with intestinalization is an irregular surface with patchy pink and pale areas (Figures 18.6 and 18.7). A technique that has encountered much favor in Japan, but which has not been found to be very reliable in either the United States or Europe, is the spraying of the gastric mucosa with indigo carmine, toluidine blue, or methylene blue. After the metaplastic mucosa sample is washed with saline, it maintains the characteristic blue color and may be differentiated from the nonmetaplastic areas.

Histopathological features

Some metaplastic areas look like normal small intestinal epithelium with an absorptive brush border and goblet cells that produce acidic mucins (Figure 18.8); other areas are lined by a disorderly mixture of irregularly shaped goblet cells and immature intermediate cells that produce a wide spectrum of sialo- and sulfomucins. The most often used classification was proposed by Jass and Filipe: type I (brush border and no sialomucins); type II (no brush border, rare sulfomucins); type III (no brush border, cellular disarray, abundant sulfomucins). Follow-up studies have shown that repeat biopsy in the same region often shows a different type. Stains that were specifically used to determine the type of metaplasia by detecting sulfated mucins (such as high iron Diamine) are being gradually replaced by immunohistochemical stains that identify proteins associated with particular mucin-encoding genes. Although

Yamada's Atlas of Gastroenterology, Fifth Edition. Edited by Daniel K. Podolsky, Michael Camilleri, J. Gregory Fitz, Anthony N. Kalloo, Fergus Shanahan, and Timothy C. Wang.
© 2016 John Wiley & Sons, Ltd. Published 2016 by John Wiley & Sons, Ltd.
Companion website: www.yamadagastro.com/atlas

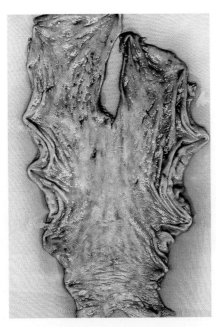

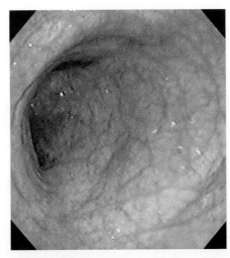

Figure 18.3 An endoscopic picture from a case similar to that depicted in Figure 18.2 with clearly visible mucosal and submucosal vessels is seen in a patient with antral atrophy. The bluish discoloration in the upper left corner is the shade of the liver seen through the thin distended gastric wall.

Figure 18.1 Total gastrectomy performed in a patient with end-stage autoimmune atrophic gastritis and multiple carcinoid tumors. The mucosa of the corpus is completely devoid of rugae, whereas the antrum maintains its normal anatomy.

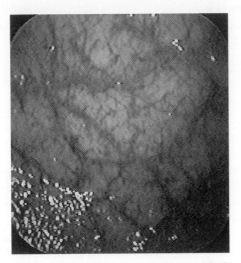

Figure 18.2 Endoscopic view of the corpus with severe atrophy. The mucosa appears thin and the underlying vasculature is prominent.

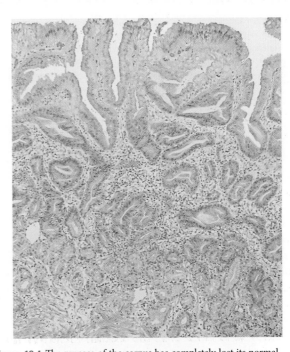

Figure 18.4 The mucosa of the corpus has completely lost its normal appearance. The normal tightly packed acid-secreting oxyntic glands have been progressively destroyed by the autoimmune inflammatory process and are replaced by mucus-secreting glands similar to those found in the distal antrum. The phenomenon is known as pyloric (or pseudopyloric) metaplasia.

more than 20 such genes have been identified, in practice only a few (*MUC1*, *MUC2*, *MUC5AC*, and *MUC6*) are used; however, the clinical relevance of mucin typing has not yet been established and is not recommended in clinical routine practice.

Helicobacter pylori gastritis

The thick mucous gel layer that normally covers the gastric mucosa often contains large numbers of curved bacteria (Figure 18.9). When in contact with the epithelium, *H. pylori* organisms

characteristically attach to surface mucous cells and cause distinctive epithelial changes: cells take irregular cuboidal shapes, reduce or lose their apical mucin droplet, and occasionally drop out, leaving small gaps that contribute to giving the epithelium a ragged, disorderly appearance (Figure 18.10).

Mucosal neutrophils are the other distinctive histological feature of *H. pylori* infection. Neutrophils are also seen in the

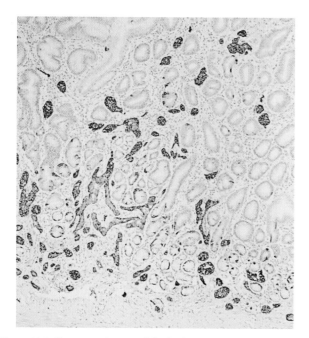

Figure 18.5 Chromogranin stain of the fundic mucosa shows severe enterochromaffin-like (ECL) cell hyperplasia and dysplasia. This is a consequence of the stimulus caused by the hypergastrinemia the patients develop in response to the low or absent acid content of the atrophic stomach. Both ECL cell hyperplasia and dysplasia are considered to be a precursor of carcinoid tumors, which frequently arise in the corpus of patients with autoimmune atrophic gastritis.

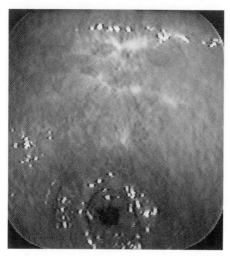

Figure 18.6 Intestinal metaplasia is usually difficult to diagnose endoscopically. Histopathological examination of biopsy specimens obtained from the flat prominent areas visible in this antrum, originally interpreted as either metaplastic or fibrotic areas (scars), showed diffuse intestinal metaplasia.

lamina propria (mixed with mononuclear cells and eosinophils), within the surface and foveolar epithelium, and in more severe cases on the mucosal surface also (Figure 18.10). After successful eradication therapy, neutrophils disappear rapidly; thus, their persistence is considered a good indicator of therapeutic

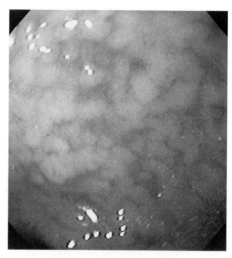

Figure 18.7 Large area of intestinal metaplasia in the antral mucosa. The appearance is characteristically pale and velvety.

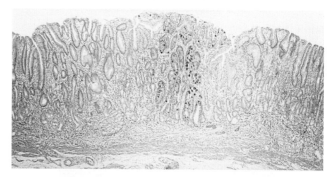

Figure 18.8 Antral mucosa with a small focus of intestinal metaplasia. Goblet cells are best visualized when Alcian blue at pH 2.5 is added to the traditional hematoxylin–eosin stain. Intestinal metaplasia is a marker for increased risk of dysplasia and adenocarcinoma. The larger the area of the gastric mucosa with atrophy (e.g., affected by metaplasia), the greater the risk for gastric cancer.

failure. The gastric mucosa infected by *H. pylori* typically also shows a mononuclear cell infiltrate (an acute-on-chronic pattern), which is often subepithelial (chronic superficial gastritis) (Figure 18.11). The intensity of mononuclear cell infiltrates declines slowly after successful eradication of the organism, and a portion of patients (estimated at 20%–30%) may retain the appearance of a chronic inactive gastritis for several years.

Detection of *Helicobacter pylori*

Helicobacter pylori infects both the antral and oxyntic mucosa, but in the cardia (narrowly defined as the transitional or antral-like mucosa found at the gastroesophageal junction) organisms may be more difficult to detect. In patients who use proton pump inhibitors *H. pylori* organisms tend to be rare or absent in the antrum and may also be more difficult to detect in the corpus, even in the presence of chronic active inflammation. In 70%–80% of gastric biopsy specimens from infected subjects, *H. pylori* organisms can be visualized by hematoxylin–eosin

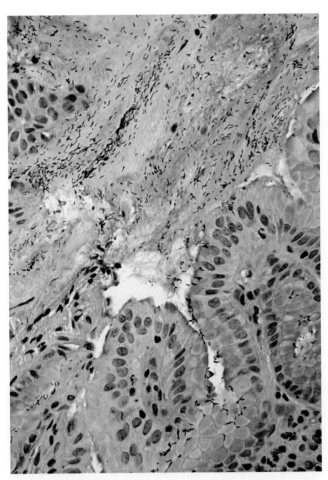

Figure 18.9 Gastric mucus with innumerable *Helicobacter pylori*. Organisms are seen both in the mucus and adhering to the antral mucosa.

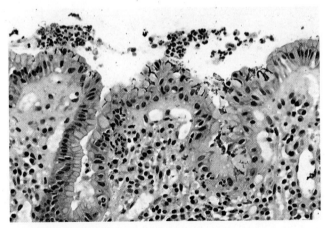

Figure 18.10 Surface epithelial damages caused by the adherence of *Helicobacter pylori*. Cells reduce or lose their apical mucin droplet, may take irregular cuboidal shapes, and occasionally drop out, leaving small gaps that give the gastric epithelium a ragged, uneven appearance.

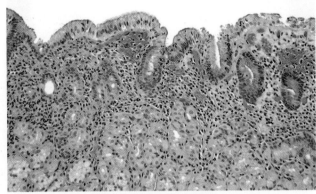

Figure 18.11 Chronic superficial gastritis in the corpus: a band of mononuclear cells separated the surface epithelium from the subjacent oxyntic glands. The surface epithelium is heavily infiltrated by neutrophils.

(H & E) stain (Figure 18.12a). In the remaining 20%–30% of cases a special stain is needed, such as Giemsa and Diff-Quik (Figure 18.12b). Another option is silver-based triple stain that simultaneously allows visualization of *H. pylori* and the morphological changes in the mucosa (see Figures 18.9, 18.10, and 18.11). Because this stain includes Alcian blue at pH 2.5, it makes detection of small foci of intestinal metaplasia easier (Figure 18.13). The increased use of proton pump inhibitors (PPIs) often leads to confusion as the reduction in gastric acidity favors overgrowth of mouth and intestinal microbiota, which are often stained by silver stains leading the pathologist to note rare organisms present, generally without other features of *H. pylori* gastritis. The typical changes induced by PPIs in the oxyntic mucosa are depicted in Figure 18.14. While these special stains are still used in some laboratories, they are being replaced by highly specific anti-*Helicobacter* immunohistochemical stains that can be run on automated stainers.

Endoscopic appearance

Hyperemia, erosions, ulcerations, hypertrophy, and atrophy may coexist in various combinations in the same stomach, juxtaposed to one another and to apparently normal areas, and none of these features has been proven useful for predicting the presence or absence of chronic *H. pylori* gastritis. Although there is no distinct endoscopic pattern of chronic *H. pylori* gastritis, the pattern of follicular gastritis (Figure 18.15) is almost invariably associated with this infection. The presence of peptic ulcers or gastric cancer, both caused by *H. pylori* gastritis, also suggests the presence of the infection.

Reactive gastropathy

The collection of endoscopic and histological features caused by chemical injury to the gastric mucosa is known as reactive (or chemical) gastropathy. This condition, which used to be found almost exclusively in patients who use aspirin or

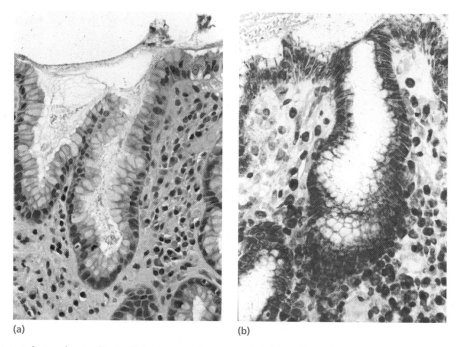

(a)   (b)

Figure 18.12 *Helicobacter pylori* can be visualized with the hematoxylin–eosin stain **(a)** as well as with inexpensive, although suboptimal, quick stains like the Giemsa **(b)**.

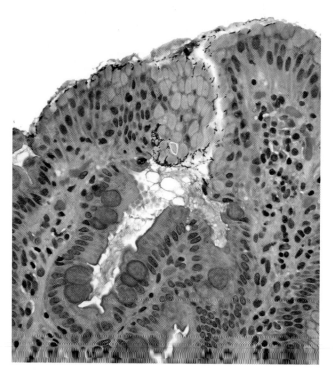

Figure 18.13 Intestinal metaplasia is highlighted in bright blue by an Alcian blue-containing silver-based triple stain for the detection of *Helicobacter pylori*. Organisms adhere to the native gastric mucosa only, apparently avoiding contact with metaplastic cells.

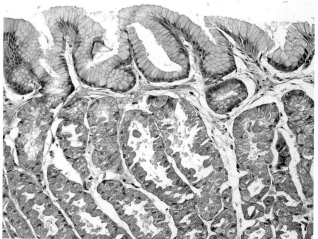

Figure 18.14 Oxyntic glands with prominent dilatations. These changes are typically associated with prolonged PPI use and may appear endoscopically as small smooth polyps.

other nonsteroidal antiinflammatory drugs (NSAIDs), has now become the most common histopathological diagnosis in gastric biopsies in the United States and is found mostly in patients with neither a history of NSAID use nor of bile reflux. While surreptitious NSAID users may account for a small portion of these patients, other factors, possibly related to diet, may be responsible for this as yet unexplained increase.

Endoscopic appearance

The mucosa of chronic NSAID users, unless they have gastric ulcers or erosions, has no distinctive appearance. Erosions due

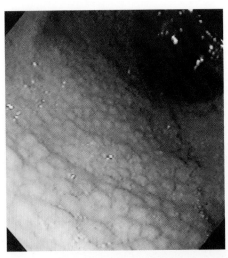

Figure 18.15 Innumerable small hemispherical elevations, many with a slightly depressed or umbilicated center, are characteristic of follicular gastritis.

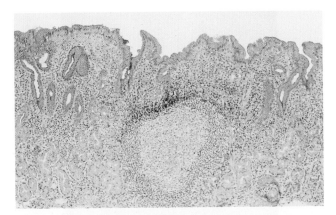

Figure 18.16 In most subjects infected with *Helicobacter pylori*, small lymphoid follicles develop in the gastric mucosa. When their diameter is smaller than the mucosal thickness they are not visible endoscopically.

to NSAID use are typically found in the antrum, often on the tops of folds. The erosions are generally multiple, and are characterized by a central depression with or without a necrotic floor, a red rim, and prominent reaction in the surrounding mucosa. Most are small (2–4 mm), but they can be more than 1 cm in diameter. Figures 18.16, 18.17, 18.18, 18.19, 18.20, and 18.21 represent NSAID-associated lesions ranging from very superficial erosions to ulcers.

Histopathology

The histopathological diagnosis of reactive gastropathy remains a challenging problem. Several mucosal changes have been associated with reactive gastropathy; however, the specificity and predictive value of any of these features is low, with many patients with *H. pylori* infection having one or more of these histological features (Figure 18.22). Superficial erosions without surrounding inflammation (Figure 18.23) are almost always caused by chemical injury, whereas the etiology of multiple inflamed erosions (Figure 18.24) is virtually impossible to determine. Thus, the pathologist can diagnose reactive gastropathy, but a firm etiological diagnosis can be made only when supportive clinical data are available and no confounding factors (e.g., *H. pylori* infection) are present.

Bile-reflux gastropathy

Postgastrectomy bile reflux may present with a syndrome characterized by burning midepigastric pain unresponsive to antacids and aggravated by eating and recumbency, sometimes accompanied by bilious vomiting, anemia, and weight loss. Endoscopic confirmation of bile reflux with characteristic histopathological findings supports the diagnosis, and corrective

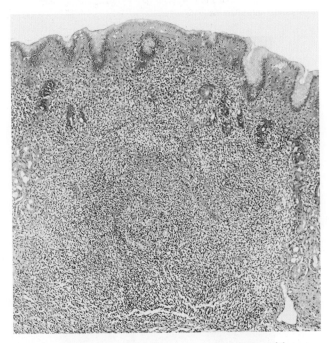

Figure 18.17 Larger lymphoid follicles increase the thickness of the mucosa and create endoscopically detectable elevations. When follicles are extremely numerous and most are large, the mucosal appearance is that of follicular gastritis.

surgery (e.g., creation of a 40- to 50-cm Roux-en-Y gastrojejunostomy) is successful in about one-half of all cases.

Endoscopic appearance

The gastric mucosa at the anastomotic site may have a polypoid appearance with congestion, edema, and friability (Figure 18.25). Superficial erosions may also be present in more proximal areas of the gastric stump.

Histopathology

The most characteristic changes include evidence of epithelial regeneration, extreme foveolar hyperplasia, edema of the lamina

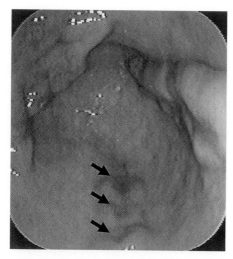

Figure 18.18 Superficial antral erosions (arrows) in a patient using nonsteroidal antiinflammatory drugs.

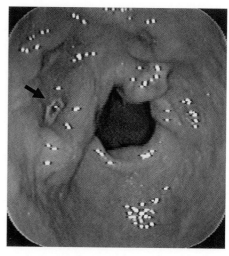

Figure 18.21 Nonsteroidal antiinflammatory drug-induced small ulcer.

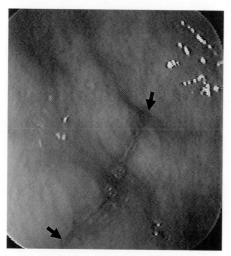

Figure 18.19 Characteristic of aspirin-induced linear erosion (extending between the two arrows).

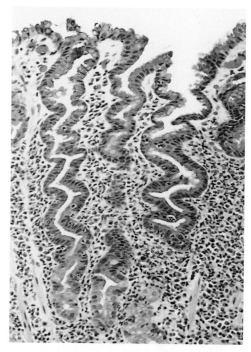

Figure 18.22 Foveolar hyperplasia is generally believed to be a characteristic histopathological finding in chemical gastropathy. This mucosal change, however, simply reflects increased epithelial turnover caused by superficial damage, and may occur in other conditions, including *Helicobacter pylori* infection. In this patient with both *H. pylori* gastritis and a history of nonsteroidal antiinflammatory drug use the etiology of the foveolar alterations cannot be determined.

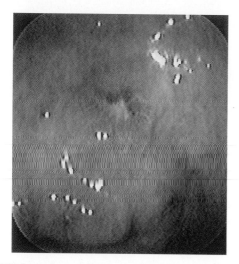

Figure 18.20 Large, deep erosion or superficial ulcer in a patient using nonsteroidal antiinflammatory drugs.

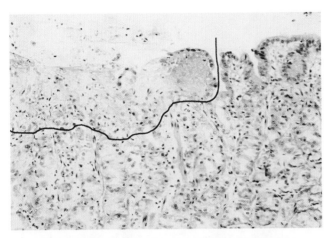

Figure 18.23 Superficial erosion of the oxyntic mucosa. The mucosa to the right and below the red line is completely normal and without inflammation. The affected portion shows hemorrhage, necrosis, and epithelial regeneration. This association of normal mucosa with an abrupt limited hemorrhagic and necrotic lesion is characteristic of chemical injury. The absence of inflammation all but excludes *Helicobacter pylori* infection.

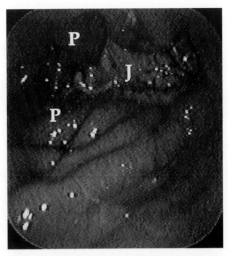

Figure 18.25 Polypoid appearance (*P*) of the gastric mucosa at the anastomotic site in a patient with Billroth II gastrojejunostomy. A portion of the jejunum (*J*) is visible, surrounded by thickened gastric mucosa.

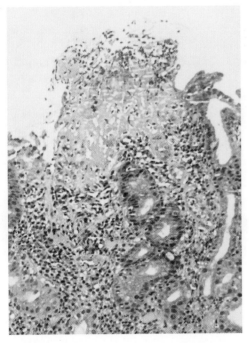

Figure 18.24 High-power view of a microerosion. The epithelium has disappeared and the uppermost part of the mucosa contains fibrin and inflammatory cells that are projected toward the lumen in a fashion that has been likened to a minuscule eruption.

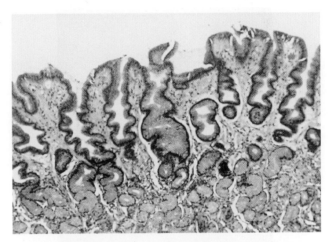

Figure 18.26 Foveolar hyperplasia without inflammation is probably caused by chemical injury.

Partial gastrectomy and carcinoma

The polypoid appearance of the distal portions of the gastric stump in postgastrectomy patients has been referred to as *gastritis cystica polyposa*. Several European and Japanese studies have reported a high prevalence of low-grade dysplasia or gastric adenocarcinoma, but these findings have not been confirmed in the United States. Since the discovery of the causative role of *H. pylori* in the pathogenesis of peptic ulcer disease, eradication therapy has largely replaced surgery and postgastrectomy gastropathy has become exceedingly rare.

Watermelon stomach

Watermelon stomach, or gastric antral vascular ectasia (GAVE) syndrome, is a rare condition of unknown etiology that is

propria, and expansion of the smooth muscle fibers into the upper third of the mucosa (Figures 18.26 and 18.27). The enhanced epithelial proliferation may cause the foveolar cells to have an increased nuclear–cytoplasmic ratio and mild to moderate architectural disarray. These findings (known to pathologists as "atypia") may be incorrectly interpreted as dysplasia or neoplasia.

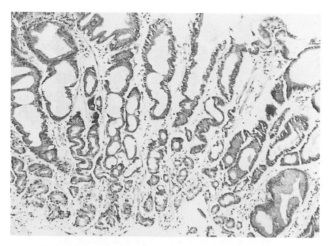

Figure 18.27 Extreme foveolar hyperplasia and dilation in a biopsy specimen from the gastric stoma in a patient with Billroth II gastrectomy. This degree of foveolar hyperplasia accounts for the juicy, polypoid aspect of the area immediately juxtaposed to the anastomotic site.

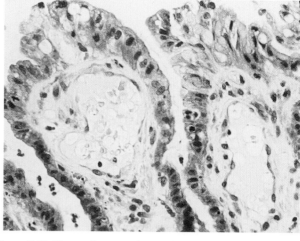

Figure 18.29 The antral mucosa shows innumerable dilated subepithelial capillaries.

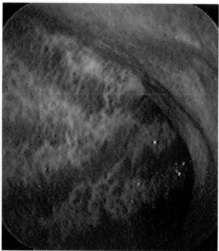

Figure 18.28 Hemorrhagic hyperemic streaks apparently converging toward the pylorus, in the antrum of a middle-aged woman with scleroderma and progressive anemia. The appearance of the streaks has been likened to the stripes of a watermelon, hence the term *watermelon stomach*.

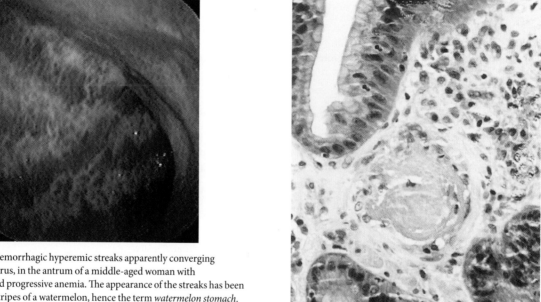

Figure 18.30 A characteristic – if not pathognomonic – finding in watermelon stomach is the presence of thrombi in the dilated superficial capillaries.

frequently associated with gastric atrophy and autoimmune and connective tissue disorders, particularly systemic sclerosis. More than 70% of reported cases have occurred in older women. Occult bleeding is seen at presentation in almost 90% of the cases, and melena or hematemesis in 60%. In most patients the chronic blood loss causes iron deficiency anemia.

Endoscopic appearance

Watermelon stomach was so named because of the "longitudinal antral folds seen converging on the pylorus, containing visible ectatic vessels resembling the stripes on a watermelon" (Figure 18.28). In other metaphors, the prominent dilated vessels have been described as resembling "a large, flat mushroom" or a "honeycomb."

Histopathology

In the antrum, the lamina propria shows smooth muscle proliferation and fibrosis, and contains markedly dilated mucosal capillaries (Figure 18.29). Fibrin thrombi are often found within the dilated capillaries (Figure 18.30).

Management

Therapeutic endoscopy, with obliteration of the dilated vessels by argon plasma coagulation, is the accepted treatment of choice and has greatly reduced the need for antrectomy.

CHAPTER 19
Tumors of the stomach

Emad M. El-Omar[1] and Chun-Ying Wu[2]
[1] Institute of Medical Sciences, Aberdeen University, Aberdeen, UK
[2] Taichung Veterans General Hospital, Taichung and National Yang-Ming University, Taipei, Taiwan

Gastric adenocarcinoma is a globally important tumor that claims the lives of thousands of patients each year. Clinically, gastric tumors are mainly diagnosed by endoscopy and confirmed by histological assessment of endoscopic biopsies. The two main histological subtypes are intestinal and diffuse (Figures 19.1 and 19.2). In countries with widespread screening programs for gastric cancer, the tumors are often diagnosed early (Figure 19.3), especially with the use of enhanced endoscopic imaging (e.g., narrow band imaging, NBI) (Figures 19.4 and 19.5). In the West, most gastric cancers are diagnosed late (Figure 19.6). The use of endoscopic ultrasound (EUS) at the time of index endoscopy is very helpful in providing immediate local staging of suspected early cancers (Figures 19.7, 19.8, 19.9, 19.10, and 19.11).

The carcinogenic pathways for gastric cancer are very well understood and represent a paradigm for infection-induced and inflammation-driven neoplasia. The initial insult in the majority of cases is caused by chronic *Helicobacter pylori* infection. Normal gastric mucosa (Figure 19.12) is transformed by the infection into a chronically inflamed niche, which progresses through stages that may include atrophic gastritis, intestinal metaplasia, gastric dysplasia (Figure 19.13), and finally intramucosal carcinoma (Figure 19.14).

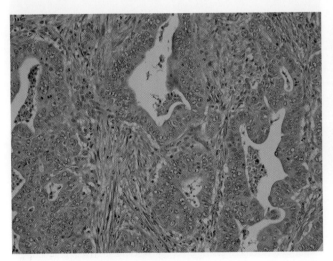

Figure 19.1 Intestinal type gastric adenocarcinoma. Source: Courtesy of Professor Graeme Murray, Aberdeen University.

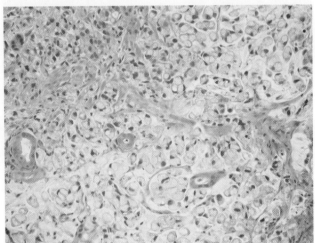

Figure 19.2 Diffuse type gastric cancer. This is characterized by lack of cellular cohesion, invasion throughout the stroma, and poor cellular differentiation. The pathognomonic feature is the presence of signet-ring cell morphology. Source: Courtesy of Professor Graeme Murray, Aberdeen University.

Yamada's Atlas of Gastroenterology, Fifth Edition. Edited by Daniel K. Podolsky, Michael Camilleri, J. Gregory Fitz, Anthony N. Kalloo, Fergus Shanahan, and Timothy C. Wang.
© 2016 John Wiley & Sons, Ltd. Published 2016 by John Wiley & Sons, Ltd.
Companion website: www.yamadagastro.com/atlas

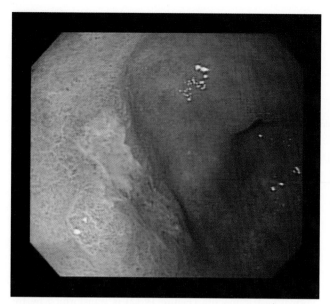

Figure 19.3 Early gastric cancer in the antrum. The patient was a 73-year-old woman. Endoscopy showed a 2-cm ulcer in the prepyloric region. Histology confirmed poorly differentiated adenocarcinoma with signet-ring cell features. The same lesion is seen with greater precision and clarity in narrow band imaging mode (as shown in Figure 19.4).

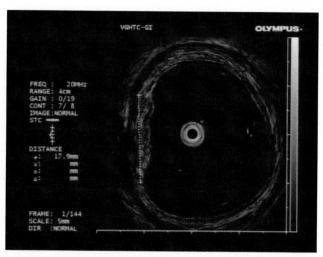

Figure 19.5 Early gastric cancer in the antrum. Endoscopic ultrasound appearance of same lesion as in Figure 19.3. The submucosa was invaded but the muscularis propria layer is intact.

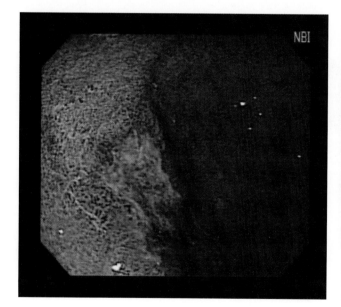

Figure 19.4 Early gastric cancer in the antrum. Narrow band imaging view of same lesion as in Figure 19.3.

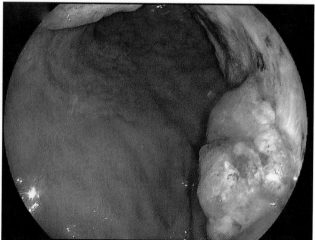

Figure 19.6 Advanced gastric cancer. Endoscopy shows a large lesion (>4 cm) at the posterior wall of the lower corpus and angualris, consistent with Bormann's type II. Histology showed moderately to poorly differentiated adenocarcinoma of the intestinal type. The tumor penetrated the serosa and metastasized to perigastric lymph nodes (2/6). Pathological tumor node metastasis (pTNM) stage pT4aN0aMa (according to the 7th edition, 2010, American Joint Committee on Cancer Staging Guidelines for Tumors/2011 CAP guideline).

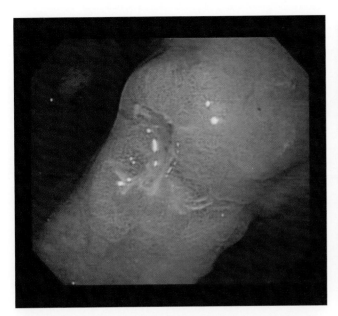

Figure 19.7 Early gastric cancer. Endoscopic findings: uneven elevated mucosal patch over angularis, with some healing ulcers. Possible adenocarcinoma in situ. Invasive carcinoma cannot be ruled out. Operative report: adenocarcinoma, intestinal type, moderately differentiated. Tumor invaded to muscularis propria. Pathological tumor node metastasis (TNM) stage: pT2N2Mx (according to the 7th edition, 2010, American Joint Committee on Cancer Staging Guidelines for Tumors / 2010 CAP guideline).

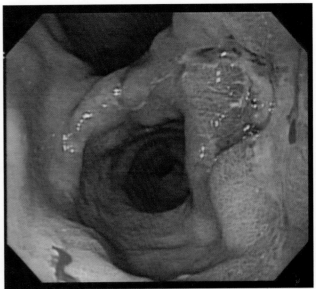

Figure 19.9 Endoscopic findings: prominent mucosal elevation with multiple ulcerations over antrum to low body, chiefly the lower curvature and posterior wall. Pathological findings: adenocarcinoma, moderately differentiated. Operative report: adenocarcinoma, intestinal type, poorly differentiated, of posterior wall of antrum. Tumor invaded to perigastric soft tissue and metastasized to perigastric lymph node (greater curvature: 0/0, lesser curvature: 1/3). Pathological tumor node metastasis (TNM) stage: pT3N2Mx (according to the 7th edition, 2010, American Joint Committee on Cancer Staging Guidelines for Tumors/ 2010 CAP guideline).

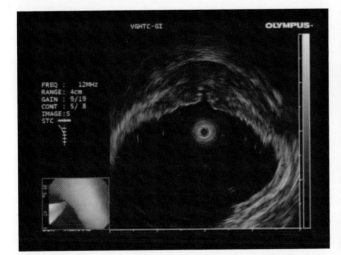

Figure 19.8 Early gastric cancer. Endoscopic ultrasound findings of the same lesion as in Figure 19.7: prominent thickening of focal gastric wall over angularis with predominantly mucosal and submucosal infiltration. The focal muscularis propria layer was also thickened and blurred. Serosal interruption was not prominent with UM3R probe.

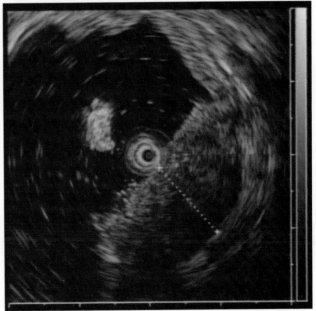

Figure 19.10 Endoscopic ultrasound findings of the same lesion as in Figure 19.9: marked thickening of the gastric wall over antrum and low body was noted with transmural infiltration.

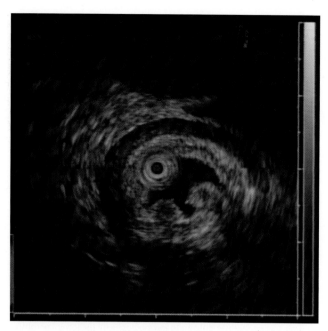

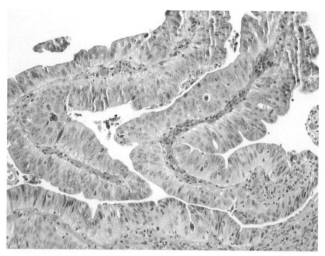

Figure 19.13 Stomach: High-grade dysplasia. Source: Courtesy of Professor Graeme Murray, Aberdeen University.

Figure 19.11 Endoscopic ultrasound findings of the same lesion as in Figure 19.9: prominent serosal invasion and penetration was noted.

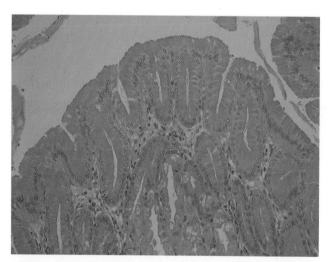

Figure 19.12 Stomach: normal gastric histology. Source: Courtesy of Professor Graeme Murray, Aberdeen University.

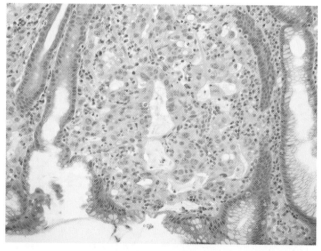

Figure 19.14 Stomach: intramucosal carcinoma. Source: Courtesy of Professor Graeme Murray, Aberdeen University.

CHAPTER 20
Miscellaneous diseases of the stomach

Tamas A. Gonda[1] and Yanghee Woo[2]
[1] Columbia University, New York, NY, USA
[2] City of Hope Medical Center, Duarte, CA, USA

In this chapter we provide examples of the different type of hiatal hernias and the possible complications associated with these conditions (Figures 20.1, 20.2, 20.3, 20.4, and 20.5). Although most of these conditions remain asymptomatic and are noted incidentally, it is important to distinguish those associated with significant complications from those that may not require an intervention.

Foreign body ingestion remains a frequently encountered emergency (Figure 20.6). There are innumerable examples of objects that have been retrieved from the human stomach. Nails and other sharp objects are some of the objects that may require immediate intervention.

We also present examples of the rare but potentially very serious presentation of a gastric volvulus and the mechanism of volvulus formation (Figures 20.7 and 20.8).

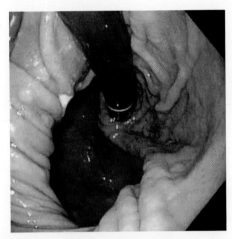

Figure 20.2 Endoscopic view in retroflexion of a large paraesophageal hernia.

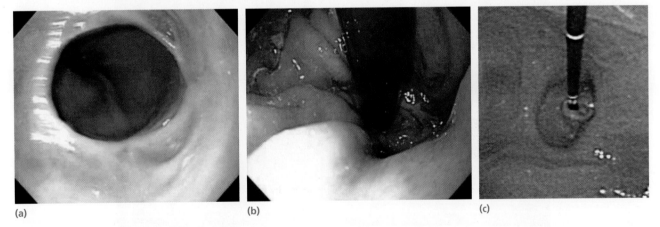

(a) (b) (c)

Figure 20.1 (a–c) Endoscopic views of hiatal hernia.

Yamada's Atlas of Gastroenterology, Fifth Edition. Edited by Daniel K. Podolsky, Michael Camilleri, J. Gregory Fitz, Anthony N. Kalloo, Fergus Shanahan, and Timothy C. Wang.
© 2016 John Wiley & Sons, Ltd. Published 2016 by John Wiley & Sons, Ltd.
Companion website: www.yamadagastro.com/atlas

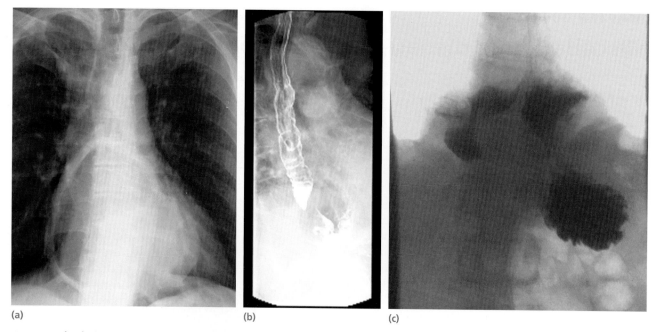

(a)   (b)   (c)

Figure 20.3 (a–c) Chest radiograph and barium esophagogram of paraesophageal hernia. Type II paraesophageal hernia where the gastroesophageal junction remains below the diaphragm. **(a)** Barium radiograph demonstrates that the entire stomach has herniated into the chest, illustrating an "upside-down" appearance.

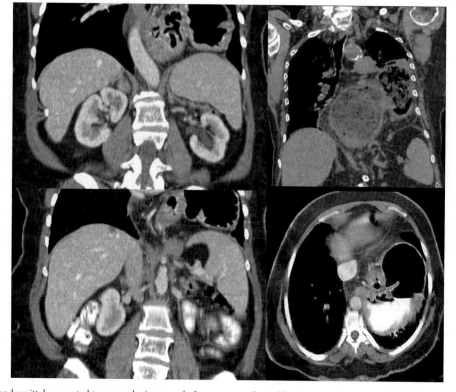

Figure 20.4 Coronal and sagittal computed tomography images of a large paraesophageal hernia containing most of the gastric body.

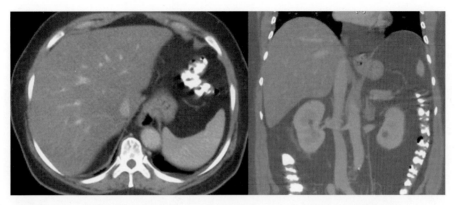

Figure 20.5 Axial and coronal images on computed tomography scan demonstrating a small sliding paraesophageal hernia.

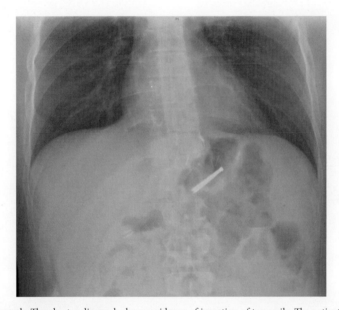

Figure 20.6 Foreign body in the stomach. The chest radiograph shows evidence of ingestion of two nails. The patient underwent urgent esophagogastroduodenoscopy and the nails were removed using endoscopic graspers. A long overtube was placed that nearly extended to the location of the nails.

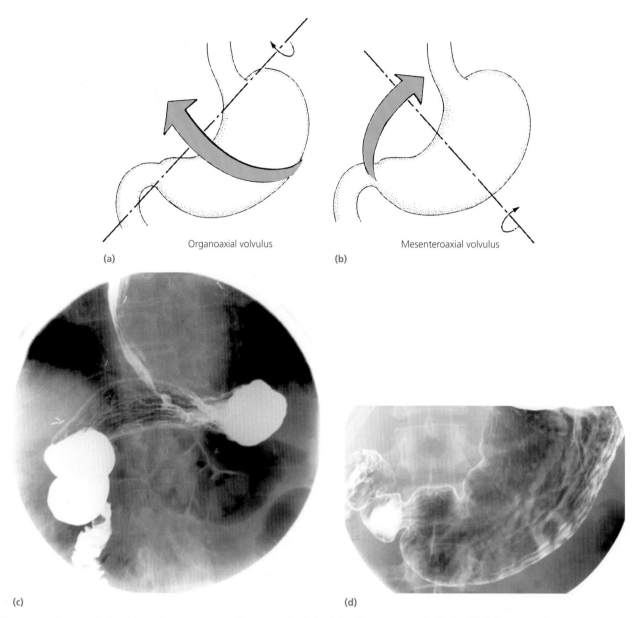

Figure 20.7 Gastric volvulus. Schematic representation of organoaxial volvulus **(a)** and mesenteroaxial volvulus **(b)**. **(c)** Barium radiograph of an organoaxial volvulus associated with a large hiatal hernia. **(d)** Barium radiograph after resolution of organoaxial volvulus (same patient as in **[c]**).

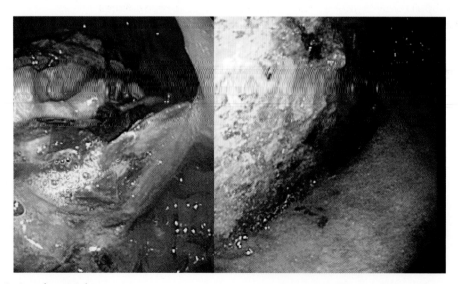

Figure 20.8 Endoscopic view of a gastric bezoar.

CHAPTER 21

Dysmotility of the small intestine and colon

Michael Camilleri,[1] Silvia Delgado-Aros,[2] and Lawrence Szarka[1]

[1] Mayo Clinic, Rochester, MN, USA
[2] Hospital del Mar, Barcelona, Spain

Motility of the digestive tract is the result of the myoelectric activity, contractile activity, tone, compliance, and transit. Normal motility of the small intestine ensures the appropriate absorption of the nutrients, propels the bolus through the intestine, and prevents bacterial overgrowth. Proper function of colonic motility is particularly important to prevent diarrhea and constipation.

Motility is controlled by the enteric nervous system (ENS), which is modulated by extrinsic nerves as well as gastrointestinal hormones and peptides. The effects of these neurons on the gut smooth muscle partly rely on interstitial cells of Cajal (ICC), which function as pacemakers in the intestinal wall. Dysfunctions in any of these components may cause intestinal or colonic dysmotility (Figure 21.1).

Diseases that affect gastrointestinal smooth muscle include primary visceral myopathies, collagen diseases, muscular dystrophies, amyloidosis, and thyroid disease (Box 21.1). Enteric nerve dysfunction occurs in primary visceral neuropathies, Hirschsprung disease, diabetes mellitus, Chagas disease, ganglioneuromatosis, paraneoplastic visceral neuropathy, and Parkinson disease. Small intestine and colonic dysmotility may be also caused by drugs (such as phenothiazines, tricyclic antidepressants, ganglionic blockers, and narcotics) and occurs among patients with mucosal diseases such as celiac disease or eosinophilic gastroenteritis. The effect of gastrointestinal hormones on the motility of the small and large intestine is manifested clinically by diarrhea in patients with carcinoid syndrome and irritable bowel syndrome. These syndromes are associated with elevated circulating levels of biogenic compounds such as serotonin, and result in rapid small intestinal or colonic transit that may partly reflect abnormal motor function or abnormal intestinal secretion.

Regardless of the underlying causes, patients with dysmotility of the small intestine and colon may experience a wide range of clinical manifestations. Patients may be asymptomatic or, at the other end of the spectrum, they may present with chronic intestinal pseudoobstruction. Between these two extremes, patients may have dyspeptic symptoms, including intermittent postprandial epigastric or periumbilical abdominal pain, bloating, nausea, vomiting, and diarrhea or constipation. Intestinal bacterial overgrowth occurs in severe cases of intestinal dysmotility and results in steatorrhea and sometimes diarrhea. Symptoms tend to occur in the postprandial period. Extraintestinal manifestations of the underlying disease may be detected among patients with the secondary causes of small intestine and colonic dysmotility.

Small intestine dysmotility seems to occur less frequently in comparison with colonic dysmotility. However, the lack of validated tests to evaluate small intestine motility makes it difficult to precisely estimate the prevalence. Novel techniques are being developed to improve measurements of the motor function of the small intestine that may help to diagnose and better estimate the prevalence of these dysfunctions. In contrast, constipation affects 12%–15% of the population, and Hirschsprung disease, the prototypic congenital colonic dysmotility, affects 1 in 5000 births. This chapter reviews primary and secondary causes of small intestine and colon motility diseases.

Primary causes

Visceral myopathies
Familial visceral myopathies

Familial visceral myopathies (FVMs) are a group of genetic diseases characterized by degeneration and fibrosis of the gastrointestinal smooth muscle and, in certain types, the urinary tract smooth muscle. There are at least three reported types of FVM based on gross lesions of the gastrointestinal tract and the pattern of inheritance (Table 21.1). Well documented mitochondrial and gene alterations exist in type II FVM, also called

Yamada's Atlas of Gastroenterology, Fifth Edition. Edited by Daniel K. Podolsky, Michael Camilleri, J. Gregory Fitz, Anthony N. Kalloo, Fergus Shanahan, and Timothy C. Wang.
© 2016 John Wiley & Sons, Ltd. Published 2016 by John Wiley & Sons, Ltd.
Companion website: www.yamadagastro.com/atlas

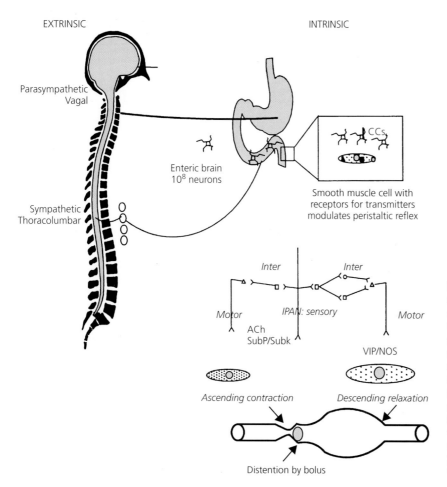

Figure 21.1 Extrinsic and enteric control of gut motility. The enteric nervous system (ENS) controls stereotypical motor functions, such as the migrating motor complex and the peristaltic reflex; enteric control is modulated by the extrinsic parasympathetic and sympathetic nerves, which respectively stimulate and inhibit nonsphincteric muscle. ACh, acetylcholine; ICCs, interstitial cells of Cajal; IPAN, intrinsic primary afferent neuron; NOS, nitric oxide synthase; Subk, substance K; SubP, substance P; VIP, vasoactive intestinal peptide. Source: Grundy D, Camilleri M. Neurogastroenterol Motil 2001;13:177. Reproduced by permission of John Wiley & Sons.

mitochondrial neurogastrointestinal encephalomyopathy syndrome (MNGIE). On routine pathological examination, the histological findings in all three types of FVM are similar and are characterized by degenerated muscle cells and fibrosis. Recognition of milder lesions may be facilitated by use of trichrome stain (Figure 21.2).Small intestinal manometric studies of patients with FVM reveal low-amplitude (usually <20 mmHg and on average <10 mmHg) intestinal contractions (Figure 21.3). Recent descriptions of type II FVM or MNGIE warrant a more detailed discussion of this entity.

Type II familial visceral myopathies

This entity forms part of a heterogeneous group of disorders that result from structural, biochemical, or genetic derangements of mitochondria. Type II FVM has an autosomal recessive inheritance and it is characterized by gastrointestinal dysmotility, ophthalmoplegia, and peripheral neuropathy; on skeletal muscle biopsy, ragged red fibers are demonstrated best on Gomori trichrome stain (Figure 21.4). Additional clinical features include lactic acidosis, increased cerebrospinal fluid protein, and leukodystrophy, which is identified by magnetic resonance imaging of the brain. Brain involvement may result in severe neurological disorders including blindness and deaf-

ness. The ubiquity of mitochondria explains the association of neuromuscular, gastrointestinal, and other nonneuromuscular symptoms that are characteristic of this syndrome. Some patients have been found to have multiple mitochondrial DNA deletions in skeletal muscle. Mitochondrial DNA contains genes that encode enzymes of the cellular oxidative phosphorylation system. Nuclear genes, however, also encode for components of this system. It is believed that mutations of nuclear DNA genes that control the expression of the mitochondrial genomes are the underlying genetic defect of this syndrome. It was proposed that a unique gene located in the long arm of chromosome 22 (22q13.32qter), distal to locus D22S1161, is responsible for this syndrome.

Childhood visceral myopathies

Two distinct forms of childhood visceral myopathies (CVM) have been recognized (Table 21.2); both forms result in small intestinal, ureteric, and bladder dilatation, but the second type has characteristic microcolon. The two diseases differ from FVM in their clinical manifestations and modes of inheritance. Degeneration and fibrosis of gastrointestinal and urinary smooth muscle can be detected in both types of CVM and result in bowel dilation (Figure 21.5), ureteropelvicaliectasis

Box 21.1 Causes of gut dysmotility.

Primary causes

Visceral myopathies
Familial visceral myopathies: type I, II (MNGIE), III
Childhood visceral myopathies: type I, II (megacystis-microcolon-intestinal hypoperistalsis)
Nonfamilial visceral myopathies
Visceral neuropathies
Familial visceral neuropathies: type I, II
Hirschsprung disease
Idiopathic nonfamilial visceral neuropathies

Secondary causes

Disease involving the intestinal smooth muscle
Collagen diseases (e.g., scleroderma, dermatomyositis, systemic lupus erythematosus, mixed connective tissue disease)
Muscular dystrophies (e.g., myotonic dystrophy, Duchenne muscular dystrophy)
Amyloidosis
Neurological diseases
Chagas disease, ganglioneuromatosis of the intestine, paraneoplastic neuropathy, Parkinson disease, spinal cord injury
Endocrine disorders
Diabetes mellitus, thyroid disease (i.e., hyperthyroidism, hypothyroidism), hypoparathyroidism
Pharmacological agents
Phenothiazines, tricyclic antidepressants, antiparkinsonian medications, ganglionic blockers, clonidine, narcotics (morphine and meperidine)
Miscellaneous intestinal disorders
Celiac disease
Radiation enteritis
Diffuse lymphoid infiltration of the small intestine
Jejunoileal bypass
Postgastrointestinal viral infection

MNGIE, mitochondrial neurogastrointestinal encephalomyopathy syndrome.

(Figure 21.6), or megacystis. The latter results from bladder degeneration (Figure 21.7).

Nonfamilial visceral myopathies

It is unclear whether cases of nonfamilial visceral myopathy among adults represent sporadic cases or unrecognized variants of FVM with a recessive pattern of inheritance. There is no histological difference between the familial and the nonfamilial forms of visceral myopathy, and both show low-amplitude contractions when investigated with intestinal manometry.

Visceral neuropathies

The ENS is a vast network of ganglionated plexuses located in the wall of the gastrointestinal tract, and it is in close contact with ICC. Their precursors originate in the neural crest. Normal migration, differentiation, and subsequent survival or maintenance of the precursor cells of the ENS has been demonstrated to be crucial for the normal function of the intestine. Different genetic defects in migration, differentiation, and maintenance of enteric neurons have been identified as causes of gut dysmotility (Table 21.3). These include: abnormalities of *RET*, the gene that encodes for the tyrosine kinase (Trk) receptor; the endothelin B system (which tends to retard development of neural elements, thereby facilitating colonization of the entire gut from the neural crest); SOX-10 (a transcription factor that enhances maturation of neural precursors); and c-KIT, which is a marker for ICCs. The protooncogene c-*Kit* encodes a transmembrane Trk receptor c-Kit. Activation of this receptor is responsible for the development of the ICCs. Disturbances in these mechanisms result in dysmotility syndromes, such as Hirschsprung disease, Waardenburg syndrome (pigmentary defects, piebaldism, neural deafness, and megacolon), and idiopathic hypertrophic pyloric stenosis. Figure 21.8 demonstrates some of the mutations in the Trk receptor that have been reported in gut dysmotility associated with familial or sporadic medullary

Table 21.1 Classification of familial visceral myopathies.

Characteristics	Type I	Type II (MNGIE)	Type III
Mode of transmission	Autosomal dominant	Autosomal recessive; isolated cases	Autosomal recessive
Gross lesions	Esophageal dilation, megaduodenum, redundant colon, and megacystis	Gastric dilation, slight dilation of the entire small intestine with numerous diverticula	Marked dilation of the entire digestive tract from the esophagus to the rectum
Microscopic changes	Degeneration and fibrosis of both muscle layers		
Clinical manifestations			
Age at onset	After the first decade	Teens	Middle age
Percentage symptomatic	<50%	>75%	>75%
Symptoms of CIP	Variable severity	Severe plus pain	Classic CIP
Extra-GI manifestations	Megacystis, uterine inertia, and mydriasis	Ptosis and external ophthalmoplegia, muscle pain, peripheral neuropathy, and deafness	None observed
Treatment, prognosis	Prognosis good with or without surgery	No effective medical or surgical treatment; prognosis poor	No effective medical or surgical treatment; prognosis poor

CIP, chronic intestinal pseudoobstruction; GI, gastrointestinal; MNGIE, mitochondrial neurogastrointestinal encephalomyopathy syndrome.

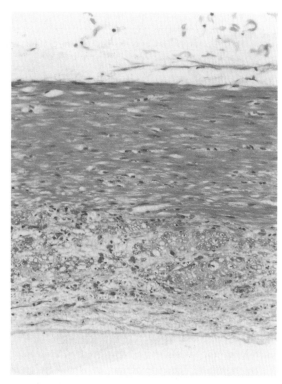

—1 min—
I 30 mmHg

I
II
III
IV
V

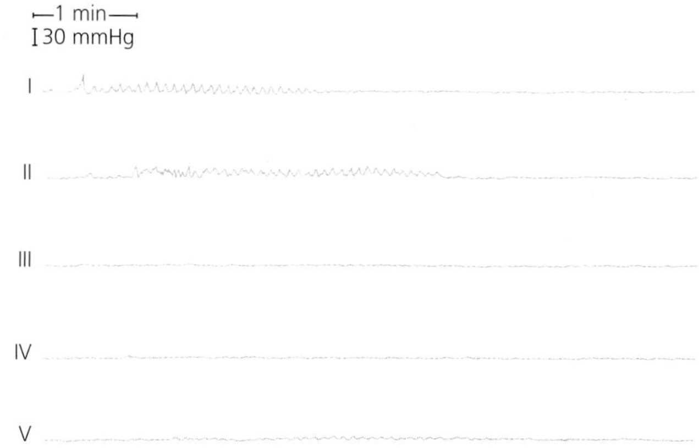

Figure 21.3 Jejunal manometric record of a patient with type I familial visceral myopathy reveals weak contractions (amplitude <30 mmHg) of phase 3. Five tracings are shown and each is 5 cm apart. Phase 3 contractions were detected in only tracings I and II but not at other locations because of the weakness of contractions at these locations.

Figure 21.2 High-power view of histology of muscularis propria of small intestine. The circular muscle (above) appears relatively normal while the longitudinal muscle shows gross vacuolar degeneration. Many of the vacuoles contain fragments of degenerate muscle cells. H and E × 400. Source: Rodrigues CA, Shepherd NA, Lennard-Jones JE, et al. Familial visceral myopathy: a family with at least six involved members. Gut 1989;30:1285. Reproduced with permission of BMJ Publishing Group Ltd.

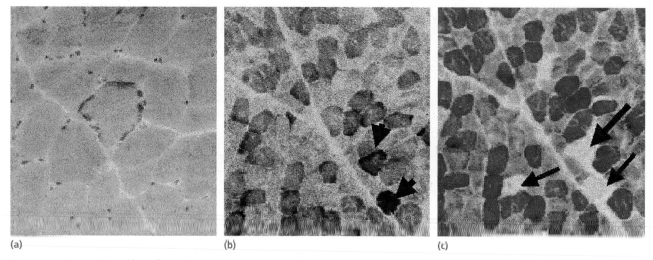

(a)　　　　　　　　(b)　　　　　　　　(c)

Figure 21.4 Histological and histochemical studies of skeletal muscle biopsy from a patient with mitochondrial myopathy. **(a)** Note the ragged red fibers characterized by the subsarcolemmal location of giant mitochondria in a few fibers, and the paucity of mitochondria in other fibers. **(b)** On histochemical analysis, a few fibers are succinate dehydrogenase positive (ragged blue appearance [arrowheads]). **(c)** The same fibers do not express cytochrome c oxidase (arrows), suggesting a defect in the respiratory enzyme chain that results in mitochondrial dysfunction and systemic acidosis. Source: Mueller LA, Camilleri M, Emslie-Smith AM. Mitochondrial neurogastrointestinal encephalomyopathy: manometric and diagnostic features. Gastroenterology 1999;116:959. Reproduced with permission of Elsevier.

Table 21.2 Classification of childhood visceral myopathies.

Characteristics	Type I	Type II (megacystis-microcolon-intestinal hypoperistalsis)
Mode of transmission	Autosomal recessive (?)	Autosomal recessive (?)
Gross lesions	Dilation of entire GI tract	Short, malrotated small intestine and malfixation of microcolon
Microscopic changes	Degeneration and fibrosis of GI and urinary smooth muscle cells	Vacuolar degeneration of GI and urinary smooth muscle cells
Clinical manifestations		
Age of onset	Infancy and young childhood	Infancy
Gender	Both	Predominantly female
Symptoms	Constipation, distention ± CIP	Obstipation, intestinal pseudoobstruction
Extra-GI manifestations	Megacystis and megaureters	Megacystis and megaureters
Treatment, prognosis	No effective medication; prognosis poor	No effective treatment; prognosis poor

CIP, chronic intestinal pseudoobstruction; GI, gastrointestinal.

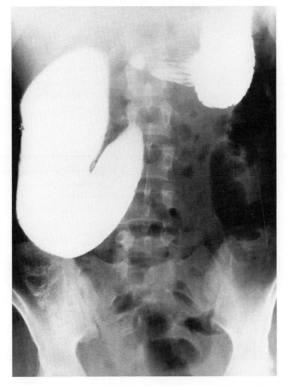

Figure 21.5 Upper gastrointestinal radiograph from a patient with type I familial visceral myopathy demonstrates severe megaduodenum.

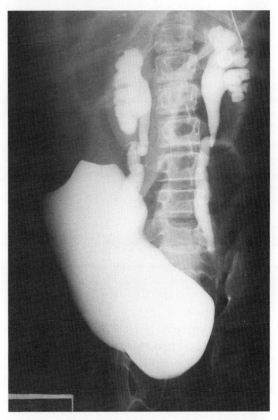

Figure 21.6 An intravenous pyelogram of a child with type I childhood visceral myopathy shows megacystis and bilateral ureteral pyelocaliectasis. Source: Bonsib SM, Fallon B, Mitros FA, et al. Urological manifestations of patients with visceral myopathy. J Urol 1984;132:1112. Reproduced with permission of Elsevier.

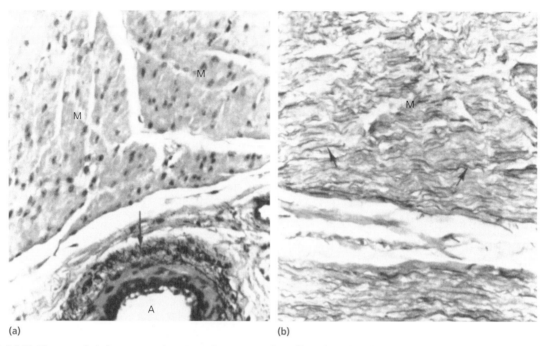

(a)   (b)

Figure 21.7 (a) Bladder muscularis from a control specimen demonstrates elastic fibers (arrow) in the adventitia of a small artery (A). No elastic fibers are present within muscle bundles (M). **(b)** Bladder muscularis from a type I childhood visceral myopathy patient demonstrates numerous, parallel, coarse, wavy, elastic fibers (arrows) within muscle bundles (M). Verhoeff–van Gieson stain; original magnification ×325. Source: Bonsib SM, Fallon B, Mitros FA, et al. Urological manifestations of patients with visceral myopathy. J Urol 1984;132:1112. Reproduced with permission of Elsevier.

Table 21.3 Genetic defects identified in different causes of gut dysmotility.

Dysmotility: prevalence genetic defect	Phenotype	Associated non-GI disease	Dysmotility: prevalence in phenotype
RET/GDNF	Hirschsprung	None in humans	20%–50% *RET*, 5% *GDNF*
ET-3/ET-B	Hirschsprung or megacolon	Waardenburg–Shah	5%–10% Hirschsprung
SOX-10	Hirschsprung	Waardenburg–Shah	?
C-KIT	?CIP/Hirschsprung	None	?

CIP, chronic intestinal pseudoobstruction; GI, gastrointestinal.

carcinoma of the thyroid, multiple endocrine neoplasia type 2A or B (Figure 21.9), and Hirschsprung disease.

The effects of motor neurons on the gastrointestinal and colonic muscle cells are relayed, at least in part, via the ICCs, which are electrically coupled to the muscle (Figures 21.10 and 21.11). They have receptors for the inhibitory transmitters (vasoactive intestinal peptide [VIP] and nitric oxide [NO]), and for the excitatory tachykinin transmitters. Because they generate physiological slow waves in the gastrointestinal tract, ICCs have also been recognized as the pacemaker cells of the gut. Slow waves are the rhythmic oscillations of the membrane potential that characterize the electrical activity of gut muscle. Slow waves are the rate-limiting step for contractile function in the smooth muscle cells. Contraction typically occurs when there is superimposition of spike potential on the slow waves.

The relevance of these functions of ICCs as neuromodulators and "pacemakers" of the gut is highlighted by the several exam-

ples of gut motility dysfunction associated with anomalous ICCs. A smaller number of ICCs were found in slow-transit constipation (Figure 21.12), and abnormal distribution of these cells have been found in Hirschsprung disease. Variants of enteric neuropathic dysmotility, such as hypoganglionosis, immature ganglia, neuronal intestinal dysplasia, and infantile pyloric stenosis, as well as in chronic and transient intestinal pseudoobstruction also have been observed. A diminished number, altered networks, and altered ultrastructural features of gastric ICCs have been demonstrated in diabetic mice with gastroparesis (Figure 21.13) and in patients with gastroparesis.

Visceral neuropathy may result in bowel dilation (Figure 21.14), although this is generally less frequent or less severe than in visceral myopathy. In Hirschsprung disease, the aganglionic segment is permanently contracted, causing dilation proximal to it (Figure 21.15). Intestinal manometry is characterized by normal-amplitude contractions with evidence of

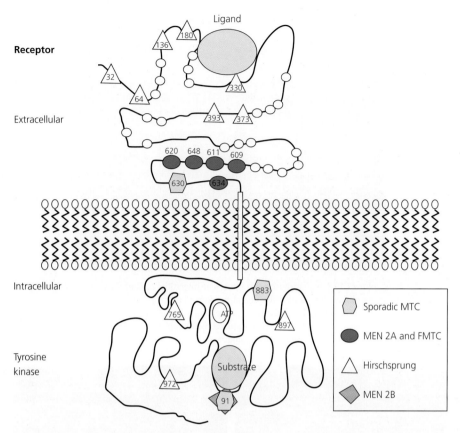

Figure 21.8 Tyrosine kinase receptor with examples of mutations associated with specific genetic disorders. ATP, adenosine triphosphate; (F) MTC, (familial) medullary carcinoma of the thyroid; MEN, multiple endocrine neoplasia.

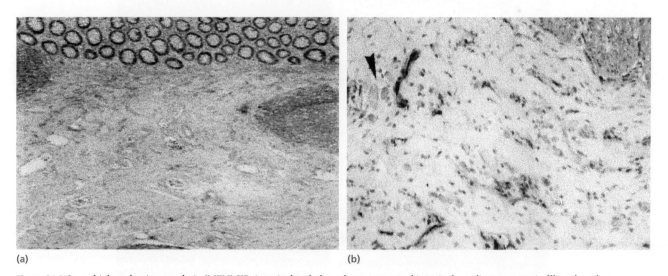

(a)   (b)

Figure 21.9 In multiple endocrine neoplasia (MEN) IIB, intestinal pathology shows transmural intestinal ganglioneuromatosis filling the submucosa (a), and the myenteric plexus (b). Note thick nerve trunks embedded with mature neurons (arrowhead). Source: Smith VV, Eng C, Milla PJ. Intestinal ganglioneuromatosis and multiple endocrine neoplasia type 2B: implications for treatment. Gut 1999; 45:143. Reproduced with permission of BMJ Publishing Group Ltd.

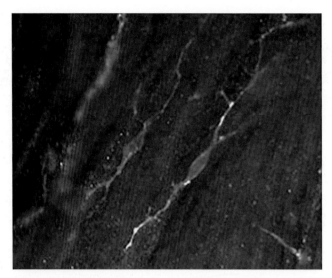

Figure 21.10 Circular muscle intramuscular interstitial cells of Cajal in tissue obtained from the left colon at the start of a laparoscopic hemicolectomy. Source: Farrugia G. Interstitial cells of Cajal in health and disease. Neurogastroenterol Motil 2008;20(Suppl 1):54. Reproduced with permission of John Wiley & Sons.

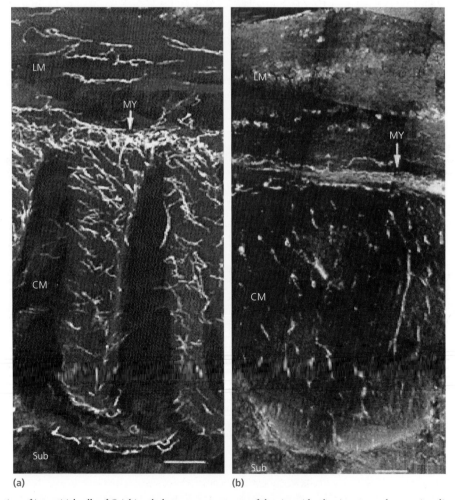

(a)   (b)

Figure 21.11 Distribution of interstitial cells of Cajal in whole transverse mounts of the sigmoid colon in a normal-appearing disease-control section of the sigmoid colon **(a)** and the sigmoid colon of a patient with slow-transit constipation **(b)**. CM, circular muscle; LM, longitudinal muscle; MY, myenteric plexus; Sub, submucosal plexus. Source: He CL, Burgart L, Wang L, et al. Decreased interstitial cell of Cajal volume in patients with slow-transit constipation. Gastroenterology 2000;118:14. Reproduced with permission of Elsevier.

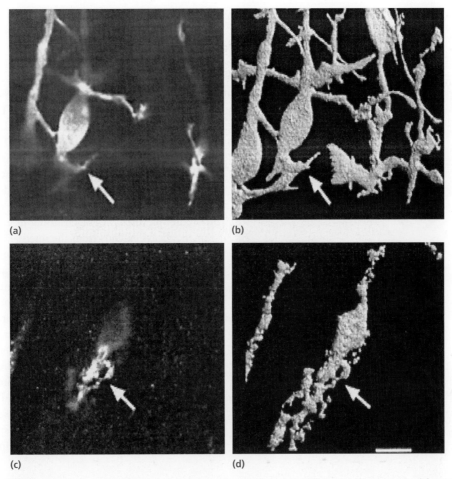

Figure 21.12 High-magnification confocal microscopy of the interstitial cells of Cajal (ICCs) from human sigmoid colon: **(a)** and **(c)** are single slices, **(b)** and **(d)** are reconstructions of 20 consecutive single slices; **(a)** and **(b)** are from healthy-appearing disease-control colons (note multiple fine processes and the network of interconnecting ICCs); **(c)** and **(d)** are from a patient with slow-transit constipation. Note the irregular markings and loss of fine processes (bar = 10 μm). Source: He CL, Burgart L, Wang L, et al. Decreased interstitial cell of Cajal volume in patients with slow-transit constipation. Gastroenterology 2000; 118:14. Reproduced with permission of Elsevier.

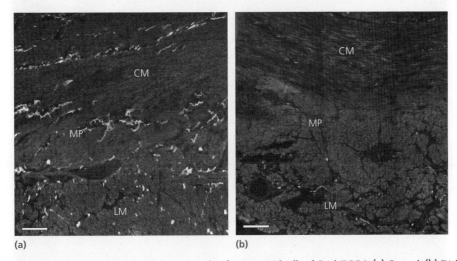

Figure 21.13 Representative images for Kit immunoreactivity as a marker for interstitial cells of Cajal (ICCs). **(a)** Control. **(b)** Diabetic gastroparesis with decreased ICCs. CM, circular muscle; MP myenteric plexus; LM, longitudinal muscle. Scale bar = 100 μm. Source: Grover M, Farrugia G, Lurken MS, et al.; NIDDK Gastroparesis Clinical Research Consortium. Cellular changes in diabetic and idiopathic gastroparesis. Gastroenterology 2011;140:1575. Reproduced with permission of Elsevier.

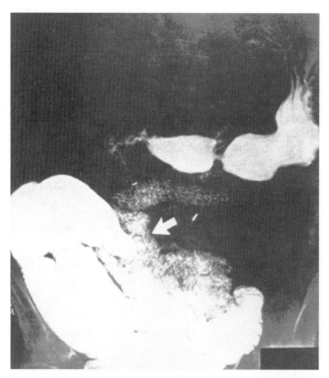

Figure 21.14 Small bowel radiograph from a patient with type I familial visceral neuropathy shows a normal stomach, duodenum, and proximal jejunum, but a dilated distal small bowel (arrow). Source: Mayer EA, Schuffler MD, Rotter JI, et al. Familial visceral neuropathy with autosomal dominant transmission. Gastroenterology 1986;91:1528. Reproduced with permission of Elsevier.

incoordination in, for example, the propagation of fasting migrating motor complexes (MMCs), or recurrence of MMC-like activity in the first postprandial hour.

Familial visceral neuropathies

Familial visceral neuropathies (FVNs) are a group of genetic diseases characterized by degeneration of the enteric nervous system. Two distinct phenotypes, I and II, have been distinguished, which are summarized in Table 21.4.

Hirschsprung disease (congenital megacolon)

Aganglionosis is caused by arrest of the caudal migration of cells from the neural crest, which is destined to develop as the gut's intramural plexuses. In Hirschsprung disease, the aganglionic segment always extends from the internal anal sphincter for a variable distance proximally; in most instances, it stays within the rectum and sigmoid colon ("classical type"), although involvement of very short segments and longer segments or the entire colon have also been described. The genetic disorders resulting in altered development of the neural crest in Hirschsprung disease have been discussed in detail above (see Table 21.3). The defect occurs once in every 5000 live births and is in some cases familial, with an overall incidence of 3.6% (about 1 in 30) among siblings of index cases. Although most children have major manifestations before the second month of life, very short segment aganglionosis may not cause severe symptoms until after infancy. Mucosal suction biopsy can rule out the disease if submucosal ganglia are present. However, the absence

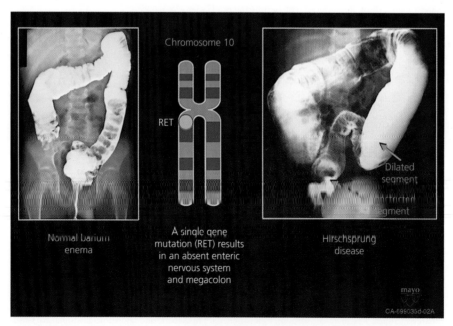

Figure 21.15 Barium enema in a normal child contrasted with megacolon and narrow segment of Hirschsprung disease.

Table 21.4 Classification of familial visceral neuropathies.

Characteristics	Type I	Type II
Mode of transmission	Autosomal dominant	Autosomal recessive
Gross lesions	Dilation of lengths of small intestine, often distal small bowel; megacolon; gastroparesis in ~25% of patients	Hypertrophic pyloric stenosis, dilated short small intestine, malrotation of small intestine
Microscopic changes	Degeneration of argyrophilic neurons and decreased numbers of nerve fibers	Deficiency of argyrophilic neurons and increased neuroblasts
Clinical manifestations		
Age of onset	Any age	Infancy
Percentage symptomatic	>75%	100%
Symptoms	~67% CIP	All CIP
Extra-GI manifestations	None	±Malformation of CNS, patent ductus arteriosus
Treatment, prognosis	No effective medical or surgical treatment; prognosis fair	No effective medical or surgical treatment; prognosis poor

CIP, chronic intestinal pseudoobstruction; CNS, central nervous system; GI, gastrointestinal.

of ganglion cells does not establish the diagnosis, and a deep or full-thickness biopsy from at least 3 cm proximal to the pectinate line should be obtained. Ganglia may be absent from the deep and superficial submucosal layers for even longer distances, and myenteric ganglia may also be absent in normal infants over that distance proximal to the internal sphincter. A very short aganglionic segment may be missed by biopsy and radiographs. In these cases, the absence of internal sphincter relaxation in response to rectal distention (e.g., by balloon) may help to confirm the diagnosis. However, distention of a balloon in a dilated rectum (for example in patients with chronic constipation or megarectum) may be associated with a false-positive result, because the intrarectal balloon may not sufficiently distend the rectum to elicit the reflex relaxation of the internal anal sphincter.

Idiopathic nonfamilial visceral neuropathies (chronic neuropathic intestinal pseudoobstruction of idiopathic variety)

Damage to the myenteric plexus can occur for a variety of different reasons, including chemical exposure, drug use, and viral infections. Patients with idiopathic nonfamilial visceral neuropathy may have dysmotility at any level of the gastrointestinal tract and present with features of chronic intestinal pseudoobstruction; a useful screening test is a solid-phase gastric emptying test. The intestine may be dilated but shows active, nonperistaltic contractions. Histological examination of the myenteric plexus shows a reduction in the total number of neurons; the remaining neurons may be enlarged with thick, clubbed processes. An increase in the number of Schwann cells and hypertrophy of the muscularis propria may also be observed. In patients with colonic inertia, the ICCs are reduced in number and are morphologically abnormal. The precise mechanism and neurotransmitter deficiencies of this disorder are unclear. Box 21.2 summarizes information from a number of studies in the

---

Box 21.2 Colonic neuropathy in slow transit constipation. Source: De Giorgio R, Camilleri M. Human enteric neuropathies: morphology and molecular pathology. Neurogastroenterol Motil 2004;16:515. Reproduced with permission of John Wiley & Sons.

Histological and immunohistochemical findings

Decreased number or abnormal appearance of silver staining neurons or axons

Increased number of variably sized nuclei within ganglia

Decreased colonic VIP nerves

Decreased neurofilament staining in myenteric plexus in 75% of patients

17/29 entire colon affected

12/29 segmental involvement

Increased number of PGP 9.5 reactive nerve fibers in muscularis layer of ascending and descending colon

Decreased total nerve density in myenteric plexus

Decreased VIP and increased NO positive neurons

Decreased substance P nerves in 7/10 patients

Decreased VIP nerves in 4/7 patients

Decreased substance P in mucosa and submucosa of rectal biopsies

Increased VIP, substance P and galanin in ascending colon

Increased VIP and galanin in transverse colon

Increased VIP and neuropeptide Y in descending colon myenteric plexus

Decreased VIP in submucosa

Decreased tachykinin (substance P) and enkephalin fibers in circular muscle

Decreased colonic total neuron density

Decreased VIP and NO neurons in myenteric plexus

Decreased VIP neurons in submucous plexus

Decreased enteroglucagon and 5-HT cells in mucosa

Decreased cell secretory indices of enteroglucagon and somatostatin cells

Decreased volume of interstitial cells of Cajal and neurons in circular muscle

5-HT, 5-hydroxytryptamine; NO, nitric oxide; PGP 9.5, protein gene product 9.5; VIP, vasoactive intestinal peptide.

literature regarding histological changes that have been found in patients with motility disorders, such as chronic intestinal pseudoobstruction or slow transit constipation, severe enough to warrant subtotal colectomy. Box 21.3 summarizes the literature pertaining to specific disorders of neurotransmitters in disease. In less severe cases, differentiation from constipation-predominant irritable bowel syndrome may be difficult, especially when the gut is not dilated. Features of intestinal manometry mimic those of familial and secondary neuropa-

thies (Figure 21.16). In slow-transit constipation, colonic manometry shows a reduction in high-amplitude propagated sequences or contractions (which are associated with mass movements in the colon)

Secondary causes

Several systemic diseases may involve the digestive tract and result in intestinal dysmotility, although gastrointestinal manifestations rarely are the presenting feature. These secondary dysmotilities include diseases involving the intestinal smooth muscle, that is collagen diseases (such as scleroderma, dermatomyositis, systemic lupus erythematosus, and mixed connective tissue disease) (Figure 21.17), muscular dystrophy, and amyloidosis. Secondary intestinal dysmotility may also occur in diseases with associated neurological derangement (diabetic neuropathy, Chagas disease, Parkinson disease, neurofibromatosis, and paraneoplastic visceral neuropathy), endocrine disorders (diabetes mellitus, thyroid and parathyroid disease), drug-induced conditions (by phenothiazines, tricyclic antidepressants, antiparkinsonian drugs, ganglionic blockers, and narcotics), and miscellaneous diseases (celiac disease, radiation enteritis, immunoproliferative disorders, jejunoileal bypass, and sequela of gastrointestinal viral infections) (Figure 21.18).

Box 21.3 Pathological features of enteric neuromuscular. disease. Source: De Giorgio R, Camilleri M. Human enteric neuropathies: morphology and molecular pathology. Neurogastroenterol Motil 2004;16:515. Reproduced with permission of John Wiley & Sons.

Aganglionosis
Neuronal intranuclear inclusions and apoptosis
Neural degeneration
Intestinal neuronal dysplasia
Neuronal hyperplasia and ganglioneuromas
Mitochondrial dysfunction: syndromic and non-syndromic
Inflammatory neuropathies: cellular and humoral mechanisms
Neurotransmitter disorders
Interstitial cell pathology

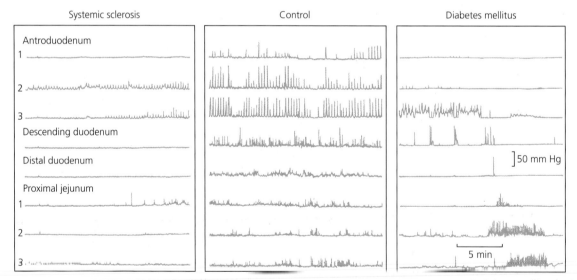

Figure 21.16 Altered postprandial intestinal manometric tracing in a patient with scleroderma (left) and in a patient with diabetes mellitus (right). Note the low amplitude of contractions typical of a myopathic disorder in the left panel, and the normal amplitude but abnormal pattern typical of a neuropathic disorder in the right panel. The antral hypomotility, excessive pyloric tonic and phasic pressure activity, and the persistence of the migrating motor complex during the postprandial period are typical features of enteric nerve dysfunction. Source: Camilleri M. Medical treatment of chronic intestinal pseudo-obstruction. Pract Gastroenterol 1991;15:10. Reproduced with permission of Practical Gastroenterology.

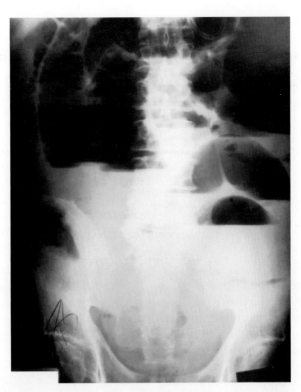

Figure 21.17 Plain abdominal radiograph of a patient with scleroderma and intestinal pseudoobstruction demonstrates dilated loops of small bowel with air–fluid levels.

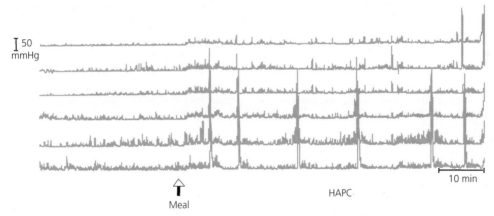

Figure 21.18 High-amplitude pressure contractions recorded in the left side of the colon after a meal in a patient with diarrhea caused by extrinsic neuropathy. Source: Choi MG, Camilleri M, O'Brien MD, et al. A pilot study of motility and tone of the left colon in patients with diarrhea due to functional disorders and dysautonomia. Am J Gastroenterol 1997;92:297. Reproduced with permission of John Wiley & Sons.

CHAPTER 22

Bacterial, viral, and toxic causes of diarrhea, gastroenteritis, and anorectal infections

Gail A. Hecht,[1] Jerrold R. Turner,[2] and Phillip I. Tarr[3]

[1] Loyola University Medical Center, Maywood, IL, USA
[2] University of Chicago, Chicago, IL, USA
[3] Washington University, St. Louis, MO, USA

The spectrum of organisms that can infect and cause disease in the human colon includes bacteria, viruses, and protozoa. Reviewed in this chapter are the bacterial and viral pathogens of the large intestine. Although the symptoms associated with infection by enteric bacterial pathogens are essentially indistinguishable (including abdominal pain, diarrhea, and fever), the range of pathological appearances is somewhat more varied. For example, colonic biopsies of *Campylobacter* colitis often have features similar to those seen in inflammatory bowel disease, including crypt abscesses (Figure 22.1), but typically lack changes associated with chronicity.

Figures 22.2 and 22.3 portray the results of cholera infection and equipment used by patients to cope with the symptoms. Infection with enterohemorrhagic *Escherichia coli* (EHEC) typically induces histopathology that overlaps with ischemic colitis (Figure 22.4). The colon can be quite severely affected, as demonstrated by contrast and computed tomography studies of affected children (Figure 22.5) and by the colon at laparotomy. (Figure 22.6). Gastroenterologists need to be cognizant of the clinical progression of this infection, as patients can present at multiple different points during their illness, although it is most often the bloody diarrhea that prompts evaluation (Figure 22.7). The histological features of colitis associated with enteroinvasive colitis and *Shigella* are typically identical (Figure 22.8). This stems from the fact that the genes conferring the invasive phenotype are identical for these two pathogens. Despite these highlighted differences, colonic histology is usually not specific enough to conclusively determine the causative agent. The one exception to this statement is *Clostridium difficile*-associated pseudomembranous colitis. *C. difficile* holds the title of the

number one cause of healthcare-associated diarrhea because hospitals and long-term care facilities serve as reservoirs, and establishment of infection in the colon by this spore-forming pathogen is dependent upon disruption of the resident colonic microflora by antibiotics (Figure 22.9). Although the diagnosis of *C. difficile*-associated colitis is usually determined by assays that identify the presence of toxin A or B in the stool, the gross appearance of pseudomembranes seen at sigmoidoscopy, as are evident quite vividly following resection (Figure 22.10), and the characteristic histological volcano lesions (Figure 22.11) are virtually pathognomonic for this infection. If a barium enema is performed, which is not recommended, then the presence of pseudomembranes may be demonstrated (Figure 22.12).

Infections of the anus and rectum are most commonly seen in homosexual men and heterosexual women who engage in anoreceptive intercourse. Primary anorectal syphilis appears as a chancre of the squamous epithelial lining of the anal canal or rectum (Figure 22.13). Condyloma lata represents the secondary phase of syphilis (Figure 22.14). Biopsy of anorectal lesions from patients infected with *Treponema pallidum* may reveal spirochetes (Figure 22.15). However, nonpathogenic spirochetes can also reside in the rectum, thus reducing the significance of this finding.

More commonly seen are condyloma acuminata (anal warts) caused by infection with human papillomavirus. These verrucous lesions are generally easy to differentiate from the flat, fleshy lesions of condyloma lata, but histology easily distinguishes between the two and is recommended to confirm the diagnosis (Figure 22.16).

Yamada's Atlas of Gastroenterology, Fifth Edition. Edited by Daniel K. Podolsky, Michael Camilleri, J. Gregory Fitz, Anthony N. Kalloo, Fergus Shanahan, and Timothy C. Wang.
© 2016 John Wiley & Sons, Ltd. Published 2016 by John Wiley & Sons, Ltd.
Companion website: www.yamadagastro.com/atlas

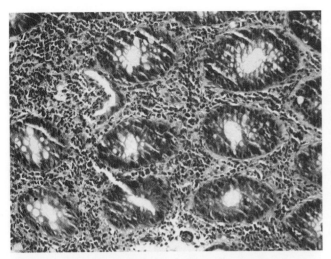

Figure 22.1 Photomicrograph of colonic mucosal biopsy from a patient with *Campylobacter jejuni* colitis. Note the presence of crypt abscesses, crypt destruction, and lamina propria infiltrates of neutrophils, eosinophils, and lymphocytes. These features can overlap with those present in inflammatory bowel disease. However, the uniform spacing and shape of the crypts, that is a lack of architectural distortion, suggests that an alternative diagnosis, such as an infectious process, should be considered. Source: Courtesy of Dr. Neal S. Goldstein, William Beaumont Hospital, Royal Oak, MI.

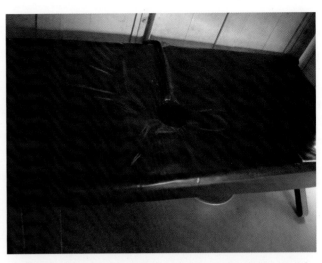

Figure 22.3 Cholera cot. Mattress covered with non-absorbable material to permit collection of high-volume enteric effluent, as is produced during cholera infection. Source: Courtesy of Matlab Hospital of the International Centre for Diarrhoeal Diseases Research, Bangladesh.

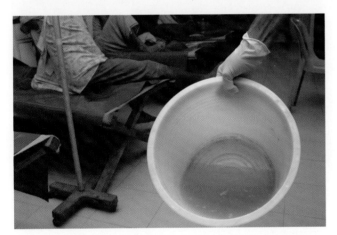

Figure 22.2 Classic rice water cholera stools. Liquid stool collected over 1 h from an adult with *Vibrio cholerae*. In the 5 h since this 54-kg man was admitted, he produced 5 liters of rice water stool. Source: Courtesy of Matlab Hospital of the International Centre for Diarrhoeal Diseases Research, Bangladesh.

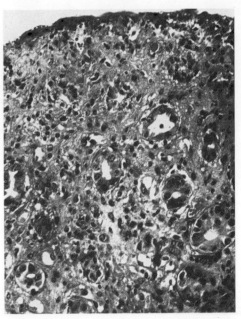

Figure 22.4 This colonic mucosal biopsy from a patient with *Escherichia coli* O157:H7 colitis demonstrates superficial epithelial atrophy with crypt cell hyperplasia. These features overlap with those of ischemic colitis. Source: Courtesy of Dr. Neal S. Goldstein, William Beaumont Hospital, Royal Oak, MI.

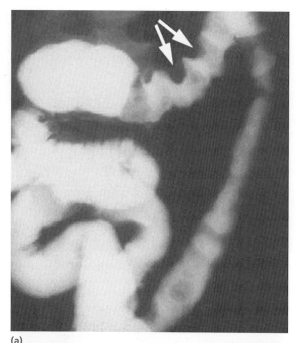

(a)

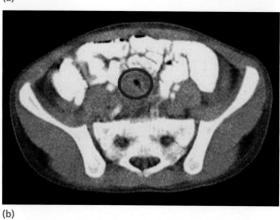

(b)

Figure 22.5 Radiographic features of *Escherichia coli* O157:H7 infection.
(a) Radiograph after barium enema with thumbprinting appearance of
mucosa (arrows), suggesting colonic edema, in a patient who
subsequently developed hemolytic–uremic syndrome (HUS).
(b) Computed tomography of the pelvis of an 8-year-old boy on the
eighth day of an *E. coli* O157:H7 infection. Note severely thickened colon
(circled). This infection did not progress to HUS.

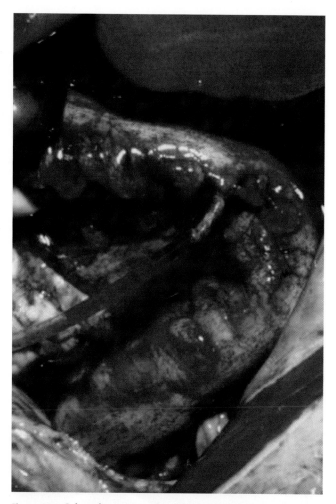

Figure 22.6 Colon of patient acutely infected with *Escherichia coli*
O157:H7. Note marked hyperemia of serosal surface. Source: Courtesy of
Dr. David Tapper, Seattle Children's Hospital.

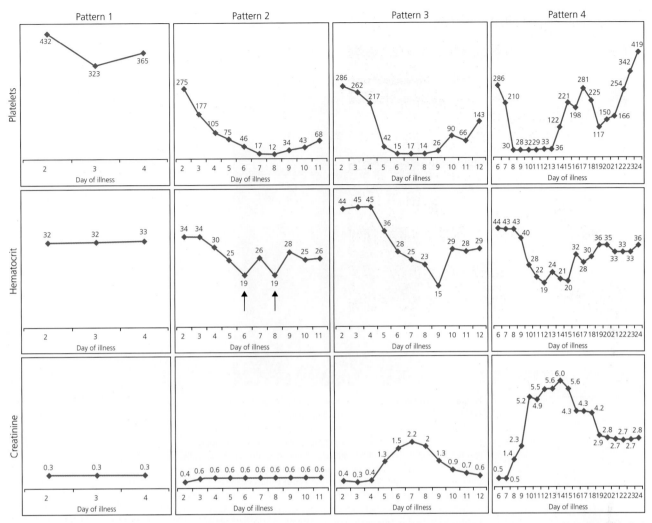

Figure 22.7 Progression of *Escherichia coli* O157:H7 infections in children. *E. coli* O157:H7 infections tend to follow a quite predictable pattern. We find that it is helpful to make clinical judgments based on stage of illness, in consideration of trends in laboratory tests. Pattern 1 (uncomplicated) accounts for ~70% of cases. The platelet count falls slightly before rising, remains constant, or actually rises, between determinations. In ~25% of cases, the platelet count falls to <150,000/mm^3, but the hematocrit remains >30%. Pattern 2 represents substantial vascular injury but no azotemia, and occurs in 5–10% of patients. Hemolysis required two red cell transfusions (arrows). This pattern is sometimes termed partial HUS, but we do not believe this designation is appropriate. Pattern 3 (5–10% of cases) exemplifies non-oligoanuric HUS, defined by a platelet count <150,000/mm^3, hematocrit <30% with smear evidence of intravascular red cell destruction, and creatinine >upper limit of normal for age. These patients continue urinating, and rarely need dialysis. Pattern 4 (10–15% of cases) is anuric HUS, which has a worse short and long term prognosis.

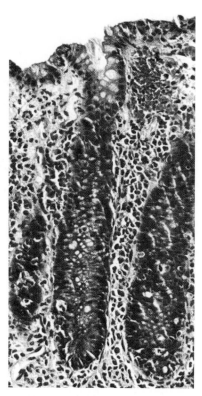

Figure 22.8 This colonic mucosal biopsy from a patient with enteroinvasive *Escherichia coli* colitis demonstrates pronounced infiltration of surface and crypt epithelium by neutrophils. The lamina propria also contains numerous neutrophils with admixed eosinophils and fewer lymphocytes and plasma cells. Some apoptotic epithelial cells can also be appreciated and can be present in even greater numbers in more severe cases. The clinical and pathological features can be indistinguishable from *Shigella* infection. The uniform spacing and shape of the crypts helps to exclude inflammatory bowel disease. Source: Courtesy Dr. Neal S. Goldstein, William Beaumont Hospital, Royal Oak, MI.

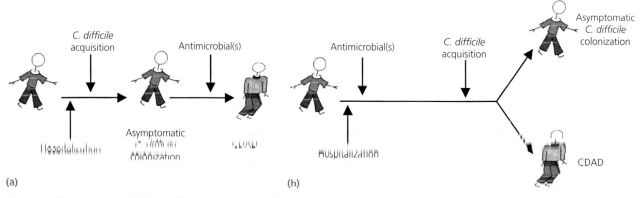

(a) (h)

Figure 22.9 Hypotheses by which hospitalized patients acquire *Clostridium difficile* and the associated diarrhea. **(a)** Depiction of the initial hypothesis that hospitalized patients become colonized with *C. difficile* and upon exposure to antimicrobial agents develop the symptoms that typify this infection. More recently, a revised hypothesis has been put forth and is shown in **(b)**. In this case, the hospitalized patient may be exposed to *C. difficile* throughout the course of stay but is not susceptible to colonization until antibiotics are introduced. At that point, true acquisition of the organism occurs and host factors, such as the level of antibody production to the organism or its toxins, determines which patients will become colonized but remain asymptomatic and which will manifest the associated symptom of diarrhea. CDAD, *Clostridium difficile*-associated diarrhea. Source: Adapted from Johnson S, Gerding D. Clin Infect Dis 1998;26:1027. Reproduced with permission of Oxford University Press.

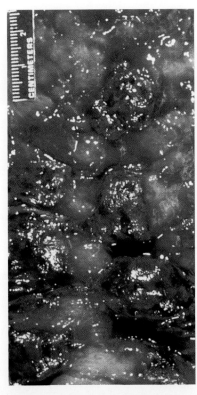

Figure 22.10 Gross appearance of *Clostridium difficile* pseudomembranous colitis. This photo shows the severe, nearly confluent, pale pseudomembranes that are typical of severe *C. difficile* pseudomembranous colitis. The pseudomembranes are composed of purulent debris and contrast sharply against the surrounding dark edematous mucosa.

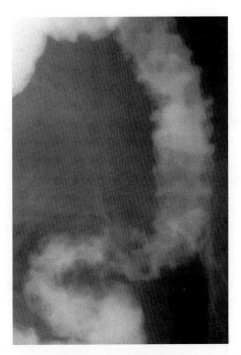

Figure 22.12 Radiograph of a barium enema performed on a patient with *Clostridium difficile*-induced pseudomembranous colitis. Note the presence of multiple filling defects within the colonic mucosa, which represent pseudomembranes and mucosal edema.

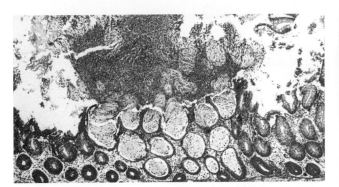

Figure 22.11 Histological appearance of *Clostridium difficile* pseudomembranous colitis. This photomicrograph shows a classic type II volcano-like eruption with a mushroom-shaped cloud of adherent inflammatory exudate.

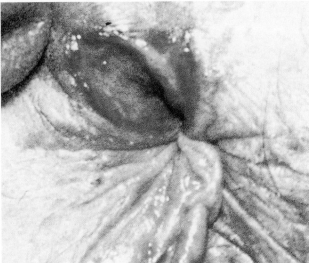

Figure 22.13 Primary syphilitic chancre of the anus. Such lesions occur in homosexual men and heterosexual women who engage in anoreceptive intercourse. Anorectal syphilitic chancres may be asymptomatic or painful, usually upon defecation.

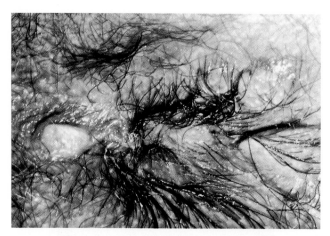

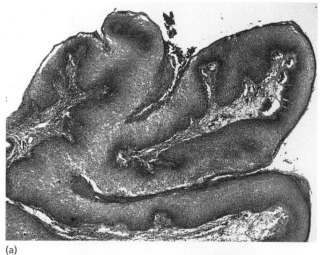

(a)

Figure 22.14 Condyloma lata of the anorectal area, shown here, represent the secondary stage of syphilis. Condyloma lata appear as smooth, moist, fleshy lesions, which can secrete a discharge that is highly infectious. Condyloma lata are distinguishable from the verrucous anal warts or condyloma acuminata caused by infection with human papillomavirus.

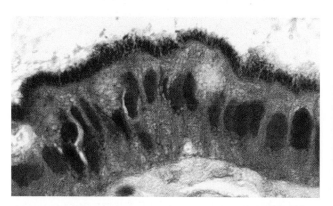

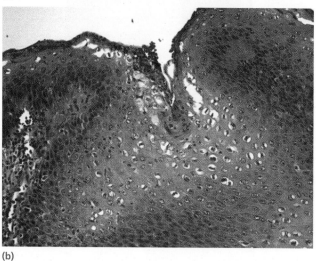

(b)

Figure 22.15 High-power photomicrograph of rectal spirochetosis showing the typical apical layer of spirochetes that stain dark blue on standard hematoxylin and eosin stain. The organisms are oriented parallel to the microvilli and, by electron microscopy, can be seen to interdigitate between the microvilli. Rectal spirochetes may represent *Treponema pallidum* or nonpathogenic organisms, diminishing the significance of such a finding.

Figure 22.16 Condyloma acuminatum of the anal region. The low-power view **(a)** shows the typical papillomatous growth pattern of this lesion. The higher magnification photomicrograph **(b)** demonstrates the typical vacuolization of koilocytotic human papillomavirus-infected squamous cells.

CHAPTER 23

Chronic infections of the small intestine

George T. Fantry,[1] Lori E. Fantry,[1] Stephen P. James,[2] and David H. Alpers[3]

[1] University of Maryland School of Medicine, Baltimore, MD, USA
[2] National Institute of Diabetes and Digestive and Kidney Diseases, Bethesda, MD, USA
[3] Washington University School of Medicine, St. Louis, MO, USA

There are four chronic infections of the small intestine that occur in immunocompetent hosts: Whipple disease, tropical sprue, tuberculosis, and histoplasmosis. Other chronic infections of the small intestine are seen primarily among immunocompromised hosts and include mycotic infections such as aspergillosis, candidiasis, and mucormycosis, and *Mycobacterium avium* complex (MAC) occurring among patients with acquired immunodeficiency syndrome (AIDS). The last infection may mimic the histopathological findings of Whipple disease.

Whipple disease is a rare syndrome caused by infection with *Tropheryma whipplei*. The most important step in the evaluation of Whipple disease is to have a high degree of suspicion in the appropriate clinical setting. The challenge is to establish the correct diagnosis while avoiding the temptation to overdiagnose the disease. The diagnostic procedure of choice is endoscopic small intestine mucosal biopsy. The disease is usually diffuse but can be patchy; therefore, multiple (four to six) biopsy specimens should be obtained. The characteristic duodenal appearance consists of thickened mucosal folds coated with a yellow granular material or 1- to 2-mm yellow plaques that may be diffuse or patchy (Figure 23.1).

The appearance with periodic acid–Schiff (PAS) staining often is sufficient to establish the diagnosis of Whipple disease for most patients (Figures 23.2, 23.3, 23.4, and 23.5); however, it can be confirmed with electron microscopic demonstration of the bacilli (Figure 23.6). Occasional macrophages are found in the normal intestinal lamina propria. These macrophages usually stain faintly PAS positive, but the inclusions are not sickle shaped as in Whipple disease. There are three clinical entities in which the presence of numerous PAS-positive macrophages in the intestinal lamina propria may be misleading: AIDS with MAC infection, systemic histoplasmosis, and macroglobulinemia. Macroglobulinemia can be differentiated from Whipple disease because of the faintly staining, homogeneously

PAS-positive macrophages, and histoplasmosis can be differentiated by the large, PAS-positive, rounded, encapsulated *Histoplasma* organisms. More care must be taken in differentiating the histopathological findings in the intestinal mucosa of patients with Whipple disease from those in patients with AIDS and MAC infection. In MAC infection, the lamina propria is packed with macrophages containing MAC, which when stained with hematoxylin and eosin and PAS stain clearly resemble those seen in Whipple disease. However, MAC bacilli are acid fast, easily cultured, and have an electron microscopic appearance that is quite different from that of Whipple bacilli (Figure 23.7). The diagnosis of MAC is easily established among persons with human immunodeficiency virus (HIV) infection. *T. whipplei* infection has not been reported among persons with HIV infection. Studies have suggested that the polymerase chain reaction may be a helpful confirmatory test for patients believed to have Whipple disease. In very rare instances the diagnosis of Whipple disease has been established in the absence of intestinal involvement. In these cases the diagnosis was established with electron microscopic demonstration of bacilli in cerebrospinal fluid, brain biopsy specimens, or peripheral lymph nodes.

Considerable caution is required in the interpretation of gastric and rectal biopsy findings. PAS-positive macrophages frequently are present in the normal gastric and rectal mucosa, and in many diseases of the stomach and rectum. The stomach often contains faintly PAS-positive, lipid-containing macrophages (lipophages), whereas the rectal mucosa usually contains strongly PAS-positive muciphages and pigment-containing macrophages (Figure 23.8). Electron microscopic demonstration of Whipple bacilli in these tissues usually is necessary to establish the diagnosis.

Barium studies of the small intestine usually are abnormal in Whipple disease and may reveal a characteristic but nonspecific finding of marked thickening of the mucosal folds (Figure 23.9). These findings usually are more prominent in the duodenum

Yamada's Atlas of Gastroenterology, Fifth Edition. Edited by Daniel K. Podolsky, Michael Camilleri, J. Gregory Fitz, Anthony N. Kalloo, Fergus Shanahan, and Timothy C. Wang.
© 2016 John Wiley & Sons, Ltd. Published 2016 by John Wiley & Sons, Ltd.
Companion website: www.yamadagastro.com/atlas

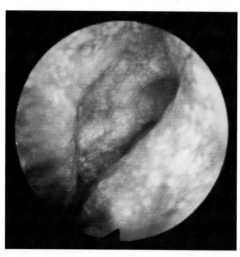

Figure 23.1 Characteristic duodenoscopic appearance of the duodenum of an untreated patient with Whipple disease. The folds are thickened and are covered with small yellowish-white plaques. This endoscopic appearance may be the first clue to the diagnosis.

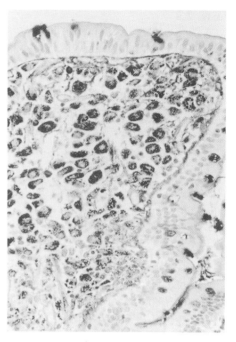

Figure 23.3 Periodic acid–Schiff and hematoxylin stain of the same villus as in Figure 23.2 shows prominence of the macrophages with this stain (original magnification ×200). Source: Courtesy of Dr. John E. Stone.

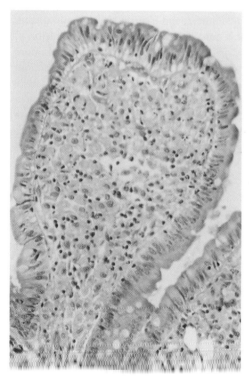

Figure 23.2 Characteristic appearance of a hematoxylin and eosinstained intestinal villus in Whipple disease. The macrophages, although abundant throughout the lamina propria, are rather inapparent (original magnification ×200). Source: Courtesy of Dr. John E. Stone.

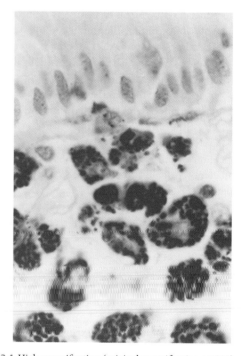

Figure 23.4 High-magnification (original magnification ×1000) photograph of macrophages stained with periodic acid–Schiff in the intestinal mucosa in Whipple disease. Note the characteristic rounded and sickle-shaped inclusions in the macrophages. This appearance alone is highly suggestive of the diagnosis.

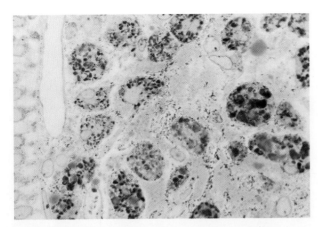

Figure 23.5 High-magnification (original magnification ×750) photograph of a toluidine blue-stained section of a plastic-embedded specimen of intestinal mucosa in Whipple disease. Characteristic macrophage inclusions and numerous extracellular bacilli are present throughout the lamina propria.

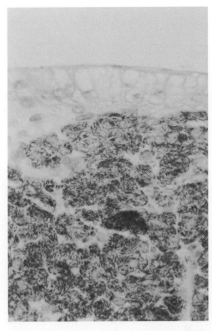

Figure 23.7 High-magnification (original magnification ×1000) photograph of an acid-fast stained intestinal villus in *Mycobacterium avium* complex infection in acquired immunodeficiency syndrome. Exclusively intracellular, very large bacilli are present. Whipple bacilli are much smaller, largely extracellular, and not acid fast. Source: Courtesy of Dr. Wilfred M. Weinstein.

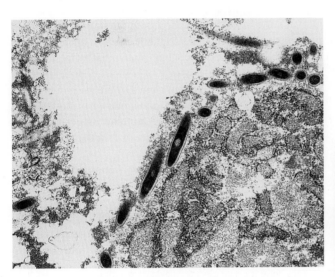

Figure 23.6 Electron micrograph of a duodenal biopsy specimen from a patient with Whipple disease shows the cytoplasm of a macrophage, with positive results at periodic acid–Schiff staining, and its surrounding extracellular space. Note the numerous bacilli with characteristic cell walls and pale central nuclei just outside the macrophage. Source: Fantry GT, James SP. Whipple's disease. Dig Dis 1995;13:108.

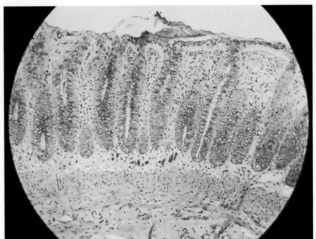

Figure 23.8 Periodic acid–Schiff and hematoxylin stain of a rectal biopsy specimen from a healthy person. Prominent macrophages are just below the crypts and above the muscularis mucosae. This finding is a frequent cause of confusion; however, the rectum and colon are very rarely involved in Whipple disease (original magnification ×100).

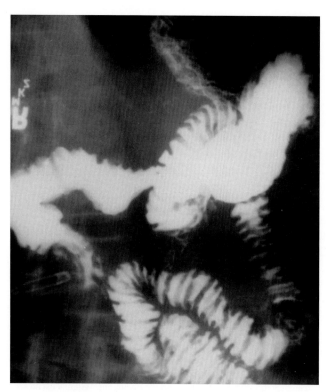

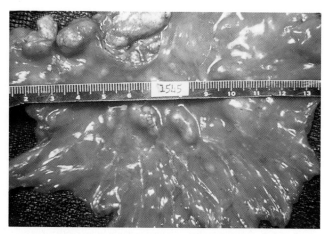

Figure 23.10 Autopsy image of the mesentery and nodes of a patient with Whipple disease shows marked thickening of the mesentery and a striking degree of adenopathy.

Figure 23.9 Radiograph shows coarsened folds in the duodenum and jejunum of an untreated patient with Whipple disease. Source: Courtesy of Dr. John E. Stone.

and proximal jejunum and less prominent in the distal jejunum; the ileum is spared. In addition to marked thickening of the proximal small bowel, abdominal computed tomographic scanning often reveals marked mesenteric, paraaortic, and retroperitoneal adenopathy (Figure 23.10).

Three specific chronic bacterial infections of the small intestine are caused by *Yersinia* (*Y. enterocolitica* and *Y. pseudotuberculosis*), *Mycobacterium tuberculosis*, and *Histoplasma capsulatum*. *Yersinia* penetrates the lamina propria and causes submucosal thickening that can mimic Crohn's disease (Figure 23.11). Histologically, there are massively enlarged lymphoid follicles with prominent germinal centers (Figure 23.11).

Intestinal tuberculosis is most common in patients with active pulmonary disease and is caused by swallowed organisms that cross the mucosa of the bowel segments rich in lymphoid tissue, that is the ileum and cecum. Figure 23.12 shows tuberculosis in the ileocecal region, where nearly all gastrointestinal infections occur. The tissue response can be either hypertrophic (Figure 23.12b), ulcerative, or a combination of both. When tuberculosis becomes disseminated (miliary tuberculosis), tubercles are found on the serosal surface of the bowel.

Histoplasmosis is originally a pulmonary infection that most often becomes generalized, as in immunocompromised patients. The causative organism can affect both the small or large intestine and the liver, although symptoms are most often attributed to small bowel disease (crampy abdominal pain, diarrhea, anemia, malabsorption). Figure 23.13a shows nodular ulcerated lesions. This ulceration is accompanied by intense mononuclear cell infiltration, possibly with granuloma formation (Figure 23.13b), in those patients who are immunocompetent enough to mount a response. Oval yeast forms of 2–3 μm may be visualized in macrophages (Figure 23.14).

Aspergillosis affects only severely immunocompromised patients, including those with AIDS, those undergoing organ transplantation or immunosuppressive chemotherapy, and premature infants. The small intestine is involved in about 5% of patients with disseminated aspergillosis. *Aspergillus* grows by branching and longitudinal extension of wide (2–5 μm) Y-shaped, branching, septate hyphae. Clinical disease is produced by vascular invasion and necrosis (Figure 23.15).

Candida species are the fourth most common organisms isolated from the blood of hospitalized patients and are normal colonizers of the gastrointestinal tract. These organisms are commonly associated with esophageal disease in immunocompromised patients but rarely cause disease of the small intestine. Persons at highest risk include those with AIDS, chronic mucocutaneous conditions, or malignancies, and those taking immunosuppressive agents. The most common lesions associated with *Candida* are single or multiple ulcerations. Because *Candida* is a normal colonizer of the entire gastrointestinal tract, diagnosis requires biopsy evidence of invasion (Figure 23.16).

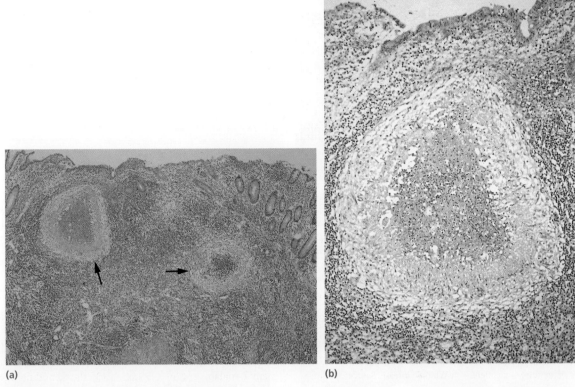

(a) (b)

Figure 23.11 *Yersinia* enterocolitis; **(a)** and **(b)** demonstrate the presence of the prominent necrotizing granulomas that characterize *Yersinia* when it presents in a typical fashion. Two granulomas (arrows) are shown in (a). The overlying epithelium appears atrophic and ulcerated. (b) Higher magnification showing palisading histiocytes without foreign body giant cells. The entire granuloma is surrounded by a prominent cuff of lymphocytes. Source: Fenoglio-Preiser CM, Noffsinger AE, Stemmermann GN, et al. Nonneoplastic lesions of the small intestine. In: Gastrointestinal Pathology: An Atlas and Text, 2nd edn. Philadelphia: Lippincott-Raven, 1999. Reproduced with permission of Wolters Kluwer Health.

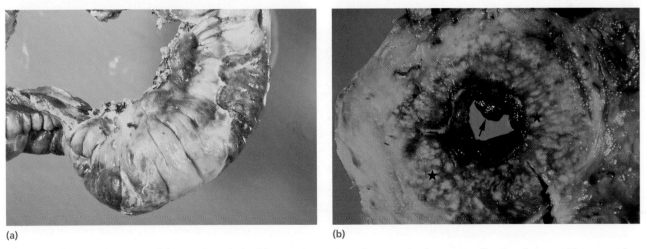

(a) (b)

Figure 23.12 Ileocecal tuberculosis. **(a)** Gross photograph of the resection specimen demonstrating the presence of an ileocolectomy with transmural inflammation. It is difficult to delineate the exact ileocecal valve area. The serosal tissues are markedly congested and edematous and show fibrinous adhesions. **(b)** Cross-section through the specimen demonstrating transmural necrosis and replacement of the intestinal wall by numerous granulomas, several of which are indicated by stars. Source: Fenoglio-Preiser CM, Noffsinger AE, Stemmermann GN, et al. Nonneoplastic lesions of the small intestine. In: Gastrointestinal Pathology: An Atlas and Text, 2nd edn, 1999. Reproduced with permission of Wolters Kluwer Health.

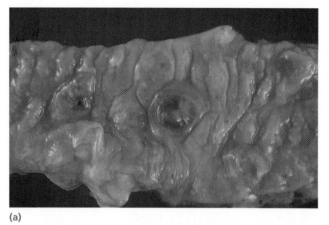

(a)

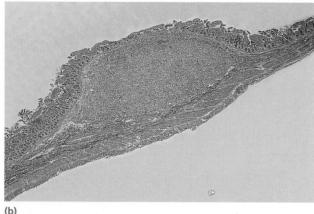

(b)

Figure 23.13 **(a)** Histoplasmosis. Intestinal resection specimen showing nodular ulcerated lesions located diffusely throughout the bowel wall, obliterating the normal mucosal fold pattern. **(b)** Histological section of the lesion shown in (a) indicating the presence of a submucosal granuloma. Source: Fenoglio-Preiser CM, Noffsinger AE, Stemmermann GN, et al. Nonneoplastic lesions of the small intestine. In: Gastrointestinal Pathology: An Atlas and Text, 2nd edn, 1999. Reproduced with permission of Wolters Kluwer Health.

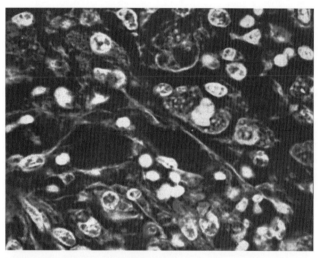

Figure 23.14 Light microscopic appearance of oval yeast forms of *Histoplasma capsulatum* within macrophages from a patient with disseminated histoplasmosis. High-power magnification. Source: Shull HJ. Human histoplasmosis: a disease with protean manifestations, often with digestive system involvement. Gastroenterology 1953;25:582. Reproduced with permission of Elsevier.

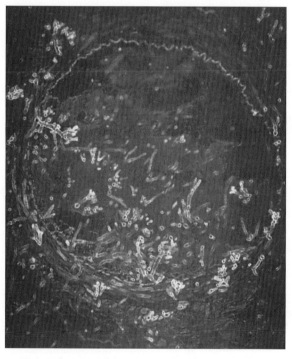

Figure 23.15 Light microscopic appearance of *Aspergillus* organisms showing vascular invasion. Source: Prescott RJ, Harris M, Banerjee SS. Fungal infections of the small and large intestine. J Clin Pathol 1992;45:806. Reproduced with permission of BMJ Publishing Group Ltd.

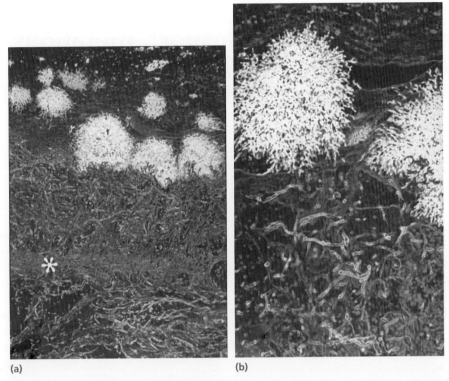

(a) (b)

Figure 23.16 Light microscopic appearance of *Candida* organisms on the surface of infarcted bowel mucosa with *Aspergillus* hyphae in the underlying mucosa and submucosa. **(a)** Low magnification; **(b)** high magnification (Grocott–Gomori methenamine–silver stain). Source: Prescott RJ, Harris M, Banerjee SS. Fungal infections of the small and large intestine. J Clin Pathol 1992;45:806. Reproduced with permission of BMJ Publishing Group Ltd.

CHAPTER 24

Disorders of epithelial transport, metabolism, and digestion in the small intestine

Richard J. Grand

Boston Children's Hospital, Boston, MA, USA

Phenotypically, disorders of intestinal epithelial transport demonstrate similar symptoms irrespective of the specific molecular basis of the defect in absorption. Symptoms include abdominal distension and/or pain, flatulence, and diarrhea. These disorders are usually classified by the specific nutrient that is malabsorbed, and many of them are quite rare. For some, clinical tests are available that may yield clues to the specific diagnosis. These will be discussed in this chapter.

Lactose malabsorption

Lactose malabsorption may occur whenever the level of small intestinal lactase is compromised either as a consequence of genetically regulated reductions in the expression of lactase enzyme or secondary to small intestinal injury (e.g., viral infection, Giardiasis, celiac disease, and other insults). During intestinal development, fetal lactase mRNA and enzyme activity reach mature levels in the third trimester of gestation, and remain relatively constant until age 3–5 years. Subsequently, in the majority of the world's population, lactase levels then fall by about 85%–90% and remain low thereafter (known as lactase nonpersistence). In contrast, in peoples of Northern European ancestry and in localized groups elsewhere, lactase activity remains at the infantile level for life (known as lactase persistence). Lactase nonpersistence has also been called "lactase deficiency" or "adult hypolactasia," terms which are no longer in use. In a rare syndrome, congenital lactase deficiency, the enzyme fails to develop, and affected infants exposed to lactose immediately after birth develop severe watery diarrhea and failure to thrive. Although lactose nonpersistence leads to intestinal complaints of varying intensity, known as lactose intolerance, it is not strictly speaking a disease. Symptoms are induced by the osmotic effects of nonabsorbed lactose, increased intraluminal fluid, and increased intestinal transit. Lactic acid produced in the colon by colonic flora may exacerbate symptoms. This phenomenon is also the basis for the lactose breath hydrogen test (Figure 24.1). The simplest screening test to identify lactase nonpersistence is withdrawal of dietary milk and milk products. Should this maneuver produce confusing results, the next screening test should be a breath hydrogen test (Figure 24.1). Breath hydrogen content of greater than 10–20 ppm over baseline after ingestion of a lactose load consisting of 2 g/kg body weight up to 25 g is considered diagnostic for lactose malabsorption.

Cystic fibrosis

Cystic fibrosis is the most commonly occurring lethal genetic disorder in the world, and is associated predominantly with pulmonary and pancreatic disease but may affect multiple organs. With modern treatment programs, most affected people survive to adulthood (median age of survival is currently about 40 years). Effects on extrapulmonary organs, including the intestine, are variable. Intestinal symptoms are caused by the presence of thick mucus produced by altered chloride secretion (Figure 24.2) with prominent goblet cells and luminal retention of mucus (Figure 24.3). These pathophysiological changes can produce intestinal obstruction known as meconium ileus in infants and the distal intestinal obstruction syndrome in older patients (Figure 24.4). Gastric, small intestinal, and colonic mucosal changes are also seen due to the effects of abnormal mucus production (Figures 24.5 and 24.6).

Abetalipoproteinemia

A number of genetic disorders in lipoprotein synthesis and function are now known to cause hypo- or abetalipoproteinemia. The intestinal phenotype seen in affected patients is a

Yamada's Atlas of Gastroenterology, Fifth Edition. Edited by Daniel K. Podolsky, Michael Camilleri, J. Gregory Fitz, Anthony N. Kalloo, Fergus Shanahan, and Timothy C. Wang.
© 2016 John Wiley & Sons, Ltd. Published 2016 by John Wiley & Sons, Ltd.
Companion website: www.yamadagastro.com/atlas

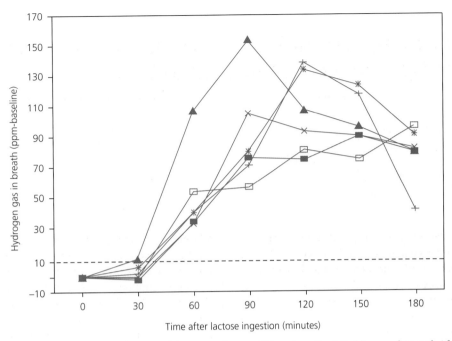

Figure 24.1 Lactose breath hydrogen tests in four persons with lactose intolerance. Values above the dotted line are abnormal. After an overnight fast, a basal breath sample is obtained, and lactose (2 g/kg body weight) is administered in water. Breath is sampled every 30 min for 3 h and analyzed for hydrogen content in a dedicated gas chromatograph (in this study, a Quinton instrument [Quinton Instruments, Bothell, WA] was used). The peak in breath hydrogen occurs between 90 and 120 min in the subjects and remarkably similar curves are seen for all four subjects. It is customary to obtain a concomitant symptom chart to correlate breath hydrogen excretion with subjective symptoms.

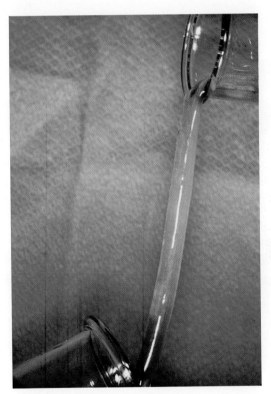

Figure 24.2 Duodenal mucus from a patient with cystic fibrosis obtained by means of intraduodenal intubation. Extremely viscid mucus retains its elastic properties even when poured from flask to flask.

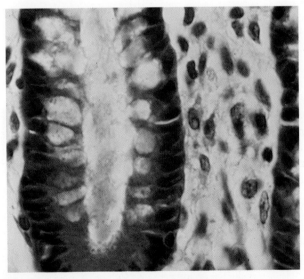

Figure 24.3 Ileal biopsy specimen from a patient with cystic fibrosis at operation for distal intestinal obstruction syndrome (periodic acid–Schiff stain). Prominent and enlarged goblet cells and retained mucus are present in the crypt lumen. This appearance is virtually pathognomonic of cystic fibrosis.

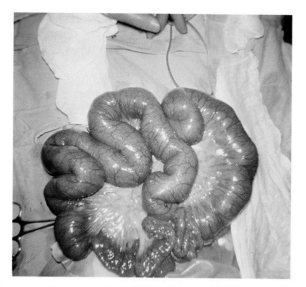

Figure 24.4 Photograph obtained at operation shows distal intestine of an adolescent patient with cystic fibrosis and distal intestinal obstruction. Terminal ileum is enlarged with impacted retained mucoid material, which failed to pass with nonoperative therapy. When surgical intervention is necessary, it is often sufficient to milk the retained intestinal contents distally. It is usually unnecessary to perform enterotomy or resection.

marked reduction in lipid transport, leading to retention of lipid in enterocytes (Figure 24.7).

Sucrase–isomaltase deficiency

Of all the disorders of congenital carbohydrate absorption, the altered cellular events associated with sucrase–isomaltase deficiency have been best characterized. Seven genetic forms of this disorder have been defined, five of them leading to absent functional sucrase or isomaltase. Examples of the first three of these molecular abnormalities described are shown in Table 24.1. Clinical symptoms are characteristic of carbohydrate malabsorption, as noted above for lactase nonpersistence. A presumptive diagnosis of sucrase deficiency can be made after a clinical response to sucrose exclusion from the diet. The diagnosis can be confirmed by means of breath hydrogen testing after administration of 2 g/kg body weight (maximum 25 g) oral sucrose (Figure 24.8), or by means of mucosal disaccharidase assays that show low sucrase activity in biopsy specimens with normal mucosal histological features. Some patients with this condition lack any isomaltase activity. The associated decreased maltase activity is attributable to the fact that sucrase–isomaltase accounts for a substantial amount of normal maltose hydrolysis.

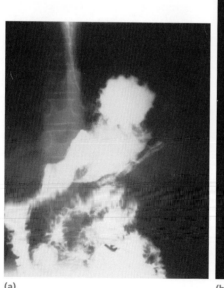

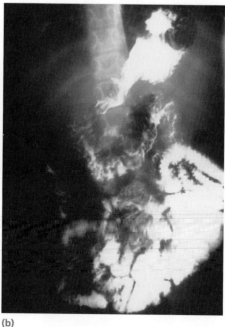

(a)   (b)

Figure 24.5 Upper gastrointestinal barium series with small bowel follow-through shows a 9-year-old patient with newly diagnosed cystic fibrosis. **(a)** The gastric and duodenal mucosa are nodular, thickened, and irregular. **(b)** The small intestine has a thickened, irregular mucosa with scattered nodularity.

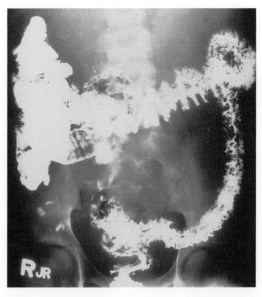

Figure 24.6 Barium enema radiograph of a 9-year-old patient with newly diagnosed cystic fibrosis. Spiculations, thickening, and irregularity of the mucosa are depicted. The nodularity is readily visible.

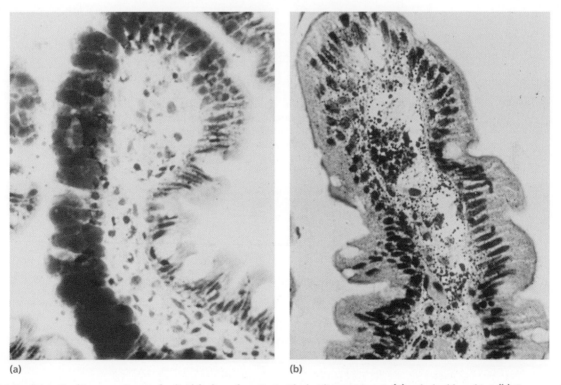

(a)   (b)

Figure 24.7 Small intestine biopsy specimens after lipid feeding of a patient with abetalipoproteinemia **(a)** and a healthy subject **(b)**. Frozen sections were stained with Oil red O. Among patients with abetalipoproteinemia, lipid cannot be transported out of the enterocyte, and it accumulates intracellularly in large droplets, stained red here. Among healthy persons, lipid is transported into the lymphatic vessels, where it exists in small droplets.

Table 24.1 Types of sucrase–isomaltase deficiency. Data from Naim HY, Roth J, Sterchi EE, et al. Sucrase–isomaltase deficiency in humans. Different mutations disrupt intracellular transport, processing, and function of an intestinal brush border enzyme. J Clin Invest 1988;82:667.

	Type I	Type II	Type III
Forms of sucrase–isomaltase detected	High mannose ($M_r = 212\,000$) ± complex ($M_r = 245\,000$) in reduced amounts	High mannose ($M_r = 210\,000$) Sucrase ($M_r = 45\,000$)	High mannose ($M_r = 210\,000$) Complex ($M_r = 245\,000$) Isomaltase ($M_r = 151\,000$)
Immunolocalization defect	Not studied Incomplete trimming reaction in endoplasmic reticulum	Golgi Transport arrested in Golgi apparatus	Brush border Sucrase enzymatic active site altered

M_r, relative molecular mass.

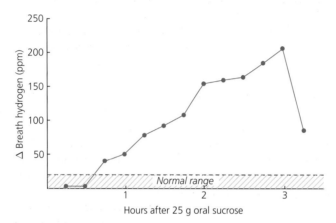

Figure 24.8 Breath hydrogen response to sucrose of a patient with sucrase–isomaltase deficiency. A marked increase in breath hydrogen level follows ingestion of 25 g of sucrose. The hydrogen production reflects colonic fermentation of the unabsorbed disaccharide.

CHAPTER 25

Short bowel syndrome

Richard N. Fedorak, Leah M. Gramlich, and Lana Bistritz
University of Alberta, Edmonton, AB, Canada

The term "short bowel syndrome" refers to the clinical consequences and pathophysiological disorders associated with a malabsorptive state resulting from the removal of a large portion of the small and/or large intestine. A related term, "intestinal failure", describes a situation where a significant portion of the small intestine is not present or does not function normally. This can occur when a large portion of the small intestine has been surgically removed resulting in short bowel syndrome, a newborn has an abnormal intestine, or in cases of intrinsic bowel disease, such as Crohn's disease or motility disorder. Parenteral nutrition is necessary for patients with intestinal failure so that they can meet their fluid, macro- and micronutrient, and electrolyte needs.

The degree of nutrient and nonnutrient malabsorption that occurs in a patient with short bowel syndrome and/or intestinal failure is a consequence of a number of factors: the extent and site of the resected or diseased intestine; the presence or absence of an ileocecal valve; the condition of the remaining intestine; the degree of adaptation of the residual small intestine; and the potential impact of underlying disease(s) (Box 25.1). It is thus possible that the removal of similar lengths of small intestine might cause short bowel syndrome to develop in one person but not in another.

Diarrhea is inevitable for patients who have had extensive small intestinal resection and have developed short bowel syndrome. Diarrhea and fluid and electrolyte loss is multifactorial and often involves one or more of the following causes: reduction of absorptive surface area, decrease in intestinal transit time, hormone-mediated intestinal hypersecretion, increase in the osmolality of intestinal contents, and bacterial overgrowth. Rational and judicious use of varying antidiarrheal therapies can significantly limit fluid and electrolyte losses and reduce or even eliminate the requirements for parenteral nutrition (Table 25.1).

In addition to the severe losses of fluid and electrolytes, micronutrient deficiencies (Figure 25.1) and systemic complications (e.g., gallstones (Figure 25.2), enteric hyperoxaluria, renal calculi (Figure 25.3; Box 25.2), and bacterial overgrowth) are likely to occur. Almost all patients with short bowel syndrome at one time or another need parenteral nutrition, or intravenous fluid and electrolyte therapy. Although the need for parenteral nutrition and electrolyte therapy may be transient, intermittent, or chronic, it is often life-sustaining therapy. Tables 25.2–6, and Boxes 25.3 and 25.4 provide examples of total parenteral nutrition order forms, component composition, and suggested monitoring blood work and additive routines for the adult population. Tables 25.7–25.11 provide similar information for pediatric patients. Figures 25.4 and 25.5 provide algorithms for managing vitamin D insufficiency and deficiency, respectively.

Once parenteral nutrition is initiated for short bowel syndrome patients it often becomes life sustaining, requiring lifetime home parenteral nutrition therapy. The complications of home parenteral nutrition therapy tend to be related to the central venous catheter (Table 25.12). While some patients are susceptible to recurrent problems, most have very few complications.

Quality of life for patients receiving home parenteral nutrition is generally reasonable and evidence indicates that a plateau occurs after 3–5 years (Table 25.13). The 1 year survival rate of patients receiving home parenteral nutrition is approximately 95% for the young Crohn's disease patient; however, this survival rate decreases dramatically in the elderly patient and over time (Table 25.14).

Intestinal transplantation has become a life-saving treatment that can be considered for patients with irreversible intestinal failure who cannot be maintained on parenteral nutrition. Figure 25.6 describes an algorithm for patients with intestinal failure and the management that should be considered in defining those individuals for intestinal transplantation. Figure 25.7 represents intestinal transplant graft and patient survival data by era of transplant from the intestinal transplant registry.

Yamada's Atlas of Gastroenterology, Fifth Edition. Edited by Daniel K. Podolsky, Michael Camilleri, J. Gregory Fitz, Anthony N. Kalloo, Fergus Shanahan, and Timothy C. Wang.
© 2016 John Wiley & Sons, Ltd. Published 2016 by John Wiley & Sons, Ltd.
Companion website: www.yamadagastro.com/atlas

Box 25.1 Factors influencing short bowel syndrome.

Extent of intestine removed
Site of intestine removed
Presence of an ileocecal valve
Extent of intestinal adaptation
Underlying disease(s)

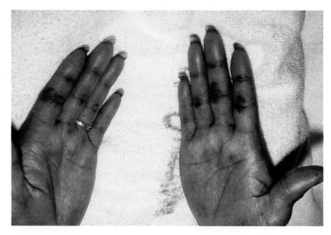

Figure 25.1 Acral skin lesions of a patient receiving home total parenteral nutrition without supplemental zinc.

Table 25.1 Antidiarrheal therapies.

Drug	Dosage	Adverse effects	Comments
Opiate agonists			
Opium and belladonna suppository	One q12h PRN	Sedation, potentially addictive, nausea, dry mucous membranes	60–65 mg opium, 15–16 mg belladonna
Opium (Diban)	One q4h PRN	Sedation, nausea, potentially addictive	Capsule: 12 mg opium, 52 g hyoscyamine, 10 g atropine, 3 g scopolamine, 300 mg attapulgite, 71 mg pectin
Opium camphor (paregoric)	Varies depending on concentration	Sedation, nausea, potentially addictive	May not be generally available
Codeine	30 mg–60 mg q4h PRN	Sedation, nausea, potentially addictive	Tablet: 15 mg or 30 mg; solution: 30 mg/mL or 60 mg/mL
Diphenoxylate atropine sulfate (Lomotil, generics)	5 mg initially then 2.5 mg after each loose bowel movement to a maximum of 20 mg/day	Sedation, abdominal cramps, dry skin and mucous membranes (from atropine), some addiction potential	Capsule: 2.5 mg diphenoxylate, 0.025 mg atropine
Loperamide (Imodium, generics)	2 mg after each loose bowel movement to a maximum of 16 mg/day	Sedation, abdominal cramps	Capsule: 2 mg; solution: 2 mg/10 mL. After oral administration absorption is poor, ~40% excreted unabsorbed in feces
α_2-Adrenergic agonists			
Clonidine (Catapres, generics)	0.1 mg–0.6 mg q12h	Centrally medicated sedation and hypotension	Tablets: 0.1 mg and 0.2 mg
Somatostatin			
Octreotide (Sandostatin)	50 μg–500 μg q8–12h	Pain at injection site, diarrhea, abdominal pain	Ampules: 50 μg, 100 μg, and 500 μg; multidose vial: 200 and 1000 μg/mL
Sandostatin LAR depot	10–30 mg q4 weeks intragluteally	Pain at injection site, diarrhea, abdominal pain	Ampules: 10 mg, 20 mg, and 30 mg
Bulking agents			
Psyllium (Fibrepur, Metamucil, generics)	1 tsp (5 g–6 g) q12h	Inhaled psyllium powder may cause allergic reaction	Products in which psyllium has been mixed with laxatives need to be avoided
Cholestyramine resin (Questran, generics)	4 g q12h	Nausea, fat-soluble vitamin deficiency with long term use, may bind other drugs in GI tract	One packet: 4 g; should not be taken dry must be mixed with fluids; no oral drugs 1 h before or 4 h after
			Useful in patients with residual colon to prevent bile-salt induced secretory diarrhea

GI, gastrointestinal.

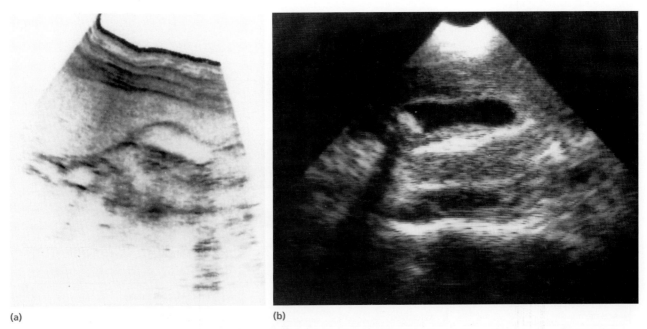

(a)   (b)

Figure 25.2 Ultrasound scans of the gallbladder of a 35-year-old woman with severe short bowel syndrome after multiple resections for Crohn's disease. **(a)** Ultrasound scan before home total parenteral nutrition (TPN) shows no stones. **(b)** Ultrasound scan after 2 years of home TPN demonstrates stones and sludge. The patient needed a cholecystectomy for symptomatic cholelithiasis.

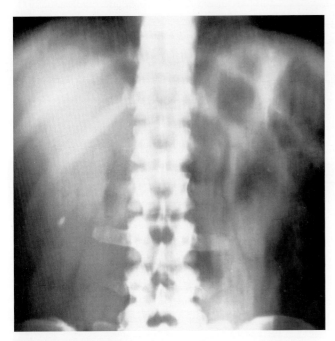

Figure 25.3 Nephrotomogram of a patient after resection of all but 100 cm of small intestine because of midgut volvulus with infarction showing bilateral renal calculi. The patient had hyperoxaluria (urinary oxalate excretion 70 mg/day). Analysis of a surgically extracted stone showed that it was composed of calcium oxalate.

Box 25.2 Foods that contain high oxalate concentrations.

Apples	Cola	Plums
Asparagus	Collard greens	Potatoes
Bananas	Concord grapes	Rhubarb
Beets	Cranberries	Spinach
Brussel sprouts	Green beans	Strawberries
Cabbage	Mustard greens	Tea
Carrots	Oranges	Tomatoes
Celery	Peaches	Turnip greens
Cherries	Pears	
Chocolate	Peas	

Centers performing large numbers of intestinal transplants are reporting 1 year graft and patient survival rates of 90% and 70%, respectively.

A recent development in the treatment of short bowel syndrome is the use of lipid emulsions. In our practice, we use Clinoleic™ (a soybean and olive oil emulsion) initially and SMOFlipids (soybean/medium-chain triglycerides/olive/fish oils) in those with cholestasis. Omegaven (an omega-3 fatty acid emulsion based on fish oils) is used as a rescue therapy in patients with advanced parenteral nutrition cholestasis. Table 25.15 highlights the composition of common lipid emulsions.

Preliminary evidence suggests a therapeutic role of teduglutide (a glucagon-like peptide 2 analogue) to wean short bowel patients off of chronic parenteral nutrition. However, more work needs to be done to assess long-term efficacy and identify suitable patients most likely to respond. Thus, the exact role for teduglutide within clinical practice is unclear at this time.

Table 25.2 Sample adult TPN orders.

Patient weight _____ kg

〰️ Central administration 〰️ Peripheral administration

Components	Recommended requirements	24 hour intake (g)	Energy provided (kcal)	24 hour volume (mL)	Rate (mL/h)	Pharmacy use only
Amino acids (as 10%)	1–1.5 g/kg/24 h				███	
Dextrose (as D70W)	2–4 mg/kg/min				███	
Additional volume[1]	150 mL minimum	███	███		███	
Total amino acid dextrose solution (mL)	███	███	███	███		
Lipid (as 20%)	1 g/kg/24 h	███	███			
Total fluid volume	30 mL/kg/24 h	███	███		███	
Total energy (kcal)	25–30 kcal/kg/24 h	███	███	███	███	

Volume for additives and/or free water.[1]

Additives[5]	Recommended requirements	Total 24-hour intake
Acetate (mmol)	As required	
Calcium (mmol)	5–15 mmol/day	
Magnesium (mmol)	4–8 mmol/day	
Multiple vitamin soln[3]	10 mL/day	
Phosphate (mmol)	15–30 mmol/day	
Potassium (mmol)[1]	30–80 mmol/day	
Sodium (mmol)[1]	60–150 mmol/day	
Trace element soln[4]	1 mL/day	
Vitamin K (mg)	10 mg/week	

Zinc (mg)	Additional as required
Folic acid (mg)	Additional as required
Ranitidine/famotidine (circle one)	As required
Heparin (units)	As required
Insulin, human regular (units) novolin/humulin (circle one)[2]	As required
Other (specify)	

1. Sodium and potassium will be added as chloride salts unless otherwise indicated.
2. Patient must reach glucose hemostasis for at least 48 hours.
3. See Table 25.3.
4. See Table 25.6.
5. See Box 25.3.

*Cycled administration (if appropriate).
Cycle over _____ hours at _____ mL/h Start time _____ Stop time _____ Decrease rate to _____ ml/h Start time _____
~~~~~~~~~~~~~~~~~~~ device dependent.

Duration of order: *Maximum 96 hours.*
Date ordered _____ Date to be reordered _____

Nutrition support service signature _____ Physician signature _____

Bag number				
Nursing initials				
Date				

Table 25.3 Intravenous multiple vitamins: 12-component composition for use by adults.

Component	Amount per 10 mL
Biotin (μg)	60
D-panthenol (mg)	15
Folic acid (mg)	0.4
Niacinamide (mg)	40
Vitamin A (IU)	3300
Vitamin B-1, thiamine (mg)	3.0
Vitamin B-12, cyanocobalamin (μg)	5.0
Vitamin B-2, riboflavin (mg)	3.6
Vitamin B-6, pyridoxine (mg)	4.0
Vitamin C (mg)	100
Vitamin D (IU)	200
Vitamin E (IU)	10

Table 25.4 Intravenous trace element composition for use by both adults and children.

Component	Amount per 1 mL
Chromium	10 μg
Copper	1 mg
Manganese	0.5 mg
Selenium	60 μg
Zinc	5 mg

Table 25.5 Suggested daily intravenous intake of vitamins for adults.

Vitamin	RDA adult range
Ascorbic acid (mg)	45
Biotin (μg)	150–300[a]
Folacin (μg)	400
Niacin (mg)	12–20
Pantothenic acid (mg)	6–10[a]
Riboflavin (mg)	1.1–1.8
Thiamin (mg)	1.0–1.5
Vitamin A (IU)	4000–5000[b]
Vitamin B-12 (cyanocobalamin) (μg)	3
Vitamin B-8 (pyridoxine) (mg)	1.6–2.0
Vitamin D (IU)	400
Vitamin E (IU)	12–15

[a] Recommended daily allowance (RDA) not established; amount considered adequate in usual dietary intake.
[b] Assumes 50% intake as carotene, which is less available than vitamin A.
Results do not include requirements of pregnancy or lactation.

Table 25.6 Suggested daily intravenous intake of trace elements for adults.

Trace element	Stable adult	Adult in acute catabolic state[a]	Stable adult with intestinal losses[a]
Chromium	10–15 μg		
Copper	0.5–1.5 mg		
Manganese	0.15–0.8 mg		
Selenium	40–80 μg		
Zinc	2.5–4.0 mg	Additional 2.0 mg	Add 17.1 mg/kg of stool or ileostomy output

[a] Frequent monitoring of blood levels for these patients is essential to provide proper dosage.

Box 25.3 Additive equivalents for use in both adult and pediatric total parenteral nutrition solutions.

1 g dextrose = 3.4 kcal
1 g fat = 9 kcal
1 g nitrogen = 6.25 g protein
1 g protein = 4 kcal
20% lipid: 1 mL = 2 kcal
Amino acid = 100 mOsm/g
Calcium gluconate: 1 mEq = 0.5 mmol Ca^{2+} = 216 mg Ca^{2+}
Dextrose = 50 mOsm/g
Magnesium sulfate: 1 mEq = 0.5 mmol Mg^{2+} = 125 mg Mg^{2+}
Potassium acetate: 1 mEq = 1 mmol K^+
Potassium chloride: 1 mEq = 1 mmol K^+
Potassium phosphate: 1 mL = 4.4 mmol K^+ and 3 mmol P
Sodium acetate: 1 mEq = 1 mmol Na^+
Sodium phosphate: 1 mL = 4 mmol Na^+ and 3 mmol P

Box 25.4 Suggested routine bloodwork for adults and children (6 months to 14 years) on total parenteral nutrition.

Initial: CBC, electrolytes, magnesium, phosphorus, calcium, albumin, PT (INR), PTT, creatinine, urea, glucose
Biweekly: CBC, sodium, potassium, CO_2, creatinine, urea, glucose
Weekly (as appropriate): alkaline phosphatase, albumin, ALT, bilirubin, magnesium, phosphorus, calcium, PT (INR), PTT
Others as needed: 24-h urine for electrolytes and nitrogen balance, cholesterol, triglycerides

ALT, alanine aminotransferase; CBC, complete blood count; INR, international normalized ratio; PT, prothrombin time; PTT, partial thromboplastin time.

Table 25.7 Sample pediatric TPN order form.

Patient weight _____ kg   Height _____ cm
〰 Central administration   〰 Peripheral administration (*Maximum 12.5% dextrose concentration*)

Components	24 hour intake (g)	Energy provided (kcal)	24 hour volume (mL)	Rate (mL/h)	Pharmacy use only
Additional volume[1]	███	███		███	
Amino acids (as 10%)				███	
Dextrose (as D70W)				███	
Lipid (as 20%)					
Total amino acid-dextrose solution (mL)	███				
Total energy (kcal)	███	███	███	███	
Total volume	███	███	███	███	

Volume for additives and/or free water.[1]

Additives[4]	Recommended requirements	Total 24-hour intake
Acetate (mmol)	For correction of acidemia	
Calcium (mmol)	0.5–1 mmol/kg/day	
Heparin (units)	As required	
Magnesium (mmol)	0.3–0.5 mmol/kg/day	
Multiple vitamin solution, pediatric[2]	5 mL/day	
Phosphate (mmol)	0.5–1 mmol/kg/day	
Potassium (mmol)[1]	1–3 mmol/kg/day	
Sodium (mmol)[1]	2–3 mmol/kg/day	
Trace element soln[3]	0.02 mL/kg to a maximum of 1 mL/day	

1. Sodium and potassium will be added as chloride salts unless otherwise indicated.
2. See Table 25.8.
3. See Table 25.11.
4. See Box 25.3.

Duration of order: *Maximum 96 hours*.
Date ordered _____   Date to be reordered _____

Nutrition support service signature _____ Physician signature _____

Bag number					
Nursing initials					
Date					

Table 25.8 Intravenous multiple vitamin composition for use by children aged from 6 months to 14 years.

Component	Amount per 5 mL
Biotin (μg)	20
D-panthenol (mg)	5
Folic acid (mg)	0.14
Niacinamide (mg)	17
Vitamin A (IU)	2300
Vitamin B-1, thiamin (mg)	1.2
Vitamin B-12, cyanocobalamin (μg)	1
Vitamin B-2, riboflavin (mg)	1.4
Vitamin B-6, pyridoxine (mg)	1
Vitamin C (mg)	80
Vitamin D (IU)	400
Vitamin E (IU)	7
Vitamin K (μg)	200

Table 25.9 Suggested protein, fat, and energy requirements for children.

Age	Gender	Protein requirements (g/kg/day)	Fat requirements (g/kg/day)	Energy requirements[a]
0–2 months	Both	2.2	1–3 (initiate at 1 g/kg/d)	100–200 kcal/kg/day
3–4 months	Both	1.5		95–100 kcal/kg/day
6–8 months	Both	1.4		95–97 kcal/kg/day
9–11 months	Both	1.4		97–99 kcal/kg/day
1–3 years	Both	1.2		13.5 kcal/cm/day
4–6 years	Both	1.1	1–3 (initiate at 1 g/kg/d)	17 kcal/cm/day
7–9 years	M	1.0		17.5 kcal/cm/day
	F	1.0		15 kcal/cm/day
10–12 years	M	1.0		17.5 kcal/cm/day
	F	1.0		15.5 kcal/cm/day
13–15 years	M	1.0	2 (initiate at 1 g/kg/d)	17.5 kcal/cm/day
	F	0.9		14 kcal/cm/day
16–18 years	M	0.9		18.5 kcal/cm/day
	F	0.9		13 kcal/cm/day

[a] Actual energy requirements may vary by 20%–30% depending on stress and activity factors.

Table 25.10 Suggested daily intravenous intake of vitamins for children.

Vitamin	Term infants and children (dose per day)
Lipid soluble	
A (μg)[a]	700
D (μg)[c]	10
E (mg)[b]	7
K (μg)	200
Water soluble	
Ascorbic acid (mg)	80
Biotin (μg)	20
Folate (μg)	140
Niacin (mg)	17
Pantothenate (mg)	5
Pyridoxine (mg)	1.0
Riboflavin (mg)	1.4
Thiamin (mg)	1.2
Vitamin B-12 (μg)	1.0

[a] 700 μg vitamin A = 2300 IU.
[b] 7 mg vitamin E (α-tocopherol) = 7 IU.
[c] 10 μg vitamin D = 400 IU.

Table 25.11 Suggested daily intravenous intake of trace elements in children.

Element	Infants (μg/kg/day)		Children (μg/kg/day)
	Preterm	Term	
Chromium[b]	0.20	0.20	0.20 (5)
Copper[a]	20	20	20 (300)
Iodide	1.0	1.0	1.0 (70)
Manganese[a]	1.0	1.0	1.0 (50)
Molybdenum[a]	0.25	0.25	0.25 (5)
Selenium[b]	2.0	2.0	2.0 (30)
Zinc	400	250 < 3 months	50 (5000)[c]
		100 > 3 months	

[a] Omit for patients with obstructive jaundice.
[b] Omit for patients with renal dysfunction.
[c] Values in parentheses are maximum number of micrograms per day.

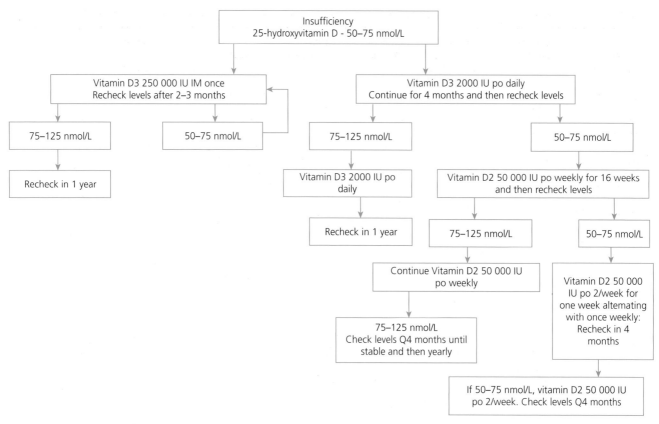

Figure 25.4 Vitamin D supplementation algorithm – insufficiency.

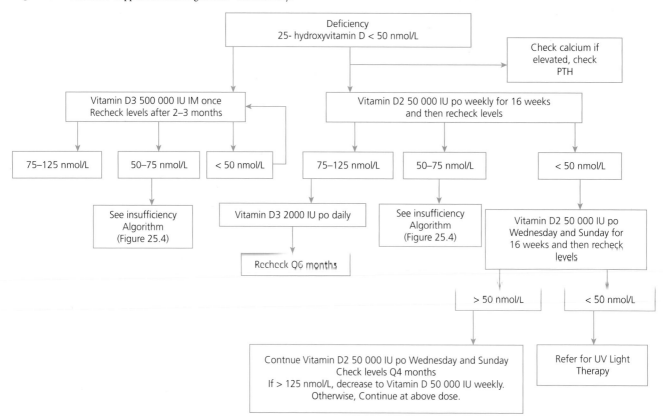

Figure 25.5 Vitamin D supplementation algorithm – deficiency.

Table 25.12 Complications of home parenteral nutrition (January 2004–October 2014; episodes per catheter year unless indicated; [95% CI]).

Study (1st author, publication year)	Catheter sepsis	Catheter sepsis (episodes per patient year)	Catheter occlusion	Central vein thrombosis	Liver/biliary problems	Metabolic bone disease	Other
Dibb, 2014	0.14	–	–	–	–	–	–
Higuera, 2014	0.01	–	0.00	0.00	0.05	0.17	–
Elfassy, 2013	0.79	0.74	–	–	–	–	–
Gillanders, 2012	0.97	–	0.13	–	–	–	–
Wiskin, 2011	–	0.01	–	–	–	–	–
Elriz, 2011	–	–	–	–	0.02	–	0.01 Mortality
Mohammed, 2011	–	8.74	–	–	–	–	–
Santarpia, 2010	0.62	0.66	–	–	–	–	–
Elphick, 2009	–	–	–	–	–	–	0.13 Muscle cramps
Colomb, 2007	–	0.44	–	–	0.09[a]	–	–
Dray, 2007	–	–	–	–	Cholelithiasis 0.5[a]; biliary complications 0.77[a]	–	–
Marra, 2007	0.85	1.17	–	0.06	–	–	–
De Burgoa, 2006	–	1.41[a]	0.17[a]	–	–	–	–
Raman, 2006	–	–	–	–	–	0.81[a]	–
Shirotani, 2006	0.30 (0.18, 0.47)	0.24 (0.14, 0.38)	0.03 (0.00, 0.09)	0.02 (0.00, 0.09)	–	–	–
Ugur, 2006	0.48	–	–	0.02	–	–	–
Hoda, 2005	–	0.36	–	0.08[a]	0.04[a]	–	–
Ireton-Jones, 2005	0.13	–	0.24	–	–	–	–

[a]Episodes per patient year.

Table 25.13 Quality of life for patients receiving home parenteral nutrition (January 2004–October 2014).

Study (1st author, publication year)	Who values	Instrument used	Profile or index	Index scores	Best QOL or outcome	Worst QOL or outcome	Comments
Chambers, 2006	Patient	SF-36, EQ5D	Index	QOL scores rose significantly within the first 6 months of HPN	Mental health, emotional role were same as normative data after 6 months of HPN	Body pain, general health, physical component did not significantly improve	All QOL scores at discharge were lower than normative data
Huisman-de Waal, 2006	Patient	Interviews	Profile	–	Psychosocial issues, physical problems, dependence, patient–care provider issues	One-third endorsed incapability due to physical limitations	Underlying theme expressed by respondents: loss, longing, and grief
Pironi, 2006	Patient	SF-36	Index	Physical functioning 2.3 and role 1.5; pain 1.0; health 1.2; vitality 0.5; social 0.9; emotional 0.7; mental 0.0	–	–	HPN subjects had poorer physical health scores compared with ITx
Gottrand, 2005	Patient, parents, siblings, doctor	Validated questionnaires; type dependent upon age	Index	No significant difference between QOL scores for all ages vs healthy children	Parents rated child's QOL higher vs doctors	Parents of HPN infants scored child's QOL lower than parents of healthy infants	Unlike adult HPN patients, pediatric QOL for HPN patients is not lower than their healthy counterparts
Orrevall, 2005	Patient, family	Semistructured interview	Profile	–	Acceptable: improved strength, activity, sense of relief, and security	Restrictive family life and social contacts	HPN benefits outweigh negative aspects
Persoon, 2005	Patient	Nonvalidated questionnaire and interview	Profile	–	–	Severe depression (65%) and fatigue (63%)	Low QOL associated with fatigue, sleeping disorders, anxiety, depression, and social impairment

HPN, home parenteral nutrition; QOL, Quality of life

Table 25.14 Survival rates when receiving home parenteral nutrition (January 2004–October 2014)

Study (1st author, publication year)	Benign underlying disease	Malignant underlying disease (including AIDS)
Higuera, 2014	10 year survival 65%	Cancer: mean survival 1.0 year
Bonifacio, 2007	1 year survival 90.2%; 3 year survival 87.8%; 5 year survival 82.9%	–
Colomb, 2007	2 year survival 97%; 5 year survival 89%; 10 year survival 81%	–
Lloyd, 2006	1 year survival 86%; 3 year survival 77%; 5 year survival 73%; 10 year survival 71%	–
Ugur, 2006	–	Cancer: mean survival 1.0 year (0.2–2.4)
Gavazzi, 2005	5 year survival: radiation enteritis, 90%	–
Hoda, 2005	–	Cancer: median time to death 5 months (range 1–154 months)
Duerksen, 2004	–	Gastric or colon cancer: variable survival rate of 27–433 days; 67% survived for longer than 60 days
Vantini, 2004	1 year survival 95%; 4 year survival 79%; 6 year survival 66%. Survival better in patients with >50 cm small bowel ($P < 0.05$) or in those starting HPN > age 45 ($P < 0.02$)	–

AIDS, acquired immunodeficiency syndrome.

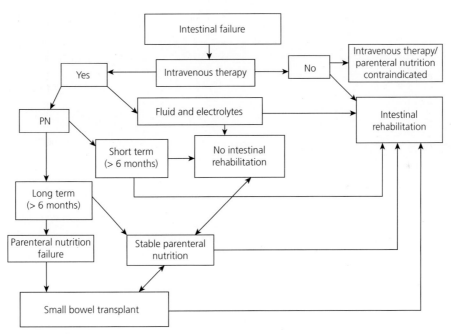

Figure 25.6 Algorithm for intestinal failure.

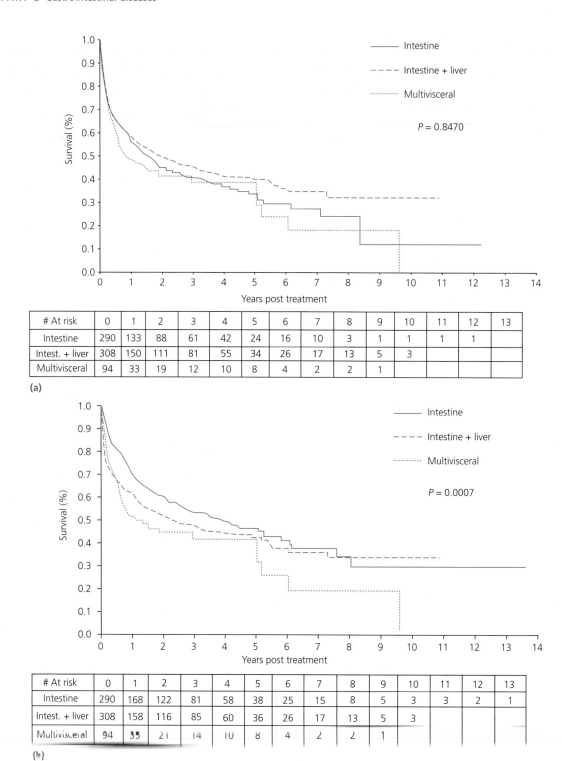

(a)

(b)

Figure 25.7 Intestinal transplant graft **(a)** and patient **(b)** survival by era of transplant.

Table 25.15 Composition of common lipid emulsions.

Product	Intralipid	Liposyn II	ClinOleic	SMOF lipid	Omegaven
Manufacturer	Baxter Healthcare/ Fresenius Kabi	Hospira	Baxter Healthcare/ Parenteral S.A.	Fresenius Kabi	Fresenius Kabi
Oil source (g)					
Soybean	10	5	2	3	0
Safflower	0	5	0	0	0
MCT	0	0	0	3	0
Olive oil	0	0	8	2.5	0
Fish oil	0	0	0	1.5	10
α-Tocopherol (mg/l)	38	NR	32	200	150–296
Phytosterols (mg/l)	348 ± 33	383	327 ± 8	47.6	0
Fat composition (g)					
Linoleic	5.0	6.5	0.9	2.9	0.1–0.7
α-Linoleic	0.9	0.4	0.1	0.3	<0.2
EPA	0	0	0	0.3	1.28–2.82
DHA	0	0	0	0.05	1.44–3.09
Oleic	2.6	1.8	2.8	2.8	0.6–1.3
Palmitic	1.0	0.9	0.7	0.9	0.25–1.0
Stearic	0.35	0.34	0.2	0.3	0.05–0.2
Arachidonic	0	0	0.03	0.05	0.1–0.4

Values in Omegaven group represent means. Data provided by each manufacturer.
DHA, docosahexanoic acid; EPA, eicosapentaenoic acid; MCT, medium chain triglyceride; NR, not reported.

CHAPTER 26

Tumors of the small intestine

Barbara H. Jung[1] and Maria Rosario Ferreira[2]
[1] University of Illinois at Chicago, Chicago, IL, USA
[2] Northwestern University, Feinberg School of Medicine, Evanston, IL, USA

Tumors of the small intestine originate from epithelial, neuroendocrine, or mesenchymal cells. Overall, they are rare and account for only about 2% of all primary gastrointestinal tumors. Adenocarcinoma used to be the most common type of primary small intestinal cancer, but it is now being surpassed by small intestinal carcinoids. The mesenchymal gastrointestinal stromal tumors (GISTs), as well as primary small bowel lymphomas, are less common. Given their anatomic location in a difficult to reach part of the bowel, small intestinal tumors pose a significant challenge in regards to diagnosis and management; malignant tumors have often spread by the time of diagnosis. Both benign and malignant small bowel tumors are associated with significant morbidity and mortality, and more mechanistic insight is needed to advance therapeutic measures. This chapter summarizes our current knowledge on the various types of small intestinal tumors.

A 51-year-old man underwent an upper endoscopy for evaluation of dyspeptic symptoms. The exam was otherwise unremarkable except for a submucosal lesion identified in the duodenal bulb (Figure 26.1a). An endoscopic ultrasound was performed which revealed features consistent with hamartoma (Figure 26.1b). This was subsequently removed with endoscopic mucosal resection and the specimen is seen in Figure 26.1c.

A 61-year-old woman presented with iron deficiency anemia and had an initial negative evaluation with an esophagogastroduodenoscopy and colonoscopy. She then had a video capsule endoscopy revealing a jejunal lesion, in addition to several jejunal arteriovenous malformations (AVMs). An enteroscopy was performed and showed a jejunal tubulovillous adenoma (Figure 26.2), which was removed with endoscopic mucosal resection. The anemia improved after iron therapy, but eventually recurred, requiring repeat evaluation with enteroscopy. No further adenomas were identified but there were several AVMs that were cauterized, after which the anemia resolved.

A 73-year-old man presented with abdominal discomfort, gradually worsening over three months, associated with anorexia, early satiety, and weight loss of 20 pounds. Physical exam was unremarkable. An esophagogastroduodenoscopy revealed a mass in the third portion of the duodenum with biopsies consistent with adenocarcinoma. The patient underwent surgical resection (Figure 26.3a). Pathology confirmed adenocarcinoma (Figures 26.3b,c), the margins of resection were clear, however three of seven lymph nodes examined were positive for adenocarcinoma. The patient did well initially after resection, and received adjuvant chemotherapy with 5-fluorouracil. However, several months later there was evidence of metastatic disease in the liver and peritoneum and the patient died 18 months after the initial diagnosis.

A 44-year-old woman underwent an esophagogastroduodenoscopy for evaluation of abdominal pain. A nodular lesion was identified in the third portion of the duodenum (Figure 26.4a), with biopsies consistent with carcinoid. The patient underwent surgical resection (Figure 26.4b), the specimen is seen in Figure 26.4c. Pathology examination revealed carcinoid (Figures 26.4d,e), with positive chromogranin stain (Figure 26.4f). There was no evidence of metastatic spread to lymph nodes or distally. The patient did well and was alive with no evidence of disease after 3 years.

A 59-year-old man was admitted to the hospital with melena for 2–3 days, and anemia with indices consistent with iron deficiency. A colonoscopy was negative and an esophagogastroduodenoscopy did not reveal a source of acute or chronic blood loss. The patient had recurrence of melena and an enteroscopy was performed, revealing a submucosal mass with central depression, and ulceration in the third portion of the duodenum (Figure 26.5a). Surgical resection was performed the specimen is seen in Figures 26.5b–d. Pathology was consistent with GIST (Figures 26.5e,f). The patient did well after with no further gastrointestinal bleeding, and resolution of the

---

Yamada's Atlas of Gastroenterology, Fifth Edition. Edited by Daniel K. Podolsky, Michael Camilleri, J. Gregory Fitz, Anthony N. Kalloo, Fergus Shanahan, and Timothy C. Wang.
Companion website: www.yamadagastro.com/atlas

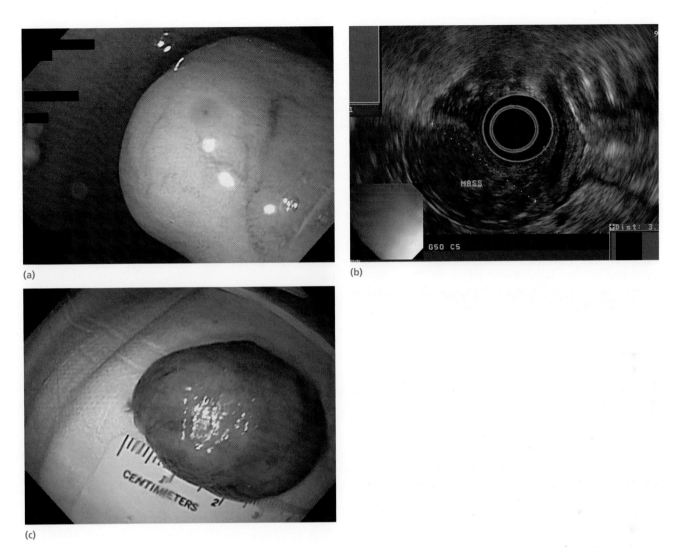

(a)

(b)

(c)

Figure 26.1 (a) Duodenal hamartoma, endoscopic view. **(b)** Endoscopic ultrasound. **(c)** Gross specimen after endoscopic mucosal resection.

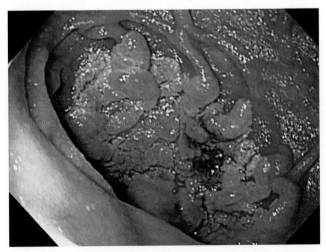

Figure 26.2 Jejunal tubulovillous adenoma, endoscopic view.

anemia of iron deficiency. He had no evidence of recurrence two years later.

A 78-year-old man presented with a several month history of abdominal pain, crampy, associated with anorexia and 30 pound weight loss. He also noted some subjective fever and night sweats. An esophagogastroduodenoscopy was unremarkable. A CT scan of the abdomen revealed thickening of the wall of a proximal segment of jejunum. Enteroscopy revealed a polypoid lesion in the proximal jejunum with biopsies consistent with B cell lymphoma. Initial staging did not reveal involvement beyond the small bowel. The patient underwent surgical resection, yielding the specimen shown in Figure 26.6a; pathology was consistent with B cell lymphoma (Figure 26.6b), including positive staining for CD 20 (Figure 26.6c). At the time of resection several of the lymph nodes exhibited involvement with lymphoma. The patient received adjuvant chemotherapy but the

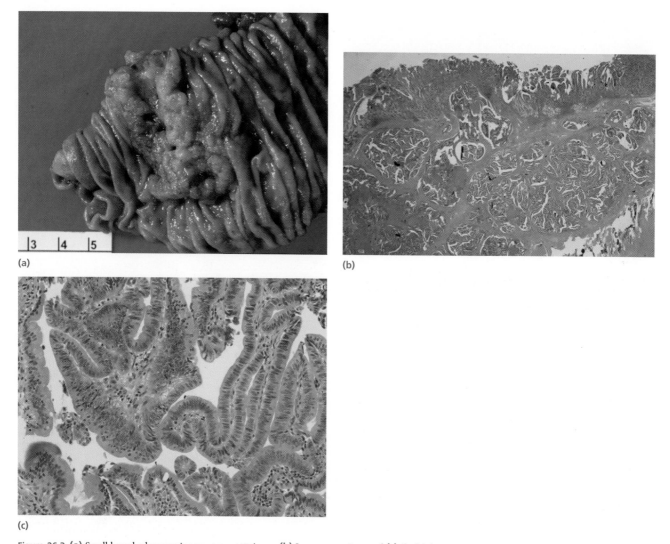

(a)

(b)

(c)

Figure 26.3 (a) Small bowel adenocarcinoma, gross specimen. (b) Low power view, and (c) the high power view.

disease progressed and he eventually died approximately 2 years after the initial diagnosis.

A 54-year-old woman presented with vague mid abdominal discomfort over a period of several months. Thickening of a segment of jejunal wall was revealed on a CT scan of the abdomen. Enteroscopy revealed an ulcerated mass, with biop-

sies consistent with follicular lymphoma. Staging for extra intestinal involvement was negative. The patient underwent surgical resection (Figure 26.7a), with pathology confirming follicular lymphoma (Figure 26.7b). There was no lymph node involvement. The patient received no further treatment and was well without evidence of recurrence 3 years later.

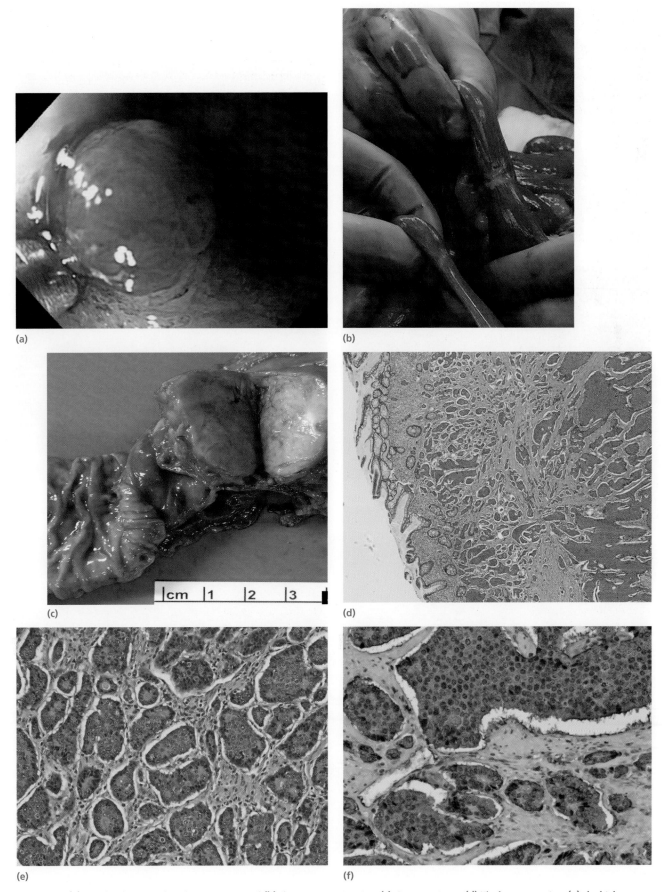

Figure 26.4 (a) Duodenal carcinoid, endoscopic view, and **(b)** the intraoperative view. **(c)** Gross specimen. **(d)** The low power view, **(e)** the high power view, and **(f)** high power view with chromogranin stain.

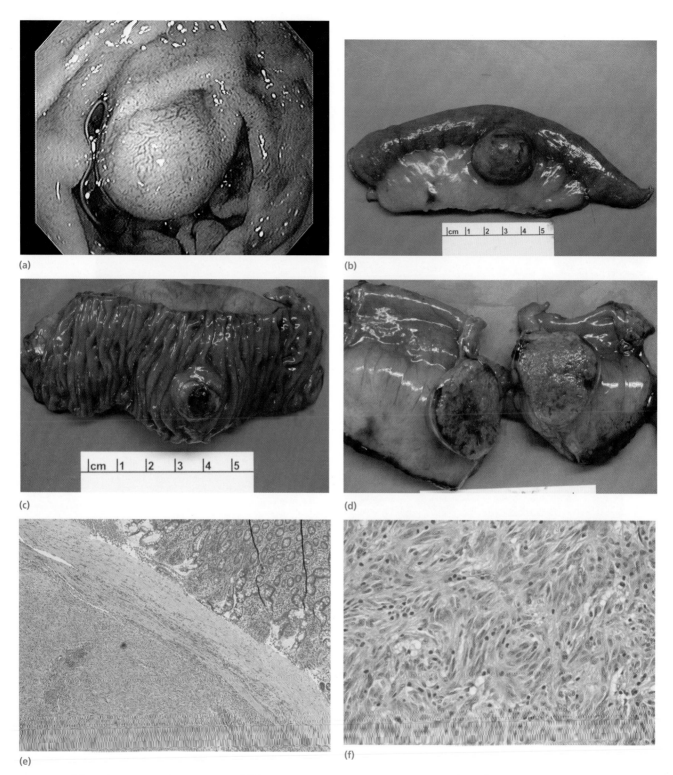

(a)

(b)

(c)

(d)

(e)

(f)

Figure 26.5 (a) Duodenal GIST, endoscopic view, and (b) gross specimen, peritoneal view. (c) Gross specimen, lumen view and (d) gross specimen, cross sectioned. (e) The low power view, and (f) the high power view.

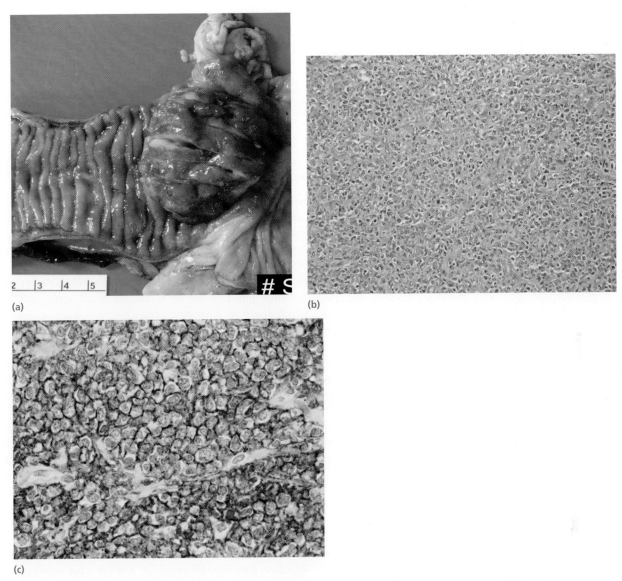

Figure 26.6 (a) Small bowel B cell lymphoma, gross specimen. **(b)** The high power view, and **(c)** the high power view with CD20 stain.

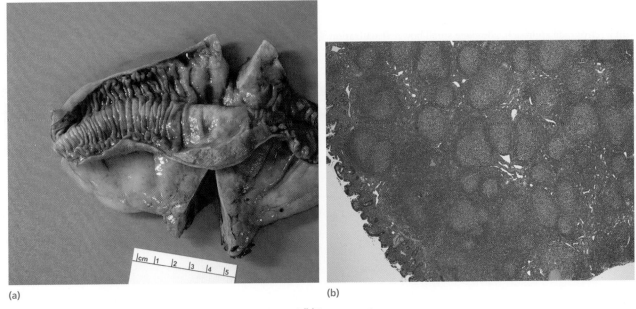

Figure 26.7 (a) Small bowel follicular lymphoma, gross specimen, and **(b)** low power view.

CHAPTER 27

Miscellaneous diseases of the small intestine

Marc S. Levin

VA St. Louis Health Care System and Washington University School of Medicine in St. Louis, St. Louis, MO, USA

Ulcers of the small intestine

There are many causes of ulcers of the small intestine (Table 27.1). Primary (idiopathic) small bowel ulcers are diagnosed when other identifiable causes of small bowel ulcers are eliminated. Seventy-five percent are located in the middle to distal ileum. Symptomatic complications include bleeding, perforation, and obstruction. The ulcers vary in size from 0.3 to 5 cm and usually have sharp, demarcated borders. The diagnosis sometimes is made with radiological studies, such as small bowel follow-through (Figure 27.1), enteroclysis, or more commonly computed tomography (CT) or magnetic resonance (MR) enterography (i.e., distension of small bowel loops achieved perorally without intubation). Advances in endoscopic techniques allow improved visualization of the small bowel mucosa, leading to more frequent identification of small bowel pathology. Push enteroscopy is a useful adjunct for the diagnosis of small intestine lesions in the proximal third of the small intestine. With the advent of wireless capsule endoscopy, visual images can be captured from the entire small bowel, though localization of abnormal findings is not always accurate. Wireless capsule endoscopy is superior to push enteroscopy and enteroclysis for the detection of small intestinal ulcers because it allows evaluation of almost the entire small bowel mucosa. When findings on wireless capsule endoscopy need further evaluation, deep small bowel enteroscopy for diagnosis, biopsies, and therapeutic interventions is now possible using single balloon, double balloon, or spiral techniques. When combined with a retrograde approach, complete small bowel visualization can sometimes be achieved. Intraoperative enteroscopy with laparotomy or laparoscopy remains a valuable adjunct in difficult cases, or when findings on other tests suggest the need for resection of a diseased small bowel segment.

Therapy is dictated by the severity of complications. Perforation and bleeding usually necessitate surgical resection.

Many medications have been known to cause ulcers and strictures of the small intestine (Table 27.2), and among them

nonsteroidal antiinflammatory drugs (NSAIDs) are recognized as common causes. Although the exact pathogenesis is unknown, increased intestinal permeability is believed to increase susceptibility to lumenal macromolecules, bacteria, and toxins. NSAID-mediated cyclooxygenase inhibition is not believed to play an important role in the pathogenesis. NSAID-associated intestinal injury primarily affects the distal small intestine, which leads to diagnostic confusion with Crohn's disease. Therapy includes discontinuation of the offending agent whenever possible. Surgical intervention may be needed for symptomatic strictures or intestinal perforation. When an acceptable alternative medication is unavailable, use of prodrugs such as sulindac or nabumetone may lessen intestinal toxicity.

Other medications implicated as ulcerogens include enteric-coated potassium chloride, ferrous salts (Figure 27.2), digoxin, corticosteroids, sodium polystyrene sulfonate (Kayexalate), cytarabine and other chemotherapeutic agents, and clofazimine. Parenteral gold therapy has been associated with enterocolitis characterized by edema and ulceration of the ileum. Ischemic damage can result from drugs that interfere with autonomic regulation of vascular supply to the bowel (see Table 27.2; Figure 27.3), or with the coagulation process, resulting in intravascular thrombus formation (Figure 27.4). On the other hand, anticoagulants can cause ulceration from intramucosal and transmural hematoma formation with mucosal pressure necrosis (Figure 27.5). Drug smugglers sometimes ingest packets of illicit drugs for transport to avoid detection (body packer, Figure 27.6), the rupture of which can result in overwhelming toxicity from the drug and often death of the smuggler.

Behçet syndrome is associated with intestinal ulceration among less than 1% of patients. These patients have multiple deep ulcers, often bleeding or penetrating, in the ileocecal region. Microthrombosis and vasculitis with intestinal ischemia can result in intestinal ulceration in systemic lupus erythematosus. Mesenteric vasculitis with small bowel ischemia and stricture formation has been reported in rheumatoid arthritis,

Yamada's Atlas of Gastroenterology, Fifth Edition. Edited by Daniel K. Podolsky, Michael Camilleri, J. Gregory Fitz, Anthony N. Kalloo, Fergus Shanahan, and Timothy C. Wang.
© 2016 John Wiley & Sons, Ltd. Published 2016 by John Wiley & Sons, Ltd.
Companion website: www.yamadagastro.com/atlas

Table 27.1 Causes of small intestine ulceration.

Infectious	Tuberculosis, typhoid, cytomegalovirus infection, syphilis, parasitic infestation, strongyloidosis hyperinfection, *Campylobacter* infection, yersiniosis
Toxic	Acute jejunitis (β-toxin-producing *Clostridium perfringens*), arsenic
Inflammatory	Crohn's disease, systemic lupus erythematosus with high serum antiphospholipid levels, diverticulitis
Mucosal lesions	Gluten-sensitive enteropathy (jejunoileitis)
Tumors	
Primary	Malignant histiocytosis, lymphoma
Secondary	Adenocarcinoma, melanoma, Kaposi sarcoma
Vascular	Mesenteric insufficiency, giant cell arteritis, vasculitis, vascular abnormality, amyloidosis (ischemic lesion)
Hyperacidic	Zollinger–Ellison syndrome, Meckel diverticulum, stomal ulceration
Metabolic	Uremia
Drugs	Potassium chloride, nonsteroidal antiinflammatory drugs, antimetabolites
Radiation	Therapeutic, accidental
Idiopathic	Primary ulcer, Behçet syndrome

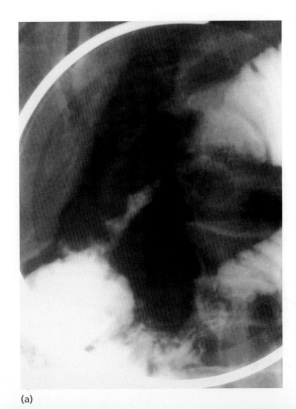

(a)

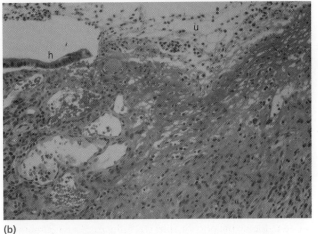

(b)

Figure 27.1 **(a)** Small bowel follow-through image of a patient who sought treatment with clinical features obstruction of the small intestine shows intestinal spasm associated with ulceration and dilation of the proximal segment. The patient underwent exploratory laparotomy and resection of the affected bowel segment. **(b)** Histopathological section of the resected segment of small bowel shows ulceration (u) with epithelialization of the healing edge (h). A nifedipine capsule was found in the vicinity of the ulcer at operations, raising the possibility of a causative association. Source: **(a)** Courtesy of Dr. Dennis Balfe; **(b)** courtesy of Dr. Paul Swanson.

scleroderma, polyarteritis nodosa (Figure 27.7), Henoch–Schönlein purpura, Wegener granulomatosis (Figure 27.8), giant cell arteritis, Churg–Strauss syndrome, and Sézary syndrome. Spasm of the mesenteric arteries (see Figure 27.3), sometimes induced by drugs such as ergot or cocaine, can cause mesenteric ischemia and result in ulceration if prolonged. Thrombosis of the mesenteric veins resulting from many conditions, including hypercoagulable states and collagen vascular diseases, can cause transmural hemorrhage, mucosal ulceration, or even perforation of the bowel (see Figure 27.4). Angiodysplasia consists of ectatic submucosal blood vessels with a thin, overlying mucosal layer (Figure 27.9), the erosion or rupture of which can result in ulceration and gastrointestinal bleeding. Radiation damage to the intestine can result in fibrosis of the submucosal layers and vascular insufficiency with the formation of intraepithelial telangiectasia (Figure 27.10). Stricture formation can result in bowel obstruction, sometimes necessitating surgical intervention.

Chronic ulcerative jejunoileitis (CUJ) is a rare clinical syndrome. It occurs most frequently among patients with longstanding gluten-sensitive enteropathy in the sixth or seventh decade of life. It is characterized by malabsorption, abdominal pain, and multiple nonmalignant ulcers of the small intestine. Villous atrophy, which is believed to be related to infiltration by activated T cells, usually is present. Mucosal ulceration, crypt

Table 27.2 Drug-induced small bowel disease.

Mechanism	Drugs implicated
Erosive damage	Nonsteroidal antiinflammatory drugs, potassium chloride
Ischemic damage	
Hypotension	Antihypertensives, diuretics
Direct vasoconstriction	Norepinephrine, dopamine, vasopressin
Decreased splanchnic blood flow	Digoxin
Increased sympathetic stimulation	Cocaine
Vasospasm	Ergot compounds
Arterial/venous thrombosis	Oral contraceptives
Hematoma formation	Anticoagulants
Motility disorders	
Pseudoobstruction	Anticholinergics, phenothiazines, tricyclic antidepressants, opioids, verapamil, clonidine, cyclosporine
Neurotoxicity	Vincristine
Narcotic bowel syndrome	Narcotics
Malabsorption	
Interference with intralumenal digestion	Tetracycline, cholestyramine, mineral oil, aluminum and magnesium hydroxide
Increased intestinal transit	Prokinetic agents, cathartics
Mucosal injury	Colchicine, neomycin, methotrexate, methyldopa, allopurinol, mefenamic acid
Direct inhibition of absorption	Sodium aminosalicylate, thiazide diuretics
Inhibition of epithelial cell turnover	
Erosive enteritis	Methotrexate, 5-fluorouracil, actinomycin D, doxorubicin, cytosine arabinoside, bleomycin, vincristine, ara-C, interleukin-2

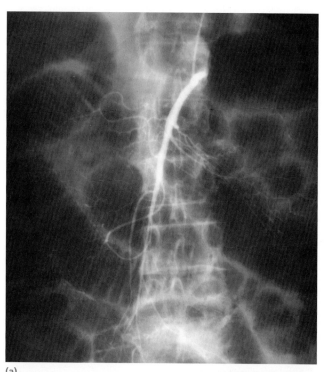

(a)

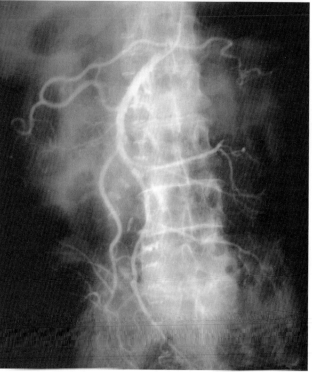

(b)

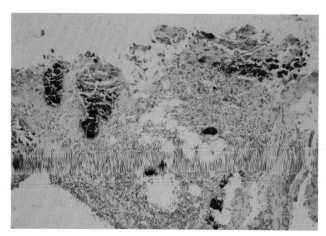

Figure 27.2 Prussian blue stain shows iron deposition in an ulcer of the terminal ileum. Iron tablets were thought to be the cause of small bowel ulceration and occult gastrointestinal bleeding in this patient. Source: Courtesy of Dr. Paul Swanson.

Figure 27.3 **(a)** Mesenteric arteriogram of a patient with abdominal pain and ileus shows spasm of the superior mesenteric circulation. Prolonged spasm of the mesenteric vessels can lead to vascular insufficiency and intestinal ulceration. **(b)** Repeat arteriography after intraarterial infusion of papaverine shows relief of the spasm and ileus and restoration of normal blood flow to the intestine. Source: Courtesy of Dr. Daniel Picus.

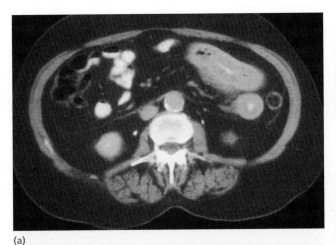

(a)

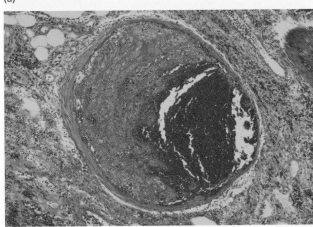

(b)

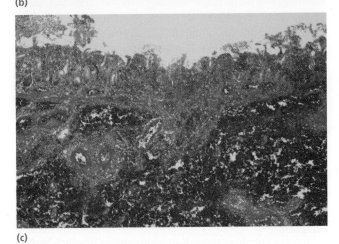

(c)

Figure 27.4 (a) Computed tomographic scan of a patient with superior mesenteric venous thrombosis shows a thickened loop of small bowel. This can cause mucosal sloughing with ulceration and intestinal perforation that necessitates exploratory laparotomy and bowel resection. **(b)** Section through the superior mesenteric vein shows acute and organizing thrombus within the lumen. **(c)** Section through surgically resected segment of bowel shows transmural hemorrhage and acute inflammation with focal epithelial necrosis. Source: **(a)** Courtesy of Dr. Dennis Balfe; **(b, c)** courtesy of Dr. Paul Swanson.

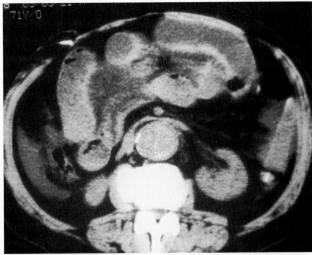

Figure 27.5 Abdominal computed tomographic scan of a patient who took an overdose of warfarin demonstrates bowel hemorrhage. The intestinal wall appears thickened because of the presence of intramural hematomas. Required therapeutic interventions included correction of coagulopathy and surgical resection of the affected bowel segments. Source: Courtesy of Dr. Dennis Balfe.

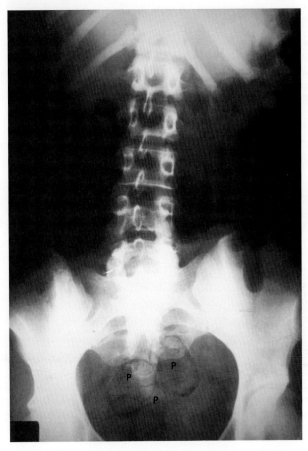

Figure 27.6 Plain radiograph of the abdomen of a drug smuggler shows multiple packets (P) of illicit drugs in the bowel lumen. Body-packer syndrome occurs when rupture of the drug-containing packets causes severe drug toxicity. Source: Courtesy of Dr. Dennis Balfe.

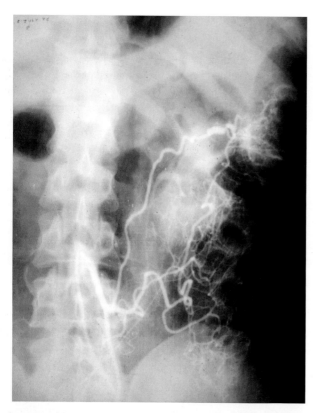

Figure 27.7 Mesenteric arteriogram of a patient with polyarteritis nodosa shows beaded appearance of the medium-sized arteries. Vasculitis of the arteries supplying the bowel can lead to intestinal ulceration. Angiography of other vessels, including the renal arteries, can show aneurysmal dilation. Source: Courtesy of Dr. Dennis Balfe.

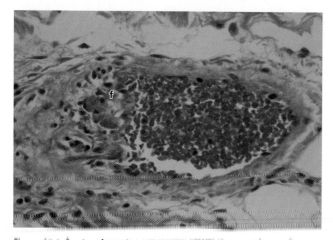

Figure 27.8 Section through a mesenteric artery shows evidence of vasculitis and fibrinoid necrosis (f) involving the arterial wall. This patient with Wegener granulomatosis had bowel ischemia, ulceration, and gastrointestinal bleeding that necessitated surgical resection of the affected bowel segment. Source: Courtesy of Dr. Paul Swanson.

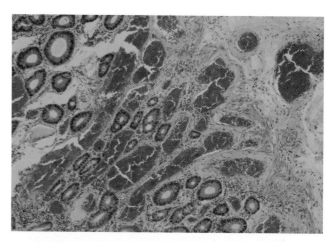

Figure 27.9 Section through angiodysplasia of the small intestine shows typical thickened and ectatic vasculature involving mucosa and submucosa (red). Rupture or erosion of the mucosa over areas of angiodysplasia can result in ulceration and gastrointestinal bleeding that can be difficult to localize. Intraoperative enteroscopy sometimes is necessary to identify the segment of bowel that needs surgical resection. Source: Courtesy of Dr. Paul Swanson.

hyperplasia, and an inflammatory cell infiltrate also occur and result in malabsorption and protein-losing enteropathy. Other symptoms include midepigastric pain, weight loss, and complications of ulceration, including small bowel obstruction, bleeding, and perforation. The diagnosis should be considered in the care of patients with long-standing gluten-sensitive enteropathy with worsening malabsorption despite continued compliance with a gluten-free diet. Biopsies of the small intestine are essential to establish the diagnosis. Although oral steroids and surgical resection of severely affected bowel have been tried, no specific therapy has been shown to modulate the course of CUJ. Data suggest that CUJ may be an important risk factor for the development of enteropathy-associated T-cell lymphoma (Figure 27.11).

Necrotizing enterocolitis

Acute jejunitis is largely a disease of nonindustrialized nations. Outbreaks are most frequent in communities in which poor nutrition and poor food hygiene are prevalent. *Clostridium perfringens* type C has been established as the causative organism. The illness is characterized by bloody diarrhea, fever, and abdominal pain. Nonocclusive small intestinal ischemia results in necrosis of varying severity. Successful treatment involves

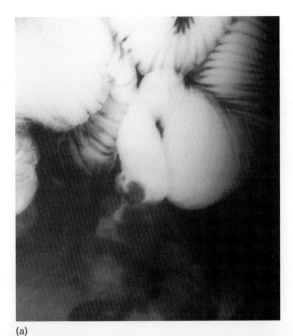

(a)

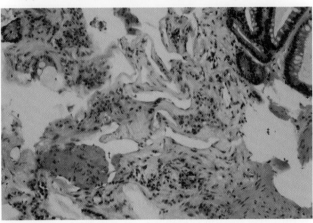

(b)

Figure 27.10 (a) Intestinal stricture with food impaction and dilation of proximal segment in a patient who had received radiation therapy for lymphoma. This patient had clinical features of small bowel obstruction and underwent surgical resection of the affected segment.
(b) Histopathological section of the surgically resected segment shows fibrosis of the lamina propria (f) with mucosal telangiectasis (t), a common finding with radiation-induced intestinal injury. Source:
(a) Courtesy of Dennis Balfe; **(b)** courtesy of Dr. Paul Swanson.

early recognition, antibiotics, and surgical resection of severely affected bowel segments.

Neonatal necrotizing enterocolitis (NEC) is a disorder of unknown causation. It affects premature infants and low-birth-weight neonates. It is characterized by focal or diffuse small intestine ulceration and necrosis (Figure 27.12). Pathogenic etiological factors implicated include prematurity, intestinal ischemia, infectious agents, and initiation of enteral nutrition. There is a high prevalence among infants whose mothers used cocaine during pregnancy, suggesting a pathogenic role of hypoxic and ischemic injury. Although no organism has been consistently identified with NEC, a pathogenic role for bacteria is suggested by the occurrence of epidemics within intensive care units.

Protein-losing gastroenteropathy

The defining characteristic of protein-losing gastroenteropathy (PLGE) is hypoproteinemia resulting from gastric or intestinal loss of plasma proteins in abnormal amounts. A number of intestinal disorders have been implicated in the pathogenesis (Box 27.1; Figures 27.13 and 27.14; see Figure 27.11). The diagnosis is established with documentation of excessive intestinal protein losses by means of measuring fecal α_1-antitrypsin clearance. There is no specific therapy for PLGE, and management of the primary condition is the only effective remedy.

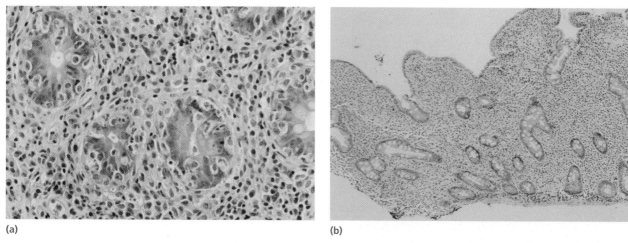

(a)   (b)

Figure 27.11 (a) Infiltration of a segment of small bowel with large atypical lymphoid cells consistent with enteropathy-associated T-cell lymphoma in a patient with refractory celiac disease. This condition can present with malabsorption, ulceration of the intestine, and protein-losing enteropathy. **(b)** Monotonous plasma cell infiltration of small bowel mucosa in a patient with α-heavy-chain disease, which can also result in malabsorption and protein-losing enteropathy. Source: Courtesy of Dr. Paul Swanson.

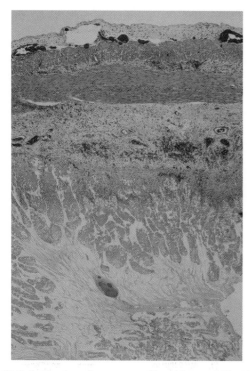

Figure 27.12 Section through a segment of bowel from a child with necrotizing enterocolitis shows submucosal hemorrhage, epithelial necrosis and an acute inflammatory cell infiltrate. Source: Courtesy of Dr. Paul Swanson.

Box 27.1 Causes of protein-losing enteropathy.

Increased interstitial pressure
  Congenital intestinal lymphangiectasia
  Mesenteric lymphatic obstruction
    Tuberculosis
    Sarcoidosis
    Lymphoma
    Retroperitoneal fibrosis
Increased central venous pressure
  Constrictive pericarditis
  Congestive heart failure
Ulcerative disease
  Erosive gastritis or enteritis
  Helicobacter pylori associated gastritis
  Neoplasia: carcinoma or lymphoma
  Crohn's disease
  Pseudomembranous enterocolitis
  Acute graft-versus-host disease
Nonulcerative disease
  Giant hypertrophic gastropathy (Ménétrier disease)
  Atrophic gastritis
  Eosinophilic gastroenteritis
  Collagenous colitis
  Polyposis syndromes (e.g., Cronkhite–Canada, Peutz–Jeghers, and
    juvenile polyposis)
  Hypertrophic hypersecretory gastropathy
  Viral enteritides
  Bacterial overgrowth
  Parasitic diseases (e.g., malaria, giardiasis, schistosomiasis, helminth
    infections)
  Cystic fibrosis
  Whipple disease
  Allergic enteritis
  Eosinophilic gastroenteritis
  Gluten-sensitive enteropathy
  Tropical sprue
  Systemic lupus erythematosus

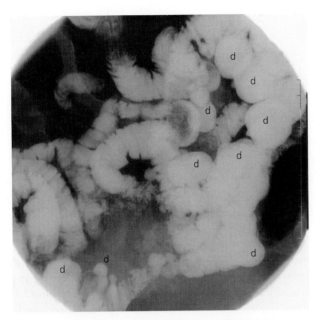

Figure 27.13 Images from small bowel follow-through series show multiple, large diverticula (d) of the small bowel. This patient had malabsorption caused by bacterial overgrowth. Treatment included long-term antibiotic therapy and correction of nutritional and vitamin deficiencies.

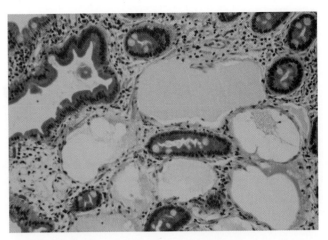

Figure 27.14 Intestinal lymphangiectasia can present as malabsorption and protein-losing enteropathy. Section shows lakes of ectatic lymphatic vessels within the lamina propria of the small intestine. Source: Courtesy of Dr. Paul Swanson.

CHAPTER 28

Ulcerative colitis: clinical manifestations and management

William F. Stenson,[1] William J. Tremaine,[2] and Russell D. Cohen[3]
[1] Washington University School of Medicine, St Louis, MO, USA
[2] Mayo Clinic College of Medicine, Rochester, MN, USA
[3] University of Chicago Medical Center, Chicago, IL, USA

Pathology

The classic gross appearance of ulcerative colitis is circumferential, continuous inflammation starting at the rectum and then progressing proximally; there is often a sharp demarcation between abnormal mucosa distally and normal mucosa proximally, although some patients have the entire colon uniformly involved (Figure 28.1). The involved segments are diffusely abnormal, often with a gradation of inflammation less severe proximally (i.e., perhaps just mild edema in the cecum to submucosal hemorrhage in the transverse colon) to more severe distally, with frank ulceration in the rectum. Sometimes the ulcerations can be seen only in histological sections but, in other cases, large distinct ulcerations may be seen in the gross specimen.

At histological examination, the inflammatory infiltrate in ulcerative colitis usually extends down no further than the muscularis mucosae. The inflammatory infiltrate includes both neutrophils, a sign of acute inflammation, and macrophages and lymphocytes, signs of more chronic inflammation. Crypt abscess (Figure 28.2), a collection of neutrophils in a colonic crypt, is characteristic of ulcerative colitis but also is seen in other diseases, including Crohn's colitis, infectious colitides, acute ischemic colitis, diverticular colitis, acute radiation colitis, and nonspecific colitis. Crypt branching (Figure 28.3) occurs in many patients with ulcerative colitis and persists even when the disease is inactive and the mucosal inflammation has resolved. Crypt branching may also be seen in Crohn's colitis, but is uncommon in other disease processes. Inflammatory polyps in ulcerative colitis may be filiform (Figure 28.4), or they may be broad based and sessile. Often they are covered with a whitish cap of exudate (Figure 28.5).

It is possible to screen for patients at an increased risk for colorectal carcinoma in ulcerative colitis by identifying areas of colonic dysplasia (Figure 28.6). Dysplastic mucosa can be villiform owing to the proliferation of epithelial cells. At low-power microscopic examination, low-grade dysplasia is marked by enlarged goblet cells and atypical hyperchromatic nuclei, whereas high-grade dysplasia is characterized by more marked nuclear pleomorphism and pseudostratification of the nuclei. Under higher-power magnification, low-grade dysplasia shows hyperchromatic cells with preservation of nuclear polarity, whereas high-grade dysplasia shows complete loss of nuclear polarity. Biopsy screening for dysplasia may reveal carcinoma in situ. Adenocarcinoma of the colon occurs with increased frequency in ulcerative colitis (Figure 28.7) and Crohn's colitis.

Extraintestinal manifestations

The most common extraintestinal manifestation in patients with ulcerative colitis is an inflammatory arthritis, typically presenting as fluctuating, asymmetric joint swelling of large and small joints, affecting both the axial and appendicular skeletons. Ankylosing spondylitis may be seen in conjunction with inflammatory bowel disease, often HLA-B27+. Common dermal manifestation of both ulcerative colitis and Crohn's colitis are pyoderma gangrenosum (Figures 28.8 and 28.9), marked by sharply defined areas of ulceration with serpiginous borders, and erythema nodosum, which presents as red, raised, tender nodules, typically on the extensor surfaces of the body. Ophthalmalogical events include episcleritis, uveitis, and iritis; the latter is a potentially serious ophthalmological complication of ulcerative colitis and Crohn's disease, accompanied by conjunctival injection (Figure 28.10). Aphthous stomatitis may also be seen in patients with ulcerative colitis, although it is more commonly associated with Crohn's disease. Hepatobiliary manifestations includes primary sclerosing cholangitis (PSC), which

Yamada's Atlas of Gastroenterology, Fifth Edition. Edited by Daniel K. Podolsky, Michael Camilleri, J. Gregory Fitz, Anthony N. Kalloo, Fergus Shanahan, and Timothy C. Wang.

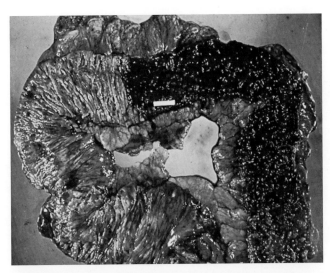

Figure 28.1 Colectomy specimen from a patient with ulcerative colitis demonstrates sharp demarcation in the midtransverse colon between involved and uninvolved mucosa. Source: Courtesy of Dr. Ira Kodner.

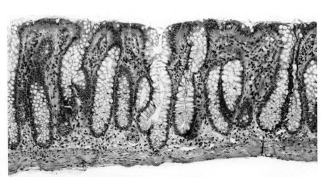

Figure 28.3 Histology of quiescent ulcerative colitis, with branched colonic crypts but no active inflammatory infiltrate. Source: Courtesy of Dr. John Hart, Chicago, IL.

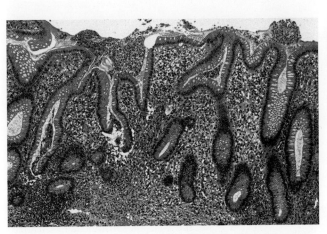

Figure 28.2 Histology of active ulcerative colitis, with distorted colonic crypts, inflammatory infiltrates, and crypt abscesses. Source: Courtesy of Dr. John Hart, Chicago, IL.

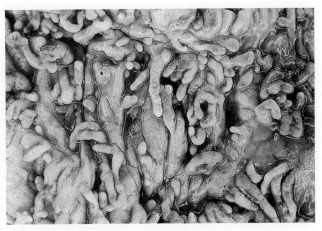

Figure 28.4 When inflammatory polyps assume the filiform appearance seen here, they are readily recognizable grossly; when smaller in numbers and rounded, they can be confused with adenomas or hyperplastic polyps. Source: Mitros FA. Atlas of Gastrointestinal Pathology. London: Gower, 1988. Copyright ©1988 Elsevier.

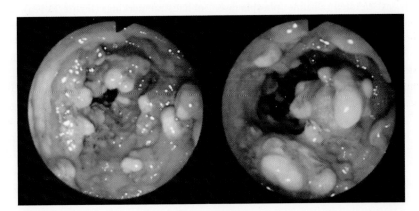

Figure 28.5 Multiple pseudopolyps in ulcerative colitis. Their surface is smooth and glistening. Detailed view of exudate creating whitish caps. Source: Silverstein FE and Tytgat GNJ. Gastrointestinal Endoscopy, 3rd edn. London: Mosby-Wolfe, 1997. Copyright ©1997 Elsevier.

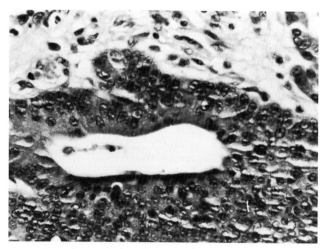

Figure 28.6 High-grade dysplasia with nuclear stratification, nuclear and cellular pleomorphism, and loss of nuclear polarity. Source: Courtesy of Dr. David Lacey.

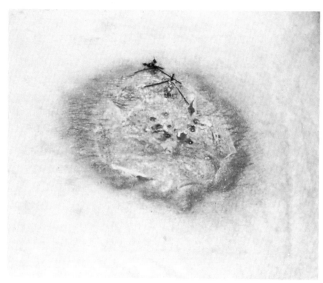

Figure 28.8 Pyoderma gangrenosum. Source: Courtesy of Dr. Ira Kodner.

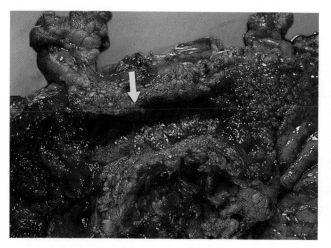

Figure 28.7 Adenocarcinoma (arrow) in a patient with ulcerative colitis. Source: Courtesy of Dr. Ira Kodner.

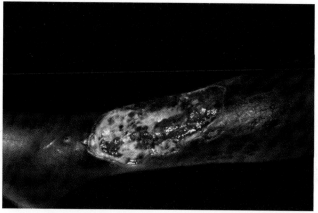

Figure 28.9 Severe pyoderma gangrenosum of the lower extremity. Note that the deep ulceration has reached the bone.

can be seen in approximately 5% of inflammatory bowel disease (IBD) patients (although 70%–90% of PSC patients have IBD). Pericholangitis manifests as elevated alkaline phosphatase without structural alteration of the ducts apparent on imaging and may be more common and represent the very earliest phase of PSC. The urogenital system is not excluded from this list either; oxalate kidney stones are more common, although this should raise the question of possible Crohn's disease rather than ulcerative colitis in some cases.

Radiology

Plain radiographs are helpful in establishing the diagnosis of toxic megacolon, which is characterized by dilation of a colonic segment, typically the transverse colon (Figure 28.11). Double-contrast studies identify early changes in ulcerative colitis that

would not be seen with full-column studies. Early changes in ulcerative colitis include mucosal edema, granularity, and loss of haustral markings (Figure 28.12a). As the disease progresses, ulcerations develop with penetration of the mucosal layer (Figure 28.12b). Undermining of the mucosal layer gives the characteristic appearance of collar-button ulcers (Figure 28.13).

Although ulcerative colitis tends to involve the left colon more than the right, the inflammatory process may affect the cecum and result in severe narrowing. The terminal ileum is affected among about 10% of patients with pancolitis. Involvement of the terminal ileum is manifested radiographically with thickening of the mucosal folds, spasm, and irritability. The ileocecal valve in ulcerative colitis tends to be gaping, as opposed to its position in Crohn's disease, in which it tends to be narrowed.

Computed tomography (CT) imaging in ulcerative colitis is characterized by circumferential wall thickening with

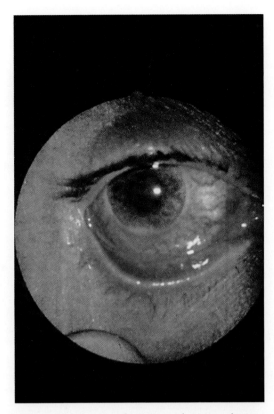

Figure 28.10 Marked conjunctival injection. A hypopyon also is present. Source: Misiewicz JJ, Forbes A, Price A, et al. Atlas of Clinical Gastroenterology, 2nd edn. London: Wolfe, 1994. Copyright ©1994 Elsevier.

enlargement of the mucosal folds; in patients with pancolitis, this will involve the entire colon, but those with less extensive disease will have a correlating finding on CT scan. The different densities of the colonic lumen and inflamed wall may result in a "target sign" on cross-sectional imaging; many cases may also show proliferation of the perirectal fat (Figure 28.14).

Magnetic resonance imaging (MRI) is often used in lieu of CT scans in patients less than age 50 years with IBD due to concerns of repeated exposure to ionizing radiation. Inflammation limited to the mucosal and submucosal layers may be nicely defined in patients with ulcerative colitis. Abdominal ultrasound, endoscopic ultrasound, and radionucleotide imaging have occasional but limited roles In patients with ulcerative colitis.

Endoscopy

In quiescent ulcerative colitis, there is distortion of vascular markings without edema or erythema (Figure 28.15). In mildly and moderately active disease, there is edema and erythema granularity and distortion of vascular markings (Figures 28.16 and 28.17).

In severe ulcerative colitis, the mucosa is friable, erythematous, and edematous with ulceration (Figure 28.18). Although the severity of inflammation seen endoscopically may lessen as one moves proximally in the colon in ulcerative colitis, the degree of inflammation at a given level is uniform through the entire circumference of the colon. Thus, ulceration in ulcerative colitis almost always occurs in areas of diffuse edema and erythema. The mucosa surrounding ulcerations may become so edematous that the result is a coarsely nodular deformity (Figure 28.19). With the exception of patients with uniformly severe

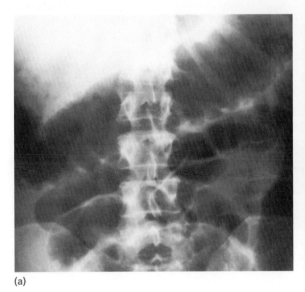

(a)

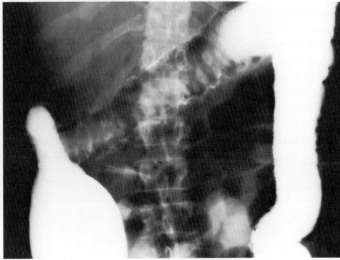

(b)

Figure 28.11 Toxic megacolon. **(a)** Plain radiograph shows colonic dilation. **(b)** Contrast radiograph reveals large ulceration. Source: Courtesy of Dr. Dennis Balfe.

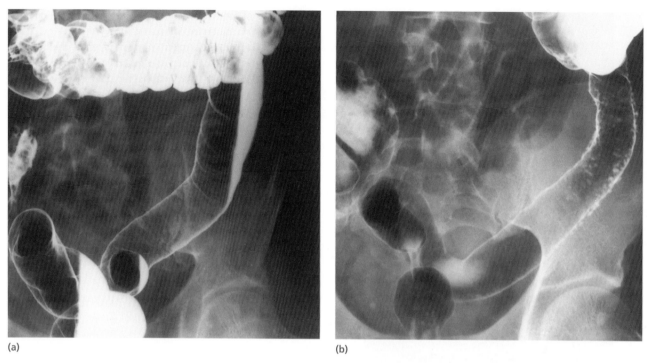

(a)

(b)

Figure 28.12 Progression of ulcerative colitis in the sigmoid and descending colon. **(a)** Colon of a patient with mild ulcerative colitis. There is mucosal edema, granularity, and loss of haustral markings. **(b)** Two years later, there is shortening of the colon and mucosal ulcers. Numerous collar-button ulcers are present in the descending colon. Source: Courtesy of Dr. Dennis Balfe.

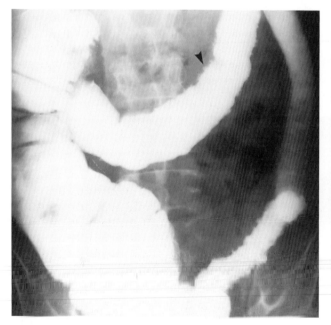

Figure 28.13 Ulcerative colitis extending to midtransverse colon with collar-button ulcerations in profile (arrowhead). Source: Courtesy of Dr. Dennis Balfe.

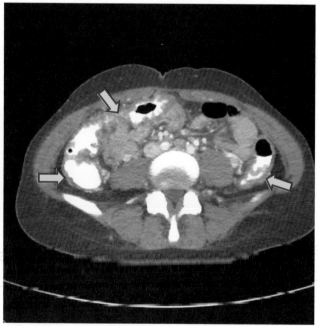

Figure 28.14 Computed tomography scan of a patient with panulcerative colitis. The arrows indicate colonic bowel wall thickening.

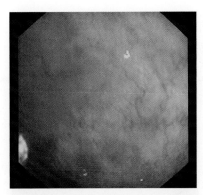

Figure 28.15 Quiescent (inactive) ulcerative colitis in a 39-year-old woman with ulcerative pancolitis for 11 years, now asymptomatic. There is distortion of the vascular markings but no granularity, edema, friability, mucous exudate, or ulcerations.

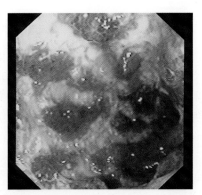

Figure 28.18 Severely active ulcerative colitis in a 54-year-old woman with left-sided ulcerative colitis for 7 years. There is marked ulceration. At least half of the surface area depicted is denuded by ulcers, and there are intervening areas of edematous granular mucosa.

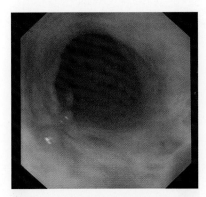

Figure 28.16 Mildly active ulcerative colitis with pseudopolyps. Same patient as in Figure 28.15, 1 year after the endoscopic examination in Figure 28.15, with a mild flare in symptoms. The disease is responding to prednisone 20 mg daily and mesalamine 4 g daily. There are two small pseudopolyps; the mucosa is mildly granular and erythematous, and the vascular markings are distorted.

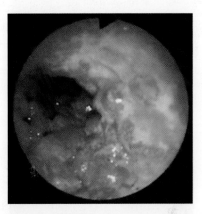

Figure 28.19 Coarsely nodular deformity of mucosal contour in ulcerative colitis. Mucosa is intensely erythematous and friable. Source: Silverstein FE and Tytgat GNJ. Gastrointestinal Endoscopy, 3rd edn. London: Mosby-Wolfe, 1997. Copyright ©1997 Elsevier.

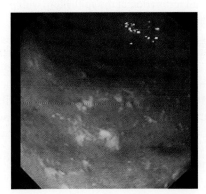

Figure 28.17 Moderately active ulcerative colitis in a 19-year-old woman with ulcerative pancolitis for 2 years. The patient has continuing symptoms despite oral mesalamine 4 g daily and prednisone 40 mg daily. Moderate granularity, edema, and mucus exudate is demonstrated.

pancolitis, the more proximally one moves in the colon, the less severe the endoscopic changes are likely to be. Sometimes there is sharp demarcation between normal and inflamed tissue (Figure 28.20). It is important to intubate the terminal ileum and obtain multiple biopsies of the small intestine in any patient with diarrhea or suspected IBD. As some patients with ulcerative colitis may have mild inflammation just above the ileocecal valve, endoscopic visualization and histological sampling 10–20 cm proximal to this point is advised to exclude Crohn's disease.

Pseudopolyps can occur in ulcerative colitis of any degree of activity (Figures 28.21, 28.22, and 28.23; see Figure 28.16); these vary from a few millimeters to several centimeters in length and width. They may be filamentous, bridging with connections to the colon at two or more locations, and they may be uninflamed or inflamed in appearance.

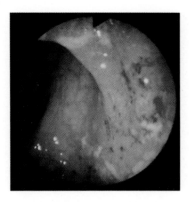

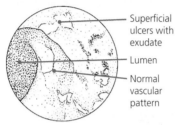

Superficial
ulcers with
exudate

Lumen

Normal
vascular
pattern

Figure 28.20 Sharp transition from normal to inflamed bowel is discernible at the rectosigmoid junction. Erythema and superficial ulceration of diseased mucosa contrast to the normal vascular pattern. Source: Silverstein FE and Tytgat GNJ. Gastrointestinal Endoscopy, 3rd edn. London: Mosby-Wolfe, 1997. Copyright ©1997 Elsevier.

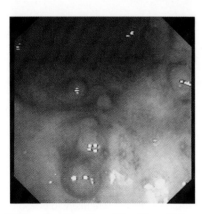

Figure 28.21 Mildly active ulcerative colitis with multiple pseudopolyps. This 54-year-old woman (same patient as in Figure 28.18) about 1 year later after a course of topical 5-ASA (mesalamine) and prednisone 60 mg daily tapered and discontinued 9 months previously. There is mild granularity and erythema, the vascular markings are distorted, and multiple small pseudopolyps are seen.

Figure 28.24 shows sequential endoscopic studies of a patient with severe pancolitis. At the first colonoscopy (Figure 28.24a), there was almost universal ulceration with only a few islands of remaining mucosa. In Figure 28.24b, the mucosa is beginning to heal, and less ulcer and more epithelium are seen. In Figure 28.24c, there is further regression of ulcers with pseudopolyp

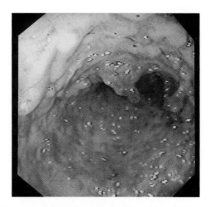

Figure 28.22 Long-standing ulcerative colitis with scarring and pseudopolyps. A 25-year-old man had a 9-year history of ulcerative colitis. The patient is now asymptomatic with azathioprine 150 mg daily and mesalamine 2.4 g daily. There is scarring and loss of the normal vascular markings. Two small pseudopolyps are present.

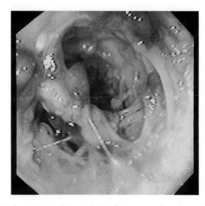

Figure 28.23 Ulcerative colitis with bridging pseudopolyps. A 25-year-old man has had ulcerative colitis for 9 years (same patient as in Figure 28.22) and the disease is asymptomatic with azathioprine 150 mg daily and mesalamine 2.4 g daily. Endoscopic picture shows bridging pseudopolyps in the transverse colon.

formation. Full restoration of the epithelium with persistence of pseudopolyps is shown in Figure 28.24d.

Dysplasia is most often found either when carcinoma is present in the colon or when the patient is at an increased risk for a future carcinoma. Pancolonoscopy with surveillance biopsies (four quadrant every 10 cm) or chromoendoscopy is recommended every 2 years after 8 years of pancolitis annually after 15 years. Confirmed flat dysplasia (i.e., incidentally found on mucosal biopsy in the absence of an obvious small polyp) is considered an indication for proctocolectomy. Age-appropriate patients who have small simple adenomas entirely removed, without surrounding dysplasia, may continue with surveillance colonoscopies every 6–12 months [6]. When dysplasia is associated with a larger polypoid mass or other endoscopic abnormality, the lesion is called a *dysplasia-associated lesion or mass* (DALM) (Figure 28.25). Identification of a DALM is an

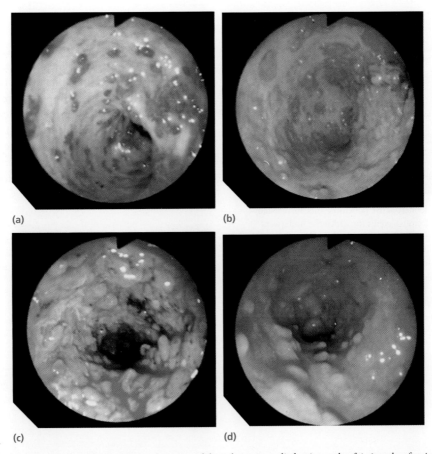

Figure 28.24 Sequential study of severe pancolitis. Massive ulceration of the colon was studied at intervals of 4–6 weeks after institution of medical therapy. **(a)** View of the proximal sigmoid shows extensive ulceration before therapy. Some islands of remaining mucosa are visible. **(b)** Regression of inflammation and early reepithelialization. **(c)** Ulcers are regressing with pseudopolypoid elevation of nonulcerated mucosal islands. **(d)** Full reepithelialization and pseudopolypoid transformation characterize healing. Source: Silverstein FE and Tytgat GNJ. Gastrointestinal Endoscopy, 3rd edn. London: Mosby-Wolfe, 1997. Copyright ©1997 Elsevier.

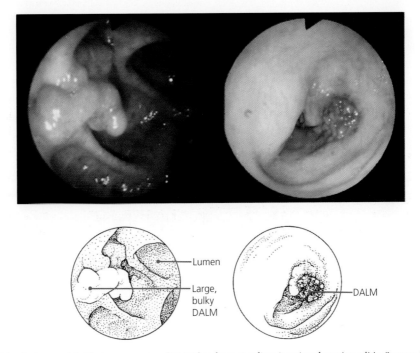

Figure 28.25 Examples of dysplasia-associated lesions or masses (DALM) in long-standing, inactive ulcerative colitis. Source: Silverstein FE and Tytgat GNJ. Gastrointestinal Endoscopy, 3rd edn. London: Mosby-Wolfe, 1997. Copyright ©1997 Elsevier.

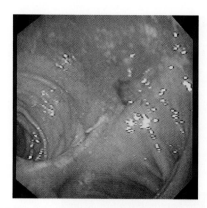

Figure 28.26 Mild to moderately active pouchitis. This 36-year-old woman has a history of ulcerative colitis for which she underwent colectomy with ileal J pouch–anal anastomosis 2 years previously. She had recurrent liquid stools and cramping discomfort relieved with bowel movements. Endoscopic image of the pouch, with views of the afferent limb of the neoterminal ileum in the left portion of the field and the blind end of the J pouch in the inferior aspect of the field, shows mucous exudate, superficial ulceration, and friability of the pouch mucosa but not of the mucosa in the neoterminal ileum.

indication for resection because of the very high probability of an associated malignant tumor.

Ulcerative colitis can be treated surgically with total procto-colectomy and construction of an ileal pouch with an ileoanal anastomosis. Pouchitis (inflammation of the ileal pouch) occurs among some patients after this procedure. The endoscopic features of pouchitis include erythema, edema, mucous exudate, and superficial ulceration (Figure 28.26). Patient with chronic recurrent pouchitis, inflammation in the afferent ileal limb of the pouch, or the formation of fistulas from the pouch 6 or more months after surgery should be investigated for possible Crohn's disease.

CHAPTER 29

Crohn's disease: clinical manifestations and management

Gil Y. Melmed and Stephan R. Targan
Cedars-Sinai Medical Center, Los Angeles, CA, USA

Introduction

Crohn's disease is characterized by relapsing and remitting chronic intestinal inflammation in a genetically susceptible host. It is closely related to ulcerative colitis, but is distinguished by key features including anatomic disease location and clinical expression. The clinical manifestations of Crohn's disease are varied, as inflammation may involve any part of the digestive tract, may include noncontiguous segments of inflammation (i.e., "skip lesions") with intervening normal segments of bowel, and can lead to fibrostenosing and perforating complications from transmural inflammation. Most commonly, Crohn's disease affects the terminal ileum and colon, but can involve any portion of the GI tract from the mouth to the anus. "Involvement" or "disease" refer to the presence of inflammation that can be visualized radiographically, endoscopically, and histologically.

About 20% of patients have isolated colonic involvement, which may present similarly to ulcerative colitis. About 30% of patients with Crohn's disease have inflammation confined to the small bowel. Perianal disease manifests in about 25% of patients with Crohn's disease, and is usually associated with inflammation in the distal colon or in the small bowel.

There are several ways to measure Crohn's disease activity, including clinical symptoms, biological parameters of inflammation, endoscopy, and imaging. One of the most common clinical scoring systems is the Crohn's Disease Activity Index (CDAI), which has been the most commonly used primary measure of disease activity for clinical trials for over 30 years (Table 29.1).

Endoscopy

Colonoscopic findings of Crohn's disease include various manifestations of inflammation, including erythema, erosions, ulceration, and stricturing. Ulcers are characterized morphologically as aphthous, linear, or stellate (Figures 29.1 and 29.2). There are several instruments that have been developed for clinical trials to score Crohn's endoscopic disease activity. The most commonly used indices include the Crohn's Disease Endoscopic Index of Severity (CDEIS) and the Simple Endoscopic Score (SES), which correlate highly with one another and score the presence, size, and extent of ulceration and inflammation in the ileum and individual colonic segments (Table 29.2). In addition to inflammation, colonoscopy can also identify healing of the mucosa, which can look normal or can display areas of scarring suggestive of prior inflammation (Figure 29.3). Polypoid lesions in patients with Crohn's disease should be biopsied to assess for dysplasia, although benign inflammatory polyps of no malignant potential are commonly seen in areas of active or prior inflammation (Figure 29.4). A stricture is an area of narrowing, or stenosis, that may be due to fibrosis, inflammation/edema, or both (Figure 29.5).

Capsule endoscopy is a relatively new technology that can identify small bowel Crohn's disease with a high degree of accuracy. Capsule endoscopy is highly sensitive for the detection of small intestine mucosal lesions that could be missed on barium studies or even cross-sectional enterography studies, and can be useful for disease diagnosis, particularly when conventional endoscopy and colonoscopy are not diagnostic in the appropriate clinical setting (Figures 29.6 and 29.7).

Histology

At the time of endoscopic evaluation, biopsies for histopathological evaluation can be helpful to establish the diagnosis, discriminate between Crohn's and ulcerative colitis, exclude certain infections such as cytomegalovirus (Figure 29.8), and assess for dysplasia or malignancy. Noncaseating granulomata are considered pathognomonic for Crohn's disease in this setting, although they are only seen in about 15% of patients with Crohn's disease (Figure 29.9). Typically, a full assessment

Yamada's Atlas of Gastroenterology, Fifth Edition. Edited by Daniel K. Podolsky, Michael Camilleri, J. Gregory Fitz, Anthony N. Kalloo, Fergus Shanahan, and Timothy C. Wang.
© 2016 John Wiley & Sons, Ltd. Published 2016 by John Wiley & Sons, Ltd.
Companion website: www.yamadagastro.com/atlas

of the extent and severity of inflammation requires a combination of colonoscopic and histological findings together with small bowel imaging, which can assess for Crohn's inflammation and stricturing more proximal than the reach of the colonoscope. Furthermore, there can be disparities between endoscopic and histological findings, due to the focal/patchy nature of the disease both endoscopically and histologically.

Radiographic aspects of Crohn's disease

Historically, the mainstay of diagnostic radiological evaluation of Crohn's disease has been barium small bowel follow through (SBFT). However, over the past decade or so, the development of cross-sectional imaging modalities (computed tomography [CT] and magnetic resonance imaging [MRI]) with enterography protocols have largely replaced SBFT for the routine evaluation of known and suspected Crohn's disease. These modalities are first-line imaging techniques that can rapidly and accurately identify areas of mucosal inflammation, fibrostenotic and penetrating complications, and many extraintestinal manifestations of Crohn's disease. Furthermore, they may be used to detect changes in inflammation and response to treatment. Barium SBFT is still useful in some situations, including the evaluation of complex fistula tracts and for the evaluation of

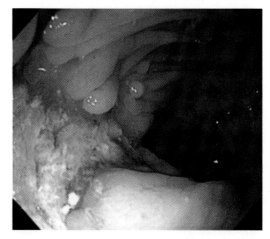

Figure 29.1 Colonoscopic ulceration in Crohn's disease. This is a long, deep, linear ulcer characteristic of severe endoscopic inflammation.

Table 29.1 The Crohn's Disease Activity Index has been used to determine health status in clinical trials for patients with Crohn's disease. Most approved medications for Crohn's disease have relied on the CDAI for the determination of eligibility and endpoints. Source: Best WR, Becktel JM, Singleton JW, Kern F, Jr. Development of a Crohn's disease activity index. National Cooperative Crohn's Disease Study. Gastroenterology 1976;70:439.

Average over the prior 7 days	Multiplier
Number of liquid bowel movements	×2
Abdominal pain (0 = none, 1 = mild, 2 = moderate, 3 = severe)	×5
General well being	×7
Extraintestinal manifestations (1 point each for arthritis, iritis/uveitis, erythema nodosum/pyoderma gangrenosum, aphthous stomatitis, anal fissure/fistula, fever)	×20
Use of antidiarrheal agents (0 = none, 1 = yes)	×30
Abdominal mass (0 = none, 2 = doubtful, 3 = definite)	×10
Hematocrit % (males 47 hematocrit, females 42 hematocrit)	×6
Total score	

CDAI score interpretation: <150 clinical remission, 150–220 mild disease, 220–450 moderate to severe disease, >450 severe disease.

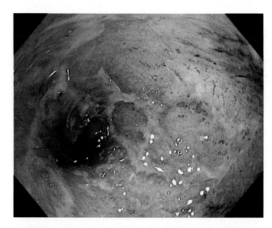

Figure 29.2 Colonoscopic ulceration in Crohn's disease. This is a serpiginous ulcer characteristic of moderate to severe endoscopic inflammation.

Table 29.2 The Simple Endoscopic Score for Crohn's disease (SES-CD). The total SES-CD score is the sum of the numbers for the five bowel segments (ileum, right colon, transverse colon, left colon, and rectum). This is a commonly used scoring index to assess inflammation in clinical trials. Data from Sipponen T, Nuutinen H, Turunen U, Farkkila M. Endoscopic evaluation of Crohn's disease activity: comparison of the CDEIS and the SES-CD. Inflamm Bowel Dis 2010;16:2131.

	0	1	2	3
Presence and size of ulcers	None	Aphthous ulcers (less than 0.5 cm)	Large ulcers (0.5–2 cm)	Very large ulcers (>2 cm)
% ulcerated surface	None	<10%	10%–30%	>30%
Affected surface	None	<50%	50%–75%	>75%
Presence of narrowing	None	Single, traversable	Multiple, traversable	Cannot be traversed

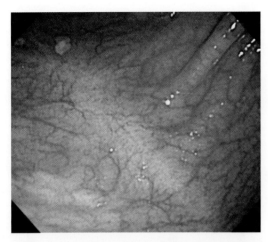

Figure 29.3 Endoscopy can identify areas of prior ulceration which have healed, such as this scar demonstrating complete mucosal healing of a long, linear ulcer.

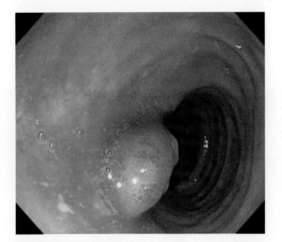

Figure 29.4 Inflammatory polyps (or "pseudo" polyps) can be seen in areas of active or prior inflammation in Crohn's disease. They have no malignant potential.

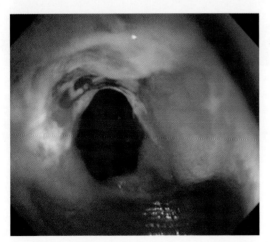

Figure 29.5 Longstanding inflammation can lead to stenosis, or stricturing, such as shown here on colonoscopy. This tight stricture could not be passed using a colonoscope, and required balloon dilation.

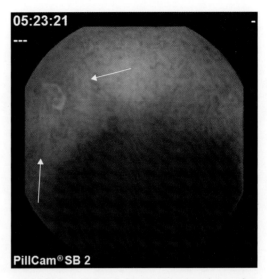

Figure 29.6 Multiple small bowel ulcerations (such as the one shown here) were seen in the mid-small bowel of this 27-year-old woman with unexplained abdominal pain and weight loss. Endoscopy and colonoscopy were normal.

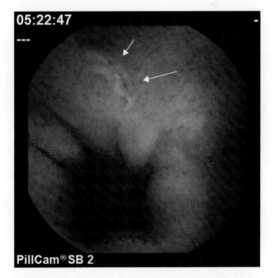

Figure 29.7 Multiple small bowel ulcerations (such as the linear ulcer shown here) were seen in the mid-small bowel of this 27-year-old woman with unexplained abdominal pain and weight loss. Endoscopy and colonoscopy were normal.

obstruction (Figure 29.10). In addition, it remains a mainstay in the absence of access to CT or MRI technologies.

Enterography studies (CTE and MRE) are distinguished from routine cross-sectional techniques in that they require adequate distension of the small bowel to identify and characterize mucosal inflammation. Intravenous contrast is also administered during these studies, in order to identify areas of mucosal hyperenhancement suggestive of active inflammation. Typical findings of active inflammation using enterography protocols include the "comb sign," which refers to engorgement of the vasa recta and the "target sign," which refers to the trilaminar

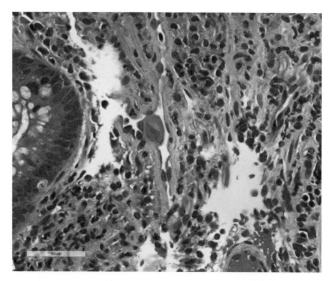

Figure 29.8 Cytomegalovirus can complicate Crohn's and ulcerative colitis. Its histological appearance is characterized by inclusion bodies, seen here on hematoxylin and eosin staining of colonic mucosal biopsies. Source: Courtesy of Dr. Maha Guindi, Department of Anatomic Pathology, Cedars-Sinai Medical Center.

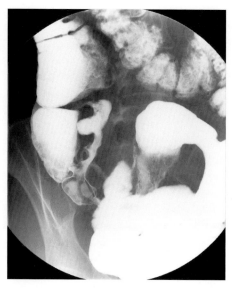

Figure 29.10 Barium small-bowel follow-through demonstrating a stricture at the terminal ileum, with proximal small bowel dilation. Source: Courtesy of Dr. Cindy Kallman, Department of Radiology, Cedars-Sinai Medical Center, Los Angeles, CA.

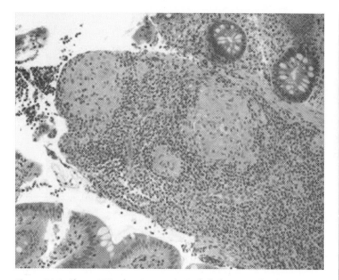

Figure 29.9 About 15% of patients with Crohn's disease will exhibit noncaseating granulomata in inflamed or uninflamed mucosa. These histopathological collections of macrophages are characteristic for Crohn's disease.

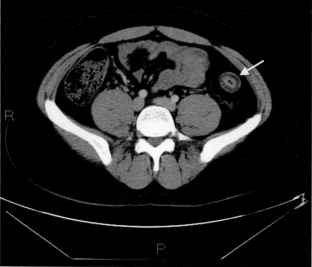

Figure 29.11 CT enterography. Seen in cross section, the "target sign" is produced by the small inner ring of bright mucosal enhancement, which suggests severely active inflammation, separated from the outer ring of muscular and serosal enhancement by a low-density layer of submucosal fat deposition consistent with inflammation of a more chronic nature. Source: Courtesy of Dr. Cindy Kallman, Department of Radiology, Cedars-Sinai Medical Center, Los Angeles, CA.

enhancement of the layers of the bowel wall including enhancing mucosa (bright), submucosal edema (dark), and enhancing serosa (bright) (Figures 29.11 and 29.12).

Both CTE and MRE can identify small bowel inflammation with a high degree of accuracy. However, there are several factors to consider when selecting one cross-sectional imaging modality over the other. CTE offers rapid image acquisition and is generally less expensive than MRE. Because of the speed in which images are acquired, motion artifact is minimized. In contrast, MRE offers high-quality images without exposure to ionizing radiation, and is more sensitive to identifying soft tissue abnormalities including fistulae and perianal complications. Furthermore, MRE protocols acquire multiple images of the same location at different time points that may allow for

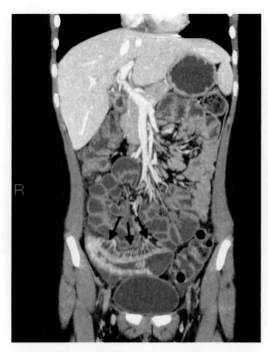

Figure 29.12 CT enterography. Increased mesenteric vascularity with prominent vasa recta (black arrows) at the mesenteric border of the affected segment produce the "comb sign," which is highly specific for acute inflammation. Source: Courtesy of Dr. Cindy Kallman, Department of Radiology, Cedars-Sinai Medical Center, Los Angeles, CA.

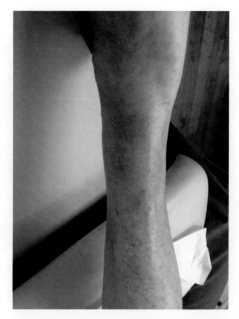

Figure 29.13 Erythema nodosum is a painful, red and often raised lesion on the legs that may occur in the setting of intestinal inflammation as well as several other inflammatory conditions. This lesion resolved within 48 hours of initiation of systemic corticosteroids to treat active Crohn's disease.

clarification of areas of questionable distension or enhancement. Advances in both of these technologies will undoubtedly yield improvements including lower radiation doses for CTE and shorter acquisition times for MRE.

Extraintestinal manifestations and complications

Extraintestinal manifestations of Crohn's disease can include eye inflammation (iritis, uveitis, episcleritis), joint involvement (axial or peripheral arthritis, sacroileitis), skin manifestations (pyoderma gangrenosum, erythema nodosum, and others), and biliary involvement (primary sclerosing cholangitis). These extraintestinal manifestations may be present in up to 25% of patients, may sometimes even be the initial symptom, and may precede bowel inflammation and the diagnosis of Crohn's or ulcerative colitis by months or even years.

Ocular

Extraintestinal manifestations of Crohn's disease can involve inflammation in every part of the eye, including episcleritis, keratitis, conjunctivitis, and more serious uveitis and scleritis. Eye manifestations occur in up to 6% of patients with Crohn's disease. Episcleritis involves injection of the conjunctiva, usually in association with disease activity, and does not threaten visual

acuity. It may present with otherwise asymptomatic conjunctival erythematous injection, or with eye pain, burning, or irritation. In contrast, scleritis is painful, and involves the deeper layers of the eye. If untreated, scleritis can lead to permanent visual loss. Infliximab is effective in treatment of scleritis. Patients with Crohn's disease who present with eye pain or redness should be promptly referred for ophthalmological evaluation.

Skin

Skin lesions are found in up to 20% of patients with Crohn's disease, and can be classified as reactive, associated, drug related, or intrinsic to the disease. The most common reactive skin lesion is erythema nodosum (EN), occurring in about 5% of patients. EN is characterized by painful, raised, red lesions, usually on the legs (Figure 29.13). EN is not specific to IBD, and usually improves with treatment of the underlying bowel inflammation. It can occur before worsening GI symptoms manifest a flare of the underlying CD. Pyoderma gangrenosum (PG) occurs in up to 2% of patients with IBD, and manifests as a sterile ulcer with raised edges, and may exhibit pathergy upon biopsy or debridement (Figure 29.14 and 29.15). Treatment for PG involves treatment of the underlying inflammatory bowel disease (IBD) although anti-TNF agents, cyclosporine, and other medical therapies may be effective for the treatment of PG even in the absence of IBD.

In addition to skin manifestations of inflammation, several medications used to treat Crohn's disease can manifest adverse

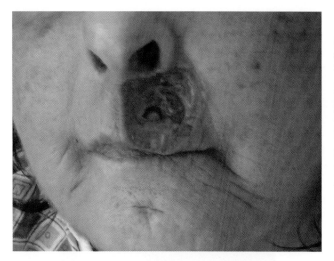

Figure 29.14 Pyoderma gangrenosum is an ulcerated skin lesion with violaceous edges that often correlates with underlying inflammatory bowel activity. Shown here is a large facial lesion with full-thickness ulceration demonstrating underlying dentition. This lesion healed completely with treatment including cyclosporine, intravenous γ-globulin, and hyperbaric oxygen.

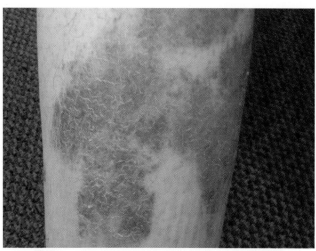

Figure 29.16 Atypical psoriasis in a patient on anti-TNF therapy. These lesions developed on both legs 7 months after initiation of anti-TNF therapy in a patient with Crohn's colitis, and disappeared gradually with discontinuation of the drug. Anti-TNF-associated psoriasis has a high likelihood of recurrence with a second anti-TNF agent.

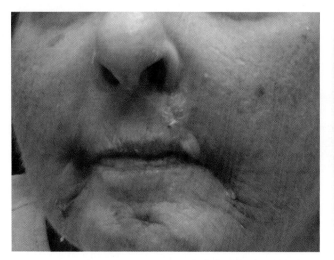

Figure 29.15 The lesion shown in Figure 29.14 healed after surgical closure of the fascial defect followed by intensive medical therapy with cyclosporine, intravenous γ-globulin, and hyperbaric oxygen therapy.

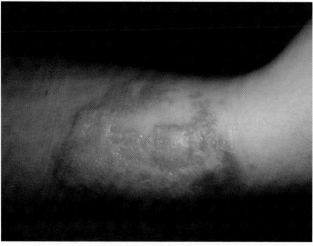

Figure 29.17 Infections must be considered in immunocompromised patients with Crohn's disease presenting with skin lesions, such as this fungal infection seen in a patient on anti-TNF therapy and azathioprine.

reactions in the skin. These include atypical psoriatic reactions (Figure 29.16) and fungal infections (Figure 29.17) in patients treated with anti-TNF agents.

Pyostomatitis vegetans is an oral lesion characterized by pustules and ulcerations along the lips, buccal mucosa, and gingiva, and is quite specific to IBD. In contrast, oral aphthous lesions are common even among the general population, but are more common among patients with Crohn's disease (Figure 29.18). These painful erosions or ulcers can be treated with topical corticosteroid solutions, but usually resolve with treatment of the underlying Crohn's disease.

Perianal disease

Perianal Crohn's disease is a frequently encountered devastating complication of Crohn's disease that causes significant morbidity and can have a profound impact on quality of life. Nonfistulizing perianal manifestations include anal fissures, skin tags, anal ulceration, and strictures. Anal fissures are tears at the anal canal that can occur de novo or in the setting of Crohn's disease (Figure 29.19). The prevalence of anal fissures among patients with Crohn's disease has been reported to be as high as 35%. Anal fissures can be treated medically, with sitz baths (to relax the anal sphincter muscles) and topically applied

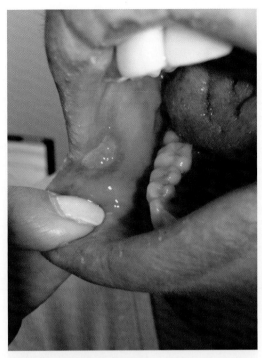

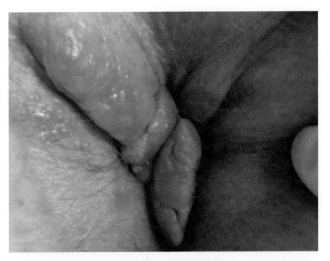

Figure 29.20 Perianal manifestations of Crohn's disease can include large, inflamed skin tags as shown here. These "elephant" tags can be painful, and fluctuate in size in association with underlying disease activity.

Figure 29.18 Aphthous oral ulcers in Crohn's disease. Painful oral lesions can be symptomatically treated with topical corticosteroids, along with treatment of the underlying bowel inflammation.

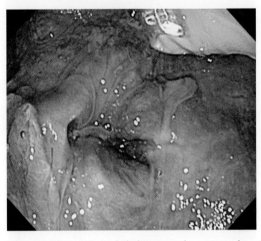

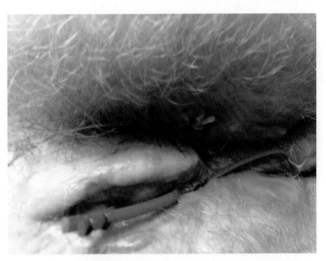

Figure 29.21 Perianal fistulae can result in abscess formation if healing occurs externally before the internal opening is closed. Placement of a seton during examination under anesthesia allows for uniform healing and drainage.

Figure 29.19 Anal fissures in Crohn's disease can be acute or chronic, as seen here in this patient with a healing chronic anal fissure characterize by a mucosal defect and underlying ulceration at the anal canal.

vasodilators, including 0.4% nitroglycerin ointment or 2% diltiazem cream (to promote blood flow to the sphincter muscles).

Anal skin tags can occur de novo, but are quite common among patients with Crohn's disease with a prevalence of 40%–70%. Skin tags may associate with fissures and fistulae, and may change in size in association with inflammatory activity. While often soft and asymptomatic, they may become

indurated, edematous, firm, and painful (Figure 29.20). These manifestations will usually subside with medical treatment of underlying Crohn's disease activity. Surgical removal of skin tags in patients with Crohn's disease is generally not recommended due to risks of poor wound healing.

Perianal fistulae occur in about 20% of patients with Crohn's disease in population-based studies. They can be associated with perianal abscesses, and examination under anesthesia is usually recommended for fistula evaluation and placement of a noncutting seton that will allow for uniform tract healing and drainage, and prevent recurrent abscess formation (Figure 29.21).

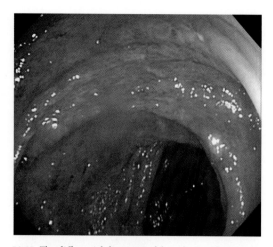

Figure 29.22 The differential diagnosis of ileocolonic inflammation includes acute, infectious enterocolitis, which may be misdiagnosed as Crohn's disease. This patient presented with 1 week of bloody diarrhea, right lower quadrant pain, and CT findings of severe ileal and right colonic wall thickening. Colonoscopy (shown here) demonstrated intense, patchy erythema, edema, and erosions. Cultures subsequently identified *Salmonella* group D and symptoms subsequently resolved with no long-term sequelae.

Differential diagnosis

The differential diagnosis of Crohn's disease includes infections, malignancies, drug-associated, and functional gastrointestinal disorders. Infections for which patients presenting with diarrhea should be considered include *Clostridium difficile*, enteric bacterial infections, and parasitic infections including giardiasis and amoebiasis. Bacterial infections such as *Salmonella*, *Shigella*, *Yersinia*, and *Campylobacter* infections may additionally present with inflammation and wall thickening of the terminal ileum that can look like Crohn's disease on cross-sectional imaging (e.g., CTE) or colonoscopy (Figure 29.22). However, in order to distinguish Crohn's disease from an acute infection, evidence of chronic (as opposed to just acute) inflammation should be sought on histopathology of biopsy specimens.

Postoperative Crohn's disease

The likelihood of eventual surgery in patients with Crohn's disease is significant, with 50%–70% of patients requiring surgery over 5–20 years after diagnosis, although this number may be decreasing over time. Endoscopic evidence of recurrence can precede clinical recurrence by months or years, and endoscopic recurrence rates of 70%–90% have been reported as early as 1 year after surgery. The endoscopic findings at the time of this assessment can be graded using the Rutgeerts classification on a 0 through 4 scale and correlate strongly with risk of future clinical recurrence (Table 29.3; Figures 29.23, 29.24, and 29.25). It is therefore recommended that patients who undergo

Table 29.3 The Rutgeerts score is used to grade the severity of inflammation of the distal ileum after a resection with an ileocolonic anastomosis, and provides prognostic information for the likelihood of clinical recurrence. Source: Rutgeerts P, Geboes K, Vantrappen G, Beyls J, Kerremans R, Hiele M. Predictability of the postoperative course of Crohn's disease. Gastroenterology 1990;99:956. Reproduced with permission of Elsevier.

Endoscopic findings	Score	Likelihood of clinical recurrence within 5 years
No aphthous ulcers	0	0%–10%
Less than 5 aphthous ulcers	1	0%–10%
More than 5 aphthous ulcers, with normal intervening mucosa or skip areas of larger lesions less than 1 cm	2	20%–40%
Diffuse aphthous ileitis	3	70%–90%
Diffuse ileal inflammation with large ulcers, nodules, or stenosis	4	90%–100%

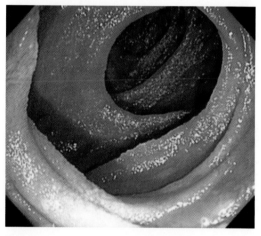

Figure 29.23 Rutgeerts score i0, demonstrating no anastomotic inflammation and very low risk of clinical recurrence.

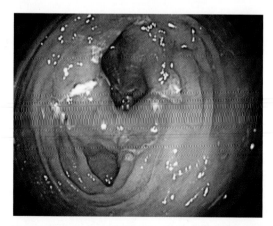

Figure 29.24 Rutgeerts score of i3, demonstrating multiple ulcerations on the ileal side of the ileocolonic anastomosis. This appearance is associated with a 50%–70% risk of clinical recurrence within the next 5 years.

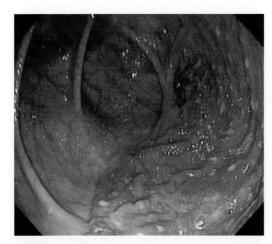

Figure 29.25 The anastomosis is widely patent, but clearly demonstrates multiple ulcers on the ileal (but not colonic) side of the anastomosis. This was classified as Rutgeerts i3, with a 50%–70% risk of clinical recurrence within 5 years.

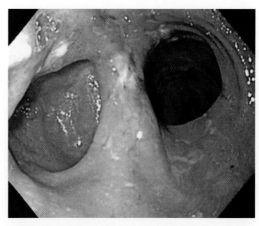

Figure 29.26 Crohn's disease can occur de novo after ileal pouch–anal anastomosis, and can be characterized by severe inflammation and ulceration of the pouch and afferent limb. Shown here are several large ulcerations in the proximal J-pouch, extending into the afferent limb. Note the characteristic "owl's eyes" seen when looking toward the top of the J-pouch, with the efferent (left) and afferent (right) limbs representing the "eyes" and the suture line in between.

ileal or ileocolonic resection have a colonoscopy 6 to 12 months after surgery in order to evaluate the anastomosis and stage the degree of endoscopic recurrence on the i0 through i4 scale even if clinically well, without symptoms. Patients with scores of i2 or higher have an increased risk of clinical recurrence and future surgery, and therefore should be considered for escalation of medical therapy with the goal of modifying the natural course of disease progression.

Crohn's of the ileal pouch

The procedure of choice for the definitive treatment of medically refractory ulcerative colitis or ulcerative colitis with dysplasia is total proctocolectomy with ileal pouch–anal anastomosis (IPAA), or J-pouch. A minority of these patients with what has heretofore appeared to be ulcerative colitis will develop de novo Crohn's disease involving the ileal pouch and/or proximal small bowel (Figure 29.26). The diagnosis of Crohn's disease after IPAA generally is made in the presence of ulceration above the pouch in the afferent limb, or the presence of a fistula not thought to be a postoperative complication (i.e., arising more than 3 months after takedown of the temporary diverting ileostomy.

Crohn's disease involving the ileal pouch has a poor prognosis, with up to 50% of affected patients requiring ileal diversion, with or without pouch resection.

CHAPTER 30

Polyps of the colon and rectum

Daniel C. Chung and John J. Garber III
Massachusetts General Hospital and Harvard Medical School, Boston, MA, USA

A polyp is any abnormal protrusion of the mucosa into the bowel lumen. In contrast to the more proximal intestine, the colon is a common site of benign and malignant polyps. The detection and treatment of adenomatous polyps through routine screening and early detection markedly improves survival. Because a large number of polypoid lesions in the large intestine can appear very similar to adenomas and adenocarcinomas, it is important to combine endoscopic and histological features to try to distinguish benign from malignant polyps and nonadenomas from adenomas. A radiological approach can also be utilized to identify large polyps (Figure 30.1). In this selection of images we have included several variants of adenomas, which are likely to be encountered at some point by the endoscopist, including an adenoma associated with a fibrosing desmoplastic response (Figure 30.2), an adenoma displaying the typical features of high-grade dysplasia (Figure 30.3), which is a term sometimes used interchangeably with intramucosal carcinoma (Figure 30.4), and an uncommonly encountered malignant polyp (Figure 30.5), which is an adenomatous polyp in which a focus of carcinoma penetrates through the muscularis mucosae. Because the colon is also the site of a large number of benign polyps of diverse etiology, we have also included typical examples of several commonly encountered nonadenomatous polyps, including inflammatory fibroid polyps (Figure 30.6), psuedopolyps, which are most often encountered in the setting of chronic inflammation (Figure 30.7), and hamartomatous polyps (Figure 30.8), which are disorganized tissue growths composed of normal tissue elements. Hamartomatous polyps tend be pedunculated and they are often friable and bleed easily.

Yamada's Atlas of Gastroenterology, Fifth Edition. Edited by Daniel K. Podolsky, Michael Camilleri, J. Gregory Fitz, Anthony N. Kalloo, Fergus Shanahan, and Timothy C. Wang.
Companion website: www.yamadagastro.com/atlas

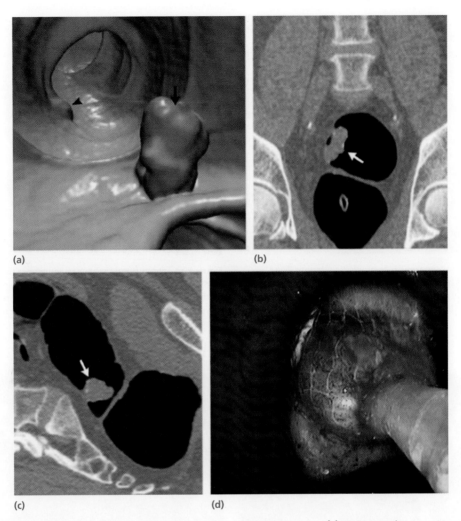

(a)

(b)

(c)

(d)

Figure 30.1 Comparison of computed tomographic colonography (CTC) and optical colonoscopy. **(a)** CTC image showing a 33-mm lobulated rectal polyp (arrow) as well as a 13-mm polyp (arrowhead) near the rectosigmoid junction. Coronal **(b)** and sagittal **(c)** CTC images confirm the presence and soft-tissue composition of the polyp (arrows). Same-day optical colonoscopy **(d)** shows the endoscopic capture of the polyp immediately before resection. Pathological evaluation revealed a tubulovillous adenoma with high-grade dysplasia. Source: Kim DH, Pickhardt PJ, Taylor AJ, et al. CT colonography versus colonoscopy for the detection of advanced neoplasia. N Engl J Med 2007;357:1403–12. Reproduced with permission of the Massachusetts Medical Society.

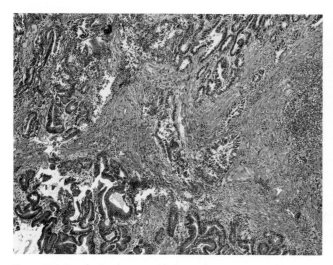

Figure 30.2 Dysplastic adenoma with desmoplastic response. The adenoma has induced fibrosis of the surrounding stroma and nests of tumor cells become surrounded by the desmoplastic response. Source: Courtesy of Lawrence R. Zukerberg, MD, Massachusetts General Hospital.

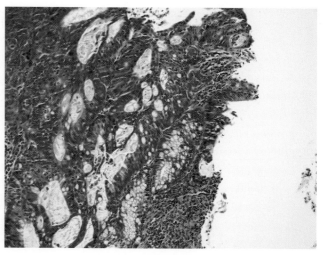

Figure 30.4 Intramucosal carcinoma. Sometimes this term is used interchangeably with high-grade dysplasia. The characteristic histology is of high-grade nuclear and architectural atypia. Source: Courtesy of Lawrence R. Zukerberg, MD, Massachusetts General Hospital.

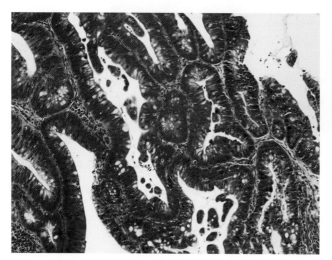

Figure 30.3 Adenomatous polyp with high-grade dysplasia. The features of high-grade dysplasia include stratification of nuclei and increased nuclear pleomorphism, with some nuclei extending into the apical half of the cytoplasm. Increased crypt complexity and cribiforming are also apparent. Source: Courtesy of Lawrence R. Zukerberg, MD, Massachusetts General Hospital.

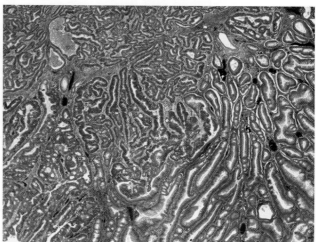

Figure 30.5 Malignant polyp. An adenomatous polyp that contains a focus of carcinoma penetrating through the muscularis mucosae is termed a malignant polyp. Source: Courtesy of Lawrence R. Zukerberg, MD, Massachusetts General Hospital.

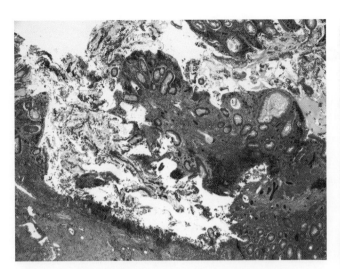

Figure 30.6 Inflammatory fibroid polyp. These polyps are found infrequently in the colon, and more often in the right colon. The pathological features include fascicles or whorls of myofibroblasts and histiocytes. There is often a plasmacytic inflammatory infiltrate and stromal fibrosis. Source: Courtesy of Lawrence R. Zukerberg, MD, Massachusetts General Hospital.

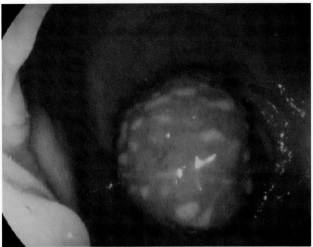

Figure 30.8 Endoscopic appearance of hamartomatous polyp. Hamartomatous polyps are disorganized tissue growths that are composed of the cellular elements known to normally reside within that tissue. They are frequently pedunculated, smooth, and cherry-red, and are often friable and tend to bleed easily.

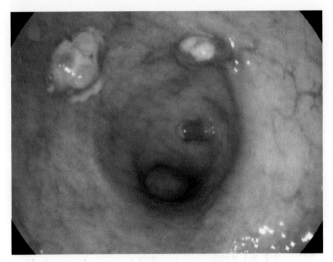

Figure 30.7 Endoscopic appearance of pseudopolyps. Multiple pseudopolyps in the colon of a patient with longstanding ulcerative colitis. Note the polyps occurring in the background of luminal narrowing, loss of haustral folds, and loss of normal vascular pattern.

CHAPTER 31

Malignant tumors of the colon

Jay Luther and Andrew T. Chan
Massachusetts General Hospital and Brigham and Women's Hospital, Harvard Medical School, Boston, MA, USA

Despite improved screening modalities and therapeutic options, colorectal cancer remains a prevalent disease that carries significant morbidity and mortality. Globally, colorectal cancer is the second most common cancer; at current rates, one in five individuals will develop colorectal cancer during their lifetime. Our understanding of risk factors for the development of colorectal cancer is broadening. In addition to traditional risk factors such as age and sex, emerging data highlight the potential importance of lifestyle factors, such as diet, to cancer incidence (Figure 31.1). Genetic determinants of colorectal cancer development are also critical, perhaps best illustrated by hereditary colorectal cancer syndromes known to be associated with single-gene mutations (Table 31.1), including familial adenomatous polyposis (Figure 31.2), serrated polyposis syndrome (Figure 31.3), Cowden syndrome (Figure 31.4), and Peutz–Jeghers syndrome (Figure 31.5). The most common hereditary colorectal cancer syndrome, Lynch syndrome, accounts for one in every 20 colorectal cancers and is characterized by tumors that exhibit loss of DNA mismatch repair proteins and regions of DNA microsatellite instability. Nonetheless, a significant proportion of sporadic colorectal cancers also arise through noninherited, epigenetic inactivation of mismatch repair proteins (Figure 31.6, Table 31.2).

The differential diagnosis of colonic lesions is broad, and includes inflammatory masses and polyps (Figure 31.7), tumors metastatic to the colon (Figure 31.8), submucosal lesions (Figure 31.9), diverticulitis, lymphoma, infection, ischemia, endometriosis, and anatomical defects (such as a volvulus). Neuroendocrine tumors can also arise within the large bowel, most commonly as carcinoid tumors in the rectum (Figure 31.10). With the advent of more sophisticated endoscopic techniques, small neuroendocrine tumors can be resected endoscopically. In all cases, appropriate tissue sampling is critical to define the presence of malignancy and degree of differentiation, both of which are needed to plan appropriate therapy.

Improvements in endoscopic imaging techniques have also facilitated more accurate diagnosis and staging of other colorectal tumors. For example, endoscopic endosonographic characterization of depth of penetration has markedly improved staging of rectal adenocarcinoma, which has important implications for treatment (Figure 31.11). Furthermore, endosonography allows for better tissue sampling, especially in identifying less common causes of rectal disease, such as squamous cell carcinoma of the rectum (Figure 31.12).

Yamada's Atlas of Gastroenterology, Fifth Edition. Edited by Daniel K. Podolsky, Michael Camilleri, J. Gregory Fitz, Anthony N. Kalloo, Fergus Shanahan, and Timothy C. Wang.
© 2016 John Wiley & Sons, Ltd. Published 2016 by John Wiley & Sons, Ltd.
Companion website: www.yamadagastro.com/atlas

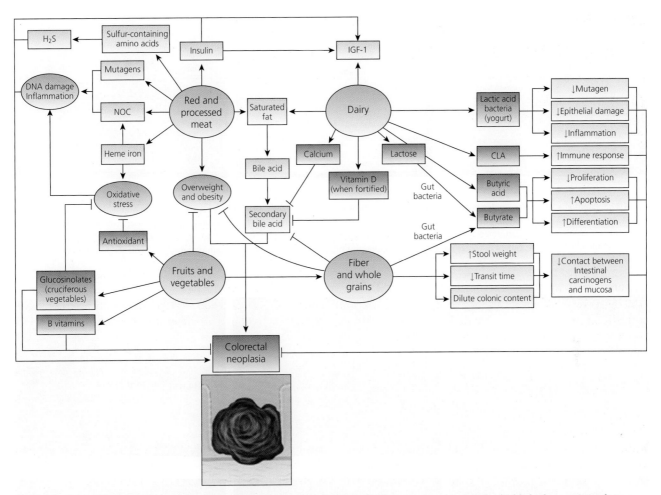

Figure 31.1 The association of food and nutrients with colorectal cancer development. There are emerging data that highlight the association between consumption of certain dietary patterns, foods, and nutrients with risk for colorectal cancer. Experimental studies have suggested several potential mechanisms by which these factors may have biological plausibility. For example, consumption of red meat has been associated with a higher risk for colorectal cancer, possibly through production of heterocyclic amines, which increase oxidative stress and injure cells. Conversely, fiber supplementation has been associated with a decreased risk for colorectal cancer. Although many mechanisms for this association have been hypothesized, growing evidence suggests that fiber may influence the composition and function of the gut microbiome. In turn, the gut microbiome modulates levels of metabolic byproducts such as butyrate with cancer preventive properties. CLA, conjugated linoleic acid; NOC, N-nitroso compound. Source: Song M, Garrett WS, Chan AT. Nutrients, foods and colorectal cancer prevention. Gastroenterol 2015;148:1244. Reproduced with permission of Elsevier.

Table 31.1 Hereditary colorectal syndromes.

Syndrome	Pattern of Inheritance	Lifetime colorectal cancer risk	Noncolorectal cancer Associated cancers	Median Age of Onset (years)	Gene(s) implicated
Lynch	Autosomal dominant	52.2%–68.7%	Endometrial, ovarian, gastric, pancreatic, sebaceous gland tumors, brain, kidney, bile ducts	Early 60s	MSH2, MLH1, MSH6, PMS2, Ep CAM
Familial Adenomatous Polyposis (FAP)	Autosomal dominant	100%	Ampullary, thyroid, pancreas, CNS	40	APC
Attenuated FAP	Autosomal dominant	69%	Ampullary, thyroid, pancreas, CNS (less likely than FAP)	56	APC
MUTYH-associated polyposis	Autosomal recessive	80%	Similar to FAP	50	MYH
Peutz-Jeghers syndrome	Autosomal dominant	39%	Pancreas, breast, small bowel, gastric	45	LKB1/STK11
Juvenile polyposis	Autosomal dominant	10%–38%	Gastric, duodenal	34	MADH4, BMPR1A, ENG
PTEN Hamartoma (Cowden syndrome)	Autosomal dominant	Very low	Breast, thyroid, uterus	Unclear	PTEN

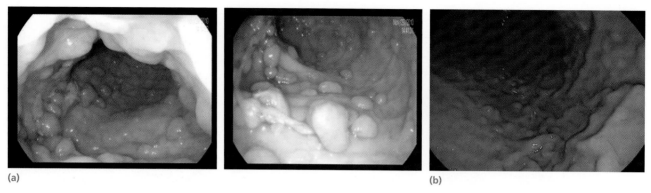

(a)   **(b)**

Figure 31.2 Familial adenomatous polyposis. A 17-year-old woman presented with diarrhea. **(a)** Colonoscopy revealed innumerable adenomas consistent with familial adenomatous polyposis. Genetic testing showed an *APC* mutation (3927del5). A total colectomy with ileoanal pouch anastomosis was subsequently performed. **(b)** Upper endoscopy revealed multiple gastric polyps with pathology consistent with fundic gland polyps with low-grade dysplasia. The patient is being monitored with upper endoscopy every 6 months and examination of her ileoanal pouch annually.

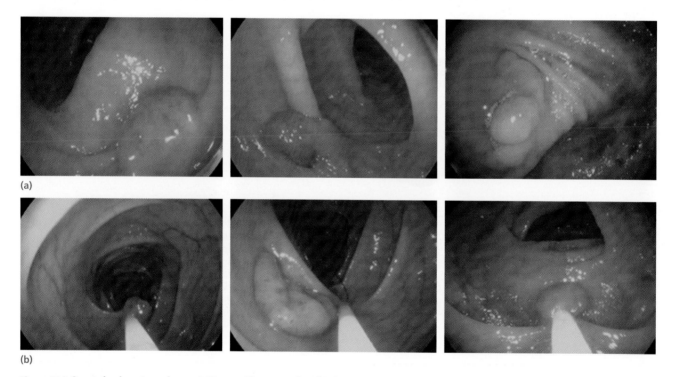

(a)

(b)

Figure 31.3 Serrated polyposis syndrome. A 53-year-old man was found to have 25 polyps on screening colonoscopy, mostly in the proximal ascending colon **(a)** and transverse colon **(b)**. Pathological evaluation from polyp specimens revealed numerous sessile serrated adenomas. Genetic testing for Lynch syndrome, familial adenomatous polyposis, and attenuated familial adenomatous polyposis did not reveal a pathogenic mutation. Based on these findings, a clinical diagnosis of serrated polyposis syndrome was made. Although no single germline mutation has been causatively linked to serrated polyposis syndrome, the condition is characterized by typical somatic changes, including tumors that are CpG island methylator phenotype (CIMP) high) and activating BRAF mutations. Given the high risk for subsequent development of colorectal adenocarcinoma, annual surveillance colonoscopy is generally recommended.

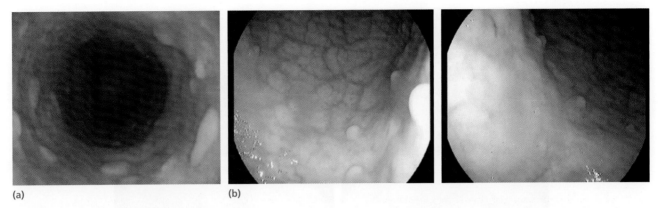

(a)   (b)

Figure 31.4 Cowden syndrome. A 14-year-old underwent upper endoscopy and colonoscopy following the identification of two hamartomas in her breast. **(a)** Upper endoscopy revealed the presence of glycogen acanthosis in the esophagus, which are benign lesions characterized by their whitish-gray and nodular appearance in the background of normal-appearing esophageal mucosa. **(b)** Multiple colonic hamartomas were identified on colonoscopy. Glycogen acanthosis and hamartomas are common features of Cowden syndrome, which is characterized by *PTEN* mutations. In this patient, genetic testing revealed a frameshift mutation in *PTEN* resulting in a premature truncation of the PTEN protein by introducing a stop signal 26 amino acids downstream of codon 231.

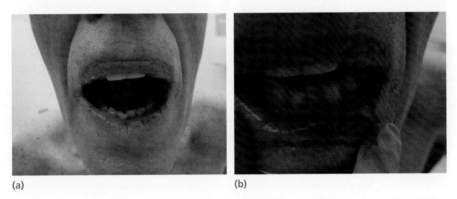

(a)   (b)

Figure 31.5 Mucocutaneous pigmentation in a Peutz–Jeghers syndrome patient. **(a, b)** A patient was referred for gastrointestinal genetics evaluation given the findings of brown macules on his lips, a history of colonic polyps, and family history of pancreatic cancer. Genetic testing revealed a mutation in *STK11*, confirming the diagnosis of Peutz–Jeghers syndrome. The flat brown spots found in this patient are caused by pigment-laden macrophages, and most commonly occur in the perioral region, although they also can be found on the palms and soles. Malignant transformation of these lesions, which can fade over time, is exceedingly rare, although routine dermatological follow-up is recommended.

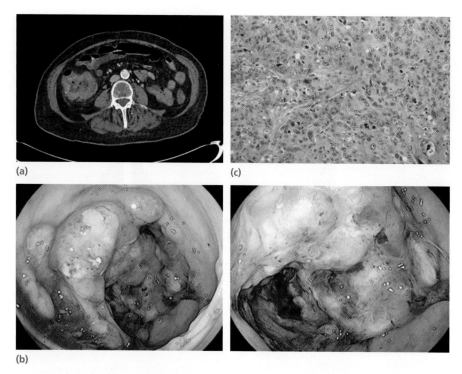

Figure 31.6 Microsatellite instability high (MSI-H) colonic adenocarcinoma in an elderly woman with hematochezia. An 81-year-old woman presented to the emergency department with progressively worsening shortness of breath and rectal bleeding. **(a)** Computed tomography imaging of the abdomen revealed a large, ulcerated mass in the proximal ascending colon. Colonoscopy confirmed the imaging findings by identifying an 8-cm, partially obstructing, ulcerated and friable lesion in the ascending colon, biopsies of which confirmed a diagnosis of colonic adenocarcinoma **(b)**, which was poorly differentiated **(c)**. The patient underwent a right hemicolectomy for T4aN2AM0 disease, electing to forgo adjuvant chemotherapy due to age and comorbidities. Molecular analysis of her tumor revealed loss of expression of the MLH1 and PMS2 DNA mismatch repair (MMR) proteins. Accounting for approximately 15% of cases, colorectal cancers that arise due to deficient MMR are also classified as MSI-H due to the accumulation of insertion/deletion mutations within microsatellite DNA regions. MSI-H cancers can result either from germline mutations in a MMR gene (*MLH1, MSH2, MSH6, PMHS2*), the basis of the Lynch syndrome, or through promoter hypermethylation of *MLH1* which causes gene inactivation. Such sporadic MSI cancers are enriched with BRAF-activating somatic V600E mutations. This patient's cancer demonstrated promoter hypermethylation and the presence of a BRAF V600E mutation (Table 31.2). Taken together, these findings suggest a sporadic MSI-H tumor, which appear to be more commonly seen in the proximal colon of elderly women.

Table 31.2 Analysis of the colonic adenocarcinoma described in Figure 31.6.

	MSH2	MSH6	MLH1	PMS2	BRAF
IHC analysis	+	+	−	−	N/A
PCR analysis	N/A	N/A	+ hypermethylation	M/A	+ V600E

MSI, microsatellite instable; IHC, immunohistochemical; PCR, polymerase chain reaction.

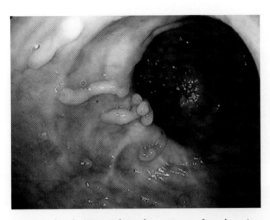

Figure 31.7 Pseudopolyps mimicking the presence of a polyposis syndrome. Patients with chronic inflammation of the intestine, as seen with inflammatory bowel disease (IBD), can develop numerous colonic pseuodopolyps. These pseudopolyps represent raised areas of non-neoplastic colonic mucosa that result from repeated cycles of ulceration and are believed to harbor no malignant potential. Accordingly, no surveillance is needed for these lesions. However, in the context of longstanding IBD, distinction from a malignant neoplasm can be challenging.

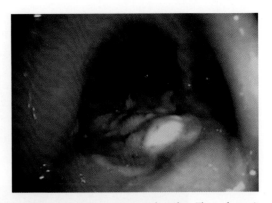

Figure 31.8 Metastatic ovarian cancer to the colon. The endoscopic appearance of metastatic lesions to the gastrointestinal tract is highly variable. However, the mucosa around the periphery of an ulcerated metastatic lesion will likely appear normal without the edema, erythema, friability, or an exophytic pattern more typically seen for primary adenocarcinoma of the gastrointestinal tract.

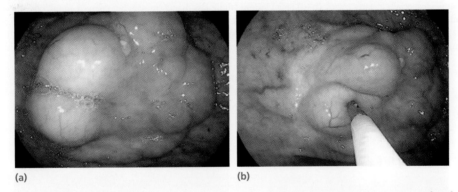

(a)   (b)

Figure 31.9 A cecal lipoma mimicking colorectal cancer. **(a)** A 75-year-old woman undergoing screening colonoscopy was found to have a 4-cm cecal mass. **(b)** Gentle probing of the lesion with biopsy forceps caused dimpling within the mass. Multiple biopsies were taken yet no abnormality was found. Given concern for malignancy, the mass was removed surgically. Pathological evaluation identified the lesion as a cecal lipoma. The differential diagnosis of a mass lesion in the colon includes malignancy (adenocarcinoma, lymphoma, neuroendocrine tumors, metastatic tumors, and Kaposi sarcoma), benign tumors (such as a lipoma), inflammatory masses (inflammatory bowel disease-related masses, tuberculosis, amebiasis, schistosomiasis, mucomycosis, and viral lesions), diverticulitis, endometriosis, and ischemic colitis.

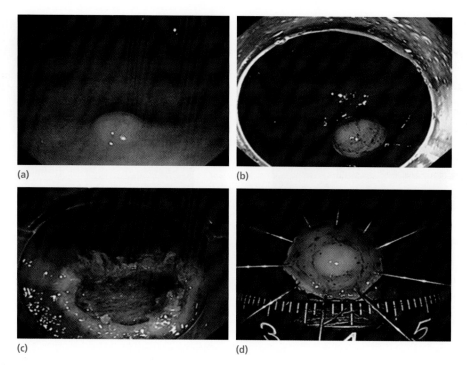

(a) (b)

(c) (d)

Figure 31.10 A rectal carcinoid removed using endoscopic submucosal dissection. **(a)** Rectal carcinoid tumors typically present as yellowish "collar button" submucosal nodules, especially at early stages. **(b–d)** Small lesions (those less than 2 cm) can be removed endoscopically with the use of endoscopic submucosal dissection. Notably, the majority of patients with rectal carcinoid do not develop the carcinoid syndrome. Source: Goto O, Uraoka T, Horii J, Yahagi N. Expanding indications for ESD: submucosal disease (SMT/carcinoid tumors). Gastrointest Endosc Clin N Am 2014;24:169. Reproduced with permission of Elsevier.

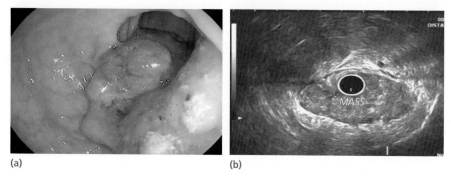

(a) (b)

Figure 31.11 Staging of rectal adenocarcinoma with rectal ultrasound. A 57-year-old man presented with hematochezia. A hypoechoic mass was found in the rectum. The mass was encountered at 12 cm from the anal verge. **(a)** The mass was partially circumferential, encompassing 40% of the lumen. The endosonographic borders were well defined. **(b)** There was sonographic evidence suggesting invasion through the muscularis propria (layer 4) without breakthrough into the perirectal fat. This is staged as a T3N0 rectal adenocarcinoma.

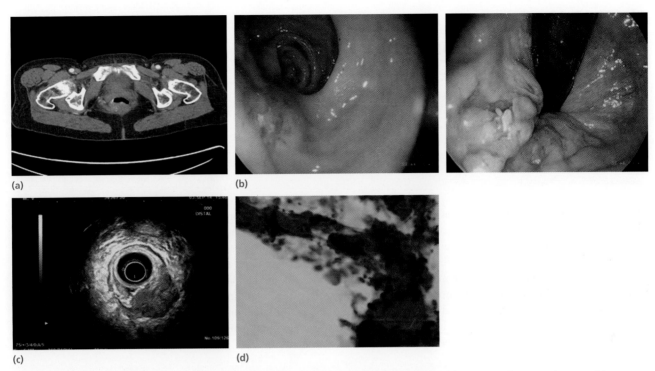

(a)

(b)

(c)

(d)

Figure 31.12 Anorectal squamous cell carcinoma. A 64-year-old woman presented with hematochezia. **(a)** A computed tomography scan of the abdomen identified a 3-cm rectal mass. Flexible sigmoidoscopy was performed and revealed a submucosal mass with a small area of central ulceration 5 cm from the anal verge. This was nonbleeding and did not compromise the lumen. **(b)** On retroflexion, the anorectal junctional mucosa appeared nodular and villous in appearance. **(c)** Radial and linear endoscopic ultrasound showed a hypoechoic lesion measuring 3 cm in maximal dimensions and was transmural in appearance, without any evidence of lymphadenopathy. **(d)** Fine-needle aspiration under Doppler guidance was performed, with rapid onsite evaluation revealing squamous cell carcinoma.

CHAPTER 32

Polyposis syndromes

Randall W. Burt,[1] Mary P. Bronner,[1] and Kory W. Jasperson[2]
[1] University of Utah, Salt Lake City, UT, USA
[2] Ambry Genetics, Aliso Viejo, CA, USA

The gastrointestinal polyposis syndromes are a set of distinct diseases considered together because they each express multiple polypoid lesions of the gastrointestinal tract. The syndromes are defined in terms of pathological and clinical characteristics. Genetic testing now often allows an even more precise diagnosis and categorization. The syndromes are important to recognize because they each exhibit both benign and malignant complications that must be managed appropriately. The conditions are sufficiently common that all GI-related specialists will deal with them. Furthermore, because endoscopically recognized gastrointestinal lesions are central to the diagnosis and management of patients with each of the polyposis syndromes, gastroenterologists are often the primary physicians caring for polyposis patients and families. The conditions and their clinical characteristics are summarized in Tables 32.1 and 32.2. Figures 32.1–32.23 demonstrate typical endoscopic and histological findings of the syndromes.

Yamada's Atlas of Gastroenterology, Fifth Edition. Edited by Daniel K. Podolsky, Michael Camilleri, J. Gregory Fitz, Anthony N. Kalloo, Fergus Shanahan, and Timothy C. Wang.

Table 32.1 Distinguishing features of the characteristic polyposis syndromes.

Syndrome	Gene (frequency that gene mutation is found)	CRC risk (mean age of diagnosis)	Polyp histology	Polyp distribution	Mean age of GI symptom onset	Other disease manifestations	
						Benign	Malignant
Familial adenomatous polyposis[a] (FAP)	APC (70%–90%)	100% (39 years), AFAP 69% (58 years)	Adenomatous, except stomach: fundic gland polyps	Stomach: 23%–100% Duodenum: 50%–90% Jejunum: 50% Ileum: 20% Colon: 100%	35.8 years AFAP 52 years	Desmoid tumors, epidermoid cysts, fibromas, osteomas, CHRPE, adrenal adenomas, dental abnormalities, pilomatrixomas, nasal angiofibromas	Duodenal or periampullary: 3%–5% life-time risk Rare: pancreatic, biliary, thyroid, gastric, CNS, hepatoblastoma, small bowel
MUTYH-associated polyposis (MAP)	MUTYH recessive inheritance (16%–40% if 15–100 adenomas and 7.5%–12.5% if >100 adenomas but not FAP)	93-fold increased risk (48 years)	Adenomatous, hyperplastic, sessile serrated	Stomach: 11% Duodenum: 17% Colon: usually	Not determined	Sebaceous gland adenomas and epitheliomas, lipomas, CHRPE, osteomas, desmoid tumors, epidermoid cysts, and pilomatrixomas	Duodenal 4%, sebaceous gland carcinoma
Serrated polyposis syndrome (SPS)	Possibly inherited, increased expression with smoking	Up to 50% or greater in some studies (63 years)	Hyperplastic, sessile serrated, traditional serrated adenomas, adenomatous	Colon	48 years	None	Unknown
Peutz–Jeghers syndrome (PJS)	STK11 (80%–94%)	39% (46 years)	Peutz–Jeghers, Adenomatous	Stomach: 24% Small bowel: 96% Colon: 27% Rectum: 24%	22–26 years	Mucocutaneous melanin pigment spots	Pancreatic 36%, gastric 29%, small bowel 13%, breast 54%, ovarian 21%, uterine 9%, lung 15%, testes 9%, cervix 10%
Juvenile polyposis syndrome (JPS)	SMAD4, BMPR1A (up to 60%)	Up to 68% (34 years)	Juvenile, Adenomatous	Stomach: 14% Duodenum: 7% Small bowel: 7% Colon: 48%	18.5 years	Hypertelorism, 20% congenital abnormalities in sporadic type	Stomach and duodenum combined up to 21% Pancreatic increased
PTEN hamartoma tumor syndrome (PHTS)[b]	PTEN (30%–55%)	9%–16%	Juvenile, adenomatous, lipomas, inflammatory, ganglioneuromas, lymphoid hyperplasia	Esophagus: 66% Stomach: 75% Duodenum: 37% Colon: 66%	Not determined	Macrocephaly, Lhermitte–Duclos disease, trichelemmomas, oral papillomas, cutaneous lipomas, macular pigmentation of the glans penis, autism spectrum disorder, esophageal glycogenic acanthosis, multinodular goiter, vascular anomalies	Breast 85%, thyroid 35%, kidney 34%, endometrium 28%, melanoma 6%

[a] FAP, familial adenomatous polyposis, includes Gardner syndrome, two-thirds of Turcot syndrome cases, and attenuated FAP.
[b] Includes Cowden syndrome, Bannayan–Riley–Ruvalcaba syndrome, and adult Lhermitte–Duclos disease.
AFAP, attenuated familial adenomatous polyposis; CHRPE, congenital hypertrophy of the retinal pigment epithelium; CNS, central nervous system.

Table 32.2 Additional conditions that exhibit gastrointestinal polyposis.

Category	Condition	Cause	Polyp histology	GI areas affected	Other disease manifestations		
					Benign	Malignant	
Polyposis syndromes with neural polyp histology	Neurofibromatosis type 1 (NF1)	Mutations of *NF1* gene, autosomal dominantly inherited	Neurofibromas and ganglioneuromas	Small bowel > stomach > colon	Café-au-lait spots, Cutaneous neurofibromas, axillary/inguinal freckling, Lisch nodules, optic glioma, pheochromocytoma	Malignant peripheral nerve sheath tumors, breast, GIST, other rare malignancies
	Multiple endocrine neoplasia type 2B (MEN 2B)	Mutations of *RET* proto-oncogene, autosomal dominantly inherited	Ganglioneuromas	Lips to anus, but most common in colon and rectum	Pheochromocytoma, parathyroid adenoma, marfanoid body habitus	Medullary thyroid carcinoma, nearly 100% risk
	Isolated intestinal neurofibromatosis	Unknown	Neurofibromas	Colon > upper GI tract	None	None
Polyposis syndromes with inflammatory polyps	Inflammatory bowel disease	Crohn's disease and ulcerative colitis	Pseudopolyps	Colon	As in inflammatory bowel disease	As in inflammatory bowel disease
	Mucosal prolapse syndrome	Unknown, possibly internal prolapse	Inflammatory polyps with smooth muscle	Rectosigmoid, possibly other areas of colon and stomach	None	None
Polyposis conditions arising from lymphoid tissue	Nodular lymphoid hyperplasia (NLH)	Isolated > Immunodeficiency > lymphoma	Hyperplasia of lymphoid nodules	Small bowel, stomach, colon	Related to underlying disease	
	Multiple lymphomatous polyposis (MLP)	A type of mantle cell lymphoma	Multiple malignant lymphomatous polyps	Small bowel and colon > stomach > esophagus	None	None
	Immunoproliferative small intestinal disease (IPSID)	Most cases from *Campylobacter jejuni* infection	Plasma cell proliferation	Small bowel	Malabsorption, progression to lymphoplasmacytic and immunoblastic lymphoma if not treated in early stages	

Table 32.2 (*Continued*)

Category	Condition	Cause	Polyp histology	GI areas affected	Other disease manifestations	
					Benign	**Malignant**
Miscellaneous rare polyposis syndromes and conditions	Constitutional mismatch repair deficiency syndrome (CMMRDS)	Biallelic mutations (recessive inheritance) in *MLH1*, *MSH2*, *MSH6*, or *PMS2*	Adenomatous	Colon, other GI reported	Café-au-lait macules, axillary/ inguinal freckling, and Lisch nodules	Hematological, brain: endometrial, small bowel, ureter/ renal pelvis, sarcomas various other rare malignancies
	Hereditary mixed polyposis syndrome (HMPS)	Autosomal dominantly inherited, linked to duplication 40 kb upstream of the *GREM1* gene locus at chromosome 15q13.3-q14	Atypical juvenile, adenomatous, hyperplastic	Colon	None	Colon
	Cronkhite–Canada syndrome (CCS)	Possibly infectious	Juvenile polyps, adenomatous	Stomach to anus	Skin hyperpigmentation, hair loss, nail atrophy, hypogeusia	Colon up to 25%, possibly stomach
	Gorlin syndrome (GS)	Mutations of *PTCH* gene, autosomal dominantly inherited	Hamartoma	Only gastric reported	Mandibular bone cysts, pits of palms and soles, macrocephaly, congenital anomalies	Multiple basal cell carcinomas, medulloblastoma
	McCune–Albright syndrome (MAS)	Postzygotic activating mutations in the *GNAS* gene, not inherited	Peutz–Jeghers	Duodenal and other GI locations	Café-au-lait macules, perioral freckling, polyostotic fibrous dysplasia of bone, various endocrinopathies	None
	Leiomyomatosis polyposis	Not known	Leiomyoma	Colon, other GI locations	None	None
	Lipomatous polyposis	Not known	Lipoma, adenomatous	Colon, other GI locations	Peritoneal lipomas	None
	Lymphangiomas polyposis	Not known	Lymphangioma	Colon	None	None
	Pneumatosis cystoides intestinalis	Many associations	Inflammatory and air spaces	Colon and other GI locations	None	None

GIST, gastrointestinal stromal tumor.

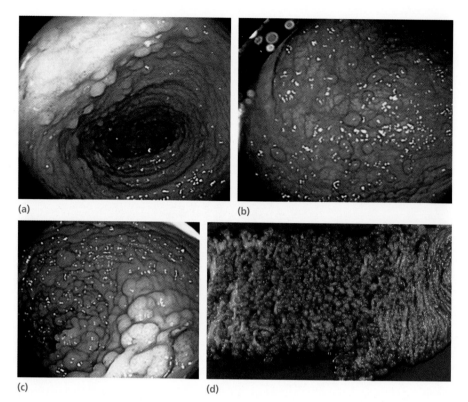

Figure 32.1 The colon in familial adenomatous polyposis. **(a–c)** colonoscopic images. **(d)** Section of colon demonstrating fully developed familial adenomatous polyposis. Source **(d)**: Bronner MP. Gastrointestinal inherited polyposis syndromes. Mod Pathol 2003;16:359.

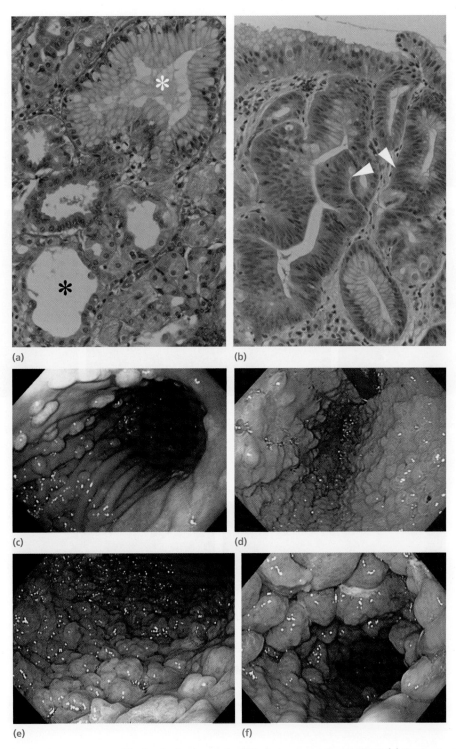

Figure 32.2 Histological and endoscopic images of fundic gland polyps in familial adenomatous polyposis (FAP). **(a)** Fundic gland polyp with foveolar dysplasia. This gastric fundic gland polyp reveals the diagnostic dilated oxyntic or fundic glands (black *), lined by normal parietal cells with eosinophilic cytoplasm and chief cells with hematoxyphilic cytoplasm. Also shown is a dilated mucinous gland (white *), which can also be variably present in fundic gland polyps. **(b)** The surface of this fundic gland polyp shows foveolar surface cells with low-grade dysplasia, characterized by epithelial cells with enlarged, hyperchromatic, and mildly irregular nuclei that maintain their nuclear polarity (the long axes of the crowded nuclei maintain a perpendicular orientation to the basal lamina). Dysplastic fundic gland polyps are a common (~40% prevalence) and highly specific finding of FAP, because surface dysplasia is rarely observed in sporadic-type fundic gland polyps arising out of either proton pump inhibitor therapy or incidental sporadic gastric fundic gland polyps. **(c–f)** Endoscopic images of gastric fundic gland polyposis in FAP with increasing severity. Source: **(a, b)** Bronner MP. Gastrointestinal inherited polyposis syndromes. Mod Pathol 2003;16:359.

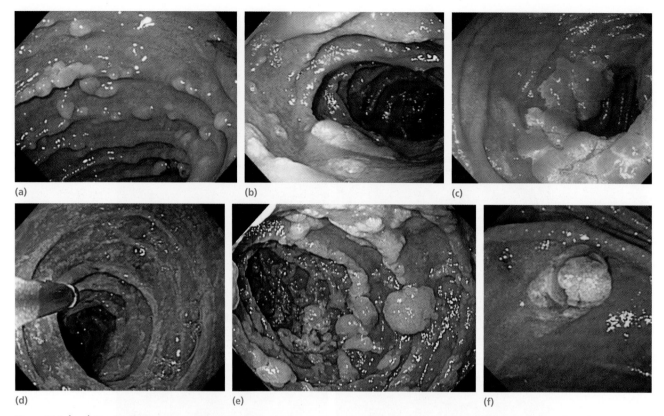

Figure 32.3 (a–e) Duodenal adenomatous polyposis with increasing severity in familial adenomatous polyposis. **(f)** Duodenal papilla with adenomatous enlargement in a familial adenomatous polyposis patient. Source **(f):** Courtesy of Jewel Samadder, MD.

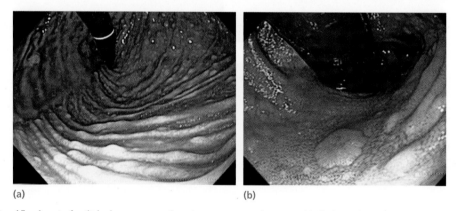

Figure 32.4 (a, b) "Pouch" polyps in familial adenomatous polyposis, post proctocolectomy with ileal pouch–anal anastomosis. Many of the polyps in **(a)** are lymphoid hyperplasia, while others are adenomas.

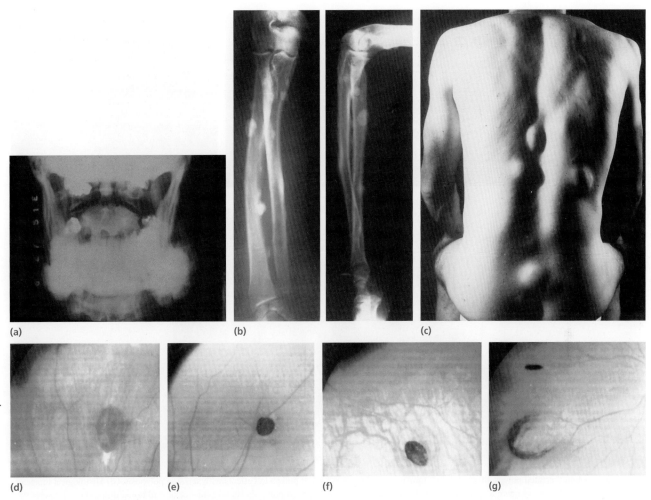

(a) (b) (c)

(d) (e) (f) (g)

Figure 32.5 Extraintestinal findings of familial adenomatous polyposis. **(a)** Large bilateral osteomas at the angle of the mandible, which is one of the most common locations for these benign lesions. They also occur commonly on the forehead and occiput, but may occur on any area of the skull and any bone of the body. **(b)** Multiple osteomas of the leg and forearm. **(c)** Cutaneous fibromas on a patient with familial adenomatous polyposis. These may occur anywhere on the cutaneous surface. They often occur before puberty and may grow to several centimeters in diameter. **(d–g)** Congenital hypertrophy of the retinal pigment epithelium. Several examples of the retinal pigment that are observed in pedigrees with familial adenomatous polyposis who exhibit *APC* gene mutations between exons 4 and 9. Although such lesions are common in the general population, the presence of bilateral or more than four retinal lesions is quite specific for familial adenomatous polyposis. Source: **(b, c)** Gardener EJ, Burt RW, Freston JW. Gastrointestinal polyposis: syndromes and genetic mechanisms. West J Med 1980;132:488. Reproduced with permission of BMJ Publishing Group Ltd. Source: **(d–g)** Traboulsi EI, Krush AJ, Gardner EJ, et al. Prevalence and importance of pigmented ocular fundus legions in Gardner's syndrome. N Engl J Med 1987; 316:661. Reproduced with permission of the Massachusetts Medical Society.

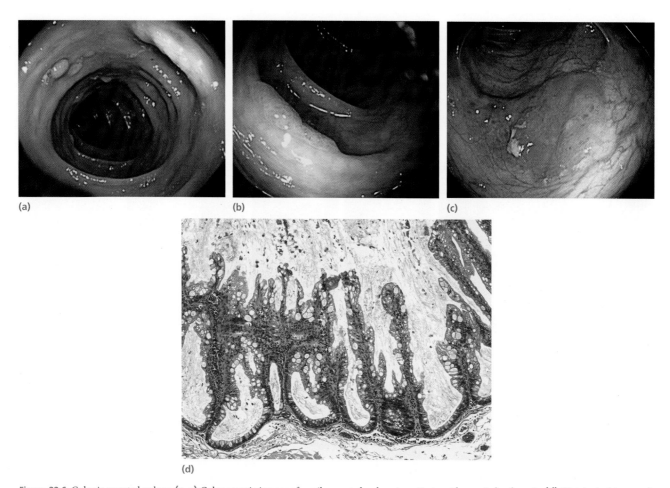

(a) (b) (c)

(d)

Figure 32.6 Colonic serrated polyps. **(a–c)** Colonoscopic images of sessile serrated polyps in patients with serrated polyposis. **(d)** Histological image of a sessile serrated polyp, also known as a sessile serrated adenoma. This sessile serrated polyp shows no evidence of traditional dysplasia and reveals the characteristic although nondiagnostic morphology. The morphology seen here is commonly shared in part by simple hyperplastic polyps, making it less reproducible as a diagnostic criterion. Large polyp size (greater than 1 cm) and right-sided colonic location are more reproducible diagnostic features. The characteristic morphology as seen here consists of serrated or jagged/ saw-toothed glandular epithelial profiles that extend through the full mucosal thickness of the polyp to also include the polyp base, accompanied by variable cystic dilatation of the serrated glands and lateral extension of the basal-most crypts along the muscularis mucosae (sometimes likened to "boot"-shaped basal crypts). Source: **(d)** Courtesy of Mary Bronner.

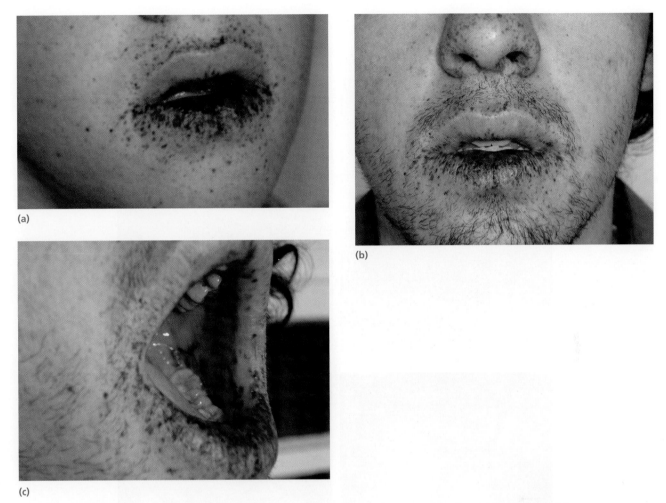

(a)

(b)

(c)

Figure 32.7 (a–c) Perioral, lip, and buccal pigmentation of Peutz–Jeghers syndrome. Source: Courtesy of Dr. Asadur J. Tchekmedyian.

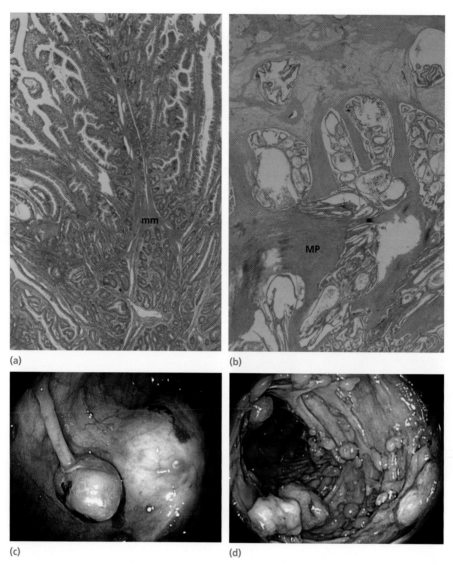

Figure 32.8 **(a, b)** Histological images of Peutz–Jeghers polyps. **(a)** This Peutz–Jeghers hamartomatous small intestinal polyp illustrates the typical arborizing, branching muscularis mucosae (labeled as "mm") extending well up into the head of the polyp. The polyp epithelium is composed of otherwise normal and nondysplastic small intestinal villi. **(b)** Peutz–Jeghers polyps, as shown here, commonly demonstrate benign misplaced epithelium that extends deep to the mucosa and into outer layers of the bowel wall, mimicking invasive carcinoma. Benign misplaced epithelium in these polyps can be exuberant and extend into and even transmurally through the muscularis propria (labeled as "MP"). This benign process is distinguished from carcinoma by the fact that the epithelial cells are bland and not dysplastic and that the epithelium is accompanied by benign mucosal lamina propria (not recognizable at this low magnification), which carcinoma never takes with it upon invading deep to the mucosa. **(c, d)** Colonoscopic images of Peutz–Jeghers syndrome polyposis. Source: **(a, b)** Bronner MP. Gastrointestinal inherited polyposis syndromes. Mod Pathol 2003;16:359.

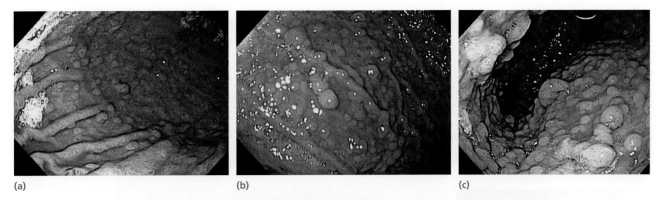

Figure 32.9 (a–c) Endoscopic images of gastric hamartomatous polyposis in Peutz–Jeghers syndrome with increasing severity.

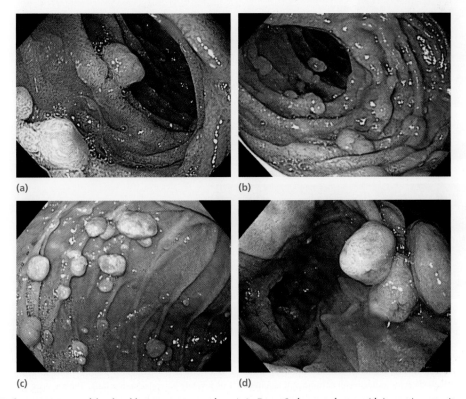

Figure 32.10 (a–d) Endoscopic images of duodenal hamartomatous polyposis in Peutz–Jeghers syndrome with increasing severity.

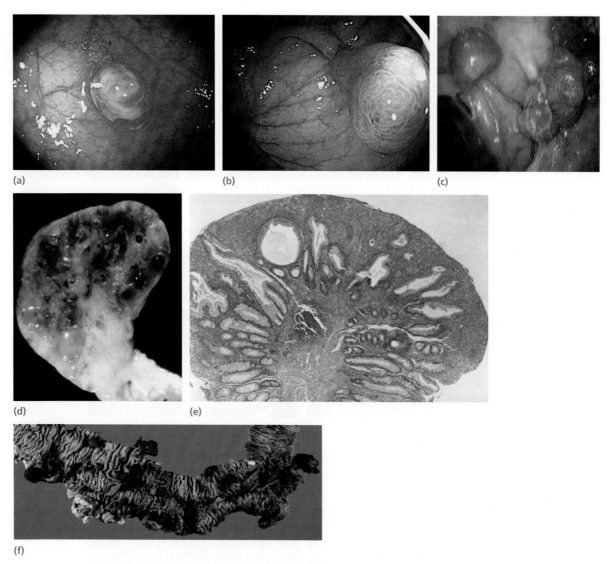

Figure 32.11 Colonic polyposis in juvenile polyposis syndrome. **(a–c)** Colonoscopic images. **(d)** Bisected gross view of a sporadic juvenile/ inflammatory polyp illustrating the classic smooth polyp surface with numerous cystic spaces within the polyp head. The cystic spaces, also referred to as mucus retention cysts, consist of dilated glands filled with mucin and variable inflammation. **(e)** Histological image of a juvenile polyp demonstrating the usual features of an inflamed and edematous lamina propria (a variable aspect of these polyps), along with crypt architectural distortion, including dilated, irregular, and branched crypts indicative of chronic mucosal injury. This juvenile polyp lacks dysplasia. The presence or absence of dysplasia is an important feature to evaluate in juvenile polyps, given the high risk of neoplasia in the juvenile polyposis syndrome arising out of the juvenile polyps themselves. The simple nondysplastic juvenile polyp, shown here, is histologically *identical* to other types of inflammatory polyps of the gastrointestinal tract. Accordingly, many pathologists prefer the nonspecific name of "inflammatory polyp" over "juvenile polyp" to emphasize the inability for histology alone to differentiate juvenile polyposis inflammatory polyps from those of idiopathic inflammatory bowel disease, Cowden disease, tuberous sclerosis, and the most common by far of all causes, the incidental inflammatory polyp caused by local and insignificant mucosal trauma. **(f)** Resected colon illustrating fully developed juvenile polyposis, with the classical variably sized to quite large, many centimeter-sized polyps with multilobulated, irregular, and nodular surfaces. Hereditary juvenile polyposis polyps commonly reveal this multilobulated appearance, especially in the larger polyps. This is not typically observed in sporadic or incidental inflammatory/juvenile type polyps, which normally have very smooth surfaces that are classically eroded as well. **(d–f)** Source: Bronner MP. Gastrointestinal inherited polyposis syndromes. Mod Pathol 2003;16:359.

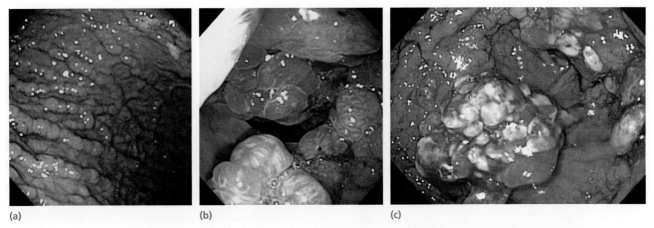

(a)   (b)   (c)

Figure 32.12 (a–c) Endoscopic images of giant gastric hamartomatous polyposis of juvenile polyposis syndrome when a *SMAD4* gene mutation is etiological.

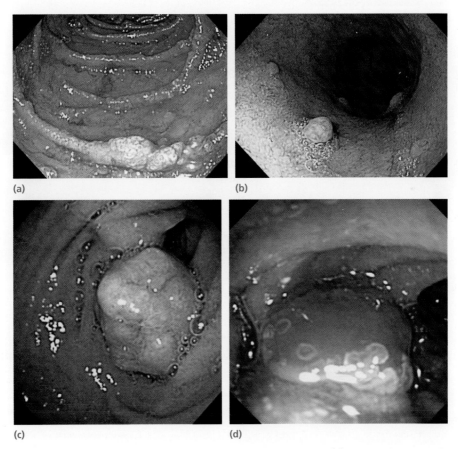

(a)   (b)

(c)   (d)

Figure 32.13 (a–c) Endoscopic images of duodenal hamartomatous polyposis in juvenile polyposis. **(d)** Jejunal polyp in juvenile polyposis.

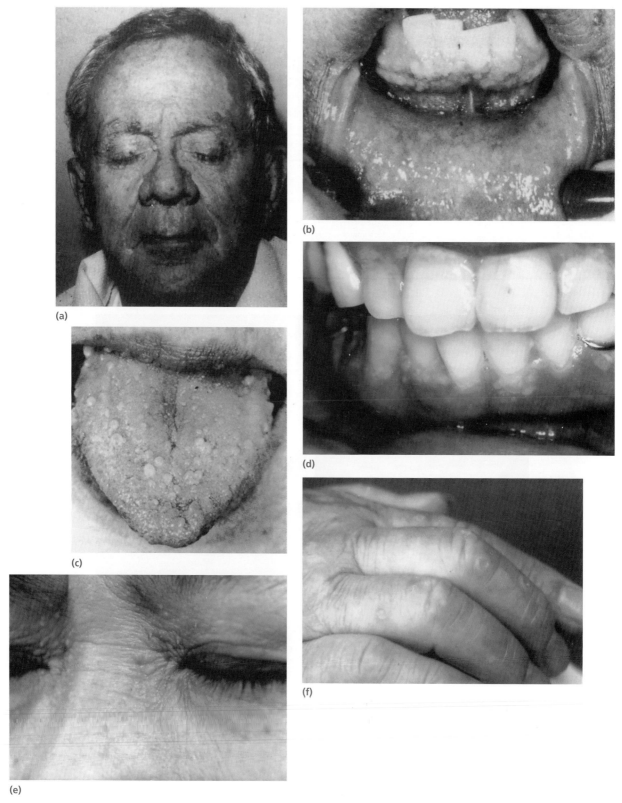

Figure 32.14 Cutaneous and mucosal lesions of Cowden syndrome. **(a)** Face of a patient with Cowden syndrome demonstrating central papules. **(b)** Labial mucosa and gingiva showing cobblestone papules. **(c)** Tongue with typical papules. **(d)** Fibromas on the gingiva. **(e)** Trichilemmomas of the face. **(f)** Hyperkeratosis of the digits. Source: **(d–f)** Courtesy of Dr. Kyosuke Ushio. Source: Sogol PB, Sugawara M, Gorden HE, et al. Cowden's disease: familial goiter and skin haematomas. West J Med 1983;139:324.

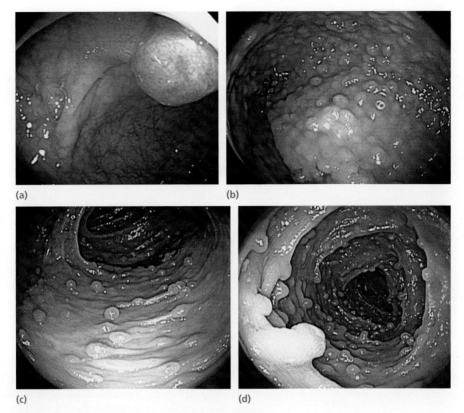

Figure 32.15 **(a–d)** Colonoscopic images of colonic polyposis in Cowden syndrome.

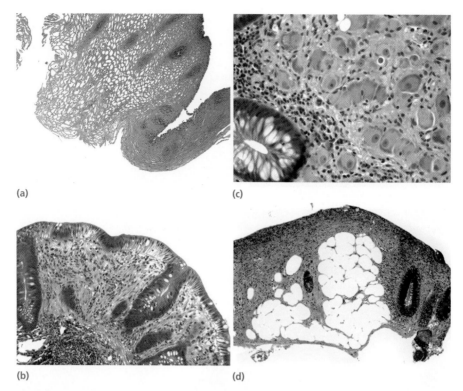

(a)

(c)

(b)

(d)

Figure 32.16 (a–d) Histological images of lesions in Cowden syndrome. This composite of four polyps demonstrates the salient histological polyps of Cowden syndrome that occur throughout the gastrointestinal tract. **(a)** Esophageal glycogenic acanthosis showing a thickened squamous epithelium containing cytoplasmic glycogen denoted by the clear cytoplasmic vacuoles in the squamous cells. **(b)** Smooth muscle hamartoma characterized by spindled smooth muscle cells replacing the lamina propria. **(c)** Ganglioneuromatous polyp showing a collection of lamina propria ganglion cells containing regular round to oval nuclei with prominent nucleoli and the characteristic hematoxyphilic Nissl substance within these neuronal cell bodies. **(d)** Colonic mucosal lipoma with abundant mature adipose tissue within the lamina propria. Source: Courtesy of Mary Bronner.

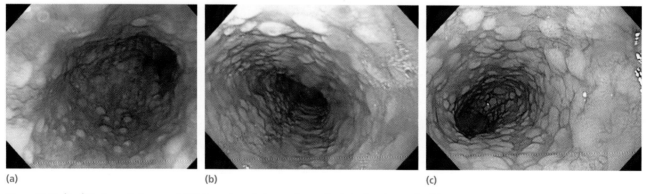

(a)　　　　　　　　　　　　　　　　(b)　　　　　　　　　　　　　　　　(c)

Figure 32.17 (a–c) Endoscopic images of diffuse esophageal glycogenic acanthosis in Cowden syndrome

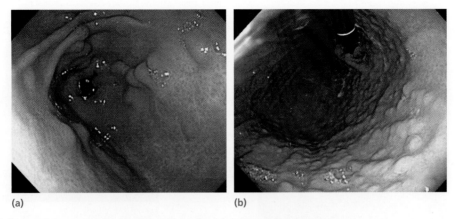

Figure 32.18 (a, b) Endoscopic images of gastric hamartomatous polyposis in Cowden syndrome.

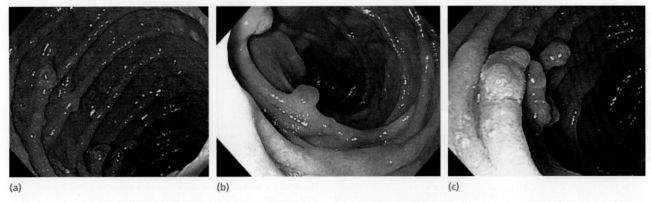

Figure 32.19 (a–c) Endoscopic images of duodenal hamartomatous polyposis in Cowden syndrome.

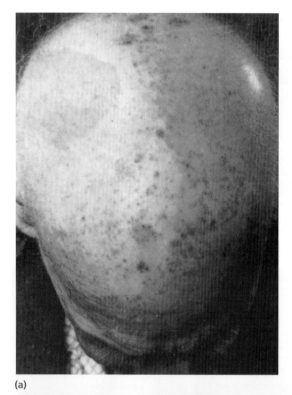

(a)

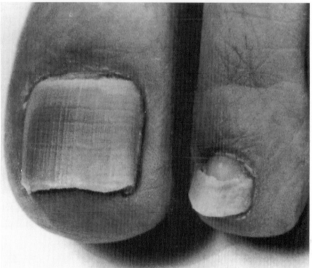

(b)

Figure 32.20 Cronkhite–Canada syndrome. **(a)** Scalp showing almost total alopecia. **(b)** Onychodystrophy of the toenails with lines of separation from the normal nail. Source: Russell DM, Bhathal PS, St John DJB. Complete remission in Cronkhite–Canada syndrome. Gastroenterology 1983;85:180. Reproduced with permission of Elsevier.

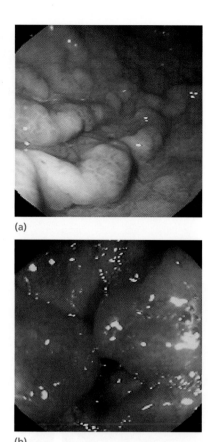

(a)

(b)

Figure 32.21 Endoscopic views of a patient with Cronkhite–Canada syndrome. The patient presented with dysgeusia, alopecia, onychodystrophy, and diarrhea. **(a)** Stomach. **(b)** Colon: the largest polyp is a pedunculated adenomatous polyp; all other polyps shown exhibited histology typical of Cronkhite–Canada lesions. Source: Courtesy of Dr. Edward L. Krawitt.

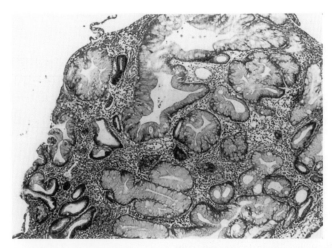

Figure 32.22 Colonic polyp from a patient with Cronkhite–Canada syndrome. The polyp demonstrates cystically dilated glands with abundant generous, edematous, and inflamed lamina propria. The polyps of Cronkhite–Canada syndrome are very similar to those of juvenile polyposis. Intervening mucosa in Cronkhite–Canada syndrome, however, is abnormal, with edema and inflammation of the lamina propria. Source: Malhotra R. Cronkhite–Canada syndrome associated with colon carcinoma and adenomatous changes in C-C polyps. Am J Gastroenterol 1988;83:722. Reproduced with permission of John Wiley & Sons.

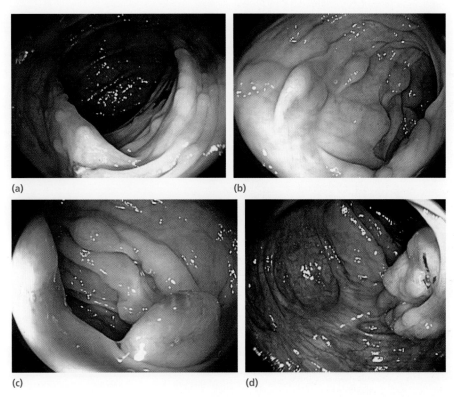

Figure 32.23 **(a)** Colonic lymphoid hyperplasia. **(b, c)** Rectosigmoid polyposis in mucosal prolapse syndrome. **(d)** Colonic pneumatosiscystoides intestinalis.

CHAPTER 33

Colorectal cancer screening

Uri Ladabaum
Stanford University School of Medicine, Stanford, CA, USA

These images illustrate key concepts related to colorectal cancer screening and surveillance in average-risk and higher-risk persons (Figures 33.1–33.10). They also illustrate the spectrum of colorectal neoplasia that is encountered in the course of colorectal cancer screening and surveillance.

Yamada's Atlas of Gastroenterology, Fifth Edition. Edited by Daniel K. Podolsky, Michael Camilleri, J. Gregory Fitz, Anthony N. Kalloo, Fergus Shanahan, and Timothy C. Wang.
© 2016 John Wiley & Sons, Ltd. Published 2016 by John Wiley & Sons, Ltd.
Companion website: www.yamadagastro.com/atlas

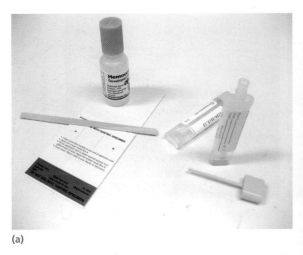
(a)

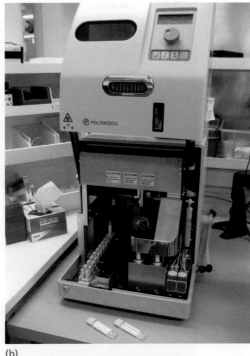
(b)

Figure 33.1 Guaiac-based fecal occult blood tests (gFOBTs) and fecal immunochemical tests (FITs) are used to screen stool for occult blood that could signal the presence of colorectal neoplasia. **(a)** Wooden sticks are used to apply smears of stool on gFOBT test card windows (left), which are then developed using a peroxide-containing developer (small bottle, left) and read by looking for color change. Some FITs use brushes or sticks to collect stool into vials (right). **(b)** FITs that can be processed by machines with high throughput are favored for population-based screening.

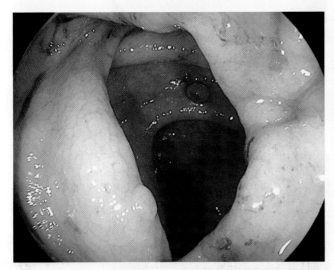

Figure 33.2 In persons found to have colorectal neoplasia at screening colonoscopy, the most common findings are one or two small adenomas. Seen here are one small adenoma on the near fold on the left, and a second adenoma on a superior fold more proximally in the colon (farther away in the image). Although it is logical to assume that larger and advanced adenomas were once small adenomas, the natural history of small adenomas is not well known. Surveillance guidelines in the USA have evolved towards longer intervals after removal of one to two small adenomas. Currently, surveillance at 5–10 years is recommended. European guidelines identify patients with one to two small adenomas as low risk, and recommend returning to regular screening.

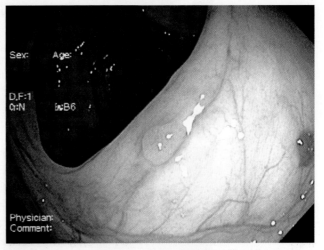

Figure 33.3 This small adenoma that developed behind a fold was seen only during retroflexion in the ascending colon. Note the colonoscope in the left upper portion of the figure, seen on retroflexion. The pooled estimates for the miss rate for 1 to 5-mm adenomas in tandem colonoscopy studies is 26% (95% CI 21%–30%).

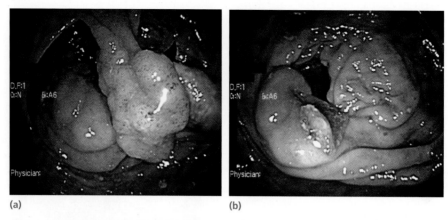

(a)   (b)

Figure 33.4 (a) In this patient, a large pedunculated polyp was seen resting on the ileocecal valve during colonoscope insertion. **(b)** After cecal inspection, which involved washing and insufflation, the polyp fell behind a fold and proved difficult to find again. The polyp was found and snare polypectomy was performed, but this case illustrates that the pooled estimate for the miss rate for $\geq$10-mm adenomas in tandem colonoscopy studies is 2.1% (95% CI 0.3%–7.3%).

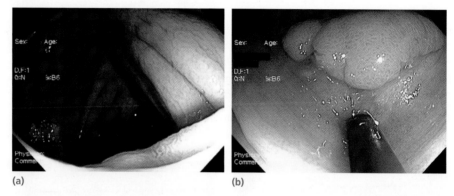

(a)   (b)

Figure 33.5 (a) The edge of a sessile lesion on the proximal side of this patient's ileocecal valve (bottom right) could have been mistaken for ileum. The lesion was not seen at all with the colonoscope tip in the cecum, with maximal deflection towards the ileocecal valve. Retroflexion in the cecum was not successful. **(b)** Exposure behind the ileocecal valve with the aid of an injection needle catheter revealed the distal portion of a large sessile lesion that proved to be a 3-cm tubulovillous adenoma. Lesions like this, either missed or incompletely resected, may account for a large fraction of interval, or postcolonoscopy, colorectal cancers – which are more likely to be proximal compared with noninterval colorectal cancers.

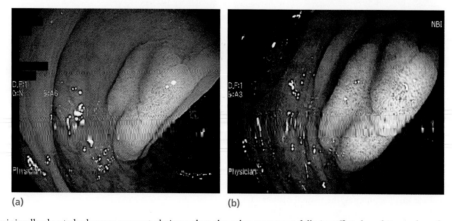

(a)   (b)

Figure 33.6 (a) This minimally elevated adenoma was not obvious when the colon was more fully insufflated, and it may have been more difficult to detect without a high-definition colonoscope. **(b)** Narrow-band imaging demonstrated the typical features of adenomas: browner color relative to the background color, and a surface pattern consisting of oval, tubular, or branched white structures surrounded by brown vessels. Note the previously snared pedunculated polyp lying in the left upper quadrant of (b), prior to retrieval with a net.

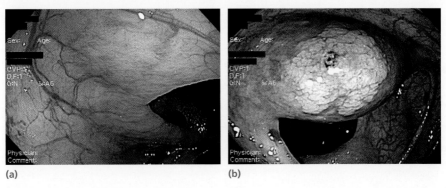

(a)   (b)

Figure 33.7 **(a)** A thin film of stool initially hid this subtle, flat sessile serrated adenoma in the ascending colon (top). Note how the colonic vessels became indistinct as they reached the edges of this lesion. **(b)** Injection with saline and indigo carmine in preparation for snare resection revealed the lesion more clearly, and highlighted its edges. Sessile serrated adenomas may progress to carcinoma through an epigenetic hypermethylation mechanism.

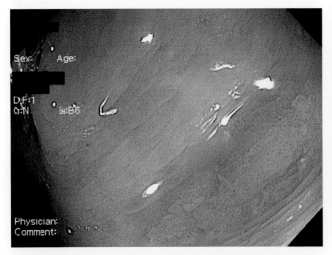

Figure 33.8 A thin film of yellow-tinged mucus highlighted this subtle sessile serrated adenoma (right lower portion of figure). Washing this film may make it more difficult to see these lesions. Sessile serrated adenomas are more common in the proximal colon than in the distal colorectum. Failure to detect or completely remove these lesions may explain in part the lower protective benefit of screening colonoscopy in the proximal colon compared with the distal colorectum.

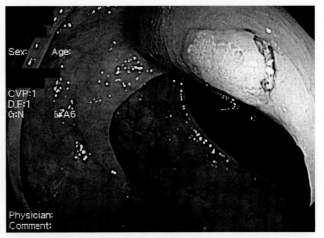

Figure 33.9 This benign-appearing sessile polyp (seen here after injection with saline and indigo carmine in preparation for snare resection) was an invasive, moderately differentiated adenocarcinoma. This ascending colon lesion was found at surveillance colonoscopy in a woman who carried her family's mutation in the *MSH2* gene, which is diagnostic of Lynch syndrome. The patient's sister had a history of proximal colon cancer. Immunohistochemistry on the resected lesion showed absence of the *MSH2* and *MSH6* gene products, with intact staining for the *MLH1* and *PMS2* gene products – the typical pattern expected in colorectal cancers developing in carriers of an *MSH2* germline mutation.

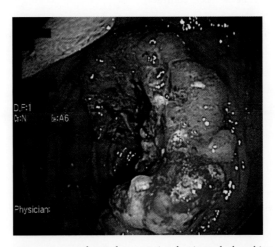

Figure 33.10 This sigmoid colorectal adenocarcinoma was not detected at screening, but instead when this patient developed moderate hematochezia after being placed on warfarin. The patient was a 73-year-old man who had never undergone colorectal cancer screening. In addition to this colonic mass, several large polyps were also found at colonoscopy (the edge of one is seen in the left upper portion of the figure). It is likely that screening with guaiac-based fecal occult blood test (gFOBT), fecal immunochemical test (FIT), sigmoidoscopy, or colonoscopy a few years earlier could have detected the premalignant lesion that ultimately developed into this invasive adenocarcinoma, or detected this malignancy at an earlier stage. It is conceivable that even earlier screening would have found at least one significant adenoma, and that subsequent surveillance in this patient could have led to cancer prevention or early detection.

CHAPTER 34

Anorectal diseases

Adil E. Bharucha[1] and Arnold Wald[2]

[1] Mayo Clinic College of Medicine, Rochester, MN, USA
[2] University of Wisconsin, Madison, WI, USA

This chapter provides a visual review of anorectal anatomy, functions, and pathologies. We begin with a coronal section of the anorectum, which highlights the orientation of the anal sphincters and pelvic floor muscles (Figure 34.1). Common instruments for anorectal examinations more frequently used by a colorectal surgeon than a gastroenterologist are shown in Figure 34.2. The equipment used for rigid proctosigmoidoscopy is shown in Figure 34.2a. Because symptomatic internal hemorrhoids are one of the most common lesions seen by the practicing gastroenterologist, we have elected to show a photograph of the simplest, most widely used instrument for management of internal hemorrhoids, the Barron-type rubber band ligator with its ancillary equipment (see Figure 34.2c).

Hemorrhoids are the most common anal lesions seen in practice; therefore, pictures of external and different degrees of internal hemorrhoids are critical to any atlas on anal disorders (Figures 34.3, 34.4, 34.5, 34.6, 34.7, and 34.8). Hemorrhoids may be treated using a variety of nonsurgical techniques. One modality is banding using a ligator device attached to the tip of an endoscope (Figure 34.9). Examples of an anorectal abscess, the classification of anorectal fistulae, rectal prolapse, solitary rectal ulcer, and chronic anal fissure are shown in Figures 34.10, 34.11, 34.12, 34.13, and 34.14. These important lesions are all best diagnosed by means of simple inspection. Figures 34.15 and 34.16 depict normal anorectal and pelvic floor motion during defecation and when subjects squeeze (i.e., contract)

their pelvic floor muscles. Figures 34.17–34.27 illustrate the techniques for digital rectal examination and encapsulate the pathophysiology of fecal incontinence. Anorectal manometry discloses a variety of disturbances in fecal incontinence (Table 34.1). Figures 34.28, 34.29, and 34.30 summarize the cardinal clinical features of syndromes associated with functional anorectal pain. Finally, we show examples of carcinoma of the anus (Figures 34.31 and 34.32). One fairly subtle lesion is Bowen disease (cutaneous squamous cell carcinoma in situ), which may be confused with the anal lesions of dermatitis and psoriasis.

Table 34.1 Manometric patterns of fecal incontinence.

	IAS weakness	EAS trauma	Neurogenic	
			Peripheral	Central
Resting P	↓	NI	NI	NI
Squeeze P	NI	↓	↓	↓
PRM	NI	NI	↓	↓
Sensation	NI	NI	NI	↓

Internal and anal sphincter (IAS, EAS) dysfunctions manifest as reduced anal resting and squeeze pressures (P), respectively. Peripheral neurogenic injury may result in external sphincter weakness and, if the sacral roots are affected, also cause puborectalis (PRM) weakness. Central neurogenic injury also affects rectal sensation. NI, normal.

Yamada's Atlas of Gastroenterology, Fifth Edition. Edited by Daniel K. Podolsky, Michael Camilleri, J. Gregory Fitz, Anthony N. Kalloo, Fergus Shanahan, and Timothy C. Wang.
© 2016 John Wiley & Sons, Ltd. Published 2016 by John Wiley & Sons, Ltd.
Companion website: www.yamadagastro.com/atlas

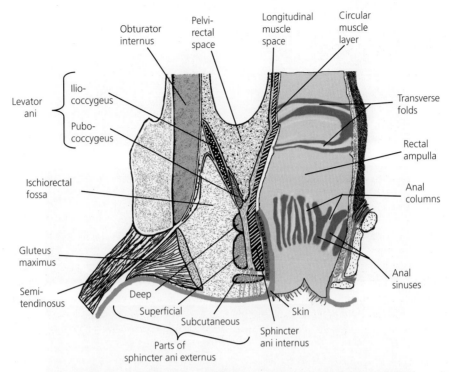

Figure 34.1 Diagram of a coronal section of the rectum, anal canal, and adjacent structures. The pelvic barrier includes the anal sphincters and pelvic floor muscles. Source: Bharucha AE. Fecal incontinence. Gastroenterology 2003;124:1672. Reproduced with permission of Elsevier.

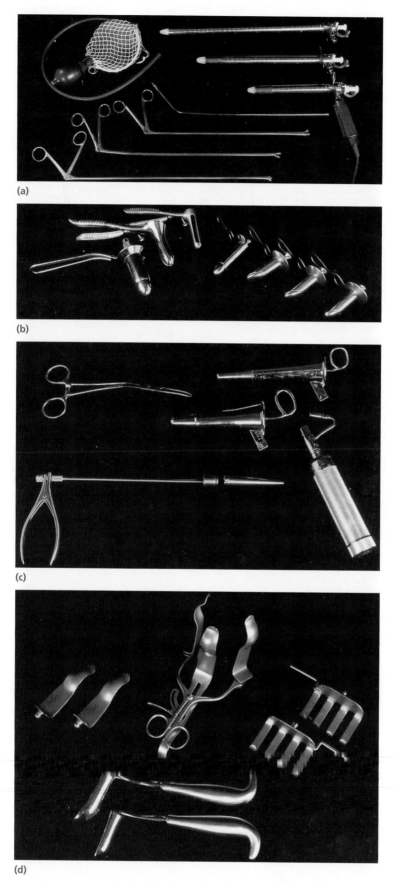

Figure 34.2 Instruments for anorectal examinations. **(a)** Equipment necessary for performance of rigid proctosigmoidoscopy with internal light source and air insufflator, interchangeable proctoscopes with light source, suction wand, and assorted biopsy forceps. **(b)** Instruments which require an external light source. Left to right: Fansler proctoscope, Pratt rectal speculum, Sims rectal speculum, Buie–Hirschman anoscope, and Hirschman anoscopes (small, medium, and large). Disposable anoscopes are also commonly used (not shown). **(c)** Instruments for rubber-band ligation of internal hemorrhoids. Barron-type ligator with grasping forceps, and device for loading bands (left). Welch–Allyn self-illuminated anoscope with large and small specula (right). **(d)** Anal retractors. Top to bottom: Parks' anal retractor with interchangeable blades, Ferguson–Moon anal retractor, and Hill–Ferguson anal retractor.

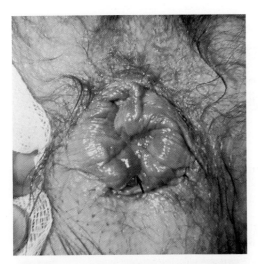

Figure 34.3 First-degree (nonprolapsing) internal hemorrhoid (arrow) and external hemorrhoids.

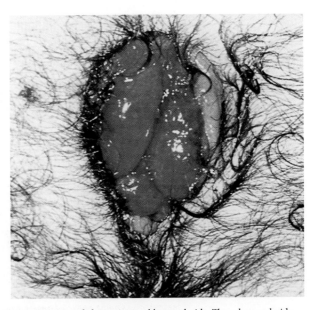

Figure 34.5 Second-degree internal hemorrhoids. These hemorrhoids prolapse but are spontaneously reducible.

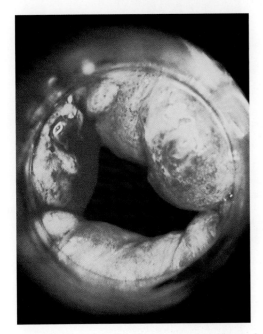

Figure 34.4 Anoscopic appearance of first-degree internal hemorrhoids.

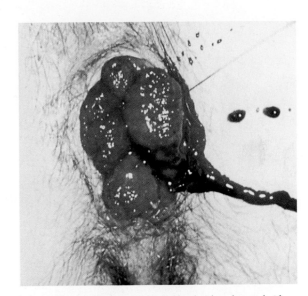

Figure 34.6 Third-degree internal hemorrhoids. These hemorrhoids prolapse and require manual reduction. Spontaneous bleeding is apparent.

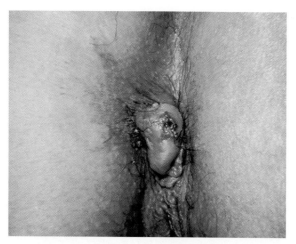

Figure 34.7 Thrombosed external hemorrhoid with cutaneous ulceration and superficial necrosis. Source: Rios Magrina E. Color Atlas of Anorectal Diseases. Philadelphia: WB Saunders, 1980. Reproduced with permission of Elsevier.

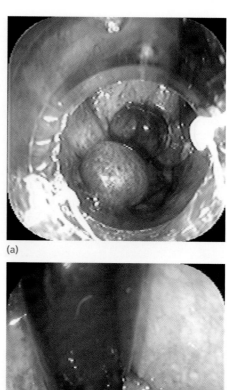

(a)

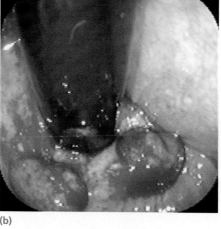

(b)

Figure 34.9 (a) A view through the endoscope after placing bands on two separate internal hemorrhoids using a multibanding ligator device attached to the instrument tip. **(b)** A retroflexed endoscopic view of banded internal hemorrhoids.

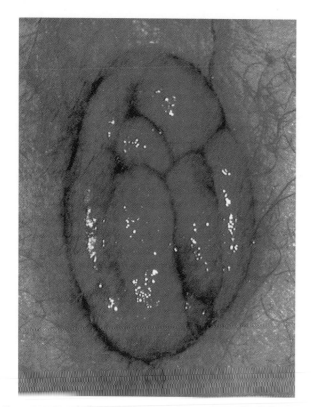

Figure 34.8 Fourth-degree (nonreducible) internal hemorrhoids. Source: Rios Magrina E. Color Atlas of Anorectal Diseases. Philadelphia: WB Saunders, 1980. Reproduced with permission of Elsevier.

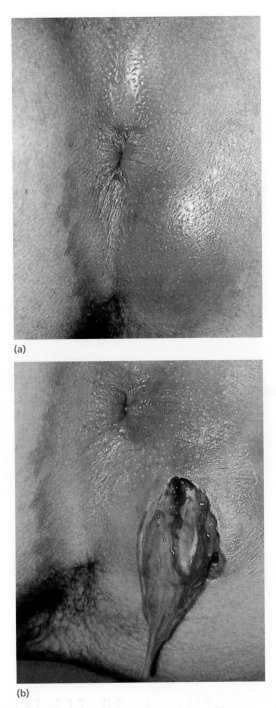

(a)

(b)

Figure 34.10 Anorectal abscess. **(a)** A ripe ischiorectal abscess in the left posterior quadrant. **(b)** The same abscess expressing pus immediately after incision. Source: Suppurative processes. In: Rios Margrina E. Atlas of Therapeutic Proctology. Philadelphia: WB Saunders, 1984. Reproduced with permission of Elsevier.

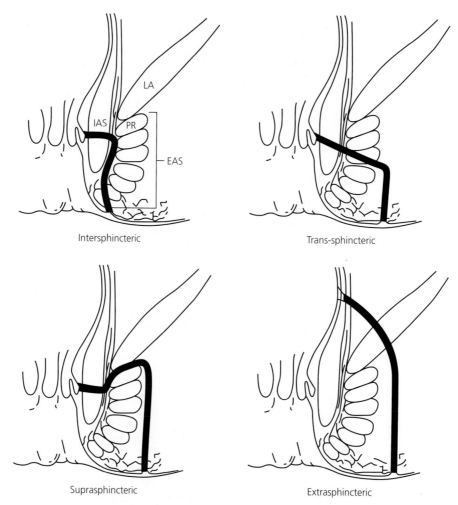

Figure 34.11 Classic location of several fistulas and their relationship to pelvic musculature depicted schematically. Anorectal anatomy: PR, puborectalis; LA, levator ani; IAS, internal anal sphincter; EAS, external anal sphincter.

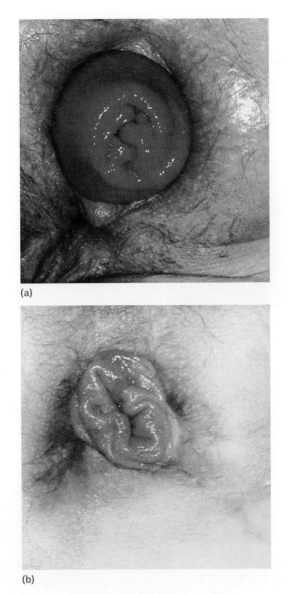

(a)

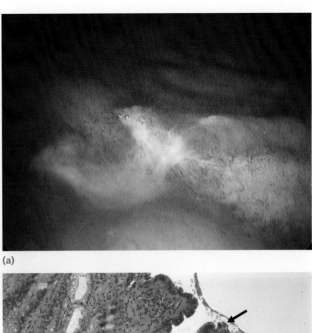

(a)

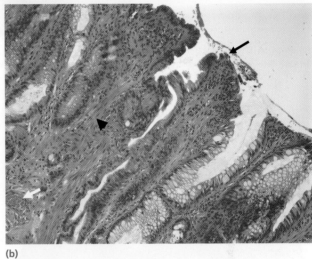

(b)

(b)

Figure 34.12 Rectal prolapse. **(a)** Complete rectal prolapse.
(b) Incomplete rectal prolapse. Source: Rios Magrina E. Color Atlas of
Anorectal Diseases. Philadelphia: WB Saunders, 1980. Reproduced with
permission of Elsevier.

Figure 34.13 Solitary rectal ulcer; **(a)** gross and **(b)** microscopic
appearance. Observe the hyperplastic mucosa with a surface erosion
(black arrow), vascular congestion (white arrow), and hyperplastic
muscle fibers between the crypts (black arrowhead). Source: **(a)** and
(b) Courtesy of Dr. Deepak Gopal, University of Wisconsin School of
Medicine and Public Health and Dr. Thomas Smyrk, Department of
Pathology, College of Medicine, Mayo Clinic, Rochester, MN, respectively.

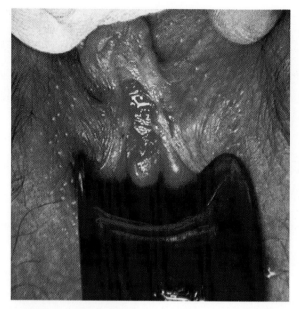

Figure 34.14 Typical appearance of a chronic anal fissure triad consisting of a sentinel pile (top), the fissure itself, and a hypertrophic papilla. Source: Rios Magrina E. Color Atlas of Anorectal Diseases. Philadelphia: WB Saunders, 1980. Reproduced with permission of Elsevier.

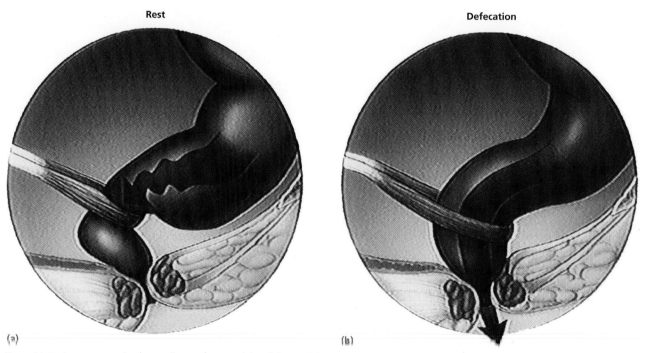

Figure 34.15 Anorectum and puborectalis muscle at rest (a) and during defecation (b). The puborectalis and anal sphincters relax allowing opening of the anal canal and perineal descent during defecation.

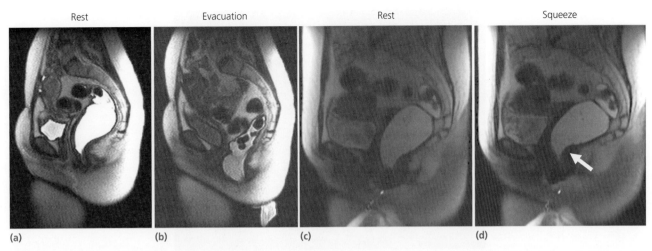

Rest   Evacuation   Rest   Squeeze

(a)   (b)   (c)   (d)

Figure 34.16 (a, b) Sagittal dynamic magnetic resonance images of normal puborectalis relaxation, perineal descent (2.6 cm), and opening of the anal canal during rectal evacuation in an asymptomatic subject. **(c, d)** During squeeze, the anal canal was elevated upward and anteriorly by pelvic floor contraction. Observe increased indentation (white arrow), reflecting contraction of the puborectalis muscle on the posterior rectal wall during squeeze (i.e., contraction of pelvic floor muscles). Source: Bharucha AE. Phenotypic variation in functional disorders of defecation. Gastroenterology 2005;128:1199. Reproduced with permission of Elsevier.

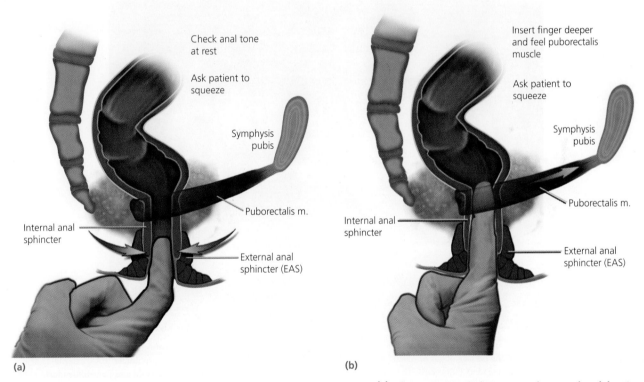

(a)   (b)

Figure 34.17 Digital examination of the anorectum of an adult with fecal incontinence. **(a)** When patient is asked to squeeze, the strength and duration of the contraction of the external anal sphincter (arrows) may be assessed after resting tone has been assessed. **(b)** The examining finger is then advanced and oriented posteriorly to assess the puborectalis muscle. When the patient is asked to squeeze, the contraction of the puborectalis muscle is felt as an anterior and upward tug as the muscle shortens (arrow). Simultaneously, the external anal sphincter contracts to increase the pressure in the anal canal. Source: Wald A. Fecal incontinence in adults. N Engl J Med 2007;356:40. Reproduced with permission of the Massachusetts Medical Society. Courtesy of Dr. Arnold Wald and Jerry Schoendorf, MAMS.

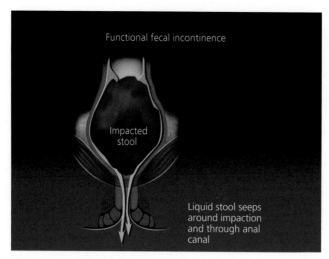

Figure 34.18 In functional fecal incontinence, impacted stool in the rectum reflexively inhibits the tone of the internal anal sphincter, which is responsible for most of the resting tone in the anal canal. This allows liquid stool to seep around the impaction and escape through the anal canal. Source: Wald A and Schoendorf J. Rome III: The functional GI disorders slide set. Courtesy of Dr. Arnold Wald and Jerry Shoendorf, MAMS.

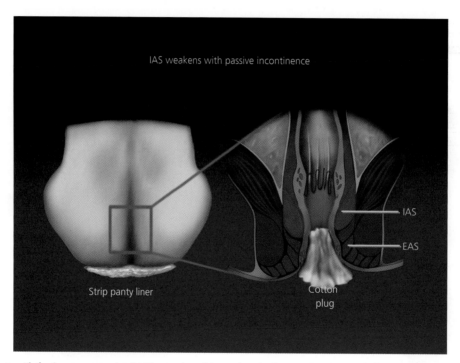

Figure 34.19 In patients with fecal seepage associated with a weakened internal anal sphincter, the placement of a cotton plug in the anal canal creates a physical and absorbent barrier to the passage of gas or fluid or its involuntary amelioration. the problem. IAS, internal anal sphincter; EAS, external anal sphincter. Source: Wald A and Schoendorf J. Rome III: The functional GI disorders slide set. Courtesy of Dr. Arnold Wald and Jerry Shoendorf, MAMS.

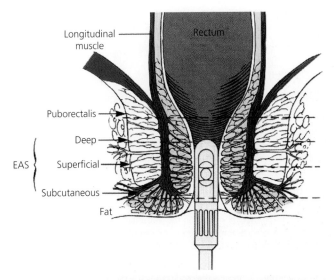

Figure 34.20 Illustration of a 360-degree anal sonographic probe shown in relationship to relevant anorectal anatomy. This technique is very reliable, although operator dependent, for evaluation of the internal anal sphincter but is less reliable for external anal sphincter and puborectalis muscle anatomy when assessing for structural causes of fecal incontinence. EAS, external anal sphincter. Source: Wald A and Schoendorf J. Rome III: The functional GI disorders slide set. Courtesy of Dr. Arnold Wald and Jerry Shoendorf, MAMS.

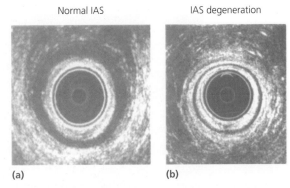

Figure 34.21 Axial sonographic views of the sphincter muscles of the anal canal. **(a)** A structurally intact, concentric hypoechogenic internal anal sphincter (IAS). **(b)** A structurally intact but very thin internal anal sphincter associated with low resting anal canal pressures, characteristic of some patients with passive incontinence. Lateral to the internal anal sphincter is a concentric ring of mixed echogenicity representing the external anal sphincter. Source: Wald A and Schoendorf J. Rome III: The functional GI disorders slide set. Courtesy of Dr. Arnold Wald and Jerry Shoendorf, MAMS.

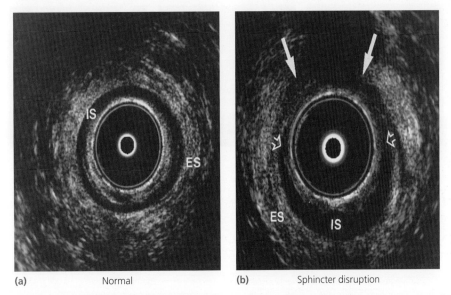

Figure 34.22 (a) Axial views of the anal canal illustrating normal internal anal sphincter (IS) and external anal sphincter (ES). **(b)** There is anterior disruption of both the IS (short arrows) and ES (long arrows) characteristic of traumatic tear during childbirth.

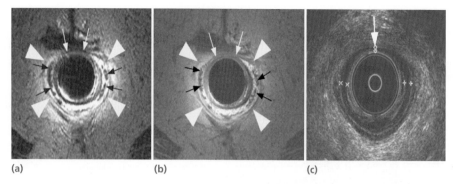

(a) (b) (c)

Figure 34.23 Endoanal fast spin-echo T2-weighted **(a)** and spin-echo T1-weighted **(b)** magnetic resonance (MR) images demonstrate marked atrophy of the external anal sphincter (arrowheads) in a 75-year-old incontinent patient, making the internal anal longitudinal muscle prominent (black arrows). Corresponding endoanal ultrasound images **(c)** identified patchy thinning of the internal sphincter also seen on the MR images (white arrows), but not external sphincter atrophy. Source: Bharucha AE, Fletcher JG, Harper CM, et al. Relationship between symptoms and disordered continence mechanisms in women with idiopathic fecal incontinence. Gut 2005;54:546. Reproduced with permission of BMJ Publishing Group Ltd.

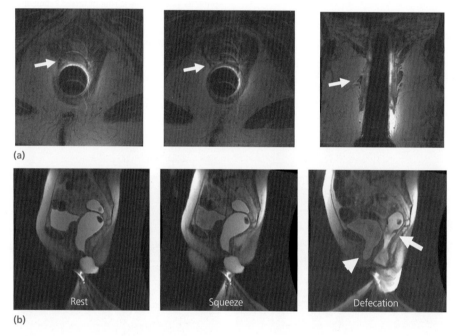

(a)

Rest Squeeze Defecation

(b)

Figure 34.24 Endoanal and dynamic magnetic resonance (MR) proctogram in a 70-year-old woman with urinary and fecal incontinence. **(a)** Endoanal MR images show partial tear and atrophy of the right puborectalis (arrow). Dynamic rest and squeeze images **(b)** show lift of the levator posteriorly, but little anterior or upward movement of the anorectal junction, consistent with puborectalis injury. Observe a cystocele (white arrowhead) and a small rectal intussusception (white arrow) during defecation.

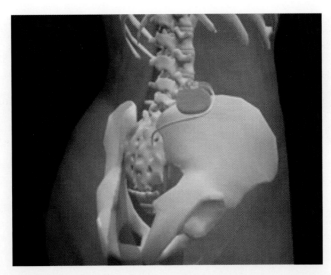

Figure 34.25 Illustration of a sacral nerve stimulator shown with relevant anatomy. A permanent electrical stimulator electrode is placed into a sacral nerve root via one of the sacral foramina. The nerve is selected as the one that produces optimal stimulation of the external anal sphincter. Shown here is the electrode in place and connected to a permanently implanted pulse generator which delivers a continuous stimulation.

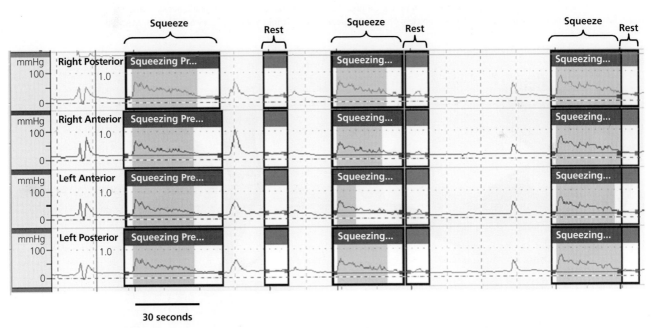

Figure 34.26 Anal sphincter pressures assessed on three separate occasions by four circumferentially oriented transducers stationed at 1 cm from the anal verge; transducers were located in separate quadrants. The maximum squeeze pressure is the highest pressure recorded by all four transducers during one of three maneuvers; the average squeeze pressure is calculated by averaging pressures across all four maneuvers. In this example, resting and squeeze pressures were comparable in all four quadrants. Source: Bharucha AE. Outcome measures for fecal incontinence: Anorectal structure and function. Gastroenterology 2004;126:S90. Reproduced with permission of Elsevier.

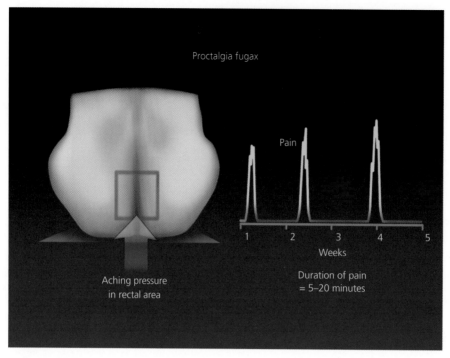

Figure 34.27 Characteristic location and pain pattern in proctalgia fugax. Typically, patients are asymptomatic between discrete episodes of rectal pain which last less than 60 min before disappearing completely. Source: Courtesy of Dr. Arnold Wald and Jerry Schoendorf, MAMS.

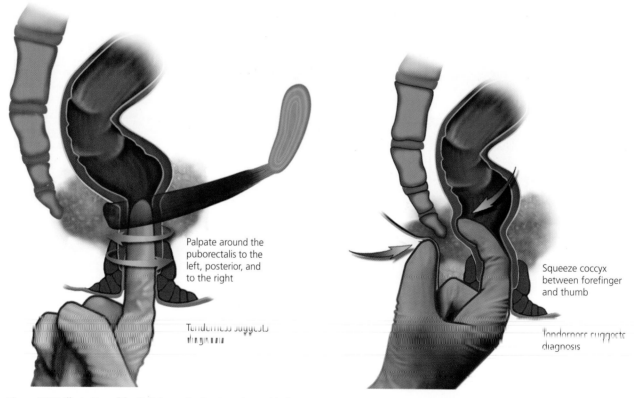

Figure 34.28 Illustration of the digital examination in patients with chronic proctalgia syndrome. There is often palpable tenderness of the puborectalis/levator muscles as the examining finger moves posteriorly to anteriorly. Tenderness is often asymmetric and most commonly found on the left side. Source: Wald A and Schoendorf J. Rome III: The functional GI disorders slide set. Courtesy of Dr. Arnold Wald and Jerry Shoendorf, MAMS.

Figure 34.29 Anorectal examination in patients with coccygodynia. The key to the diagnosis is the reproduction of the pain when the coccyx is manipulated between the examining finger and the thumb. Source: Wald A and Schoendorf J. Rome III: The functional GI disorders slide set. Courtesy of Dr. Arnold Wald and Jerry Shoendorf, MAMS.

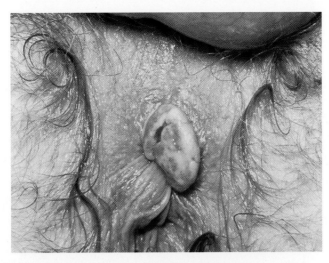

Figure 34.30 Squamous cell carcinoma of the anus. Source: Courtesy of Dr. Karen Guice.

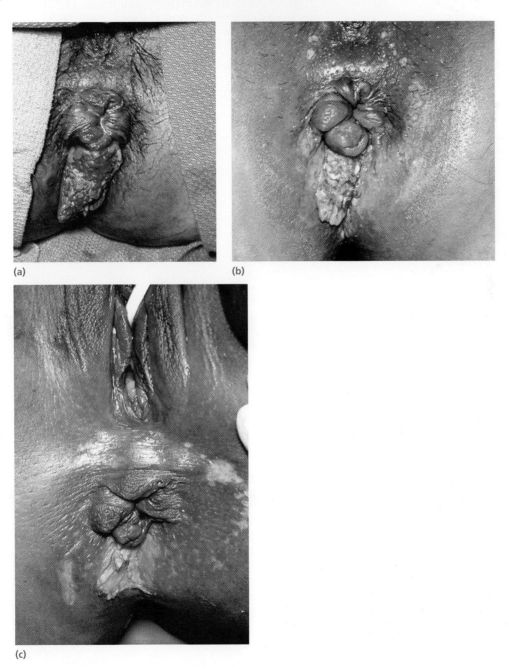

(a)

(b)

(c)

Figure 34.31 Large perianal squamous cell carcinoma just posterior to the anus. (a) Bulky tumor at the time of initial diagnosis. (b) The same tumor 3 weeks later, after partial treatment with radiation therapy and chemotherapy. (c) Complete disappearance of tumor 3 months after diagnosis and a full course of radiation therapy and chemotherapy. Source: Courtesy of Dr. Karen Guice.

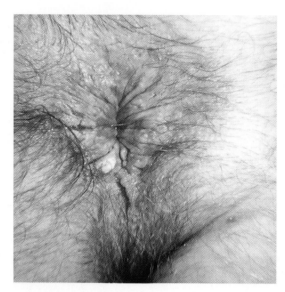

Figure 34.32 Bowen disease (cutaneous squamous cell carcinoma in situ) of the anus. The lesion has a scaly, plaque-like appearance. Source: Courtesy of Dr. Richard Burney.

CHAPTER 35

Acute pancreatitis

Hana Algül and Roland M. Schmid II
Technical University of Munich, Munich, Germany

In the United States, more than 200 000 hospital admissions per year are due to acute pancreatitis leading to more than $2 billion in expense annually. Seventy to eighty percent of acute pancreatitis patients develop mild and uncomplicated acute pancreatitis, while 20%–30% will develop more severe symptoms with concomitant multiple organ failure. Fifty percent of these patients die as a consequence of this disease. The two most common risk factors for acute pancreatitis are gallstone disease and excessive alcohol use. Microscopically, patients undergoing severe acute pancreatitis (SAP) develop extensive necrosis along with diffuse hemorrhage of the entire gland, while interstitial edema and infiltration of immune cells together with fat necrosis inside and outside of the pancreas define the typical features of mild acute pancreatitis (Figure 35.1).

Multiple organ failure in SAP is a consequence of the systemic activation of the immune system, known as systemic inflammatory response syndrome (SIRS). The clinical and pathological features of SIRS mimic those of sepsis; however, efforts to identify infecting organisms in many patients with SIRS have failed (Box 35.1). Although this syndrome is typically seen in individuals with sepsis, SIRS also occurs in patients with acute sterile inflammation in the pancreas. Major and early complications during SAP include acute lung injury, and kidney and hemodynamic failure. The pathophysiology of SAP with multiple organ failure is poorly understood. Researchers have long hypothesized that SAP results from activation of digestive enzymes within the pancreas, a process called autodigestion. Indeed, inherited mutations in genes encoding for digestive enzymes are present in at least some patients with hereditary pancreatitis. However, these patients develop chronic pancreatitis rather than SAP. As a result, an alternate hypothesis has been formulate to propose that that systemic complications during acute pancreatitis result from uncontrolled activation of the immune system (Figure 35.2).

In an attempt to identify predictors of complicated acute pancreatitis, several association studies linking cytokines and chemokines with acute pancreatitis severity have been conducted. These identified serum levels of interleukin-6 (IL-6) and the IL-6-dependent acute phase protein C-reactive protein (CRP) as the most reliable parameters for SAP. Recent findings suggest that IL-6 is not only a predictor of SAP but plays a significant role in its pathogenesis. Activation of transcription factors such as nuclear factor-κB (NF-κB) and Stat3 results in production of factors that promote distant organ failure. While excessive stimulation of the immune system (hyperinflammatory status, SIRS) accounts for the early systemic complication, compensatory antiinflammatory response syndrome (CARS) contributes to the local and septic problems in the late phase (Figures 35.3 and 35.4). IL-10 may be among the important factors contributing to this antiinflammatory response, as observed in animal models. The hypoinflammatory status of CARS might facilitate superinfections of extensive necrosis and septic complications (Figure 35.3).

Successful management of pancreatitis depends on prediction of the severity of disease and the identification of patients who are at risk for local and systemic complications. The absence of rebound tenderness and/or guarding, normal hematocrit level, and normal serum creatinine level were the best predictors of a mild course or harmless acute pancreatitis (HAP) score (Box 35.2). Recognized markers of the risk of SAP include new scoring systems such as the bedside index of severity of acute pancreatitis (BISAP) or single parameters, including elevated blood glucose, blood urea nitrogen (BUN), and hematocrit (Figure 35.5; Tables 35.1, 35.2, and 35.3). Among values that measure SIRS, CRP, IL-6, and its soluble IL-6 receptor were reliably linked to SAP. Agitation, confusion, hypoxemia, and lack of improvement within 48 h are signs suggesting deterioration. Patients older than 55 years are also at higher risk of undergoing a severe inflammation of the pancreas.

The association between elevated haematocrit and poor outcome is of particular interest. Compromised hemodynamic function and hypoperfusion with elevated BUN, decreased mean arterial pressure, and increased lactate play a critical role in the development of SAP, promoting pancreatic inflammation.

Yamada's Atlas of Gastroenterology, Fifth Edition. Edited by Daniel K. Podolsky, Michael Camilleri, J. Gregory Fitz, Anthony N. Kalloo, Fergus Shanahan, and Timothy C. Wang.
© 2016 John Wiley & Sons, Ltd. Published 2016 by John Wiley & Sons, Ltd.
Companion website: www.yamadagastro.com/atlas

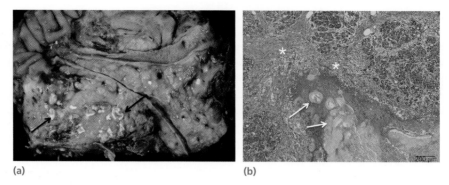

Figure 35.1 Macroscopic **(a)** and microscopic **(b)** appearance of acute pancreatitis. Note the fat necrosis within the pancreas (arrows). Strong infiltration and accumulation of immune cells are detectable around pancreatic lobules in acute pancreatitis (*).

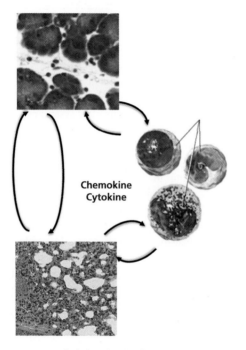

Figure 35.2 Immune cells linking local inflammation to systemic complications.

Box 35.1 Criteria to define systemic inflammatory response syndrome (SIRS).

SIRS defined by presence of two or more criteria:

Core temperature: <36°C or >38°C
Heart rate: >90 beats/min
White blood count: <4000 or >12000/mm³
Respirations: >20/min or P_{CO_2} >32 mgHg

Box 35.2 Identification of mild harmless acute pancreatitis.

HAP (harmless acute pancreatitis) score

No rebound tenderness and/or guarding
Normal hematocrit level (male ≤40%; female ≤39.6%)
Normal serum creatinine level
Specificity: 96.3%–97.0%
Positive predictive value: 98.0%–98.7%

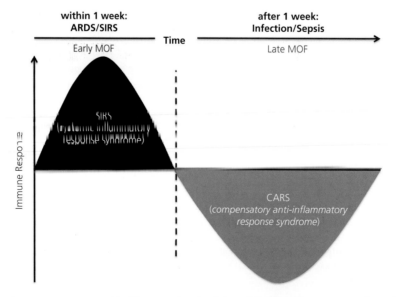

Figure 35.3 Immune response in severe acute pancreatitis. After excessive stimulation of the immune system, a paralysis of the immune system occurs during the course of acute pancreatitis. ARDS, adult respiratory distress syndrome; MOF, multiorgan failure.

Early appropriate volume resuscitation plays a critical role in management.

The most common risk factors for acute pancreatitis in adults are gallbladder disease (usually due to concomitant choledocholithiasis) and chronic or excessive alcohol consumption. Other important causes include hypertriglyceridemia, drugs (e.g.,

azathioprine, thiazide, and estrogens), trauma from endoscopic retrograde cholangiopancreatography (ERCP), hypercalcemia, abdominal trauma, various infections, ischemia, and hereditary causes (Table 35.4). In about 15% of patients the cause remains unknown after thorough investigation, although this should become less common as factors of genetic predisposition, environmental susceptibility, and autoimmunity are elucidated.

Autoimmune pancreatitis (AIP) has become an important differential diagnostic consideration in patients with otherwise

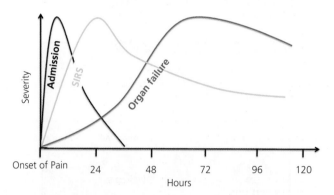

Figure 35.4 Sequence of events in acute pancreatitis. SIRS, systemic inflammatory response syndrome.

Table 35.1 Symptoms of acute pancreatitis. Source: Data from Banks PA, Freeman ML; Practice Parameters Committee of the American College of Gastroenterology. Practice guidelines in acute pancreatitis. Am J Gastroenterol 2006;101:2379.

Symptoms	
Band-like abdominal pain	90%
Vomiting	80%
Paralytic (sub-)ileus	70%
Fever	60%
"Rubber belly"	60%

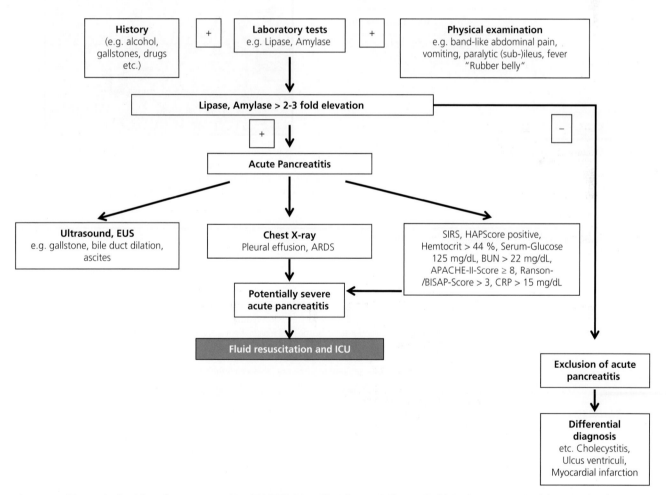

Figure 35.5 Diagnostic algorithm of acute pancreatitis. APACHE, Acute Physiology and Chronic Health Evaluation; ARDS, adult respiratory distress syndrome; BISAP, Bedside Index of Severity of Acute Pancreatitis; BUN, blood urea nitrogen; EUS, endoscopic ultrasound; HAP, harmless acute pancreatitis; ICU, intensive care unit; SIRS, systemic inflammatory response syndrome.

Table 35.2 Identification of severe acute pancreatitis.

Parameter	Score
BUN >25 mg/dL	1
Impaired mental status	1
SIRS	1
Age >60 years	1
Pleural effusion	1

BISAP score	Mortality (%)
0	0.2
1	0.6
2	2
3	5–8
4	13–19
5	22–27

BISAP, Bedside Index of Severity of Acute Pancreatitis; BUN, blood urea nitrogen; SIRS, systemic inflammatory response syndrome.

Table 35.3 Parameters and scores to classify mild and severe acute pancreatitis.

Parameters/scores	Form of pancreatitis
HAP score	mild
Hematocrit >44%	severe
Serum glucose >125 mg/dL	severe
BUN >22 mg/dL	severe
APACHE II score ≥8	severe
Ranson/BISAP score >3	severe
CRP >15 mg/dL	severe

APACHE, Acute Physiology and Chronic Health Evaluation; BISAP, Bedside Index of Severity of Acute Pancreatitis; BUN, blood urea nitrogen; CRP, C-reactive protein; HAP, harmless acute pancreatitis.

unexplained recurrent inflammation of the gland. First reported by Sarles et al. in 1961, the term "autoimmune pancreatitis" was coined for a steroid-responsive, mass-forming pancreatitis associated with increased gamma globulin (hypergammaglobulin) or gamma globulin 4 (IgG4) and elevated autoantibody titers (Figure 35.6).

Two distinct subtypes of AIP were recognized, which have been named types 1 and 2; lymphoplasmacytic sclerosing

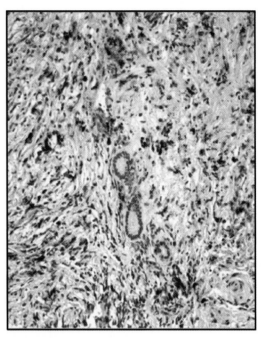

Figure 35.6 Accumulation of IgG4-positive cells in type 1 autoimmune pancreatitis, with predominant lymphoplasmacytic infiltrate.
Source: Courtesy of Professor Klöppel and Professor Esposito, Technical University of Munich.

Table 35.4 Etiology of acute pancreatitis.

Most common causes	Comments
Gallstones and microlithiasis	Impaction of stones in the bile duct, the most common cause
Alcohol abuse	The second most frequent cause
Drugs	Various and numerous drugs are known to induce pancreatitis
ERCP	Iatrogenic induced pancreatitis
Hyperlipidemia	Usually with extremely elevated triglyceride levels (>1000 mg/dL)
Hypercalcemia	As a result of hyperparathyroidism or tumor-associated hypercalcemia
Genetic	Mutations in cationic trypsinogen (*PRSS1*), *SPINK1*, *CTRC*, or *CFTR*
Autoimmune pancreatitis	"Sausage-shaped" pancreas in CECT, elevation of IgG4
Infections	Bacteria (*Mycoplasma*, *Legionella*, etc.), viruses (mumps, coxsackievirus, cytomegalovirus, herpes simplex virus, varicella simplex virus), parasites (*Ascaris*, *Cryptosporidium*, *Toxoplasma*, etc.) and fungi (*Aspergillus*)
Idiopathic	Approximately in 15%–20% of cases
Pancreas divisum	A potential cause; stenosis of the papilla minor could contribute to recurrent acute pancreatitis
Sphincter of Oddi dysfunction	Obstruction of the pancreatic duct
Cystic fibrosis	Rare cause
Trauma	Clear history
Vasculitis	In some patients with systemic vasculitis
Pancreatic tumors	IPMN, pancreatic cancer, cystic lesions (serous cystic adenomas, etc.)

CECT, contrast-enhanced computed tomography; ERCP, endoscopic retrograde cholangiopancreatography; IPMN, intraductal papillary mucinous neoplasia.

pancreatitis is the histological pattern seen in type 1 (Figures 35.7 and 35.8) and idiopathic duct centric pancreatitis is the histological pattern seen in type 2 (Figure 35.9). The two subtypes share many common features; however, one of the key distinctions between the two diseases is that whereas type 2 AIP seems to be a pancreas-specific disorder, type 1 is a multiorgan disease in which the pancreas is only one of the many organs affected, the pancreatic affliction being called AIP; Figure 35.10 indicates involvement of the biliary system which is termed IgG4 sclerosing cholangitis (IgG4-SC). Diffuse enlargement of the pancreas and effacement of the lobular contour of the pancreas in imaging of the pancreas, the so-called "sausage-like" appearance, is a typical finding in AIP (Figures 35.11 and 35.12). As fibroinflammatory changes involve the peripancreatic adipose tissue, a capsule-like rim surrounding the pancreas is specifically detected in some AIP patients. Although typical features of AIP (narrow stricture of more than one-third the length of the pancreatic duct, lack of upstream dilatation from

the stricture, multiple strictures, side branches arising from the stricture site) have been defined by ERCP, its role in the diagnostic algorithm is uncertain (Figures 35.13, 35.14, and 35.15). Corticosteroids are the treatment of choice in the acute flair of AIP1 or IgG4-SC (Figures 35.10, 35.13, and 35.14).

Pancreas divisum is the most common congenital anatomic variation of the pancreatic ductal anatomy and occurs in approximately 10% of the population (Figure 35.16). The normal pancreas develops from the fusion of dorsal and ventral pancreatic buds during fetal development. In up to 90% of individuals the ducts of both the dorsal and ventral buds fuse along with the parenchymal fusion, resulting in the main pancreatic duct draining the whole pancreas via the major papilla. In pancreas divisum, the fusion of dorsal and ventral pancreatic buds during the fetal development does not occur and the dorsal duct drains the majority of the pancreas via the minor papilla and the ventral duct drains only a small proportion of the pancreas (inferior portion of the head) via the major papilla. The most

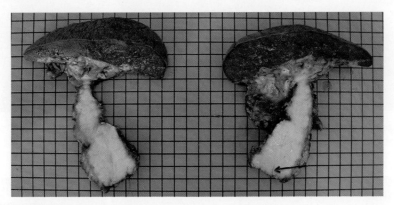

Figure 35.7 Longitudinal dissection of a pancreas with autoimmune pancreatitis type 1. Note the thin pancreatic duct (arrow). Source: Courtesy of Professor Klöppel, Technical University of Munich.

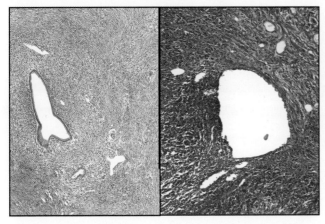

Figure 35.8 Histomorphology of autoimmune pancreatitis type 1 showing classical swirling or storiform fibrosis. Source: Courtesy of Professor Klöppel and Professor Esposito, Technical University of Munich.

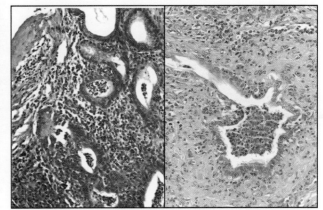

Figure 35.9 Histomorphology of autoimmune pancreatitis type 2 with granulocyte epithelial lesions. Source: Courtesy of Professor Klöppel and Professor Esposito, Technical University of Munich.

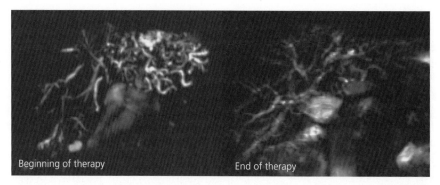

Figure 35.10 Autoimmuncholangitis in a patient with type 1 autoimmune pancreatitis regressing and improving under corticosteroid therapy.

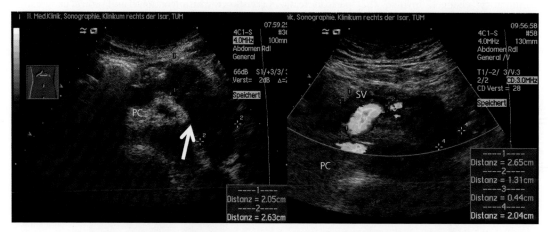

Figure 35.11 Ultrasound image of autoimmune pancreatitis type 2; pancreatic tail enlargement (arrows). The pancreas is enlarged and hypoechoic. PC, portal confluence; SV, spenic vein.

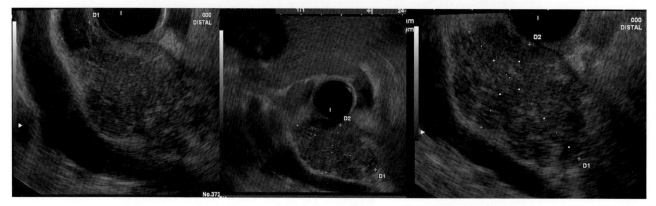

Figure 35.12 Endoscopic ultrasound images of autoimmune pancreatitis in the same patient. In addition to the enlargement, the pancreas is hypoechoic and heterogeneous.

likely mechanism for this is the presence of a small and stenotic minor papilla orifice in some individuals. This leads on to high dorsal ductal pressure during active secretion, resulting in inadequate drainage and ductal distension. This presumably causes recurrent acute pancreatitis, chronic pancreatitis, and pancreatic-type abdominal pain without biochemical or radiological evidence of pancreatitis (Figure 35.17).

A similar mechanism is proposed for patients with recurrent acute pancreatitis and sphincter of Oddi dysfunction (SOD). ERCP with manometry has been recommended to exclude SOD; a basal pressure of 40 mmHg or greater sustained for at least 30 seconds is considered abnormal. A number of studies suggest a prevalence rate for SOD of 30%–45% in unexplained acute pancreatitis, making it the most common cause of

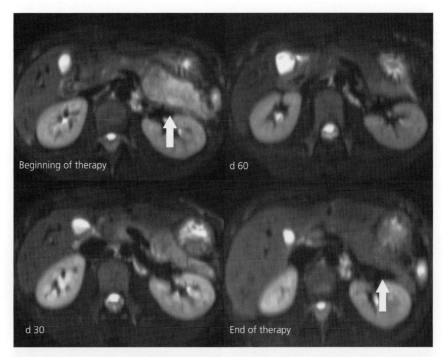

Figure 35.13 Magnetic resonance images demonstrating regression of pancreatic tail enlargement (arrow) in a patient with autoimmune pancreatitis type 2. Duration of treatment with corticosteroids is indicated. Source: Courtesy of Professor J. Gaa, Technical University of Munich.

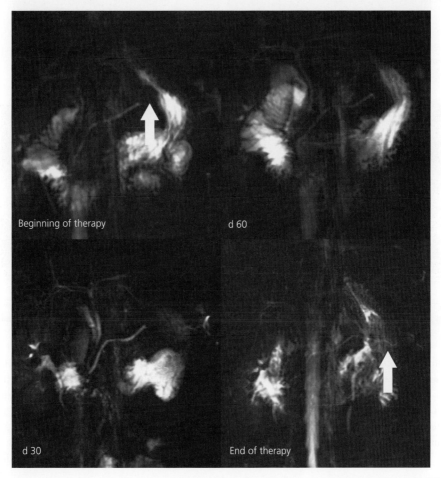

Figure 35.14 Magnetic resonance images demonstrating pancreatic duct in the tail (arrows) after therapy. Source: Courtesy of Professor J. Gaa, Technical University of Munich.

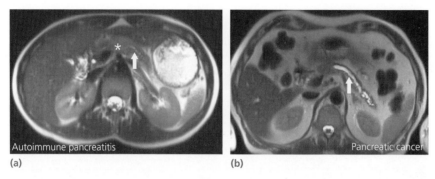

Figure 35.15 **(a)** Prestenotic dilation of the pancreatic duct (arrow) is missing in a patient with autoimmune pancreatitis in the cauda (*). **(b)** Conversely, pancreatic cancer results in strong dilatation of the main duct in the pancreas (arrow). Source: Courtesy of Professor J. Gaa, Technical University of Munich.

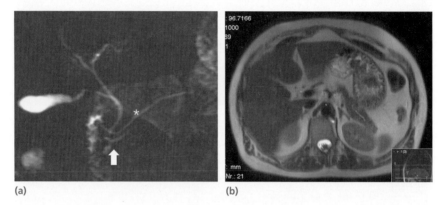

Figure 35.16 Magnetic resonance cholangiopancreatography in a patient with a pancreas divisum. **(a)** The dorsal (arrow) and ventral ducts (*) do not communicate with each other and fail to fuse. **(b)** Morphology of the pancreas tail is completely normal.

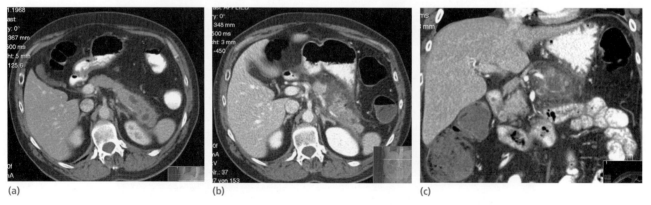

Figure 35.17 Acute pancreatitis in a patient with pancreas divisum (same patient as in Figure 35.26). (a, b) The CT scan shows edematous pancreatitis with focal heterogeneous low attenuation area in pancreas tail. (c) The pancreas is surrounded by fluid collections with nonhomogeneous enhancement

pancreatitis identified in this group. Therapy of SOD is biliary sphincterotomy or a combination of biliary and pancreatic sphincterotomy.

Patients with SOD are at high risk for development of acute pancreatitis after ERCP. This type of acute pancreatitis is called post-ERCP pancreatitis. The incidence of acute pancreatitis associated with therapeutic ERCP is 1.6%–5.4% (mild approximately 2.3%, moderate approximately 2.8%, and severe approximately 0.4%). While diagnostic ERCP is continuously replaced by magnetic resonance cholangiopancreatography (MRCP) and endoscopic ultrasound (EUS), therapeutic ERCP has still an important role in pancreatic (Figure 35.18) and biliary diseases. Further important risk factors for ERCP-associated acute pancreatitis include female gender, past

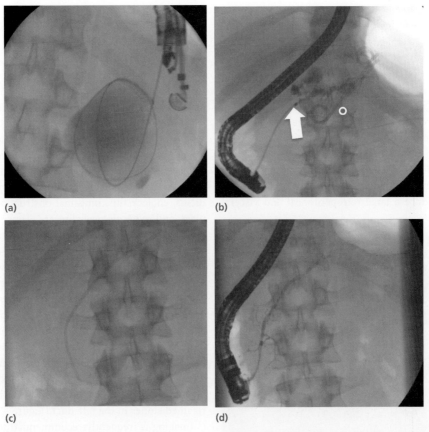

Figure 35.18 (a) EUS-guided puncture and drainage of the fluid accumulation in patient with pancreatic duct trauma (same patient as in Figure 35.43). **(b)** Endoscopic retrograde cholangiopancreatography (ERCP) showing duct rupture in the neck of the pancreas (arrow). Temporary stenting of the rupture is shown in **(c)**. **(d)** ERCP in the same patient after a period of 3 months of endoscopic therapy.

history of post-ERCP pancreatitis, precut, difficult cannulation, endoscopic papillary balloon dilation, and performance of pancreaticography (Figure 35.19).

The diagnosis of acute pancreatitis is primarily based on at least two of the following criteria: (1) acute abdominal pain; (2) evidence of elevation of lipase and/or amylase in the serum at least three times greater than the upper limit of normal; and (3) characteristic findings of acute pancreatitis on transabdominal ultrasonography or contrast-enhanced computed tomography (CECT) and less commonly magnetic resonance imaging (MRI).

The cardinal symptom of abdominal pain is present in about 95% of patients and typically radiates in a band-like manner to the lower thoracic region of the back. The pain tends to be steady but is exacerbated by eating or drinking. With biliary pancreatitis, the pain may be more localized to the right upper quadrant and more variable in intensity over time because of the contribution of biliary colic. Cullen's and Turner's signs have long been known to be associated with retroperitoneal bleeding and indicate SAP. Cullen's sign arises from the spread of retroperitoneal blood into the falciform ligament and subsequently to subcutaneous umbilical tissues through the connective tissue

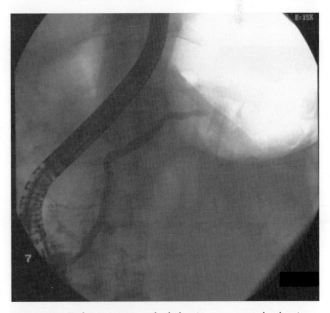

Figure 35.19 Endoscopic retrograde cholangiopancreatography showing normal pancreatic duct.

covering of the round ligament. In contrast, Turner's sign is produced by hemorrhagic fluid spreading from the posterior pararenal space to the lateral edge of the quadratus lumborum muscle and thereafter to the subcutaneous tissues by means of a defect in the fascia of the flank. Abdominal compartment syndrome is defined as an increase of intraabdominal pressure of more than 20 mmHg, which is associated with occurrence of organ failure (Figures 35.20 and 35.21). The incidence of abdominal compartment syndrome among patients with SAP ranges from 23% to 56%. The mechanisms involved in the development of abdominal compartment syndrome include increased capillary permeability, hypoalbuminemia, and volume overload, which produce a large retroperitoneal and visceral

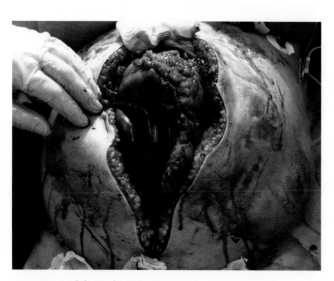

Figure 35.20 Abdominal compartment syndrome with surgical decompression.

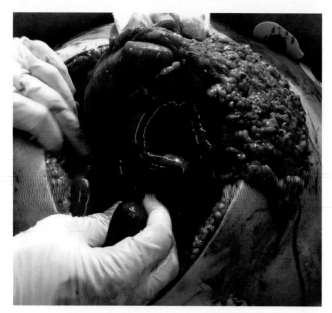

Figure 35.21 Intestinal ischemia in acute pancreatitis.

edema. Surgical decompression by midline laparotomy provides the most effective treatment of this complication.

Serum amylase generally rises within a few hours after the onset of symptoms and returns to normal within 3–5 days. In some patients, amylase activity is still normal on admission. Conversely, amylase concentrations might be high in the absence of acute pancreatitis in individuals with macroamylasemia (a syndrome characterized by the formation of large molecular complexes between amylase and abnormal immunoglobulins), in patients with decreased glomerular filtration, in diseases of salivary glands, and in extrapancreatic abdominal diseases associated with inflammation, including acute appendicitis, cholecystitis, intestinal obstruction or ischemia, peptic ulcer, and gynecological diseases. Thus, when serum amylase concentration is high and clinical presentation is not consistent with acute pancreatitis, nonpancreatic causes of hyperamylasemia should be examined. In patients with acute pancreatitis serum lipase remains elevated for a longer period of time than amylase, which can be helpful in patients with a delayed presentation. Furthermore, lipase is more pancreas specific than amylase. The biochemical markers of a biliary etiology of acute pancreatitis include an alanine aminotransferase elevation of more than three times the upper range of normal and a serum total bilirubin greater than 3 mg%. In such cases transabdominal ultrasound, EUS, or MRCP can be helpful in confirming retained stones in the bile duct (Figure 35.22).

Imaging is frequently recommended to confirm the clinical diagnosis, ascertain the cause, and grade the extent and severity of acute pancreatitis (Table 35.5). Radiography, upper gastrointestinal series, and ultrasound are of limited value in the diagnosis of acute pancreatitis. Abdominal radiography might show localized ileus in severe pancreatitis (Figure 35.23). In one-third of patients, chest radiography shows abnormalities such as elevation of one hemidiaphragm and pleural effusions, pulmonary infiltrates, or both (Figure 35.24). On abdominal ultrasound, bowel gases often mask focal hypoechoic areas within the pancreas. Abdominal ultrasound is helpful in detecting cholelithiasis and biliary obstruction. Unlike EUS, the sensitivity of abdominal ultrasound in detecting biliary sludge or choledocholithiasis is very low.

Assessment for potential of gallstone-induced acute pancreatitis should be given top priority because of its management implications (Figure 35.25). ERCP/sphincterotomy should be performed immediately (within 24 h) in patients with gallstone-induced acute pancreatitis if a complication of cholangitis is

Table 35.5 Computed tomography severity index (CTSI) and its correlation with mortality in acute pancreatitis.

CTSI	Morbidity (%)	Mortality (%)
0–3	8	3
4–6	35	6
7–10	92	17

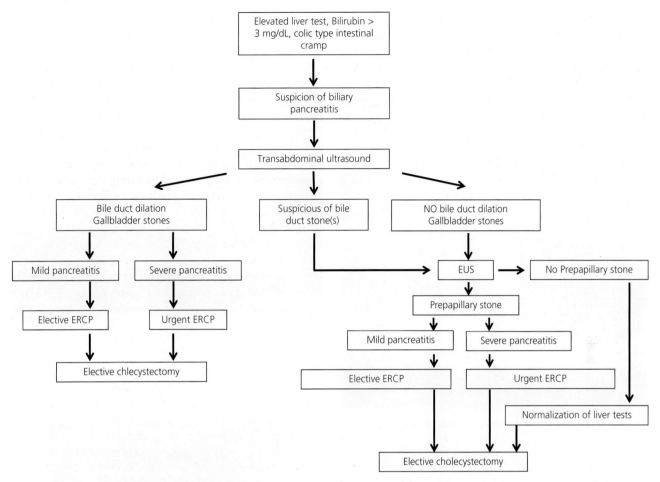

Figure 35.22 Diagnostic algorithm of acute biliary pancreatitis. ERCP, endoscopic retrograde cholangiopancreatography; EUS, endoscopic ultrasound.

present or suspected (Figures 35.26, 25.27, and 35.28). Metaanalysis failed to demonstrate a significant reduction in severity and mortality for ERCP in patients with acute biliary pancreatitis undergoing urgent ERCP. The treatment for bile duct stones with the use of ERCP/sphincterotomy *alone* is not recommended in cases of gallstone-induced pancreatitis with gallbladder stones. Cholecystectomy for gallstone-induced acute pancreatitis should be performed using a laparoscopic procedure after resolution of acute pancreatitis.

Plain films of the abdomen and lung should be considered, if an intestinal perforation is suspected and if free air is found a CT should be performed (Figure 35.29). If the diagnosis of acute pancreatitis is established by abdominal pain and by increased levels of pancreatic enzyme activities, a CECT scan is not usually required for diagnosis in the emergency room or on admission to the hospital for three reasons: (1) while local complications may be identified during the early phase, it is generally not necessary to document local complications by imaging during the first week if the course is uncomplicated; (2) CECT 5–7 days after admission is more reliable in establishing the presence and extent of pancreatic necrosis (Figure 35.30); and (3) in any case no treatment for peripancreatic fluid

collections or pancreatic necrosis are generally warranted sooner.

CT currently plays an important role in imaging of patients with acute pancreatitis, the identification of complications (Figures 35.31, 35.32, 35.33, and 35.34; Box 35.3), and assessing the response to treatment. The revision of the Atlanta classification in 2012 presented a standardized template for reporting CT images (Tables 35.6 and 35.7; Box 35.4). Fluid collections that develop in the early phase of pancreatitis are termed acute peripancreatic fluid collections (APFC). Most APFC are sterile and resolve spontaneously, but can persist beyond 4 weeks. The latter APFC can uncommonly develop into pancreatic pseudocysts. However, leakage of pancreatic ducts commonly results in pseudocyst formation. Pancreatic pseudocysts are collections surrounded by a well-defined wall without solid material or detritus (Figure 35.35). In contrast, a collection of variable amounts of fluid and necrotic tissue is called an acute necrotic collection (ANC). ANC occurs in necrotizing pancreatitis and is distinct from APFC. Early, it may be difficult to differentiate APFC from ANC because both types of collections appear as areas with fluid density. After the first week, distinction between these two types of collections is usually possible. When a

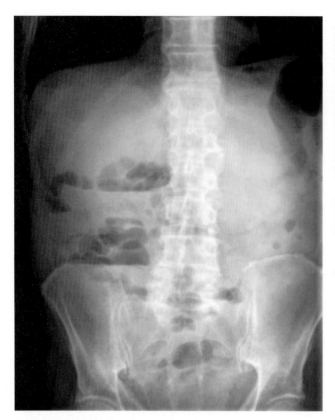

Figure 35.23 Paralytic ileus in a patient with acute pancreatitis.

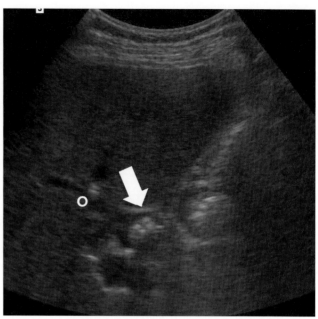

Figure 35.25 Ultrasound of the bile duct showing a large stone within the lumen (arrow) and dilation of the intrahepatic duct (circle).

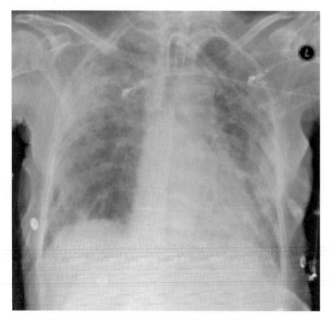

Figure 35.24 Adult respiratory distress syndrome (ARDS) in a patient with acute pancreatitis.

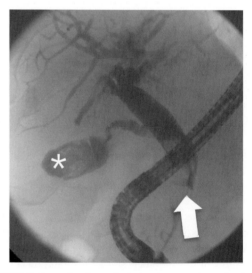

Figure 35.26 Endoscopic retrograde cholangiopancreatography showing bile stones in the main duct (arrow) and gallbladder (*).

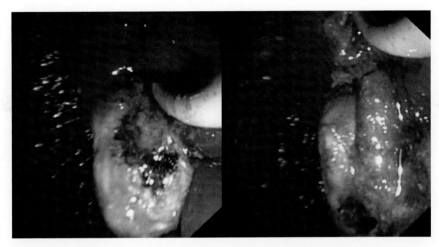

Figure 35.27 Endoscopic view of a large bile duct stone, which was removed after sphincterotomy by means of a balloon.

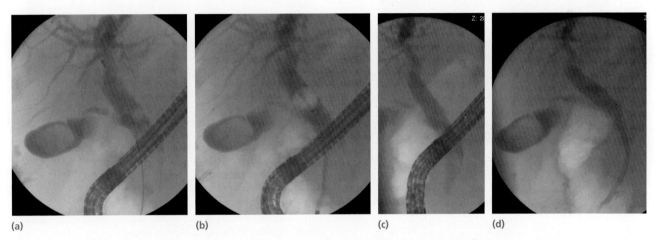

(a)   (b)   (c)   (d)

Figure 35.28 Endoscopic retrograde cholangiopancreatography showing different techniques to remove impacted bile stones; **(a)** dormia basket opened or **(b)** balloon inflated proximal of the stone. **(c)** Successful removal of the stone and **(d)** insertion of a plastic stent.

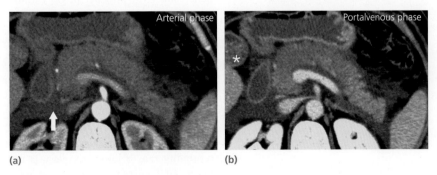

(a)   (b)

Figure 35.29 Contrast-enhanced CT scanning is accepted as the gold standard for grading and follow-up of acute pancreatitis. It is essential to examine multiphasic studies using CT in order to detect and calculate parenchymal necrosis. Cholelithiasis (*) and edematous (arrow) pancreas tissue with peripancreatic fluid areas are shown in anterior pararenal space at **(a)** arterial and **(b)** portal venous phases.

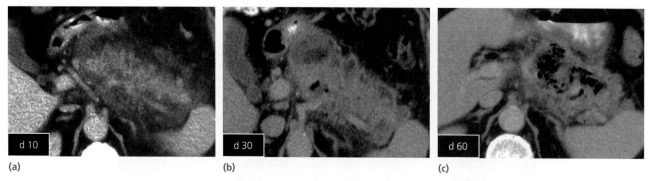

(a) (b) (c)

Figure 35.30 CT images demonstrating the sequence of acute peripancreatic and pancreatic necrosis in a patient with severe acute pancreatitis: **(a)** day 10 with acute peripancreatic fluid collections; **(b)** day 30 with acute necrotic collections; **(c)** day 60 with walled-off necrosis.

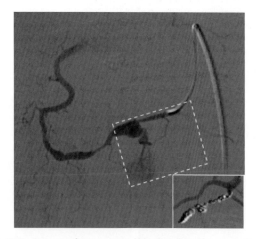

Figure 35.31 Angiographic imaging of bleeding from the arteria lienalis before and after (inset) transarterial coil embolization.

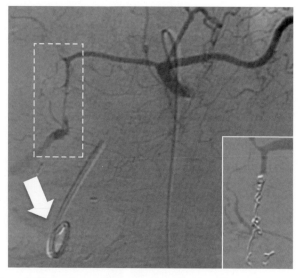

Figure 35.33 Angiographic imaging of bleeding from the arteria gastroduodenalis before and after (inset) transarterial coil embolization. A pigtail was placed in the pancreatic duct (arrow).

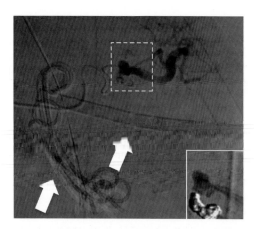

Figure 35.32 Angiographic imaging of bleeding from the arteria pancreaticoduodenalis inferiore before and after (inset) transarterial coil embolization. Next to the bleeding, transgastric and percutaneous drainages are shown (arrows).

contrast-enhancing wall of reactive tissue develops around necrotic pancreatic areas, the collection is termed walled-off necrosis; this usually occurs 4 weeks after onset of necrotizing pancreatitis. The presence of gas within the collection seen on CECT is suspicious for superinfection (Figure 35.36). Fine needle aspiration is useful for ascertain diagnosis and to obtain a specimen for culture.

EUS-guided drainage procedures have currently become the preferred option for drainage in symptomatic peripancreatic or pancreatic fluid collections, as an alternative to surgical, percutaneous, or conventional endoscopic transmural drainage (Figure 35.37). EUS-guided drainage is less invasive than surgery and therefore does not require general anesthesia. The morbidity rate is lower, recovery is faster, and the costs are lower. EUS-guided drainage can avoid local complications related to percutaneous drainage (Figures 35.38 and 35.39). Because the endoscope is placed adjacent to the fluid collection,

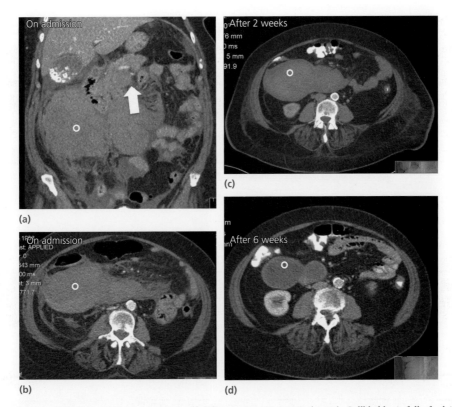

Figure 35.34 Acute intraabdominal bleeding (circle) in a patient with biliary acute pancreatitis (arrow). Gallbladder is full of calcified stones. **(a, b)** The intraabdominal bleeding stopped spontaneously. **(c, d)** After 2 and 6 weeks the intraabdominal hematoma nearly resolved, with liquidation after 8 weeks.

Box 35.3 Computed tomography (CT) grading of acute pancreatitis according to Balthazar et al. 1990.

Staging

A Normal
B Focal or diffuse enlargement of gland
C As B plus involvement of peripancreatic fat
D Single, ill-defined fluid collection
E Two or more ill-defined fluid collections and/or intrapancreatic gas

Degree of necrosis

0%
<33% of pancreas
33% to ≤50% of pancreas
≥50% of pancreas
Maximum

Staging score + degree of necrosis score = CT severity index

Source: Data from Balthazar EJ, Robinson DL, Megibow AJ, et al. Acute pancreatitis: value of CT in establishing prognosis. Radiology 1990;174:331.

Box 35.4 Classification of acute pancreatitis.

Grades of severity:

Mild acute pancreatitis
Moderately severe acute pancreatitis
Severe acute pancreatitis

Source: Data from Banks PA, Bollen TL, Dervenis C, et al. Classification of acute pancreatitis–2012: revision of the Atlanta classification and definitions by international consensus. Gut 2013;62:102.

it can have direct access to the fluid cavity, in contrast to percutaneous drainage which traverses the abdominal wall. Complications such as bleeding, inadvertent puncture of adjacent viscera, secondary infection, and prolonged periods of drainage with resultant pancreaticocutaneous fistulae may be avoided. The only difference between EUS and non-EUS-guided drainage is the initial step, namely gaining access to the pancreatic fluid collection. All the subsequent steps are similar, that is

Table 35.6 Management of selected local complications of acute pancreatitis.

Complication	Imaging	Management
APFC (acute peripancreatic fluid collection)	CT scan	Conservative management
ANC (acute necrotic collection)	CT scan	Conservative management
WON (walled-off necrosis)	CT scan	Percutaneous/endoscopic drainage and necrosectomy, surgical necrosectomy if indicated
Pancreatic pseudocyst	CT scan or EUS	Endoscopic or surgical drainage, if indicated
Pancreatic fistula	ERCP, CT scan, MRCP	Pancreatic duct stenting, somatostatin, surgery
Pseudoaneurysm formation	CECT, angiography, MRA	Angiographic embolism of feeding artery

EUS, endoscopic ultrasound; CECT, contrast-enhanced computed tomography; MRA, magnetic resonance angiography; MRCP, magnetic resonance cholangiopancreatography.

Table 35.7 Forms of pancreatitis with associated fluid collections. Source: Data from Thoeni RF. The revised Atlanta classification of acute pancreatitis: its importance for the radiologist and its effect on treatment. Radiology 2012;262:751.

	Form of pancreatitis	Fluid collections
<4 weeks after onset	Edematous pancreatitis	Acute peripancreatic fluid collections sterile infected
<4 weeks after onset	Necrotizing pancreatitis	Acute necrotic collection parenchymal necrosis sterile infected peripancreatic necrosis sterile infected parenchymal and peripancreatic necrosis sterile infected
>4 weeks after onset	Edematous pancreatitis	Pancreatic pseudocysts sterile infected
>4 weeks after onset	Necrotizing pancreatitis	Walled-off necrosis sterile infected

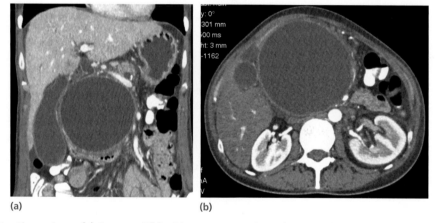

(a) (b)

Figure 35.35 Pancreatitis with pseudocyst. **(a)** Corona and **(b)** axial reconstruction obtained 6 weeks after pancreatitis. The pseudocyst has a well-defined rim representing the capsule.

insertion of guidewires with fluoroscopic guidance, balloon dilatation of the cystogastrostomy, and insertion of transmural stents or nasocystic catheters. With the introduction of the EUS scope equipped with a large operative channel that permits drainage of the APFCs in "one step," EUS-guided drainage has been increasingly carried out in many tertiary care centers and has expanded the safety and efficacy of this modality. While the nature of the APFCs determines the outcome of this procedure, EUS-guided drainage with multiple plastic stents remains technically challenging (Figure 35.40). Small-diameter plastic stents easily occlude, especially with fluid collections containing debris. Stent occlusion may therefore result in infection and delayed resolution of necrotic tissue. Novel large-diameter fully-covered self-expanding metal stents have been developed to overcome these limitations and seem to be a valuable tool to sufficiently treat pancreatic necrosis (Figures 35.37 and 35.41). Surgical debridement of necrotic tissue should be delayed because demarcation between viable and nonviable tissue is difficult during the first 2 weeks of SAP. Moreover, surgical necrosectomy within the first weeks is associated with high mortality rates (up to 65%). Figure 35.42 provides an overview over the algorithmic management of necrotizing pancreatitis. ERCP together with EUS-guided drainage are effective in treating pancreatic duct disruption, which is mostly seen on

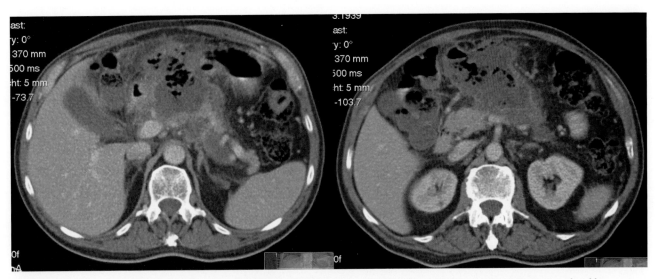

Figure 35.36 Contrast-enhanced CT scan of a large infected walled-off necrosis 4 weeks after the onset of pancreatitis. Pancreas is replaced by low-attenuation collection with a well-defined rim and multiple pockets of gas.

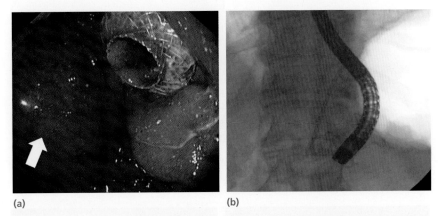

(a)   (b)

Figure 35.37 **(a)** Endoscopic image of an Axios stent placed in the stomach to drain pancreatic necrosis. Pus has drained from the stent (arrow). **(b)** Radiological image shows how the endoscope is pushed forward over the stent next to a transgastric pigtail.

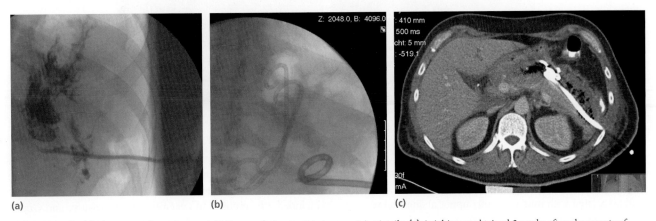

(a)   (b)   (c)

Figure 35.38 **(a, b)** Placement of percutaneous drainage catheters next to transgastric pigtails. **(c)** Axial image obtained 2 weeks after placements of catheters show larger residual walled-off necroses with air bubbles, indicative of incomplete drainage and infection.

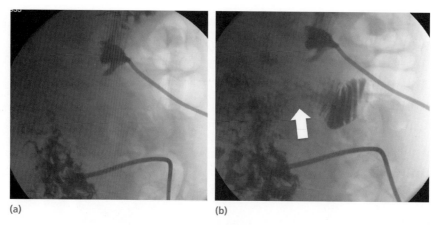

Figure 35.39 **(a)** Application of contrast agent over a percutaneous catheter showing walled-off necrosis in a patient with necrotizing pancreatitis. **(b)** After a few seconds the contrast agent spills over to the jejunum (arrow) suggesting a fistula that connects the carve to the small bowel.

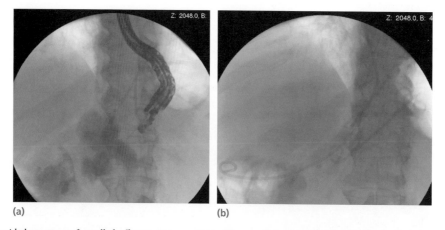

Figure 35.40 **(a)** EUS-guided puncture of a walled-off necrosis in a patient with necrotizing pancreatitis. **(b)** Wire-guided placement of transgastric pigtails to drain the necrotic tissue.

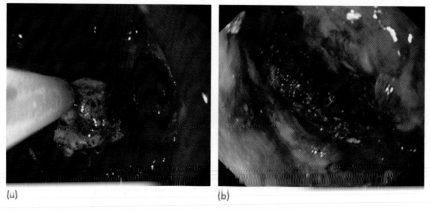

Figure 35.41 **(a)** Transgastric necrosectomy over an Axios stent. **(b)** View into the necrotic "cave" with granulated tissue and remnants of debris.

MRI-scan or endoscopic retrograde cholangiopancreaticography (Figures 35.18, 35.43, and 35.44). Pancreatic trauma is rare and associated with injury to other upper abdominal viscera.

While prophylactic antibiotics are not effective in reducing the incidence of peripancreatic or pancreatic infection in patients with necrotizing pancreatitis, the indication for antibiotics is well-documented infection. Empiric antibiotics should include both aerobic and anaerobic Gram-negative and Gram-positive microorganisms. Fungal infections are often present in these patients, and antifungal coverage or even prophylaxis

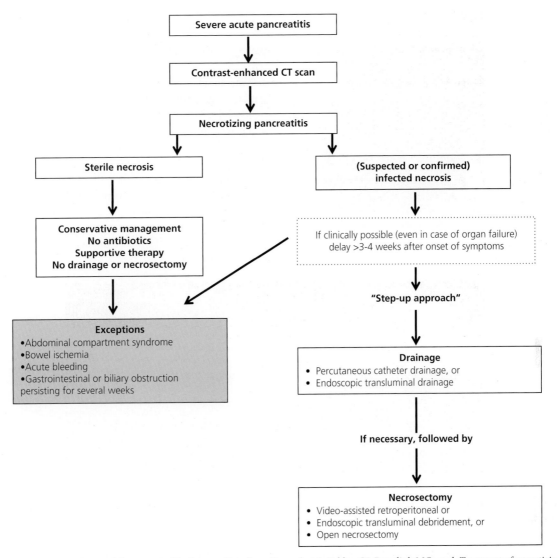

Figure 35.42 Management of necrotizing pancreatitis. Source: Data from Brunschot S, Bakker OJ, Besselink MG, et al. Treatment of necrotizing pancreatitis. Clin Gastroenterol Hepatol 2012;10:1190.

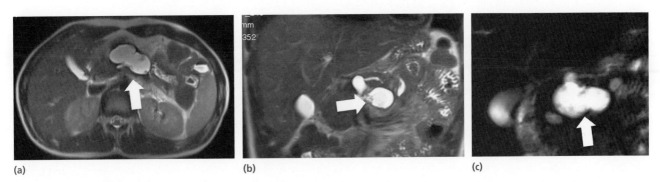

Figure 35.43 (a, b) Magnetic resonance images and **(c)** cholangiopancreatography in a patient with a pancreatic duct trauma. All images show peripancreatic secretion accumulation (arrow) and rupture in the neck of the pancreas.

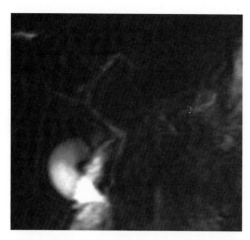

Figure 35.44 Magnetic resonance cholangiopancreatography in the same patient as in Figures 35.18 and 35.43 with a pancreatic duct trauma. Normal morphology of the pancreatic duct.

should be considered, especially if multiple risk factors for invasive candidiasis are present. Antibiotics should be given to all patients with biliary pancreatitis and cholangitis irrespective of whether urgent ERCP is undertaken.

Nutritional support plays an important role in the care of patients with SAP. In the past, parenteral nutrition seemed to be ideal for eliminating the stimulation of pancreatic secretion while preventing deterioration of nutritional status and progression to protein energy malnutrition. The concept of pancreatic rest has evolved over the years. Over the past decade, evidence suggests that enteral nutrition, rather than parenteral nutrition, significantly reduces infectious morbidity, the need for surgical intervention, and mortality in predicted SAP. Furthermore, there is evidence suggesting that the early initiation of enteral nutrition may have a favorable impact on clinical outcomes in patients with SAP.

CHAPTER 36

Chronic pancreatitis

Joachim Mössner,[1] Albrecht Hoffmeister,[1] and Julia Mayerle[2]

[1] University Hospital of Leipzig, Leipzig, Germany
[2] University Hospital, Ernst-Moritz-Arndt-University of Greifswald, Greifswald, Germany

Introduction

Chronic pancreatitis is a disease in which pancreatic parenchyma is replaced by fibrotic tissue as a result of recurring inflammation. Abdominal pain is the leading symptom in patients with chronic pancreatitis. Complications include formation of pseudocysts, pancreatic duct stenosis, duodenal stenosis, vascular complications, biliary obstruction, malnutrition, and a chronic pain syndrome. Chronic pancreatitis is also a risk factor for the development of pancreatic cancer. Overall, chronic pancreatitis reduces both quality of life and life expectancy.

The most common cause of an acute exacerbation of pancreatitis is continued alcohol abuse or dietary transgressions. Acute exacerbation of chronic pancreatitis manifests in two forms, irrespective of underlying etiology: acute interstitial edematous pancreatitis (75%–85%) with a mortality of below 1%, and acute hemorrhagic necrotizing pancreatitis (15%–25%) with a mortality between 10% and 24%. At the time of admission into the hospital, it is often difficult to differentiate between the majority of patients with a mild and uncomplicated course (about 80%) and those patients who will experience a severe course associated with multiple organ complications (about 20%).

Diagnosis of the disease and its complications by imaging procedures

A transabdominal ultrasound scan is usually appropriate as the initial imaging modality (Figures 36.1, 36.2, 36.3, and 36.4). Contrast-enhanced ultrasound (CEUS) is often a reliable method to detect pancreatic necrosis (Figure 36.4). This procedure does not expose the patient to radiation and can be applied irrespective of renal function. There are no studies that have directly compared contrast-enhanced computed tomography (CECT) and CEUS. In cases of infected necrosis and impairment of visualization by ultrasound scan due to bowel gas, CT is still the imaging procedure of choice. If signs of pancreatitis are equivocal, that is inhomogeneous gland but normal diameter of the pancreatic duct, in the context of continued clinical suspicion, endoscopic ultrasound (EUS) should be performed (Figure 36.5). CT and magnetic resonance imaging (MRI) as well as magnetic resonance cholangiopancreatography (MRCP) are supplementary diagnostic techniques, especially for equivocal pancreatic changes, such as differential diagnosis between tumor and inflammation, or clarifying whether surgery may be an option (Figures 36.6 and 36.7). MRCP should be performed to obtain more detailed information about the pancreatic ductal system if necessary (Figure 36.8). Diagnostic endoscopic retrograde cholangiopancreatography (ERCP) has been largely replaced by MRCP, given the lack of procedure-related complications with noninvasive imaging. ERCP is usually performed when an endoscopic intervention is planned (Figure 36.9). The presence of pancreatic atrophy or severe pancreatic duct abnormalities usually leads to a more conservative approach (Figure 36.10). In IgG4-positive autoimmune pancreatitis in combination with autoimmune cholangitis, biopsy of the papilla of Vater may be sufficient for diagnosis (Figure 36.11).

Complications are frequent in patients with chronic pancreatitis, and pseudocysts are among the most common findings. Compression of the duodenum or gastric outlet by a pseudocyst leads to pain and postprandial vomiting (Figures 36.3 and 36.12). An inflammatory mass of the pancreatic head may also cause pain and jaundice (Figure 36.13). Obstruction of the outflow of exocrine secretions either by an inflammatory mass, calcified protein plaques in pancreatic ducts, or narrowing of ducts by inflammatory scars usually causes chronic pain. Gastric varices, especially in the fundus, may develop due to thrombosis of the portal vein or splenic vein. These varices can rupture and cause life-threatening bleeding. Figure 36.14 demonstrates varices of the gastric fundus caused by severe compression of the splenic vein by a large pseudocyst in the pancreatic tail. The inflammatory processes may lead to a fistula, which can connect to the small or large bowel and cause short bowel syndrome. It can also connect with the pleura and cause pleural effusions (Figure 36.15). Very rare complications in chronic pancreatitis

Yamada's Atlas of Gastroenterology, Fifth Edition. Edited by Daniel K. Podolsky, Michael Camilleri, J. Gregory Fitz, Anthony N. Kalloo, Fergus Shanahan, and Timothy C. Wang.

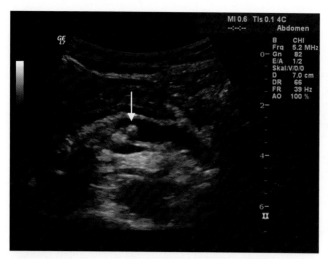

Figure 36.1 Pancreatic duct dilation and pancreatic duct stone. Transabdominal ultrasound: dilated main pancreatic duct and protein plug within the duct (arrow).

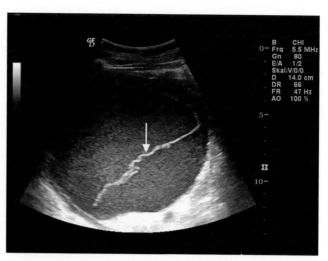

Figure 36.3 Pancreatic pseudocyst. Transabdominal ultrasound: round, echo-poor liquid structure divided by a septum (arrow).

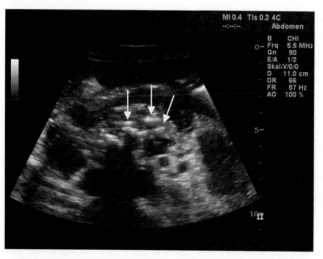

Figure 36.2 Pancreatic calcifications. Transabdominal ultrasound: acoustic reflections due to pancreatic parenchymal calcifications (arrows).

include severe upper gastrointestinal hemorrhage due to an aneurysm of the splenic artery, which lies immediately behind the pancreas and is caused by the pancreatic inflammation (Figure 36.16a). Necrotizing pancreatitis can cause bleeding due to erosion into vessels such as the gastroduodenal artery (Figure 36.17a). Severe necrosis may perforate into the duodenum (Figure 36.18a,b).

Treatment of chronic pancreatitis by interventional endoscopic or radiological procedures

In the presence of an inflammatory tumor of the pancreatic head with bile duct obstruction, ERCP with insertion of a stent into the bile duct should be performed. Pancreatic duct obstructions, which can cause pain, recurrent exacerbations, maintenance of a pseudocyst, fistula, or other complications, can be treated by endoscopic dilatation and stent placement (Figure 36.19a,b). Pancreatic pseudocysts are a frequent complication of acute and chronic pancreatitis. Symptomatic pseudocysts should be treated. Under guidance of endoscopic ultrasound, pseudocysts are most often endoscopically drained into the stomach by stents (Figure 36.20a–d). When ERCP reveals a connection of the pseudocyst with the pancreatic ducts, transpapillary drainage may also be possible.

Vascular pseudoaneurysms secondary to chronic pancreatitis should be treated. Angiographic embolization is the method of choice for active hemorrhagic pseudoaneurysms (Figures 36.16b and 36.17b).

Transgastric or transduodenal endoscopic necrosectomy is a new and much less invasive therapeutic approach compared to surgery (Figure 36.21a,b).

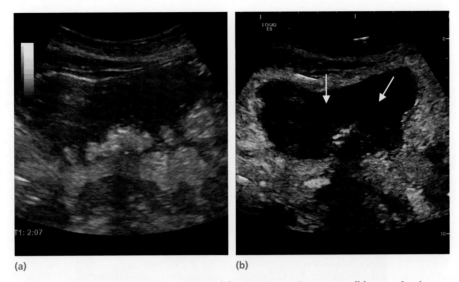

(a)   (b)

Figure 36.4 Pancreatic necrosis. Contrast-enhanced ultrasound (CEUS): **(a)** enlarged irregular pancreas; **(b)** nonperfused area resembling necrotic tissue (arrows).

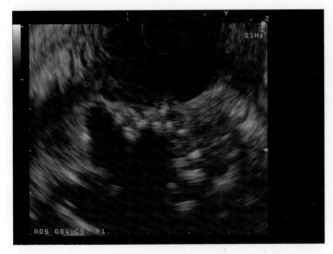

Figure 36.5 Pancreatic calcifications. Radial endoscopic ultrasound: acoustic parenchymal reflexes due to calcifications.

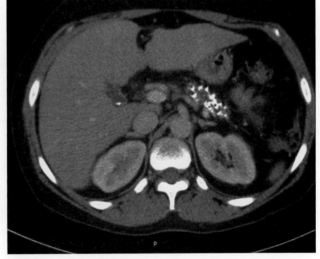

Figure 36.6 Atrophic pancreas in long-lasting chronic pancreatitis. Computed tomography: atrophic pancreas with multiple calcifications. Source: Courtesy of Thomas Kahn MD, Professor of Radiology, Institute of Radiology, University Hospitals of Leipzig.

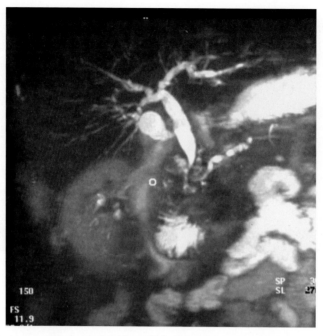

Figure 36.7 Prepapillary stenosis of the common bile duct and the duct of Wirsung. Magnetic resonance cholangiopancreatography (MRCP): slight dilatation of the common bile duct and the main pancreatic duct with tube-like narrowing in the prepapillary region due to chronic inflammation within the head of the pancreas.

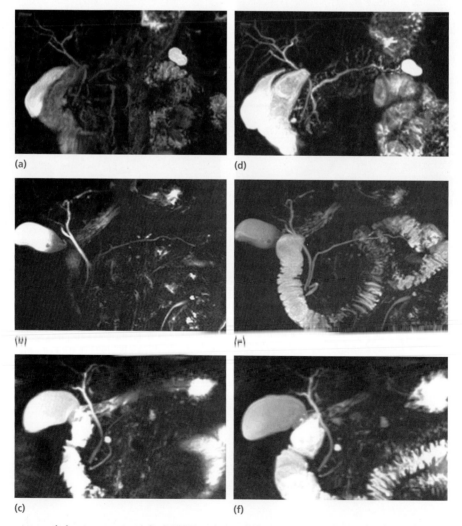

Figure 36.8 Magnetic resonance cholangiopancreatography (MRCP) secretin stimulation. Improvement of main pancreatic duct visualization after secretin stimulation **(d, e, f)**. **(a, d)** Chronic pancreatitis Cambridge II; **(b, e)** normal pancreas; **(c, f)** small cystic lesion.

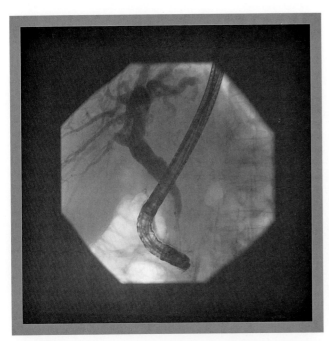

Figure 36.9 Dilatation of the common bile duct. Endoscopic retrograde cholangiography (ERC): marked dilatation of the common bile duct with rather regular tube-like narrowing within the prepapillary region.

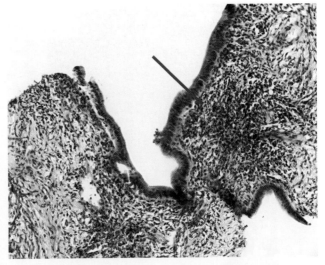

Figure 36.11 Biopsy of the papilla of Vater. Histology: dense infiltration of the papilla by lymphocytes (arrow). Source: Courtesy of Christian Wittekind MD, Professor of Pathology, Institute of Pathology, University Hospitals of Leipzig.

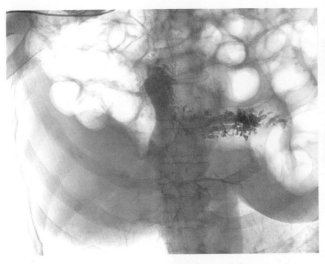

Figure 36.10 Rarefaction and dilatation of the pancreatic ducts. Endoscopic retrograde pancreatography (ERP): x-ray contrast medium injected by ERP remains in markedly dilated side branches of the ducts within the pancreatic tail. Morphology of pancreatic ducts corresponds to grade 4 according to the Cambridge classification.

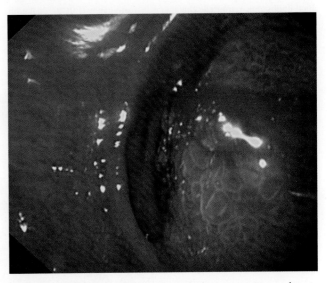

Figure 36.12 Obstruction of the gastric outlet by a pancreatic pseudocyst. Esophagogastroduodenoscopy: impression of the gastric lumen due to a pancreatic pseudocyst.

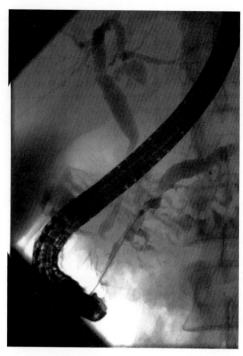

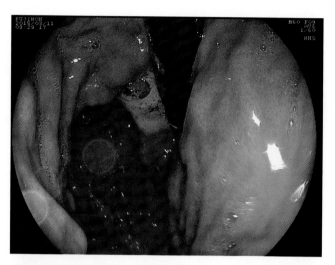

Figure 36.14 Varices within the gastric fundus. Esophagogastroduodenoscopy: the endoscope is retroflexed with view to the gastric fundus. Half-moon-like protrusions correspond to fundic varices.

Figure 36.13 Dilatation of the main pancreatic duct and the common bile duct. Endoscopic retrograde cholangiopancreatography (ERCP): dilatation of the common bile duct and marked dilatation of the main pancreatic duct; almost no side branches visualized.

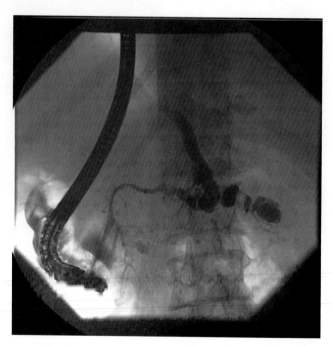

Figure 36.15 Pancreatic fistula. Endoscopic retrograde pancreatography (ERP): irregular dilated main pancreatic duct with pancreaticopleural fistula. Patient presented with dyspnea and marked left-sided pleural effusions.

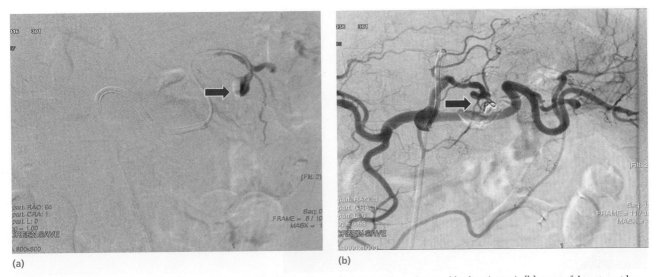

(a)

(b)

Figure 36.16 Pseudoaneurysm of splenic artery. Angiography: **(a)** small pseudoaneurysm caused severe bleeding (arrow); **(b)** successful treatment by coiling (arrow).

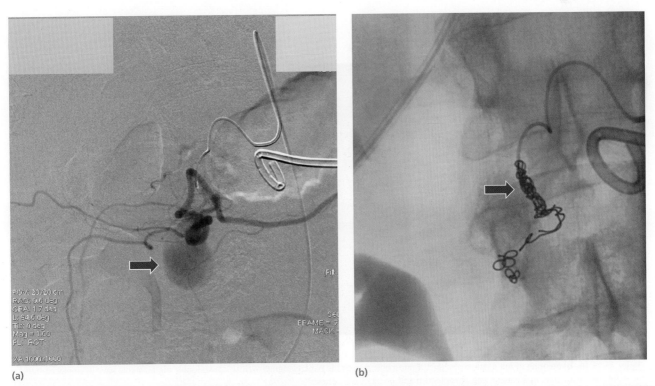

(a)

(b)

Figure 36.17 Pseudoaneurysm of gastroduodenal artery. Angiography: **(a)** proteolytic destruction of a large pseudoaneurysm (arrow) of the gastroduodenal artery caused life-threatening bleeding. **(b)** Bleeding successfully stopped by placing multiple coils before and at the end of the pseudoaneurysm (arrow).

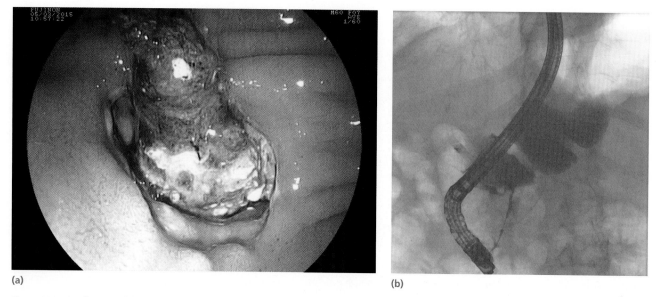

Figure 36.18 Perforation of duodenum by necrotizing pancreatitis. Duodenoscopy: **(a)** spontaneous perforation of pancreatic necrosis into the distal duodenal bulb; evacuation of pus and necrotic material. **(b)** Visualization of the necrotic cavity and fistula by endoscopic retrograde pancreatography (ERP) via the fistula.

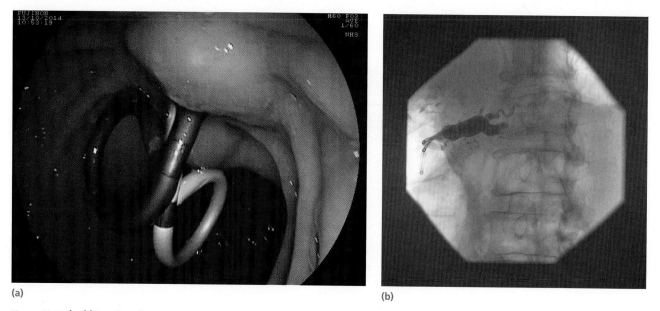

Figure 36.19 (a, b) Stenting of main pancreatic duct. Endoscopic retrograde pancreatography (ERP): two double pigtail stents have been placed into the main pancreatic duct in a patient with chronic pain and preampillary stenosis

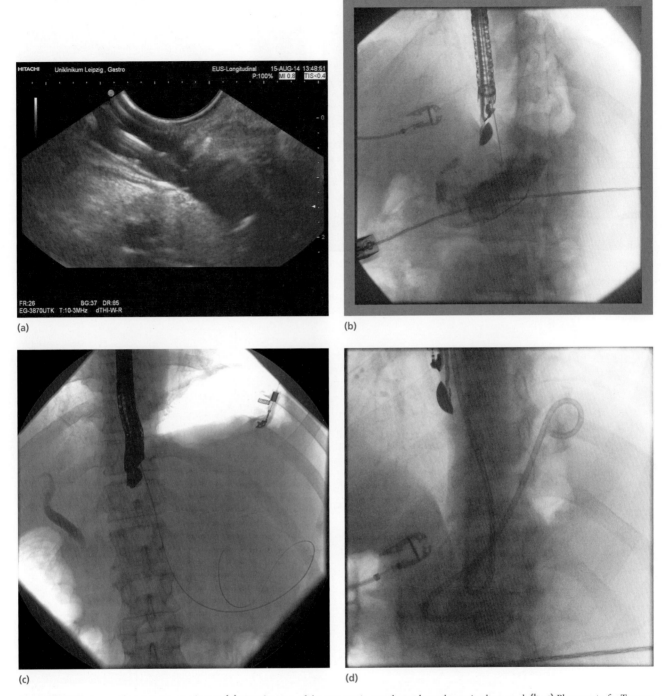

Figure 36.20 Drainage of pancreatic pseudocyst. **(a)** Visualization of the pancreatic pseudocyst by endoscopic ultrasound. **(b, c)** Placement of a Terumo wire into the pseudocyst after needle knife puncture of the gastric wall. **(d)** Transgastric placement of two double pigtails into the pseudocyst.

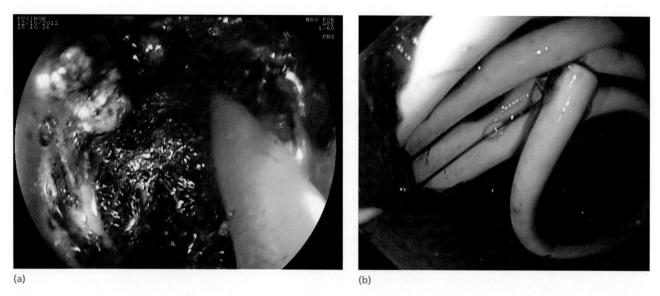

(a)

(b)

Figure 36.21 Transgastric necrosectomy. **(a)** Necrotic tissue is removed by an endoscopic transgastric approach. **(b)** Multiple double pigtail stents are placed transgastrically within the necrotic cavity to ensure both continuous drainage and repeated endoscopic transgastric approach for necrosectomy.

CHAPTER 37

Hereditary diseases of the pancreas

Carlos G. Micames[1] and Jonathan A. Cohn[2]

[1] University of Puerto Rico, Rio Piedras, Puerto Rico
[2] Duke University Medical Center, Durham, NC, USA

Cystic fibrosis (CF) is the most common inherited disease of the exocrine pancreas. It is an autosomal recessive disease caused by loss-of-function mutations of the CF gene. Typical features of CF include lung disease, pancreatic insufficiency, male infertility, and excessive salt secretion by the sweat glands. The CF gene encodes the CF transmembrane conductance regulator (CFTR), a protein which functions as a cyclic adenosine monophosphate (cAMP)-dependent anion channel and as an ion transport regulator in many epithelial tissues.

The molecular pathogenesis of CF can be understood using the CFTR structural model shown in Figure 37.1. The CFTR occurs at the luminal surface of the polarized epithelial cells that line many gastrointestinal tissues. In the pancreas and liver, CFTRs occur at the apical plasma membrane of duct cells (Figure 37.2). During normal pancreatic secretion, CFTRs contribute to the secretion of fluid and bicarbonate by duct cells (Figure 37.3).

Early features of CF pancreatic disease include blockage of the smaller ducts with eosinophilic plugs owing to insufficient dilution and alkalinization of the pancreatic juice. Pancreatic insufficiency occurs in approximately 85% of CF individuals and is usually recognized by 1 year of age. The CF pancreas is typically atrophic with prominent lobulation and progressive cystic changes, fibrosis, and fatty replacement (Figure 37.4). Similar changes occur at the microscopic level in patients with CF who have pancreatic insufficiency (Figure 37.5).

Other gastrointestinal organs are also greatly affected by CF. In the liver, steatosis is common and 2%–5% of individuals develop multilobular biliary cirrhosis (Figure 37.6). In the intestine, meconium ileus and distal intestinal obstruction syndrome (DIOS) are distinctive clinical presentations seen in patients with CF. In both conditions, the terminal ileum is blocked by impacted mucofecal material. The typical computed tomography (CT) findings of DIOS are shown in Figure 37.7. In patients with CF who do not have overt intestinal obstruction, the ileal mucosa is often partially coated with concretions consisting of inspissated mucofecal material (Figure 37.8).

Most mortality and morbidity of patients with CF is due to lung disease. Aggressive nutritional support is important for delaying the progression of lung disease in patients with CF. Many individuals with CF are malnourished and poor pulmonary function correlates closely with having a low body mass index (BMI) (Figure 37.9). It is difficult to achieve target BMI values in most individuals with CF. Clinical management usually includes pancreatic enzyme replacement therapy, a high-fat (high-calorie) diet, and vitamin supplements formulated specifically for individuals with CF.

Recently, drugs have been developed to treat CF by potentiating or correcting CFTR function. In patients with CF due to certain CFTR mutations (e.g., G551D), the first FDA-approved potentiator drug can normalize the sweat chloride test and can provide prompt and sustained improvements in pulmonary and nutritional status. Even though this drug is only indicated for a limited number of CF individuals, its dramatic effectiveness in these cases demonstrates that CFTR is a druggable target and that it is useful to individualize CF therapy based on the CFTR genotype. Thus, this example illustrates the power of a "personalized medicine" approach.

A second common inherited disease of the exocrine pancreas is hereditary pancreatitis (HP). This is an autosomal dominant disease caused by mutations of the *PRSS1* gene. This gene encodes cationic trypsinogen, the principal trypsin proenzyme in human pancreatic juice. The most common HP-causing mutation is R122H. The molecular pathogenesis of HP due to this *PRSS1* mutation can be understood using the trypsinogen structural model shown in Figure 37.10. The CT findings in HP resemble those of other forms of chronic pancreatitis (Figure 37.11). As HP causes recurrent and progressive pancreatic injury, it gradually leads to pancreatic exocrine insufficiency, diabetes mellitus, and pancreatic cancer over a period of decades (Figure 37.12).

Yamada's Atlas of Gastroenterology, Fifth Edition. Edited by Daniel K. Podolsky, Michael Camilleri, J. Gregory Fitz, Anthony N. Kalloo, Fergus Shanahan, and Timothy C. Wang.
© 2016 John Wiley & Sons, Ltd. Published 2016 by John Wiley & Sons, Ltd.
Companion website: www.yamadagastro.com/atlas

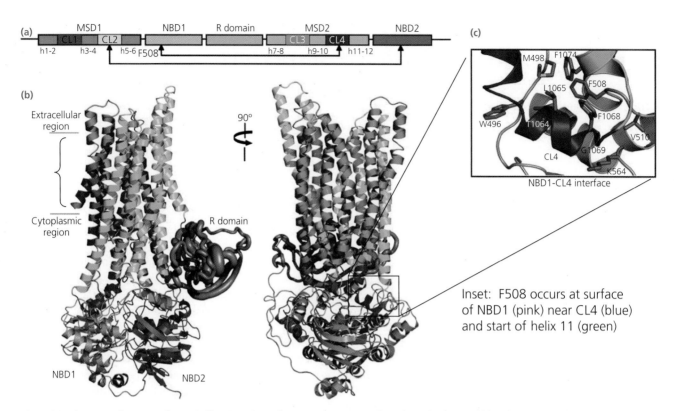

Figure 37.1 A proposed structure for cystic fibrosis transmembrane conductance regulator (CFTR). This model builds on the crystal structures of one cytoplasmic domain (NBD1) of CFTR and of a bacterial transporter related to CFTR (Sav1866). **(a)** CFTR contains two membrane-spanning domains (MSD1 and MSD2 in dark and light green), two nucleotide-binding domains (NBD1 and NBD2 in light and dark pink), and a regulatory domain (R domain, in gray). Each MSD contains six transmembrane helices (h1–h6, h7–h12) and two cytoplasmic loops (CL1–2, CL3–4). Together, the 12 helices (h1–h12) surround an aqueous pore, which forms a channel through the lipid bilayer and allows anions to passively flow through the cell membrane. Channel gating is controlled by the impact of nucleotides and cAMP-dependent signaling on the cytoplasmic NBD1, NBD2, and R domains. **(b)** This model highlights how cytoplasmic regulatory events are thought to control the structure and ion channel function of the MSD domains through NBD/CL interactions. The most common CF-causing *CFTR* mutation results in deletion of the phenylalanine normally in position 508 in the NBD1 domain of CFTR (delta F508). CFTR molecules with this mutation misfold and exhibit reduced function because of defective intracellular trafficking, instability at the cell surface, and defective ion channel gating. Based on crystallography data for NBD1 and on modeling studies for full-length CFTR, F508 occurs on the surface of NBD1 in a region where NBD1 normally interacts with the CL4 loop near the base of helix 11 **(c)**. This region contains a hydrophobic pocket where F508 probably interacts with L1065, F1068, and F1074 in CL4. Even though the deletion of F508 has little impact on the intrinsic structure of NBD1 (comparing crystal structures for the mutant and normal forms of NBD1), this mutation may cause misfolding and malfunction of full-length CFTR by disrupting the NBD1/CL4 interface. Source: Adapted from Serohijos AW, Hegedus T, Aleksandrov AA, et al. Phenylalanine-508 mediates a cytoplasmic-membrane domain contact in the CFTR 3D structure crucial to assembly and channel function. Proc Natl Acad Sci USA 2008;105:3256.

Other inherited diseases of the exocrine pancreas are rare. Among these, the most common is Shwachman–Diamond syndrome (SDS), an autosomal recessive condition caused by mutations of the *SBDS* gene. Patients with SDS usually develop pancreatic insufficiency by the age of 1 year. Common additional findings include neutropenia and growth or skeletal abnormalities. Pancreatic insufficiency in SDS results from defective development of the pancreatic acini. Typical histopathological features in the pancreas include fatty replacement of the acini with relative sparing of the pancreatic ducts and islets (Figure 37.13).

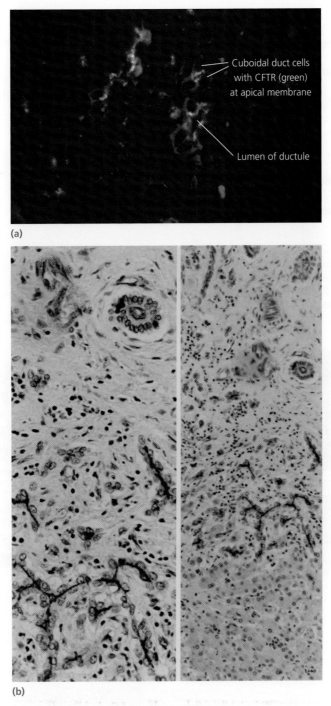

(a)

(b)

Figure 37.2 Localization of cystic fibrosis transmembrane conductance regulator (CFTR) protein in human pancreas and liver. **(a)** Double-label immunofluorescence staining of CFTR (green) and of the sodium/potassium ATPase (orange) in human pancreas. Small pancreatic ducts are surrounded by cuboidal epithelial cells which express CFTR at the apical plasma membrane and the sodium–potassium ATPase at the basolateral plasma membrane. Source: Marino CR, Matovcik LM, Gorelick FS, et al. Localization of the cystic fibrosis transmembrane conductance regulator in pancreas. J Clin Invest 1991;88:712. Reproduced with permission of the American Society for Clinical Investigation. **(b)** Immunoperoxidase staining of CFTR (brown signal) in human liver. CFTR occurs on the lumenal surface of intrahepatic bile ducts. Source: Cohn JA, Strong TV, Picciotto MR, et al. Localization of the cystic fibrosis transmembrane conductance regulator in human bile duct epithelial cells. Gastroenterology 1993;105:1857.

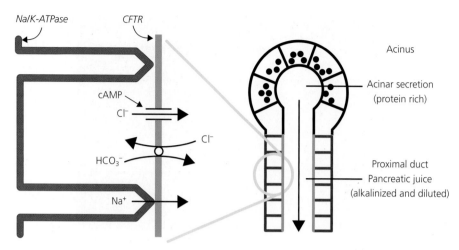

Figure 37.3 Proposed role of cystic fibrosis transmembrane conductance regulator (CFTR) during pancreatic exocrine secretion. As pancreatic juice flows through the intralobular duct, the protein-rich acinar secretions are diluted and alkalinized by the duct epithelial cells. CFTR functions at the apical plasma membrane of these cells to promote the cAMP-mediated secretion of fluid and bicarbonate into the lumen. When CFTR function at this site is reduced (e.g., in CF), inadequate dilution and alkalinization of the pancreatic juice may promote the formation of protein plugs (possibly by affecting solubility or viscosity) and thereby contribute to the ductal obstruction and progressive pancreatic insufficiency that occur in CF. Source: Adapted from Marino CR, Matovcik LM, Gorelick FS, et al. Localization of the cystic fibrosis transmembrane conductance regulator in pancreas. J Clin Invest 1991;88:712.

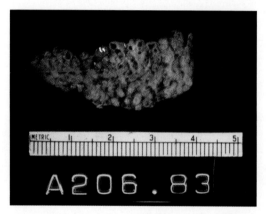

Figure 37.4 A pathological specimen of pancreas from a patient with cystic fibrosis with severe pancreatic insufficiency. This atrophic gland is fibrotic and shows prominent lobulation with cystic changes.
Source: Courtesy of Dr. Peter Durie, Hospital for Sick Children, Toronto.

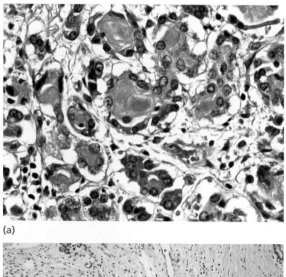

(a)

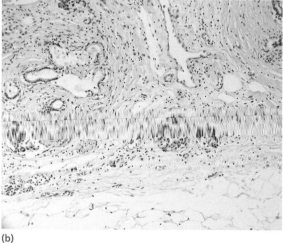

(b)

Figure 37.5 Photomicrographs of the pancreas from patients with cystic fibrosis. **(a)** Early findings include acinar atrophy and ductular plugging with inspissated eosinophilic concretions. Source: Courtesy of Dr. David Myerholz and Dr. Marcus Nashelsky, University of Iowa Medical Center. **(b)** Typical pancreatic findings with exocrine insufficiency include prominent fibrosis and fatty infiltration with relative preservation of the islets. Source: Courtesy of Dr. Alan Proia, Duke University Medical Center.

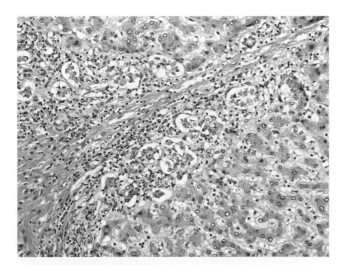

Figure 37.6 Photomicrographs of the liver from patients with cystic fibrosis showing focal biliary cirrhosis. Typical findings include focal portal and periportal fibrosis, ductular proliferation, and periductular inflammation. Steatosis and ductal plugging also are common.
Source: Courtesy of Dr. David Meyerholz and Dr. Marcus Nashelsky.

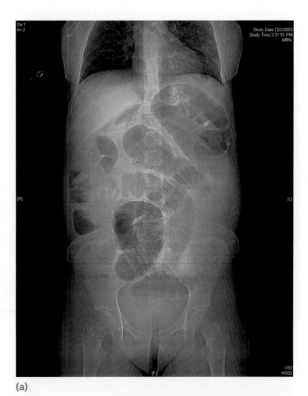

(a)

Distended small bowel with thickened bowel wall and fecal material containing small gas bubbles

Terminal ileum containing solid stool

Colon containing contrast; the lumen is not distended and the bowel wall thickness is normal

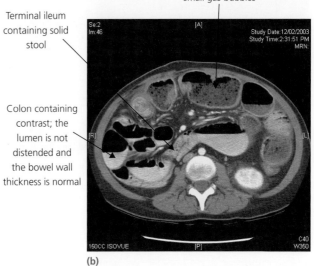

(b)

Figure 37.7 **(a)** Abdominal imaging of an adult with cystic fibrosis with distal intestinal obstruction syndrome. **(b)** The terminal ileum is filled with solid stool. Proximal to this obstruction, the small bowel is distended (note thickened bowel wall and gas bubbles in fecal material). Distal to the transition point, the colon contains contrast and is not distended.

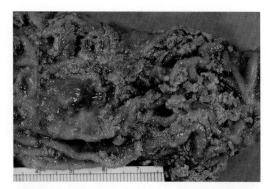

Figure 37.8 A pathological specimen of ileum from an adult with cystic fibrosis (CF) who had severe CF lung disease but who did not have overt intestinal disease. Much of the mucosal surface is covered with concretions consisting of inspissate mucofecal material. Source: Courtesy of Dr. Peter Durie.

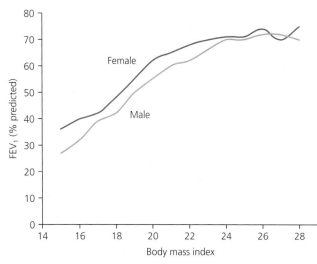

Figure 37.9 Relationship between nutritional status and lung function in adults with cystic fibrosis (CF). For patients with CF at age 20–40 years, lung function drops sharply as the body mass index falls below 22. Data like these provide the rationale for providing patients with CF with aggressive nutritional support. FEV$_1$, forced expiratory volume in 1 s.

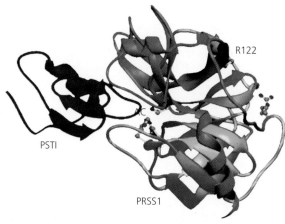

Figure 37.10 The structure of cationic trypsinogen (PRSS1) and of pancreatic secretory trypsin inhibitor (PSTI). PSTI blocks tryptic proteolysis by binding to the catalytic site of trypsinogen (AC), as shown. Mutations of the *PRSS1* and *PSTI* genes can each lead to hereditary forms of pancreatitis. The most common cause of hereditary pancreatitis is the *PRSS1* R122H mutation. R122 occurs at the trypsinogen surface as shown. If active trypsin accumulates in the pancreatic parenchyma, this potentially could cause an uncontrolled proteolytic chain reaction because additional activated trypsin can be produced by the action of trypsin on trypsinogen. To prevent this, trypsinogen normally contains an inactivating cleavage site at an accessible site on its surface (R122). Once trypsinogen is digested at R122 (e.g., by trypsin), trypsinogen can no longer be activated. In hereditary pancreatitis, the R122H mutation prevents digestion of trypsinogen at R122 and this allows active trypsin to accumulate in an uncontrolled manner. Thus, excessive activation of trypsin is thought to be the primary event causing pancreatic injury in many patients with hereditary pancreatitis. Source: Adapted from Whitcomb DC, Gorry MC, Preston RA, et al. Hereditary pancreatitis is caused by a mutation in the cationic trypsinogen gene. Nat Genet 1996;14:141.

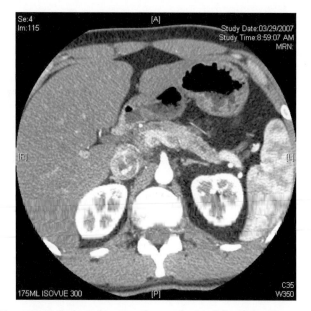

Figure 37.11 Computed tomography scan for an adult with hereditary pancreatitis. The pancreas shows changes consistent with chronic pancreatitis including mild atrophy and multiple punctate parenchymal calcifications (especially in the pancreatic head).

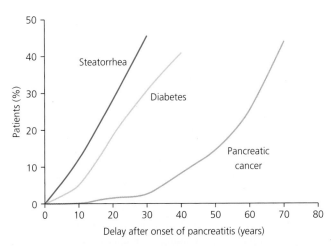

Figure 37.12 Steatorrhea, diabetes mellitus, and pancreatic cancer are common complications of hereditary pancreatitis in patients who are followed for decades. Steatorrhea and diabetes mellitus often occur two to four decades after the onset of pancreatitis, while pancreatic cancer is usually delayed by an additional two to three decades. Source: Data from Howes N, Lerch MM, Greenhalf W, et al. Clinical and genetic characteristics of hereditary pancreatitis in Europe. Clin Gastroenterol Hepatol 2004;2:252.

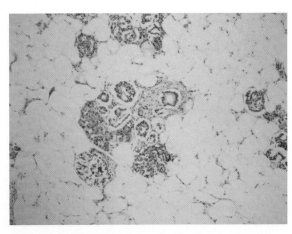

Figure 37.13 A histological section of pancreas from a patient with Shwachman–Diamond syndrome. Typical exocrine gland features include fatty replacement of acini with sparing of ducts. Many islets are preserved but have distorted architecture. Source: Courtesy of Dr. Peter Durie.

CHAPTER 38

Cystic lesions of the pancreas

James J. Farrell

Yale University, New Haven, CT, USA

Cystic neoplasms of the pancreas are found with increasing prevalence, especially in elderly asymptomatic individuals. Although the overall risk of malignancy is very low, the presence of these pancreas cysts is associated with a large degree of anxiety and further medical investigation, due to concerns about malignancy. The differential diagnosis for cystic neoplasms of the pancreas ranges from benign processes such as serous cystadenomas (Figure 38.1), to pancreatic cysts of low malignant potential such as cystic pancreatic endocrine tumors

(Figure 38.2) and solid pseudopapillary neoplasms (Figure 38.3), to the premalignant or malignant mucinous cystic neoplasms of the pancreas, including intraductal papillary mucinous neoplasms (IPMN) (Figures 38.4, 38.5, and 38.6) and mucinous cystic neoplasms (Figure 38.7). Often, the preoperative diagnosis is possible based on clinical features and imaging data, with surgical and nonsurgical management of the most common cystic neoplasms, IPMNs and MCNs, based on the recently revised Sendai guidelines.

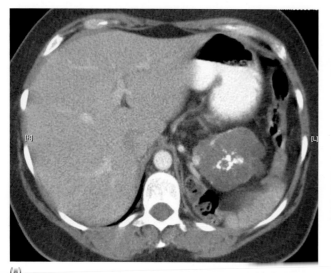

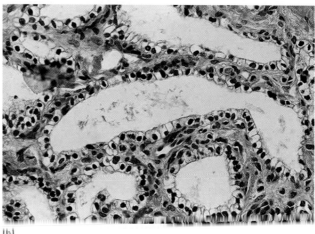

Figure 38.1 A 60-year old male with asymptomatic 3-cm pancreatic tail microcystic lesion with central stellate calcification suggestive of a classic microcystic serous cystadenoma. **(a)** CT scan showing 3-cm multicystic pancreatic tail lesion with central stellate calcification. **(b)** Histology of serous cystadenoma showing cuboidal cells, which stain positive for glycogen.

Yamada's Atlas of Gastroenterology, Fifth Edition. Edited by Daniel K. Podolsky, Michael Camilleri, J. Gregory Fitz, Anthony N. Kalloo, Fergus Shanahan, and Timothy C. Wang.
© 2016 John Wiley & Sons, Ltd. Published 2016 by John Wiley & Sons, Ltd.
Companion website: www.yamadagastro.com/atlas

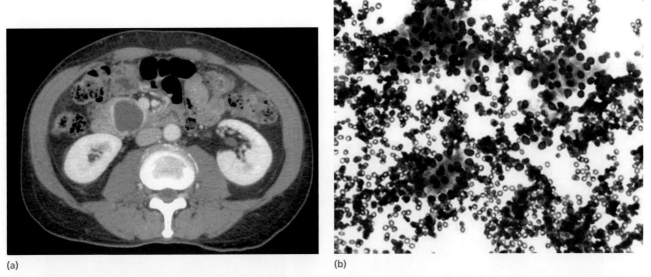

(a)

(b)

Figure 38.2 A 52-year-old male with incidental 2-cm pancreatic head cyst manifesting a hyperenhancing rim. Endoscopic ultrasound fine-needle aspiration (EUS-FNA) was performed and demonstrated pancreatic endocrine cells. At the time of surgery a cystic pancreatic endocrine neoplasm was found. **(a)** CT scan showing a 2-cm pancreatic head cyst with hyperenhancing rim. **(b)** EUS-FNA cytology showing uniform hyperchromatic cells consistent with pancreatic endocrine neoplasms.

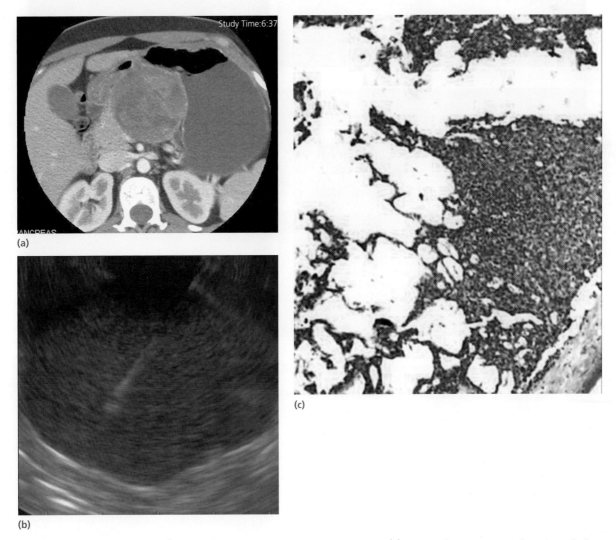

(a)

(b)

(c)

Figure 38.3 A 13-year-old female with abdominal pain and a solid pseudopapillary neoplasm. **(a)** CT scan showing a 4-cm well-circumscribed heterogeneous pancreas mass. **(b)** Endoscopic ultrasound-guided core biopsy-confirmed solid pseudopapillary epithelial neoplasm (SPEN). **(c)** Histology shows the cells oriented perpendicularly to thin vascular cores and nuclei lined up towards luminal aspect of irregular tissue crevices, consistent with pseudopapilla; PAS negative for mucin.

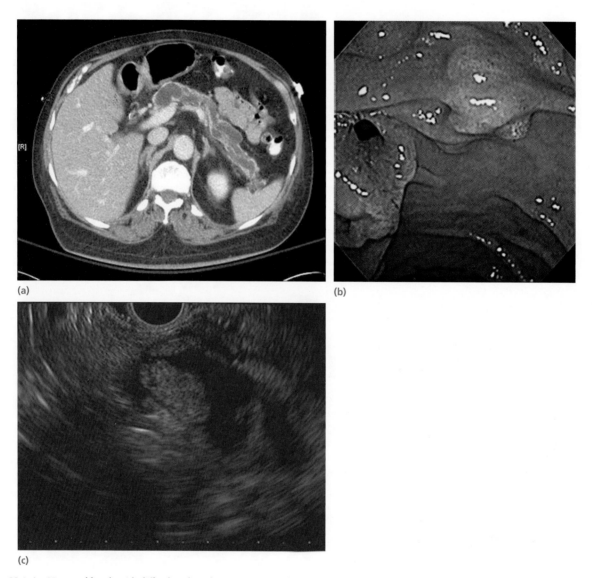

(a)

(b)

(c)

Figure 38.4 An 85-year-old male with diffusely enlarged main pancreatic duct and atrophic pancreas suggestive of main duct intraductal papillary mucinous neoplasm (IPMN). (a) CT scan shows a diffusely enlarged main pancreatic duct and atrophic pancreas suggestive of main duct IPMN. (b) Endoscopic image of gaping "fisheye" major ampulla (b.b) and prominent minor papilla (right) suggestive of main duct IPMN. (c) Endoscopic ultrasound shows a dilated main pancreatic duct with a 15-mm intraductal epithelial nodule in the head of the pancreas.

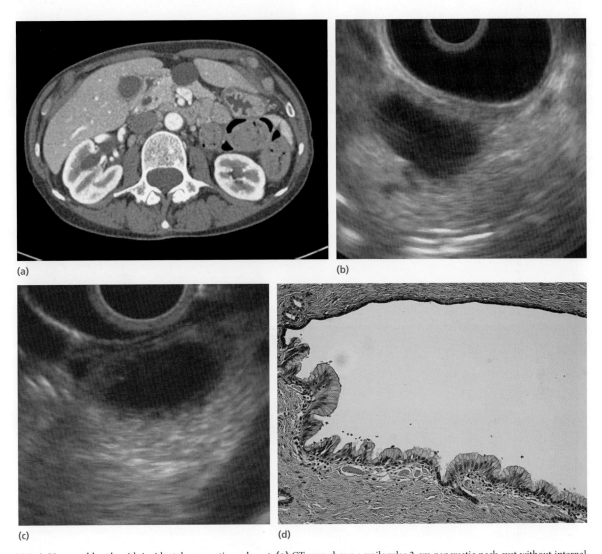

(a)

(b)

(c)

(d)

Figure 38.5 A 50-year-old male with incidental pancreatic neck cyst. **(a)** CT scan shows a unilocular 2-cm pancreatic neck cyst without internal nodules or abnormal pancreatic duct. **(b)** Endoscopic ultrasound shows branch duct communication. **(c)** Endoscopic ultrasound showing an 8-mm epithelial nodule. **(d)** Surgical resection showing intraductal papillary mucinous neoplasm (BD-IPMN) with low-grade dysplasia and gastric subtype.

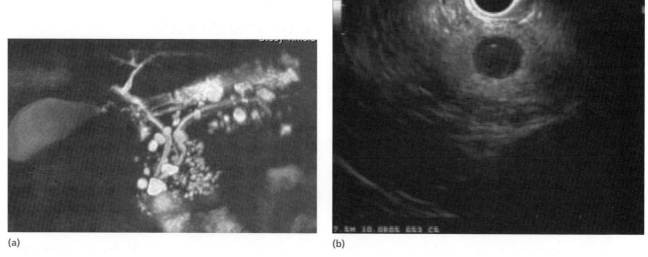

(a) (b)

Figure 38.6 A 53-year-old female with a single episode of pancreatitis and a diagnosis of multifocal intraductal papillary mucinous neoplasm (BD-IPMN). **(a)** Magnetic resonance cholangiopancreatography (MRCP) shows multiple pancreatic cysts with a normal main pancreatic duct. **(b)** Endoscopic ultrasound imaging of a 1-cm unilocular pancreatic cyst with internal mucin globule (hyperechoic edge).

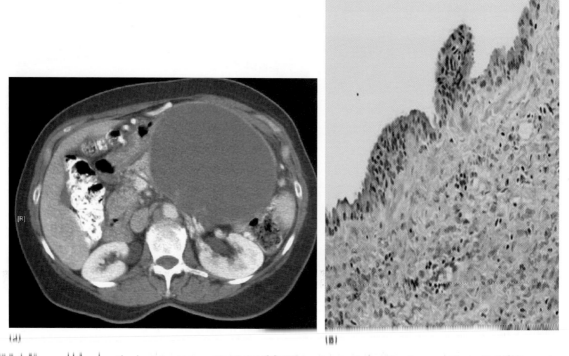

(a) (b)

Figure 38.7 A 50-year old female with a large 7-cm pancreatic tail cyst. **(a)** CT scan shows a 7-cm unilocular cyst with a well-defined capsule and eccentric wall nodularity. **(b)** Surgical resection demonstrating a mucinous cystadenoma (low grade dysplasia). Characteristic ovarian stroma is also present.

CHAPTER 39

Neuroendocrine tumors of the pancreas

Peter J. Carolan and Daniel C. Chung
Massachusetts General Hospital, Boston, MA, USA

Gastroenteropancreatic neuroendocrine tumors are a distinctive and uncommon group of tumors that arise within the diffuse neuroendocrine system of the intestine and the pancreatic islets of Langerhans. They can present with dramatic hormonal symptoms due to dysregulated production and release of endogenous and ectopic hormones. Clinical management focuses on managing the symptoms of hormone excess as well as localization and ultimately resection of the tumor mass. This chapter highlights some of the unique features of these tumors. Some tumors are associated with unusual extrapancreatic features. For example, glucagonomas can be associated with a characteristic rash (necrolytic migratory erythema, Figure 39.1). Histologically, most pancreatic neuroendocrine tumors (PNETs) are well-differentiated and exhibit sheets of homogeneous tumor cells without aneuploidy. Immunohistochemistry is a useful tool to stain for specific endogenous as well as ectopic hormones (Figure 39.2). Conventional computed tomography (CT) scans can often detect PNETs due to their hypervascular nature (Figure 39.3), but magnetic resonance imaging (MRI) has emerged as a more sensitive modality, particularly for smaller lesions (Figure 39.4). Positron emission tomography (PET) scans are not generally utilized for diagnosis or management of well-differentiated PNETs, but they can be a useful modality for poorly differentiated PNETs (Figure 39.5).

Yamada's Atlas of Gastroenterology, Fifth Edition. Edited by Daniel K. Podolsky, Michael Camilleri, J. Gregory Fitz, Anthony N. Kalloo, Fergus Shanahan, and Timothy C. Wang.
© 2016 John Wiley & Sons, Ltd. Published 2016 by John Wiley & Sons, Ltd.
Companion website: www.yamadagastro.com/atlas

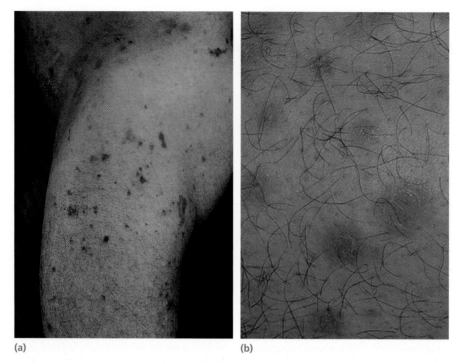

(a) (b)

Figure 39.1 Necrolytic migratory erythema in a patient with glucagonoma. Necrolytic migratory erythema is a common presentation for glucagonoma and occurs at diagnosis in 70% of cases. **(a)** The dermatitis begins in the periorofacial or intertriginous regions and then spreads more distally. **(b)** The lesions consist of erythematous macules and papules that expand into confluent plaques with superficial scale and a well-defined border. Central superficial bullae develop and rupture, forming erosions that crust and heal with hyperpigmentation. Source: (a) Wermers RA, Fatourechi V, Wynne AG, et al. The glucagonoma syndrome clinical and pathologic features in 21 patients. Medicine 1996;75:53. Reproduced with permission of Wolters Kluwer Health. (b) Pujol RM, Wang C-YE, El-Azhary RA, et al. Necrolytic migratory erythema: clinicopathologic study of 13 cases. Int J Dermatol 2004;43:12. Reproduced with permission of John Wiley & Sons.

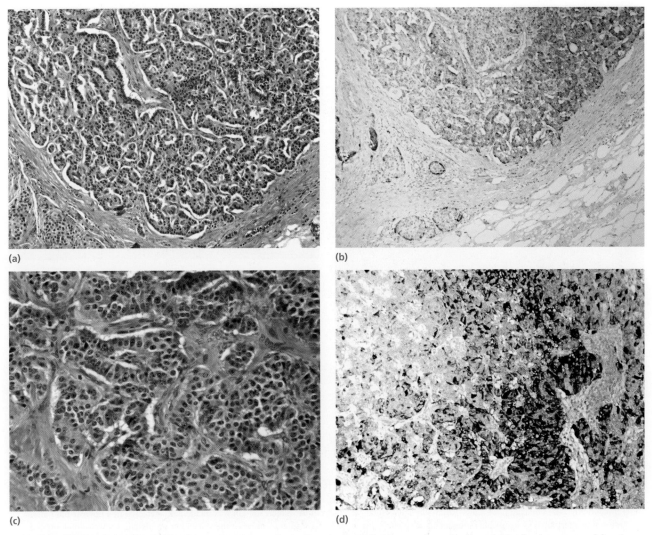

(a)

(b)

(c)

(d)

Figure 39.2 Histology of well-differentiated pancreatic neuroendocrine tumors (PNETs). Hematoxylin and eosin staining of a glucagonoma (a) and VIPoma (c) demonstrates the typical organoid growth pattern of a well-differentiated PNET. Relatively homogeneous cells are found in nesting, trabecular, or gyriform arrangements. Tumor cells are small to medium sized with eosinophilic cytoplasm and uniform, round to oval, stippled nuclei. Detecting the expression of a specific hormone such as glucagon (b) or vasoactive intestinal polypeptide (VIP) (d) is helpful in confirming the diagnosis of a functional syndrome in the presence of appropriate clinical signs and symptoms. Source: Courtesy of Dr. Vikram Deshpande, Department of Pathology, Massachusetts General Hospital.

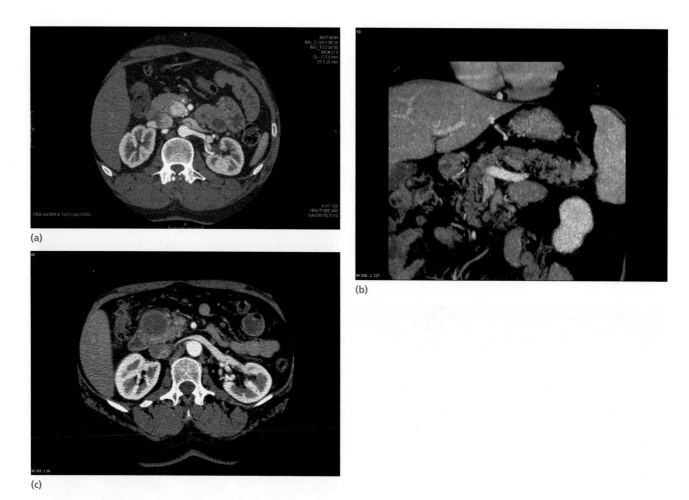

Figure 39.3 Computed tomography (CT) of neuroendocrine tumor (NET) primary lesions. **(a)** In a 33-year-old man with newly diagnosed Von Hippel-Lindau syndrome, contrast enhanced CT shows an avidly enhancing solid lesion in the uncinate process of the pancreas, due to a well-differentiated NET. **(b)** On axial CT a 2.5 × 1.8 cm lobulated enhancing mass in the pancreatic tail was incidentally detected in a 66-year-old patient. The lesion was interpreted as a possible intrapancreatic splenule due to the enhancement similar to the spleen but on histology a well-differentiated pancreatic NET was diagnosed. **(c)** A NET of the pancreatic head detected in a 47-year-old woman who presented with abdominal pain. The lesion demonstrates a purely cystic appearance and a thick, homogeneous wall. Source: Courtesy of Dr. Dushyant Sahani, Department of Radiology, Massachusetts General Hospital.

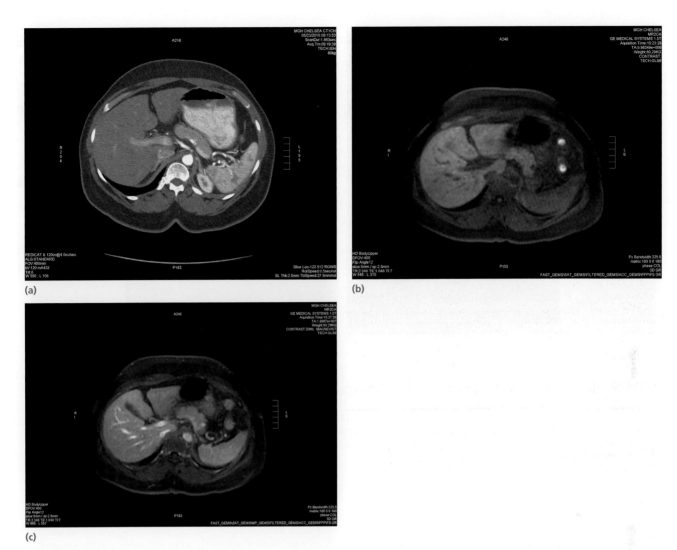

(a)

(b)

(c)

Figure 39.4 Pancreatic neuroendocrine tumor (PNET) seen on magnetic resonance imaging (MRI) but not computed tomography (CT). A 51-year-old woman presented with vague abdominal pain and weight loss. **(a)** An axial contrast enhanced multidetector CT scan acquired in the arterial phase does not clearly show any lesion within the pancreas. On axial T1-weighted fat saturation **(b)** and contrast enhanced MRI **(c)** images a small, well-defined lesion in the superior aspect of the body of the pancreas is seen. It is T1 hypointense and characterized by intense contrast-enhancement. The patient underwent a laparoscopic enucleation with the diagnosis of a non-functioning, well-differentiated, low grade PNET. Source: Courtesy of Dr. Dushyant Sahani, Department of Radiology, Massachusetts General Hospital.

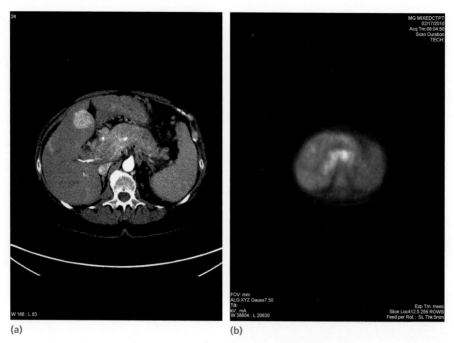

(a)   (b)

Figure 39.5 ¹⁸F-deoxyglucose (FDG) positron emission tomography computed tomography (PET-CT) of a pancreatic neuroendocrine tumor (PNET). A 61-year-old woman presented with 2 weeks of gastroesophageal reflux symptoms, abdominal pain, nausea, and diarrhea. **(a)** Axial contrast enhanced CT image demonstrated an infiltrating arterially enhancing mass involving the head, the body and the proximal part of the pancreatic tail. This lesion encases the splenic artery, invades the portal vein and leads to a partial dilatation of the main pancreatic duct. Two metastatic lesions in the liver were also seen (not shown). **(b)** In the corresponding fused PET-CT image, the FDG uptake is avid in the pancreatic lesion and moderate along the lateral margin of the hepatic lesion. FDG-PET can detect highly metabolically active tumors such as poorly differentiated PNETs that have a high proliferation rate, but is not as sensitive for slower growing well-differentiated tumors. Source: Courtesy of Dr. Dushyant Sahani, Department of Radiology, Massachusetts General Hospital.

CHAPTER 40

Gallstones

Piero Portincasa[1] and David Q.-H. Wang[2]
[1] University of Bari Medical School, Policlinico Hospital, Bari, Italy
[2] Saint Louis University School of Medicine, St. Louis, MO, USA

Classification

Gallstones are made of cholesterol monohydrate crystals, mucin, calcium bilirubinate, and protein aggregates in the biliary tree. Based on chemical composition, gallstones are divided into three types: *cholesterol*, *pigment*, and *rare* stones (Figure 40.1). The majority ($\sim$75%) of gallstones in the United States and Europe are cholesterol stones, which are usually subclassified as either pure cholesterol or mixed stones, which contain at least 50% cholesterol by weight. Pigment gallstones contain mostly calcium bilirubinate and are subclassified into two groups: black ($\sim$20%) and brown pigment stones ($\sim$4.5%). Rare stones ($\sim$0.5%) include calcium carbonate stones and fatty acid–calcium stones. The prevalence of gallstones varies from 5% to 50% in different populations and it is 10%–15% in industrialized countries (Figure 40.2).

Pathogenesis

Bile is an aqueous solution containing organic solutes, inorganic electrolytes, and trace amounts of proteins and elements (Figure 40.3). The three classes of biliary lipids are unesterified cholesterol ($>$95%), phospholipids ($>$95% lecithins), and bile acids, which are composed of primary (cholic and chenodeoxycholic acids) and secondary bile acids (derived from 7α-dehydroxylation of the primary bile acids in the liver and by intestinal bacteria in the ileum and colon: deoxycholic, lithocholic, ursodeoxycholic, sulfolithocholic, and 7α-oxo-lithocholic acids).

Cholesterol gallstones

Two lipid carriers are necessary for cholesterol solubilization in bile: micelles and vesicles (Figure 40.4). Major risk factors for cholesterol gallstones include increasing age, female gender,

pregnancy, metabolic syndrome, insulin resistance, rapid weight loss, physical inactivity, high cholesterol diet, gallbladder stasis, estrogen and oral contraceptives, diabetes mellitus, and low serum magnesium. Pathogenic mechanisms leading to the formation of cholesterol gallstones involve five defects (Figure 40.5), of which supersaturation of cholesterol in bile is predominant (Figures 40.6 and 40.7). Liver and small intestine provide the major sources of cholesterol leading to lithogenic bile. Hepatic hypersecretion of biliary cholesterol could result from increases in intestinal absorption, hepatic biosynthesis, and hepatic uptake of high-density lipoproteins (HDL) from plasma, as well as decreases in the conversion of cholesterol into bile acids and esterification of cholesterol. Cholesterol crystallization ultimately leads to the formation of solid plate-like cholesterol monohydrate crystals (Figure 40.8). Some factors act as "pronucleating" agents, including excess mucin, as found in biliary sludge, which is a precursor of gallstones. Mucin acts as a matrix for stone growth. Gallbladder stasis facilitates the precipitation and aggregation of solid cholesterol crystals (Figure 40.9). Sluggish gallbladder contractility due to impaired signal transduction might arise from excess cholesterol molecules incorporated in the gallbladder muscle cells acting as myotoxic agents. Excess cholesterol acts as a stimulant of proliferative and inflammatory changes in the mucosa and lamina propria of the gallbladder. Among intestinal factors, delayed small intestinal transit appears to be associated with increased intestinal cholesterol absorption and biliary cholesterol secretion, and impaired colonic motility is associated with increased biliary deoxycholate levels, promoting cholesterol crystallization and mucin hypersecretion. Altogether, the above-mentioned defects lead to cholesterol-supersaturated bile, with propensity to precipitation and aggregation of solid cholesterol crystals and eventually growth into stones (Figure 40.10).

Yamada's Atlas of Gastroenterology, Fifth Edition. Edited by Daniel K. Podolsky, Michael Camilleri, J. Gregory Fitz, Anthony N. Kalloo, Fergus Shanahan, and Timothy C. Wang.

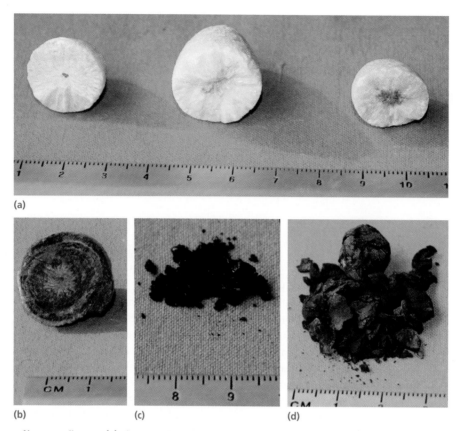

Figure 40.1 Appearance of human gallstones. **(a)** The cut surface of pure cholesterol stones with a small (left), absent (middle), and large (right) pigment center. **(b)** Mixed cholesterol stone with a concentric appearance, made of a mixture of cholesterol, bilirubin salts, and calcium. **(c)** Black pigment stones. **(d)** Brown pigment stones, partially fragmented. Source: Courtesy of P Portincasa, MD.

Pigment gallstones

Black and brown pigment gallstones form due to abnormalities in the bilirubin metabolism in the gut–liver axis (Figure 40.1). Hemolytic anemias, liver cirrhosis, cystic fibrosis, Crohn's disease, or extended ileal resection, biliary infection, vitamin B-12/folic acid deficient diets, and aging are the most common risk factors. Genetic factors play a role when *UGT1A1* mutation occurs. Black pigment stones consist of either pure calcium bilirubinate or polymer-like complexes with unconjugated bilirubin, calcium bilirubinate, calcium, and copper. A regular crystalline structure is not present. The formation of black pigment gallstones is mainly induced by hepatic hypersecretion of bilirubin conjugates (especially monoglucuronides) into bile. Unconjugated monohydroguanated bilirubin is formed by the action of endogenous β-glucuronidase, which coprecipitates with calcium because of supersaturation in bile. An increased hydrolysis rate often leads to a high concentration of unconjugated bilirubin, which markedly exceeds the solubility of bilirubin in bile. Brown pigment gallstones are primarily composed of calcium salts of unconjugated bilirubin, with varying amounts of cholesterol, pigment fraction, fatty acids, and mucin glycoproteins, as well as small amounts of bile acids, phospholipids, and bacterial residues (Figure 40.1). These stones are formed not only in the gallbladder, but also in other portions of the biliary tree, especially in intrahepatic bile ducts. The formation of brown pigment gallstones usually requires the presence of bile stasis associated with biliary infection, especially with *Escherichia coli, Clonorchis sinensis,* roundworms, and their ova.

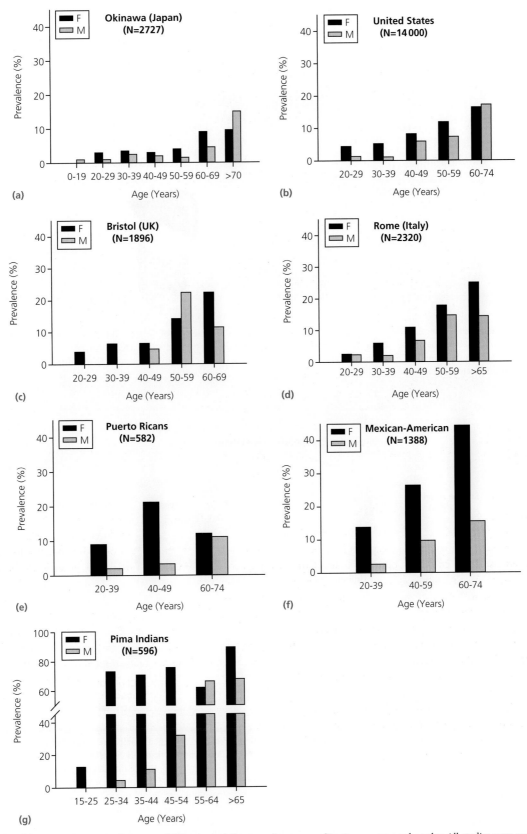

Figure 40.2 (a–g) The prevalences of gallstones in different populations are shown according to age range and gender. All studies were conducted by abdominal ultrasonography, with the exception of the one in Pima Indians (g), where cholecystography was used. Overall, the prevalence is higher in females (F) than males (M) at each age group. A high prevalence is apparent in Mexican-American females (f). Of note, Pima Indians display an extremely high prevalence (g). Source: Data from: (a) Nomura H, Kashiwagi S, Hayashi J, et al. Am J Epidemiol 1992;136:787; (b) Everhart JE, Khare M, Hill M, Maurer KR. Gastroenterology 1999;117:632; (c) Heaton IW, Braddon FEM, Mountford RA, et al. Gut 1991;32:316; (d) Attili AF, Carulli N, Roda E, et al. Am J Epidemiology 1995;141:158; (e, f) Maurer KR, Everhart JE, Ezzati TM, et al. Gastroenterology 1989;96:487; (g) Sampliner RE, Bennett PH, Comess LJ, et al. N Engl J Med 1970;283:1358.

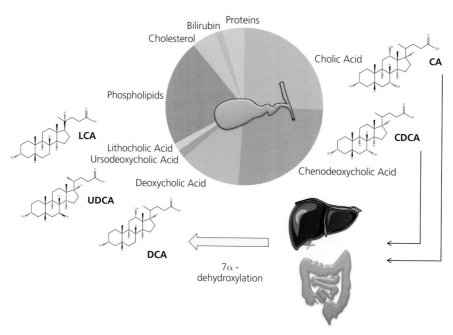

Figure 40.3 Composition of human gallbladder bile. Various components are expressed as percent of the total. Bile acids, phospholipids, and cholesterol are the three major lipids in bile. The primary bile acids are cholic acid (CA) and chenodeoxycholic acid (CDCA). After 7α-dehydroxylation in the liver and by intestinal bacteria in the ileum and colon, they are converted to the secondary bile acids deoxycholic acid (DCA), ursodeoxycholic acid (UDCA), and lithocholic acid (LCA).

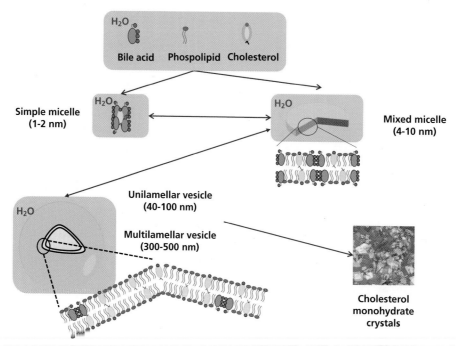

Figure 40.4 Bile is composed mainly of water (>95%). Following hepatic secretion across the canalicular membrane of hepatocytes, bile acids are found as monomers because of a low critical micellar concentration (CMC <3 mM). When CMC is higher than this cut-off value, bile acids can self-aggregate as simple micelles (~3 nm in diameter). This step increases the aqueous solubility of cholesterol. Also, simple micelles are capable of solubilizing and incorporating phospholipids to form mixed micelles (~4–8 nm in diameter). Compared to simple micelles, mixed micelles can solubilize at least three times the amount of cholesterol. With typical gallbladder lipid concentrations and compositions, simple and mixed bile acid micelles coexist in a ratio of 1 : 5. Phospholipids in an aqueous environment can self-aggregate to form stable bilayer vesicles, containing also a trace amount of bile acids, if any. A large amount of the cholesterol molecules is inserted into these bilayers of vesicles between the hydrophobic acyl chains of phospholipids. Unilamellar vesicles are larger spherical carriers in which even more cholesterol is solubilized. The ratio of unilamellar vesicles to micelles depends on the bile acid and phospholipid concentrations of bile, which is greatest in bile with low bile acid and high phospholipid concentrations. Furthermore, at low bile acid concentrations and high phospholipid concentrations, these biliary phospholipids often form larges multilamellar layers of vesicles. High concentrations of bile acids can dissolve these vesicles to form mixed micelles. When mechanisms of cholesterol solubilization fail, excess cholesterol starts precipitating as insoluble anhydrous/monohydrate crystals, the first step in cholesterol gallstone formation. Source: Adapted from Di Ciaula A, Wang DQ, Bonfrate L, Portincasa P. Current views on genetics and epigenetics of cholesterol gallstone disease. Cholesterol 2013;2013:298421.

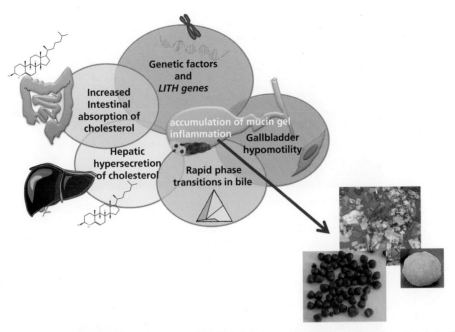

Figure 40.5 Five defects lead to cholesterol gallstone formation. *LITH* genes and their contributions to the formation of cholesterol gallstones are being investigated. Hepatic hypersecretion of biliary cholesterol leads to unphysiological supersaturation of gallbladder bile with cholesterol. At the small intestinal enterocyte level, absorption of cholesterol is enhanced. As a consequence, accelerated phase transitions of cholesterol in bile occurs, which is facilitated by prolonged gallbladder stasis due to impaired gallbladder motility, and immune-mediated gallbladder inflammation, as well as hypersecretion of mucins and accumulation of mucin gel in the gallbladder lumen. In bile, growth of solid plate-like cholesterol monohydrate crystals to form gallstones is a consequence of persistent hepatic hypersecretion of biliary cholesterol together with enhanced gallbladder mucin secretion and incomplete evacuation due to sluggish gallbladder contractility. Source: Adapted from Di Ciaula A, Wang DQ, Bonfrate L, Portincasa P. Current views on genetics and epigenetics of cholesterol gallstone disease. Cholesterol 2013;2013:298421.

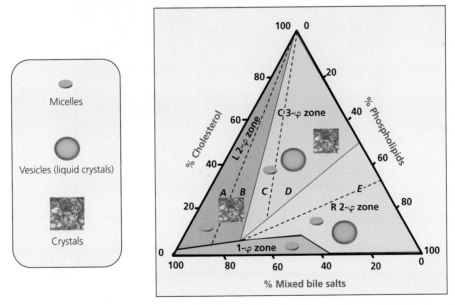

Figure 40.6 The ternary mixed bile salt-cholesterol-phospholipid phase diagram shows the different pathways of cholesterol crystallization in bile. Each zone contains different cholesterol carriers. The one-phase (φ) zone under the saturation curve contains only micelles, and represents the bile being unsaturated with cholesterol. Above, three other zones exist with cholesterol supersaturation: a right two-phase (R 2-φ) zone containing saturated micelles and vesicles; a central three-phase (C 3-φ) zone containing saturated micelles, vesicles, and solid cholesterol crystals; and a left two-phase (L 2-φ) zone containing saturated micelles and solid cholesterol crystals. Cholesterol precipitation is rapid in bile with high concentrations of bile acids. However, at increasing amounts of phospholipids, cholesterol may reside in vesicles with phospholipids, and cholesterol crystallization is slower or absent. Source: Adapted from Di Ciaula A, Wang DQ, Bonfrate L, Portincasa P. Current views on genetics and epigenetics of cholesterol gallstone disease. Cholesterol 2013;2013:298421.

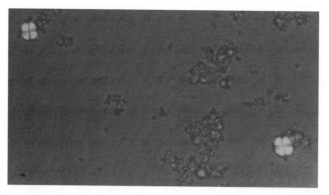

Figure 40.7 Photomicrographs of fused liquid crystals with Maltese-cross birefringence and focal conic textures observed in gallbladder bile of mice. Magnification ×1600 by polarizing light microscopy. Similar structures can be observed in human gallbladder bile. Source: Wang DQ, Paigen B, Carey MC. Phenotypic characterization of Lith genes that determine susceptibility to cholesterol cholelithiasis in inbred mice: physical-chemistry of gallbladder bile. J Lip Res 1997;38:1395.

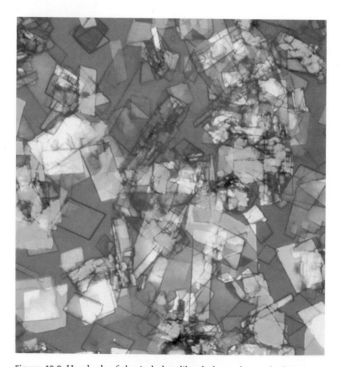

Figure 40.8 Hundreds of classical plate-like cholesterol monohydrate crystals are observed in bile by polarizing light microscopy. Typical plates have 79.2° and 100.8° angles. Source: Wang DQ, Paigen B, Carey MC. Phenotypic characterization of Lith genes that determine susceptibility to cholesterol cholelithiasis in inbred mice: physical-chemistry of gallbladder bile. J Lip Res 1997;38:1395 (Inset).

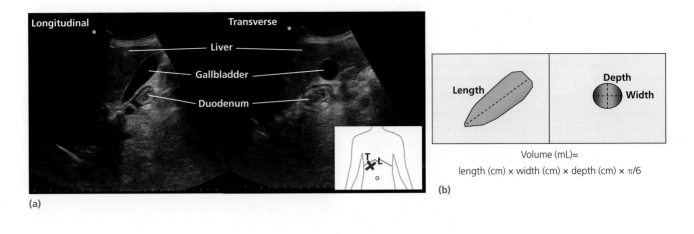

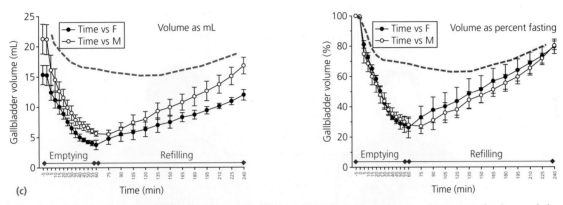

Figure 40.9 Functional ultrasonography study of gallbladder motility detects gallbladder stasis in response to a given stimulus (i.e., meal, drug, or cholecystokinin). **(a)** Scans of the gallbladder are taken in the fasting state and at several time points after a standard caloric test meal containing appropriate lipid content. The gallbladder appears pear-shaped in the longitudinal scan (inlet, L), and circular in the transversal scan (inlet, T). There is a typically anechoic content surrounded by a thin wall (<3 mm) in the fasting state. **(b)** Mathematical algorithm employed for the measurement of gallbladder volume, according to the "ellipsoid" formula. The estimated fasting volume in this case is 22 mL. **(c)** Time-dependent changes in gallbladder volumes reported as absolute values (mL) or as percent of fasting volume. Depending on the composition of the meal and duration of the exam, the emptying or the emptying/refilling phase are quantified. Graphs show gallbladder emptying in response to a mixed meal containing 19 g fat (F = females, M = males). The red dashed line indicates a slower and incomplete gallbladder emptying in a patient with cholesterol gallstones. Source: Courtesy of F Minerva, MD and P Portincasa, MD.

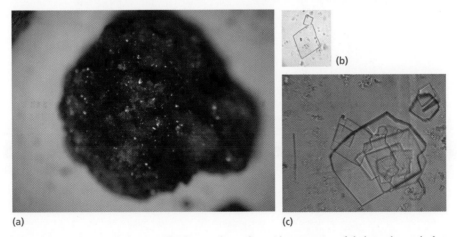

Figure 40.10 (a) Pure cholesterol stone (≈0.5 cm) showing a bright morular surface with aggregation of cholesterol monohydrate crystals. **(b)** A 10 μm rhomboidal cholesterol monohydrate crystal is observed by light microscopy in human gallbladder bile, with a smaller twin crystal growing laterally. **(c)** A large (10–60 μm) aggregate of overlapped cholesterol monohydrate crystals is shown beside a smaller aggregate (≈10 μm). Some plates show a typical notched corner. On the left, a needle-like crystal (presumably anhydrous cholesterol) is shown (≈20 μm in length).

Diagnosis

Gallstones are discovered incidentally during a different diagnostic work-up in asymptomatic patients or when the typical biliary colicky pain (Figure 40.11) or complications emerge (Box 40.1). Besides the clinical presentation, imaging studies include abdominal ultrasonography (Figures 40.12 and 40.13), computed tomography (CT) (Figures 40.14 and 40.15), magnetic resonance cholangiopancreatography (MRCP) (Figures 40.16 and 40.17), and cholescintigraphy. Oral cholecystography is no longer used, while the plain x-ray film of the right hypochondrium might detect calcified gallstones (Figure 40.18). Endoscopic retrograde cholangiopancreatography (ERCP) is usually performed when biliary drainage is required due to choledocholithiasis (Figure 40.19).

Box 40.1 Complications of gallstones.

Acute cholecystitis
Chronic cholecystitis
Gallbladder empyema
Mucocele of the gallbladder
Gangrenous – emphysematous cholecystitis
Gallbladder perforation – cholecystenteric fistulae – gallstone ileus
Gallbladder cancer
Choledocholithiasis – cholestatic jaundice
Acute cholangitis
Mirizzi syndrome
Acute biliary pancreatitis
Porcelain gallbladder
Gallbladder carcinoma

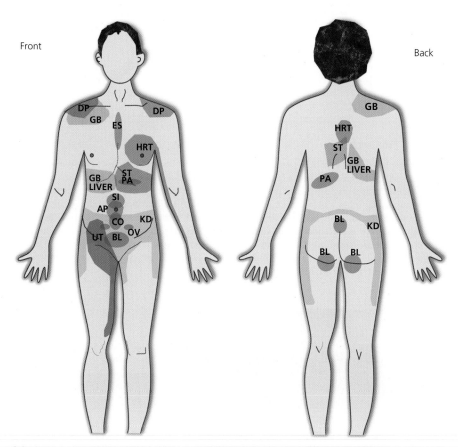

Figure 40.11 Differential diagnosis between hepatobiliary pain (in green) and other areas of referred abdominal pain. AP, appendix; BL, bladder; CO, colon; DP, diaphragm; ES, esophagus; GB, gallbladder; HRT, heart; KD, kidney; OV, ovary; PA, pancreas; SI, small intestine; ST, stomach; UT, (right) ureter.

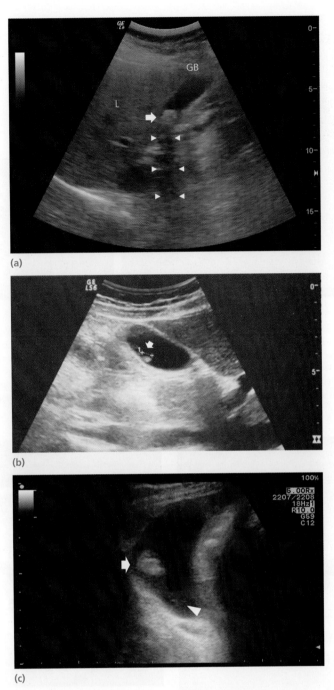

(a)

(b)

(c)

Figure 40.12 (a) Ultrasonographic appearance of gallstones. A 1-cm, mobile echogenic spot is seen (arrow) with a posterior acoustic shadowing (arrowheads). The 1-cm scale is shown on the right. L, liver; GB, gallbladder. **(b)** Ultrasonographic appearance of gallbladder polyp. Within the gallbladder, taken on a longitudinal transabdominal scan, a single 6.2-mm hyperechogenic spot is seen (arrow). Echogenicity does not change with position and there is no posterior acoustic shadow (differential diagnosis with gallstones). **(c)** A 20-mm polyp (arrow) is detected in the gallbladder which also contains sludge in the fundus (arrowhead). Source: (a) Courtesy of P Portincasa, MD; (b) courtesy of M Lorusso, MD; (c) courtesy of VO Palmieri, MD.

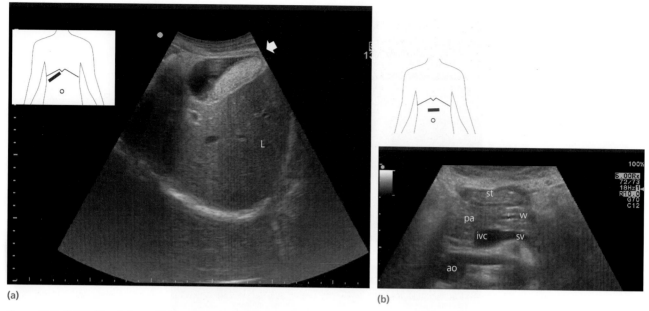

(a)

(b)

Figure 40.13 Gallbladder sludge and biliary pancreatitis. **(a)** Ultrasonographic appearance of gallbladder sludge. Within the gallbladder taken on a longitudinal transabdominal scan, finely echogenic, dense, gravity dependent, slowly mobile, biliary sludge is seen occupying 60% of the lumen (thick arrow). The thickness of the gallbladder wall is not increased. **(b)** On a transverse abdominal scan at the epigastric region, a dilated (3 mm) pancreatic duct of Wirsung (normally not detected on ultrasound) is seen. The duct is surrounded by a nonhomogeneous pancreas, suggesting chronic recurrent pancreatitis due to the effect of the sludge with consequent stasis. ao, aorta; ivc, inferior vena cava; L, liver; pa, pancreas; st, stomach; sv, splenic vein; w, duct of Wirsung. The 1-cm scale is shown on the vertical and horizontal axes (a) and on the vertical axis (b). Source: Courtesy of F Minerva, MD.

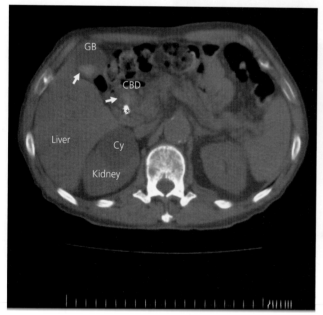

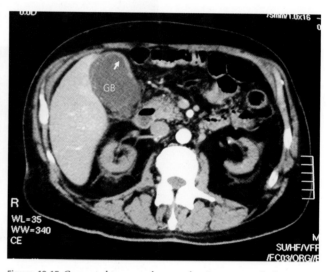

Figure 40.15 Computed tomography scan showing acute acalculous cholecystitis in an HIV-positive patient. The gallbladder (GB) is enlarged, and shows a thickened wall (arrow). No gallstones are visible. Source: Courtesy of M Rabon, MD.

Figure 40.14 Computed tomography scan showing multiple radiopaque stones in the gallbladder (GB) and in the common bile duct (CBD) (arrows). The asterisk indicates a radiopaque endoprosthesis positioned within the enlarged CBD and close to the stones. A large cyst (Cy) is incidentally found in the right kidney. Source: Courtesy of VO Palmieri, MD and G Palasciano, MD.

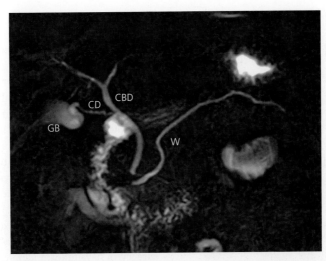

Figure 40.16 Normal magnetic resonance cholangiopancreatography (MRCP). CD, cystic duct; CBD, common bile duct; GB, gallbladder; W, duct of Wirsung. Source: Courtesy of A Scardapane, MD.

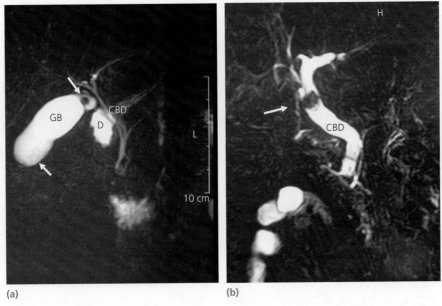

(a)   (b)

Figure 40.17 Magnetic resonance cholangiopancreatography (MRCP) in patients with recurrent episodes of biliary colic. (a) Arrows indicate one stone within the gallbladder infundibulum and small multiple stones in the fundus. (b) The arrow indicates one stone within the proximal common bile duct. CBD, common bile duct; D, duodenum; GB, gallbladder. Source: Courtesy of P Portincasa, MD.

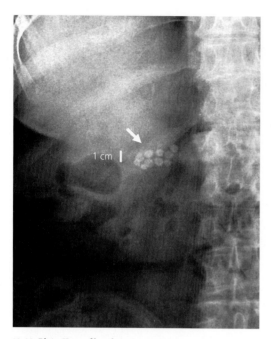

Figure 40.18 Plain X-ray film showing 10 radiopaque oval images in the right hypochondrium due to calcified gallstones (arrow); size 0.5–0.8 cm. Source: Courtesy of P Portincasa, MD.

Management

Distinct guidelines have been developed for therapeutic approaches to gallstones (Figure 40.20). Gallstones remain asymptomatic in the vast majority of patients and in this setting expectant management is the best choice. Prophylactic chole-cystectomy is only warranted in specific conditions (Table 40.1). In symptomatic patients, first-line therapy of the uncomplicated biliary colic requires medical attention and analgesia. Elective (laparoscopic, small-incision, or open) cholecystectomy is the gold standard treatment of "symptomatic and uncomplicated" gallstones. The procedure is safe, has reduced costs, and is defin-itive in nature (Figure 40.21). Oral litholysis with (tauro-) ursodeoxycholic acid is reserved for the few patients who cannot undergo surgery because of the overall operative risk, or refuse surgery, or have mild/moderate symptoms and stones amenable to dissolution. However, when complications develop, specific approaches are required (Figures 40.22–40.30).

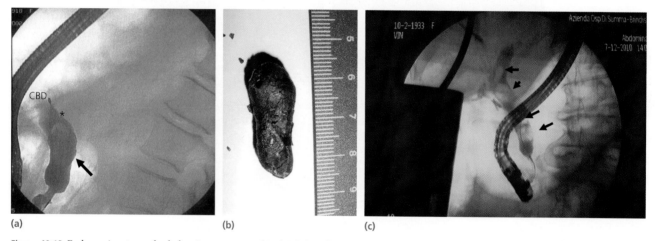

(a)   (b)   (c)

Figure 40.19 Endoscopic retrograde cholangiopancreatographic (ERCP) study in a 78-year-old woman who underwent cholecystectomy 8 years earlier. The patient developed the typical Charcot's triad (pain in the right hypochondrium, fever, and obstructive jaundice). **(a)** A large oval stone (arrow) is shown in a dilated common bile duct (CBD). The wire basket used for stone extraction is visible (asterisk). **(b)** A large (30 × 10 × 10 mm) brown pigment stone was extracted. **(c)** A dilated common bile duct containing several stacked stones (arrows). Source: (a, b) Courtesy of O Caputi-Jambrenghi, MD); (c) courtesy of B Santoro, MD.

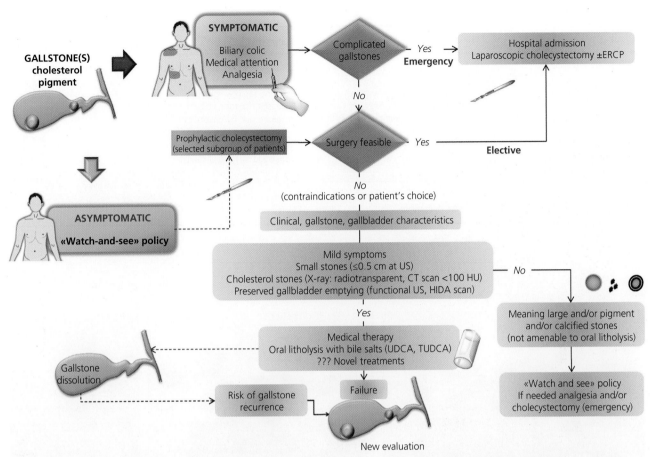

Figure 40.20 Current management of gallstones. The initial decision is independent of gallstone composition (cholesterol-enriched stones or pigment stones) and size, but rather depends on presence/absence of typical biliary symptoms or complications. In asymptomatic patients and according to current guidelines, the best choice is the expectant management (watch-and-see policy). In symptomatic gallstone patients with or without complications, following immediate medical attention and treatment of pain, cholecystectomy is the best choice. When surgery is not possible (i.e., surgical risk, patient's choice, or mild symptoms), a careful evaluation of stone type, size, and gallbladder function is required to plan the medical treatment only in a subgroup of patients with uncalcified small cholesterol-enriched stones in a functioning gallbladder with a patent cystic duct. The overall recurrence risk should be considered after successful gallstone dissolution. Large, or pigment, or calcified (radiopaque) gallstones are not amenable to oral litholysis. CT, computed tomography; ERCP, endoscopic retrograde cholangiopancreatography; HIDA, ^{99m}Tc-N-(2,6-dimethylacetanilide)-iminodiacetic acid; HU, Hounsfield unit (an arbitrary unit of x-ray attenuation used for CT scans). Each voxel is assigned a value on a scale in which air has a value of -1000; water $= 0$; compact bone $= +1000$); TUDCA, tauroursodeoxycholic acid; UDCA, ursodeoxycholic acid; US, abdominal ultrasonography.

Table 40.1 Indications for "prophylactic" cholecystectomy.

Group	Comment
Children with gallstones	Because of exposition to the long-term physical presence of stones
Morbid obese patients prior to bariatric surgery	High risk to form cholesterol gallstones and to become symptomatic during rapid weight loss
Controversial in gallstone-free patients, asymptomatic gallstone patients	
Patients with large gallstones (i.e., greater than 3 cm)	Increased risk for gallbladder cancer
A "porcelain" gallbladder or gallbladder polyps rapidly growing or larger than 1 cm	Increased risk for gallbladder cancer
Asymptomatic gallstones (even small) and gallbladder polyps (even <1 cm)	High risk of gallbladder cancer
Native Americans with gallstones	Increased risk for gallbladder cancer
Gallstone patients with sickle cell anemia	Formation of calcium bilirubinate gallstones due to chronic hemolysis
	Patients may become symptomatic with recurrent episodes of abdominal pain
Coexistence of small gallstones and gallbladder dysmotility	Increased risk of pancreatitis

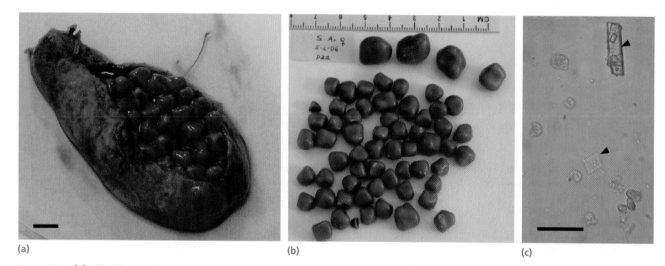

(a)   (b)   (c)

Figure 40.21 **(a)** A freshly excised human gallbladder is shown after cholecystectomy. Hundreds of pure cholesterol stones are still moistened with green bile. Bar = 1 cm. **(b)** After cleansing, gallstones appear multifaceted with smooth surface and angles. **(c)** At light microscopy, cholesterol monohydrate crystals are visible in bile (arrowheads). Bar = 50 μm. Source: Courtesy of P Portincasa, MD.

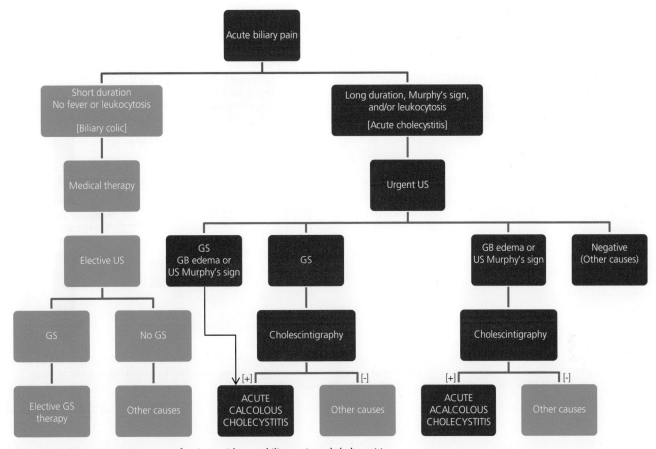

Figure 40.22 Diagnostic management of patients with acute biliary pain and cholecystitis.
After onset of acute biliary pain (biliary colic), a careful evaluation with clinical, laboratory, and imaging tests is necessary for differential diagnosis between the simple biliary colic (left part of the algorithm) and acute cholecystitis (right part of the algorithm). In the latter, the presence of leukocytosis and longer pain duration are justified by the ongoing gallbladder inflammation. Associated symptoms (e.g., fever, nausea, and vomit) are present. Acute cholecystitis, a condition at high risk of complications, requires urgent treatment. GB, gallbladder; GS, gallstones; US, abdominal ultrasound; [−], absent; [+], present. Source: Adapted from Zakko and Afdhal 2013. Pathogenesis, clinical features, and diagnosis of acute cholecystitis. In: UpToDate, Basow DS (ed). UpToDate, Waltham, MA 2013. Reproduced with permission of Wolters Kluwer Health. Copyright © 2013 UpToDate, Inc. For more information visit www.uptodate.com.

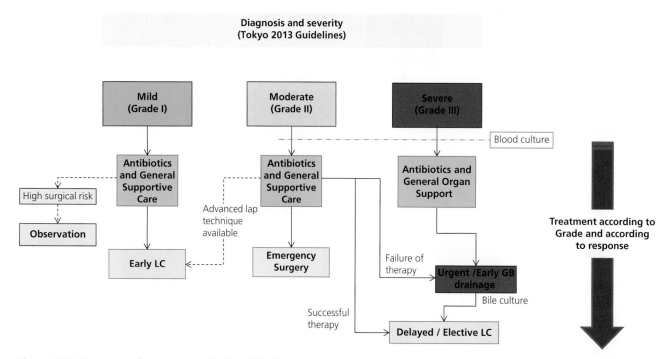

Figure 40.23 Management of acute cholecystitis. GB, gallbladder; Lap, laparoscopic; LC, laparoscopic cholecystectomy. Source: Adapted from Miura F, Takada T, Strasberg SM, et al. TG13 Flowchart for the diagnosis and treatment of acute cholangitis and cholecystitis. J Hepatobiliary Pancreat Surg 2013;20:47. Reproduced with permission of the Journal of Hepato-Biliary-Pancreatic Sciences.

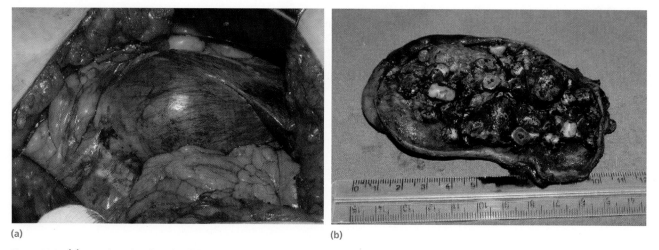

(a)   (b)

Figure 40.24 **(a)** An enlarged, inflamed gallbladder due to acute cholecystitis with empyema is shown at laparotomy. **(b)** After cholecystectomy, several cholesterol gallstones are found in the gallbladder lumen. Due to the inflammatory process, the mucosa is disrupted and the wall is thickened. Source: Courtesy of A. Margari, MD.

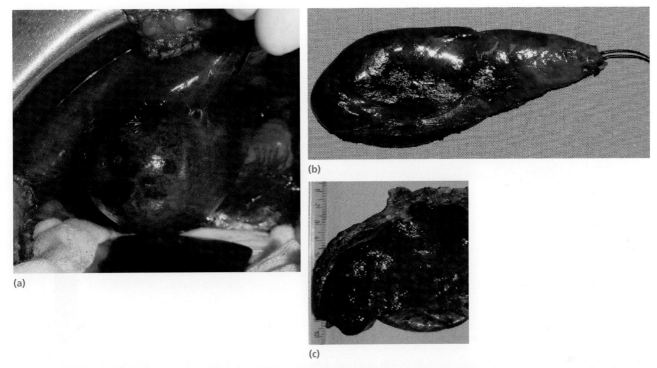

(a)

(b)

(c)

Figure 40.25 Gangrenous cholecystitis at laparotomic cholecystectomy. **(a)** Enlarged, inflamed gallbladder with necrotic areas at the serosal surface. **(b)** Excised gallbladder shows several necrotic areas at the serosal surface. **(c)** The lumen appears inflamed with necrotic areas and thickened wall. Source: Courtesy of A Margari, MD.

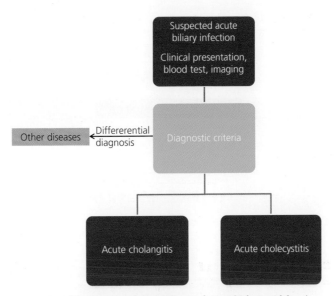

Figure 40.26 Management of acute biliary infection (Tokyo guidelines). Source: Adapted from Miura F, Takada T, Strasberg SM, et al. TG13 Flowchart for the diagnosis and treatment of acute cholangitis and cholecystitis. J Hepatobiliary Pancreat Surg 2013;20:47. Reproduced with permission of the Journal of Hepato-Biliary-Pancreatic Sciences.

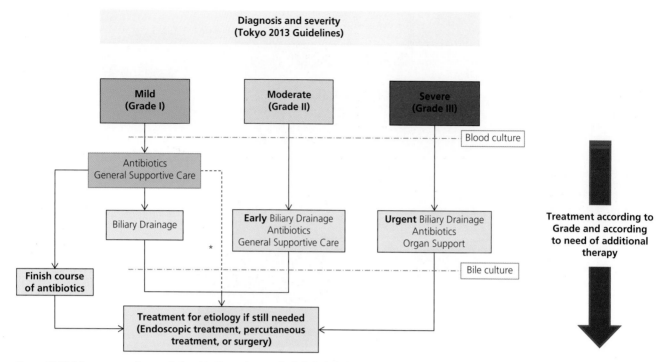

Figure 40.27 Management of acute cholangitis. For patients with choledocholithiasis, treatment for etiology might be performed simultaneously, if possible, with biliary drainage. * The principle of treatment for acute cholangitis consists of antimicrobial administration and biliary drainage including treatment for etiology. Source: Adapted from Miura F, Takada T, Strasberg SM, et al. TG13 Flowchart for the diagnosis and treatment of acute cholangitis and cholecystitis. J Hepatobiliary Pancreat Surg 2013;20:47. Reproduced with permission of the Journal of Hepato-Biliary-Pancreatic Sciences.

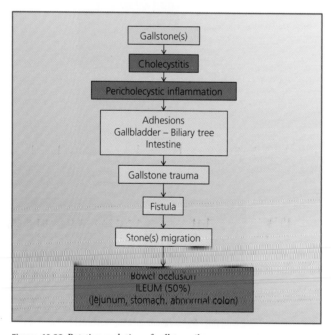

Figure 40.28 Putative evolution of gallstone ileus.

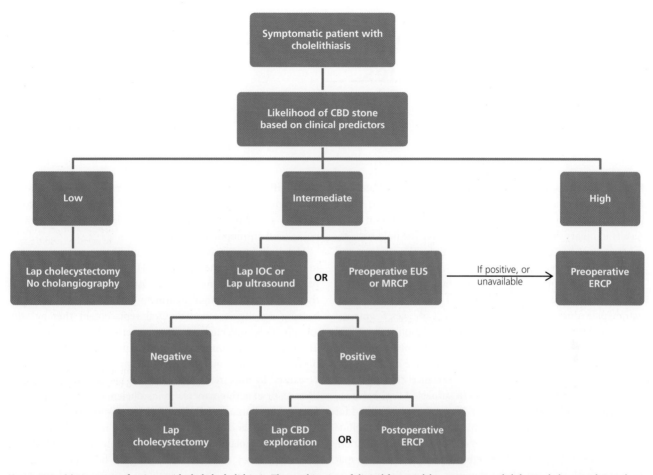

Figure 40.29 Management of patients with choledocholithiasis. The combination of clinical features, laboratory tests, and abdominal ultrasound contribute to define the predictors into very strong (bile duct stone, cholangitis, and hyperbilirubinemia), strong (dilated bile duct and hyperbilirubinemia), and moderate (other abnormal liver biochemical tests, age >55 years, and gallstone pancreatitis). By grouping the predictors, patients are stratified into three different levels of risk of having choledocholithiasis (low, intermediate, and high). This status dictates the subsequent therapeutic approach. Laparoscopic cholecystectomy with intraoperative cholangiography ± postoperative ERCP is the most cost-effective approach. CBD, common bile duct; ERCP: endoscopic retrograde cholangiopancreatography; EUS: endoscopic ultrasound; IOC: intraoperative cholangiogram; Lap, laparoscopic; MRCP: magnetic resonance cholangiopancreatography. Source: American Society for Gastrointestinal Endoscopy (ASGE) Standards of Practice Committee. The role of endoscopy in the evaluation of suspected choledocholithiasis. Gastrointest Endosc 2010;71:1. Reproduced with permission of Elsevier.

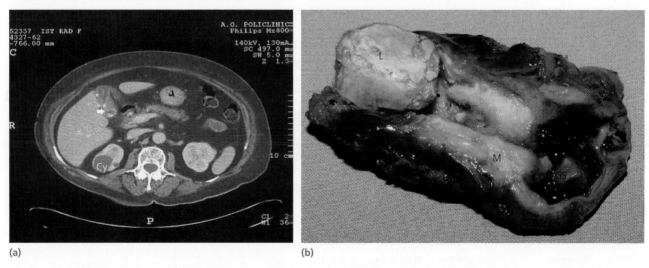

(a)

(b)

Figure 40.30 Gallbladder carcinoma. (a) Computed tomography scan shows a gallbladder with thickened wall (*), dense bile (**), and a calcified gallstone in the fundus (arrow). A cyst (Cy) is incidentally found in the right kidney. (b) Macroscopic examination of the opened gallbladder (9 × 3 × 2.5 cm in size) shows a thickened wall due to chronic cholecystitis. At the level of the corpus, a hard grey mass (2.5 cm in size) is visible (M). A large (1 cm) whitish node is evident in the neck (L). A 0.5-cm stone is visible in the fundus (GS). Histological examination of the mass disclosed a gallbladder adenocarcinoma with intravascular invasion, and calcium deposition. The tumor extends transmurally to the serosa and to the hepatic side. The lymph node showed the presence of metastasis. Classification TNM: T3 N1 Mx. Source: Courtesy of A Margari, MD.

CHAPTER 41

Primary sclerosing cholangitis and other cholangiopathies

Russell H. Wiesner and Kymberly D.S. Watt
Mayo Clinic, Rochester, MN, USA

Primary sclerosing cholangitis (PSC) is a chronic cholestatic liver disease characterized by inflammation and fibrosis of the intra- and extrahepatic bile ducts. Disease progression often results in biliary cirrhosis and hepatic failure. The only successful treatment has been liver transplantation. The etiology and etiopathogenesis remain poorly understood.

The diagnosis of PSC is made by cholangiography (Figure 41.1). Intrahepatic duct involvement is nearly universal with extrahepatic duct sparing occurring in 20% of cases. Segmental bile duct fibrosis with subsequent saccular dilation with normal intervening areas results in the characteristic beaded pattern frequently noted on the cholangiogram. The use of abdominal computed tomography or magnetic resonance cholangiopancreatography for accurate detection of suspected PSC has been increasingly useful (Figure 41.2a,b). Liver biopsy is required for staging disease severity of PSC; histological findings include periductal fibrosis with inflammation, bile duct proliferation, and ductopenia (Figure 41.3a,b). Fibroobliterative cholangiopathy (Figure 41.4) is considered the most diagnostic finding on liver biopsy but is present in only about 10% of biopsies obtained in PSC patients. Explant findings often reveal liver fibrotic reactions surrounding the large bile ducts (Figure 41.5).

The recognition of elevated serum hepatic biochemistries consistent with cholestasis in a male patient with concurrent inflammatory bowel disease (IBD) is strongly suggestive of PSC. IBD, most commonly chronic ulcerative colitis, occurs in 70%–80% of patients with PSC. In those PSC patients who undergo proctocolectomy, the formation of peristomal varices with severe bleeding can be a major complication and a cause of significant morbidity (Figure 41.6). In such cases a surgical portocaval shunt or a transjugular intrahepatic portal shunt (TIPS) procedure has been effective. In addition, pouchitis following proctocolectomy seems to be more frequent and more severe in PSC patients than in patients with ulcerative colitis alone (Figure 41.7).

The differential diagnosis of PSC includes biliary obstruction from choledocholithiasis, stricture, or malignancy, primary biliary cirrhosis, autoimmune pancreatitis, recurrent pyogenic cholangitis, fungal cholangitis, acquired immunodeficiency syndrome cholangiopathy, choledochal cysts, cystic fibrosis, primary portal hypertension, intrahepatic hepatocellular carcinoma, and eosinophilic cholangitis.

Metabolic bone disease, most commonly osteoporosis, is seen in relation to PSC patients (Figure 41.8). Approximately 50% of patients have osteopenia, whereas osteoporosis develops in less than 10% of cases. Initial treatment with calcium and weight-bearing activity is essential. Oral replacement therapy with vitamin D is indicated if measured serum levels are reduced. The use of bisphosphonates has been proven to be effective in preventing bone mineral loss. When present, steatorrhea may be caused by impaired small intestinal bile acid delivery, celiac disease, or exocrine pancreatic insufficiency. Malabsorption of fat-soluble vitamins A, D, E, and K is common in patients with advanced PSC and usually responds to oral replacement therapy.

Bacterial cholangitis is most commonly associated with a previous history of biliary tract surgery, bile duct calculi, or dominant stricture. Therapy includes empiric broad-spectrum intravenous antibiotics and biliary decompression when clinically indicated. Dominant strictures occur in 15%–20% of PSC patients (Figure 41.9a,b). Clinical manifestations include progressive jaundice, symptoms of bacterial cholangitis, and dark urine. Diagnosis and therapy include endoscopic or radiological approaches to dilate the dominant stricture and often provide significant and clinical improvement. Of note, there appears to be an increased incidence of gallbladder cancer associated with gallstones in patients with PSC.

The most serious complication of PSC is the development of cholangiocarcinoma. Primary anatomic sites of involvement include the hilum (75% of cases), intrahepatic ducts (16%), and the gallbladder (8%). Risk factors include advanced age, long duration of IBD, advanced hepatic disease, cigarette smoking, colorectal neoplasia, or carcinoma. Confirming the diagnosis of cholangiocarcinoma in PSC is challenging. The distinction between benign and malignant biliary strictures with cross-sectional imaging and cholangiography can be helpful in making the diagnosis (Figure 41.10a,b). Serum tumor

Yamada's Atlas of Gastroenterology, Fifth Edition. Edited by Daniel K. Podolsky, Michael Camilleri, J. Gregory Fitz, Anthony N. Kalloo, Fergus Shanahan, and Timothy C. Wang.
© 2016 John Wiley & Sons, Ltd. Published 2016 by John Wiley & Sons, Ltd.
Companion website: www.yamadagastro.com/atlas

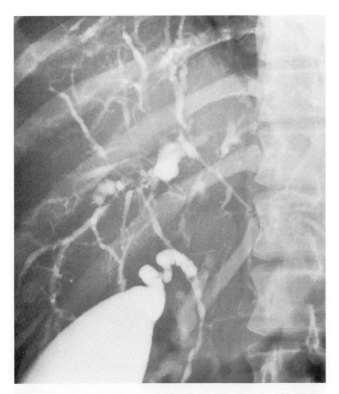

Figure 41.1 Cholangiogram showing beading and irregularity of both the intra- and extrahepatic biliary tract, typical of primary sclerosing cholangitis.

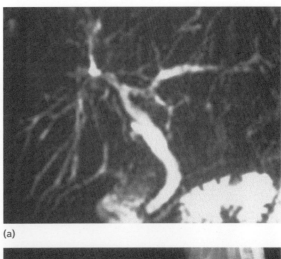

(a)

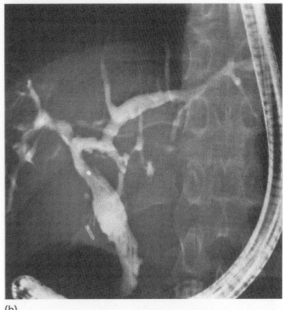

(b)

Figure 41.2 (a) Typical changes of primary sclerosing cholangitis on magnetic resonance cholangiography: diffuse changes throughout the intra- and extrahepatic bile ducts are seen without evidence of a dominant stricture or filling defect. **(b)** Images of primary sclerosing cholangitis seen on the corresponding endoscopic retrograde cholangiogram. As is seen, magnetic resonance cholangiography gives a better visualization of the peripheral branches of the biliary tree, not seen on this particular endoscopic retrograde cholangiogram. Source: Angulo P, Pearce DH, Johnson CD, et al. Magnetic resonance cholangiography in patients with biliary disease: its role in primary sclerosing cholangitis. J Hepatol 2000;33:520. Reproduced with permission of Elsevier.

markers, including carbohydrate antigen 19-9 and carcinoembryonic antigen, remain insensitive for detecting early stage disease. Rarely, bile duct dysplasia or carcinoma can be diagnosed on liver biopsy (Figure 41.11). At least one report has suggested that positron emission tomography (PET) scanning can be helpful in diagnosing cholangiocarcinoma in the presence of PSC (Figure 41.12). The use of biliary cytology, digital image analysis, and fluorescence in situ hybridization (FISH) studies can also be useful in diagnosing cholangiocarcinoma in patients with PSC (Figures 41.13 and 41.14a,b). Some studies also suggest that the use of cholangioscopy can be helpful in distinguishing between malignant and benign dominant bile duct strictures in patients with PSC (Figure 41.15a,b).

Finally, the only known successful therapy for PSC is liver transplantation; PSC is the fourth most common indication for liver transplantation in the United States. Survival rates ranging between 90% and 95% at 1 year and 83% and 88% at 5 years have been reported. Long-term graft survival is affected by a higher incidence of rejection in hepatic artery thrombosis. An increasing body of evidence suggests that PSC can recur after liver transplantation in up to 30% of cases (Figure 41.16). To date, there is no recognized effective medical therapy that appears to alter disease progression. Multiple therapies studied include antifibrotic agents, anticupric agents, and immunosuppressive agents, all of which have been proven unsuccessful in

preventing disease progression. Three randomized, placebo-controlled trials with ursodeoxycholic acid (UDCA) have also failed to show significant improvements in histology and survival. Of note, secondary causes of sclerosing cholangitis often reveal radiological and histological findings that are similar to those of PSC (Figure 41.17).

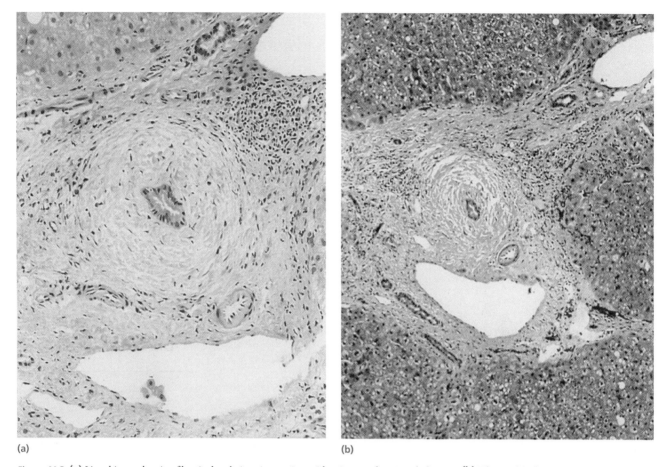

(a)

(b)

Figure 41.3 **(a)** Liver biopsy showing fibrotic duct lesions in a patient with primary sclerosing cholangitis. **(b)** Fibrotic duct lesion in a patient with primary sclerosing cholangitis. Tissue sample was stained with Mason trichrome.

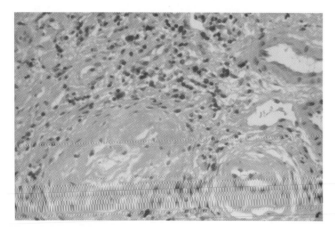

Figure 41.4 Liver biopsy showing obliterative duct lesion with only the ghost of a previous bile duct remaining.

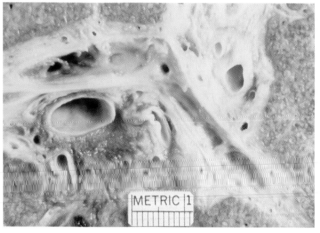

Figure 41.5 Explant liver with intense fibrosis surrounding the biliary tract, which is typical of primary sclerosing cholangitis.

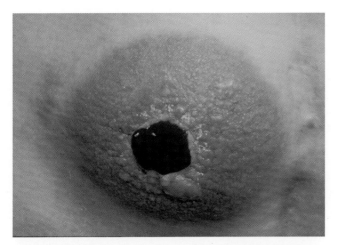

Figure 41.6 Abdominal photograph of a severe abdominal peristomal varix in a patient with primary sclerosing cholangitis with a history of chronic ulcerative colitis who underwent total proctocolectomy and ileostomy.

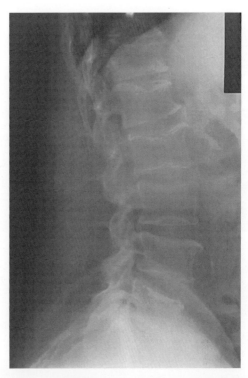

Figure 41.8 Spine radiograph of a patient with severe osteoporosis, a finding seen in 25% of patients with primary sclerosing cholangitis who undergo liver transplantation. Because of available therapies at this time, early diagnosis is important.

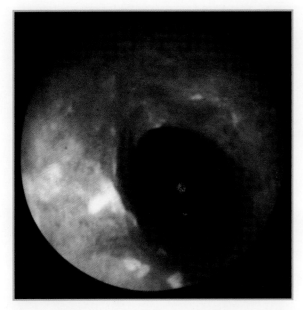

Figure 41.7 Pouchitis in a patient who has undergone proctocolectomy and ileorectal pouch anastomosis. This is seen more frequently and is more severe in patients with primary sclerosing cholangitis than in patients with ulcerative colitis alone.

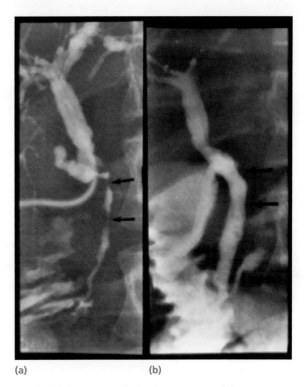

(a)   (b)

Figure 41.9 Cholangiogram of a dominant stricture of the common hepatic bile duct before **(a)** and after **(b)** dilation.

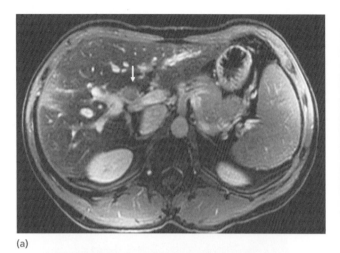

(a)

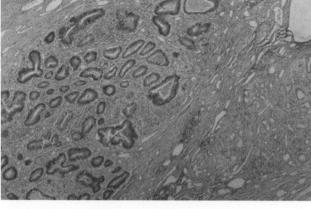

Figure 41.11 Liver biopsy showing severe dysplasia and bile duct carcinoma in a patient with primary sclerosing cholangitis.

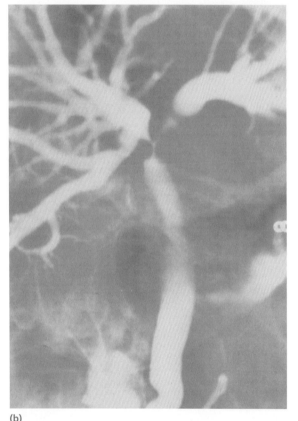

(b)

Figure 41.10 **(a)** Magnetic resonance cholangiogram showing a dominant stricture of the right hepatic duct with a tumor mass (arrow) in a patient with primary sclerosing cholangitis. (b) Cholangiogram of a hilar lesion typical of cholangiocarcinoma in a patient with long-standing chronic ulcerative colitis.

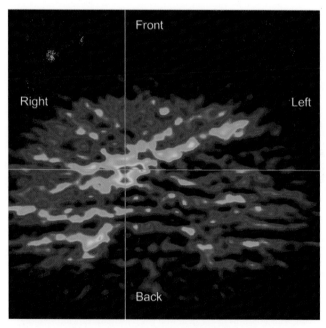

Figure 41.12 A positron emission tomography study demonstrating a perihilar irregularity in a patient with primary sclerosing cholangitis, which represented an infiltrating cholangiocarcinoma. Source: Prytz H, Keiding S, Bjornsson E, et al. Dynamic FDG-PET is useful for detection of cholangiocarcinoma in patients with PSC listed for liver transplantation. Hepatology 2006;44:1572. Reproduced with permission of John Wiley & Sons.

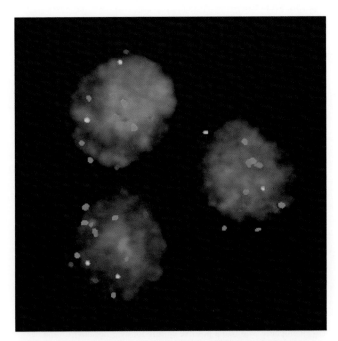

Figure 41.13 Fluorescence in situ hybridization (FISH) study showing cysts positive for polysomy with two or more copies for two or more of the four probes utilized. This is typical of malignant cells. Source: Moreno-Luna LE, Gores GJ. Advances in the diagnosis of cholangiocarcinoma in patients with primary sclerosing cholangitis. Liver Transpl 2006;17:515. Reproduced with permission of John Wiley & Sons.

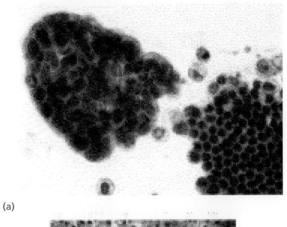

(a)

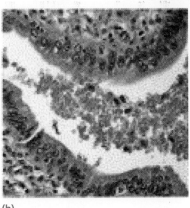

(b)

Figure 41.14 (a) Cytological specimen from a patient with primary sclerosing cholangitis showing low-grade dysplasia. (b) Epithelium from the resected main bile duct from the same patient, again showing low-grade dysplasia.

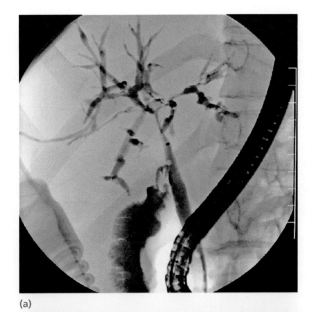

(a)

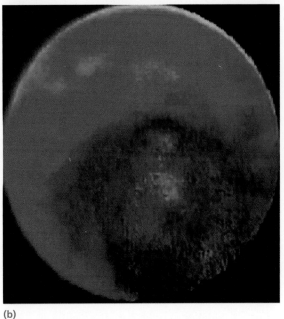

(b)

Figure 41.15 (a) Cholangiogram in a patient with cholangiocarcinoma showing bilateral intrahepatic ductal dilation and irregularity along with a high-grade irregular stricture of the proximal extrahepatic bile duct. Source: Tischendorf J, Krüger M, Trautwein C, et al. Cholangioscopic characterisation of dominant bile duct stenoses in patients with primary sclerosing cholangitis. Endoscopy 2006;38:665. Reproduced with permission of Thieme Publishing Group. (b) Cholangioscopy showing an intraductal polypoid mass in the stenotic segment of the cholangiogram noted above.

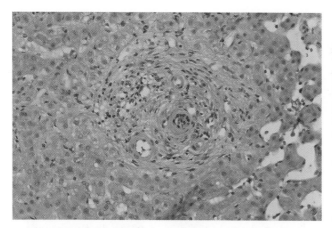

Figure 41.16 Liver biopsy that shows early recurrence of primary sclerosing cholangitis in a patient who underwent liver transplantation for primary sclerosing cholangitis 5 years previously. An early fibrotic obliterative duct lesion is present.

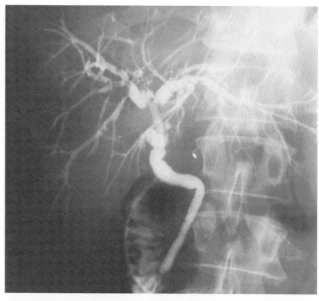

Figure 41.17 Patient with acquired immune deficiency syndrome cholangiopathy who had a positive culture for cytomegalovirus and *Cryptosporidium*: the findings are indistinguishable from cholangiographic findings in primary sclerosing cholangitis.

CHAPTER 42

Cystic diseases of the liver and biliary tract

James L. Buxbaum[1] and Shelly C. Lu[2]

[1] Los Angeles County Medical Center and University of Southern California, Los Angeles, CA, USA
[2] Cedars-Sinai Medical Center, Los Angeles, CA, USA

Biliary cysts are cystic dilatations that occur anywhere in the biliary system. They mainly afflict children and young adults. Most biliary cysts are congenital. Todani et al. proposed the most widely used classification of biliary cysts. Most common are type I choledochal cysts. Type II are diverticulum cysts found anywhere in the extrahepatic ducts, type III are choledochocele cysts, type IV are multiple cysts in the intrahepatic and extrahepatic ducts, and type V are intrahepatic bile duct cyst (single or multiple).

Clinical presentation of biliary cysts depends on the patient's age. In infancy, jaundice vomiting, failure to thrive, and hepatomegaly are often found. The classic clinical triad (pain, jaundice, and a palpable abdominal mass) has been reported in 11%–63% of large series. In patients older than 2 years of age, the most common presentation is chronic and intermittent pain. Recurrent pancreatitis, cholangitis, and ductal stones are frequently encountered. Older patients may present with carcinoma of the biliary tract, the most dire complication of biliary cysts (Figure 42.1).

Diagnosis of biliary cysts requires a high index of suspicion. Percutaneous transhepatic cholangiography (PTC) and endoscopic retrograde cholangiopancreatography (ERCP) provide the most detailed exams (Figures 42.2, 42.3a, 42.4, 42.5a, and 42.6). In infants, ultrasonography and hepatobiliary scintigraphy provide a sound basis for diagnosis (Figures 42.3b and 42.7). Ultrasonography is an excellent screening tool but provides little anatomical or functional information (Figure 42.7). Hepatobiliary scintigraphy provides information about excretory patterns (Figure 42.3b) and is excellent for postoperative patient follow-up. Computed tomography is superior to ultrasonography in older patients but does not always demonstrate the relationship of the cyst to the biliary tree. Magnetic resonance cholangiopancreatography (MRCP) is an attractive alternative to ERCP or PTC and shows the relationship of the cyst to the surrounding ductal system (Figure 42.8).

Presence of an anomalous pancreaticobiliary ductal union (Figure 42.4), in which the common bile duct enters the pancreatic duct at a right angle abnormally far from the ampulla of Vater, occurs commonly in association with choledochal cysts. This abnormal anatomy impairs normal sphincteric function at the pancreaticobiliary junction, which may lead to reflux of pancreatic juice into the bile duct causing injury and cystic malformation.

Cholangiography is the best means of diagnosis (Figure 42.5a). Typically the distal common bile duct appears "clubbed". Emptying of contrast material is often delayed. Choledochoceles are easily distinguished from duodenal diverticuli and duodenal duplication cysts by filling during cholangiography but not during upper gastrointestinal contrast studies (Figure 42.5b). Sarris and Tsang proposed a further anatomic classification of choledochoceles (Figure 42.9), which is useful for guiding therapy. Choledochoceles may be amenable to endoscopic sphincterotomy. The treatment of choice for the remainder of choledochal cysts is operative excision. For intrahepatic cyst (i.e., type IVA and V) treatment depends on the degree of involvement. When segmental cystic disease is confined to one lobe (more often the left lobe), then lobectomy is usually curative. Ultimately, if attacks of cholangitis are frequent and quality of life poor, hepatic transplantation may be the best therapeutic option. Histology of the cyst wall typically demonstrates extensive fibrous tissue with a lack of muscle and biliary epithelium (Figure 42.10).

Type V is Caroli disease (Figure 42.6). There is a simple type and a type associated with congenital hepatic fibrosis, known as Caroli syndrome. In addition to intrahepatic cystic dilatation, congenital hepatic fibrosis, cirrhosis, portal hypertension, and esophageal varices are frequently seen. It is often associated with the renal abnormalities of autosomal recessive and is also known as polycystic kidney disease. Congenital hepatic fibrosis refers to a unique congenital liver histology characterized by bland

Yamada's Atlas of Gastroenterology, Fifth Edition. Edited by Daniel K. Podolsky, Michael Camilleri, J. Gregory Fitz, Anthony N. Kalloo, Fergus Shanahan, and Timothy C. Wang.
© 2016 John Wiley & Sons, Ltd. Published 2016 by John Wiley & Sons, Ltd.
Companion website: www.yamadagastro.com/atlas

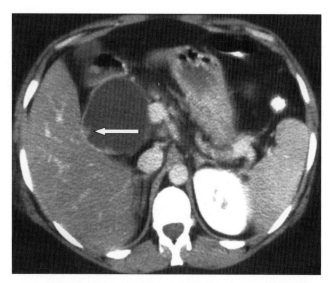

Figure 42.1 Choledochal cyst with cholangiocarcinoma. Cystic dilatation of the common bile duct with irregularities in the wall (arrow) consistent with cholangiocarcinoma. Source: Courtesy of Dr. Randall Radin, Department of Radiology, LAC/USC Medical Center.

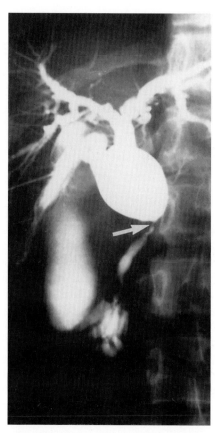

Figure 42.2 Choledochal cyst – type IA. Mild stenosis (arrow) of the common bile duct immediately distal to the cyst contributes to the slight intrahepatic ductal distension.

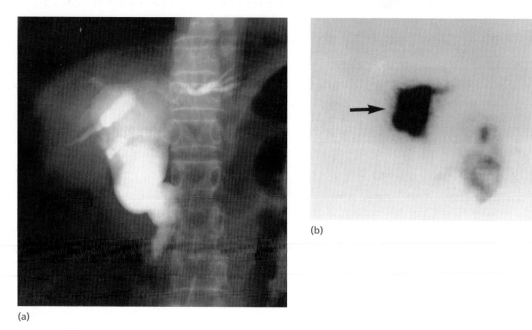

(a)

(b)

Figure 42.3 Choledochal cyst – type IC. **(a)** Diffuse enlargement of the common bile duct with distal tapering. **(b)** Radionuclide scan with activity predominantly in the cyst (arrow) and left hepatic duct. Bowel activity indicates patency of the common bile duct.

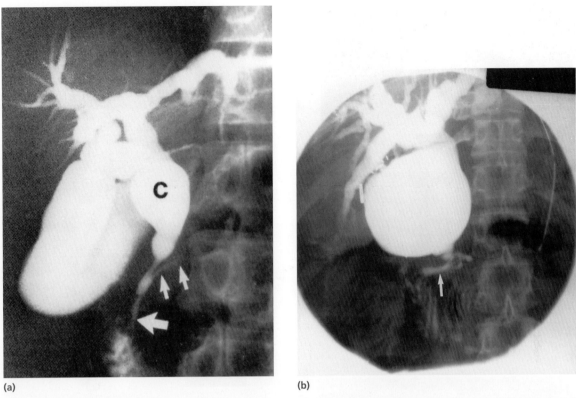

(a)　　　　　　　　　　　　　　　　　　　　(b)

Figure 42.4 Choledochal cyst – anomalous ductal relationship. **(a)** Cystic enlargement of the common bile duct (C) with associated dilatation of the common hepatic and intrahepatic ducts. The abnormal junction of the pancreatic (small arrows) and common bile ducts and the long common channel (large arrow) are displayed. **(b)** A large cyst involves the common hepatic and common bile duct accompanied by intrahepatic ductal dilatation. A long common channel (arrow) results from the abnormally high junction with the pancreatic duct.

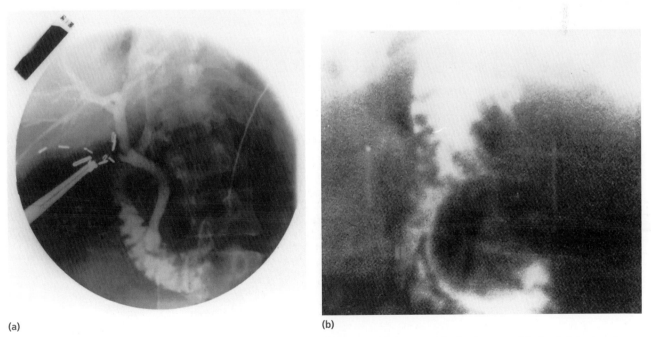

(a)　　　　　　　　　　　　　　　　　　　　(b)

Figure 42.5 Choledochocele – type III cyst. **(a)** Cholangiography reveals a club-shaped enlargement of the distal common bile duct bulging into the duodenum. **(b)** Upper gastrointestinal series reveals a smoothly rounded filling defect in the second portion of the duodenum.

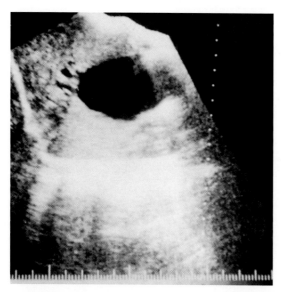

Figure 42.6 Caroli disease – type V cyst. T-tube cholangiography demonstrates cystic dilatation of multiple intrahepatic bile ducts representing type V biliary cyst.

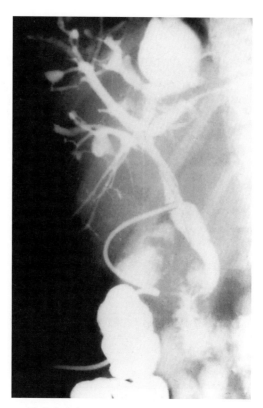

Figure 42.7 Choledochal cyst – sonographic findings. The anechoic mass with enhanced through transmission is characteristic of a cystic structure. Note one and possibly two ducts entering the cephalic aspect of the cyst. Absence of dilation of the bile ducts proximal to the cystic mass is typical for most type I cysts.

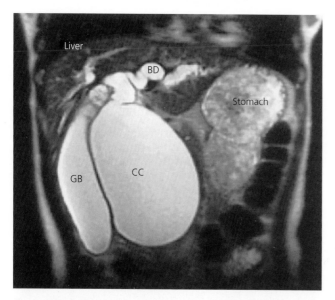

Figure 42.8 Magnetic resonance cholangiopancreatography (MRCP) of a choledochal cyst. Coronal T2-weighted fast spin-echo MRCP performed on a 16-year-old female patient presenting with right upper quadrant pain, jaundice, and amylasemia shows a very dilated segment of the common bile duct compatible with a choledochal cyst identical to the arm in of the cystic duct. The intrahepatic ducts are normal in size and shape. BD, bile duct; CC, choledochal cyst; GB, gallbladder. Source: Courtesy of Dr. Fergus Coakley, Department of Radiology, UCSF.

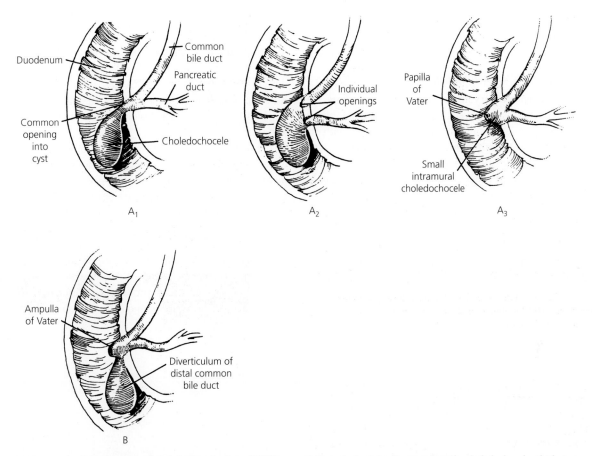

Figure 42.9 Proposed subclassification of choledochoceles (type III biliary cyst). Type A, the ampulla opens into the choledochocele which, in turn, communicates with the duodenum via another small opening. Type A is subclassified into: A_1, the pancreatic and common bile duct share a common opening into the cyst (33%) of cases); A_2, the openings are distinct (4% of cases); A_3, the choledochocele is small and entirely intramural (25% of cases); and type B, the ampulla opens directly into the duodenum with the choledochocele communicating with the distal common bile duct (21% of cases). Source: Kaplowitz N (ed.) Liver and Biliary Diseases; 1992. Reproduced with permission of Lippincott Williams and Wilkins.

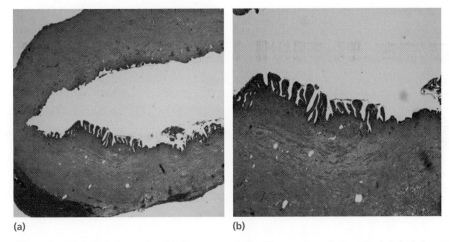

(a) (b)

Figure 42.10 Pathological features of choledochal cyst. A surgical specimen obtained by resection of a type IV choledochal cyst shows **(a)** extensive fibrous but minimal muscle tissue in the cyst wall, and **(b)** paucity of biliary epithelium lining the cyst lumen. Source: Courtesy of Dr. Para Chandrasoma, Department of Pathology, LAC/USC Medical Center.

portal fibrosis, hyperproliferation of interlobular bile ducts within the portal areas with variable shapes and sizes of bile ducts, and preservation of normal lobular architecture (Figure 42.11).

Biliary cysts are distinct from polycystic liver disease (PLD), which is a rare hepatobiliary fibropolycystic disorder characterized by the progressive development of fluid-filled biliary epithelial cysts in the liver that do not communicate with the biliary tree. The most common form of PLD coexists with autosomal dominant polycystic kidney disease (ADPKD); however PLD can occur without renal involvement as in isolated polycystic liver disease (PCLD) (Figure 42.12). In 21% of PCLD patients, mutations in *PRKCSH* or *SEC63* are found. These genes encode for proteins in the endoplasmic reticulum that are involved in quality control, translocation, and folding of newly synthesized glycoproteins. The hepatic cysts are rarely detected before puberty, but approximately 80% of the patients with renal cysts have liver cysts by the fifth decade of life. They are more prevalent and prominent in women, and increase dramatically in number and size through the child-bearing years.

Most patients with PLD are asymptomatic. The cysts range in size from <1 mm to >10 cm and may be diffuse or involve only one lobe. The most common presenting symptom is abdominal pain, with or without distention. Complications of PLD include hepatic cyst hemorrhage, rupture, or infection.

Abdominal ultrasound and CT scans are excellent in the detection of hepatic cysts. MRCP can also be a useful modality for better visualizing intrahepatic ductal dilatations and distinguishing PLD from other lesions such as biliary hamartomas and Caroli disease.

There is no approved medical therapy for PLD. However, with better understanding of the pathogenesis of PLD, targeted medical therapies are being developed. Encouraging results using somatostatin analogues have been obtained and the clinical criteria for this form of treatment are being defined. For dominant cyst (>5 cm), aspiration sclerotherapy may be suitable. Surgical fenestration of hepatic cysts, involving the deroofing of as many cysts as possible, can be performed through open laparotomy or by laparoscopy. Patients with severely symptomatic PLD and significant comorbid conditions or diffuse liver involvement by small cysts may benefit from orthotopic liver transplantation.

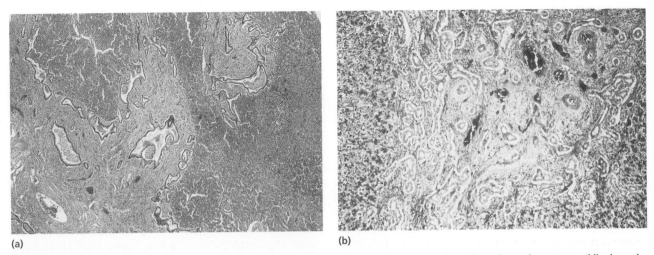

(a)

(b)

Figure 42.11 Congenital hepatic fibrosis. A 27-year-old female presented with periodic right upper quadrant discomfort and persistent mildly elevated alkaline phosphatase levels. A liver biopsy was done which showed: **(a)** the liver parenchyma is normal but the portal areas show prominent portal fibrosis without inflammation; the interlobular bile ducts are numerous, dilated and some contain inspissated bile (hematoxylin & eosin stain, low power); and **(b)** marked portal fibrosis as demonstrated by trichrome staining. Note the sharp demarcation of the fibrotic area from the parenchyma (trichrome stain, high power). Source: Courtesy of Dr. Gary Kanel, Department of Pathology, Rancho Los Amigos Medical Center.

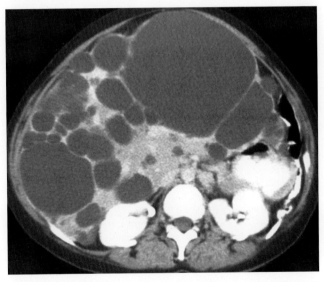

Figure 42.12 Polycystic liver disease. Small and large cysts fill the liver of a patient without polycystic kidneys. Source: Courtesy of Dr. Randall Radin, Department of Radiology, LAC/USC Medical Center.

CHAPTER 43
Tumors of the biliary tract

Tushar Patel

Mayo Clinic, Jacksonville, FL, USA

Tumors of the biliary tract comprise of a heterogeneous and diverse group, which includes both benign and malignant conditions that develop within the biliary tract (Boxes 43.1, 43.2, 43.3, and 43.4). These can occur throughout the biliary tract, from the ampulla of Vater to the intrahepatic ductules, and including the gallbladder. Biliary tract tumors vary in their presentation, natural history, and management.

Benign tumors of the biliary tract are uncommon and usually present as biliary tract strictures or masses within the lumen of the bile duct that can mimic and need to be distinguished from malignancies. Benign tumors of the gallbladder may present as luminal masses that need to be distinguished from gallstones or malignancies.

The main types of biliary tract cancers are: (1) cholangiocarcinomas, arising from the intrahepatic or extrahepatic bile ducts; (2) gallbladder cancer, arising from the gall bladder and cystic duct; and (3) ampullary cancers, arising from biliary epithelia at the ampulla of Vater. Cholangiocarcinomas are anatomically classified into intrahepatic, perihilar, and distal cholangiocarcinoma (Figure 43.1). These three types of cholangiocarcinoma need to be distinguished as separate tumor types as they vary in their clinical presentation, behavior, and molecular pathogenesis. Selected features on diagnostic imaging are shown in Figures 43.1–43.7. Suggested approaches for the diagnosis and management of these cancers are outlined in Figures 43.8, 43.9, and 43.10.

Box 43.1 Benign tumors of the biliary tract.

Benign tumors of the intrahepatic and extrahepatic biliary tract
Bile duct adenoma
Biliary papillomatosis
Biliary cystadenoma
Granular cell tumor
Rare: mesenchymal tumors, e.g., leiomyoma, lipoma, neurofibroma, paraganglioma
Benign tumors of the gall bladder
Cholesterol polyp/cholesterolosis
Inflammatory polyp
Adenomyomatosis /adenomatous hyperplasia/adenomyoma
Xanthogranulomatous cholecystitis
Gall bladder adenoma
Rare: cystadenoma, papillomatosis, heterotopia, mesenchymal tumors

---

Box 43.2 Biliary tract cancers.

Intrahepatic cholangiocarcinoma
Perihilar cholangiocarcinoma
Distal cholangiocarcinoma
Gallbladder cancers
Ampullary cancers
Rare: cystadenocarcinomas, mixed hepatocellular–cholangiocellular cancers

---

Yamada's Atlas of Gastroenterology, Fifth Edition. Edited by Daniel K. Podolsky, Michael Camilleri, J. Gregory Fitz, Anthony N. Kalloo, Fergus Shanahan, and Timothy C. Wang.
© 2016 John Wiley & Sons, Ltd. Published 2016 by John Wiley & Sons, Ltd.
Companion website: www.yamadagastro.com/atlas

Box 43.3 Risk factors for biliary tract cancers.

General
  Cirrhosis
  Obesity
  Diabetes
  Alcohol
  Smoking
Infectious
  Opisthorchis viverrini
  Clonorchis sinensis
  Hepatitis C
  Hepatitis B
Congenital or anatomical changes
  Bile duct cystic disease
  Caroli disease
  Congenital hepatic fibrosis
  Anomalous pancreatic–biliary duct
  Biliary–enteric anastomosis
Inflammatory
  Primary sclerosing cholangitis
  Hepatolithiasis
  Gallstones or biliary tract stones
Toxins and chemicals
  Thorotrast
  Dioxin
  Vinyl chloride
  Nitrosamines
  Asbestos
  Organic solvents

The contribution of several of these risk factors for specific types of biliary cancers has not been confirmed.

Box 43.4 Malignant neoplasms of the gallbladder.

Epithelial origin
  Adenocarcinoma
  Squamous cell carcinoma
  Oat cell carcinoma
Mesenchyal origin
  Embryonal rhabdomyosarcoma
  Leiomyosarcoma
  Malignant fibrous histiocytoma
Others
  Lymphoma
  Carcinoid
  Carcinosarcoma
  Melanoma
  Various others

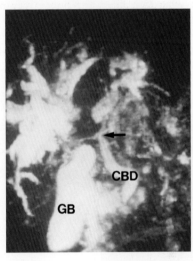

Figure 43.2 Magnetic resonance cholangiogram showing extrahepatic and intrahepatic biliary tract. Narrowing of the bile duct produced by a hilar tumor is shown (arrow). CBD, common bile duct; GB, gallbladder. Source: Courtesy of Dr. Joseph T. Ferrucci, Department of Radiology, Boston University School of Medicine.

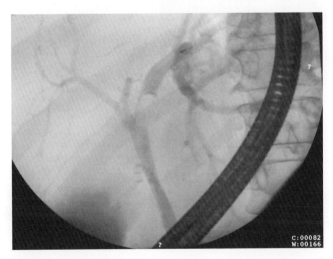

Figure 43.1 Endoscopic retrograde cholangiogram showing a bullet-shaped filling defect in the left hepatic duct. At surgery, this was found to be a tumor embolus from an intrahepatic cholangiocarcinoma. This patient presented with pancreatitis, presumably caused by such an embolus. Source: Callery MP, Strasberg SM, Doherty GM, et al. J Am Coll Surg 1997;185:33. Reproduced with permission of Elsevier.

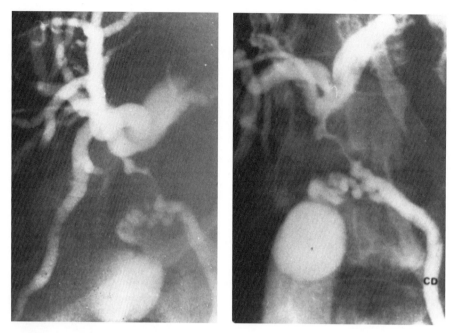

Figure 43.3 Cholangiogram shows a perihilar cholangiocacrinoma. The intrahepatic bile ducts are dilated whereas the size of the common bile duct (CD) is normal.

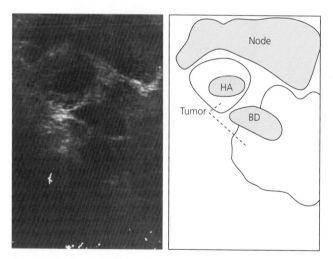

Figure 43.4 Laparoscopic ultrasonogram showing encasement of the hepatic artery (HA) and bile duct (BD). An enlarged lymph node that contains tumor is also seen.

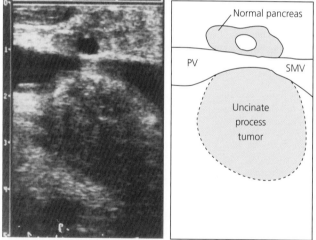

Figure 43.5 High-resolution laparoscopic ultrasound image demonstrating a 2.5 to 3-cm inhomogeneous hypoechoic mass that abuts the superior mesenteric vein (SMV) and portal vein (PV) posteriorly behind the neck of the pancreas, which itself appears to be normal. No evidence of actual vascular invasion is seen. At laparotomy, a lesion in the uncinate was removed. (Source: Gullery MP, Strasberg SM, Doherty GM, et al. J Am Coll Surg 1997;185:33. Reproduced with permission of Elsevier.)

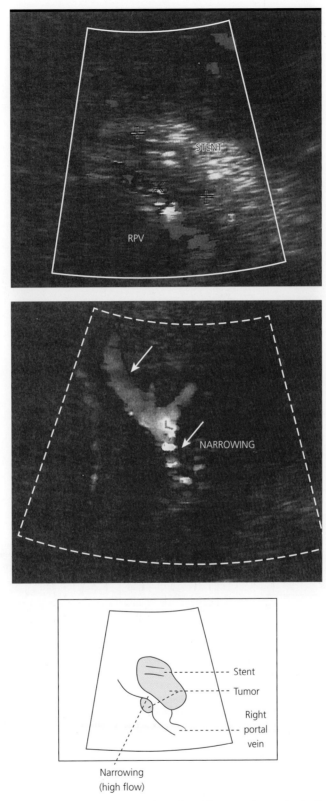

Figure 43.6 Doppler ultrasonograms showing encasement of right portal vein (RPV) by tumor. A stent that had been placed through the tumor can also be seen. Color flow Doppler studies can indicate venous compression by demonstrating regions of higher-velocity flow in such regions.

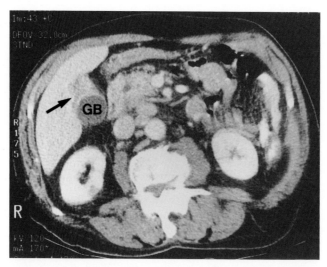

Figure 43.7 Computed tomography scan of patient with carcinoma of the gallbladder (GB) showing invasion of hepatic parenchyma (arrow).

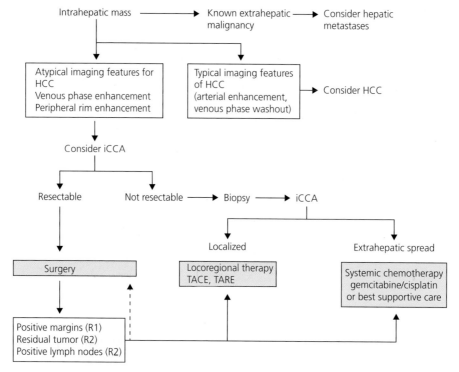

Figure 43.8 Diagnosis and management of intrahepatic cholangiocarcinoma (iCCA). For unresectable disease, a biopsy should be obtained to confirm the diagnosis. For localized disease, treatment with locoregional approaches such as transarterial chemoembolization (TACE), transarterial radioembolization (TARE), or systemic therapy can be considered. HCC, hepatocellular carcinoma.

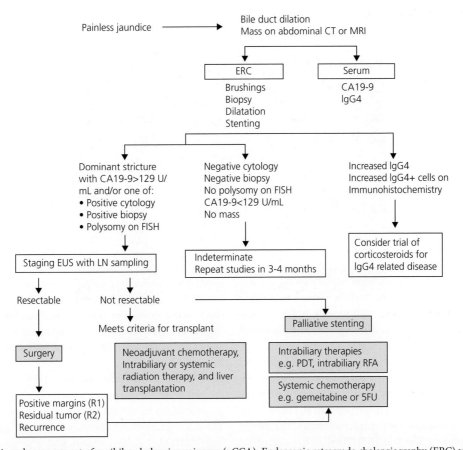

Figure 43.9 Diagnosis and management of perihilar cholangiocarcinoma (pCCA). Endoscopic retrograde cholangiography (ERC) with tissue sampling should be performed. If diagnostic for malignancy, a staging endoscopic ultrasound (EUS) should be considered for sampling lymph nodes (LN). EUS fine needle aspiration of the tumor should not be attempted in patients who are potential candidates for transplantation because of the risk of seeding. Surgical resection may be considered for localized resectable disease. If unresectable, and does not meet criteria for transplantation, intrabiliary photodynamic therapy (PDT) or radiofrequency ablation (RFA) may be attempted. Systemic chemotherapy with gemcitabine, or if performance status is poor with 5-fluorouracil (5FU), regimens could be considered for unresectable advanced or recurrent disease. FISH, fluorescence in situ hybridization.

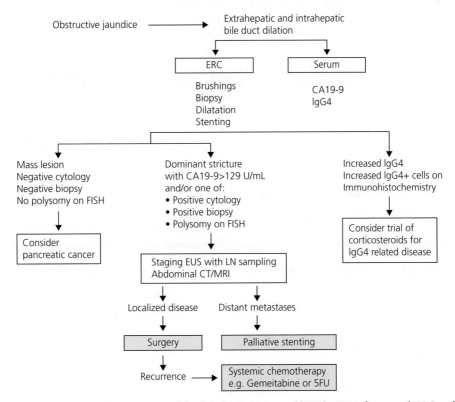

Figure 43.10 An approach to the diagnosis and management of distal cholangiocarcinoma (dCCA). 5FU, 5-fluorouracil; ERC, endoscopic retrograde cholangiography; EUS, endoscopic ultrasound; FISH, fluorescence in situ hybridization; LN, lymph node.

CHAPTER 44

Acute viral hepatitis

Marc G. Ghany and T. Jake Liang
National Institutes of Health, Bethesda, MD, USA

Acute viral hepatitis is a syndrome characterized by a constellation of clinical, biochemical and pathological features following primary infection of the liver by viruses that cause injury to hepatocytes. Five hepatotrophic viruses, A, B, C, D, and E, account for over 90% of cases. Although the hepatotrophic viruses are found worldwide (see Figures 44.1, 44.2, 44.3, 44.4, and 44.5); the prevalence varies greatly from region to region and their individual distribution is partly dependent on their mode of transmission. Hepatitis A virus (HAV) and hepatitis E virus (HEV) are transmitted enterically while hepatitis B, C and D are transmitted via the percutaneous/permucosal routes. The liver is the primary site of infection and replication of hepatotrophic viruses. Four, (HAV, hepatitis C virus, (HCV), hepatitis D virus (HDV) and HEV) are single stranded RNA viruses and hepatitis B virus (HBV) is a partially double stranded, DNA virus.

The genomic organization of HAV is shown in Figure 44.6. The replication process of HAV has been inferred from studies of other picornaviruses. Entry of the virus into the host is mediated by a cell surface receptor, a mucin-like Class 1 integral membrane glycoprotein. Viral entry is followed by uncoating, and initiation of viral protein synthesis. Viral RNA synthesis proceeds from negative to positive strand and occurs in the cytoplasm. Viral assembly follows a sequence similar to that of picornaviruses in a cellular membrane compartment.

The infectious HBV virion (Dane particle) has a 42 nm spherical, double shelled structure, consisting of a lipid envelope containing HBsAg which surrounds an inner nucleocapsid. The hepatitis B core antigen (HBcAg) complexes with viral-encoded polymerase and viral DNA genome to form the nucleocapsid. The genome of hepatitis B virus is a partially double stranded circular DNA of approximately 3.2 kbp. The viral genome encodes four overlapping open reading frames (ORF) from which 4 mRNA transcripts are derived and code for 7 viral proteins (see Figure 44.7 for details). HBV replicates through a RNA intermediate and this process is summarized in Figure 44.8.

The HCV has a positive-sense, single-strand RNA genome of approximately 9.6 kb in length with a single large open reading frame and highly conserved untranslated regions (UTR) at the 5' and 3' ends. The genomic organization is summarized in Figure 44.9. HCV replicates in the cytoplasm, in a membrane-associated compartment. The replication process is illustrated in Figure 44.10.

HDV requires coinfection with HBV for replication. Delta antigen is the inner ribonucleoprotein component of a subviral particle that is enveloped by the hepatitis B virus surface antigen. The ribonucleoprotein complex consists of small (SHDAg) and large (LHDAg) delta antigens and a single-stranded circular RNA genome of 1.7 kb in length which has extensive self-complementation to form a rod-like structure (Figure 44.11). The antigenome is synthesized from the genomic RNA and is the template for HDV mRNA encoding the delta antigens. The antigenome also serves as the template for genome synthesis. The HDV genome utilizes host RNA polymerase II to carry out RNA directed RNA synthesis that is dependent on the small delta antigen. Both genomic and antigenomic RNAs possess ribozyme activities that catalyze RNA self-cleavage and self-ligation. Transcription and replication are integrated into a single process using a double rolling circle mechanism. After entry into cells, HDV genome serves as a template for replication, resulting in the production of multimeric antigenomes. Nascent antigenomes, through their intrinsic ribozyme activities, form circular monomeric RNAs, that, in turn, serve as templates for the production of HDV genomes. Alternatively, the elongating product can be cleaved and released as polyadenylated mRNAs, which then direct delta antigen synthesis. HDV assembly begins with the association of the delta antigens with the newly synthesized genome to yield a ribonucleoprotein complex (RNP). The RNP is transported from nucleus to cytoplasm, presumably mediated by the nucleocytoplasmic shuttling function of delta antigens. The LHDAg of the RNP interacts with HBsAg to facilitate assembly. Large delta antigen is required

Yamada's Atlas of Gastroenterology, Fifth Edition. Edited by Daniel K. Podolsky, Michael Camilleri, J. Gregory Fitz, Anthony N. Kalloo, Fergus Shanahan, and Timothy C. Wang.

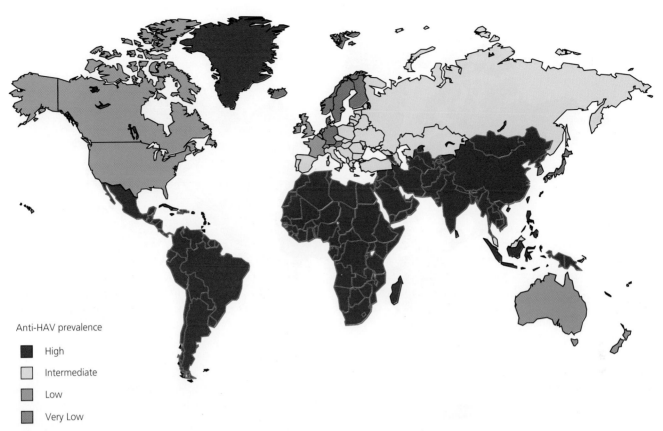

Anti-HAV prevalence

■ High

□ Intermediate

▨ Low

▨ Very Low

Figure 44.1 Worldwide prevalence of hepatitis A virus infection.
The prevalence of HAV can be can be characterized globally by areas of high, intermediate, low or very low levels of endemicity. The levels of endemicity closely correlate with hygienic and sanitary conditions of each geographic area.

for particle assembly while small delta antigen is copackaged but not required for particle formation.

The HEV genome is a single-strand, positive-sense RNA of approximately 7.5 kb. The genome is organized into three over-lapping open reading frames (ORF 1–3) flanked by noncoding regions (Figure 44.12). Replication of HEV has not been char-acterized. The mechanisms of viral attachment, entry, and uncoating are unknown.

During primary infection, the initial pathway of antiviral immune response is largely unknown. Initial viral infection is associated with activation of innate immunity in the liver. Rec-ognition of infected hepatocytes by resident natural killer (NK) and/or natural killer T (NKT) cells results in activation of these cells and induction of antiviral cytokines including interferons. This phase of innate immunity leads to the initial control of viral replication. Since this antiviral response is likely associated with a noncytopathic mechanism, little or no hepatocellular injury is evident. Innate immunity also plays a critical role in the activa-tion of the adaptive immunity including humoral and cellular responses. Induction of a humoral immune response with pro-duction of neutralizing antibodies prevents viral spread and leads to subsequent elimination of circulating viruses. For HBV, the antibody response to the envelope proteins is a T cell-dependent process.

Cell-mediated immunity (CMI), the other limb of the immune response, is critical for the long-term control of viral infections including the hepatitis viruses. In acute HBV infec-tion, individuals can mount a vigorous, multi-specific, and polyclonal cellular immune response to HBV. In contrast, chronically infected patients have a weak or barely detectable anti-HBV response. This is true for both CD4 and CD8 responses. During acute hepatitis B, a vigorous HLA Class II-restricted, CD4+, helper T cell response to multiple epitopes of HBc/eAg predominates in virtually all patients. By helping B cells produce neutralizing antienvelope antibodies and activat-ing HBV-specific CTLs, this CD4+ T helper population may direct the initial antiviral response.

In most viral infections, the activation of virus-specific CD8+ cytotoxic T lymphocytes is critical for viral clearance. Patients acutely infected with HBV develop a strong, polyclonal, HLA Class I-restricted CTL response that is directed against multiple epitopes in all viral proteins. This response persists for many years after recovery from acute HBV infection.

The molecular and cellular mechanisms of viral clearance and hepatocellular injury have been studied in great detail for HBV infection (see Figure 44.13). CD8+, Class I-restricted HBsAg-specific CTLs target the liver through interaction between the HBV-specific T cell receptors and the antigen-presenting HLA

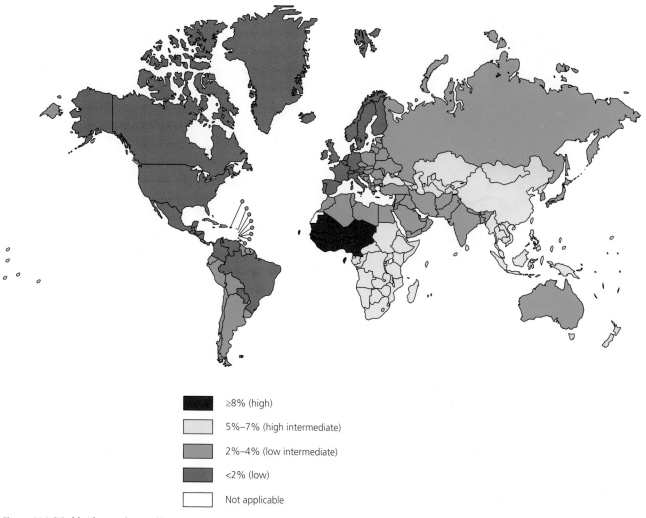

Figure 44.2 Worldwide prevalence of hepatitis B infection.
Approximately 45% of the world's population lives in regions that are high (≥8%) or high intermediate (5%–7%) endemicity for hepatitis B infection. The prevalence of hepatitis B surface antigen (HBsAg) is declining in many of these areas due to the introduction of mandatory vaccination programs. In areas of low intermediate endemicity such as the Middle East, Eastern Europe, and the Mediterranean Basin, the prevalence of HBsAg ranges from 2% to 4%. Approximately 43% of the world's population lives in regions of low endemicity. In regions of low endemicity, such as North America, Western Europe, Australia, and parts of South America, the prevalence of HBsAg is less than 2%.

Class I molecules on the hepatocytes and cause scattered apoptosis of hepatocytes. By secreting cytokines including interferons, the CTLs recruit a variety of antigen-nonspecific inflammatory cells into the liver, resulting in more extensive necroinflammatory injury of the liver. The predominant infiltrating effector cells are macrophages, which probably mediate the majority of hepatocellular injury. The CTLs, although not primarily responsible for the majority of hepatocellular injury, initiate the cascade of immunological events leading to hepatitis. They also play a role in elimination of infected hepatocytes through noncytolytic inhibition of HBV gene expression and viral replication. The detection of virus-specific CD4 and CD8 cells in the peripheral blood and liver of chronically infected individuals suggests a pathogenic relationship between the indolent cellular immune response and necroinflammatory liver disease associated with chronic hepatitis. Therefore, vigorous CMI response leads to

viral clearance, whereas ineffective CMI response results in chronic hepatocellular injury.

Following infection, the hepatotrophic viruses give rise to similar clinical, biochemical and pathological features. Serologic testing is the only reliable way to determine the infecting agent (see Figures 44.14, 44.15, 44.16, 44.17, 44.18, and 44.19). The incubation period differs for each virus ranging from 2 weeks to 6 months. The clinical course ranges from an asymptomatic illness to fulminant hepatitis and is typified by three phases, prodromal, symptomatic and convalescent, lasting from 6 weeks to 6 months. Approximately 20% of cases present with jaundice. The primary biochemical abnormality is an acute rise in serum alanine and aspartate aminotransferases, markers of hepatocellular necrosis, to greater than 2.5 times the upper limit of normal; more commonly to greater than 10 times the upper limit of normal. The basic pathological lesion is an acute

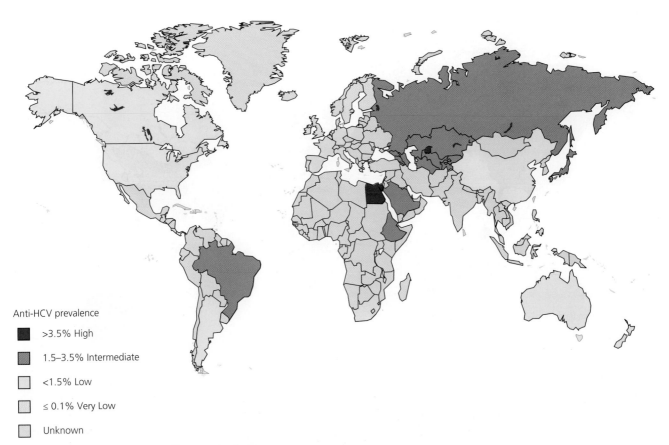

Figure 44.3 Worldwide prevalence of hepatitis C infection.
Worldwide the prevalence of anti-HCV is fairly consistent ranging from 1.2–3.8% (average 2.8%). Central and East Asia and North Africa/Middle East are estimated to have a high prevalence (>3.5%); South and South East Asia, Sub-Saharan Africa, Andean, Central and Southern Latin America, Caribbean, Oceania, Australisia and Central, Eastern, and Western Europe have intermediate prevalance (1.5–3.5%); Asia Pacific, tropical Latin America and Northern America have low prevalence (<1.5%).

Anti-HCV prevalence

- >3.5% High
- 1.5–3.5% Intermediate
- <1.5% Low
- ≤ 0.1% Very Low
- Unknown

inflammation of the entire liver. The severity can range from mild, involving a few hepatocytes, to moderate, to massive necrosis, involving almost all hepatocytes (see Figures 44.20, 44.21, and 44.22). The classic pathological features of acute viral hepatitis are swollen hepatocytes, apoptotic hepatocytes (acidophil bodies), and the presence of inflammatory cells within the hepatic lobule, predominantly lymphocytes and macrophages, which result in distortion of the normal liver architecture.

HAV and HEV generally do not lead to chronic infection in an immunocompetent host and development of antibody protects against reinfection for HAV. Persistent HEV infection has been noted in solid organ transplant patients under immunosuppression. HBV, HCV and HDV have the propensity to cause chronic infection and are associated with an increased risk of hepatocellular carcinoma. Effective and safe vaccines exist for the prevention of infection with HAV, HBV and HEV. Vaccination against HAV and HBV are recommended in the pre and post exposure setting and for persons with HCV-related chronic liver disease. Institution of risk behavior modifications is the only effective way to prevent HDV superinfection in persons with chronic hepatitis B. No vaccine exists for HCV and strategies for preventing infection include screening of blood products

and risk behavior modification. Improving hygiene, providing safe drinking water and proper cooking of meats should lower the risk of HEV infection.

Treatment of acute viral hepatitis is supportive with the aim to maintain adequate nutrition, hydration and monitoring for the development of fulminant hepatitis. Antiviral therapy is rarely indicated especially for HAV and HEV where the course is benign and recovery the rule. Most adults with acute HBV infection recover spontaneously. Specific antiviral therapy can be considered in persons who fail to clear HBV after 12 weeks or who appear to be progressing to fulminant hepatitis.. Household and sexual contacts of persons with acute HBV infection should receive HBIG and HBV vaccine. Treatment of acute hepatitis C should be considered because of the high propensity to develop chronic hepatitis. The optimal timing of treatment is unknown. A period of monitoring HCV RNA for at least 12 to 16 weeks is recommended to allow for spontaneous clearance before starting treatment. Subjects with interleukin 28B (IL28B) genotype CC have a higher rate of spontaneously clearance compared to those with IL28 genotype CT or TT. Specific antiviral therapy can be considered in patients who fail to clear HCV after the observation period.

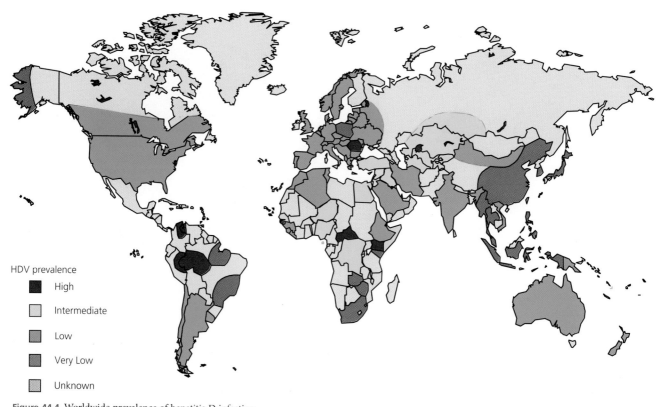

Figure 44.4 Worldwide prevalence of hepatitis D infection.
The prevalence of HDV mimics that of HBV due to its dependency on HBV for its lifecycle. However, areas of discordance exist, such as China where the rate of HDV infection is low but HBV infection high. The reasons for this finding are not known.

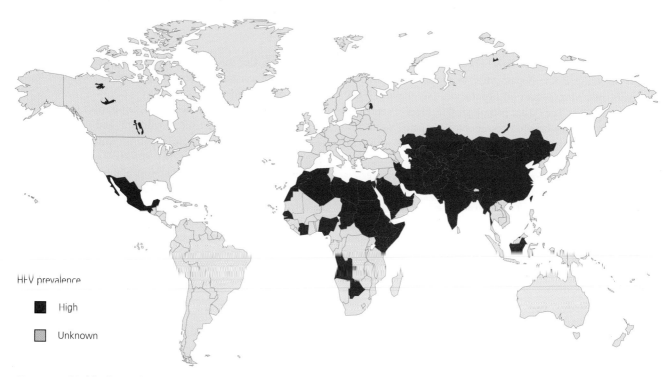

Figure 44.5 Worldwide prevalence of hepatitis E infection. Prevalence of anti-HEV in the red highlighted areas is estimated to be >2.5%–25%. In lightly shaded areas, prevalence of anti-HEV is unknown but estimated to range from 0%–2.5%.

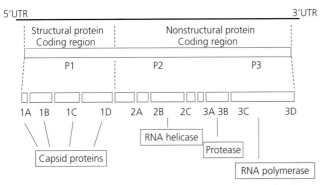

Figure 44.6 Structure of the hepatitis A virus and genetic organization. The top line represents the hepatitis A virus RNA genome. The HAV has a linear, positive-sense, single stranded RNA genome of approximately 7.5 kb. Translation of the genome yields a single polyprotein, divided into 3 main functional domains (P1, P2 and P3) from which nine or more individual viral proteins are cleaved. The three major capsid proteins form protomers that then assemble into pentamers that require the action of pX, an 8-kDa carboxy-terminal extension of VP1. Pentamers subsequently self-assemble into an icosahedral capsid that packages the viral genome and is released from cells wrapped in cellular membranes (eHAV).

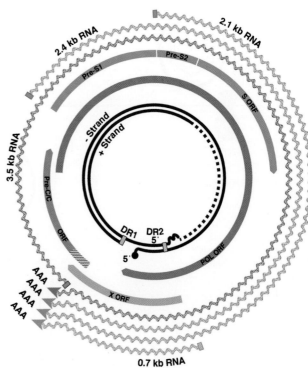

Figure 44.7 Genome structure and organization of hepatitis B virus. The hepatitis B virus open reading frames: preC and C (precore and core proteins), P (polymerase protein), preS1, preS2, and S (L, M, and S surface envelope proteins), and X protein are shown. The viral genome structure is composed of the full length (-)-DNA strand and variable length (+)-DNA strand (solid followed by dashed line). The polymerase protein is covalently attached to the 5′ of the (-) strand and a capped oligoribonucleotide (spiral line) to the (+) strand. Direct repeats 1 and 2 (small rectangular boxes) are shown on the genome. The outer lines represent the four transcripts, all terminating at a common polyadenylation site. The S open reading frame (ORF) encodes the viral surface envelope proteins, the HBsAg, and comprises the pre-S1, pre-S2, and S regions. The core gene consists of precore and core regions; separate initiation codons give rise to the hepatitis B e antigen (HBeAg) and the viral nucleocapsid (HBcAg). The polymerase ORF encodes the polymerase protein, which is involved in encapsidation and initiation of negative strand synthesis. The polymerase has multiple functions including reverse transcriptase activity and catalyzes genome synthesis as well as RNAse H activity which degrades pregenomic RNA and facilitates replication. The HBX protein is translated from the X transcript (0.7 kb) and is a viral protein with pleotrophic functions that plays an integral role in the viral life cycle.

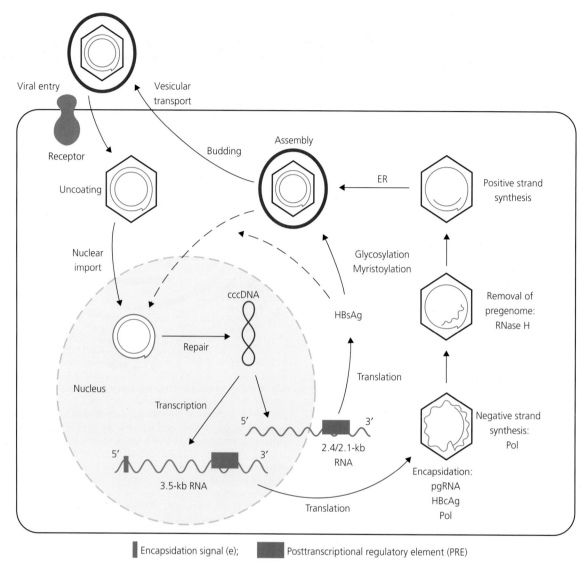

Figure 44.8 Replication of hepatitis B virus. Infectious virions attach to hepatocytes via the preS1 domain of the L protein. The sodium taurocholate cotransporter polypeptide (NTCP) has been recently identified to be the HBV receptor. Upon entering, the nucleocapsid is delivered to the nucleus and the viral genome is repaired to the covalently closed circular form (cccDNA). Viral transcripts are translated in the cytoplasm, and the core and polymerase proteins interact with the genomic length RNA to form the nucleocapsids. Reverse transcription occurs, and the mature virions are assembled in the endoplasmic reticulum, where they acquire the surface proteins. The virion is then secreted via vesicular transport. The encapsidation signal and posttranscriptional regulatory element on the HBV transcripts are shown as rectangular boxes.

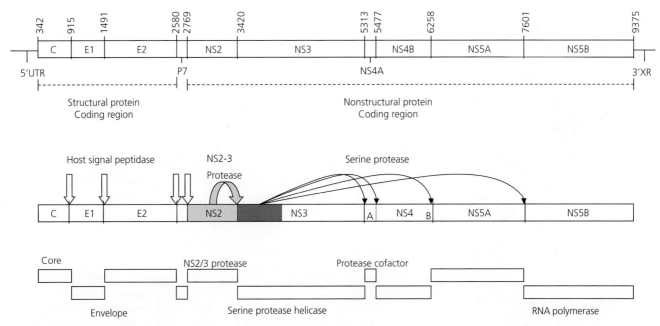

Figure 44.9 Genome organization of hepatitis C virus. The 5′ and 3′ untranslated regions (UTR) flanking a polyprotein ORF are shown at the top. Numbering refers to nucleotide positions of genes, based on the sequence of a HCV genotype 1a infectious clone. The HCV polyprotein of approximately 3000 amino acids is processed co- and posttranslationally by cellular and viral proteases to produce the individual gene products. Cellular proteases in the endoplasmic reticulum catalyze the cleavage of the structural proteins, while viral encoded proteases cleave the nonstructural proteins. The middle panel shows HCV polyprotein processing with cleavage sites of host signal peptidase (open arrows), NS2-3 protease (gray arrow) and NS3 serine protease (thin arrows). The processed HCV proteins are shown at the bottom. The highly conserved core protein is the putative viral nucleocapsid and encompasses the first 191 amino acids of the polyprotein. The E1 and E2 are envelope glycoproteins with C-terminal hydrophobic transmembrane domains. The NS2 region encodes a metalloproteinase. The NS2-3 protease mediates autocatalytic cleavage between the NS2 and NS3. The NS3 region encodes a multifunctional protein with a N-terminal serine protease and a C-terminal RNA helicase and nucleotide triphosphatase (NTPase). The NS3 protease, distinct from the NS2-3 protease activity, is involved in processing the downstream polyprotein. The NS4A interacts with and acts as a cofactor for the NS3 protease. The function of NS4B is unknown. The NS5A may play a role in the replication complex. The NS5B is the RNA dependent RNA polymerase that mediates viral replication.

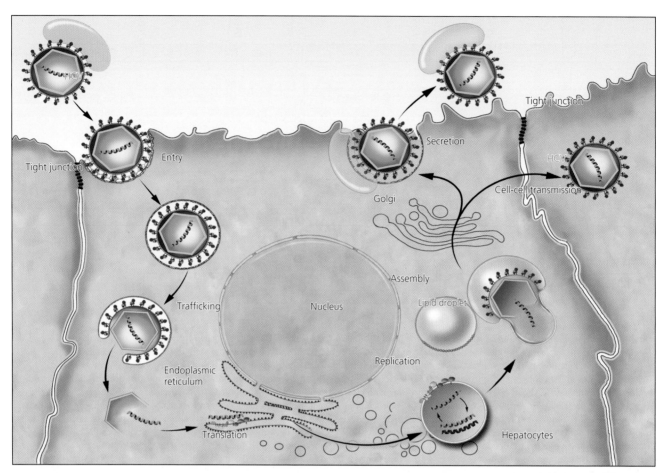

Figure 44.10 Replication of hepatitis C virus. The virion attaches and enters the hepatocyte and is internalized via clathrin-mediated endocytosis. Initial attachment to the cell is via an interaction with the low density lipoprotein receptor and glycosaminoglycans present on heparan sulphate proteoglycans. Five cell surface molecules are also required for entry and include: CD81, scavenger receptor Class B member 1, claudin 1, occludin and the cholesterol absorption receptor Niemann–Pick C1-like 1. The viral genome is then directed to a membranous component in the perinuclear ER region and serves as template for HCV protein synthesis. The nonstructural proteins form a replication complex with the genomic RNA and direct RNA replication (to negative and then positive strands). The structural proteins, which are retained in the ER, interact with the progeny genomes and assemble into virions. The virions are then secreted via an unknown exocytotic pathway, probably involving lipoprotein and not passing through the Golgi compartment.

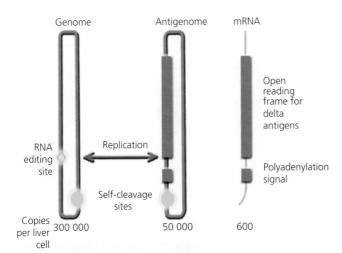

Figure 44.11 Genomic organization of hepatitis D virus. The RNA genome has a rod-like structure and contains a RNA editing and a self-cleavage site (circle). The antigenome is synthesized from the genomic RNA and is the template for HDV mRNA encoding the delta antigens. The antigenome also serves as the template for genome synthesis. The estimated copy numbers of the RNA species in the infected liver.

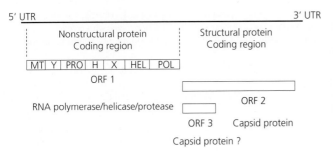

Figure 44.12 Genomic organization of hepatitis E virus. The genome is organized into three overlapping open reading frames flanked by 5′ and 3′ noncoding regions and a 3′ polyadenylation. The ORF 1 appears to encode the nonstructural gene products: MT (methyl transferase), X and Y (unknown functions), Pro (protease), Hel (helicase), H (proline rich hinge region), Pol (RNA-dependent RNA polymerase). ORF 2 codes for the capsid, and ORF 3 codes for a protein with possible nucleocapsid function.

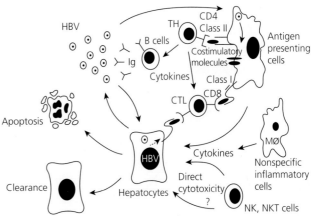

Figure 44.13 The immunopathogenesis of hepatitis B (see text for details).

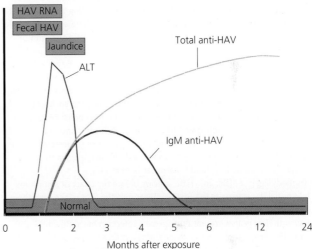

Figure 44.14 Serologic course of acute hepatitis A. Hepatitis A virus can be detected in stool before the onset of clinical symptoms by electron microscopy (EM) and polymerase chain reaction (PCR). Persons are therefore infectious during the incubation period. Levels of virus fall and become almost undetectable with the onset of symptoms and the peak of the alanine aminotransferase (ALT) level. Antibody to HAV (anti-HAV) first becomes detectable during this period. The initial antibody response is IgM anti-HAV; levels usually peak at 3 months following acute exposure and rapidly decline to undetectable by month 5 or 6. Occasionally IgM anti-HAV may remain detectable for up to 1 year or longer. IgG anti-HAV is also present at low levels during acute infection but levels rise as IgM anti-HAV begin to fall. IgG anti-HAV persists for life and confers protection against re-infection. Thus diagnosis of acute hepatitis A rests on the demonstration of IgM anti-HAV in serum. IgG anti-HAV is a marker of past infection. However, commercial assays for total anti-HAV measure both IgM and IgG and therefore are not helpful in diagnosing acute infection.

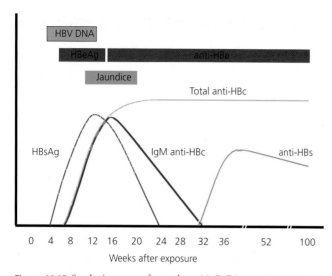

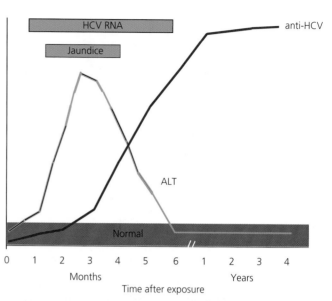

Figure 44.15 Serologic course of acute hepatitis B. Diagnostic tests are available for most of the HBV antigens and corresponding antibodies. The presence or absence of each of these antigens and antibodies serologically defines the stage of illness as acute, chronic or recovered. Detection of HBsAg in serum is the serologic hallmark of HBV infection. It usually appears in serum 1–10 weeks after acute exposure and 2–6 weeks before the onset of symptoms. It is detectable in both acute and chronic sera. HBeAg is the next viral antigen to appear in serum soon after HBsAg. Its presence correlates with other markers of viral replication such as HBV DNA and it is a useful marker of infectivity. HBcAg is not detectable in serum but can be demonstrated in liver tissue. With the onset of symptoms, HBeAg and HBV DNA levels may become undetectable and the level of HBsAg also begins to decline. HBsAg may persist in the convalescent phase but should disappear by 6 months.
Antibody against HBc, anti-HBc appears before the onset of symptoms. IgM anti-HBc is usually the first to appear and the titer peaks with the onset of symptoms but declines to undetectable levels within 6 months. IgG anti-HBc is also present during acute infection but unlike IgM anti-HBc, remains elevated lifelong and is a marker of past infection. Thus diagnosis of acute HBV infection is made by the demonstration of HBsAg and IgM anti-HBc in serum. During the convalescent phase, HBsAg disappears and antibodies to HBsAg, anti-HBs, appear. Therefore loss of HBsAg, HBeAg and development of anti-HBs indicates recovery from acute infection and immunity against re-infection. Rarely all markers of HBV infection, HBsAg, HBeAg and HBV DNA are cleared from serum before the development of anti-HBs. If testing is performed during this period, IgM anti-HBc may be the only marker to indicate HBV infection and this "serologically silent" period is referred to as the window period.

Figure 44.16 Serologic course of acute HCV infection. Following exposure to HCV, the virus can be detected within 2 weeks in serum and liver using sensitive PCR assays. An antibody response can be demonstrated as early as week 4 but more commonly by week 12 coinciding with the onset of clinical symptoms. Anti-HCV usually persists for life but may disappear in up to 25% of persons who recover spontaneously. Anti-HCV does not confer immunity against reinfection.

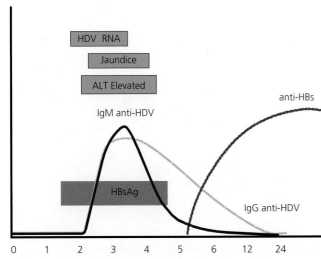

Figure 44.17 Serologic course of HDV coinfection. Acute hepatitis D infection occurs in two settings: simultaneously with acute hepatitis B infection – co infection or following exposure in a patient with chronic HBV infection – superinfection. The serologic course is different in each instance. In acute coinfection, markers of HBV are usually evident before HDV is detected. HDVAg and HDV RNA can be detected in serum before the peak in ALT level; however these are research tests and not commercially available. IgM anti-HDV can be detected by week 4 following exposure but is often weak and may disappear before the development of IgG anti-HDV. IgG anti-HDV is usually delayed for several weeks following exposure and in some cases is only present transiently during convalescence. Therefore, both acute and convalescent sera should be tested for anti-HDV. Following recovery, levels of anti-HDV may decline to undetectable and no serologic markers of HDV may remain. Thus some cases may be diagnosed as acute HBV infection alone. The presence of IgM anti-HBc, which is associated with acute HBV infection is an important marker for distinguishing HDV coinfection from superinfection. Thus the diagnosis of HDV coinfection is determined by the presence of IgM anti-HDV, HBsAg and IgM anti-HBc.

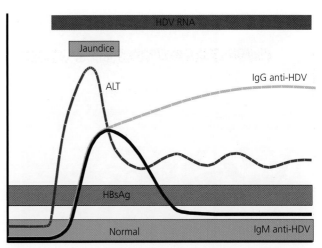

Figure 44.18 Serologic course of HDV superinfection. The incubation period of HDV superinfection is usually shorter than for coinfection. HDV RNA and HDVAg are present during the incubation period and symptomatic phase. The titer of HBsAg usually falls when HDVAg appears in serum. Most cases of HDV superinfection result in chronic infection and HDV RNA and HDVAg persist in serum. In contrast to HDV coinfection, IgM and IgG anti-HDV are both present during the symptomatic phase of infection and persist indefinitely. IgM anti-HBc is usually absent or present in low titer. Thus diagnosis of acute HDV superinfection rests on the detection of anti-HDV and HBsAg and the absence of IgM anti-HBc.

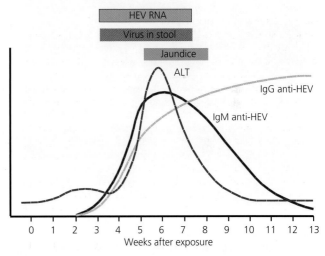

Figure 44.19 Serologic course of HEV infection. Following acute exposure to the virus, viral excretion is detectable within 2 weeks in serum and stool. Similar to HAV infection virus levels are highest during the incubation phase and begin to decline with the onset of symptoms. Both IgM and IgG antibody are elicited during acute infection. IgM anti-HEV is detectable within 2 weeks of exposure and peaks with the onset of symptoms and ALT levels. It disappears rapidly over 4–5 months. IgG anti-HEV is present during the acute illness and remains elevated for several years and then levels begin to decline. Current assays for anti-HEV vary widely in their sensitivity and false negatives can result in diagnostic error.

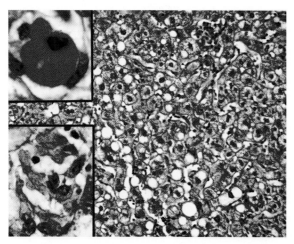

Figure 44.20 Acute viral hepatitis. The biopsy demonstrates typical features of acute viral hepatitis with a mild inflammatory infiltrate, ballooning degeneration, scattered acidophil bodies and mild lobular disarray. Upper left insert shows a high power view of an acidophil body with densely eosinophilic, irregularly shaped cytoplasm and pyknotic nucleus. Lower left insert shows a high power view of the inflammatory infiltrate. There are lymphocytes, pigmented macrophages and occasional plasma cells. Mild steatosis is present. (Hematoxylin and eosin stain used.)

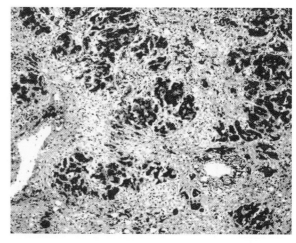

Figure 44.22 Acute viral hepatitis with submassive necrosis. There is almost complete involvement of the acini with extensive loss of parenchyma. Islands of hepatocytes are seen, separated by reticulin and inflammatory cells that form bridges. (Hematoxylin and eosin stain used.)

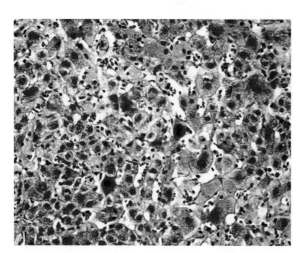

Figure 44.21 Acute viral hepatitis, moderate severity. Note ballooned hepatocytes together with scattered acidophil bodies (towards the center of biopsy). There is a moderate inflammatory infiltrate. (Hematoxylin and eosin stain used.)

CHAPTER 45

Chronic hepatitis B viral infection

Robert G. Gish

Stanford University, Palo Alto, CA and
Hepatitis B Foundation, Doylestown, PA, USA

Hepatitis B viral (HBV) infection remains one of the most common chronic infections in the world. In addition, chronic HBV accounts for one of the most devastating and common cancers in the world, hepatocellular carcinoma, which is now the second leading cause of liver cancer worldwide. The lifetime risk of death caused by HBV is approximately 30% in individuals who are chronically infected (Figure 45.1). Unfortunately, most patients with chronic hepatitis B remain undiagnosed because of the lack of population screening. If a diagnosis of chronic HBV infection is made, often little intervention takes place because of the lack of symptoms in most patients and a lack of knowledge of the rapidly evolving therapies available for HBV infection, which can result in viral control in up to 95% of patients. It is important for all practitioners to understand that HBV infection is suppressible and controllable in many patients although no curative therapy is yet available. Viral suppression can markedly improve long-term outcomes and decrease the rate of death, cirrhosis, liver transplant, and liver cancer. Understanding all aspects of HBV disease is essential to the management of this complex problem. The physician managing HBV infection must be a liver specialist, virologist, radiologist, clinician, pathologist, and oncologist, combined. Each practitioner must understand the natural history of the various forms of chronic hepatitis B infection and recognize the multiple ways in which a patient may present (Figure 45.1). Each patient group with chronic HBV infection is quite heterogeneous in the initial presentation, serological, genotype (Figure 45.2) and quantitative nucleic acid test pattern, as well as clinical course. Each patient needs to be monitored for changes in liver enzymes (ALT/AST), liver function tests (albumin, INR, and bilirubin), and serological status and viral replication (HBV DNA by PCR) at least every 6 months. This monitoring process allows interventions to take place for those patients who have ongoing replication and those who clinically manifest with progressive liver disease. Ultrasound testing every 6 months for patients with cirrhosis, family history of liver cancer, African ancestry, or elevated HCC biomarker(s), as well as those who have carried HBV infection for more than 40–50 years, will help in the early identification of patients who develop hepatocellular carcinoma. Liver biopsy or elastography should be considered in all patients with elevated liver enzymes who have HBV and have indeterminate laboratory tests for significant fibrosis or may have additional diseases such as fatty liver. Understanding the scoring system for liver fibrosis and inflammation, and applying this system to the liver biopsy for each patient who has had a liver biopsy is important to reproducibly stage the patient's liver disease. Currently, with the advent of noninvasive tests such as elastography, liver biopsy is performed or needed in a distinct minority of patients. The elastography, imaging, blood test, and/or biopsy information can be used to counsel patients about the chances of developing cirrhosis, cancer, the need for transplant, and the risk of disease transmission, as well as the possibility of identifying additional diagnoses.

A 26-year-old man who had a history of more than 50 sexual partners presented with elevated liver enzymes that normalized after 1 month of follow-up. The serum liver enzyme levels were markedly elevated again 3 months later. The patient underwent a liver biopsy and had active liver disease with positive core and surface antigen immunoperoxidase stains as well as grade 3 inflammation and stage 3 fibrosis (Figure 45.3a–d). The patient was treated with interferon therapy but could not tolerate interferon due to the severe fatigue associated with the treatment. Interferon treatment was subsequently discontinued. The patient's liver tests normalized for 4 months and serum levels of HBV DNA were 2000 IU/mL. After this 4-month interval there was a sudden increase in liver enzymes and the serum level of HBV DNA increased to more than 10 million IU/mL. Entecavir (0.5 mg orally per day) was initiated. There was a subsequent rapid decrease in liver enzyme levels and the serum HBV DNA became undetectable after 6 months of therapy. The patient's serum became negative for hepatitis B early antigen (HBeAg) at 14 months and positive for anti-HBe at month 16.

Yamada's Atlas of Gastroenterology, Fifth Edition. Edited by Daniel K. Podolsky, Michael Camilleri, J. Gregory Fitz, Anthony N. Kalloo, Fergus Shanahan, and Timothy C. Wang.
© 2016 John Wiley & Sons, Ltd. Published 2016 by John Wiley & Sons, Ltd.
Companion website: www.yamadagastro.com/atlas

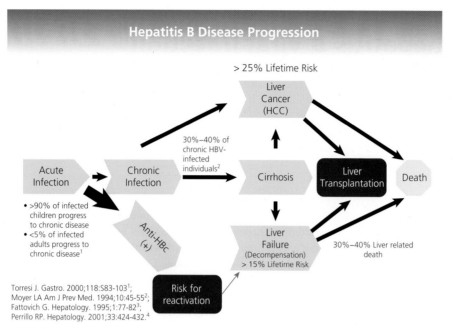

Figure 45.1 Natural history of chronic hepatitis B. Source: Courtesy of W. Ray Kim, MD.

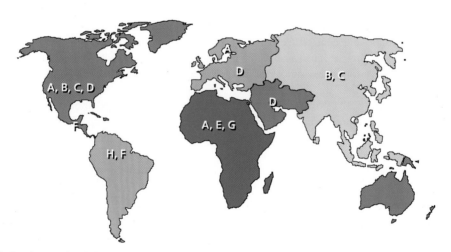

Figure 45.2 Worldwide distribution of eight hepatitis B virus (HBV) genotypes, based on the complete HBV genome.

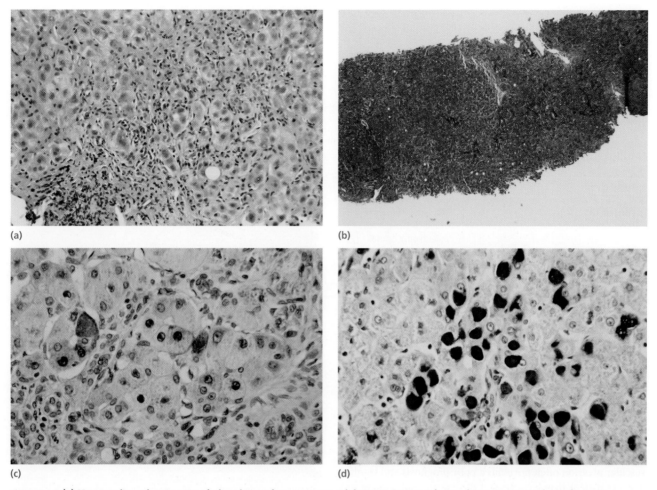

Figure 45.3 (a) Hematoxylin and eosin stain of a liver biopsy from a patient with hepatitis B virus infection demonstrating grade 3 inflammation. **(b)** Trichrome staining demonstrating stage 3 fibrosis. **(c)** Immunoperoxidase staining for hepatitis B core antigen. **(d)** Immunoperoxidase staining for hepatitis B surface antigen.

The serum levels of liver enzymes were normal and HBV DNA was negative 2 years after entecavir therapy was initiated and subsequently entecavir was stopped 1 year after HBeAg sero-conversion. Table 45.1 outlines the suggested patient groups for observation or treatment.

A 35-year-old Romanian woman who was infected with HBV and hepatitis D virus (HDV) presented with jaundice, ascites, and encephalopathy. She rapidly developed coma within the ensuing 6 weeks and underwent a liver transplant. A liver biopsy was performed 6 months before her clinical presentation with rapidly progressive liver disease in her transplanted liver. The patient died of recurrent HDV infection and liver failure after the liver transplant despite hepatitis B immunoglobulin therapy and adequate serum levels of immunoglobulin. Liver tissue photomicrographs are shown in Figure 45.4a–c and demonstrate hematoxylin and eosin, trichrome, and delta antigen staining, respectively.

A 23-year-old woman with chronic HBV infection after a liver transplant developed a rapidly progressive liver disease in the transplanted liver, with jaundice and liver dysfunction. Liver biopsy results indicated fibrosing cholestatic hepatitis (Figure 45.5a,b) and positive in situ HBV DNA stain throughout the liver tissue. The clinical course in this patient was modified by the addition of a nucleoside analogue, lamivudine. Her jaundice, ascites, and abnormal coagulation tests corrected to normal within 3 months of initiating antiviral therapy. She remains well 8 years later and a liver biopsy shows early cirrhosis but no evidence of progression by physical examination or by liver synthetic abnormalities.

A 45-year-old man presented with chronic HBV infection and cirrhosis, and waited 2 years before undergoing a liver transplant for evolving liver failure. The patient had a known hepatoma at the time of liver transplant, which was a single lesion, less than 5 cm in diameter, without evidence of vascular invasion by four-phase computed tomography. After the liver transplant, the explant and tumor (Figure 45.6a) were examined microscopically in detail by the pathologist and the tumor was found to have microvascular invasion (Figure 45.6b). The

Table 45.1 Management of chronic hepatitis B virus (HBV) infection. Source: Modified from Gish RG. Clin Liver Dis 2005;9:541. Reproduced with permission of Elsevier.

HBV DNA level	ALT activity	
	<17–25 U/L[a]	>17–25 U/L
<2000 IU/mL for HBeAg(−); <20000 IU/mL for HBeAg(+)	Observe[b]	Perform biopsy or treat[c]
>2000 IU/mL for HBeAg(−) >20000 IU/mL for HBeAg(+)	Treat if active HBV infection on liver biopsy	Treat: HBeAg(+): ≥6 months after eAg seroconversion; HBeAg(−): prolonged treatment (≥24 months) beyond NAT negative[d] Consider biopsy or use noninvasive fibrosis testing such as elastography

[a] Upper limit of normal for a person with a normal body mass index.
[b] Treat any patient with cirrhosis who is NAT positive, refer to specialist.
[c] Rule out fatty liver and other causes of chronic liver disease.
[d] Consider 3–5 years.
ALT, alanine aminotransferase; HBeAg, hepatitis B early antigen; NAT, nucleic acid testing, such as polymerase chain reaction, branched DNA, transcription-mediated amplification.

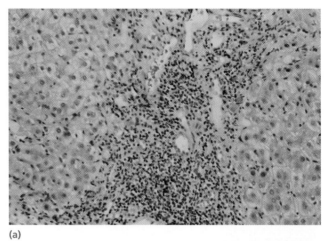

(a)

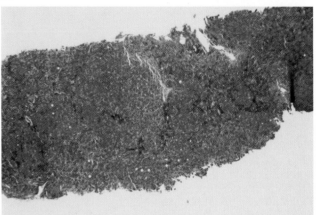

(b)

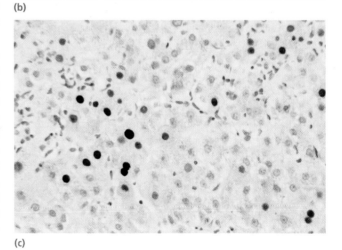

(c)

Figure 45.6 (a) Hematoxylin and eosin stain of a liver biopsy specimen demonstrating grade 3 inflammation. (b) Trichrome staining demonstrating stage 3 fibrosis. (c) Immunoperoxidase staining for hepatitis delta antigen

patient died 1 year later of brain metastasis. The finding of vascular invasion often portends a poor prognosis and signifies that the patient may have stage 4 disease and subsequent risk for disseminated cancer.

Fortunately, the incidence of acute HBV infection has been decreasing in the USA during the last two to three decades (Figure 45.7). With the introduction of neonatal vaccination and screening of pregnant mothers throughout the world, there is a clear expectation that not only will early deaths due to hepatocellular carcinoma decline but also that the incidence of end-stage liver disease caused by HBV will also decrease, with a subsequent fall in the demand for liver transplantation for chronic HBV infection. The mandate for occupational safety, vaccination of adolescents, and education of individuals involved in high-risk activities are also very important public health policies to prevent new infections and change the epidemiology of this disease.

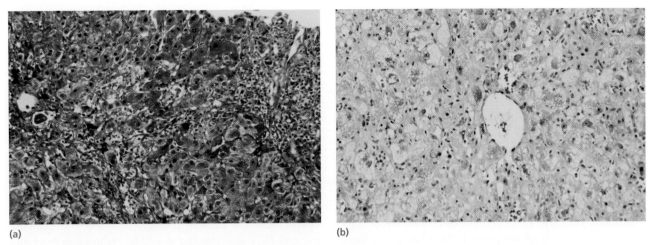

(a)   (b)

Figure 45.5 **(a)** Fibrosing cholestatic hepatitis (trichrome stain). **(b)** Fibrosing cholestatic hepatitis (hematoxylin and eosin stain).

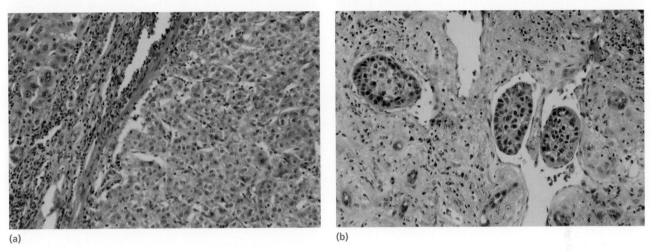

(a)   (b)

Figure 45.6 **(a)** Liver cancer (hepatoma, hepatocellular carcinoma). **(b)** Liver cancer invading a blood vessel.

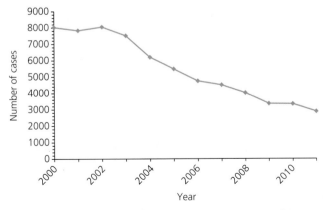

Figure 45.7 Reported number of acute hepatitis B cases in United States, 2000–2011. Source: National Notifiable Disease Surveillance System (NNDSS).

CHAPTER 46

Hepatitis C virus infection

Raymond T. Chung[1] and Andrew Tai[2]

[1] Massachusetts General Hospital and Harvard Medical School, Boston, MA, USA
[2] University of Michigan and VA Ann Arbor Healthcare System, Ann Arbor, MI, USA

Hepatitis C virus (HCV) is an enveloped positive-sense, single-stranded RNA virus of the genus Hepacivirus in the family Flaviridae (Figure 46.1). Among the 10 mature viral proteins are several that are targets for antiviral therapeutic agents, including the NS3/4A serine protease, the NS5A nonstructural protein, and the NS5B RNA-dependent RNA polymerase.

HCV infects hepatocytes (Figure 46.2), leading in many chronically infected individuals to a typical histopathological pattern of a mononuclear portal tract infiltrate with interface hepatitis (Figure 46.3). In many individuals, chronic HCV infection leads to progressive hepatic fibrosis and ultimately cirrhosis, which is associated with an elevated risk of hepatocellular carcinoma and liver failure (Figure 46.4).

In the United States, populations with increased HCV seroprevalence have been identified (Box 46.1) and should be offered anti-HCV antibody testing. An individual with a positive anti-HCV antibody test should be evaluated to determine whether chronic infection is present and, if so, antiviral therapy should be considered (Figure 46.5). Table 46.1 summarizes diagnostic tests for HCV infection, including anti-HCV antibody testing, HCV RNA testing, and HCV genotyping. Several classes of direct-acting antiviral (DAA) drugs targeting viral proteins (Table 46.2) have led to interferon-free regimens for the treatment of chronic HCV infection. In situations where DAAs are not available, treatment with peginterferon and ribavirin can be considered; Box 46.2 lists contraindications to the use of peginterferon and ribavirin.

Yamada's Atlas of Gastroenterology, Fifth Edition. Edited by Daniel K. Podolsky, Michael Camilleri, J. Gregory Fitz, Anthony N. Kalloo, Fergus Shanahan, and Timothy C. Wang.
© 2016 John Wiley & Sons, Ltd. Published 2016 by John Wiley & Sons, Ltd.
Companion website: www.yamadagastro.com/atlas

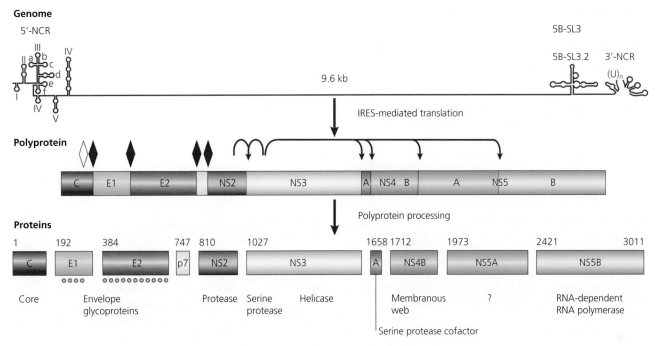

Figure 46.1 Genetic and polyprotein organization of HCV. HCV is encoded by a single-stranded, 9.6-kilobase RNA genome flanked by 5′ and 3′ noncoding regions (NCRs), depicted at the top of the diagram. A single large polyprotein precursor (middle) is generated by translation of the positive-sense RNA; translation initiation occurs at an internal ribosome entry site (IRES) located at the 5′ NCR. The HCV polyprotein is then cleaved by the endoplasmic reticulum signal peptidase (black diamonds), signal peptide peptidase (open diamond), and the HCV NS2 and NS3/4A viral proteases (arrows) to release the 10 mature viral proteins (bottom). Numbers indicate the amino acid position relative to the HCV H strain (genotype 1a, GenBank accession number AF009606). Source: Moradpour D, Penin Fand Rice CM. Replication of hepatitis C virus. Nat Rev Microbiol 2007;5:453. Reprinted with permission of Macmillan Publishers Ltd.

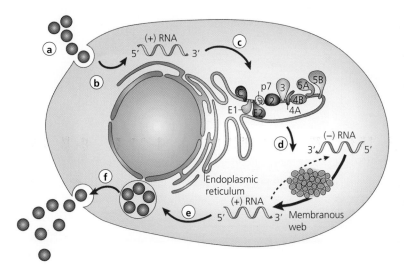

Figure 46.2 Life cycle of HCV infection. Cell entry of HCV (a) requires the host receptors CD81, scavenger class B type 1 receptor (SR-B1), claudin-1, and occludin. After virus internalization and uncoating (b), the positive-sense RNA genome is translated at the endoplasmic reticulum to a single polyprotein, which is processed to release the 10 mature viral proteins (c). HCV induces the formation of an altered host membrane compartment called the membranous web (d), where a negative-sense RNA intermediate is transcribed and used as a template for the production of positive-sense HCV genomes. HCV virions are then assembled at or in the vicinity of cellular lipid droplets (e), followed by secretion of assembled virions through the endoscopic reticulum and Golgi apparatus (f), where the envelope proteins E1 and E2 become glycosylated. Source: Moradpour D, Penin Fand Rice CM. Replication of hepatitis C virus. Nat Rev Microbiol 2007;5:453. Reprinted with permission of Macmillan Publishers Ltd.

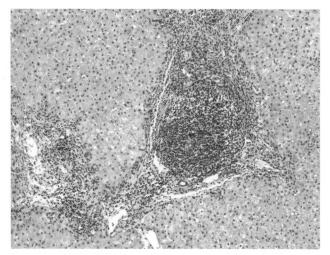

Figure 46.3 Typical histology of HCV-infected liver. This micrograph (100×) of a hematoxylin and eosin-stained liver biopsy specimen depicts the typical mononuclear portal tract infiltrate seen in chronic HCV infection. The mononuclear infiltrate is composed predominantly of lymphocytes, which often forms aggregates or even distinct lymphoid follicles with germinal centers, and occasional plasma cells and eosinophils. There may be evidence of interlobular bile duct damage. Interface hepatitis, formerly known as "piecemeal necrosis," is characterized by chronic inflammation extending beyond the limiting plate of the portal tract and is also seen in this micrograph. Lobular activity can consist of acidophil bodies, chronic inflammation, and occasional epithelioid-cell granulomas; confluent necrosis is not typically seen. An increase in stainable iron is often found, although hepatic iron content is not quantitatively elevated in the majority of cases. Another common finding in chronic HCV infection, not well seen in this micrograph, is hepatic steatosis, particularly with genotype 3 infection. Source: Courtesy of Dr. Joseph Misdraji, Massachusetts General Hospital, Boston, MA.

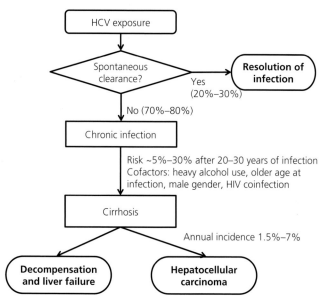

Figure 46.4 Natural history of HCV infection. This figure illustrates the possible outcomes of HCV exposure. Up to 30% of exposed individuals may spontaneously clear their infection, while 70%–80% develop chronic HCV infection. The estimated risk of progression to cirrhosis varies significantly depending on the population studied; some of the cofactors believed to accelerate fibrosis progression are shown. Once advanced fibrosis/cirrhosis develops, then the patient is at increased risk of developing hepatocellular carcinoma and/or liver failure, which is manifested clinically by decompensated cirrhosis (e.g., ascites, portal hypertensive gastrointestinal bleeding, jaundice, and/or hepatic encephalopathy).

Box 46.1 Recommendations for HCV testing in high-risk populations.

All adults born between 1945 and 1965
People who have ever injected illegal drugs, even only once
HIV-infected individuals
History of receiving clotting factor concentrates produced before 1987
Any history of chronic hemodialysis
Unexplained abnormal alanine aminotransferase levels
History of receiving blood, blood product transfusion, or organ transplant before 1992
Children born to HCV-positive mothers
Healthcare, emergency medical, and public safety workers after percutaneous or mucosal exposure to HCV-positive blood

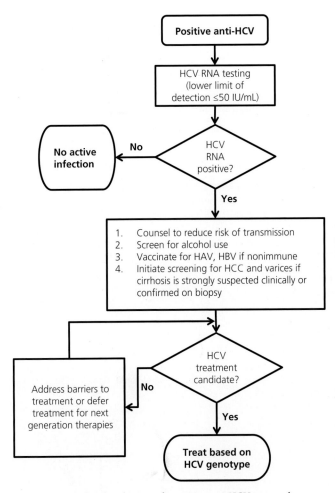

Table 46.1 Diagnostic tests for HCV infection.

Test	Clinical application
Anti-HCV EIA (enzyme immunoassay)	Detects anti-HCV antibodies Screening test of choice for HCV infection, but does not distinguish between resolved (spontaneously cleared or successfully treated) and active infection
RIBA (recombinant immunoblot assay)	Historically used to confirm a positive anti-HCV EIA result Like anti-HCV EIA, does not distinguish between active and resolved infection Largely supplanted by HCV RNA testing, but may be useful to evaluate a suspected false-positive anti-HCV EIA result
Qualitative HCV RNA	Reports the absence or presence of detectable HCV RNA Can be used to confirm active infection following a positive anti-HCV EIA, or to evaluate for HCV clearance on or following antiviral therapy Historically more sensitive than first-generation quantitative HCV RNA assays, but has been largely replaced by highly sensitive quantitative assays with lower limits of detection of ≤ 50 IU/mL
Quantitative HCV RNA	Highly sensitive quantitative assays with lower limits of detection of ≤ 50 IU/mL Can be used to confirm active HCV infection and to monitor HCV RNA levels during and following antiviral therapy
HCV genotyping	Used to determine the genotype and, in some assays, the subtype in an HCV-infected individual Essential for determining an antiviral regimen and duration of therapy Not necessary if the patient is not a treatment candidate
Quantitative core antigen immunoassay	Detects HCV core antigen levels in serum or plasma Correlates with HCV RNA levels and may be useful to confirm HCV infection and to guide treatment in resource-constrained settings where routine HCV RNA testing is not feasible

Figure 46.5 Suggested evaluation of a positive anti-HCV test result. Because anti-HCV does not distinguish between active and resolved infection, the next step is to confirm the presence of active infection using a sensitive HCV RNA test. If the HCV RNA is undetectable, then the patient does not have active HCV infection. On the other hand, if infection is confirmed, further evaluation is suggested. In rare instances, during acute HCV infection, HCV RNA may become transiently undetectable, so longitudinal HCV RNA testing is advisable under these circumstances. HCC, hepatocellular carcinoma.

Table 46.2 Classes of direct-acting antiviral (DAA) therapies.

Viral target	Examples	Barrier to resistance	Comments
NS3/4A serine protease			
First-generation	Telaprevir, boceprevir	Low	Genotype-selective
Second-generation	simeprevir, paritaprevir, faldaprevir, asunaprevir, grazoprevir, danoprevir, vedroprevir	Moderate due to higher potency	
NS5A	Ledipasvir, daclatasvir, ombitasvir, GS-5816, elbasvir, ACH-3102	Low	High potency; some with broad activity against multiple genotypes
NS5B RNA-dependent RNA polymerase			
Nucleos(t)ide inhibitors	Sofosbuvir, mericitabine	High (low genetic barrier but high fitness cost as resistance mutations impair replication)	Generally have broader activity against multiple genotypes
Nonnucleoside inhibitors	Dasabuvir, beclabuvir, tegobuvir, ABT-072, GS-9669, setrobuvir	Low	Genotype-selective

Box 46.2 Contraindications to HCV treatment with peginterferon and ribavirin.

Peginterferon
  Uncontrolled psychiatric illness
  Decompensated cirrhosis outside of the pretransplant setting
  Comorbidities that significantly limit life expectancy
  Nonadherence to prior therapy or with pretreatment appointments
  Uncontrolled autoimmune disorders such as autoimmune hepatitis
    or psoriasis
  Solid organ transplant recipient (other than liver)
  Ongoing alcohol abuse or dependence
  Ongoing injection drug use (relative contraindication)
Ribavirin (if contraindicated, peginterferon monotherapy can be
  considered)
  Glomerular filtration rate (GFR) <50 mL/min or chronic hemodialysis
  Inability to tolerate anemia (e.g., severe cardiopulmonary disease)
  Pregnancy, planned pregnancy in patient or partner, or
    unwillingness to comply with contraception during therapy and
    for 6 months after completion of therapy

CHAPTER 47

Drug-induced liver disease

Frank V. Schiødt[1] and William M. Lee[2]

[1] Bispebjerg Hospital, Copenhagen, Denmark
[2] University of Texas Southwestern Medical Center, Dallas, TX, USA

Drug-induced liver injury (DILI) has become an important topic as it often determines the success or failure of new, potentially valuable agents. In recent years, careful attention to hepatic injury during phase III trials has reduced the number of drugs withdrawn after approval by FDA or by EMEA, its European counterpart. Drugs can cause hepatotoxicity in either a dose-dependent, or a dose-independent (idiosyncratic) fashion. Both types of drug-induced liver injury are very frequent causes of acute liver failure with hepatic encephalopathy and coagulopathy (Figure 47.1), although the proportion of cases of acute liver failure caused by drugs varies greatly worldwide (Table 47.1 and Figure 47.2).

Idiosyncratic drug reactions occur rarely (in 1:10000–1:100000 persons using the specific drug). Enzyme polymorphisms in one of the cytochrome P450 (CYP) or other genes undoubtedly play a role in many susceptible patients. However, the clinical role and value of pharmacogenetics are just beginning to emerge.

Acetaminophen (paracetamol) exemplifies a drug which is hepatotoxic in a dose-dependent manner. Acetaminophen is extremely safe when taken within the recommended doses (4 g/day), but doses of 8–10 g/day may cause severe liver necrosis. Figure 47.3 describes the metabolic pathways of acetaminophen. The highly reactive metabolite N-acetyl-p-benzoquinone imine (NAPQI) is responsible for its toxicity. NAPQI can bind covalently to cellular proteins and cause blebbing and later lysis of the hepatocyte. Acetaminophen-induced acute liver failure develops within days after ingestion of the overdose. Biochemical characteristics include very high aminotransferase levels (5000–25000 IU/L), and often also an elevated creatinine level because of a concomitant, direct nephrotoxic effect of acetaminophen. Liver transplantation is not frequently performed for patients with acetaminophen-induced acute liver failure because the disease progresses too rapidly, or medical, or social contraindications preclude transplantation. In addition, the spontaneous (transplantation free) survival rate is better (approximately 70%) than for other causes of acute liver failure, and liver transplantation is not needed for most patients. Cases of acetaminophen toxicity can be missed if the patient is encephalopathic on arrival or does not admit to use of acetaminophen. In these instances, a newly developed assay that can measure acetaminophen protein adducts is effective in identifying the "smoking gun" (Figure 47.4).

Idiosyncratic drug-induced liver injury differs from acetaminophen-induced acute liver failure in a number of ways, including a slower onset of symptoms and lower spontaneous (transplantation free) survival rates. Biochemical differences are also apparent in lower aminotransferase and creatinine levels and higher bilirubin levels. Unlike acetaminophen, most idiosyncratic reactions do not appear to be dose related. As they occur very rarely (1:10000–1:100000 exposures), there must be some genetic predisposition to explain an altered metabolic pathway (Figure 47.5), or host response. One theory is that the initial alteration in cell proteins leads to the release of cytokines (the danger hypothesis, Figure 47.6), which augment the initial pattern of injury. The mechanisms that result in damage to liver cells in cases of idiosyncratic toxicity are varied, as are the effects on the liver. Figure 47.7 describes some of the mechanisms that may be involved in this damage. As with acetaminophen, it is likely that drugs that cause significant liver injury lead to highly reactive intermediates that bind irreversibly to cell proteins, leading to formation of haptens that can then provoke an immune attack mediated by cytotoxic T cells and possibly B cells (autoantibody formation) as well. The rarity of DILI indicates that there is likely something distinctive about the patient who reacts to an agent that most people tolerate. Recently, attention has been focused on determining the genetic basis for this uniqueness via genome-wide association studies (GWAS). Figure 47.7 demonstrates a Manhattan plot, indicating single nucleotide polymorphisms on chromosome 6 that represent HLA haplotypes, confirming the immune nature of most drug reactions. Table 47.2 indicates some of the haplotypes that have

Yamada's Atlas of Gastroenterology, Fifth Edition. Edited by Daniel K. Podolsky, Michael Camilleri, J. Gregory Fitz, Anthony N. Kalloo, Fergus Shanahan, and Timothy C. Wang.
© 2016 John Wiley & Sons, Ltd. Published 2016 by John Wiley & Sons, Ltd.
Companion website: www.yamadagastro.com/atlas

been identified for various drugs. The color-coding demonstrates that some HLA markers are common to more than one drug. In spite of some success with GWAS, the genomic signature for most drugs continues to be elusive.

Idiosyncratic drug-induced hepatotoxicity has been described for a large number of drugs. Implicated agents include antibiotics (including isoniazid as the most commonly recognized), nonsteroidal agents, seizure medications, and a miscellaneous group. The proportion of drug-induced liver disease varies greatly among drug classes as evidence of class effect. The majority of reactions are directed against hepatocytes, but biliary injury and combined hepatocyte-biliary injury or damage to specific organelles can produce the different disease patterns observed (Figure 47.8). Figure 47.9 displays some of the different histological patterns of acute liver failure caused by drugs. One important issue is that of establishing causality. This is usually limited to a process of guilt by association, establishing

that the drug was given in an appropriate time interval in relation to the hepatic injury and that other causes were excluded (Box 47.1)

A number of drugs have been approved after careful clinical trials only to be subsequently severely restricted or withdrawn by the US Food and Drug Administration (FDA) following identification of toxic reactions that had been unrecognized in the approval process (Table 47.3 and Figure 47.10). This is because, once approved, the exposure is much greater and the prescribing pattern much broader than that observed in the approval trial. A rare reaction (e.g. 1:50 000) is unlikely to be

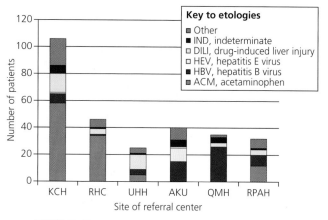

Figure 47.2 Prevalence of different etiologies of acute liver failure around the world as indicated by the number of patients seen at large referral centers over a 1 year period. Acetaminophen and drug-induced liver injury predominate in developing countries while viral hepatitis is observed in Asia and the developing world.

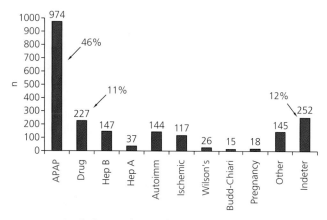

Figure 47.1 Graph showing the prevalence of different etiologies in the registry of the US Acute Liver Failure (ALF) Study Group from 1998 to 2014 (n = 2172 patients). There has been a significant increase in the number of cases of acetaminophen poisoning since 1998. These very often involve narcotic–acetaminophen combinations.
APAP, acetaminophen.

Table 47.1 The presumed etiology of acute liver failure in different parts of the world.

	ACM (%)	HAV (%)	HBV (%)	Drug (%)	Shock (%)	Indeterminate (%)	Other (%)
Argentina 1996–2001 (n = 83)	0	8	22	14	0	25	31
Denmark 1973–1990 (n = 160)	19	2	31	17	3	15	13
France 1972–1990 (n = 502)	2	4	44	15	7	18	11
India 1987–1993 (n = 423)	0	2	31	5	0	0	62
Japan 1992–1999 (n = 38)	0	3	18	0	0	71	8
United Kingdom 1993–1994 (n = 342)	73	2	2	2	3	8	9
United States 1994–1996 (n = 295)	20	7	10	12	3	15	33
United States 1998–2006 (n = 1033)	46	3	7	12	4	15	13

ACM, acetaminophen; drug, idiosyncratic drug reactions; HAV, hepatitis A virus; HBV, hepatitis B virus; shock, ischemic hepatitis.
All studies have cases of hepatitis A and hepatitis B, whereas acetaminophen-induced acute liver failure is a feature of studies in Western countries.
Idiosyncratic drug reactions typically constitute 12%–17% of cases, with India, Japan, and the United Kingdom reporting fewer cases.

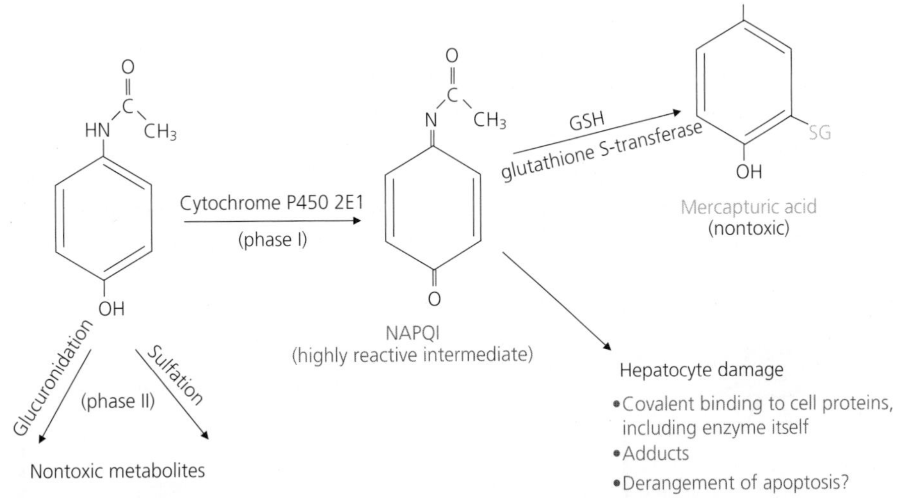

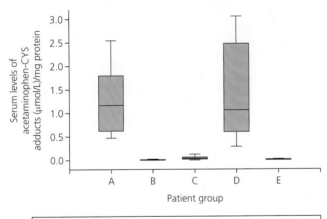

Figure 47.3 The metabolic pathways of acetaminophen. The major hepatic pathways include glucuronidation and sulfation (left), which yield nontoxic water-soluble conjugates that are excreted by the kidney (top right). A second pathway involves the cytochrome P450 (CYP) system, especially CYP2E1, by which acetaminophen is metabolized to the highly reactive metabolite N-acetyl-p-benzoquinone imine (NAPQI), which may bind covalently with hepatic proteins and cause cellular necrosis (lower right). The toxic effect of NAPQI is eliminated by binding to the natural antidote glutathionine (GSH), yielding mercapturic acid, a nontoxic, water-soluble excretion product. N-acetylcysteine serves as an antidote by replenishing glutathione. Alcohol may enhance toxicity by induction of CYP2E1 or by depleting hepatic glutathione stores.

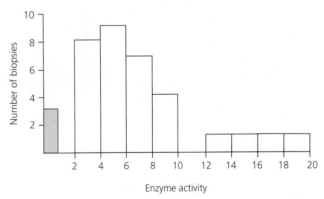

Figure 47.5 Genetic polymorphisms occur in cytochrome P450 (CYP450) enzymes. In this example, debrisoquine hydroxylase, CYP2D6, is present in several forms that differ greatly in their enzyme activity from nil to very high levels. These naturally occurring differences explain why individuals may metabolize drugs very differently.

Key
A, patients with acute liver failure (ALF) secondary to known acetaminophen overdose
B, patients with ALF due to nonacetaminophen causes
C, patients with acetaminophen overdose but no ALF
D, patients with ALF of indeterminate etiology and detectable serum adducts
E, patients with ALF of indeterminate etiology and negative adducts

Figure 47.4 Serum levels of acetaminophen-CYS adducts in patient groups. The boxes represent the 25th–75th interquartile range and the horizontal line represents the median. The extremes of the population are represented by the endmarks.

identified during an approval trial involving 5000 patients. Evidence of elevation of aminotransferase levels in a significant number of patients combined with any elevation of bilirubin often serves to elevate concern for FDA reviewers assessing phase III trials submitted as the basis for approval. Experience shows that if jaundice attributable to the drug in question is observed in any patients during the trial, then with larger numbers of patient exposures there is likely to be hepatic failure in ∼10% of those developing jaundice. This is sometimes referred to as "Hy's Law" in honor of Hyman Zimmerman, the father of the study of drug-induced liver injury (Figure 47.11). A final word: drug toxicity from herbal medications is also common and ranks near to drug toxicity from antibiotics in frequency (Figure 47.12). Studies are difficult to perform but it appears that herbal medication-related toxicity is increasing in this country, and currently represents 20% of all DILI in a recent study.

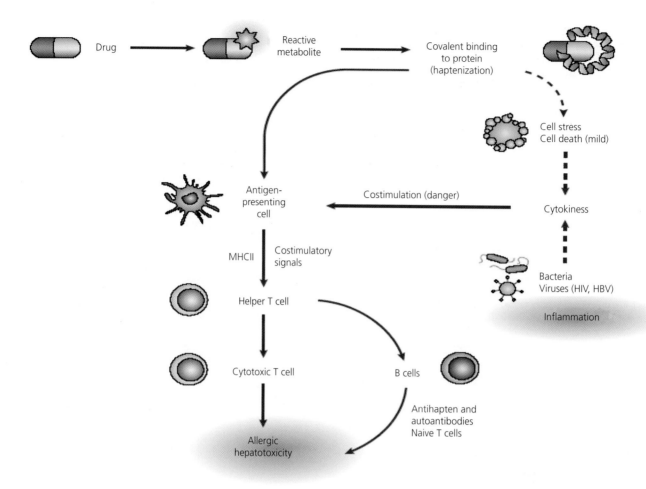

Figure 47.6 The danger hypothesis proposes that covalent binding to cell proteins (see (c) and (d) in Figure 47.8) initiates cytokine responses that then augment the injury to the cell in certain settings.
HBV, hepatitis B virus; HIV, human immunodeficiency virus; MHCII, major histocompatibility complex II.

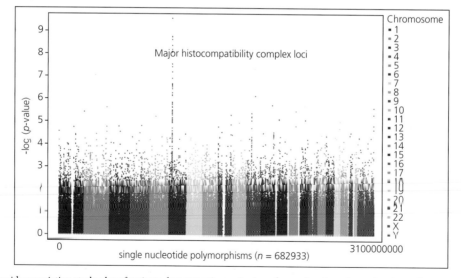

Figure 47.7 Genome wide association study plot of patients demonstrating aminotransferase elevations due to lumiracoxib, a nonsteroidal antiinflammatory agent. Nearly a million comparisons are made using a gene chip technique. The y-axis is –log10 p values for the specific single nucleotide polymorphisms ISNPs) that are unique to patients when compared with unaffected controls and the x-axis represents the chromosomes. The large number of decimal places reflects that significance is only obtained at a level of $p < 0.000000001$ because of nearly a million comparisons.

Table 47.2 MHC haplotypes associated with specific drug-related injury events. Note that certain haplotypes are common to more than one drug as indicated by color coding.

HLA Haplotype	Drug reaction	Drug
HLA B*1502	Stevens/Johnson/TEN	Carbamazepine
DRB1*0701/DQA1*02	Hepatotoxicity	Ximelagatran
DQA1*02	Hepatotoxicity	Lumiracoxib
DRB1*1501/DQA1*0102	Mixed hepatotoxicity	Amoxicillin-clavulanate
HLA B*5701	Hypersensitivity/hepatotoxicity	Abacavir
DRB1*0701/HLA B*5701	Hepatotoxicity	Flucloxacillin

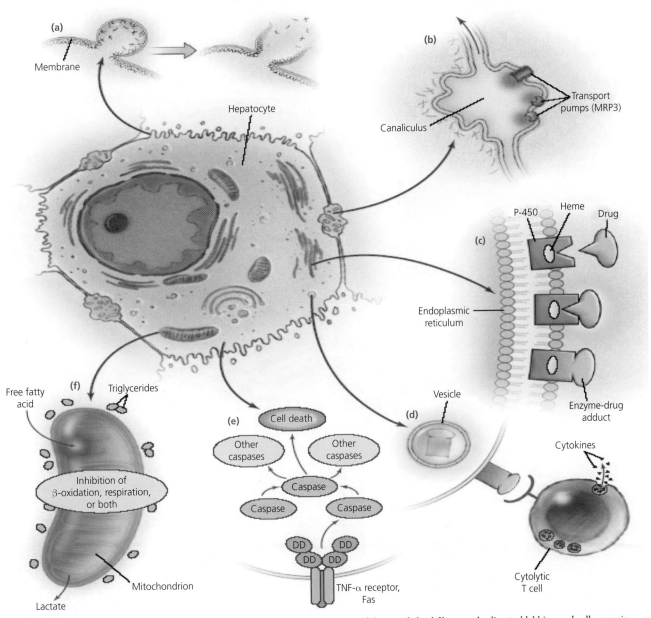

Figure 47.8 Proposed mechanisms of liver cell injury due to drugs. **(a)** Disruption of the cytoskeletal filaments leading to blebbing and cell necrosis. **(b)** Damage to biliary canalicular transport mechanisms causes cholestasis. **(c)** Highly reactive intermediates that bind to cell proteins lead to hapten formation. **(d)** These neoantigens can be transported to the cell surface and evoke a cytotoxic immune response or autoantibody formation. **(e)** Apoptotic mechanisms can also take place. **(f)** Mitochondrial disruption leads to accumulation of microvesicular fat in hepatocytes as well as lactic acid formation due to anaerobic metabolism.

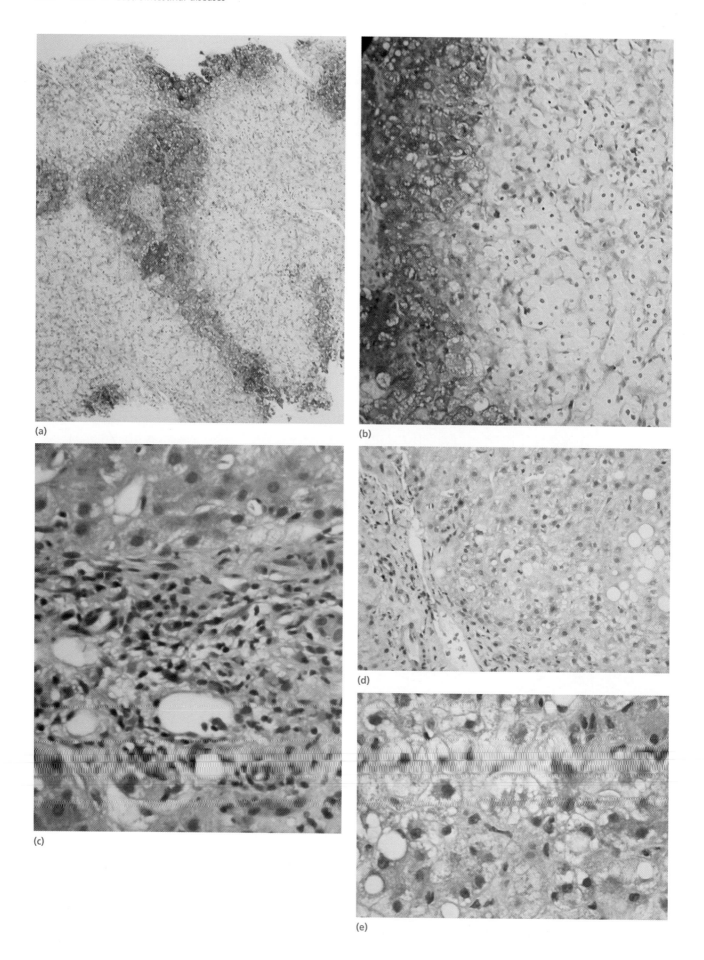

(a)

(b)

(c)

(d)

(e)

Figure 47.9 A variety of histological patterns of acute liver injury are caused by drugs. **(a)** Characteristic pattern of acetaminophen toxicity with acute necrosis-apoptosis of zones 2 and 3 (centrilobular region), with sparing of zone 1 (periportal region) (periodic acid-Schiff [PAS] stain; original magnification ×60). **(b)** Close-up view showing pattern of glycogen depletion and pyknotic nuclei in zones 2 and 3 (PAS stain; original magnification ×300). **(c)** Bile duct injury and eosinophilia in a patient with mixed cholestatic-hepatocellular injury caused by trimethoprim-sulfamethoxazole (Hematoxylin and Eosin [H & E] stain; original magnification ×240). **(d)** Diffuse cellular unrest with cell swelling and necrosis in a patient with fatal hepatitis caused by sulfasalazine (H & E stain; original magnification ×100). **(e)** Close-up view of cells with prominent ballooning degeneration in the same patient as shown in **(d)** (H & E stain; original magnification ×500).

Box 47.1 Components of the Roussel Uclaf causality assessment method (RUCAM).

Points awarded for the following categories:
1 Time of onset
2 Course
3 Risk factors (age, alcohol)
4 Concomitant drugs
5 Search for non drug causes
6 Previous information on hepatotoxicity of the drug
7 Response to readministration

- Components of most causality assessment methods (CAMs) are similar.
- CAMs are efforts to codify the practice of "guilt by association."
- The most significant components are temporal relationship and exclusion of other causes.
- Most drugs cause injury at a delay from the initial dose (latency).
- The usual interval is 5–90 days, with drug reactions being very rare after 6 months of continuous ingestion.
- Response to rechallenge with a medication is seldom used as it is risky; however, it may be the most reliable evidence that a drug is implicated.
- It is undertaken only in extreme situations when the value and uniqueness of the drug are evident.

Table 47.3 Regulatory actions due to nonallergic hepatotoxicity.[a]

Drug	Use	Regulatory action
Acetaminophen	Analgesic	Warnings
Bromfenac	Analgesic	Withdrawn
Felbamate	Anticonvulsant	Restricted use
Leflunomide	Immunomodulator	Warnings
Nefazodone	Antipsychotic	Warnings
Nevirapine	Antiviral (HIV)	Warnings
Pemoline	Central nervous system stimulant	Restricted use
Pyrazinamide	Antituberculosis	Warnings
Rifampin	Antituberculosis	Warnings
Terbinafine	Antifungal	Warnings
Tolcapone	Parkinson disease	Restricted use
Troglitazone	Diabetes	Withdrawn
Trovafloxacin	Antibiotic	Restricted use
Valproic acid	Anticonvulsant	Warnings
Zafirlukast	Asthma	Warnings

[a] Ximelagatran, anticoagulant, never approved; telithromycin, antibiotic, restricted use.
Source: Data from Kaplowitz N. Idiosyncratic drug hepatotoxicity. Nat Rev Drug Disc 2005;4:489.

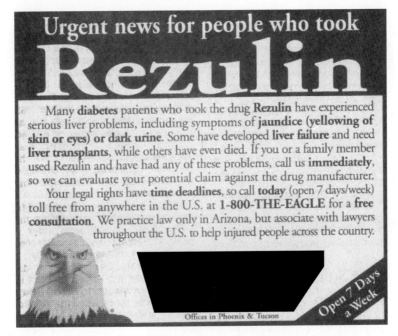

Figure 47.10 Rezulin was approved by the US Food and Drug Administration (FDA) in 1999, only to be withdrawn more than 3 years later after more than 50 deaths, or liver transplants. There are other ramifications to drug withdrawals as this nationally publicized advertisement indicates.

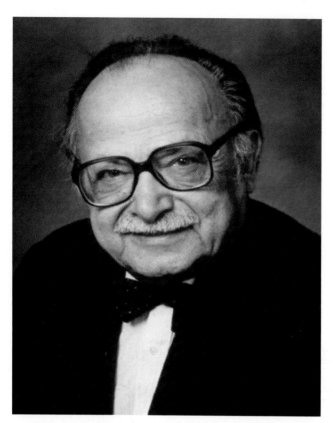

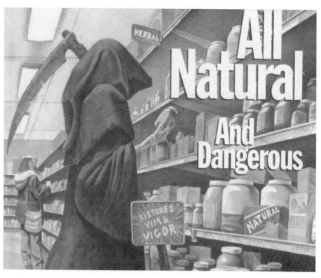

Figure 47.12 Health foods are not always healthy. After antibiotics, herbal medications are the second most common "drug class" implicated in hepatotoxicity. There is limited quality control of nutraceuticals and herbs. In addition, patients often take excessive doses because of their implied promise of safety, and take a variety of herbs simultaneously. Assessing causality in this setting is particularly difficult.

Figure 47.11 Hyman Zimmerman, MD, 1917–99, is the father of the field of drug-induced hepatotoxicity. "Hy's Law" suggests that if jaundice is observed in a clinical trial, the drug is likely to cause more severe toxicity when larger numbers of patients are exposed – once ten patients are jaundiced, one will be observed to have acute liver failure.

CHAPTER 48
Autoimmune hepatitis

Richard Taubert and Michael P. Manns

Hannover Medical School, Hannover, Germany

Autoimmune hepatitis (AIH) can occur in all age groups but has a female preponderance. External stimuli such as viral infections (e.g., hepatitis E) or drugs are thought to break hepatic tolerance and trigger a chronic autoimmune response against hepatocytes in genetically predisposed individuals. After the exclusion of other causes of hepatitis, the diagnosis is based on the profile of autoantibodies (Figures 48.1 and 48.2), the histology, and a suggestive polyclonal hypergammaglobulinemia. Depending on the types of autoantibodies detected, two subtypes of AIH can be distinguished, that is the more common type 1 and the rarer type 2 (Table 48.1). As pathognomonic features are missing, two scores were introduced to facilitate the diagnosis of AIH (Table 48.2).

The natural course of the AIH can include progressive liver damage and liver-related death within months to years. Suppression of the inflammatory activity (persistent normalization of transaminases and immunoglobulins) and a low to normal histological disease activity has the best clinical outcome with respect to liver fibrosis. Along this line, an immunosuppressive therapy should be considered in all patients with significant inflammatory activity. First-line therapy is based on steroids or a combination therapy of steroids with azathioprine (Table 48.3) and can achieve a biochemical remission in about 80% of patients within weeks. After persistent biochemical remission under maintenance doses over about 2 years, the histological remission should be assessed. The withdrawal of medication should be discussed critically because relapse rates are high even in cases of a complete remission under ongoing therapy. The immunosuppressive medication dramatically improves but does not normalize survival rates. Multiple salvage therapies for refractory AIH are described but not approved in controlled trials. Due to the generally good treatment responses, AIH rarely progresses to end-stage liver disease with the need for transplantation.

Table 48.1 Comparison of autoimmune hepatitis (AIH) types. Source: Data from Gleeson D, Heneghan MA; British Society of Gastroenterology. British Society of Gastroenterology (BSG) guidelines for management of autoimmune hepatitis. Gut 2011;60:1611 and Krawitt EL. Autoimmune hepatitis. N Engl J Med 2006;354:54.

Feature	AIH type 1	AIH type 2
Characteristic autoantibodies	ANA and/or SMA (70%–80%) Anti-SLA/LP (10%–30%) pANCA (50%–96%) Negative (10%–20%)	Anti-LKM1 (up to 100%) Anti-LC1 (20%–70%)
Geographical variation	Worldwide	Worldwide
Age at presentation	All age groups	Usually childhood and young adulthood
Gender (female : male)	3–4 : 1	9 : 1
Clinical presentation	Variable	Generally severe
Histological disease at presentation	Variable (mild to cirrhosis)	More inflammation and generally advanced
Treatment failure	Rare	Common
Relapse after drug withdrawal	Variable	Common
Need for long-term maintenance	Variable	Approximately 100%

Yamada's Atlas of Gastroenterology, Fifth Edition. Edited by Daniel K. Podolsky, Michael Camilleri, J. Gregory Fitz, Anthony N. Kalloo, Fergus Shanahan, and Timothy C. Wang.
© 2016 John Wiley & Sons, Ltd. Published 2016 by John Wiley & Sons, Ltd.
Companion website: www.yamadagastro.com/atlas

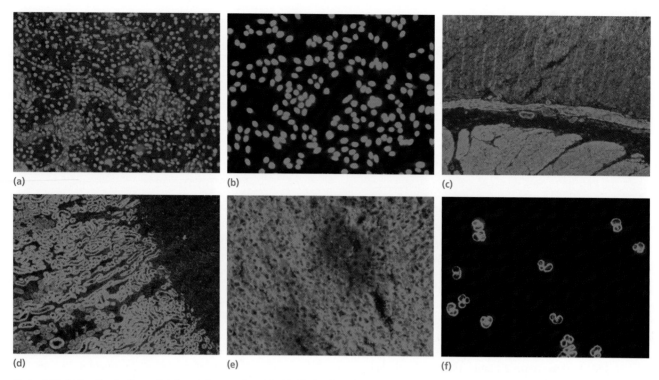

(a)
(b)
(c)
(d)
(e)
(f)

Figure 48.1 Autoantibody diagnostics for autoimmune hepatitis (AIH). Serological screening for AIH with indirect immunofluorescence pattern on rodent tissue sections (stomach, liver, kidney), human epithelial cells (HEp2 cells), and human neutrophils. **(a)** Antinuclear antibodies (ANA) stain the nuclei of, for example, kidney sections. **(b)** The ANA that are typically found in AIH homogenously staining on the nuclei of HEp2. **(c)** Antismooth muscle antibodies (SMA) stain the smooth muscles, for example of the gastric mucosa. **(d)** Antibody to liver kidney microsome (LKM 1) stain the cytoplasm of hepatocytes and the proximal renal tubules of kidney sections. **(e)** Antibodies to liver cytosol (anti-LC1) bind to hepatocytes cytoplasm but spare the centrilobular areas around the central vein. **(f)** Perinuclear staining pattern of perinuclear antineutrophil cytoplasmic antibodies (pANCA). Because pANCA in AIH-1 react with peripheral nuclear membrane components, instead of the myeloperoxidase as pANCA in rheumatoid diseases, they are alternatively denominated peripheral antinuclear neutrophil antibodies (pANNA).

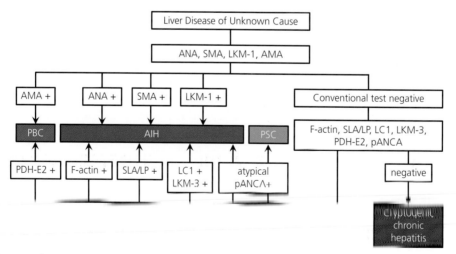

Figure 48.2 Diagnostic approach in liver disease of unknown cause. Initially, patient sera are assessed for antinuclear antibodies (ANA), smooth muscle antibodies (SMA), antibodies to liver/kidney microsome type 1 (LKM-1), and antimitochondrial antibodies (AMA). If these tests are negative, a further serological battery that includes tests for antibodies to actin (F-actin), soluble liver antigen/liver pancreas (SLA/LP), liver cytosol type 1 (LC-1), UDP-glucuronosyltransferases (LKM-3), the E2 subunits of the pyruvate dehydrogenase complex (PDH-E2), and perinuclear antineutrophil cytoplasmic antibodies (pANCA) should be obtained. The results of these two sequential serological assessments suggest the diagnosis of autoimmune hepatitis (AIH), primary biliary cirrhosis (PBC), primary sclerosing cholangitis (PSC), or cryptogenic chronic hepatitis. Source: Manns MP, Czaja AJ, Gorham JD, et al. Diagnosis and management of autoimmune hepatitis. Hepatology 2010;51:2193. Reproduced with permission of John Wiley & Sons.

Table 48.2 Diagnostic scoring systems for autoimmune hepatitis (AIH). Source: Data from Alvarez F, Berg PA, Bianchi FB, et al. International Autoimmune Hepatitis Group Report: review of criteria for diagnosis of autoimmune hepatitis. J Hepatol 1999;31:929 and Hennes EM, Zeniya M, Czaja AJ, et al. Simplified criteria for the diagnosis of autoimmune hepatitis. Hepatology 2008;48:169.

Revised scoring system	Score	Simplified scoring system	Points
Female sex	+2		
ALP : AST (or ALT) ratio			
<1.5	+2		
1.5–3.0	0		
>3.0	−2		
Serum globulins or IgG above normal		**IgG above normal**	
>2.0	+3	>1.1	+2
1.5–2.0	+2	1.0–1.1	+1
1.0–1.5	+1		
<1.0	0		
ANA, SMA or LKM-1 (IF)			
>1 : 80	+3	ANA or SMA ≥1 : 40	+1
1 : 80	+2	ANA or SMA ≥1 : 80	+2[a]
1 : 40	+1	or LKM ≥1 : 40	
<1 : 40	0	or SLA positive	
AMA positive	−4		
Viral hepatitis markers		**Viral hepatitis**	
(IgM anti-HAV, HBsAg, IgM anti-HBc, anti-HCV, and HCV-RNA)		Absence	+2
positive	−3		
negative	+3		
Hepatotoxic drug history *(recent or current)*			
positive	−4		
negative	+1		
Average alcohol intake			
<25 g/day	+2		
>60 g/day	−2		
Liver histology		**Liver histology** *(evidence of hepatitis is a necessary condition)*	
Interface hepatitis	+3	Typical AIH	+2
Predominantly lymphoplasmacytic infiltrate	+1	Compatible with AIH	+1
Rosetting of liver cells	+1		
None of the above	−5		
Biliary changes	−3		
Other changes	−3		
Other autoimmune disease(s)	+2		
Optional additional parameters			
Seropositivity for other defined autoantibodies	+2		
(pANCA, anti-LC1, anti-SLA, anti-ASGPR, anti-LP and antisulfatide)			
HLA DR3 or DR4	+1		
Response to therapy			
Complete	+2		
Relapse	+3		

Interpretation of aggregate scores		Interpretation of aggregate points	
Pretreatment			
Definite AIH	>15	Definite AIH	≥7
Probable AIH	10–15	Probable AIH	≥6
Posttreatment			
Definite AIH	>17		
Probable AIH	12–17		

[a] Addition of points achieved for all autoantibodies (maximum, 2 points).

Ab, antibody; ALP, alkaline phosphatase; ALT, alanine aminotransferase; AMA, antimitochondrial antibody; anti-LP, antiliver pancreas antibody; AST, aspartate aminotransferase; CMV, cytomegalovirus; EBV, Epstein–Barr virus; HAV, hepatitis A virus; HBsAg, hepatitis B surface antigen; HBc, hepatitis B core antigen; HCV, hepatitis C virus; HLA, human leucocyte antigen; IF, immunofluorescence; IgM, immunoglobulin M.

Table 48.3 Immunosuppressive regimen for autoimmune hepatitis in adults. Source: Manns MP, Czaja AJ, Gorham JD, et al. Diagnosis and management of autoimmune hepatitis. Hepatology 2010;51:2193. Reproduced with permission of John Wiley & Sons.

	Monotherapy	Combination therapy			
	Prednisone or prednisolone	Steroid		Azathioprine	
	(mg / day)	Prednisone or prednisolone (mg/day)	Budesonide *in noncirrhotic patients* (mg/day)	USA (mg/day)	Europe (mg/kg/day)
Week 1	60	30	9	50	1–2
Week 2	40	20	9	50	1–2
Week 3–4	30	15	6	50	1–2
Maintenance therapy	≤20	10	≤6	50	1–2
Reasons for preference	Cytopenia	Postmenopausal state			
	Thiopurin methytransferase deficiency	Osteoporosis			
	Pregnancy	Uncontrolled diabetes, hypertension, obesity			
	Malignancy	Acne			
	Expected therapy <6 month	Emotional lability			

CHAPTER 49

Primary biliary cirrhosis

Marlyn J. Mayo and Dwain L. Thiele
University of Texas Southwestern Medical School, Dallas, TX, USA

Primary biliary cirrhosis (PBC) is a chronic liver disease that is defined by its clinical presentation (Figures 49.1, 49.2, and 49.3), histological features (Figures 49.4–49.12), and serological findings. The underlying abnormality in PBC is a slowly progressive, nonpurulent inflammatory destruction of the biliary epithelial cells lining the small to medium-sized interlobular ducts.

Autoantibodies are a characteristic feature of the disease; over 90% of PBC patients have antimitochondrial antibodies (AMA) and about 50% have antinuclear antibodies (ANA). Loss of normal biliary drainage eventually leads to a clinical picture of chronic hepatic cholestasis and its potential complications (Figures 49.13 and 49.14).

Yamada's Atlas of Gastroenterology, Fifth Edition. Edited by Daniel K. Podolsky, Michael Camilleri, J. Gregory Fitz, Anthony N. Kalloo, Fergus Shanahan, and Timothy C. Wang.
© 2016 John Wiley & Sons, Ltd. Published 2016 by John Wiley & Sons, Ltd.
Companion website: www.yamadagastro.com/atlas

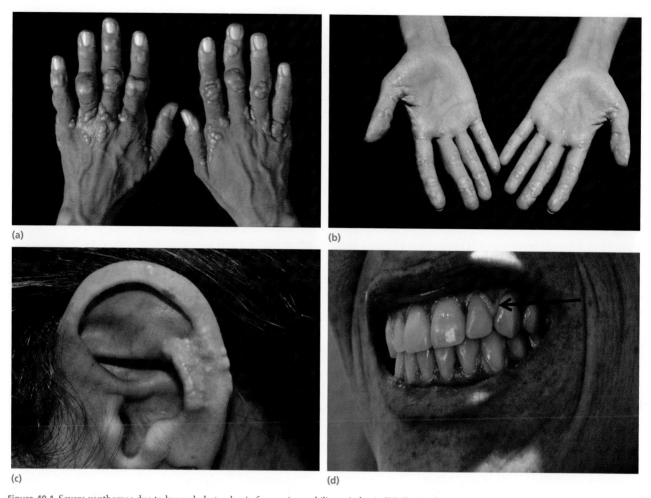

Figure 49.1 Severe xanthomas due to hypercholesterolemia from primary biliary cirrhosis (PBC). Xanthomas are most often seen around the eyes (xanthelasma), but may also develop over tendons and in palmar-digital creases. Shown here are xanthomas on the hands **(a, b)**, pinnae **(c)**, and gums **(d)** of patients with PBC. Xanthomas are more often seen in PBC patients with prolonged cholestasis but can also be seen before the onset of cirrhosis.

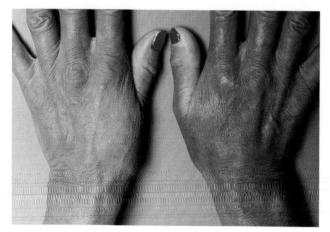

Figure 49.2 Hyperpigmentation, which results from increased melanin deposition, is more often seen in primary biliary cirrhosis (PBC) patients with prolonged cholestasis but can also be seen before the onset of cirrhosis. Pictured here is one PBC patient with asymmetric hyperpigmentation of the hands. Hyperpigmentation is most often found on the trunk and arms. Skin may also darken in areas that are repetitively scratched, which may result in a butterfly pattern of sparing in the middle of the back.

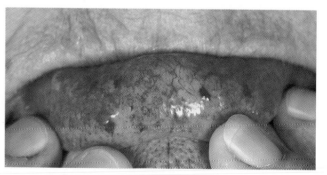

Figure 49.3 Telangiectasias are seen as part of the CREST (calcinosis, Raynaud phenomenon, esophageal dysmotility, sclerodactyly, telangiectasias) syndrome in 5%–7% of PBC patients. Telangiectasias are most commonly found on the lips (shown here) and the fingertips.

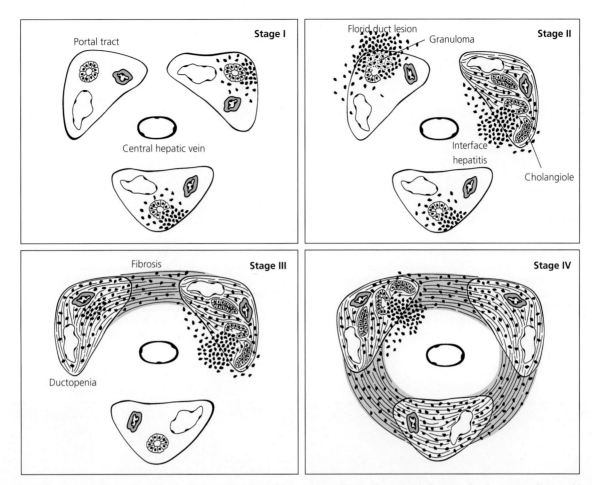

Figure 49.4 Diagrammatic illustration of the four stages of histological progression of PBC. Characteristic features of each stage are illustrated here, but the lesions are often patchy in nature. Stage I: mononuclear portal tract infiltrates, sometimes involving the bile duct. Stage II: intense mononuclear portal tract infiltrate with interface hepatitis, a florid duct lesion (granulomatous involvement of bile duct), and pseudoductular (cholangiolar) proliferation. Stage III: bridging fibrosis, mononuclear portal tract infiltrates with interface hepatitis, pseudoductular proliferation, and ductopenia. Stage IV: cirrhosis, mononuclear portal tract infiltrates with interface hepatitis, pseudoductular proliferation, and ductopenia.

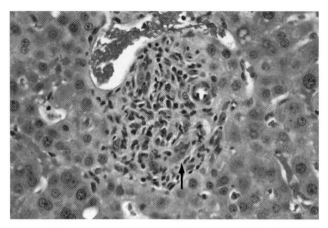

Figure 49.5 Primary biliary cirrhosis (PBC), stage I is characterized by a mononuclear cell portal infiltrate that does not extend beyond the limiting plate. The inflammatory infiltrate consists predominantly of T lymphocytes, but it may also contain plasma cells and eosinophils. The arrow points to residual biliary epithelial cells of a native bile duct destroyed by the inflammatory process. Bile duct destruction suggests the diagnosis of PBC, but may not be evident in biopsy specimens during stage I disease.

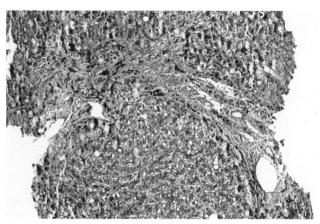

Figure 49.7 Primary biliary cirrhosis (PBC), stage III is defined by the presence of bridging fibrosis. All of the features seen in stage II PBC (see Figure 49.6) may be present, but ductopenia is more common in later stages of the disease. The diagnosis of ductopenia is often difficult to make because of lack of sufficient diagnostic material. A minimum sample of four portal tracts (with all four portal tracts containing arterioles but no ducts) or ideally 20 portal tracts (with ≥10 portal tracts containing arterioles but no ducts) are needed to make a diagnosis of ductopenia.

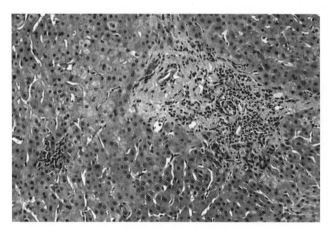

Figure 49.6 Primary biliary cirrhosis (PBC), stage II is characterized by a mononuclear cell infiltrate (predominantly of T lymphocytes, also plasma cells and eosinophils) of the portal tract that extends beyond the limiting plate. Bile ductules are usually found at the periphery of the portal tract (as opposed to the native bile ducts, which tend to be located adjacent to the portal arteriole) and they frequently have poorly defined basement membranes and lumens. Proliferation of bile ductules (pseudoducts or cholangioles) that arise from hepatic cell plates or putative stem cells under conditions of chronic cholestasis is a common feature in stage II disease. Nonsuppurative cholangitis and granulomatous and granulomatous cholangitis (see Figure 49.9) are present in about 50% of stage II PBC biopsies. Septal fibrosis and/or ductopenia (not shown in this figure) may also be present. Foci of lobular hepatitis, as noted in the right upper corner of the photomicrograph, may also be seen in primary biliary cirrhosis.

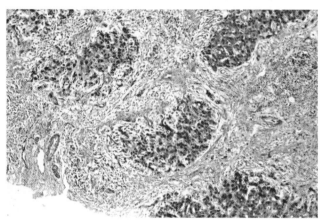

Figure 49.8 Primary biliary cirrhosis (PBC), stage IV is defined by the presence of cirrhosis. Although any of the characteristic histological features of PBC (see Figure 49.7) may be present, they may also be absent if the much of the liver has been replaced by fibrous tissue. Ductopenia is usually evident in stage IV PBC.

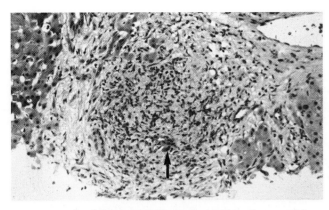

Figure 49.9 A florid duct lesion with granulomatous involvement of the bile duct (indicated by arrow) is the most specific histological finding suggestive of the diagnosis of primary biliary cirrhosis (PBC). The granulomas in PBC are often poorly defined. Portal granulomas without bile duct involvement are also seen in PBC, but lobular granulomas are much less common.

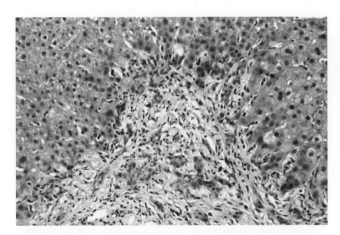

Figure 49.10 Biliary piecemeal necrosis in which there is death of periportal hepatocytes associated with an inflammatory infiltrate may also be evident in primary biliary cirrhosis. The injured hepatocytes appear swollen (feathery degeneration) as a result of cholate stasis.

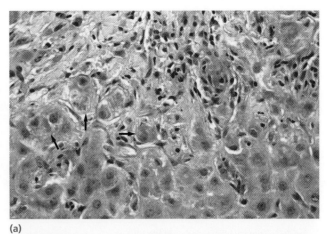

(a)

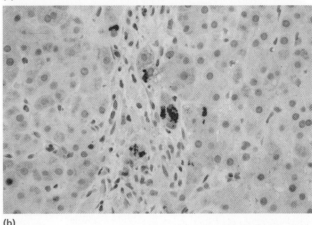

(b)

Figure 49.11 (a) Mallory bodies (arrows) may be seen in primary biliary cirrhosis (PBC). They are typically located in the periportal hepatocytes, as opposed to localization in the hepatic lobule in steatohepatitis. **(b)** Immunohistochemistry for ubiquitin (red pigment) highlights the presence of Mallory hyaline in PBC liver tissue.

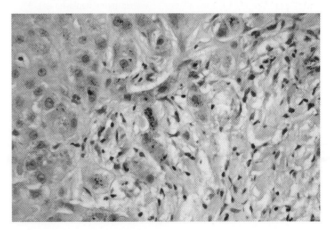

Figure 49.12 A rhodamine stain (red pigment) demonstrates copper granules in the liver of a patient with primary biliary cirrhosis. Copper accumulates in the periportal hepatocytes as cholestasis progresses. It is frequently accompanied by Mallory hyaline (see Figure 49.11) and is typically found in areas of cholate stasis (see Figure 49.10).

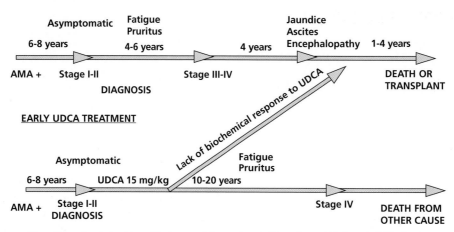

<u>NATURAL HISTORY</u>

<u>EARLY UDCA TREATMENT</u>

*Transition rates derived from Markov modeling and may differ substantially from individual cases.

Figure 49.13 The clinical course of primary biliary cirrhosis has improved over the past decade. Patients are more likely to be diagnosed at an earlier stage and to receive treatment with ursodeoxycholic acid (UDCA). Biochemical nonresponders progress faster than those who achieve significant improvement in alkaline phosphatase. AMA, antimitochondrial antibodies.

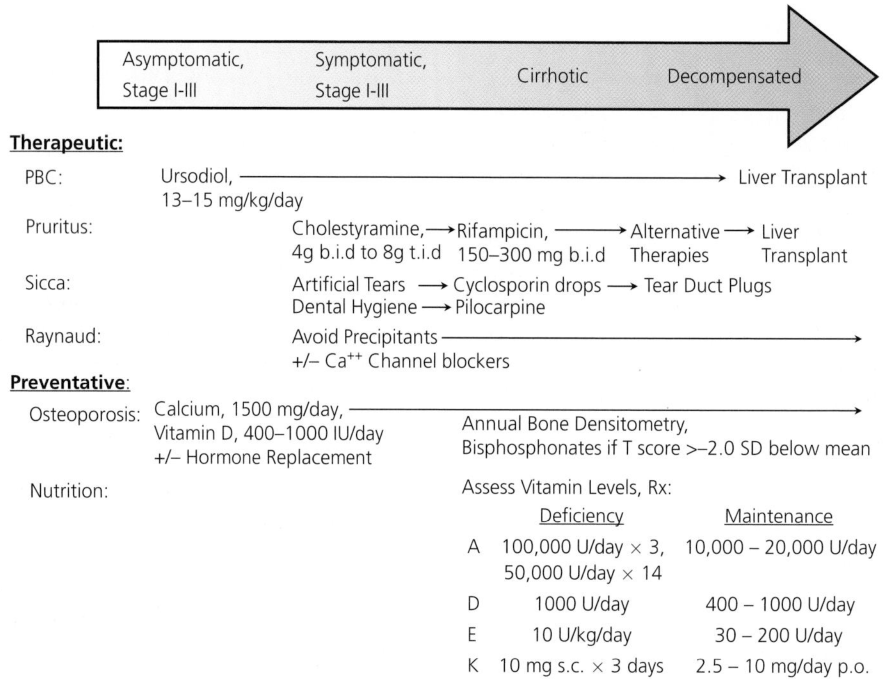

| | Asymptomatic, Stage I–III | Symptomatic, Stage I–III | Cirrhotic | Decompensated |

Therapeutic:

PBC: Ursodiol, 13–15 mg/kg/day ————————————————————→ Liver Transplant

Pruritus: Cholestyramine, 4g b.i.d to 8g t.i.d —→ Rifampicin, 150–300 mg b.i.d —→ Alternative Therapies —→ Liver Transplant

Sicca: Artificial Tears —→ Cyclosporin drops —→ Tear Duct Plugs
Dental Hygiene —→ Pilocarpine

Raynaud: Avoid Precipitants ————————————————————→
+/– Ca^{++} Channel blockers

Preventative:

Osteoporosis: Calcium, 1500 mg/day, ————————————————————→
Vitamin D, 400–1000 IU/day
+/– Hormone Replacement
Annual Bone Densitometry,
Bisphosphonates if T score >–2.0 SD below mean

Nutrition: Assess Vitamin Levels, Rx:

	Deficiency	Maintenance
A	100,000 U/day × 3, 50,000 U/day × 14	10,000 – 20,000 U/day
D	1000 U/day	400 – 1000 U/day
E	10 U/kg/day	30 – 200 U/day
K	10 mg s.c. × 3 days	2.5 – 10 mg/day p.o.

Figure 49.14 Overview of the management of primary biliary cirrhosis (PBC) and associated conditions. Complications of portal hypertension (not shown) are managed in the same manner as in other forms of cirrhosis.

CHAPTER 50

Hemochromatosis

Paul C. Adams

Western University, London, ON, Canada

Introduction

Hemochromatosis is one of the most common genetic diseases and may lead to iron accumulation in the liver (Figures 50.1 and 50.2), heart, pancreas, and endocrine organs. Early diagnosis and treatment are essential to prevent organ damage. Arthopathy (Figure 50.3) and pigmentation (Figure 50.4) are also clinical features of hemochromatosis.

Genetics

Since the discovery of the gene for hemochromatosis (*HFE*) in 1996, a simple genetic blood test has been developed, which can be done on a blood sample or stored tissue.

The C282Y mutation on chromosome 6 of the *HFE* gene is present in 93%–100% of homozygotes in pedigree studies. In less well-defined patients with iron overload the prevalence ranges from 60% to 80%. A second mutation, H63D is less common and its relationship to hemochromatosis is less well defined. There have been other iron overload diseases associated with mutations in other iron-related genes (transferrin receptor 2, hemojuvelin, hepcidin, ferroportin) (Box 50.1).

Use of the C282Y genetic test for hemochromatosis

The genetic test is most useful in a patient who is suspected clinically of having hemochromatosis (Box 50.2) or with an elevated transferrin saturation and/or serum ferritin (Figure 50.5; Box 50.3). It is also useful when investigating siblings and other family members of a C282Y homozygote. It will replace HLA typing in pedigree studies.

There have already been reports of a number of cases within hemochromatosis families that are homozygous for the C282Y mutation without iron overload. This may represent incomplete penetrance. The frequency of this phenomenon in the general population has not been clearly established. However, population studies in North America, Europe, and Australia suggest that, overall, the C282Y mutation is more common than the clinical disease. This may reflect a high degree of incomplete penetrance or underdiagnosis of the disease.

Treatment of hemochromatosis

Patients are initially treated by the weekly removal of 500 mL of blood. Patients attend an ambulatory care facility and the venesection is performed by a nurse using a kit containing a 16-gauge straight needle and collection bag. Blood is removed with the patient in the reclining position over 15–30 min. A hemoglobin test is done at the time of each venesection. If the hemoglobin decreases to less than 100 g/L the venesection schedule is modified to 500 mL every other week. Serum ferritin is measured periodically (every 3 months in severe iron overload, monthly in mild iron overload) and weekly venesections are continued until the serum ferritin is approximately 50 μg/L. Transferrin saturation often remains elevated despite therapy. After the initial iron depletion therapy, a serum ferritin is repeated 6 months later. If the ferritin is rising patients may then begin maintenance venesections three to four times per year. Iron re-accumulation is inconsistent and many patients will go for years without a rise in serum ferritin with no treatment. Chelation therapy is not used for the treatment of hemochromatosis.

Yamada's Atlas of Gastroenterology, Fifth Edition. Edited by Daniel K. Podolsky, Michael Camilleri, J. Gregory Fitz, Anthony N. Kalloo, Fergus Shanahan, and Timothy C. Wang.
Companion website: www.yamadagastro.com/atlas

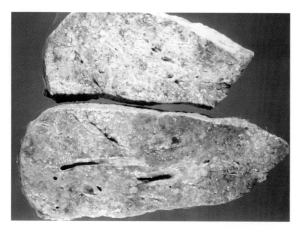

Figure 50.1 A cirrhotic liver from a patient with hemochromatosis. The upper specimen has been stained for iron, which appears blue, and illustrates the diffuse iron distribution throughout the liver. Source: Courtesy of LW Powell.

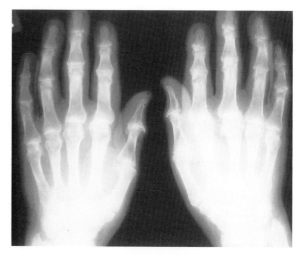

Figure 50.3 The arthropathy of the metacarpal phalangeal joints in hemochromatosis. In this case, a 55-year-old surgeon had to give up surgical practice because of severe disabling arthritis.

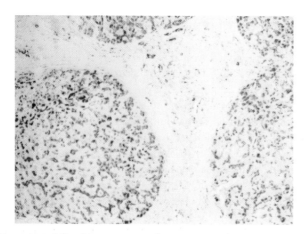

Figure 50.2 A liver biopsy specimen from an untreated C282Y homozygote with cirrhosis. The cirrhotic nodules are stained for iron (Prussian blue).

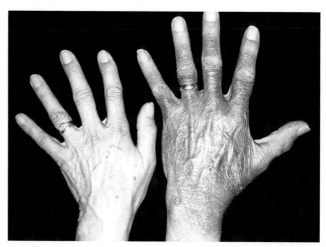

Figure 50.4 The skin pigmentation of hemochromatosis is illustrated in a hemochromatosis patient (right) compared to his wife (left).

Box 50.1 Differential diagnosis of iron overload.

HFE **related hemochromatosis**
    C282Y homozygotes (95%)
    C282Y/H63D compound heterozygotes (4%)
    H63D homozygotes (1%)
Non-*HFE* related hemochromatosis
    Juvenile hemochromatosis (hemojuvelin or hepcidin mutations)
    Transferrin receptor 2 mutation
    Ferroportin disease
Miscellaneous iron overload
    African-American iron overload
    African iron overload
    Polynesian iron overload
    Transfusional iron overload
    Insulin resistance-related iron overload
    Aceruloplasminemia
    Alcoholic siderosis
    Iron overload secondary to end-stage cirrhosis
    Porphyria cutanea tarda
    Post-portacaval shunt

Box 50.2 Interpretation of genetic testing for hemochromatosis.

C282Y homozygote: this is the classical genetic pattern, which is seen in >90% of typical cases. Expression of disease ranges from no evidence of iron overload to massive iron overload with organ dysfunction. Siblings have a 1 in 4 chance of being affected and should have genetic testing. For children to be affected, the other parent must be at least a heterozygote. If iron studies are normal, false-positive genetic testing or a nonexpressing homozygote should be considered.

C282Y/H63D compound heterozygote: this patient carries one copy of the major mutation and one copy of the minor mutation. Most patients with this genetic pattern have normal iron studies. A small percentage of compound heterozygotes have been found to have mild to moderate iron overload. Severe iron overload is usually seen in the setting of another concomitant risk factor (alcoholism, viral hepatitis).

C282Y heterozygote: this patient carries one copy of the major mutation. This pattern is seen in about 10% of the Caucasian population and is usually associated with normal iron studies. In rare cases the iron studies are high, in the range expected in a homozygote rather than a heterozygote. These cases may carry an unknown hemochromatosis mutation and liver biopsy is helpful to determine the need for venesection therapy.

H63D homozygote: this patient carries two copies of the minor mutation. Most patients with this genetic pattern have normal iron studies. A small percentage of these cases have been found to have mild to moderate iron overload. Severe iron overload is usually seen in the setting of another concomitant risk factor (alcoholism, viral hepatitis).

H63D heterozygote: this patient carries one copy of the minor mutation. This pattern is seen in about 20% of the Caucasian population and is usually associated with normal iron studies. This pattern is so common in the general population that the presence of iron overload may be related to another risk factor. Liver biopsy may be required to determine the cause of the iron overload and the need for treatment in these cases.

No *HFE* mutations: there are other iron overload diseases associated with mutations in other iron related genes (transferrin receptor 2, hemojuvelin, ferroportin, hepcidin, BMP6). There will likely be other hemochromatosis mutations discovered in the future. If iron overload is present without any *HFE* mutations, a careful history for other risk factors must be reviewed and liver biopsy may be useful to determine the cause of the iron overload and the need for treatment.

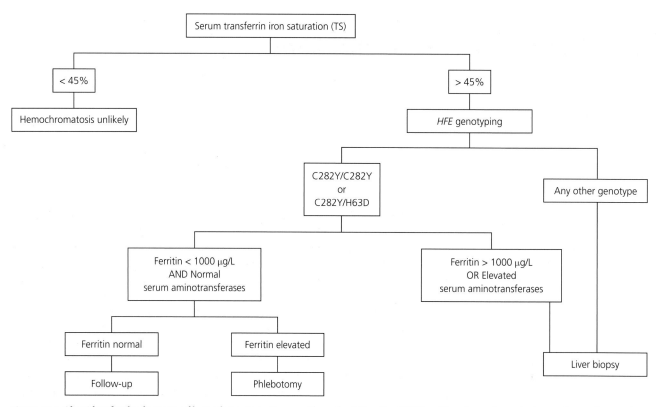

Figure 50.5 Algorithm for the diagnosis of hemochromatosis. Source: Alexander J, Kowdley KV. Hereditary hemochromatosis: genetics, pathogenesis, and clinical management. Ann Hepatol 2005;4:240. Reproduced with permission of Annals of Hepatology.

Box 50.3 Phenotypic diagnostic tests for hemochromatosis and iron overload.

Transferrin saturation is better than serum iron alone; it is available and inexpensive.. Results of this test are elevated with hemochromatosis, even in children. Thresholds for investigation vary from >45% to 62%.

  Serum ferritin is an indirect measurement of body iron stores. It increases with age in hemochromatosis. Levels can be elevated in all liver diseases and chronic inflammation.

  Liver biopsy: since the development of genetic testing, liver biopsy has gone from a diagnostic test to a prognostic test. A biopsy should be considered in the hemochromatosis patient with liver dysfunction (Figure 50.02) and in the patient with iron overload who does not have the typical genetic pattern. All types of end-stage liver disease can have mild to moderate iron overload.

  Magnetic resonance imaging: the sensitivity of this technique continues to improve. It does not replace liver histology and liver iron concentration. It can be helpful in a patient with a contraindication to liver biopsy.

CHAPTER 51
Metabolic diseases of the liver

Ronald J. Sokol and Mark A. Lovell

University of Colorado School of Medicine and Children's Hospital Colorado, Aurora, CO, USA

Metabolic liver diseases comprise a diverse group of genetic disorders in which an enzyme or transport protein is deficient or dysfunctional. Most present during childhood with symptoms of neonatal cholestasis, chronic progressive hepatic fibrosis, or a metabolic syndrome (hypoglycemia, acidosis, encephalopathy, hyperammonemia). Identification of the precise etiology is possible through molecular, biochemical, or enzymatic testing and is important in order to initiate therapy, when available, to prevent irreversible injury to the liver, brain, kidneys, or other organs. Several of the most common and important metabolic liver diseases will be summarized here and the histology of the liver histology illustrated.

α-1 antitrypsin (A1AT) deficiency is an autosomal recessive disorder in which the PIZZ or PISZ phenotype of A1AT leads to liver involvement in 10%–20% of affected individuals and emphysema that is exacerbated by exposure to cigarette smoke. The incidence of A1AT deficiency varies with ethnic group, from 1 in 800 to 1 in 2000. Mutant A1AT, which accumulates in the endoplasmic reticulum of the hepatocyte, can be detected as PAS-positive, diastase-resistant globules, and is thought to be responsible for initiating injury to the hepatocyte (Figure 51.1). There is currently no effective medical treatment for this liver disease; however, most patients do not have progressive disease. Liver transplant is required for those patient with end-stage liver disease and is curative of all manifestations of A1AT deficiency because normal circulating A1AT levels are restored after transplantation.

Wilson disease is an autosomal recessive disorder of copper storage primarily involving the liver, brain, eye, and kidney, with a frequency of 1 in 30 000. It is caused by mutations in the *ATP7B* gene, which codes for a P-type ATPase that is essential for copper transport out of the hepatocyte into bile and for incorporation of hepatic copper into ceruloplasmin, which is secreted into the systemic circulation. In Wilson disease, copper first accumulates in the liver, leading to acute or chronic hepatitis, fulminant liver failure, or cirrhosis, and then the brain, causing psychiatric symptoms and dystonic or pseudoparkinsonian symptoms. Liver lesions characteristically demonstrate steatohepatitis, glycogen-filled nuclei of periportal hepatocytes, varying degrees of portal tract inflammation, and periportal fibrosis advancing to cirrhosis (Figure 51.2); however, none of these findings are specific nor diagnostic of Wilson disease. Diagnosis is established by elevated quantitative liver copper, low plasma ceruloplasmin, elevated urine copper excretion, presence of Kayser–Fleischer rings, or by genotyping. Copper chelation and zinc therapies are effective; liver transplantation is required for acute fulminant cases and those with advanced cirrhosis unresponsive to medical therapy.

Several physical findings suggest Wilson disease. The Kayser–Fleischer ring of the cornea is a hallmark of the disease (Figure 51.3) and is a greenish-brown ring in Descemet's membrane at the periphery of the cornea on its posterior surface. It is best detected by slit-lamp examination by an experienced ophthalmologist, but can occasionally be seen by the naked eye, particularly in people with blue or green pigmentation of the iris. The ring, composed of granules rich in copper and sulfur, disappears during appropriate copper chelation therapy. Skin pigmentation may be increased, particularly on the anterior aspect of the lower leg, due to deposition of melanin (Figure 51.4). Blue lunulae of the fingernails may also occur, presumably from deposition of copper.

Glycogen storage diseases (GSD) are a heterogeneous group of defects in degradation or synthesis of hepatic and muscle glycogen. Several GSD subtypes primarily affect the liver. In GSD type I, glucose-6-phosphatase is defective, leading to massive hepatomegaly, profound fasting hypoglycemia, lactic acidosis, hyperlipidemia, hyperuricemia, and growth failure. Liver biopsy (Figure 51.5) shows swollen hepatocytes with clear cytoplasm (so called "mosaic" appearance), macrovesicular and microvesicular steatosis, and a general lack of inflammation, cell death,

Yamada's Atlas of Gastroenterology, Fifth Edition. Edited by Daniel K. Podolsky, Michael Camilleri, J. Gregory Fitz, Anthony N. Kalloo, Fergus Shanahan, and Timothy C. Wang.
© 2016 John Wiley & Sons, Ltd. Published 2016 by John Wiley & Sons, Ltd.
Companion website: www.yamadagastro.com/atlas

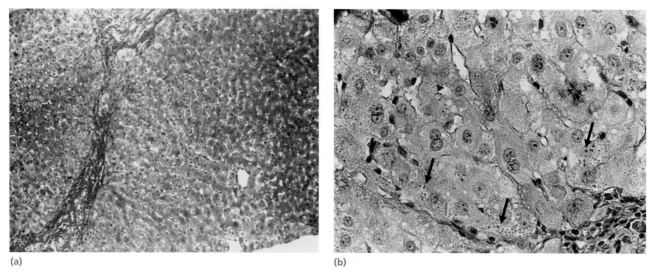

(a)

(b)

Figure 51.1 Liver biopsy of an 8-year-old boy with PIZZ phenotype of α-1-antitrypsin deficiency. **(a)** Note periportal bridging fibrosis with mild portal tract inflammation (trichrome stain, ×10). **(b)** Periodic acid–Schiff (PAS)–diastase staining reveals typical globules (arrows) of α-1-antitrypsin trapped within periportal hepatocytes (×40).

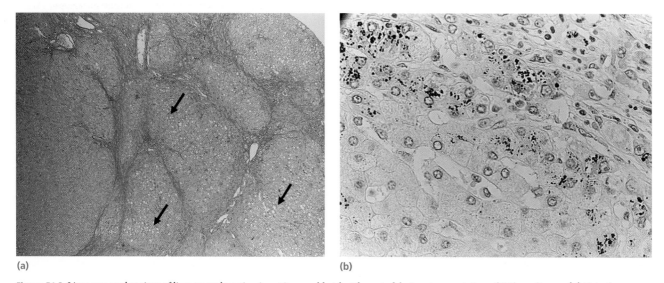

(a)

(b)

Figure 51.2 Liver removed at time of liver transplantation in a 12-year-old girl with acute fulminant presentation of Wilson disease. **(a)** Note the established cirrhosis with regenerative nodules and mild macrovesicular steatosis (arrows) (H&E stain, ×4). **(b)** Rhodanine staining reveals increased copper-associated proteins (brownish pigment) present in hepatocytes (×40).

or portal fibrosis. Treatment is aimed at maintaining normal blood sugar, and includes frequent high-starch meals, oral doses of uncooked cornstarch throughout the day, and nocturnal nasogastric tube or gastrostomy tube drip feedings of a formula high in carbohydrate or awakening every 3–4 hours at night to ingest cornstarch. GSD type IX is a generally benign disease manifested by hepatomegaly without the metabolic symptoms of type I. Liver biopsy (Figure 51.6) shows swollen hepatocytes with clear cytoplasm and varying degrees of periportal fibrosis. Occasional patients progress to develop portal hypertension.

Reye syndrome, the prototypic mitochondrial hepatopathy, is called encephalopathy with fatty degeneration of the viscera. Its onset follows a viral infection (most often influenza or varicella) with the sudden onset of vomiting and lethargy in the absence of central nervous system infection; with elevated aminotransferase, prothrombin time, and ammonia but normal bilirubin and which progresses to coma. Most patients in the United States have been exposed to salicylates during the prodromal viral illness. Liver biopsy (Figure 51.7) demonstrates diffuse, panlobular microvesicular steatosis characterized by swollen hepatocytes with central nuclei. Because the fat droplets may be so fine, the steatosis is frequently not appreciated unless special fat stains are used (Figure 51.7). There is no portal tract inflammation, although apoptotic hepatocytes are occasionally observed.

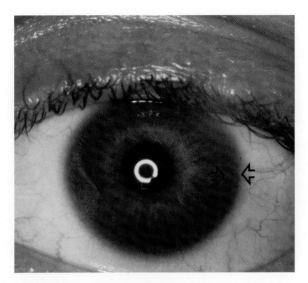

Figure 51.3 Kayser–Fleischer ring (between arrows) on cornea of a 30-year-old man with Wilson disease.

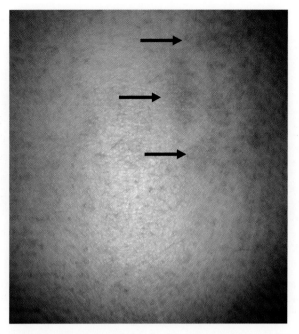

Figure 51.4 Increased brownish discoloration (arrows) of skin over tibia in a 10-year-old Cambodian boy with subfulminant Wilson disease.

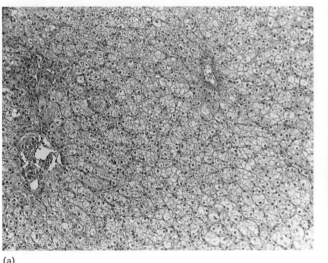

(a)

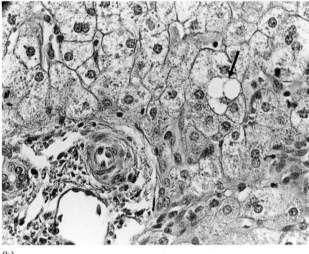

(b)

Figure 51.5 Liver biopsy from a 2-month-old Hispanic girl with glycogen storage disease type 1b. **(a)** Extensive hepatocyte ballooning with clear cytoplasm and lobular disarray are prominent. Fibrosis and portal tract inflammation are absent (H&E stain, ×10). **(b)** Macrovesicular steatosis (arrow) is also present (H&E stain, ×40).

Special stains will demonstrate a marked decrease in mitochondrial enzyme activity (e.g., succinic acid dehydrogenase) with normal microsomal enzyme activity. Electron microscopy shows markedly swollen and pleomorphic mitochondria with hypodense matrix and loss of dense bodies. The hepatopathy is accompanied by cerebral edema which becomes the primary clinical challenge in managing the patients, because the liver injury eventually fully recovers. The diminished use of aspirin products in febrile children in the early 1980s after several government warnings about the association with Reye syndrome has been associated with a marked decline in the number of cases. Some of the cases, however, are probably now being correctly diagnosed as defects of mitochondrial fatty oxidation, urea cycle defects, and related metabolic disorders, which were possibly triggered in the past by viral infections and the effect of salicylates on mitochondrial oxidative phosphorylation.

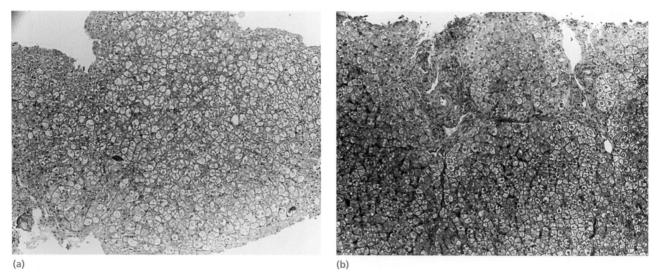

(a)   (b)

Figure 51.6 Liver biopsy from a 19-year-old man with glycogen storage disease type IX. **(a)** Note the swollen pale hepatocytes with clear cytoplasm exhibiting "mosaic" appearance (H&E stain, ×10). **(b)** Mild periportal and early bridging fibrosis is present, although there is no indication of chronic inflammation or hepatocellular death (trichrome stain, ×10).

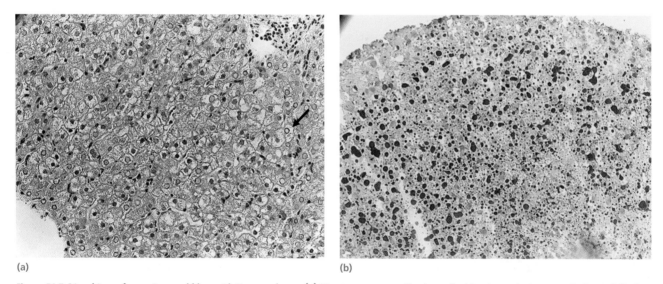

(a)   (b)

Figure 51.7 Liver biopsy from a 5-year-old boy with Reye syndrome. **(a)** Hepatocytes are swollen (arrow) with microvesicular steatosis that is difficult to discern on routine stains, absent portal tract inflammation, and no hepatocyte death. Bile ducts are normal (H&E stain, ×20). **(b)** Oil-red-O stain reveals extensive neutral lipid responsible for microvesicular steatosis (×20).

CHAPTER 52

Alcoholic liver disease

Jose Altamirano,[1] Eric S. Orman,[2] and Ramon Bataller[1,3]

[1] Institut d'Investigacions Biomèdiques August Pi i Sunyer (IDIBAPS), Barcelona, Spain
[2] Indiana University School of Medicine, Indianapolis, IN, USA
[3] University of North Carolina at Chapel Hill, NC, USA

Introduction

Alcoholic liver disease (ALD) is a leading cause of liver-related morbidity and mortality worldwide and is a major cause of death among adults with prolonged alcohol abuse. Despite its burden, the incidence, natural history and modifying factors of ALD remain largely unknown and its pathogenesis is incompletely understood. Most studies have been performed in animal models that do not reproduce the histological findings of patients with severe ALD. Recent translational studies in human samples have revealed several key molecular drivers and potential targets for therapy.

Alcohol misuse is one of the main causes of preventable disease worldwide. Mortality in people with alcohol use disorders is markedly higher than previously thought. Women have generally higher mortality risks than men. A recent report from the World Health Organization (WHO) indicates that 3.3 million deaths (6% of all global deaths) were attributable to alcohol use, and that alcohol abuse accounts for 50% of cirrhosis. In large-scale studies on the prevalence of liver fibrosis in the general population, alcohol abuse accounts for one-third of cases. Of note, many patients have more than potential cause of liver disease (e.g. obesity and alcohol abuse).

Diagnosis and management of moderate ALD

Diagnosis of alcohol abuse

The diagnosis of alcohol abuse is based on self-reporting, but collection of objective data is advisable. The AUDIT-C is an extensively validated screen for hazardous alcohol use (i.e. drinking above recommended limits, or alcohol use disorder), which consists of three questions about alcohol consumption. AUDIT-C scores ≥ 4 points for men, and ≥ 3 for women are considered positive screens based on US validation studies that compared the AUDIT-C to "gold standard" measures of unhealthy alcohol use from independent, detailed interviews (Box 52.1). Among the various biomarkers of chronic alcohol abuse, carbohydrate-deficient transferrin (CDT) appears to be the most reliable. A combined index based on gamma-glutamyltransferase (GGT), and carbohydrate-deficient transferrin (CDT) measurements (GGT-CDT) recently has been suggested to improve the detection of excessive ethanol consumption. The sensitivity of GGT-CDT (90%) in correctly classifying heavy drinkers exceeded that of CDT (63%), GGT (58%), mean corpuscular volume (MCV) (45%), aspartate aminotransferase (AST) (47%), and alanine aminotransferase (ALT) (50%), being also essentially similar for alcoholics with (93%), or without (88%) liver disease.

Moderate ALD: natural history and risk factors

ALD presents as a broad spectrum of disorders ranging from fatty liver, alcoholic steatohepatitis (ASH), progressive fibrosis, end-stage cirrhosis, and superimposed hepatocellular carcinoma. Alcoholic fatty liver (AFL) can be referred as a moderate or mild stage in the spectrum of ALD. AFL is an early response to alcohol consumption, developed in more than 90% of heavy drinkers. It is characterized by early-mild steatosis in zone 3 (perivenular) hepatocytes; it can also affect zone 2, and even zone 1 (periportal) hepatocytes when liver injury is more severe. Interestingly, only about one third of heavy drinkers with AFL will develop more severe forms of ALD, such as advanced fibrosis and cirrhosis. In patients with underlying ALD and heavy alcohol intake, episodes of superimposed alcoholic hepatitis (AH) may occur.

Several risk factors for ALD have been identified. These include sex, obesity, drinking patterns, dietary factors, nonsex-linked genetic factors, and cigarette smoking. Female sex is a well-documented risk factor for susceptibility to ALD; the

Yamada's Atlas of Gastroenterology, Fifth Edition. Edited by Daniel K. Podolsky, Michael Camilleri, J. Gregory Fitz, Anthony N. Kalloo, Fergus Shanahan, and Timothy C. Wang.
© 2016 John Wiley & Sons, Ltd. Published 2016 by John Wiley & Sons, Ltd.
Companion website: www.yamadagastro.com/atlas

Box 52.1 AUDIT-C Questionnaire for hazardous alcohol consumption.

1. How often do you have a drink containing alcohol?
   a. Never
   b. Monthly or less
   c. 2–4 times a month
   d. 2–3 times a week
   e. 4 or more times a week
2. How many standard drinks containing alcohol do you have on a typical day?
   a. 1 or 2
   b. 3 or 4
   c. 5 or 6
   d. 7 to 9
   e. 10 or more
3. How often do you have six or more drinks on one occasion?
   a. Never
   b. Less than monthly
   c. Monthly
   d. Weekly
   e. Daily or almost daily

The AUDIT-C is scored on a scale of 0–12.

Each AUDIT-C question has 5 answer choices.
   Points allotted are:
   a = 0 points, b = 1 point, c = 2 points, d = 3 points, e = 4 points

Heavy/hazardous drinking

Men >3, Women >4

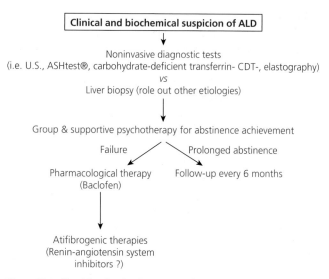

Figure 52.1 Algorithm for the diagnosis and management of moderate Alcoholic liver disease (ALD).

increased risk among women likely results from lower levels of gastric alcohol dehydrogenase, a higher proportion of body fat, and the presence of estrogens. Obesity represents another important risk factor that accelerates fibrosis progression and the development of cirrhosis in ALD. Experimental studies indicate that the synergistic effects of obesity and alcohol abuse involve the endoplasmic reticulum response to cell stress, type I macrophage activation, and adiponectin resistance. Moreover, genetic factors might also influence susceptibility to advanced ALD, however little data are available. Variations in genes that encode antioxidant enzymes, cytokines and other inflammatory mediators, and alcohol-metabolizing enzymes could have a role. Recently, variations in patatin-like phospholipase domain-containing protein 3 (PNPLA3) has showed to influence the development of advanced liver fibrosis among Mexican and Caucasian populations. Importantly, PNPLA3 polymorphisms can be considered to be the only confirmed and replicated genetic risk factor for ALD.

Finally, long-term alcohol intake causing AFL has synergistic effects with hepatitis virus B or C, nonalcoholic fatty liver disease, autoimmune liver diseases, and metabolic liver disorders (e.g. hemochromatosis) and can accelerate the progression of liver diseases.

Moderate ALD: diagnosis and treatment

In its early stages, ALD is typically a silent disease and can only be detected by laboratory tests, or imaging techniques. Some patients with early ALD can show stigmata of alcohol abuse such as bilateral parotid gland hypertrophy, muscle wasting, malnutrition, Dupuytren's sign, and signs of peripheral neuropathy. In patients with cirrhosis, most physical findings are not specific of the etiology. However, some signs such as gynecomastia and extensive spider angiomas may be more frequently seen in those with alcohol as the main cause of liver disease. The diagnosis of ALD is frequently suspected upon documentation of excess alcohol consumption, and the presence of clinical and/or biological abnormalities suggestive of liver injury. In patients with ALD, the AST/ALT ratio typically is greater than 1. This ratio is typically greater than 2 in AH and can also be found in patients with advanced cirrhosis regardless of the etiology.

Compared to patients with nonalcoholic fatty liver disease (NAFLD), few patients with ALD undergo a liver biopsy. A liver biopsy could be indicated in patients with other cofactors suspected of contributing to liver disease. In the setting of clinical trials, the assessment of liver histology by liver biopsy is recommended. The typical findings in patients with ALD include alcohol hepatocellular damage (ballooning and/or Mallory Denk bodies), an inflammatory infiltrate basically composed of when polymorphonuclear (PMN) cells that predominates in the lobules, and a variable degree of fibrosis and lobular distortion that may progress to cirrhosis.

For the assessment of liver fibrosis in patients with ALD, there are noninvasive methods including serum markers and liver stiffness measurement (Figure 52.1). Most noninvasive tests have been largely validated in patients with hepatitis C, while few studies have included patients with ALD. Thus, AST to platelet ratio index (APRI), FibroTest, Fibrometer, and Fibrosure can be useful in patients with ALD. They are useful to distinguish between mild and severe fibrosis, but have limited utility in intermediate degrees of fibrosis. Transient elastography (Fibroscan) is commonly used to assess fibrosis in patients with chronic liver disease. This device was recently approved by the Food and Drug Administration (FDA). In patients with ALD, liver stiffness correlates with the degree of fibrosis. Elevated liver stiffness values in patients with ALD and AST serum levels >100 U/L should be interpreted with caution because of the possibility of falsely elevated liver stiffness as a result of superimposed ASH. Moreover, recent alcohol consumption can also elevate liver stiffness, perhaps related to the vasodilatory effects of alcohol. Imaging techniques can also be used to assess the severity of ALD. Ultrasonography, MRI, and CT are useful to detect fatty liver, advanced fibrosis/cirrhosis as well as signs of portal hypertension. Among those methods, ultrasound is the most used due to its low cost. However, its sensitivity and specificity is low especially when steatosis is mild.

Alcohol cessation is the mainstay of therapy for patients with all stages of ALD. Behavioral therapy must be a central component of alcoholism treatment. Brief motivational interventions are encouraged in the primary-care setting. The four main parameters that should be considered and assessed when approaching these patients are: self-awareness of alcohol misuse, appropriate family/social support, underlying psychiatric disorders, and willingness to be seen by an addiction therapist. In addition, pharmacologic therapy can be considered, although their efficacy is limited. Disulfiram has been used in the past and works well, but there have been case-reports of disulfiram-induced severe hepatitis, which clearly limit its use in patients with ALD. Naltrexone was found to decrease heavy drinking in alcoholics both alone and when combined with a behavioral approach, however there is also concern for hepatotoxicity with this agent, and it has not been tested in patients with ALD. Other compounds known to prevent alcohol relapse include acamprosate, gamma-hydroxybutyric acid, and topiramate. The usefulness of all these compounds in the setting of ALD has not been adequately assessed. A more promising compound is baclofen, a derivative of GABA that binds to the GABAB receptor. Baclofen is the only agent that has been tested in patients with advanced ALD and demonstrated a significant improvement in the proportion of patients abstinent from alcohol, when compared to placebo with no hepatic side effects seen. Studies assessing the efficacy and safety of anticraving drugs in the setting of AH are warranted.

For patients that are unable to stop drinking despite the medical advice, there are no approved antifibrogenic therapies. The most promising drugs are those interfering with the reninangiotensin system (angiotensin receptor blockers or ACE inhibitors). Antioxidants can also be useful (SAMe, phosphatidylcholine, etc) yet better designed studies are required to confirm their usefulness.

Differential diagnosis and prognostic assessment in patients with alcoholic hepatitis

Patients with advanced ALD (in most cases cirrhosis) and active drinking can develop an episode of acute-on-chronic liver failure named "alcoholic hepatitis" (AH). In most alcoholic patients with this clinical syndrome, the histological analysis shows the presence of ASH, and advanced fibrosis. In its severe forms, AH carries a bad prognosis and current therapies are not fully effective.

Clinical presentation and differential diagnosis

AH should be considered as a clinical syndrome defined by the recent onset of jaundice and/or liver decompensation (i.e. ascites) in a patient with chronic alcohol abuse. Although the clinical presentation may present abruptly, it is felt to reflect an exacerbation of underlying chronic liver disease. It is important to clarify that while AH is a clinical syndrome; the existence of ASH needs to be confirmed histologically.

The hallmark of symptomatic AH is the abrupt onset and/or rapid progression of jaundice, which may be associated with fever, infection, weight loss, malnutrition, and tender hepatomegaly. In its severe form, AH may induce liver decompensation with ascites, encephalopathy, or gastrointestinal bleeding. Laboratory evaluation typically demonstrates AST levels that are elevated to 2–6 times the upper limit of normal with an AST/ALT ratio >2. Increased bilirubin and neutrophilia are also frequently observed. Serum albumin may be decreased, prothrombin time prolonged, and the international normalized ratio (INR) may be elevated. Patients with severe AH are prone to develop bacterial infection and acute kidney injury.

The existence of AH can be highly suspected based on clinical and analytical criteria, however, a definitive diagnosis requires histological confirmation by transjugular biopsy due to the coagulopathy of most patients. In most cases, advanced liver fibrosis (mainly cirrhosis) and superimposed ASH is found. ASH is defined by the coexistence of steatosis, hepatocyte ballooning and/or Mallory-Denk bodies, and an inflammatory infiltrate with PMNs. A typical finding in many patients is the presence of megamitochrondria. Importantly, canalicular and/or lobular bilirubinostasis is commonly seen in AH, especially in patients with ongoing bacterial infections.

Approximately, in 20%–25% of patients with the clinical syndrome a true ASH is not found. Other histological findings include signs if drug-induced liver disease, signs of ischemic hepatitis (especially in patients with cocaine consumption), foamy hepatic degeneration and signs of biliary obstruction (Table 52.1).

The incidence of AH remains largely unknown. A Danish population-based retrospective cohort study estimated that it ranges from 24 to 46 per million, depending on gender, and is increasing. A large study, where systematic liver biopsies were performed in 1604 alcoholic patients, found the prevalence of

AH to be approximately 20%. In symptomatic patients, including those with decompensated liver disease, the prevalence of AH is not well known, partly because most centers rely on clinical criteria rather than transjugular liver biopsy as routine practice in the diagnosis of patients with decompensated ALD.

Relying only clinical criteria alone carries a 10%–50% risk of misclassifying patients as having, or not having AH. Therefore, the recently published EASL Practical Guidelines on Alcoholic Liver Disease strongly recommends performing a liver biopsy, if available, in patients with suspected AH.

Table 52.1 Differential diagnosis of alcoholic hepatitis: Causes and characteristics for diagnosis.

Cause	Diagnosis
DILI	Hepatotoxic drug, eosinophilia, liver histology
Ischemic hepatitis	Bleeding, hypotension, cocaine, elevated ALT, histology
Malignancies	Lymphoma, metastasis, MRI, liver histology
Obstuctive jaundice	Cholestasis, pain, abdominal ultrasound, MRI
Others	Tuberculosis, autoimmune hepatitis, alcoholic foamy degeneration
Progressive ALD	More progressive liver deterioration, liver histology
Septic liver	Signs of sepsis, positive culture, histology
Steatohepatitis	Typical presentation, liver histology (80% of cases)

Prognostic assessment

The prognosis of patients with AH can be estimated using biochemical and histological criteria. Several prognostic models have been developed to identify patients with AH who are at high risk of death within 1–3 months of their hospitalization. Maddrey's discriminant function (DF) was the first score to be developed and remains the most widely used. Severe AH is defined as a DF>32 and the reported 1 month survival of untreated patients with a DF>32 ranges from 50% to 65%. Other prognostic scores, such the MELD (Model for End-Stage Liver Disease), the GAHS (Glasgow Alcoholic Hepatitis Score), and the ABIC score (age, serum Bilirubin, INR, and serum Creatinine score) have been shown utility in this setting. However, the proposed cut-offs of these scores need to be tested

(a) Alcoholic hepatitis histological score (AHHS)

	Points
Stage of fibrosis	
No fibrosis or portal fibrosis	0
Expansive fibrosis	0
Bridging fibrosis or cirrhosis	+3
Bilirubinostasis	
No	0
Hepatocellular only	0
Canalicular or ductular	+1
Canalicular or ductular plus hepatocellular	+2
PMN infiltration	
No/Mild	+2
Severe	0
Megamitochondria	
No megamitochondria	+2
Megamitochondria	0

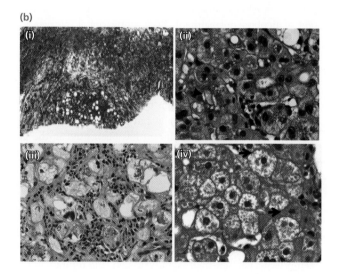

(b)

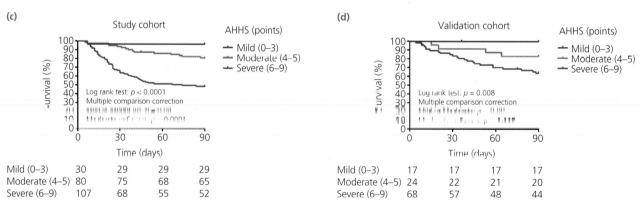

(c) Study cohort

AHHS (points)
- Mild (0–3)
- Moderate (4–5)
- Severe (6–9)

Log rank test: $p < 0.0001$
Multiple comparison correction

Mild (0–3)	30	29	29	29
Moderate (4–5)	80	75	68	65
Severe (6–9)	107	68	55	52

(d) Validation cohort

AHHS (points)
- Mild (0–3)
- Moderate (4–5)
- Severe (6–9)

Log rank test: $p = 0.008$
Multiple comparison correction

Mild (0–3)	17	17	17	17
Moderate (4–5)	24	22	21	20
Severe (6–9)	68	57	48	44

Figure 52.2 Histological findings associated with survival in alcoholic hepatitis. **(a)** Alcoholic hepatitis histological score (AHHS), **(b)** Histological features evaluated with the AHHS; **(i)** advanced fibrosis, **(ii)** ductular bilirubinostasis, **(iii)** severe polymorphonuclear (PMN) infiltration, **(iv)** megamitochondria; **(c)** Three-month survival probability of patients according to the AHHS in the study and **(d)** validation cohorts.

in populations other than those used initially for score development and the vast majority of these models only stratify patients into two categories (e.g. severe or nonsevere) and only early mortality risk is considered. As a result, a proportion of patients may not meet the criteria for severe AH, and die at time points longer than 1 month (i.e. up to 6 months). The ABIC score permit to stratify patients with AH in three subgroups with different mortality at day 90.

The most widely used scoring system to evaluate the response to therapy (e.g. corticosteroids) is the Lille Model. The Lille Model determines prognosis on the basis of response or nonresponse to prednisolone and incorporates the serum bilirubin at baseline and at day 7. A recent meta-analysis was able to categorize patients as complete responders, partial responders, or null responders and was able to predict the 6 month survival of each group using two new cut-offs of the Lille score . Another factor that predicts mortality in AH is the development of acute kidney injury (AKI), defined as an absolute increase of serum creatinine of 0.3 mg/dL, or a 50% increase above baseline. AKI is associated with a marked decreased in 90 day survival. Interestingly, patients with systemic inflammatory response syndrome (SIRS) at admission developed AKI in much higher proportions and SIRS was also associated with decreased 90 day survival.

Recently, a histological scoring system capable of predicting short-term survival in patients with AH was evaluated in a multicenter trial. The resulting Alcoholic Hepatitis Histological Score (AHHS) comprises 4 parameters that are independently associated with patients' survival: fibrosis stage, PMN infiltration, type of bilirubinostasis and presence of megamitochondria. By combining these parameters in a semiquantitative manner, we were able to stratify patients into low-, intermediate-, or high-risk for death within 90 days (Figure 52.2).

CHAPTER 53

Nonalcoholic fatty liver disease

M. Shadab Siddiqui and Arun J. Sanyal
Virginia Commonwealth University, Richmond, VA, USA

Introduction

Nonalcoholic fatty liver disease (NAFLD) is the most common cause of abnormally elevated aminotransferases. NAFLD encompasses a spectrum of disorders characterized by intrahepatic fat accumulation (simple hepatic steatosis) accompanied by varying degrees of hepatic necroinflammatory activity and hepatic fibrosis (nonalcoholic steatohepatitis or NASH) through to cirrhosis. NAFLD is considered the hepatic manifestation of the metabolic syndrome and is associated with increased mortality, particularly cardiovascular disease (CVD) related mortality. Steatohepatitis can progress to cirrhosis in 15%–25% of patients and, with the projected increase in its prevalence, NASH is poised to become the leading indication for liver transplantation in the United States.

Histological presentation

The diagnosis of NAFLD can be made using imaging methods such as a CT scan or MRI-based technologies. However, the distinction between fatty liver and NASH can only be made by a liver biopsy. Hepatic steatosis is predominantly macrovesicular in nature where individual hepatocytes have their cytoplasm replaced with a large fat vacuole pushing the nucleus to the side (Figure 53.1). Other histological findings that are typically seen in NASH include cytological ballooning (Figure 53.2), megamitochondria (Figure 53.3), Mallory hyaline (Figure 53.4), and predominantly lobular inflammation (Figure 53.5). Hepatic fibrosis is typically pericellular in nature (Figure 53.6). Frequently, inflammation surrounds affected hepatocytes (Figure 53.7). Fibrosis can also be portal in location (Figure 53.8). Progressive fibrosis leads to central fibrosis, to portal and central fibrosis, then central bridges, and eventually cirrhosis (Figures 53.8, 53.9, and 53.10). Steatohepatitis is defined by steatosis, ballooning, and inflammation, usually in a centrilobular location

(Figure 53.11). Other histological findings include pigment-laden macrophages (Figure 53.12), acidophil bodies (Figure 53.13), lipogranulomas (Figure 53.14), and glycogen nuclei (Figures 53.15 and 53.16). Iron overload has been reported inconsistently (Figure 53.17).

Pathophysiology

The pathophysiology of NAFLD is multifactorial and incompletely understood but appears to be closely related to insulin resistance and lipotoxicity. Insulin resistance and caloric excess drive hepatic steatosis (Figure 53.18). Additionally, oxidative stress, mitochondrial injury, cytokines, adipokines, and metabolic endotoxemia likely contribute to cellular injury and fibrosis progression. The intestinal microbiome appears to play a central role in the pathogenesis of NAFLD by affecting adipocytes, insulin resistance, and hepatic steatosis.

Clinical presentation

Patients with NAFLD are usually asymptomatic, although general malaise or fatigue appears to be the most prevalent complaint in symptomatic individuals. Mild elevations in serum aminotransferase are the first clues to underlying NAFLD. The presence of other common liver diseases, including viral hepatitides and cholestatic liver diseases, are ruled out serologically. The diagnosis is confirmed on liver biopsy in the absence of any significant alcohol consumption (less than 20 g/day in women and less than 30 g/day in men).

The most common physical finding in subjects with NAFLD is obesity, present in majority of patients in the USA. Hepatomegaly and abnormal fat distribution are present in up to a quarter of patients with NAFLD. Patients with underlying insulin resistance might also have acanthosis nigrans. In

Yamada's Atlas of Gastroenterology, Fifth Edition. Edited by Daniel K. Podolsky, Michael Camilleri, J. Gregory Fitz, Anthony N. Kalloo, Fergus Shanahan, and Timothy C. Wang.

Grade 1: 5%–33%   Grade 2: 34%–66%   Grade 3: >67%

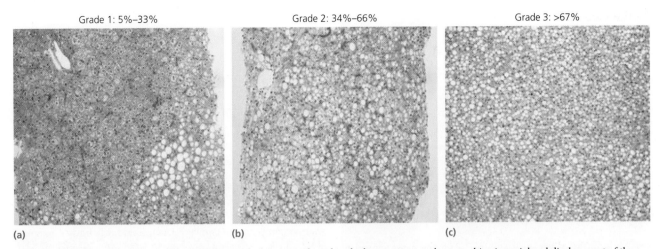

(a)   (b)   (c)

Figure 53.1 Macrovesicular hepatic steatosis with a single, large vacuole within the hepatocyte cytoplasm resulting in peripheral displacement of the nucleus. The extent of steatosis is graded based on the percentage of total hepatocytes that are involved: **(a)** grade 1 is defined as 5%–33% of parenchymal involvement by steatosis; **(b)** grade 2 is 34%–66%; **(c)** grade 3 is >67% (hematoxylin and eosin stain; original magnification × 20). Source: Courtesy of David E. Kleiner, MD. Histology definition and scoring system are based on the NASH Clinical Research Network criteria.

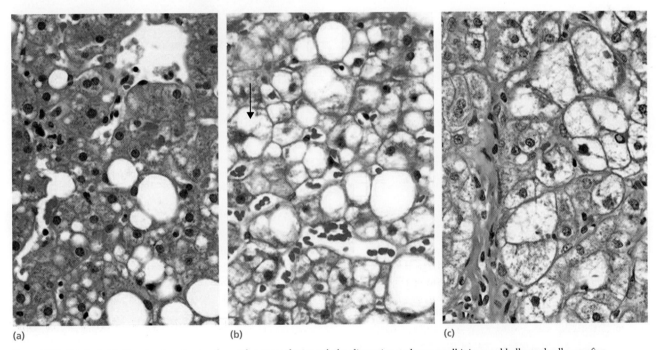

(a)   (b)   (c)

Figure 53.2 Cytological ballooning is a structural manifestation of microtubular disruption and severe cell injury and ballooned cells are often intermixed in areas of steatosis. The ballooned cells are swollen and enlarged (two times normal size), with a pale cytoplasm, which appears finely granular or reticulated. **(a)** Mild steatosis without ballooning degeneration. **(b)** This field shows a ballooned cell (arrow) with the characteristics of a scalloped margin, filamentous appearing intracytoplasmic material, and an accentuated nuclear membrane and prominent nucleoli. **(c)** More prominent ballooning injury (H&E stain; original magnification × 40). Source: Courtesy of David E. Kleiner, MD. Histology definition and scoring system are based on the NASH Clinical Research Network criteria.

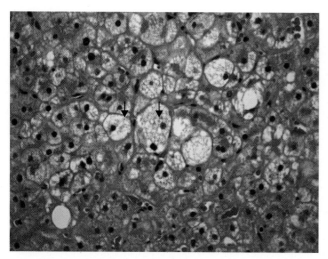

Figure 53.3 Membranes of paired mitochondria fuse and defuse to form megamitochondria as illustrated here (arrows). They appear as hepatocellular, cytoplasmic, discrete eosinophilic bodies, often 3 to 10 μm in diameter and have a globoid or, less often, needle-like shape (H&E stain; original magnification × 40). Source: Courtesy of David E. Kleiner, MD. Histology definition and scoring system are based on the NASH Clinical Research Network criteria.

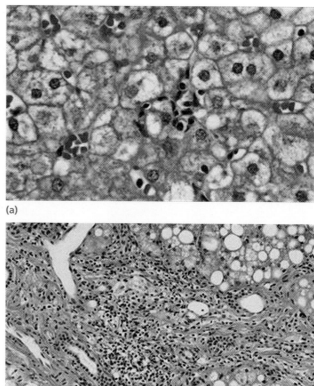

(a)

(b)

Figure 53.5 Inflammation. **(a)** A small cluster of inflammatory cells consisting mainly of lymphocytes is seen. The extent of lobular inflammation is scored as follows: score of 0 is defined as no inflammatory foci; score of 1 indicates fewer than two foci per 200 × field; score of 2 indicates two to four foci per 200 × field; and a score of 3 indicates greater than four foci per 200 × field. **(b)** Greater than minimal portal inflammation with predominantly lymphocytes infiltration is also seen, although neutrophils, eosinophils, and plasma cells may be present as the disease activity progresses (H&E stain; original magnification × 40). Source: Courtesy of David E. Kleiner, MD. Histology definition and scoring system are based on the NASH Clinical Research Network criteria.

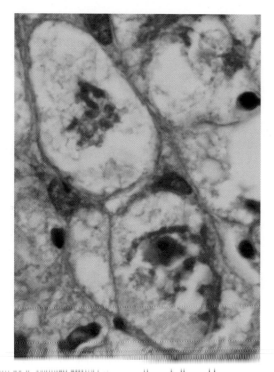

Figure 53.4 Mallory hyaline is seen within a ballooned hepatocyte at the center of the field. On routine H&E stained sections, it is recognized as intracytoplasmic, perinuclear eosinophilic material that ranges in shape from short coarsely clumped masses to elongated rope-like cords (H&E stain; original magnification × 40). Source: Courtesy of David E. Kleiner, MD. Histology definition and scoring system are based on the NASH Clinical Research Network criteria.

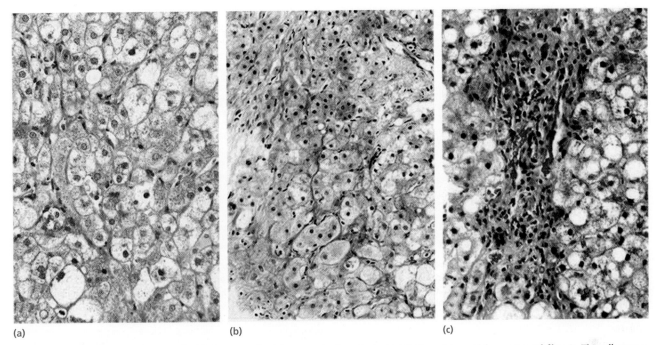

(a)   (b)   (c)

Figure 53.6 Pericellular fibrosis stage 1. **(a, b)** The Masson's trichrome stain for collagen highlights perisinusoidal or periportal fibrosis. The collagenous tissue (shown in blue) surrounds individual hepatocytes, producing a chicken-wire appearance. (**c**) In another field, the pericellular fibrosis is noted around several ballooned hepatocytes (Masson trichrome stain; original magnification × 40). Source: Courtesy of David E. Kleiner, MD. Histology definition and scoring system are based on the NASH Clinical Research Network criteria.

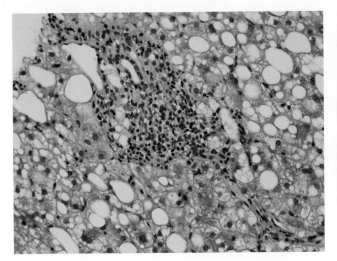

Figure 53.7 This photograph illustrates extensive inflammation with polymorphonuclear leukocytes and lymphocytes surrounding some hepatocytes with both macro- and microvesicular steatosis (H&E stain; original magnification × 40). Source: Courtesy of David E. Kleiner, MD. Histology definition and scoring system are based on the NASH Clinical Research Network criteria.

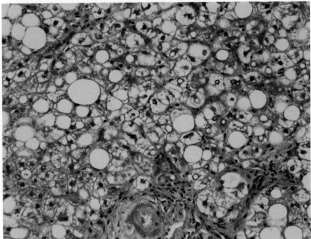

Figure 53.8 Portal fibrosis. Progressive injury in NASH results in portal fibrosis, as shown here. This field illustrates fibrous expansion of portal fields with fibrosis extension along the terminal centracinar portal vein (Masson trichrome stain; original magnification x 40). Source: Courtesy of David E. Kleiner, MD. Histology definition and scoring system are based on the NASH Clinical Research Network criteria.

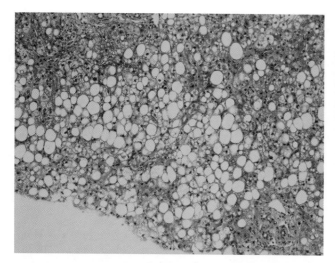

Figure 53.9 Bridging fibrosis. This field illustrates an early stage 3 bridging fibrosis. Note the condensed reticulin connecting two portal tracts (Masson trichrome stain; original magnification × 40). Source: Courtesy of David E. Kleiner, MD. Histology definition and scoring system are based on the NASH Clinical Research Network criteria.

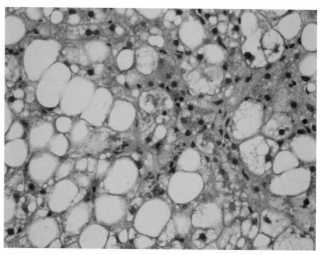

Figure 53.11 Patterns of NASH as evidenced by the presence of hepatic steatosis, lobular inflammation with lymphocytic infiltration, and hepatocellular ballooning (H&E stain; original magnification × 40). Source: Courtesy of David E. Kleiner, MD. Histology definition and scoring system are based on the NASH Clinical Research Network criteria.

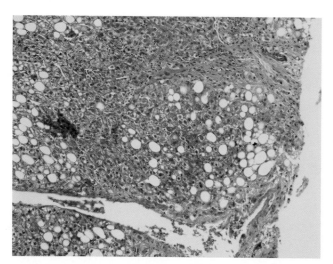

Figure 53.10 Cirrhosis in evolution. Extensive fibrosis with distortion of overall architecture and formation of a regenerative nodule surrounded by dense fibrous tissue. Note the absence of a central vein or portal tracts within the regenerative nodule (Masson trichrome stain; original magnification × 40). Source: Courtesy of David E. Kleiner, MD. Histology definition and scoring system are based on the NASH Clinical Research Network criteria.

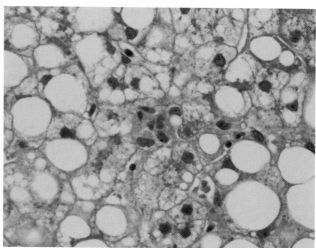

Figure 53.12 Pigment-laden macrophages are seen at the center of the field (H&E stain; original magnification × 40). Source: Courtesy of David E. Kleiner, MD. Histology definition and scoring system are based on the NASH Clinical Research Network criteria.

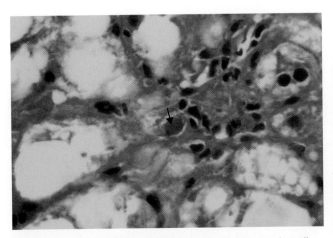

Figure 53.13 Acidophil body (arrow) is seen as well-demarcated, small eosinophilic cytoplasmic globules, either anuclear or possessing nuclear fragments lying within the lobules, sinusoids, or in periportal areas. In addition to cytological ballooning, hepatocellular injury in NASH may also manifest as apoptotic (acidophil) bodies (H&E stain; original magnification × 40). Source: Courtesy of David E. Kleiner, MD. Histology definition and scoring system are based on the NASH Clinical Research Network criteria.

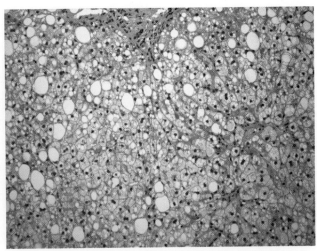

Figure 53.15 Histology highlighting the hepatic glycogenesis and macrovesicular steatosis. The hepatocytes are enlarged by accumulating glycogen, resulting in compression of sinusoids. In addition, mild macrovesicular steatosis is present (H&E stain; original magnification × 40). Source: Courtesy of David E. Kleiner, MD. Histology definition and scoring system are based on the NASH Clinical Research Network criteria.

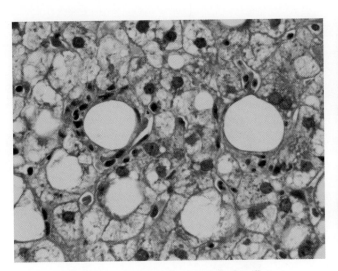

Figure 53.14 Formation of lipogranuloma around a fat cell. Lipogranulomas often occur in NASH although such finding is neither specific for nor diagnostic of steatohepatitis. They result from the rupture of a lipid-laden hepatocyte that eventually leads to the development of a foreign-body type granulomatous reactive response. They are composed of steatotic hepatocyte surrounded by mononuclear cells, Kupffer cells, and occasionally eosinophil (H&E stain; original magnification × 40). Source: Courtesy of David E. Kleiner, M.D. Histology definition and scoring system are based on the NASH Clinical Research Network criteria.

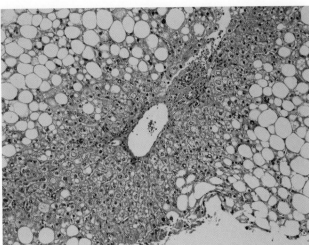

Figure 53.16 Numerous glycogenated hepatocyte nuclei are seen as clear nuclear inclusion, enlarged nuclei with a prominent nuclear membrane. This is often seen in patients with diabetes mellitus and is a common finding in NASH (H&E stain; original magnification × 40). Source: Courtesy of David E. Kleiner, MD. Histology definition and scoring system are based on the NASH Clinical Research Network criteria.

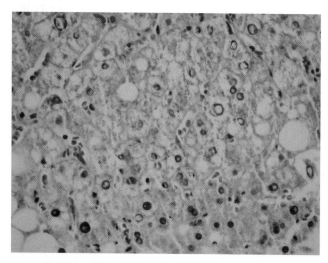

Figure 53.17 Iron overload in NAFLD. A Prussian blue iron stain demonstrates the blue granules of hemosiderin in hepatocytes (Prussian blue stain; original magnification × 40). Source: Courtesy of David E. Kleiner, MD.

individuals presenting with advanced fibrosis or cirrhosis, spider angiomatas, palmar erythema, ascites, and hepatic encephalopathy can occur but do not differentiate NASH from other causes of cirrhosis. NASH is associated with an approximately 4% annual mortality following development of cirrhosis (Figure 53.19). It is also associated with an increased risk of hepatocellular cancer (Figure 53.20).

Treatment

The mainstay of treatment of NAFLD remains lifestyle induced modifications to help achieve sustained weight loss. Although a number of pharmacological agents have been investigated, no specific therapy has been shown to produce a durable histological response. The current treatment of NAFLD involves weight loss (lifestyle or surgical), tight control of other features of metabolic syndrome, and pharmacological therapy in selected individuals (i.e., vitamin E in nondiabetic subjects with steatohepatitis).

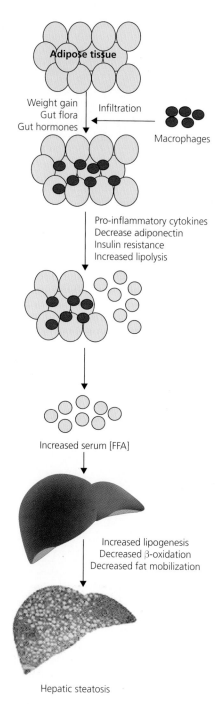

Figure 53.18 Mechanism of hepatic steatosis in nonalcoholic fatty liver disease. Infiltration of adipose tissue by macrophages results in a decrease serum adiponectin and an increase in proinflammatory cytokines. These proinflammatory adipokines worsen insulin resistance, particularly at the level of adipose tissue. Adipose tissue insulin resistance leads to incomplete suppression of lipolysis, resulting in increased serum free fatty acid (FFA) concentrations. The increase free fatty acid load to the liver promotes de novo lipogenesis and, in conjunction with decreased β-oxidation and fat mobilization, results in hepatic steatosis.

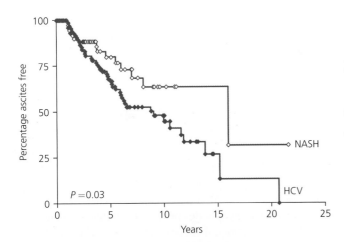

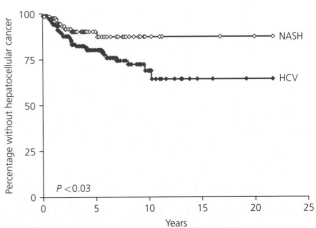

Figure 53.19 The natural history of cirrhosis due to nonalcoholic steatohepatitis (NASH): ascites. The probability of developing ascites and decompensation in those with cirrhosis caused by NASH is less than that seen in subjects with cirrhosis due to hepatitis C (HCV). Source: Sanyal AJ, Banas C, Sargeant C, et al. Similarities and differences in outcomes of cirrhosis due to nonalcoholic steatohepatitis and hepatitis C. Hepatology 2006;43:682. Reproduced with permission of John Wiley & Sons.

Figure 53.20 The natural history of cirrhosis due to nonalcoholic steatohepatitis (NASH): hepatocellular cancer. Subjects with cirrhosis due to NASH can develop hepatocellular cancer but the cancer risk appears to be somewhat lower than that seen in those with hepatitis C (HCV). Source: Sanyal AJ, Banas C, Sargeant C, et al. Similarities and differences in outcomes of cirrhosis due to nonalcoholic steatohepatitis and hepatitis C. Hepatology 2006;43:682. Reproduced with permission of John Wiley & Sons.

CHAPTER 54
Hepatic fibrosis

Don C. Rockey
Medical University of South Carolina, Charleston, SC, USA

This chapter provides additional images of interest in the area of liver fibrosis, and includes images spanning basic science concepts to clinical concepts.

The cellular basis of hepatic fibrosis

A number of effector cells have been identified as critical to the fibrogenic response; these include portal fibroblasts, fibrocytes (derived from the bone marrow), mesenchymal cells derived from hepatocytes through epithelial–mesenchymal transition (EMT), and hepatic stellate cells (Figure 54.1). Considerable controversy exists as to the importance of EMT in hepatic fibrogenesis. Stellate cells appear to be the key fibrogenic effectors in the injured liver.

Portal fibroblasts
Portal fibroblasts (Figure 54.2) appear to be most prominent in liver disease with portal based injury such as primary biliary cirrhosis, sclerosing cholangitis, or sarcoidosis. In experimental models, bile duct obstruction in particular leads to proliferation of portal fibroblasts.

Fibrocytes
The role of fibrocytes (Figure 54.3) in liver fibrogenesis is controversial. Available data clearly indicate that these CD45-positive, collagen I producing cells migrate to the liver after injury, where they appear in small numbers. While they do not appear to be a major matrix-producing cell in the liver, they appear to play a role in stimulation of stellate cell activation via inflammatory pathways.

Stellate cells
Stellate cells make up approximately 6% of the cells found in the liver and are commonly accepted as the primary extracellular matrix-producing cell in the injured liver. They are found in much larger numbers proportionally than are the other putative fibrogenic cells. A remarkable feature of hepatic stellate cells is

that they are rich in retinoid and lipids. After liver injury, they become activated; in this process, they undergo a number of striking morphological changes. These include the development of an extensive endoplasmic reticulum, the development of an intricate network of stress fibers, focal adhesions, and actin cytoskeleton. The also loose their retinoid/lipid droplets (Figures 54.4, 54.55, and 54.6).

One of the major features of hepatic stellate cells is their rich retinoid and lipid content (Figures 54.4, 54.55, and 54.56). This feature helps identify them in cultures and makes them easily identifiable. The lipid droplets in stellate cells readily take up oil red O. This diazo dye, used for staining of neutral triglycerides and lipids, can be seen in abundance in a perinuclear fashion in quiescent stellate cells (i.e., those soon after isolation). After stellate cells are grown in culture and they become activated, their lipid content declines significantly (Figures 54.4 and 54.6).

Stellate cells are enriched with a variety of intermediate filaments, including desmin, vimentin, and others (Figure 54.7).

One of the classic features of stellate cell activation is the upregulation of the smooth muscle isoform of actin (Acta2), indicating that they represent liver-specific myofibroblasts (Figure 54.8).

The robust cytoskeleton typical of stellate cells further extends to other components; for example, cell-matrix attachments such as focal adhesions are prominent (Figure 54.9). Stellate cells exhibit remarkable expression of vinculin, talin, and focal adhesion kinase (FAK) (Figure 54.9).

With stellate cell activation, a number of functions ensue. Prominent among these is enhanced motility (Figure 54.10). Stellate cell motility is likely to be important in cell movement to certain parts of the liver (e.g., stellate cells likely home to areas of increased injury and inflammation).

In addition to enhanced motility, activated stellate cells exhibit a contractile phenotype (Figure 54.11). This is likely important on a number of levels. For example, stellate cells that contract may constrict sinusoids and likely play a role in altering blood flow patterns. Further, contraction itself likely is important in stimulating the stellate cell to produce extracellular

Yamada's Atlas of Gastroenterology, Fifth Edition. Edited by Daniel K. Podolsky, Michael Camilleri, J. Gregory Fitz, Anthony N. Kalloo, Fergus Shanahan, and Timothy C. Wang.

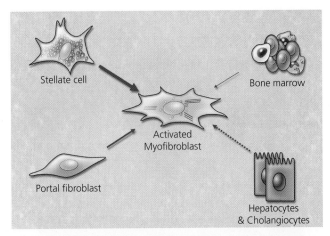

Figure 54.1 Cellular sources of matrix in liver wound healing. Shown are characteristic cells that may transition to myofibroblast-like matrix producing cells. Source: Friedman SL. Hepatic stellate cells: protean, multifunctional, and enigmatic cells of the liver. Physiol Rev 2008;88:125. Reproduced with permission of The American Physiological Society.

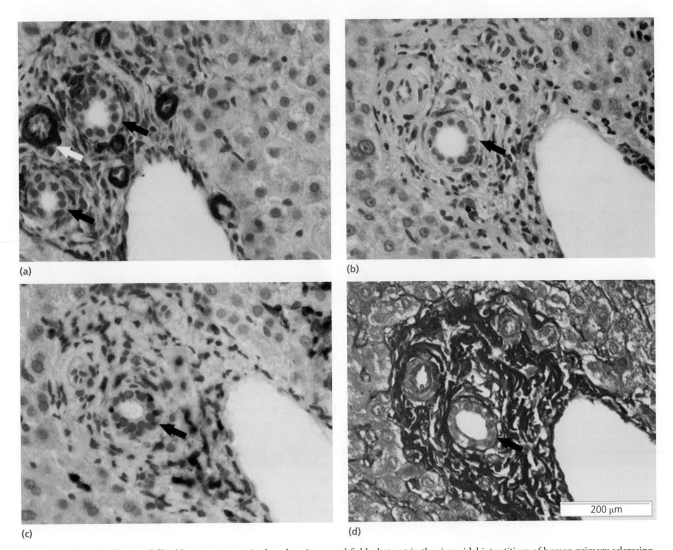

Figure 54.2 Myofibroblasts and fibroblasts are present in the sclerosing portal fields, but not in the sinusoidal interstitium of human primary sclerosing cholangitis. Immunohistochemistry to detect smooth muscle α-actin **(a)**, CD45 **(b)** and S100A4 **(c)**; **(d)** depicts picrosirius red staining, all on serial liver sections. Seen are smooth muscle α-actin-positive myofibroblasts **(a)** and infiltration of CD45-positive **(b)** and S100A4-positive **(c)** cells in the sclerosing areas around the injured bile ducts (black arrows). Smooth muscle α-actin is also found in smooth muscle cells of the portal veins and the hepatic artery (white arrow). The picrosirius red staining **(d)** shows collagen around injured bile ducts. Source: Strack I, Schulte S, Varnholt H, et al. β-Adrenoceptor blockade in sclerosing cholangitis of Mdr2 knockout mice: antifibrotic effects in a model of nonsinusoidal fibrosis. Lab Invest 2011;91:252. Reproduced with permission of Nature Publishing Group.

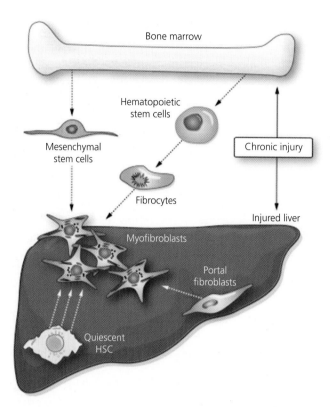

Figure 54.3 Fibrocytes from the bone marrow migrate to the liver. There, these cells transform into hepatic myofibroblasts. Although the role of mesenchymal stem cells in liver fibrosis is not well characterized due to the lack of specific markers and difficulties with their isolation, hematopoietic stem cells contribute to hepatic fibrocytes in response to liver injury. HSC, hepatic stellate cell. Source: Kisseleva T, Brenner DA. The phenotypic fate and functional role for bone marrow-derived stem cells in liver fibrosis. J Hepatol 2013;56:965. Reproduced with permission of Elsevier.

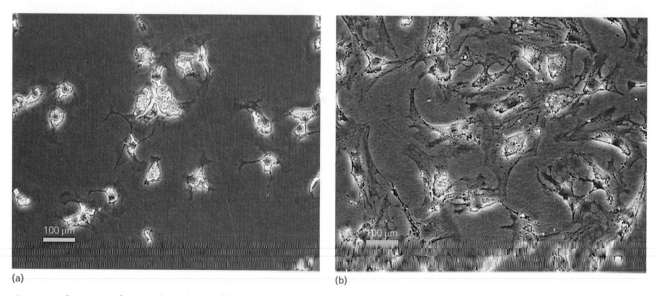

(a) (b)

Figure 54.4 Quiescent and activated stellate cells. (a) Hepatic stellate cells isolated from normal rat livers, and grown for 1 day. They appear compact, with refractile, lipid droplets readily visible in a perinuclear fashion. (b) Cells from the same cell isolation, but grown in culture in medium containing serum for 5 days. These activated cells have lost significant amounts of their lipid droplets, have grown in size with the development of long cytoplasmic extensions, and have developed large nuclei.

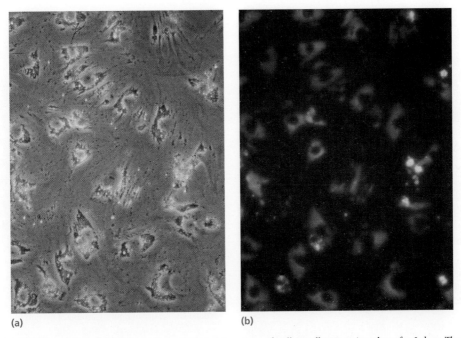

(a) (b)

Figure 54.5 Activated rat hepatic stellate cells. **(a)** Phase contrast photomicroscopy of stellate cells grown in culture for 3 days. The lipid droplets can be seen encircling the nucleus, and large amounts of cellular cytoplasm are seen extending away from the nucleus. **(b)** The same field exposed to UV light, which causes the lipid droplets to autofluoresce a light blue-white color. Each stellate cell is approximately 50 μm in diameter.

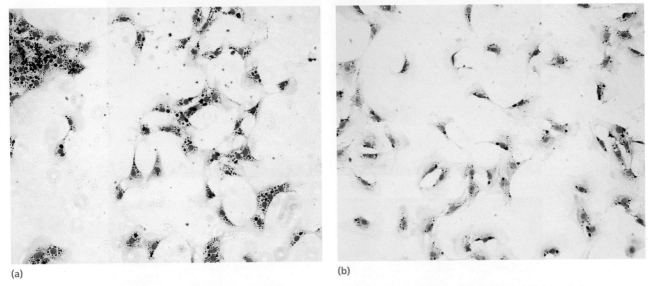

(a) (b)

Figure 54.6 **(a, b)** Oil red O staining in hepatic stellate cells. Stellate cells were isolated from normal (left) or bile duct ligated (right) male Sprague-Dawley rats and placed on plastic dishes. After 24 hours, cells were washed and exposed to oil red O for 5 minutes, then fixed with 4% paraformaldehyde. Reduced oil red O droplets can be readily appreciated in the cells from the bile duct ligated liver, consistent with their activation. Source: Courtesy of Loretta Jophlin, MD, PhD, Medical University of South Carolina, Division of Gastroenterology.

matrix. Finally, stellate cell contraction may itself cause physical distortion of the liver at a whole-organ level.

The process of stellate cell activation appears to be highly complex and is controlled by many factors, including paracrine and autocrine factors (cytokines, chemokines, peptides). Stellate cells activation in vitro appears to be primarily as a function of the physical rather than the chemical properties of the substrate (Figure 54.12). In these experiments, stellate cells require a mechanically stiff substrate, with adhesion to matrix proteins and the generation of mechanical tension, to differentiate. The findings have implications for stellate cell activation in vivo.

Stellate cells reside in the hepatic sinusoidal space of Disse (physically located between the sinusoidal endothelial cell and the hepatocyte), and as such interact with multiple other cell types, including endothelial cells, hepatocytes, macrophages, and others. Recently, it has been shown that stellate cells interact

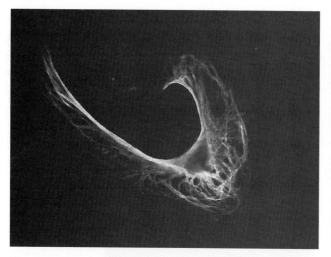

Figure 54.7 Vimentin in a stellate cell. The cell is approximately 50 μm in diameter. Source: Rockey DC, Friedman SL. Cytoskeleton of liver perisinusoidal cells (lipocytes) in normal and pathological conditions. Cytoskeleton 1992;22:227. Reproduced with permission of John Wiley & Sons.

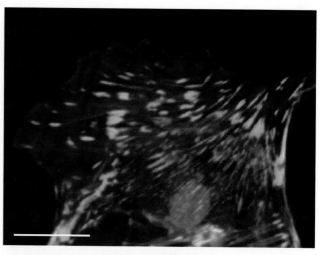

Figure 54.9 Focal adhesion expression in stellate cells. Focal adhesion kinase (green), smooth muscle a actin (Acta 2) (red), and the nucleus (blue) were detected by immunohistochemistry. Shown is an overlay image. The size bar is 5 microns. Source: Courtesy of Serhan Karvar, MD, Medical University of South Carolina, Division of Gastroenterology.

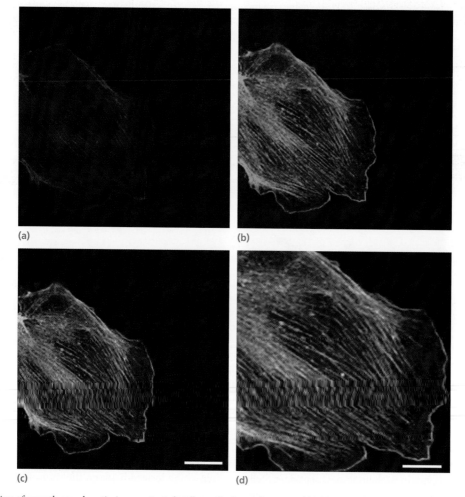

Figure 54.8 Expression of smooth muscle actin in an activated stellate cell after carbon tetrachloride (CCl₄) induced liver injury; **(a)** smooth muscle α-actin (red; *Acta2*) and **(b)** nonmuscle β-actin (green). **(c, d)** Overlays revealing colocalization of actins. **(c)** bar = 10 μm; **(d)** bar = 5 μm. Source: Rockey DC, Weymouth N, Shi Z. Smooth muscle α actin (Acta2) and myofibroblast function during hepatic wound healing. PLoS ONE 2013;8:e77166. Reproduced with permission of PLoS under the Creative Commons License.

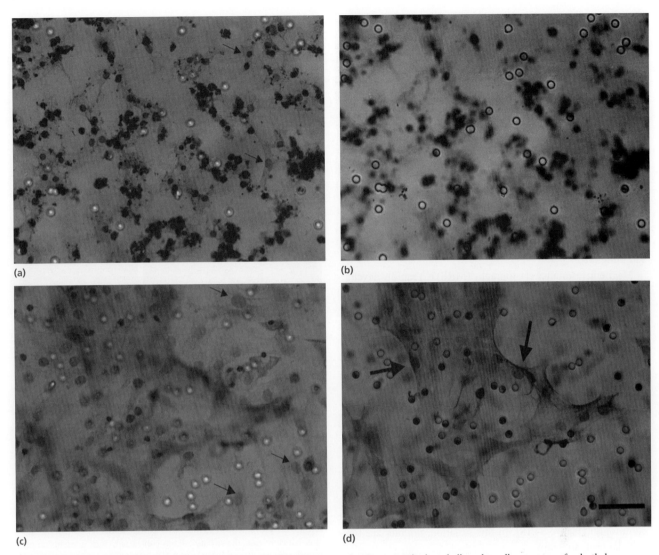

Figure 54.10 Stellate cell motility. Cells from normal and injured livers were isolated as in Methods and allowed to adhere on top of polyethylene terphthalate membranes containing 8 μm pores. In **(a)** and **(b)** are shown representative examples of cells from normal liver and in **(c)** and **(d)** are shown cells from injured liver (carbon tetrachloride). **(a)** Shows an exposure focused on the top of the membrane; **(b)** depicts the same field but focused on the bottom of the membrane. In **(a)** many cells remain compact and therefore are darkly stained; the small arrows point to cells that have begun to spread on the top of the membrane. In **(b)** no cells have passed through the membrane and therefore none are in focus. In **(c)** and **(d)** virtually all cells have spread markedly; the small arrows in **(c)** point to cells that have spread on the top of the membrane. In **(d)** the larger arrows point to cells that have migrated through the membrane. Bar = 50 μm. Source: Rockey DC, Weymouth N, Shi Z. Smooth muscle α actin (Acta2) and myofibroblast function during hepatic wound healing. PLoS ONE 2013;8:e77166. Reproduced with permission of PLoS under the Creative Commons License.

with dendritic cells; such cell–cell interactions can be prominently seen in mouse liver (Figure 54.13).

Reversion of fibrosis

Essentially all forms of fibrosis, including hepatic fibrosis, are linked to a population of effector cells that produce abnormal amounts of extracellular matrix that is deposited in parenchymal tissue and disrupts organ function. Further, available evidence suggests that fibrosis is reversible or may revert to some extent in many different organs (Figure 54.14). In the liver,

fibrosis appears to be particularly reversible, especially when the underlying disease can be eradicated. As highlighted above, hepatic stellate cells are key effectors in the liver process. Thus, the mechanism of reversion appears to be through stellate cell apoptosis, reversion of activation, or even cellular senescence.

Measurement of fibrosis

Measurement of fibrosis is important for several reasons. For one, fibrosis is important prognostically. Additionally, it is often drives treatment algorithms (for new direct-acting HCV antiviral therapy, therapy now is currently being directed primarily towards those with advanced fibrosis). For many years, measurement of fibrosis has been assessed primarily histologically, requiring liver biopsy. Recent research has begun to focus on noninvasive approaches to measurement of fibrosis, including routine laboratory tests, quantitative assays of liver function, markers of extracellular matrix synthesis and/or degradation, and radiological imaging studies. Imaging approaches are particularly attractive because they combine a noninvasive approach with the potential for high sensitivity and specificity. Transient elastography has gained considerable interest as a method to quantitate fibrosis because it appears that liver "stiffness" may accompany the fibrogenic response (see above, and Figure 54.15). The procedure is performed by obtaining multiple measurements in each patient, further reducing the potential for sampling error.

Magnetic resonance elastography (MRE) is a rapidly developing technology for quantitative assessment of the mechanical properties of tissue. MRE obtains information about liver stiffness by assessing the propagation of mechanical waves through the tissue using magnetic resonance imaging (MRI) (Figures 54.16 and 54.17). The technique is rapidly evolving, and appears to have similar, if not slightly better, sensitivity and specificity than transient elastography.

Cirrhosis

Cirrhosis has several different gross histological appearances. Although there is overlap among the various gross appearances, it has been classically taught that macronodular (or postnecrotic) cirrhosis is typical of viral hepatitis (B or C most commonly) (Figure 54.18). In this situation, nodules are typically larger than 3 mm.

Micronodular cirrhosis is typically believed to occur in patients with alcoholic or nonalcoholic steatohepatitis (Figure 54.19). Nodules in this pathological condition are usually less than 3 mm in size. The distinction between macronodular and micronodular cirrhosis is typically not clinically relevant, because hepatocyte dysfunction, portal hypertension, and clinical complications as well as fibrosis are typical of each. In fact, many patients with a variety of etiologies of cirrhosis have different sized "mixed" cirrhosis.

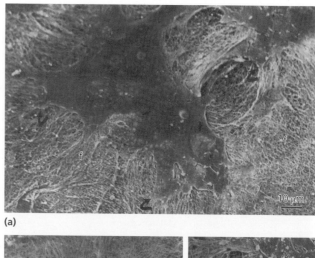

(a)

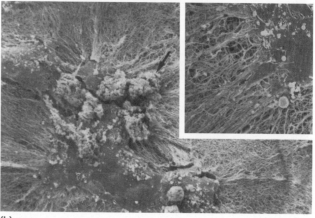

(b)

Figure 54.11 Stellate cell contraction. The image depicts scanning electron microscopy of stellate cells on a collagen lattice. In **(a)** is shown a stellate cell (middle) prior to lattice release. Cytoplasmic processes (curved arrows) are prominently extended over collage fibrils (f). In **(b)** 4 hours after lattice release, the stellate cell has contracted, causing extrusion of rounded bodies. The collagen lattice also appears denser, consistent with its contraction. In the inset, an intricate association between the stellate cell cytoplasmic cell processes and collagen fibrils is evident. **(a, b)** ×1200; inset ×3000. Source: Rockey DC, Housset CN, Friedman SL. Activation-dependent contractility of rat hepatic lipocytes in culture and in vivo. J Clin Invest 1993;92:1795. Reproduced with permission of the American Society for Clinical Investigation.

0.4 kPa　　　　　　　　1.0 kPa　　　　　　　　1.75 kPa

2.5 kPa　　　　　　　　8.0 kPa　　　　　　　　12 kPa

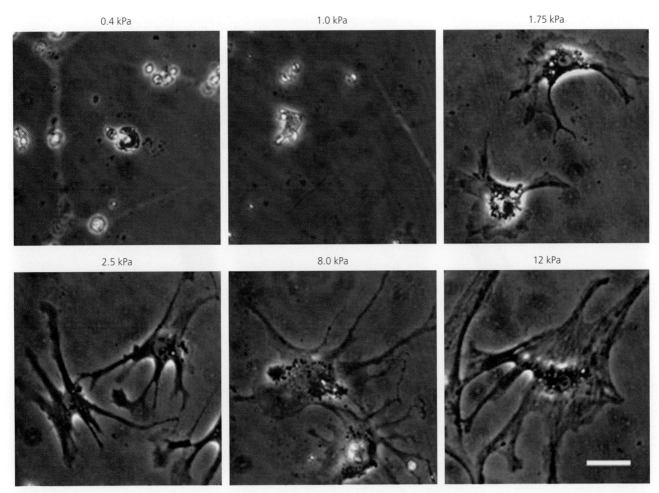

Figure 54.12 Hepatic stellate cells (HSC) demonstrate increased spreading on stiffer substrates. Phase contrast light microscopy reveals that stellate cells appear morphologically quiescent on soft supports (0.4–1.0 kPa), while those grown on stiff (8–12 kPa) polyacrylamide supports displayed an activated, myofibroblastic-like phenotype. Cells cultured on intermediate supports (1.75–2.5 kPa) showed intermediate phenotypes. Bar = 50 μm. Source: Olsen AL, Bloomer SA, Chan EP, et al. Hepatic stellate cells require a stiff environment for myofibroblastic differentiation. Am J Physiol Gastrointest Liver Physiol 2011;301:G110. Reproduced with permission of The American Physiological Society.

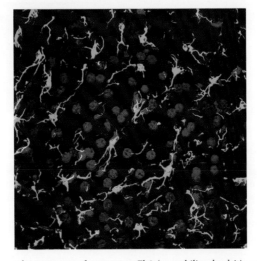

Figure 54.13 Stellate cell–cell communications. After exposure of a mouse to Flt3 (to mobilize dendritic cells), a liver section was fixed and exposed to antidesmin (green) and anti-CD11c antibody (red). Nuclei were labeled with DAPI. The image was generated in the Center for Biologic Imaging, University of Pittsburgh by Donna Stolz in collaboration with Angus Thomson and Osamu Yoshida at the TE Strarzl Transplantation Institute, University of Pittsburgh. Source: Gandhi 2015. Reproduced with permission of Elsevier and Chadrashekar Gandhi.

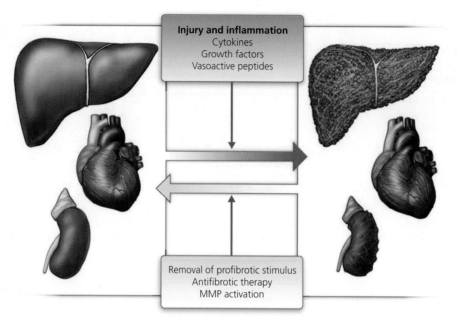

Figure 54.14 Reversion of fibrosis. Fibrosis is a remarkably plastic process in which there is dynamic interplay between extracellular matrix protein deposition and degradation. For instances in which degradation overtakes deposition, tissue fibrosis can be reversed, and may occur in many organs, suggesting consistent biological themes. Often, the removal of the inciting stimulus is sufficient, and in some instances therapeutic interventions targeting the underlying disease process may help to reverse the fibrogenic process. MMP, matrix metalloproteinase. Source: Rockey DC, Bell PD, Hill JA. Fibrosis–a common pathway to organ injury and failure. N Engl J Med 2015;372:1138. Reproduced with permission of Massachusetts Medical Society.

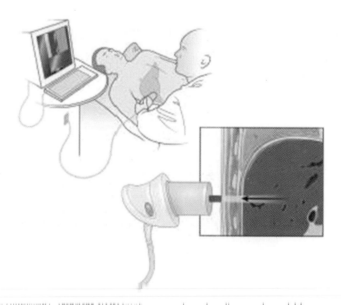

Figure 54.15 Transient elastography (fibroscan). Transient elastography uses pulse-echo ultrasound acquisitions to measure liver stiffness by "shooting" pulse echos into the liver. It is able to predict advanced fibrosis stages with high specificity. Its advantages include that it is noninvasive and simple to perform. However, it should be noted that it may be difficult to obtain accurate measurements in obese patients or those with ascites. Newer probes for use in obese patients have helped overcome this issue. Source: Rockey DC. Noninvasive assessment of liver fibrosis and portal hypertension with transient elastography. Gastroenterology 2008;134:8. Reproduced with permission of Elsevier.

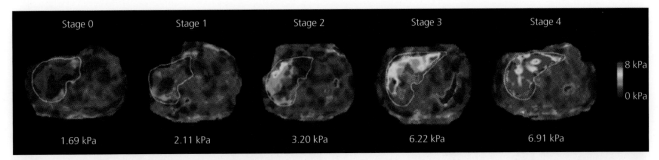

Figure 54.16 Magnetic resonance elastography (MRE). MRE stiffness maps of five patients with nonalcoholic fatty liver disease and different stages of liver fibrosis. These maps depict the spatial distribution of stiffness (in kPa) within the liver (outlined in white). As shown in the color key, the stiffness values range from near zero (dark purple) to 8 kPa (red). The histology-determined liver fibrosis stage is shown above each stiffness map, and the MRE-determined mean liver stiffness is shown below each image. Notice that the stiffness values are greater in patients with more-advanced fibrosis. Source: Loomba R, Wolfson T, Ang B, et al. Magnetic resonance elastography predicts advanced fibrosis in patients with nonalcoholic fatty liver disease: a prospective study. Hepatology 2014;60:1920. Reproduced with permission of John Wiley & Sons.

2D-MRE elastograms			
Fibrosis stage	1	3	4
Advanced fibrosis diagnosis	No	Yes	Yes
Hepatic stiffness (kPa)	2.5	3.7	5.7
2D-MRE Performance	Correct	Correct	Correct
Clinical prediction rules performance			
FIB-4	Indeterminate	Indeterminate	Indeterminate
Lok Index	Correct	Indeterminate	Indeterminate
Bonacini cirrhosis discriminant score	Correct	Wrong	Wrong
AST to ALT ratio	Correct	Wrong	Correct
NAFLD fibrosis score	Wrong	Indeterminate	Indeterminate
BARD	Wrong	Wrong	Correct
APRI	Wrong	Correct	Wrong
NASH CRN model	N/A	N/A	N/A

Figure 54.17 Two-dimensional magnetic resonance elastography (2D-MRE). Two-dimensional magnetic resonance elastograms of three patients with stiffness values of 2.5 (left), 3.7 (middle), and 5.7 (right) kPa are shown. Patients had stage 1, 3, and 4 fibrosis respectively. 2D-MRE correctly diagnosed all three patients with or without advanced fibrosis, whereas clinical prediction rules produced mixed results. AST, aspartate aminotransferase; ALT, alanine aminotransferase; NAFLD, nonalcoholic fatty liver disease; BARD, body mass index, AST:ALT, diabetes; APRI, AST to platelet ratio index; NASH CRN, Nonalcoholic Steatohepatitis Clinical Research Network. Source: Cui J, Ang B, Haufe W, et al. Comparative diagnostic accuracy of magnetic resonance elastography vs. eight clinical prediction rules for non-invasive diagnosis of advanced fibrosis in biopsy-proven non-alcoholic fatty liver disease: a prospective study. Aliment Pharmacol Ther 2015;41:1271. Reproduced with permission of John Wiley & Sons.

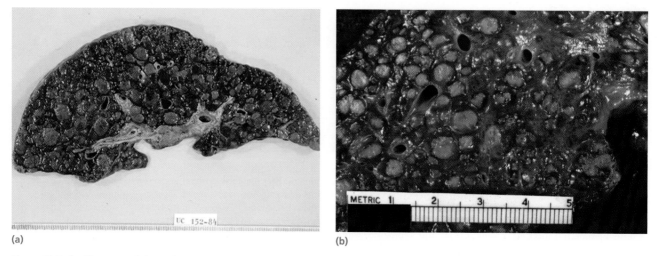

Figure 54.18 (a, b) Macronodular cirrhosis. In macronodular cirrhosis, nodules are large and variable in size. Source: www.wikidoc.org/index.php/File:Cirrhosis_017.jpg. Reproduced with permission under the Creative Commons License.

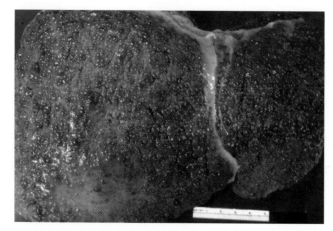

Figure 54.19 Micronodular cirrhosis. Nodules are typically small. Source: www.wikidoc.org/index.php/File:Cirrhosis_001.jpg. Reproduced with permission under the Creative Commons License.

CHAPTER 55

Approach to the patient with ascites and its complications

Guadalupe Garcia-Tsao

Yale University School of Medicine, New Haven, CT, USA

Ascites is the accumulation of fluid in the peritoneal cavity. The most common causes of ascites are cirrhosis, peritoneal malignancy, and heart failure.

In patients with cirrhosis, ascites is one of the complications that marks the transition from a compensated to a decompensated stage. Initially, ascites is "uncomplicated," that is, it responds well to diuretics and is not infected. As cirrhosis progresses and the mechanisms that lead to ascites formation worsen, ascites ceases to respond to diuretics (refractory ascites). Bacteria may infect ascites, an entity known as spontaneous bacterial peritonitis (SBP) that occurs mainly in hospitalized patients with severe liver disease. With further progression of cirrhosis, the patient with ascites may develop hyponatremia and functional renal failure (hepatorenal syndrome). The hemodynamic alterations that lead to ascites and refractory ascites are the same as those that lead to hyponatremia and hepatorenal syndrome, differing only in the degree of abnormality, with the latter complications denoting a more deranged circulatory status. The approach to a patient with ascites depends on the setting surrounding its presentation (Figures 55.1–55.19 and Tables 55.1, 55.2, 55.3, and 55.4).

Suspected ascites

In a patient with suspected ascites (by history and physical examination) the least invasive and most cost-effective method to confirm the presence of ascites is abdominal ultrasonography. This test can be accompanied by Doppler examination of the hepatic venous system; this is an important initial test to rule out the presence of hepatic vein obstruction, which is a frequently overlooked cause of ascites.

New onset ascites

In a patient with new onset ascites, the priority is to determine the etiology of ascites as this will determine its management. A diagnostic paracentesis should be the first test performed in such a patient. The serum-ascites albumin gradient (SAAG) and the ascites total protein are two inexpensive tests that, taken together, are most useful. The three main causes of ascites (cirrhosis, peritoneal pathology [malignancy or tuberculosis] and heart failure) can be easily distinguished by combining the results of SAAG (a measure of sinusoidal pressure) and ascites total protein. In cirrhosis, the SAAG is high ($>1.1\,g/dL$) and ascites protein is low ($<2.5\,g/dL$); in peritoneal disease, the SAAG is low and ascites protein is high; in heart failure, both the SAAG and the ascites protein are high. The decisive test to determine the source of ascites (sinusoidal or not) is by measuring the hepatic venous pressure gradient. When the source is likely to be peritoneal (carcinomatosis or tuberculosis), the decisive test is a laparoscopy with peritoneal biopsy, culture, and histological examination.

Cirrhotic ascites

In a patient with cirrhotic ascites, management depends on the phase of ascites at which the patient with cirrhosis is situated, from the patient with uncomplicated ascites to the patient with hepatorenal syndrome.

Therapy of cirrhotic ascites is not an emergency as the risk of death is not implicit unless the fluid is infected. The mainstay of therapy is aimed at achieving a negative sodium balance (i.e., sodium restriction and diuretics). Diuretic treatment should

Yamada's Atlas of Gastroenterology, Fifth Edition. Edited by Daniel K. Podolsky, Michael Camilleri, J. Gregory Fitz, Anthony N. Kalloo, Fergus Shanahan, and Timothy C. Wang.
© 2016 John Wiley & Sons, Ltd. Published 2016 by John Wiley & Sons, Ltd.
Companion website: www.yamadagastro.com/atlas

only be initiated in the patient with cirrhosis in whom complications, such as gastrointestinal (GI) hemorrhage, bacterial infection, and renal dysfunction, are absent or have resolved. In a patient with tense ascites who experiences not only abdominal discomfort, but also respiratory distress, a single large-volume paracentesis (LVP) should be performed prior, or concomitant to, starting diuretics. Diuretic therapy should be spironolactone based, either with spironolactone alone (initial dose of 100 mg in a single daily dose, increased to a maximum of 400 mg/day), or in combination with furosemide (range of 20–160 mg/day). Both schedules are equally effective; however, dose adjustments are needed more frequently in patients in whom treatment is initiated with combination therapy. Before considering that ascites is refractory to diuretics, it is necessary to ascertain whether the patient has adhered to the prescribed sodium-restricted diet and has restrained from using nonsteroidal antiinflammatory drugs.

Refractory ascites

First line therapy for patients with refractory ascites is serial LVP, adding albumin (6–8 g/L of ascites removed) if more than 5 L are removed at once. In patients in whom 5 L or less are being removed, a plasma volume expander can be utilized. To increase the time between paracenteses, patients should continue on maximally tolerated diuretic dose provided that the urinary sodium is >30 mEq/L. In patients requiring more than two or three LVPs per month or in those in whom ascites is loculated and cannot be entirely removed with a single LVP, evaluation for TIPS placement should be undertaken. In general TIPS should not be performed in patients with serum bilirubin >3 mg/dL, a CTP score >11, age >70 years or evidence of heart failure, as these factors are associated with a poorer survival and a poorer shunt function. Patients with refractory ascites that seem to benefit most from TIPS are those with a MELD of 15 or lower. Although studies on TIPS for refractory ascites were performed using uncovered stents, covered stents should be used because of the lower rate of shunt dysfunction and potential benefits regarding development of encephalopathy, and survival. In patients who are requiring frequent LVP and who are not TIPS candidates, a peritoneovenous shunt (PVS) should be considered. Refractory ascites is often associated with type 2 hepatorenal syndrome, a moderate renal failure (serum creatinine between 1.5 and 2.5 mg/dL), with a steady or slowly progressive course.

Hepatic hydrothorax

Hepatic hydrothorax should be treated in the same way as cirrhotic ascites, that is, the mainstay of therapy is sodium restriction and diuretics. Before determining that hydrothorax is refractory, a trial of in-hospital diuretic therapy should be attempted. In patients with refractory hepatic hydrothorax, other therapeutic options such as repeated thoracenteses, TIPS, or pleurodesis should be considered.

Spontaneous bacterial peritonitis

Spontaneous bacterial peritonitis (SBP) is the most common type of bacterial infection in hospitalized cirrhotic patients and occurs mainly in patients with low ascites protein and severe liver disease. Spontaneous bacterial peritonitis should be suspected in patients with symptoms/signs of SBP (fever, abdominal pain or tenderness, and leukocytosis) and in those with unexplained encephalopathy, jaundice, or worsening renal failure. A diagnostic paracentesis, as well as simultaneous blood and urine cultures and chest radiograph should be obtained. The diagnosis of SBP is established with an ascites polymorphonuclear leukocyte (PMN) count >250/mm³. Intravenous antibiotics proven to be effective in SBP are cefotaxime (2 g every 12 h), ceftriaxone (1–2 g every 24 h) and the combination of amoxicillin and clavulanic acid (1 mg/0.2 g every 8 h). In patients with baseline serum bilirubin >4 mg/dL and serum creatinine >1 g/dL albumin should be used to prevent renal dysfunction. The dose of albumin used is arbitrary, 1.5 g/kg of body weight during the first 6 h, followed by 1 g/kg on day 3, with a maximum of 100 g/day. Patients surviving an episode of SBP should be started on indefinite antibiotic prophylaxis (norfloxacin or ciprofloxacin 400 mg orally every day).

Acute renal failure

In hospitalized patients with cirrhosis, the most common cause of acute renal failure is prerenal (accounting for 60%–80% of the cases), resulting from any factor that will further decrease the effective arterial blood volume of the patient with cirrhosis. Therefore, it can result from:

(a) factors that cause hypovolemia, such as GI hemorrhage, overdiuresis or diarrhea;

(b) factors that worsen vasodilatation, such as sepsis, use of vasodilators and the postparacentesis circulatory dysfunction; and

(c) factors that cause renal vasoconstriction, such as nonsteroidal antiinflammatory drugs or intravenous contrast agents.

These factors account for up to 80% of the causes of prerenal failure. Hepatorenal syndrome (HRS) is a type of prerenal failure as it results from hemodynamic abnormalities (extreme vasodilatation) leading to renal vasoconstriction.

In a patient with cirrhosis who presents with an acute deterioration in renal function, as evidenced by a >50% (>1.5-fold) increase in serum creatinine, the main concern is to rule out type 1 HRS. Diuretics should be discontinued and volume expanded with albumin intravenously. Spontaneous bacterial peritonitis (a common precipitant of HRS), other bacterial infections, and GI hemorrhage should be excluded and treated if present. If creatinine does not improve or continues to worsen, the diagnosis HRS-type 1 is suspected. The main differential at this point is with acute tubular necrosis (ATN), particularly in the presence of a history of a hypotensive event. Albuminuria >50 mg/dL and urine casts suggests ATN, while FeNa equal or lower than 0.1% suggests HRS. In patients with ATN, renal function must be supported with hemodialysis until resolution of tubular function.

In patients with suspected type 1 HRS, diuretics should continue to be withheld to prevent further decreases in effective arterial blood volume. Although liver transplant is the only curative treatment for HRS, treatment with vasoconstrictors plus albumin can be used as a bridge to transplantation as this treatment leads to reversal of HRS-1 in about one-third of the patients, improving outcomes after liver transplant. The best evidence supports the use of terlipressin at a dose 0.5–2 mg intravenously every 4–6 h. Dose should probably be adjusted according to the mean arterial blood pressure (an indirect indicator of vasodilatation). This method has been used for adjusting the dose of midodrine (7.5–12.5 mg three times a day) plus octreotide (100–200 mcg s.c. three times a day). Albumin (20–40 g/day) should be administered together with the vasoconstrictor. Limited evidence favors the use of TIPS in responders to vasoconstrictors and the use of extracorporeal albumin dialysis in HRS; however, further trials are awaited.

Table 55.1 Etiology of ascites and classification by the serum-ascites albumin gradient (SAAG) and ascites protein: main etiological factors of ascites.

	SAAG	Ascites protein
Cirrhosis and/or alcoholic hepatitis	High	Low
Congestive heart failure	High	High
Peritoneal malignancy	Low	High
Peritoneal tuberculosis	Low	High

Table 55.2 Other etiologies of cirrhosis (account for <2% of all cases).

	SAAG	Ascites protein
Massive hepatic metastases	High	Low
Nodular regenerative hyperplasia	High	Low
Fulminant liver failure	High	Low?
Budd–Chiari syndrome (late)	High	Low
Budd–Chiari syndrome (early)	High	High
Constrictive pericarditis	High	High
Venoocclusive disease	High	High
Myxedema	High	High
Nephrogenous (dialysis) ascites	High	High
Mixed ascites (cirrhosis + peritoneal malignancy)	High	Variable
Pancreatic ascites	Low	High
Serositis (connective tissue disease)	Low	High
Chlamydial/gonococcal	Low	High
Biliary	Low	High?
Ovarian hyperstimulation syndrome	Low?	High
Nephrotic syndrome	Low	Low

Those assessments followed by a question mark are theoretical and have not been confirmed by data in the literature.

Table 55.3 Analysis of ascitic fluid.

Routine analysis of ascitic fluid
Gross appearance
Total protein
Albumin (with simultaneous estimation of serum albumin) so that the ascites-albumin gradient can be calculated by subtracting the ascitic fluid value from the serum value
White blood cell count and differential
Bacteriological cultures

Focused analysis of ascitic fluid
Cytology (to exclude malignant ascites)
Amylase (if pancreatic ascites is suspected)
Acid-fast bacilli smear and culture and adenosine deaminase determination (if peritoneal tuberculosis is suspected)
Glucose and lactic dehydrogenase (if secondary peritonitis is suspected in a patient with ascites PMN >250/mm3)
Triglycerides (if the fluid has a milky appearance, i.e., chylous ascites)
Red blood cell count (if the fluid is bloody)

PMN, polymorphonuclear leukocytes.

Table 55.4 Differential of ascites based on HVPG measurements.

Cause of ascites	WHVP	FHVP	HVPG
Cirrhosis	Increased	Normal	Increased
Cardiac ascites	Increased	Increased	Normal
Peritoneal malignancy or TB	Normal	Normal	Normal

FHVP, free hepatic venous pressure; HVPG, hepatic venous pressure gradient; TB, tuberculosis; WHVP, wedged hepatic venous pressure.

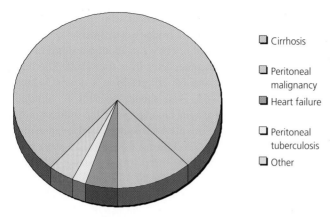

Figure 55.1 Causes of ascites. Cirrhosis is the most common cause of ascites, accounting for 80% of cases. Peritoneal malignancy, heart failure, and peritoneal tuberculosis are also common, accounting for another 15% of the cases. Less common causes of ascites include massive hepatic metastases, pancreatitis, nephrogenic ascites, and the Budd–Chiari syndrome. Of the most common causes, cirrhosis and heart failure are portal sinusoidal hypertensive causes of ascites, whereas peritoneal malignancy and tuberculosis are nonportal hypertensive causes.

☐ Cirrhosis

☐ Peritoneal malignancy

■ Heart failure

☐ Peritoneal tuberculosis

☐ Other

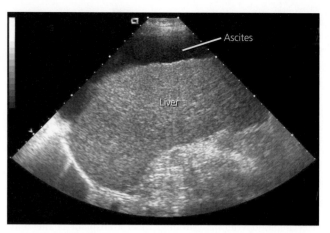

Figure 55.2 Ultrasound demonstrating the presence of ascites (dark area). Physical examination is relatively insensitive for detecting ascetic fluid, particularly when the amount is small, or the patient is obese. The initial, most cost effective and least invasive method to confirm the presence of ascites is abdominal ultrasonography. It is considered the gold standard for diagnosing ascites as it can detect amounts as small as 100 mL.

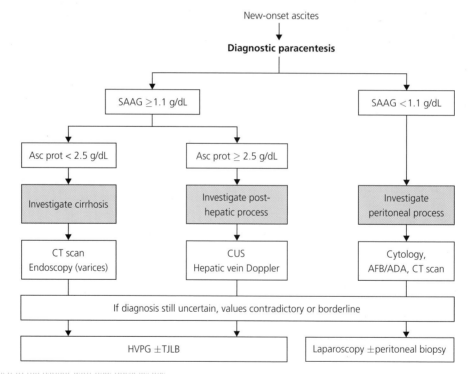

Figure 55.3 Approach to the patient with new onset ascites.
AFB, acid fast bacillus; ADA, adenosine deaminase; CT, computed axial tomography; HVPG, hepatic venous pressure gradient; SAAG, serum-ascites albumin gradient; TJLB, transjugular liver biopsy.

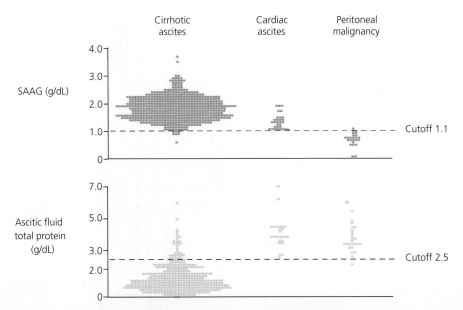

Figure 55.4 Serum–ascites albumin gradient (SAAG) and ascites protein levels help distinguish the most common causes of ascites. The three main causes of ascites (cirrhosis, right-sided heart failure and peritoneal pathology [malignancy or tuberculosis]), can be easily distinguished by combining the results of both the SAAG (top panel) and ascites total protein content (lower panel). The cutoffs for SAAG and ascites protein levels are 1.1 g/dL and 2.5 g/dL, respectively. Cirrhotic ascites is typically high SAAG and low protein; cardiac ascites is high SAAG and high protein; and ascites secondary to peritoneal malignancy is typically low SAAG and high protein. SAAG is obtained by subtracting ascites albumin from serum albumin in samples obtained almost simultaneously.

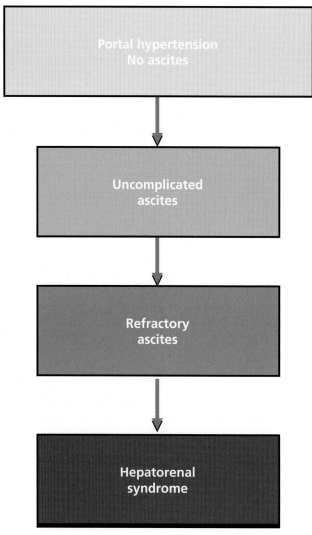

Figure 55.5 Natural history of cirrhotic ascites. The patient with cirrhosis develops portal hypertension. Initially, even though the patient has portal hypertension, it has not yet reached the minimal pressure threshold necessary for the formation of ascites. Later, and once this threshold is reached and hemodynamic alterations lead to sodium retention, the patient develops ascites, which is initially well controlled with diuretics. Later on in the natural history, the patient no longer responds to diuretics (refractory ascites) and, at its most severe, in addition to sodium retention there is renal vasoconstriction that leads to hepatorenal syndrome.

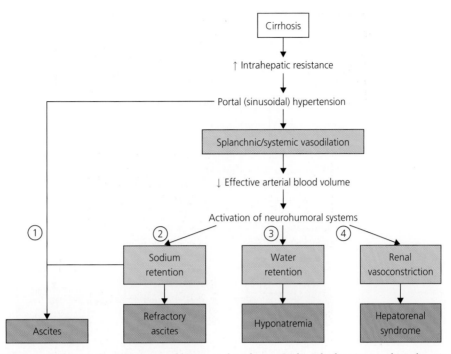

Figure 55.6 Common pathogenesis of ascites, hyponatremia, and hepatorenal syndrome. Cirrhosis leads to increased intrahepatic resistance and thereby to an increased sinusoidal pressure. In addition, portal hypertension leads to splanchnic and systemic arteriolar vasodilation, decreased effective arterial blood volume, up-regulation of sodium-retaining hormones, sodium and water retention and, consequently, plasma volume expansion. With progression of cirrhosis and portal hypertension, the systemic arteriolar resistance is more pronounced, leading to further activation of the renin–angiotensin–aldosterone and sympathetic nervous systems. The resulting increase in water and sodium retention can lead to refractory ascites and hyponatremia, whereas the increase in renal vasoconstriction can lead to a functional renal failure, the hepatorenal syndrome.

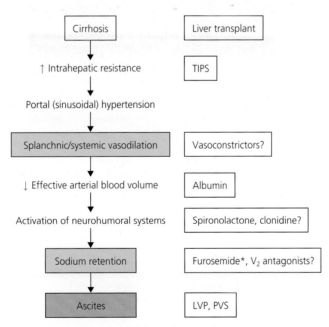

Figure 55.7 Site of action of different therapies for ascites.
*Furosemide should only be used in conjunction with spironolactone.
LVP, large-volume paracentesis; PVS, peritoneovenous shunt; TIPS, transjugular intrahepatic portosystemic shunt; V2, vasopressin type 2.

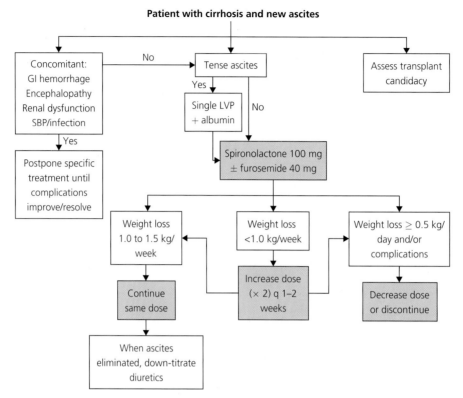

Figure 55.8 Approach to the patient with cirrhosis and uncomplicated ascites.
LVP, large-volume paracentesis

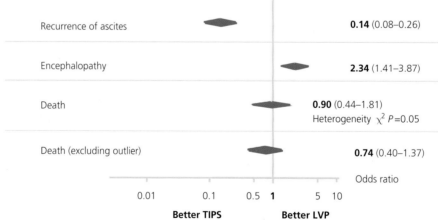

Figure 55.9 Meta-analysis of five randomized controlled trials of large-volume paracentesis (LVP) verses transjugular intrahepatic portosystemic shunt
(TIPS) for refractory ascites. This meta-analysis shows that TIPS is more effective than LVP in preventing recurrence of ascites; however, the risk of
encephalopathy was higher in patients treated with TIPS. Results on mortality were heterogeneous but once an outlier trial (Lebrec et al) was excluded
there was a slight tendency for an improvement in survival in patients treated with TIPS.
LVP, large-volume paracentesis; TIPS, transjugular intrahepatic portosystemic shunt.

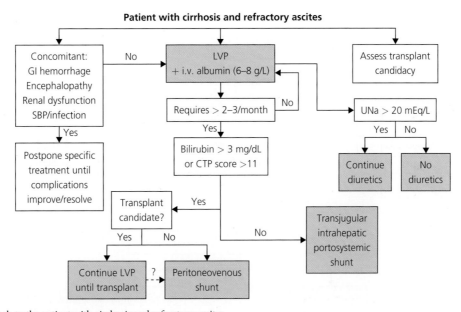

Figure 55.10 Approach to the patient with cirrhosis and refractory ascites.
CTP, Child–Turcotte–Pugh; GI, gastrointestinal; i.v., intravenous; LVP, large-volume paracentesis; SBP, spontaneous bacterial peritonitis; UNa, urinary sodium.

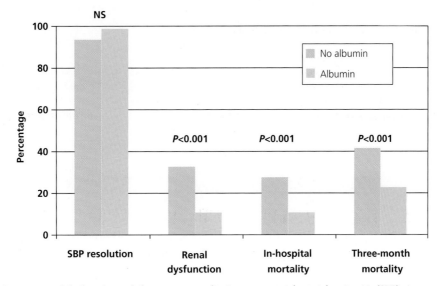

Figure 55.11 Albumin decreases renal dysfunction and short-term mortality in spontaneous bacterial peritonitis (SBP). A prospective randomized nonblinded study that compared cefotaxime plus albumin versus cefotaxime alone showed that patients who received albumin had significantly lower rates of renal dysfunction, and this was associated with a reduction in hospital mortality and 3 month mortality rates. The subgroup of patients that appear to benefit most from albumin are those with a baseline creatinine >1 g/dL, blood urea nitrogen >30 mg/dL or bilirubin >4 mg/dL.

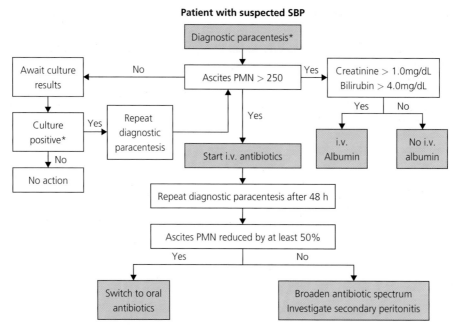

Figure 55.12 Approach to the patient with suspected SBP.
*A diagnostic paracentesis should be performed in any patient with symptoms or signs suggestive of SBP, any patient with unexplained renal dysfunction or encephalopathy, and in any hospitalized patient with cirrhosis and ascites.
i.v., intravenous; PMN, polymorphonuclear leukocytes.

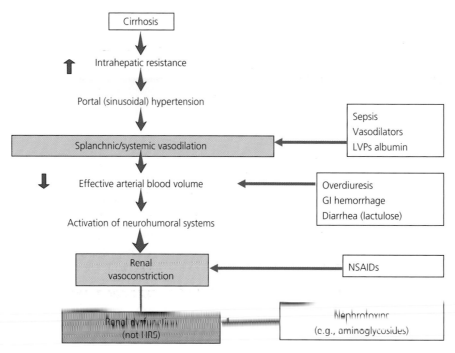

Figure 55.13 Causes of renal dysfunction in patients with cirrhosis. These causes need to be excluded before a diagnosis of hepatorenal syndrome can be established.
GI, gastrointestinal; HRS, hepatorenal syndrome; LVP, large-volume paracentesis; NSAID, nonsteroidal antiinflammatory drug.

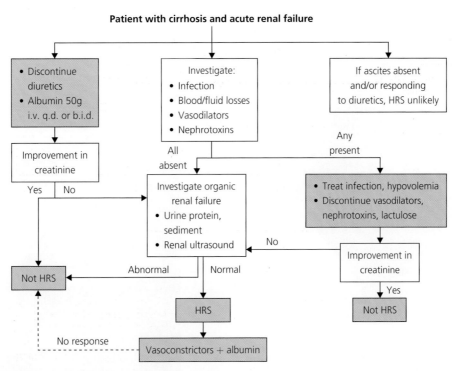

Figure 55.14 Approach to the patient with cirrhosis and acute renal failure. HRS, hepatorenal syndrome.

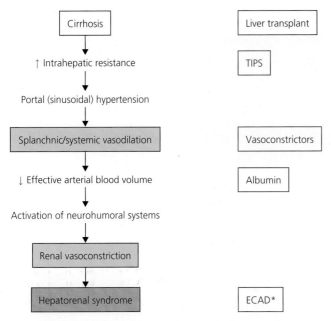

Figure 55.15 Site of action of different therapies for hepatorenal syndrome.
*ECAD stands for extracorporeal albumin dialysis, an experimental therapy that seems to improve hepatorenal system (HRS) that probably acts by decreasing the amount of circulating vasodilators.
TIPS, transjugular intrahepatic portosystemic shunt.

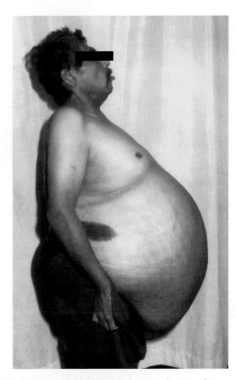

Figure 55.16 A man with alcoholic cirrhosis and ascites that was so massive it caused a gait disturbance. Source: Courtesy of TB Reynolds.

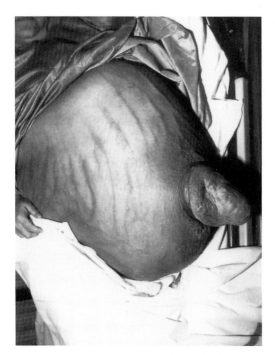

Figure 55.17 A woman with cryptogenic cirrhosis who did not seek medical attention until her umbilical hernia almost touched the floor when she was sitting. Source: Courtesy of TB Reynolds.

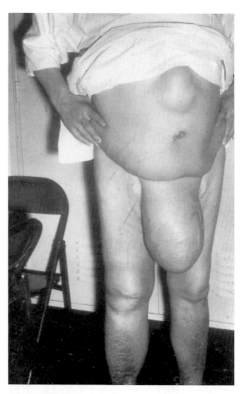

Figure 55.18 A man with large umbilical hernia and massive inguinal hernia. Source: Courtesy of TB Reynolds.

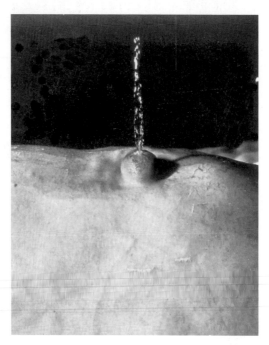

Figure 55.19 Ruptured umbilical hernia – one of the most feared complications of ascites. Source: Courtesy of TB Reynolds.

CHAPTER 56

Liver transplantation

Alyson N. Fox and Robert S. Brown, Jr.

Columbia University College of Physicians and Surgeons, New York Presbyterian Hospital, New York, NY, USA

Background

The first successful human liver transplant was performed by Thomas Starzl in 1967. Over subsequent decades, the field of liver transplantation has grown exponentially, mainly owing to advances in surgical technique and immunosuppression as well as improved management of complications and postoperative infections. Today, liver transplantation is considered to be a life-saving treatment option for patients suffering from a variety of liver diseases (Figure 56.1; Box 56.1).

According to data from the Organ Procurement and Transplantation Network, there were 6010 liver transplants performed in the United States in 2012 (Figure 56.2). The unadjusted 1-year survival after transplant was 88.2%; however, many centers report 1-year survival exceeding 90%. Although the outcomes for liver transplantation continue to improve, the field is limited by the availability of donor organs. Every year, thousands of potential recipients die while on the waiting list due to lack of available donor organs. In 2011, approximately 2456 patients died while waiting for a donor organ and 482 patients were removed from the list after being deemed too sick.

In order to alleviate wait list dropout, there has been increasing use of extended-criteria donor (ECD) organs and living donor organs. These options allow some waitlist candidates to have access to an organ despite a limited supply of ideal deceased donor grafts. ECD organs are those that confer some additional risk to the recipient, such as a risk of illness transmission or risk of initial or long-term inferior function (Box 56.2). Living donor liver transplantation emerged in the early 1990s and offers several benefits to the recipient including: access to an organ earlier in their disease course, freedom from the waitlist,

an "elective" transplant with reduced ischemic time to the organ, and a potentially healthier organ from a well-evaluated donor. Outcomes of those undergoing living donor transplants are equal to or slightly improved over those undergoing deceased donor transplants (Figure 56.3).

Organ allocation

Prior to 2002, organs were allocated based upon the Child–Turcotte–Pugh (CTP) score. The CTP score incorporates serum bilirubin, albumin, and elevation in prothrombin time (PT) above control values, and the presence of hepatic encephalopathy and ascites. One to three points are assigned for each degree of variation amongst these parameters to yield a composite score. A patient is then classified as a class A (5–6 points), B (7–9 points), or C (10–15 points). With progressive disease, CTP score increases, denoting worse survival (Table 56.1). In February 2002, the Model for End-Stage Liver Disease (MELD) score was adopted as the score by which patients are ranked on the transplant waiting list. The MELD score is a mathematically derived score that incorporates three biochemical markers of hepatic function: the serum bilirubin, International Normalized Ratio (INR), and creatinine (Figure 56.4). With worsening hepatic function, the components of the score increase, resulting in a higher MELD score and denoting increasing severity of liver disease. Using the MELD allocation schema those with the highest scores are prioritized for transplant and receive organs first, regardless of competing factors such as etiology of liver disease or list waiting time. Certain disease states are poorly represented by the MELD score and many of those cases are given MELD "exception points" in order to accurately estimate

Yamada's Atlas of Gastroenterology, Fifth Edition. Edited by Daniel K. Podolsky, Michael Camilleri, J. Gregory Fitz, Anthony N. Kalloo, Fergus Shanahan, and Timothy C. Wang.

© 2016 John Wiley & Sons, Ltd. Published 2016 by John Wiley & Sons, Ltd.

Companion website: www.yamadagastro.com/atlas

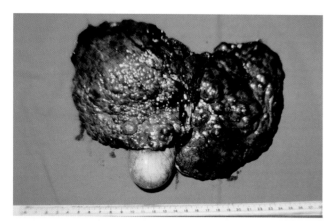

Figure 56.1 Cirrhotic liver explant. Source: Courtesy of Jean Emond, Columbia University Medical Center.

Box 56.1 Indications for liver transplantation. Source: Murray KF, Carithers RL Jr.; AASLD. AASLD practice guidelines: Evaluation of the patient for liver transplantation. Hepatology 2005;41:1407. Reproduced with permission of John Wiley & Sons.

Viralok
    Hepatitis C
    Hepatitis B
Autoimmune liver disease
Alcohol related liver disease
Inherited/metabolic liver diseases
    Hereditary hemochromatosis
    α1-Antitrypsin deficiency
    Wilson disease
    Nonalcoholic fatty liver disease
    Tyrosinemia
    Type IV glycogen storage disease
    Neonatal hemochromatosis
    Amyloidosis
    Hyperoxaluria
    Urea cycle defects
    Amino acid defects
Cholestatic liver disease
    Primary biliary cirrhosis
    Primary sclerosing cholangitis
    Biliary atresia
    Alagille syndrome
    Progressive familial intrahepatic cholestasis
    Cystic fibrosis
    Bile duct loss
Malignancy
    Hepatocellular carcinoma
    Cholangiocarcinoma
    Fibrolamellar carcinoma
    Epithelioid hemangioendothelioma
    Hepatoblastoma
    Metastatic neuroendocrine tumor
Polycystic liver disease
Vascular disorder
    Budd–Chiari syndrome
Fulminant hepatic failure

disease mortality and prioritize those affected for transplant (Box 56.3).

Transplant indications, contraindications, and evaluation

A variety of disease conditions serve as indications for liver transplantation (Box 56.1). The goal of the liver transplant evaluation is to identify the patients who will most benefit from transplant and have the best chance for long-term survival. The evaluation process is multidisciplinary and involves thorough medical, psychiatric, social, and financial screening (Figure 56.5; Box 56.4). The transplant evaluation serves to identify modifiable complications of liver disease, evaluate conditions that may impact the outcome of the transplant, and assess for potential contraindications to the procedure (Box 56.5). Once the requisite consultations and testing are completed, a committee, usually comprised of transplant hepatologists, transplant surgeons, transplant coordinators, psychiatrists, and social workers, convenes to determine who is most appropriate for listing. Once a patient is determined to be a good candidate for transplant, they are placed on the national United Network for Organ Sharing (UNOS) waiting list.

Posttransplant complications

Complications after liver transplantation can be divided into those that occur in the early postoperative period and those occurring much later (Figures 56.6 and 56.7). Early on, the major causes of morbidity and mortality are infection, bleeding, graft dysfunction, vascular and biliary complications, and rejection episodes. Years after transplant, patients are affected by chronic diseases such as obesity, diabetes, cardiovascular disease, and renal dysfunction. Additionally, solid organ transplant recipients are predisposed to posttransplant lymphoproliferative disorder (PTLD), de novo malignancies, and recurrence of their primary liver disease. Recurrent disease represents an ongoing management challenge for the transplant community. In many cases these diseases can be aggressive and ultimately cause graft failure, need for retransplant, or death.

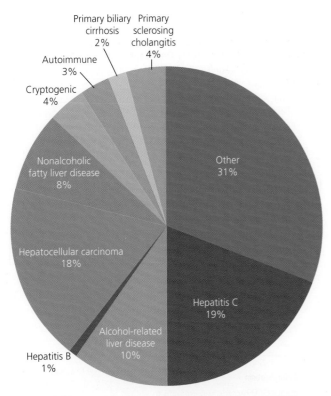

Figure 56.2 Liver transplants in the United States by diagnosis, 2012.

Pie chart segments:
- Other 31%
- Hepatitis C 19%
- Alcohol-related liver disease 10%
- Hepatitis B 1%
- Hepatocellular carcinoma 18%
- Nonalcoholic fatty liver disease 8%
- Cryptogenic 4%
- Autoimmune 3%
- Primary biliary cirrhosis 2%
- Primary sclerosing cholangitis 4%

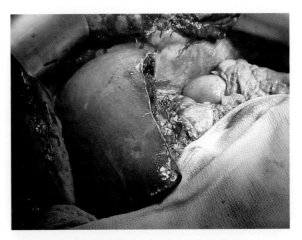

Figure 56.3 Right lobe implanted during living donor liver transplantation. Source: Courtesy of Jean Emond, Columbia University Medical Center.

Box 56.2 Extended-criteria donor organs.

Exposure to hepatitis B, C
Exposure to syphilis, HTLV I/II
Centers for Disease Control (CDC) high risk
Prior malignancy
Older age (>60 years)
Graft steatosis (≥ 30% macrosteatosis)
Split grafts
Prolonged cold ischemic time (12 h)
Donor hypotension requiring vasopressor support
Abnormal liver enzymes in donor due to cardiac arrest, hypotension, or trauma
Donation after cardiac death (DCD, previously termed nonheart beating donor)

Table 56.1 The Child–Turcotte–Pugh scoring system and patient survival at 1 and 2 years.

Parameter	Points		
	1	**2**	**3**
Encephalopathy	None	Minimal	Advanced
Ascites	None	Slight	Moderate
Bilirubin (mg/dL)	<2.0	2–3	>3.0
Albumin (g/dL)	>3.5	2.8–3.5	<2.8
PT prolongation above control (seconds)	1–4	5–6	>6

CTP class	Score	
A	5–6	
B	7–9	
C	10–15	

CTP class	Survival	
	1 year	**2 years**
A	100%	85%
B	80%	60%
C	45%	35%

CTP, Child–Turcotte–Pugh; PT, prothrombin time.

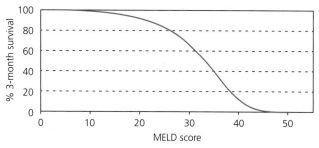

Figure 56.4 The MELD score equation: MELD = 3.78[Ln serum bilirubin (mg/dL)] + 11.2[Ln INR] + 9.57[Ln serum creatinine (mg/dL)] + 6.43. Source: Wiesner R, Edwards E, Freeman R, et al. Model for end-stage liver disease (MELD) and allocation of donor livers. Gastroenterology 2003;124:91. Reproduced with permission of Elsevier.

Box 56.3 Conditions for which Model for End-Stage Liver Disease (MELD) exception points are allocated.

Hepatocellular carcinoma within the Milan criteria (1 lesion ≤ 5 cm, or ≤ 3 lesions ≤ 3 cm)
Cholangiocarcinoma
Familial amyloidosis
Primary hyperoxaluria
Hepatopulmonary syndrome
Portopulmonary hypertension
Intractable pruritus
Budd–Chiari syndrome
Cystic fibrosis
Hereditary hemorrhagic telangiectasia
Polycystic liver disease
Recurrent cholangitis
Small-for-size syndrome following living donor liver transplantation

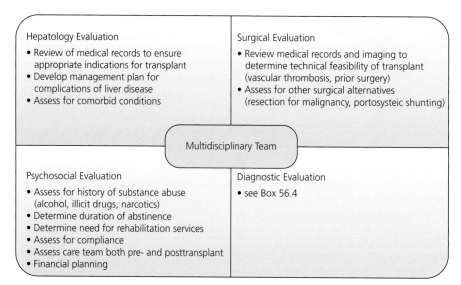

Figure 56.5 Multidisciplinary approach to liver transplant evaluation.

Box 56.4 Diagnostic evaluation for liver transplant.

Laboratory evaluation

Electrolytes, liver function tests, complete blood count, coagulation studies, hepatitis serologies, markers for autoimmune, inherited and metabolic liver diseases, blood typing with antibody screen, rapid plasma reagin, Epstein–Barr virus, cytomegalovirus, HIV testing, thyroid function studies

Radiology evaluation

Abdominal sonogram with Doppler

Contrast-enhanced abdominal imaging

Bone density scan

Computed tomography scan of the chest (if hepatocellular carcinoma)

Nuclear bone scan (if hepatocellular carcinoma)

Cardiac evaluation

Electrocardiogram

Echocardiogram (with agitated saline injection to evaluate for intrapulmonary shunting)

Nuclear stress test (if age >45 years or cardiac risk factors are present)

Coronary catheterization (if stress test is abnormal or high risk for cardiac disease)

Right heart catheterization (if elevated pulmonary pressures on noninvasive studies)

Cardiology consultation

Pulmonary evaluation

Pulmonary artery pressure testing

Chest x-ray

Pulmonary function testing

Room air arterial blood gas

Shunt fraction study if evidence of intrapulmonary shunt

Pulmonary consultation

Neurological evaluation

Carotid Doppler ultrasound imaging if age >60 years

Neuroimaging and neurology consultation if history of neurological disorder

Age-appropriate cancer screening

Pap smear

Mammogram

Colonoscopy

Prostate-specific antigen

Box 56.5 Absolute and relative contraindications to liver transplantation.

Absolute contraindications

Severe, irreversible co-morbid medical illness that adversely impacts short-term life expectancy

Severe pulmonary hypertension (PAP ≥50 mmHg)

Extrahepatic malignancy (excluding some skin cancers)

Extensive hepatocellular carcinoma or with macrovascular or lymph node invasion

Cholangiocarcinoma[a]

Uncontrolled systemic sepsis

Poor social support

Active alcohol and/or drug abuse

Unacceptable risk of recidivism

Severe uncontrolled psychiatric disease

Relative contraindications

Advanced age

Moderate pulmonary hypertension (mean PAP between 35 and 50 mmHg)

Severe hepatopulmonary syndrome with Pao_2 ≤50 mmHg

Severe obesity (body mass index ≥35)

Extensive portal vein and mesenteric vascular thrombosis

[a] Liver transplant has been performed at some centers under specific protocol.
PAP, pulmonary artery pressure.

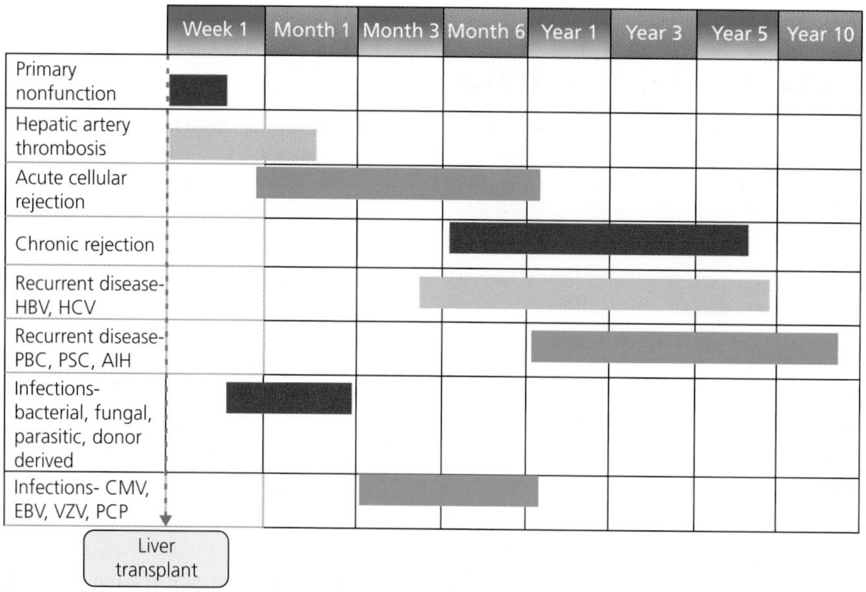

	Week 1	Month 1	Month 3	Month 6	Year 1	Year 3	Year 5	Year 10
Primary nonfunction	▇							
Hepatic artery thrombosis	▇▇▇							
Acute cellular rejection		▇▇▇▇▇▇						
Chronic rejection				▇▇▇▇▇▇				
Recurrent disease-HBV, HCV				▇▇▇▇▇▇▇▇				
Recurrent disease-PBC, PSC, AIH					▇▇▇▇▇▇▇▇			
Infections-bacterial, fungal, parasitic, donor derived	▇▇▇							
Infections- CMV, EBV, VZV, PCP		▇▇▇▇▇						

Liver transplant

Figure 56.6 Postliver transplant complications. AIH, autoimmune hepatitis; CMV, cytomegalovirus; EBV, Epstein–Barr virus; HBV, hepatitis B virus; HCV, hepatitis C virus; PBC, primary biliary cirrhosis; PCP, *Pneumocystis carinii* (*jirovecii*) pneumonia; PSC, primary sclerosing cholangitis; VZV, varicella zoster virus.

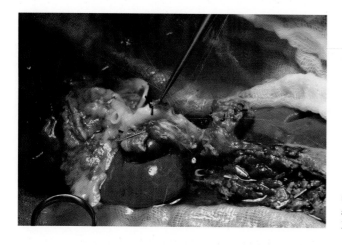

Figure 56.7 Liver transplant surgery – construction of the hepatic arterial anastomosis. Source: Courtesy of Jean Emond, Columbia University Medical Center.

To access the video for this chapter, please go to
www.yamadagastro.com/atlas

Video 56.1 Surgical technique used for laparoscopic left lobe donation. Living donor liver transplantation provides ready access to a liver allograft for those in need. Outcomes of living donor transplants are equal or superior to deceased donor grafts, yet, despite this statistic, living donation remains a poorly utilized option in the US, accounting for less than 5% of the total number of transplants annually. Source: Courtesy of Drs. Benjamin Samstein, Daniel Cherqui, and Jean Emond at New York Presbyterian Hospital.

CHAPTER 57

Hepatocellular carcinoma

Jorge A. Marrero and Amit Singal
University of Texas Southwestern Medical Center, Dallas, TX, USA

Hepatocellular carcinoma (HCC) is one of the most common solid malignancies worldwide, with the highest prevalence rates in East Asia and Africa. Although the prevalence of HCC is lower in the United States and Europe, its incidence is rapidly increasing due to the burden of advanced hepatitis C virus (HCV) and nonalcoholic fatty liver disease (NAFLD) cases (Figure 57.1). In parallel with its increasing incidence rate, HCC has one of the fastest increasing mortality rates among solid tumors in the United States (Figure 57.2). Prognosis for patients with HCC depends on tumor stage at diagnosis, with curative options only available for patients diagnosed at an early stage.

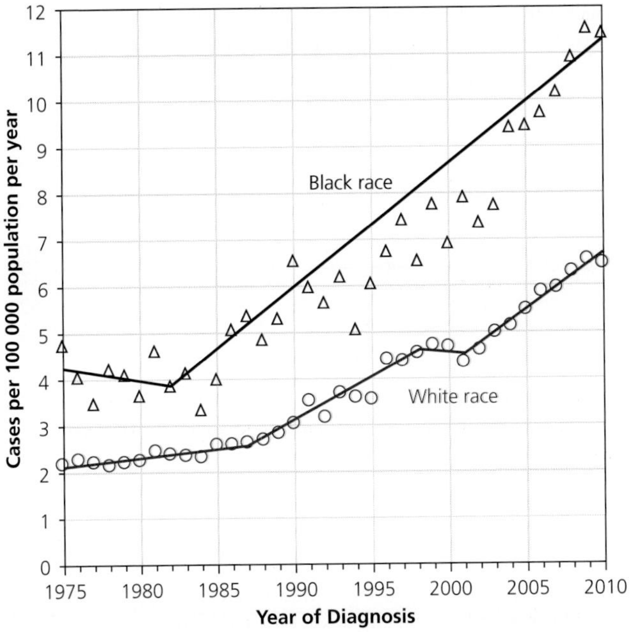

Despite the availability of efficacious surveillance tests, most HCC patients continue to be diagnosed at an advanced stage.

Abdominal ultrasound forms the backbone of HCC surveillance testing and is efficacious for early tumor detection (Figure 57.3). HCC surveillance has been associated with significantly improved rates of early tumor detection, curative treatment, and overall survival in several cohort studies. The diagnosis of HCC can be made radiographically using multiphase computed tomography (CT) or gadolinium contrast-enhanced magnetic resonance imaging (MRI) in the majority of patients (Figure 57.4). Characteristic imaging criteria for HCC include arterial phase enhancement and portal venous/delayed phase hypointensity ("washout") in a liver mass exceeding 1 cm in diameter. Although most diagnoses can be established using imaging alone, biopsy should be considered in patients with noncharacteristic imaging. Histological variants of HCC include trabecular, pseudoglandular, scirrhous, and fibrolamellar types (Figures 57.5, 55.6, 55.7, and 57.8).

Treatment decisions for patients with HCC depend on tumor burden, degree of liver dysfunction, and patient performance status. Patients with early-stage HCC should be considered for curative treatment with liver transplantation, surgical resection, or local ablative therapies. Liver transplantation is typically reserved for patients within Milan criteria (one tumor less than 5 cm or two to three lesions of less than 3 cm); however, there are increasing data evaluating expansion of these criteria. The benefit to patients beyond Milan criteria must be weighed against the impact from delaying transplantation of other patients on the waiting list (Figure 57.9). Patients who are not eligible for curative therapies should be considered for other therapies, including transarterial chemoembolization and systemic therapy, which have been shown to improve survival (Figure 57.10). Patients with significant liver dysfunction and/or poor performance status do not benefit from HCC-directed therapy and should be treated with best supportive care. With increasing availability and complexity of therapeutic options for HCC, a multidisciplinary approach is needed to provide best care.

Figure 57.1 The incidence of hepatocellular carcinoma in the United States is rapidly increasing. Source: Data from www.statecancerprofiles.cancer.gov.

Yamada's Atlas of Gastroenterology, Fifth Edition. Edited by Daniel K. Podolsky, Michael Camilleri, J. Gregory Fitz, Anthony N. Kalloo, Fergus Shanahan, and Timothy C. Wang.
© 2016 John Wiley & Sons, Ltd. Published 2016 by John Wiley & Sons, Ltd.
Companion website: www.yamadagastro.com/atlas

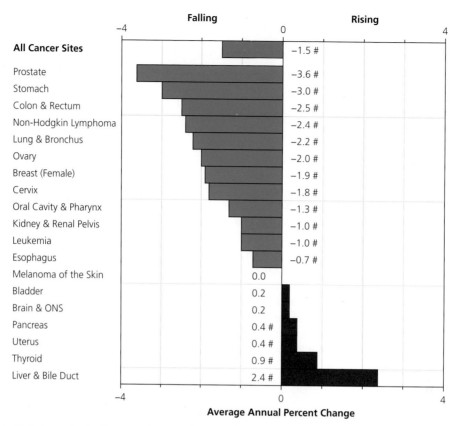

Figure 57.2 In parallel with its increasing incidence rate, hepatocellular carcinoma has the fastest growing death rate among solid tumors in the United States. # indicates annual percentage change significantly different from zero ($P < 0.05$). Source: Data from www.statecancerprofiles.cancer.gov.

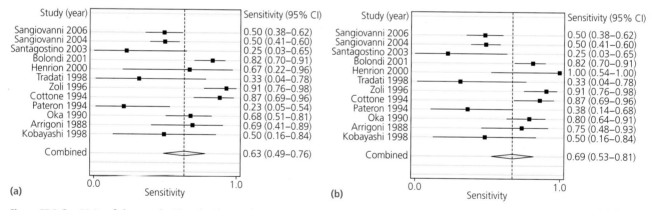

Figure 57.3 Sensitivity of ultrasound with and without α-fetoprotein (AFP) for the detection of early-stage hepatocellular carcinoma (HCC). (a) forest plot for sensitivity of ultrasound to detect early HCC. (b) forest plot for sensitivity of ultrasound with AFP to detect early HCC. Source: Singal A, Volk ML, Waljee A, et al. Meta-analysis: surveillance with ultrasound for early-stage hepatocellular carcinoma in patients with cirrhosis. Aliment Pharmacol Ther 2009;30:37. Reproduced with permission of John Wiley & Sons.

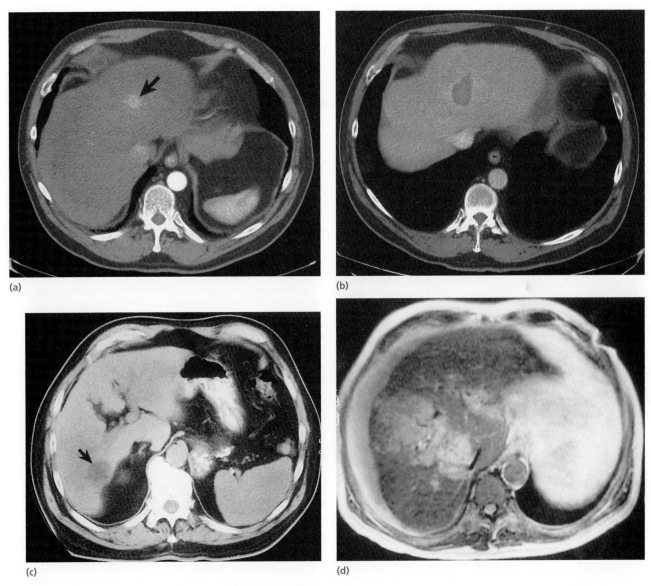

Figure 57.4 Imaging of hepatocellular carcinoma. **(a)** Computed tomography (CT) scan of a 1.8-cm small enhancing hepatocellular carcinoma (arrow). **(b)** CT image after treatment of the hepatocellular carcinoma in (a) by radiofrequency ablation. **(c)** CT image showing a hypodense hepatocellular carcinoma with a visible capsular rim (arrow). **(d)** Magnetic resonance image showing a large hepatocellular carcinoma located centrally within the liver.

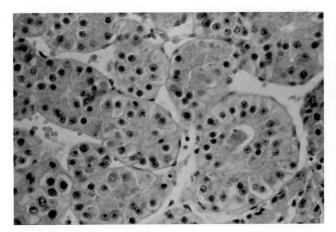

Figure 57.5 Hepatocellular carcinoma. The tumor has a mixed pseudoglandular and trabecular pattern with bile plugs. The sinusoid-like blood spaces show variable dilation.

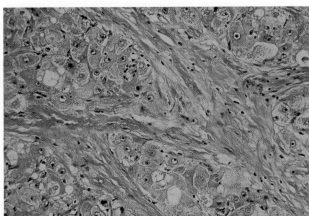

Figure 57.6 Fibrolamellar hepatocellular carcinoma is characterized by sheets of large polygonal tumor cells separated by hyalinized collagen bundles with a lamellar pattern. This variant of hepatocellular carcinoma usually affects adolescents or young adults who have no known risk factors for hepatocellular carcinoma.

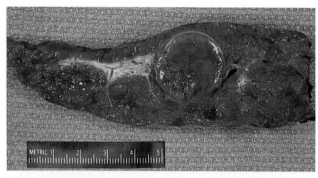

Figure 57.7 Nodular type of hepatocellular carcinoma. The tumor is expansile with a fibrous pseudocapsule. Prominent bile production gives the tumor its green color. The surrounding liver is cirrhotic, with multiple regenerative nodules.

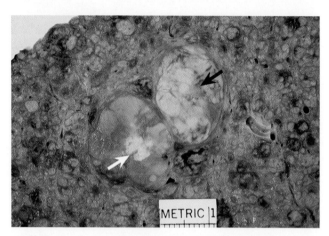

Figure 57.8 Nodule-in-nodule type of hepatocellular carcinoma. A lighter colored, higher grade focus of hepatocellular carcinoma (black arrow) has arisen within the upper right nodule and is compressing the original lower grade tumor towards the pseudocapsule. There is a small high-grade focus of hepatocellular carcinoma arising in the center of the lower left nodule (white arrow), surrounded by well-differentiated tumor.

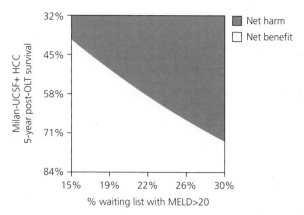

Figure 57.9 The impact of the proportion of patients with model for end-stage liver disease (MELD) scores >20 on the 5-year posttransplant survival threshold for patients with Milan-UCSF hepatocellular carcinoma (HCC). The intersection between the black and white shaded areas demonstrates the posttransplant survival at which the benefit of transplantation is outweighed by the harm caused to other patients. Source: Volk ML, Vijan S, Marrero JA. A novel model measuring the harm of transplanting hepatocellular carcinoma exceeding Milan criteria. Am J Transplant 2008;8:839. Reproduced with permission of John Wiley & Sons.

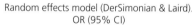
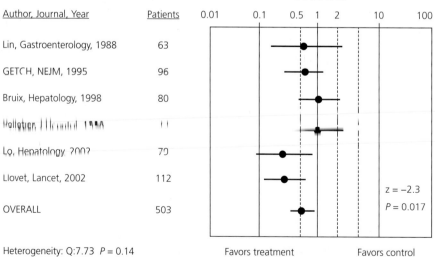

Figure 57.10 Metaanalysis of randomized controlled trials demonstrating improved 2-year survival with chemoembolization/embolization compared to conservative management for patients with unresectable hepatocellular carcinoma. Source: Llovet JM, Bruix J. Systematic review of randomized trials for unresectable hepatocellular carcinoma: chemoembolization improves survival. Hepatology 2003;37:429. Reproduced with permission of John Wiley & Sons.

CHAPTER 58

Liver abscess

Roman E. Perri and David S. Raiford
Vanderbilt University Medical Center, Nashville, TN, USA

Amebic versus pyogenic abscess

Although there is considerable overlap in the clinical presentation and imaging characteristics of amebic and pyogenic abscesses, differences in epidemiology, associated conditions, treatment, and prognosis underscore the need for the physician to distinguish these entities. Effective management depends critically upon prompt and correct definition of the abscess type.

Epidemiology

Intestinal amebiasis is a necessary prelude to hepatic amebic abscess; therefore, persons with amebic abscess typically have emigrated from or traveled to areas where intestinal amebiasis is prevalent. In contrast, the ethnicity and travel history of patients with pyogenic abscess does not differ from that of the general hospital population. Over the last few decades, biliary obstruction, both benign and malignant, has emerged as the most common etiology of pyogenic liver abscess.

Imaging modalities in diagnosis

The clinical constellation of fever, right upper quadrant discomfort, and hepatic enlargement with tenderness should prompt an imaging study early in the diagnostic assessment. Depending on the age of the patient and level of clinical suspicion for cholelithiasis or biliary obstruction, either ultrasonography (US) or computed tomography (CT) will be performed. These techniques facilitate discrimination of liver abscess from cholecystitis, bile duct obstruction, or pancreatitis. Both US and CT are sensitive for small lesions and offer precision in localizing lesions that may require percutaneous aspiration or drainage. Of note,

lesions near the dome of the right hepatic lobe may be difficult to visualize by US. Typically, on US abscesses appears as a hypoechoic lesions, sometimes with internal echoes (Figure 58.1, arrow). CT scanning will identify abscessed as low-density lesions (Figure 58.2, arrow), often with peripheral enhancement after i.v. contrast administration, and may provide better definition of extrahepatic pathology associated with pyogenic abscess (e.g., appendiceal or diverticular abscess). Although both modalities are sensitive for detecting abscesses and biliary obstruction, neither can distinguish reliably between amebic and pyogenic abscesses. Although less widely used, magnetic resonance imaging (MRI) also has high sensitivity for detection of hepatic abscess. Characteristically, liver abscesses are hypointense on T1-weighted and hyperintense on T2-weighted images and wall enhancement soon after gadolinium infusion is typical (Figure 58.3, arrow). Because CT and MRI techniques permit multiplanar imaging, these may be useful if US findings are ambiguous or when coronal or sagital images will help guide management of a lesion.

The majority of abscesses, both amebic and pyogenic, occur in the right hepatic lobe. The presence of multiple abscesses strongly suggests pyogenic infection, as does identification of concomitant biliary tract obstruction. Chest radiographs in patients with an abscess adjacent to the diaphragm may show elevation of the right diaphragm, subpulmonic effusion, and right lower lobe atelectasis or infiltrate. Note that a hepatic neoplasm may present with necrosis and secondary infection, mimicking a primary abscess.

Management

The mainstay of treatment of amebic abscess is metronidazole or tinidazole. Aspiration of an amebic abscess is indicated if there is no clinical improvement within several days or if the

Yamada's Atlas of Gastroenterology, Fifth Edition. Edited by Daniel K. Podolsky, Michael Camilleri, J. Gregory Fitz, Anthony N. Kalloo, Fergus Shanahan, and Timothy C. Wang.
Companion website: www.yamadagastro.com/atlas

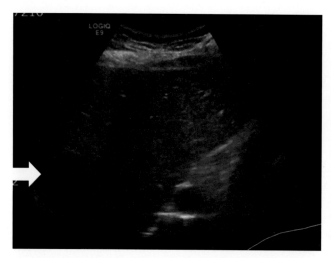

Figure 58.1 Sonographic image of a 5.3-cm hypoechoic mass in segment 8 of the liver. The mass is seen to be thick-walled and with internal echogenic debris, consistent with an hepatic abscess. This image is from a 39-year-old woman without obvious predisposing cause of her abscess. Her clinical presentation included fevers and severe right upper quadrant abdominal pain. Cultures from aspirated abscess material prior to the initiation of antibiotics grew *Streptococcus constellatus*.

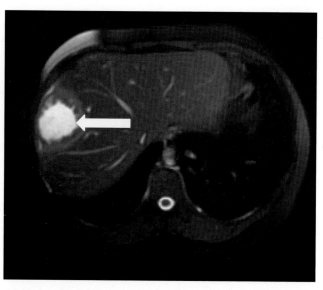

Figure 58.3 Magnetic resonance image of the abscess demonstrated in Figures 58.1 and 58.2. On T2-weighted imaging, there is marked signal intensity, and abscess wall enhancement noted after administration of gadolinium.

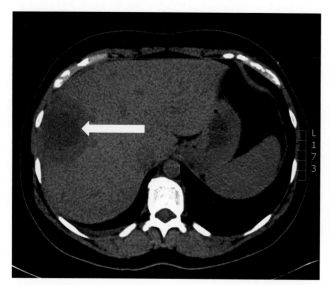

Figure 58.2 CT image of the abscess seen in Figure 58.1. A large right lobe subcapsular mass demonstrates central necrosis consistent with hepatic abscess.

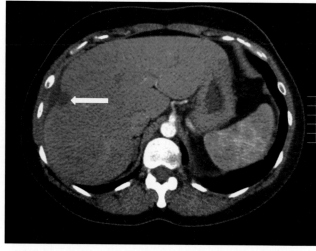

Figure 58.4 CT image of the abscess seen in Figures 58.1, 58.2, and 58.3 after 4 weeks of antibiotics and needle aspiration of the abscess. She was treated with 2 weeks of parenteral antibiotics (piperacillin/ tazobactam) followed by 2 weeks of oral antibiotics (amoxicillin/ clavulanic acid). Her fever abated quickly after initiation of antibiotics and right upper quadrant pain completely resolved after 2 weeks of antibiotic therapy.

diagnosis of amebic abscess is in doubt. After therapy with either of these tissue amebicides, treatment with a luminal amebicide such as paromomycin is warranted to eradicate amoeba within the bowel, which may be a source of relapsing or persisting infection. Surgery is not typically indicated for uncomplicated amebic abscess but may be appropriate in the rare situation of failure of medical management. US-guided percutaneous drainage is effective and may obviate the need for surgical management.

Pyogenic hepatic abscesses are treated with antibiotic therapy. Typically, broad-spectrum parenteral antibiotic therapy with effective coverage for aerobic enteric bacilli, *Streptococcus milleri* group, and enteric anaerobes is appropriate. After 2–3 weeks of parenteral antibiotic therapy, an additional 2–4 weeks of oral antibiotic therapy, directed at identified bacterial sensitivities, is appropriate. Clinical, biochemical, and radiological evaluations confirm reduction in the size of the abscess cavity (Figure 58.4, arrow). Resolution of the abscess cavity is often delayed well beyond clinical improvement and, in the absence of other clinical signs, should not form the basis for prolonged antimicrobial therapy. Antibiotic therapy alone may be insufficient to successfully treat any but the smallest (<3 cm) abscesses. Additional therapies employed to successfully treat pyogenic liver abscesses include surgical drainage, either laparoscopic or open, and interventional radiological procedures, including aspiration and drain placement. These latter procedures have proven to be effective in the management of pyogenic liver abscesses, relegating surgical procedures to second tier in the management of liver abscesses.

To access the videos for this chapter, please go to
www.yamadagastro.com/atlas

Video 58.1 Under ultrasound guidance, the radiologist inserts a needle into an abscess.

Video 58.2 Under ultrasound guidance, a wire is placed via the needle into the abscess.

Video 58.3 Under ultrasound guidance, a pigtail drainage catheter is inserted into the abscess to allow for continuous drainage of the abscess.

CHAPTER 59

Vascular diseases of the liver

Susana Seijo[1] and Laurie D. DeLeve[2]

[1] Hospital Clínic-Institut de Investigacions Biomèdiques August Pi I Sunyer (IDIBAPS), Barcelona, Spain
[2] Keck School of Medicine of USC, Los Angeles, CA, USA

This chapter provides images of Budd–Chiari syndrome, portal vein thrombosis, sinusoidal obstruction syndrome (hepatic venoocclusive disease), nodular regenerative hyperplasia, and peliosis hepatitis. These diseases are all thought to be primary vascular problems that lead to secondary changes in the hepatic parenchyma.

In Budd–Chiari syndrome, severity of liver injury will depend on the extent of the involvement of the hepatic veins, the time course over which the obstruction of the hepatic veins develops, and the duration of untreated disease. Slower development of the obstruction or occlusion allows formation of collaterals to alleviate sinusoidal congestion as the obstruction progresses. These collaterals are veins that do not follow normal hepatic veins direction and are easily detected in color Doppler ultrasound (Figure 59.1). In acute Budd–Chiari syndrome, there is perivenular and sometimes midzonal sinusoidal congestion, acute hemorrhage, and hepatocyte ischemia or drop-out. Figure 59.2 demonstrates hemorrhage within the hepatic cords, with red blood cells replacing the damaged hepatocytes. In chronic Budd–Chiari syndrome, chronic outflow obstruction may lead to bridging fibrosis between terminal hepatic venules with sparing of the portal tracts and fibrosis that obliterates the terminal hepatic venules, as demonstrated in Figure 59.3.

Portal vein thrombosis (PVT) may present with two distinct clinical scenarios, acute or chronic PVT. These represent successive stages of the same disease and have similar causes but different clinical presentation and management. Presence of hyperattenuating material in the lumen of the vein, lack of significant portoportal collaterals, and lack of signs of portal hypertension on imaging are characteristic features acute PVT (Figure 59.4). In the chronic phase of PVT, imaging shows the presence of a network of small irregular collateral vessels and the absence of the main portal vein and its main branches (Figure 59.5) Portal cholangiopathy is due to biliary abnormalities present in patients with portal cavernoma. Radiological abnormalities

such as stenosis, dilatation, angulation, or irregularity of the bile ducts are frequent. However, clinical manifestations are infrequent and seem to occur only in patients with the more severe grade of portal cholangiopathy (Figure 59.6).

Sinusoidal obstruction syndrome (SOS, previously known as hepatic venoocclusive disease) is initiated by damage to liver sinusoidal endothelial cells. Figure 59.7 demonstrates the ultrastructural changes in the sinusoid that occur prior to "clinical" evidence of disease in the experimental model, notably formation of gaps in the sinusoidal endothelial cell barrier that allow penetration of red blood cells through the gaps into the space of Disse. Figure 59.8 demonstrates the ultrastructural features of early SOS with denudation of the sinusoidal lining and loss of hepatocyte microvilli during early SOS. The histological features of early SOS shown in Figure 59.9 include subendothelial and sinusoidal hemorrhage and perivenular necrosis. Occlusion of terminal hepatic venules is not present in all patients, but is seen more commonly in patients with more severe disease. Narrowing of terminal hepatic venules in early SOS is due to subendothelial accumulation of plasma and some formed elements or frank subendothelial hemorrhage. In late SOS, there is fibrosis within perizonal sinusoids and adventitial or subendothelial fibrosis with narrowing or occlusion of the terminal hepatic veins (Figure 59.10). Unlike more subtle changes in the sinusoid, venular occlusion is easily recognized on histology and this led to the previous name, hepatic venoocclusive disease. It was because of the recognition that the disease is initiated in the sinusoid and that venular involvement is not present in a sizable minority of patients that the disease was renamed sinusoidal obstruction syndrome.

Nodular regenerative hyperplasia is currently thought to result from uneven perfusion of the liver. In areas of hypoperfusion, hepatocytes atrophy or undergo apoptosis, with reactive hyperplasia in areas in which perfusion is maintained. Impaired perfusion may occur at the level of the portal vein or

Yamada's Atlas of Gastroenterology, Fifth Edition. Edited by Daniel K. Podolsky, Michael Camilleri, J. Gregory Fitz, Anthony N. Kalloo, Fergus Shanahan, and Timothy C. Wang.
© 2016 John Wiley & Sons, Ltd. Published 2016 by John Wiley & Sons, Ltd.
Companion website: www.yamadagastro.com/atlas

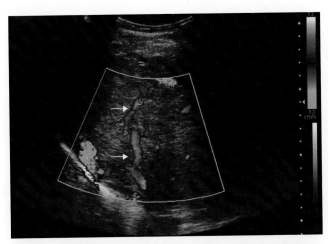

Figure 59.1 Budd–Chiari syndrome. Color Doppler ultrasound showing the absence of hepatic veins and irregular abnormal vascular structures (blue, arrows). These collaterals develop to alleviate sinusoidal congestion. Source: Courtesy of Dr. Angeles Garcia-Criado, Hospital Clinic, Barcelona.

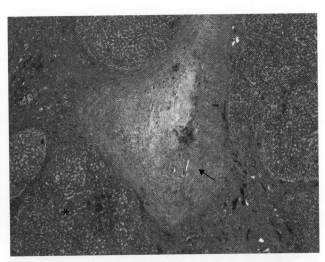

Figure 59.3 Budd–Chiari syndrome, chronic. High-power image of hematoxylin–eosin staining. A terminal hepatic venule is completely obstructed with a thickening wall vessel with fibrosis (arrow). There are nodules composed of normal-appearing hepatocytes (pink) surrounded by fibrosis (violet) (*). Source: Courtesy of Dr. Rosa Miquel, Hospital Clinic, Barcelona.

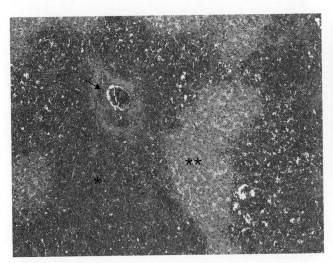

Figure 59.2 Budd–Chiari syndrome, acute. Sample from a hepatectomy showing extensive bridging hemorrhagic necrosis (*) around a central vein with a recent thrombus (arrow). Some residual patches of normal hepatocytes can be seen (**). Hematoxylin–eosin stain. Source: Courtesy of Dr. Rosa Miquel, Hospital Clinic, Barcelona.

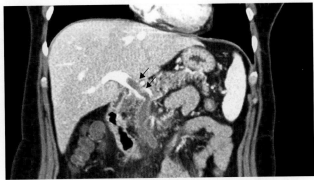

Figure 59.4 Acute portal vein thrombosis. A coronal computed tomography image demonstrates the presence of material within the portal vein trunk (arrows) that corresponds to a thrombosis. Notice the lack of endoluminal enhancement of the portal vein that extends to the superior mesenteric vein (*). The absence of collaterals suggests an acute episode of portal vein thrombosis. Source: Courtesy of Dr. Angeles Garcia-Criado, Hospital Clinic, Barcelona.

the sinusoids. Figures 59.11 and 59.12 demonstrate small regenerative nodules, which are composed of cytologically benign hepatocytes. The nodules displace portal structures and are surrounded by areas with atrophic hepatocytes. The vast majority of patients with nodular regenerative hyperplasia are asymptomatic, whereas a small subset of patients are symptomatic (mainly portal hypertension-related symptoms), with what is described as noncirrhotic idiopathic portal hypertension (INCPH). Liver features in INCPH include sinusoidal dilatation, perisinuoidal fibrosis (Figure 59.13), portal fibrosis, and/or aberrant vessels.

Patients with chronic wasting illnesses or who have been exposed to androgenic anabolic steroids or long-term azathioprine therapy may develop one or multiple peliotic lesions in the liver or spleen (Figure 59.14). The peliotic lesion consists of well-defined vascular cavities without a discrete endothelial lining. Peliosis may also be found in patients with acquired immunodeficiency syndrome (AIDS) because of infection with Bartonella species. As revealed by electron microscopy, Bartonella bacilli infect sinusoidal endothelial cells leading to disruption of the sinusoidal endothelial cell barrier, with initial sinusoidal dilation and subsequent formation of peliotic cavities.

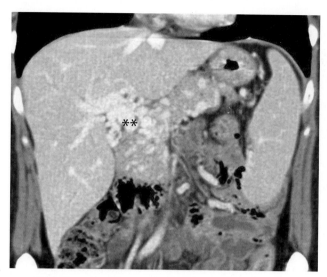

Figure 59.5 Chronic portal vein thrombosis (portal cavernoma). A coronal computed tomography image shows the presence of multiple tortuous collateral veins that bypass the thrombosed area: cavernous transformation of the portal vein (**). Source: Courtesy of Dr. Angeles Garcia-Criado, Hospital Clinic, Barcelona.

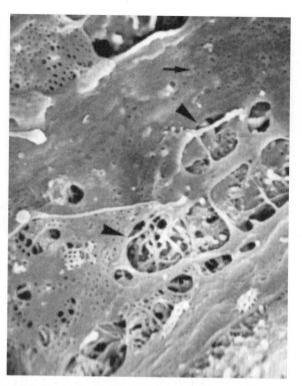

Figure 59.7 Sinusoidal obstruction syndrome (SOS), "pre-SOS." A scanning electron microscopic image (original magnification × 10 300) was taken from the rat model of SOS 1 day after administration of monocrotaline. This demonstrates changes that occur before clinical or light microscopic changes are observed in this model, that is pre-SOS: gaps in sinusoidal endothelial cells (arrowheads) that allow penetration of red blood cells into the space of Disse and loss of fenestrae organized as sieve plates (arrow). Source: Courtesy of Dr. Robert McCuskey, University of Arizona.

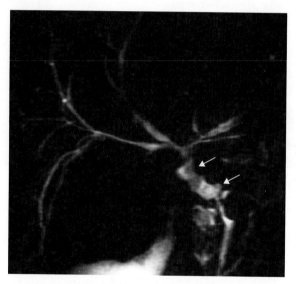

Figure 59.6 Portal cholangiopathy. Thick-slab coronal-oblique magnetic resonance cholangiopancreatography (MRCP) image. Note significant dilatation of the common biliary (CBD) duct above the stenosis (arrows) and multiple irregularities of the intrahepatic ducts. In patients with long-standing portal vein thrombosis, the cavernoma or enlarged biliary veins can produce focal stenosis on the CBD, leading to portal cholangiopathy. Source: Courtesy of Dr. Angeles Garcia-Criado, Hospital Clinic, Barcelona.

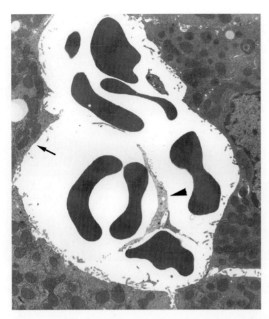

Figure 59.8 Sinusoidal obstruction syndrome (SOS), early. A transmission electron microscopy image, taken from the rat model of SOS during early SOS, demonstrates loss of sinusoidal lining and of microvilli on the hepatocyte (arrow) and a remnant of a sinusoidal endothelial cell in the lumen (arrowhead). Source: Courtesy of Dr. Robert McCuskey, University of Arizona.

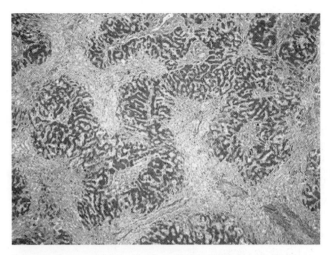

Figure 59.10 Sinusoidal obstruction syndrome (SOS), late. Marked sinusoidal and venular fibrosis is present in the perivenular zone in the liver. Source: Courtesy of Dr. Howard Shulman, Fred Hutchinson Cancer Research Center and the University of Washington.

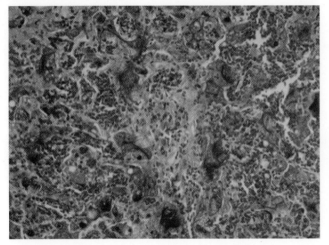

Figure 59.9 Sinusoidal obstruction syndrome (SOS), early. A photomicrograph demonstrates the changes of early SOS. Features demonstrated here are marked subendothelial and sinusoidal hemorrhage and perivenular necrosis. Source: Courtesy of Dr. Howard Shulman, Fred Hutchinson Cancer Research Center and the University of Washington.

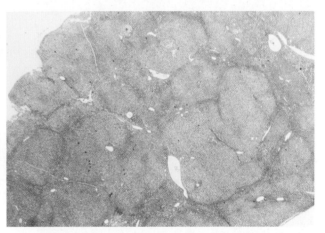

Figure 59.11 Nodular regenerative hyperplasia. A low-power photomicrograph shows small regenerative nodules ranging in size from 3 to 6 mm, displacing portal structures.

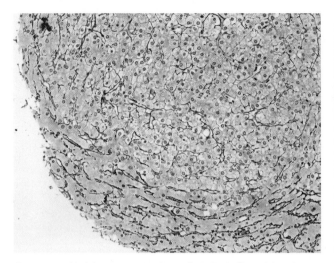

Figure 59.12 Nodular regenerative hyperplasia. Reticulin staining. At high-power magnification the hyperplasic nodule is composed of irregular trabeculae, which contains a double layer of hepatocytes. Compressed and thin trabeculae can be observed at the lower part of the image. Source: Courtesy of Dr. Rosa Miquel, Hospital Clinic, Barcelona.

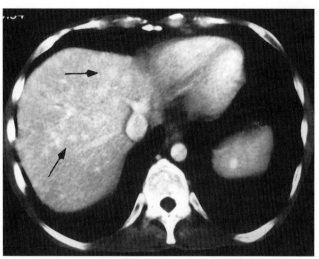

Figure 59.14 Peliosis hepatitis. A computed tomography image demonstrates multiple peliotic lesions, two of which are indicated by arrows. Source: Courtesy of Dr. Randall Radin, University of Southern California.

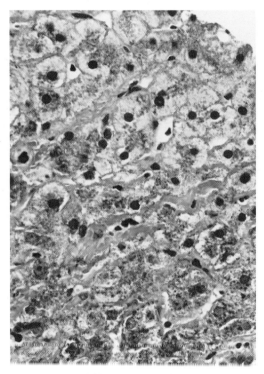

Figure 59.13 Perisinusoidal fibrosis. Collagen deposition (blue) can be observed along the sinusoidal wall. Masson's trichrome. Source: Courtesy of Dr. Rosa Miquel, Hospital Clinic, Barcelona.

CHAPTER 60

Intraabdominal abscesses and fistulae

Peter Irving and Nyree Griffin

Guy's and St Thomas' Hospital NHS Foundation Trust, London, UK

Introduction

Intraabdominal abscesses are contained areas of infection within the peritoneal cavity. They occur most commonly in recesses within the peritoneum, such as in the subphrenic space, the paracolic gutters or within the pelvis (Figure 60.1a–c). Intraabdominal abscesses form as a result of the immune response to eliminate and contain bacterial contamination of the peritoneal cavity and occur most commonly in the post-operative setting (Figures 60.2 and 60.3). Other causes include penetrating trauma, spontaneous perforation of a hollow viscus, primary or metastatic infection, inflammation (such as Crohn's disease) and ischemia. Diseases of the gastrointestinal tract such as appendicitis and diverticulitis (Figures 60.4 and 60.5), the genitourinary tract, or the hepatobiliary system and pancreas can lead to abscess formation within the abdomen.

Gastrointestinal fistulae commonly occur in association with abscesses. They are defined as abnormal communications between the gastrointestinal tract and another epithelialized surface. Fistulae can be classified by their anatomical location, by their physiological characteristics (that is, fluid output), or by their etiology. The vast majority of gastrointestinal fistulae are acquired as a result of previous abdominal surgery. Alternatively, spontaneous fistulae can occur in the setting of inflammatory disorders, such as Crohn's disease (Figure 60.6), or in relation to necrosis or malignancy (Figure 60.7).

Advances in imaging technology have revolutionized the diagnosis and assessment of intraabdominal abscesses and fistulae. The choice of investigation for imaging abscesses and fistulae depends on a number of factors relating not only to the pathology but also to available modalities and local expertise. The advent of computerized tomography (CT) which quickly and accurately outlines the contents of the peritoneal cavity and, furthermore, allows intervention to drain collections percutaneously, has resulted in this being the imaging modality of choice for assessment of intraabominal abscesses (Figures 60.3, 60.4, and 60.8). Magnetic resonance imaging (MRI) (Figures 60.9 and 60.10) and ultrasound (Figure 60.11) have the advantage of avoiding exposure to ionizing radiation. In addition, MRI is of particular use in patients with fistulae and, in specific circumstances, contrast radiography still has a role to play (Figure 60.12).

Yamada's Atlas of Gastroenterology, Fifth Edition. Edited by Daniel K. Podolsky, Michael Camilleri, J. Gregory Fitz, Anthony N. Kalloo, Fergus Shanahan, and Timothy C. Wang.
Companion website: www.yamadagastro.com/atlas

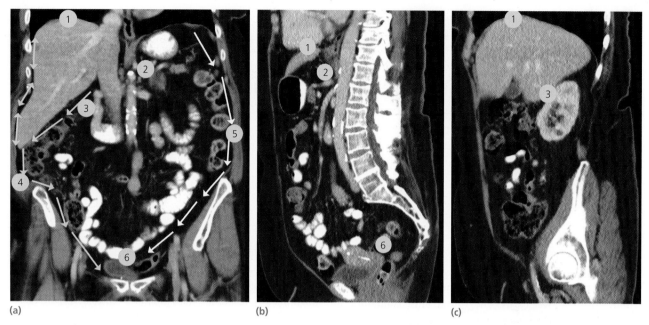

(a)   (b)   (c)

Figure 60.1 Pooling of purulent exudate can occur in dependent parts of the peritoneal cavity after diffuse peritoneal infection. As patients with peritoneal infection tend to be supine, abscesses commonly form in areas such as the para-colic gutters, the subphrenic regions, or the rectovesical pouch although the site of abscess formation will also be influenced by the primary source of infection. Peritoneal compartments in which abscesses commonly form with potential drainage pathways are shown (arrows) **(a)** coronal reformat contrast enhanced CT of the abdomen and pelvis. **(b)** Midline sagittal reformat CT of the abdomen and pelvis. **(c)** Right parasagittal reformat CT of the abdomen and pelvis. 1, Subphrenic space; 2, lesser sac; 3 subhepatic space (pouch of Morison); 4, right paracolic gutter; 5, left paracolic gutter; 6, rectouterine space in a female patient (rectovesical space in males).

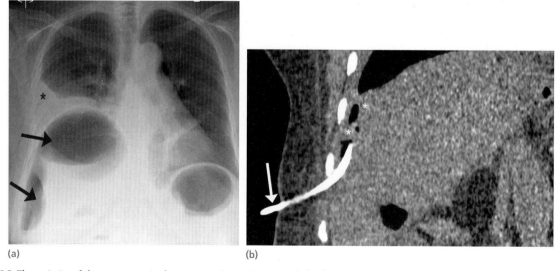

(a)   (b)

Figure 60.2 The majority of abscesses occur in the postoperative setting, particularly after gastrointestinal surgery, and usually in association with leakage from a surgical anastomosis. This is an example of a subphrenic collection post right hemicolectomy and anastomotic breakdown. **(a)** CXR shows subphrenic collection containing air fluid levels (arrows), with elevation of the right hemidiaphragm and small right pleural effusion (*). Percutaneous drainage of abscesses in the abdomen is possible in the large majority of cases with current imaging techniques. Success rates of 70% to more than 90% are described in the literature. Repeat drainage is necessary in a small proportion of patients and is generally also successful at emptying the abscess cavity allowing the avoidance of surgery in approximately 50% of cases. **(b)** Coronal reformat noncontrast CT shows final placement of the drain (arrow) with tip in the collection (*).

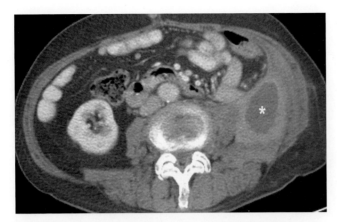

Figure 60.3 Example of postnephrectomy abscess: Axial contrast enhanced CT shows thick walled enhancing abscess with central fluid attenuation (*).

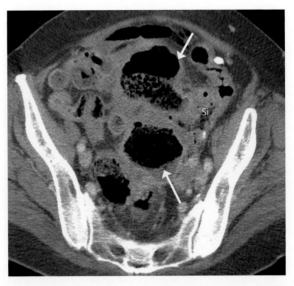

Figure 60.5 Diverticulitis is commonly complicated by abscess formation which it is normally possible to manage conservatively in the first instance. In general, abscesses less than 4 cm in size can be managed with antibiotic therapy. Drainage of diverticular abscesses is successful in up to 85% of cases; recurrence occurs in up to 40%, this being more common in abscesses of greater than 5 cm. Example of a diverticular abscess from localized perforation of diverticulum. Axial contrast enhanced CT show two large collections containing faeces and gas (arrows) on either side of the sigmoid colon (Si) which demonstrates mural hypertrophy and diverticulosis.

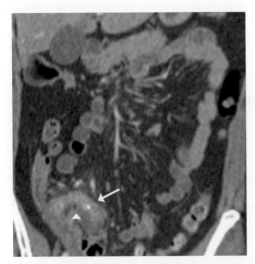

Figure 60.4 Abscess or phlegmon formation occurs in approximately 4% of patients with appendicitis and nonsurgical management is both successful in over 90% of cases and safer than immediate surgery. Coronal reformat contrast enhanced CT shows thickened appendix (arrow) with local perforation (arrowhead) and small associated collection in a patient with acute appendicitis.

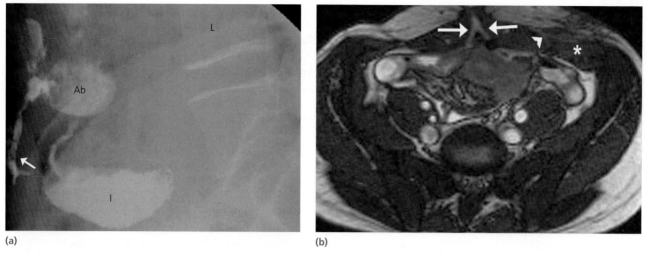

Figure 60.6 Fistulae are defined as abnormal communications between the gastrointestinal tract and another epithelialized surface, for example the skin, the genitourinary tract or another part of the gastrointestinal tract. Example of an enterocutaneous fistula in a patient with penetrating Crohn's disease: **(a)** Fistulogram in the lateral projection with lumbar spine to the right of the image (L), shows contrast introduced via a cutaneous opening (arrow) in the left side of the abdomen extends into an abscess (Ab) in the abdominal wall and then into the ileum (I); **(b)** corresponding axial True FISP MRI confirms high signal enterocutaneous fistula tracts in the midline (arrows) as well as in the left rectus muscle (arrowhead) with associated small ill defined abscess collection (*); the underlying bowel loops are thickened.

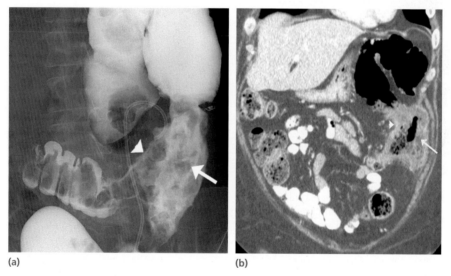

Figure 60.7 Example of a malignant fistula. **(a)** Water soluble enema, and **(b)** coronal reformat contrast enhanced CT study show irregular outline and mural thickening to the descending colon, in keeping with a primary colonic tumor with malignant fistulation (and hence early opacification) to the distal transverse colon (arrowhead). A left ureteric stent is *in situ*.

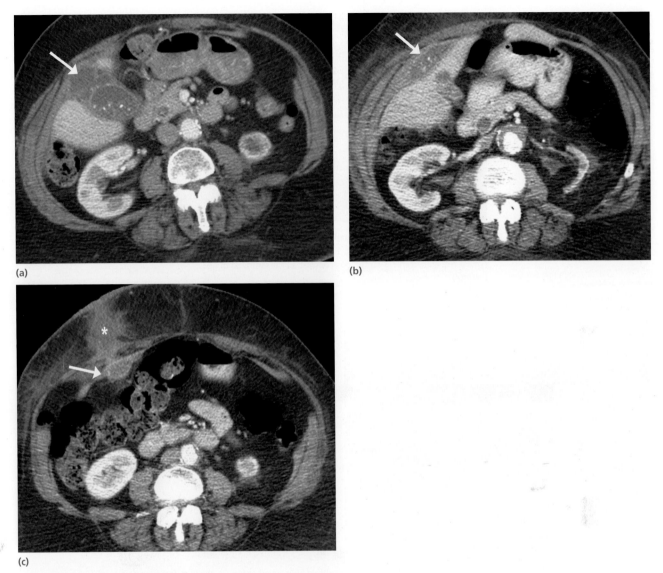

(a)

(b)

(c)

Figure 60.8 Fistulae may form spontaneously, accounting for between 15% and 25% of fistulae. Inflammatory conditions, such as Crohn's disease, pancreatitis, diverticulitis, or radiation enteritis can result in spontaneous fistula formation as many noninflammatory conditions such as malignancy, infection, and ischemia. Example of acute cholecystitis with perforated gallbladder, subcapsular liver abscess and fistula formation to the skin. **(a)** Axial contrast enhanced CT shows a collection in the gallbladder fossa (arrow). Note small gallstones within the gallbladder. **(b)** Axial contrast enhanced CT at a slightly more inferior level shows collection extends into the subcapsular space with gallstones spilling into this collection. **(c)** axial contrast enhanced CT at a further more inferior level, shows ill defined fistula tract (*) extending from abscess (arrow) to skin surface.

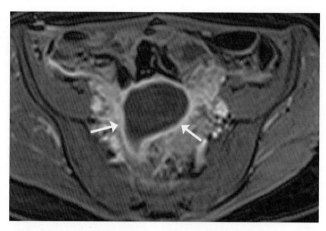

Figure 60.9 Rim enhancement is typically seen on cross-sectional imaging after injection of contrast. Example of a pelvic abscess with typical rim enhancement on the postcontrast T1 fat saturated image (arrows).

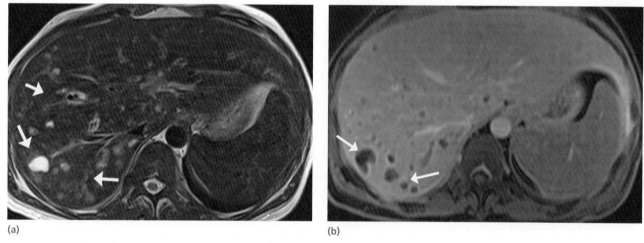

(a)   (b)

Figure 60.10 Example of liver abscesses. **(a)** Axial T2 HASTE MRI shows multiple high signal lesions in the liver (arrows). **(b)** Axial T1 fat saturated post contrast MRI shows these lesions demonstrate wall enhancement (arrows).

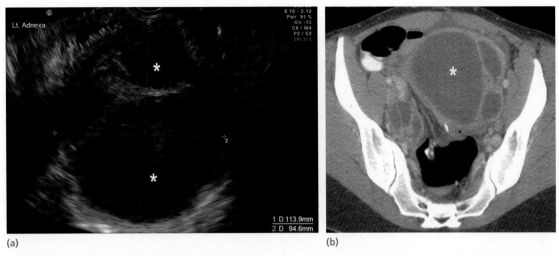

(a)　　　　　　　　　　　　　　　　　　　　(b)

Figure 60.11 Ultrasound is an inexpensive, quick, safe and noninvasive method of imaging the abdominal cavity. It is also a portable technology allowing assessment of critically ill patients at their bedside. Ultrasound can also be used to guide drainage of intraabdominal abscesses and, given its nature and the fact that it does not involve the use of ionizing radiation, allows multiple examinations to be used without concern. In addition, ultrasound is a "real-time" method of imaging, allowing the path of a needle, during ultrasound-guided drainage, to be followed as it is inserted. A further benefit is that the operator can scan in any plane, compared to CT where, conventionally, axial images are first acquired and are then reformatted to provide coronal, or sagittal images. Septations may be seen and are often better recognized on ultrasound than on CT. Example of tuboovarian abscess: **(a)** pelvic ultrasound shows large thick-walled septated adnexal cyst (*); **(b)** corresponding axial contrast enhanced CT shows large septated adnexal cyst with wall enhancement and central fluid attenuation (*).

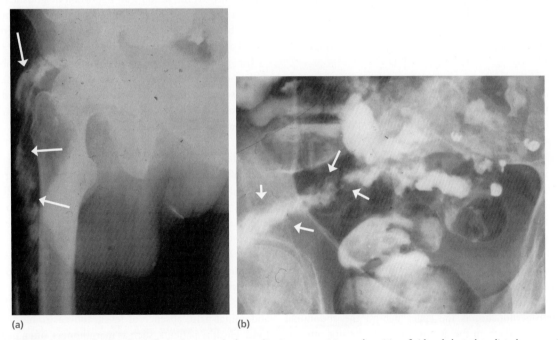

(a)　　　　　　　　　　　　　　　　　　　(b)

Figure 60.12 Enterocutaneous fistulae classically lead to a triad of complications comprising malnutrition, fluid and electrolyte disturbance, and sepsis. In addition, digestive enzymes can result in local skin damage at the external opening. Enterocutaneous fistulae can resolve with conservative management although the majority require surgical intervention. Example of an enterocutaneous fistula to the thigh in a patient with complicated penetrating Crohn's disease. **(a)** Fistulogram shows contrast opacifying a cutaneous tract (arrows) overlying the right femur and extending into the pelvis. **(b)** Water soluble enema performed in the AP projection shows contrast extending from opacified bowel loops into this cutaneous tract (arrows). Source: Images courtesy Prof Sir Miles Irving.

CHAPTER 61

Diseases of the peritoneum, retroperitoneum, mesentery, and omentum

Jennifer W. Harris, Scott D. Stevens, and B. Mark Evers

University of Kentucky, Lexington, KY, USA

The peritoneal cavity is lined by mesothelium that splits the cavity into parietal and visceral compartments. Diseases of the peritoneum include peritonitis, pseudomyxoma peritonei, and tuberculous peritonitis.

Peritonitis, an inflammation of the peritoneal linings, requires surgical intervention. The abdomen can remain open if safe closure is not possible or for a planned reoperation, using a Bogata bag as illustrated in Figure 61.1. Peritonitis can develop secondary to a gossypiboma, or retained foreign object (RFO). Derived from the Latin gossypium for "cotton" and "oma" meaning tumor, gossypiboma develop if surgical materials remain in the abdomen postoperatively (Figures 61.2 and 61.3). Tuberculous peritonitis results from spread of infection from a primary focus, usually the lung, and occurs in approximately 1% of patients. A computed tomography (CT) scan may identify thickened bowel and ascites (Figure 61.4).

Peritoneal carcinomatosis (PC) is a metastatic manifestation of gastrointestinal and pelvic carcinomas. Figure 61.5 demonstrates PC secondary to metastatic ovarian cancer. Features include ascites, peritoneal studding, and bowel obstruction (Figure 61.5).

Primary peritoneal cancer (PPC) is a rare tumor of the peritoneal lining. PPC has diffuse involvement of the peritoneum by papillary carcinoma without a primary site and grossly normal ovaries. Demonstrated are calcifications throughout the omentum and peritoneal lining (Figure 61.6).

Pseudomyxoma peritonei is another rare condition that involves the peritoneal cavity and omentum. Characteristic CT findings include scalloping of the hepatic and intestinal margins caused by extrinsic compression of ascitic spaces containing gelatinous material (Figure 61.7).

The retroperitoneum is the space behind the abdominal cavity that extends from the diaphragm to the levator ani muscle of the pelvis. Retroperitoneal diseases include retroperitoneal hemorrhage, inflammation, fibrosis, and neoplasia. Rupture of an abdominal aortic aneurysm results in retroperitoneal hemorrhage and hypovolemic shock (Figure 61.8). Retroperitoneal infections are caused by diseases surrounding abdominal organs, urinary tract, or vertebral column. Figure 61.9a,b demonstrates a retroperitoneal abscess with gas and enhancing margins due to Crohn's disease. Retroperitoneal fibrosis is an uncommon disease characterized by progressive nonspecific fibrosis of connective and adipose tissue in the retroperitoneal space (Figure 61.10). Retroperitoneal tumors arise from mesodermal, neuroectodermal, or embryonic remnants (Figure 61.11). Enlarged tumors cause hollow viscus obstruction by invasion and mass effect (Figure 61.12). Magnetic resonance imaging (MRI) has become an important diagnostic tool in the management of retroperitoneal neoplasms. It allows better definition between the mass and surrounding muscle groups and vascular structures compared to CT scanning (Figure 61.13a,b).

The mesentery or omentum may become involved in a variety of disease processes, most of which originate in adjacent visceral organs. These include inflammatory and vascular processes, mesenteric/omental cysts, and tumors (benign, malignant, and metastatic) (Box 61.1). Fibromatous proliferation of the mesentery, or mesenteric desmoid, is a rare, noninflammatory condition. The majority of these cases are associated with Gardner syndrome. These mesenteric lesions generally do not metastasize, but infiltrate surrounding structures and tend to recur locally when excised (Figure 61.14). The mesentery is sometimes the first site to manifest clinical symptoms related to systemic inflammatory diseases. Mesenteric amyloidosis is a very rare condition with symptoms including abdominal pain and distension (Figure 61.15). An omental infarction results from vascular compromise of the greater omentum. Patients present with sudden onset of abdominal pain, absence of fever, and gastrointestinal symptoms. Healthy patients such as marathoners, often present with this condition because of low omental blood flow. This condition has a nonspecific clinical presentation, and is managed nonoperatively (Figure 61.16).

Yamada's Atlas of Gastroenterology, Fifth Edition. Edited by Daniel K. Podolsky, Michael Camilleri, J. Gregory Fitz, Anthony N. Kalloo, Fergus Shanahan, and Timothy C. Wang.

© 2016 John Wiley & Sons, Ltd. Published 2016 by John Wiley & Sons, Ltd.

Companion website: www.yamadagastro.com/atlas

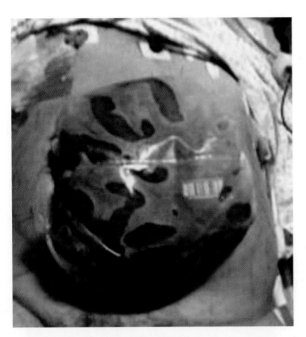

Figure 61.1 A Bogata bag is used to control abdominal contents after the development of abdominal compartment syndrome secondary to peritonitis and sepsis.

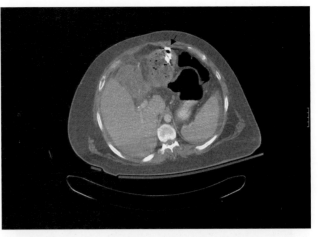

Figure 61.3 Computed tomography demonstrates a surgical sponge retained in the abdominal cavity with surrounding inflammatory reaction (arrow indicates sponge with surrounding inflammatory response).

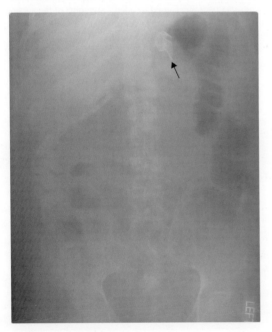

Figure 61.2 Abdominal radiograph of a patient with gossypiboma secondary to retained foreign object in the abdominal cavity (arrow indicates sponge).

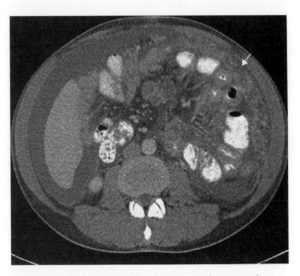

Figure 61.4 Computed tomography of a patient with peritoneal tuberculosis demonstrates mesenteric and peritoneal involvement of disease (arrow) with ascites.

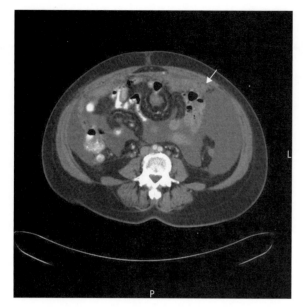

Figure 61.5 Computed tomography demonstrates diffuse peritoneal carcinomatosis with ascites and omental caking (arrow) in a patient with ovarian cancer.

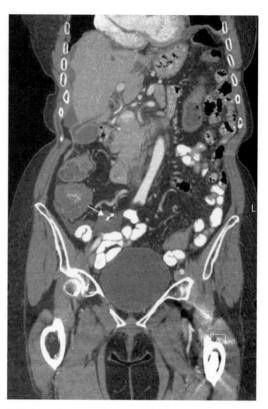

Figure 61.7 Coronal computed tomography image of a patient with pseudomyxoma peritonei caused by adenocarcinoma of the appendix demonstrates gelatinous perihepatic mass and gelatinous mass engulfing surgical clips from prior appendectomy (arrow).

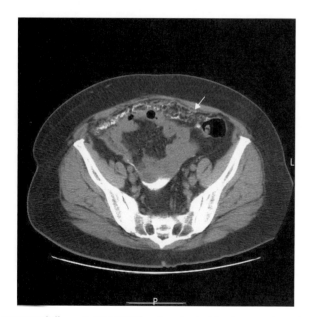

Figure 61.6 Computed tomography of a patient with primary peritoneal carcinoma demonstrates extensive calcifications involving omentum and peritoneum (arrow).

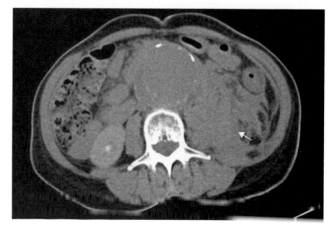

Figure 61.8 Computed tomography demonstrates a large ruptured abdominal aortic aneurysm (AAA) with adjacent retroperitoneal hematoma (arrow).

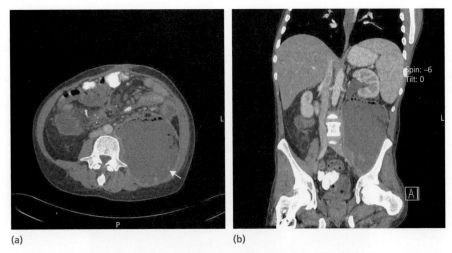

(a)   (b)

Figure 61.9 (a) Axial computed tomography (CT) demonstrates a large retroperitoneal abscess (arrow) with enhancing margins secondary to perforated viscus in a patient with Crohn's disease. **(b)** Coronal CT demonstrates this retroperitoneal abscess displacing the left kidney superiorly.

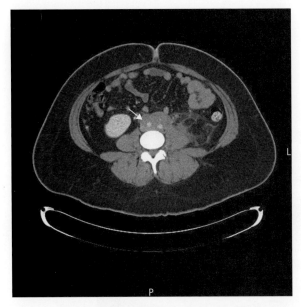

Figure 61.10 Computed tomography demonstrates preexistent retroperitoneal fibrosis (arrow) encasing the common iliac arteries in a patient who required left nephrectomy after motor vehicle trauma.

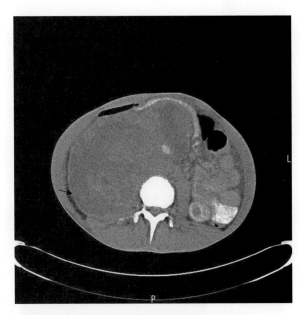

Figure 61.11 Computed tomography demonstrates metastatic nonseminomatous germ cell tumor of the right testicle that presented as a very large retroperitoneal tumor (arrow).

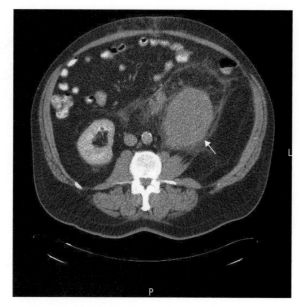

Figure 61.12 Computed tomography demonstrates left retroperitoneal spindle cell sarcoma (arrow).

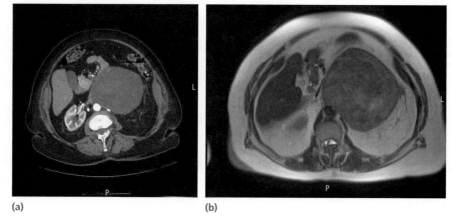

(a)

(b)

Figure 61.13 (a) Computed tomography demonstrates a large retroperitoneal benign schwannoma with mass effect. (b) Axial T2-weighted magnetic resonance image demonstrates the heterogeneous internal nature of this well-marginated mass.

Box 61.1 Classification of mesenteric and omental diseases.

Mesenteric diseases

Primary mesenteric inflammatory diseases
    Mesenteric panniculitis
    Retractile mesenteritis
Mesenteric cysts
    Embryonic and developmental cysts
    Traumatic or acquired cysts
    Neoplastic cysts
    Infective and degenerative cysts
Mesenteric tumors
    Benign tumors
        Lipoma
        Hemangioma
        Leiomyoma
        Ganglioneuroma
    Malignant tumors
        Leiomyosarcoma
        Liposarcoma
        Rhabdomyosarcoma
        Metastatic disease
    Mesenteric fibromatosis

Omental diseases

Mass lesions
    Primary tumors and cysts
    Metastatic disease
    Vascular lesions damaging blood supply
Torsion
    Primary
    Secondary: hernia, adhesion, tumor
Infarction
    Primary
    Secondary: torsion, incarceration in hernia

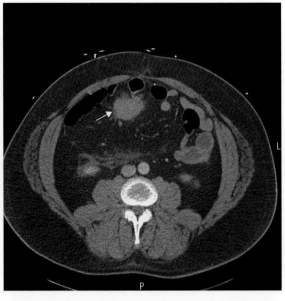

Figure 61.14 Computed tomography demonstrates a desmoid tumor in the mesentery of a patient with familial adenomatous polyposis syndrome. Note the spiculated margins of the tumor as it encroaches upon the surrounding mesentery (arrow).

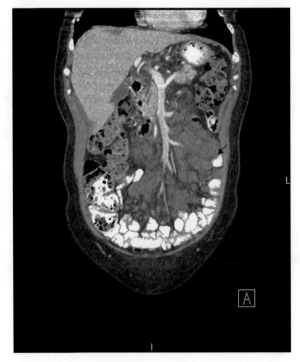

Figure 61.15 Coronal computed tomography demonstrates extensive mesenteric adenopathy (arrow) secondary to mesenteric amyloidosis in a patient with AL subtype multiple myeloma, which is associated with amyloidosis.

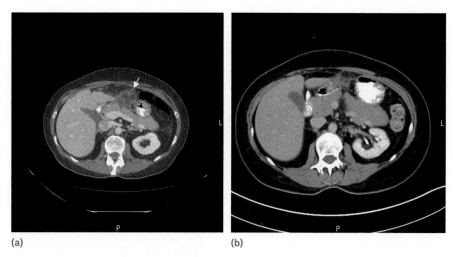

(a)   (b)

Figure 61.16 (a) Computed tomography (CT) demonstrates omental infarct anterior to the gastric antrum (arrow) imaged at the time of patient presentation due to pain. **(b)** CT demonstrates resolving area of infarction in the same patient 6 weeks later after nonoperative management.

CHAPTER 62

Obesity: treatment and complications

Louis A. Chaptini[1] and Steven Peikin[2]

[1] Yale University School of Medicine, New Haven, CT, USA
[2] Cooper University Hospital, Camden, NJ, USA

Obesity is defined as an excessive amount of body fat and correlates with body mass index (BMI), an index of the relationship between height and weight, calculated by dividing weight in kilograms by the square of height in meters. Overweight is defined as BMI between $25\,kg/m^2$ and $29.9\,kg/m^2$. Obesity is diagnosed when BMI is over $30\,kg/m^2$. Measurement of the patient's waist circumference is important to assess the abdominal distribution of adipose tissue, which by itself is associated with an increased risk of medical complications (Figure 62.1).

In the most recent data from the National Health and Nutrition Examination Survey (NHANES), the prevalence of obesity among adults in the USA was estimated at 35.7%. Figure 62.2 illustrates the change in percentage of obese adults from 1990 to 2010 in the United States.

Multiple etiological factors have been associated with the development of obesity. These include genetic, prenatal, environmental, neuroendocrine, and iatrogenic factors. Metabolic syndrome, the constellation of insulin resistance, visceral adiposity, hypertension, and dyslipidemia, is a major complication of obesity. Gastrointestinal complications are also frequent and involve multiple organ systems.

The treatment of obesity starts with lifestyle modifications (dietary and behavioral interventions in addition to physical activity) (Figure 62.3). When these fail, pharmacotherapy is offered and includes a variety of agents targeting fat absorption and appetite reduction. Bariatric surgery is recommended in patients with BMI over $40\,kg/m^2$ or above $35\,kg/m^2$ if comorbid conditions are present. Bariatric procedures can be divided into two varieties, malabsorptive and restrictive, depending on the mechanism by which weight loss is induced. Changes in gastrointestinal hormones after bariatric surgery may also contribute to weight loss. Gastroenterologists are often confronted with complications indirectly related to the surgery, such as anastomotic ulceration (Figure 62.4), band erosion, stricture, and fistula, which may require endoscopic therapy.

Although not widely available, minimally invasive endoscopic procedures for obesity constitute an attractive option, especially in patients who do not respond to lifestyle modifications and pharmacotherapy and yet are not candidates for bariatric surgery (Figures 62.5 and 62.6). Endoscopic procedures may also be indicated as bridge-to-surgery to reduce operative risks, and as metabolic procedures that have a more pronounced metabolic effect (for example on diabetes) than weight loss effect. Other potential and emerging indications in this setting include the use of endoscopic procedures as primary obesity procedures with outcomes comparable to current strategies and as revisional procedures in cases of failed bariatric surgical procedures (Table 62.1).

Table 62.1 Potential endoscopic obesity procedure categories. Source: Thompson CC. Endoscopic therapy of obesity: a new paradigm in bariatric care. Gastrointest Endosc 2010;72:497. Reproduced with permission of Elsevier.

Procedure category	Procedure aim
Early intervention	Providing weight loss or stabilization in early-stage obese patients who do not yet qualify for traditional surgery
Bridge to surgery	Reducing the obesity-related operative risk for various bariatric and nonbariatric surgeries
Metabolic	Primarily addressing comorbid illness (e.g., diabetes)
Primary	Endoscopic option for the traditional surgical population, with outcomes and risk profiles similar to those of current surgeries
Revision	Repairing failed bariatric surgical procedures

Yamada's Atlas of Gastroenterology, Fifth Edition. Edited by Daniel K. Podolsky, Michael Camilleri, J. Gregory Fitz, Anthony N. Kalloo, Fergus Shanahan, and Timothy C. Wang.
© 2016 John Wiley & Sons, Ltd. Published 2016 by John Wiley & Sons, Ltd.
Companion website: www.yamadagastro.com/atlas

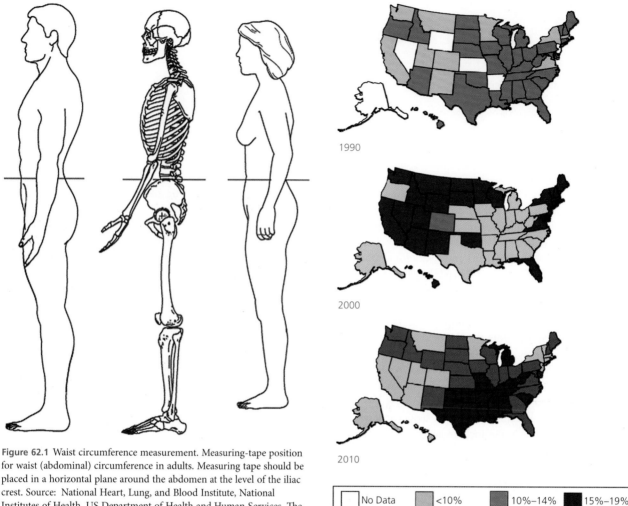

Figure 62.1 Waist circumference measurement. Measuring-tape position for waist (abdominal) circumference in adults. Measuring tape should be placed in a horizontal plane around the abdomen at the level of the iliac crest. Source: National Heart, Lung, and Blood Institute, National Institutes of Health, US Department of Health and Human Services. The Practical Guide: Identification, Evaluation, and Treatment of Overweight and Obesity in Adults, 2000.

1990

2000

2010

	No Data		<10%		10%–14%		15%–19%
	20%–24%		25%–29%		≥30%		

Figure 62.2 Maps showing the change in percentage of obese adults from 1990 to 2010 in the United States. Data of the Behavioral Risk Factor Surveillance System (BRFSS). In 2011, methodological changes were implemented to the BRFSS. These changes affect obesity prevalence estimates, and mean that data collected in 2010 and before cannot be compared to the 2011 estimates. Source: Centers for Disease Control and Prevention. The History of the Increase in State Obesity Prevalence. Available at: www.cdc.gov/obesity/data/adult.html.

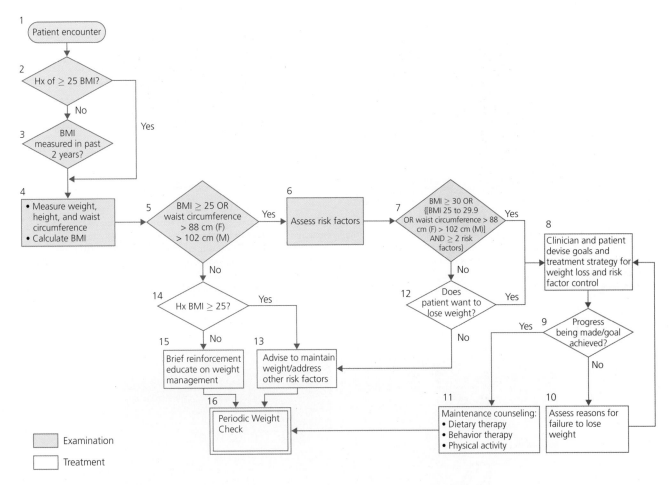

Figure 62.3 Algorithm for the diagnosis and treatment of obesity. BMI, body mass index; Hx, history. Source: National Heart, Lung, and Blood Institute, National Institutes of Health, US Department of Health and Human Services. The Practical Guide: Identification, Evaluation, and Treatment of Overweight and Obesity in Adults, 2000.

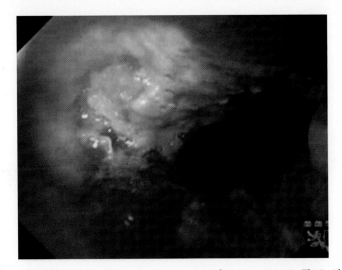

Figure 62.4 Marginal ulcer. Stomal or marginal ulceration often presents as retrosternal or epigastric pain. The incidence of stomal ulceration is between 0.6% and 16%. It is believed that ulceration may occur at any time; however, symptoms most commonly develop in the first 3 months after the procedure with a progressively decreasing incidence thereafter. The exact cause is unclear, and many factors are thought to be associated with their development, including mucosal ischemia, nonsteroidal antiinflammatory drugs, gastrogastric fistula, and *Helicobacter pylori*. Source: Obstein KL, Thompson CC. Endoscopy after bariatric surgery (with videos). Gastrointest Endosc 2009;70:1161. Reproduced with permission of Elsevier.

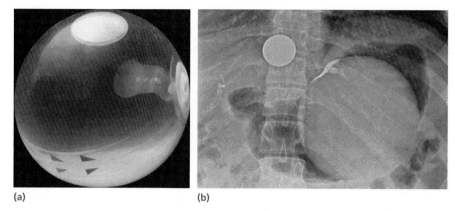

(a)   (b)

Figure 62.5 Intragastric balloon. **(a)** The BioEnterics intragastric balloon. The balloon is smooth and spherical. The arrowheads at the equator point toward the valve. The shell consists of inert, nontoxic silicone elastomer, impervious and resistant to gastric acid. The radiopaque self-sealing and repenetrable valve with its Z-shape configuration (visible inside balloon) allows adjustment of the balloon volume from 400 to 800 mL. **(b)** Plain abdominal radiograph showing balloon in body of stomach. A coin taped on the lower sternum permits follow-up comparisons of balloon size to detect premature deflation. Source: Mathus-Vliegen EMH, Tytgat GNJ. Intragastric balloon for treatment-resistant obesity: safety, tolerance, and efficacy of 1-year balloon treatment followed by a 1-year balloon-free follow-up. Gastrointest Endosc 2005;61:19. Reproduced with permission of Elsevier.

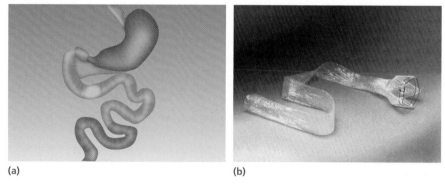

(a)   (b)

Figure 62.6 (a) Depiction of the GI Dynamics sleeve in place preventing ingested contents from contacting the mucosa of the duodenum and proximal jejunum. **(b)** The GI Dynamics DJBS (duodenojejunal bypass sleeve). It consists of a nitinol retaining device and a 60-cm plastic sleeve that prevents contact of food with bile and pancreatic secretions and the mucosa of the duodenum and proximal jejunum. The sleeve system is passed over a guidewire and then, under direct visualization, the sleeve is deployed over a deeply placed guidewire. With the sleeve in place, the retaining device is then fully deployed in the duodenal bulb to anchor the device. Source: Coté GA, Edmundowicz SA. Emerging technology: endoluminal treatment of obesity. Gastrointest Endosc 2009;70:991. Reproduced with permission of Elsevier.

CHAPTER 63

Bariatric surgery and complications

Obos Ekhaese, Danny O. Jacobs, and Russell LaForte
University of Texas Medical Branch, Galveston, TX, USA

Bariatric surgery is an increasingly complex discipline based in four basic procedures: adjustable gastric banding, sleeve gastrectomy, Roux-en-Y gastric bypass, and biliopancreatic diversion with duodenal switch. Although these basic procedures are performed with minor regional variations, the resulting anatomy and potential complications are largely the same. Both in emergency and in daily practice, gastroenterologists are increasingly encountering bariatric patients and should be able to address the most frequently encountered problems. Common endoscopic and radiographic findings are presented, including normal views for orientation and basic anatomic illustration (Figures 63.1, 63.2, and 63.3). While not exhaustive, this selection is made with an emphasis on the diagnosis of complications (Figures 63.4–63.17).

Vertical banded gastroplasty, still a primary operation in some regions, has largely been replaced by the gastric sleeve and adjustable gastric band. The main reason for its abandonment is illustrated in Figure 63.10, namely that breakdown of the gastric partition is common and results in the lost weight being regained over the first postoperative decade. The adjustable gastric band and gastric sleeve have become popular restrictive operations in its place. Several device-related complications plague the adjustable band as well; namely, band slippage (Figures 63.8 and 63.12), band erosion (Figures 63.6 and 63.13),

and megaesophagus (Figure 63.11). The gastric sleeve also has significant complications, such as stricture formation (Figure 63.9).

Gastric bypass has been and remains an extremely effective weight loss procedure. Marginal ulceration, as seen in Figure 63.4, is one common complication. Persistent ulceration can lead to stricture formation, well visualized in Figures 63.5a and 63.17. Stricture formation is readily treated endoscopically, as shown in Figure 63.5b. A more urgent complication of gastric bypass, leak formation (Figure 63.16), has also been treated endoscopically (Figure 63.7a,b).

Also presented is a super morbidly obese patient who had a biliopancreatic diversion with duodenal switch. After his operation, he had difficulty following the prescribed diet and suffered the two complications, illustrated in both Figures 63.14 and 63.15. In spite of reoperation and a difficult recovery period, this patient had excellent weight loss and full resolution of comorbidities. In bariatric surgery, one complication is all too often followed by another. Although biliopancreatic diversion with duodenal switch has a higher complication rate than the other major procedures, its greater weight loss and resolution of comorbidities make it a major option in many severely obese patients, even those patients with a body mass index below 50.

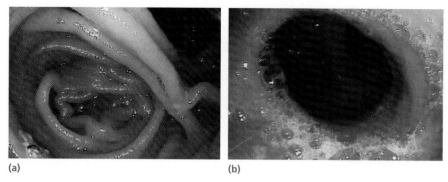

Figure 63.1 Roux-en-Y gastric bypass: **(a)** view of blind pouch of "Roux" limb; **(b)** view of gastrojejunal anastomosis (stoma) and "Roux" (alimentary) limb.

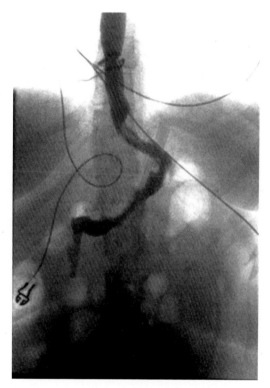

Figure 63.3 Gastric sleeve. A normal barium study is presented.

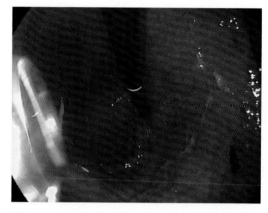

Figure 63.2 Laparoscopic adjustable gastric band. A normal retroflexed view of fundus from beneath the level of the band.

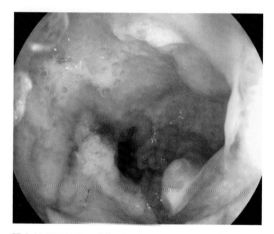

Figure 63.4 Marginal ulcer following Roux-en-Y gastric bypass. A circumferential ulcer is seen entirely on the jejunal aspect of the gastrojejunal anastomosis. This patient presented 6 weeks after Roux-en-Y gastric bypass with increasing volume depletion secondary to poor oral intake with a large marginal ulcer on endoscopy. Most marginal ulcers occur in the first several weeks after operation. Both sucralfate and a proton pump inhibitor are routinely prescribed. Misoprostol is added in some cases as well. Preoperative testing for *H. pylori* and appropriate treatment reduces the risk of marginal ulcers. For prevention, avoidance of nonsteroidal antiinflammatory drugs and tobacco in the perioperative period is also strongly recommended.

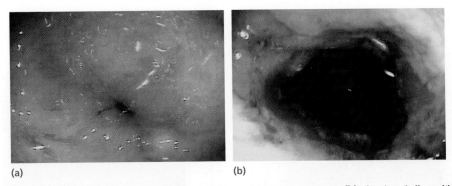

(a)   (b)

Figure 63.5 Anastomotic stricture following Roux-en-Y gastric bypass: **(a)** gastrojejunostomy stricture; **(b)** after three balloon dilatations. This patient experienced progressive postprandial nausea and vomiting 1 month postoperatively. Anastomotic strictures most often form in the early operative period. The pathophysiology is usually attributed to chronic scarring from marginal ulcerations.

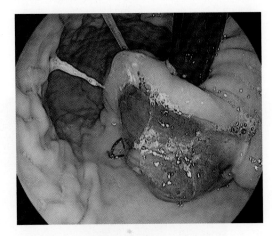

Figure 63.6 Laparoscopic adjustable gastric band erosion. A severe erosion of a gastric band is seen beneath the fundus. This patient presented with weight gain 20 months after successful adjustable gastric band placement despite increasing band volume.

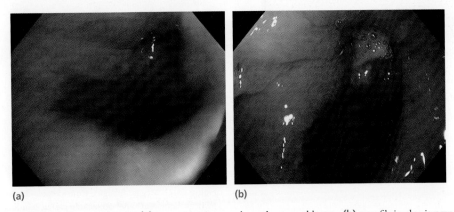

(a)   (b)

Figure 63.7 Leak following Roux-en-Y gastric bypass: **(a)** an opening is seen above the normal lumen; **(b)** gray fibrin glue is now seen filling the opening. The patient was diagnosed 5 days after Roux-en-Y gastric bypass with a leak at the gastrojejunal anastomosis. Conservative management with 6 weeks of drainage and bowel rest failed to resolve the leak. Fibrin glue placed endoscopically sealed the leak. The patient tolerated a clear liquid diet the next morning and was advanced to a regular diet per normal postoperative protocols without further incident.

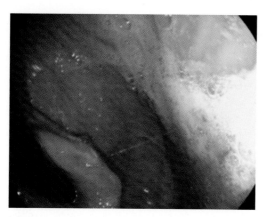

Figure 63.8 Laparoscopic adjustable gastric band slippage. Fundus dilatation is observed above the band. Six years after successful adjustable gastric band placement this patient developed heartburn unresponsive to proton pump inhibitor therapy. Barium imaging and endoscopy confirmed band slippage. The band was removed, which promptly resolved the symptoms.

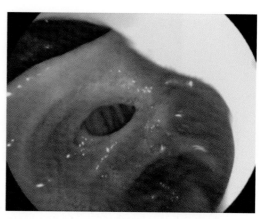

Figure 63.10 Gastrogastric fistula. A gastrogastric fistula from staple line disruption is presented. This patient, who underwent a vertical banded gastroplasty, experienced significant weight loss, which was maintained for 20 years. She then began to gain weight and have frequent heartburn. Conversion to a Roux-en-Y gastric bypass resulted in resolution of symptoms and weight loss to a body mass index of 24. The breakdown of staple lines is common after gastroplasty.

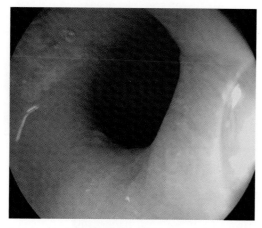

Figure 63.9 Gastric sleeve stricture. A stricture is visualized near the pylorus. This patient was unable to progress to solid food 1 month after operation due to heartburn, nausea, and vomiting. Dilation of a gastric stricture resulted in resolution of symptoms.

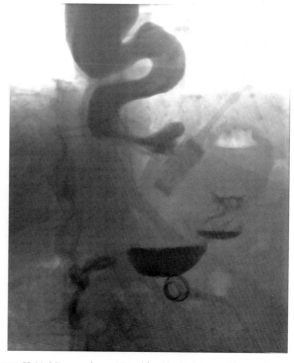

Figure 63.11 Megaesophagus. Considerable dilatation of the esophagus is evident. Four years after adjustable gastric banding this patient presented with increasing reflux unresponsive to maximum doses of proton pump inhibitors, antacids, and sucralfate. Band deflation and subsequent removal resulted in resolution of symptoms.

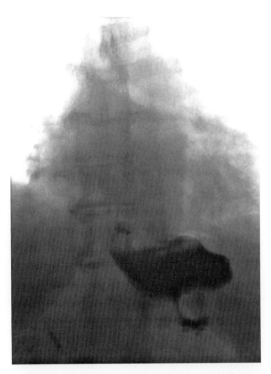

Figure 63.12 Prolapsed band. A horizontal band is noted. This patient with an adjustable gastric band had good initial weight loss. After 2 years, however, the sense of restriction subsided and the patient experienced weight regain. Conversion to Roux-en-Y gastric bypass resulted in successful weight loss.

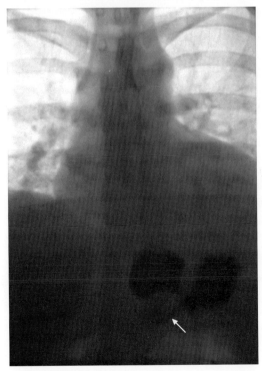

Figure 63.13 Eroded band. An arrow demonstrates medial dissection of contrast around the lower margin of this band. This patient with excellent initial weight loss began having emesis and weight regain in the second postoperative year. With removal of the band the emesis resolved, but the patient experienced a rapid return to prebanded weight.

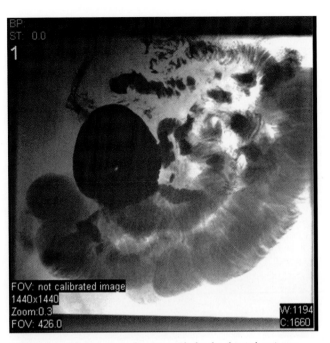

Figure 63.14 Biliopancreatic diversion with duodenal switch stricture. Dilatation of the ileoileal anastomosis and the proximal biliopancreatic limb is evident. The distal common channel is decompressed. This patient presented 2 weeks after the procedure with nausea and vomiting while not following the prescribed liquid diet. The patient did not respond to conservative management and subsequently underwent exploratory laparoscopy, lysis of adhesions, and extensive revision of the ileoileal anastomosis.

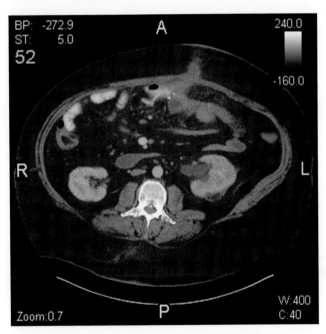

Figure 63.15 Biliopancreatic diversion with duodenal switch enterocutaneous fistula. Fat stranding is noted and fluid collection in the anterior abdominal wall communicates with small bowel. The patient shown in Figure 63.14 re-presented with drainage of succus from the anterior abdominal wall 3 weeks after the revisional procedure. A protracted postoperative course, including drainage and parenteral nutrition, resulted in eventual resolution 3 months after ileoileal anastomotic revision.

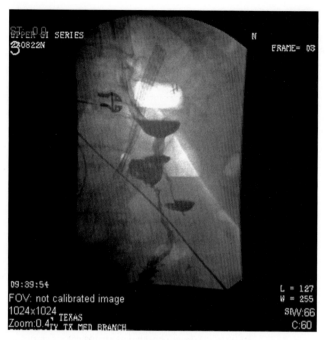

Figure 63.16 Roux-en-Y gastric bypass leak. Contrast extravasates at the stump of the Roux limb. This patient had abdominal pain and tachycardia 24 h postoperatively. An upper gastrointestinal series with iohexol contrast was performed. An enterotomy was closed in the medial aspect of the staple line on repeat laparoscopy. Symptomatic leaks must be addressed aggressively.

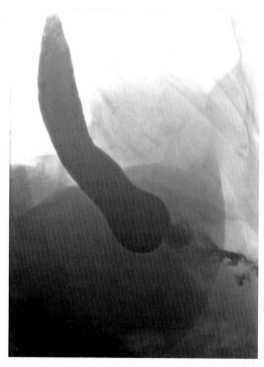

Figure 63.17 Roux-en-Y gastric bypass stricture. Profound dilation of the esophagus and stomach pouch with trickling of contrast past the anastomosis is shown. Postanastomotic decompression is also noted. This patient progressed initially to semisolid foods, but 4 weeks after Roux-en-Y gastric bypass began having intermittent, yet progressive nausea and vomiting. A contrast study was performed in clinic 7 weeks after the operation because the patient was tolerating only clear liquids.

To access the video for this chapter, please go to
www.yamadagastro.com/atlas

Video 63.1 This video shows the off-label use of a stent for treating a gastric sleeve leak. First, a guidewire is deployed and its position is confirmed with fluoroscopy. Then, a covered self-expanding Nitinol stent is carefully deployed, again with position confirmation via fluoroscopy. Contrast study should be performed prior to stent removal, at about 6 weeks at the earliest. Source: Courtesy of Dana Portenier, MD, Assistant Professor of Surgery, Duke University Medical Center.

CHAPTER 64

Complications of AIDS and other immunodeficiency states

Phillip D. Smith,[1] Nirag C. Jhala,[2] C. Mel Wilcox,[1] and Edward N. Janoff[3]

[1] University of Alabama at Birmingham, Birmingham, AL, USA
[2] Temple University, Philadelphia, PA, USA
[3] University of Colorado Health Sciences Center, Denver, Aurora, CO, and Veterans Affairs Medical Center, Denver, CO, USA

The acquired immunodeficiency syndrome (AIDS) and other cellular and humoral immunodeficiency states are associated with an array of gastrointestinal complications. The complications associated with AIDS are caused predominantly by infection. Parasitic (mainly protozoal), viral, bacterial, and fungal pathogens cause a spectrum of mucosal disease, depending on the location and severity of infection and the degree of immunosuppression induced by human immunodeficiency virus-1 (HIV-1), the causative agent of AIDS. These pathogens are considered opportunistic in immunosuppressed persons because they occur more frequently, cause more severe disease, and are associated with more prolonged or recurrent infection. Opportunistic pathogens in patients with advanced HIV-1 disease more frequently develop resistance to antimicrobial agents than do the same pathogens in immunocompetent persons. Gastrointestinal complications are also associated with allogeneic hematopoietic stem cell and solid organ transplantation. Graft-versus-host disease, which must be differentiated from infectious processes, is the most common gastrointestinal complication of hematopoietic stem-cell transplantation. Opportunistic enteric infections, particularly cytomegalovirus, also commonly complicate solid organ transplantation. This chapter focuses on endoscopic and histological features of gastrointestinal infections associated with AIDS, hepatic complications of AIDS, and intestinal involvement in graft-versus-host disease (Figures 64.1–64.14).

Yamada's Atlas of Gastroenterology, Fifth Edition. Edited by Daniel K. Podolsky, Michael Camilleri, J. Gregory Fitz, Anthony N. Kalloo, Fergus Shanahan, and Timothy C. Wang.
© 2016 John Wiley & Sons, Ltd. Published 2016 by John Wiley & Sons, Ltd.
Companion website: www.yamadagastro.com/atlas

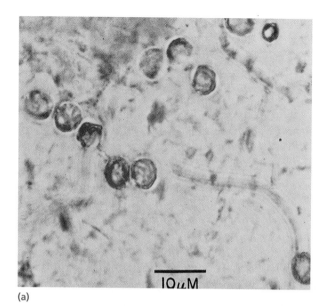

(a)

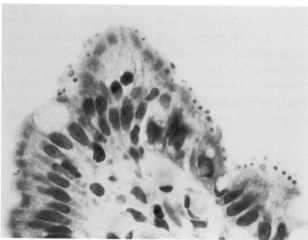

(b)

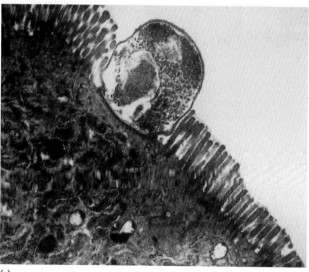

(c)

Figure 64.1 *Cryptosporidium parvum* is a parasitic protozoa that causes prolonged, often profuse, watery diarrhea among immunosuppressed persons with HIV-1 infection, particularly in the developing world. **(a)** Acid-fast stained stool specimen shows round *Cryptosporidium* oocysts 4–6μm in diameter (modified Kinyoun stain; magnification ×630). **(b)** Light microscopic image shows *Cryptosporidium parvum* lining the luminal surface of the epithelium in an intestinal biopsy specimen from a patient with chronic diarrhea (hematoxylin and eosin, magnification ×400) **(c)** Electron micrograph of an intestinal biopsy section shows a *Cryptosporidium* trophozoite that has displaced the microvilli to attach to the apical surface of an epithelial cell (magnification ×12 500). Source: Janoff EN Cryptosporidium. The Immunocompromised Host 1988;5:1. Courtesy of Dr. Phillip D. Smith (University of Alabama at Birmingham); courtesy of Dr. Ronald J Sokol (University of Colorado Denver).

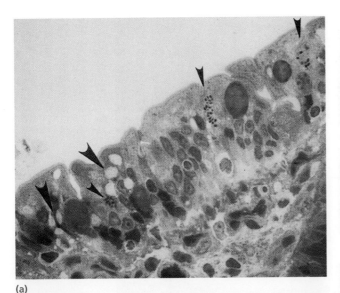

(a)

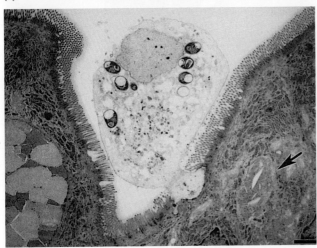

(b)

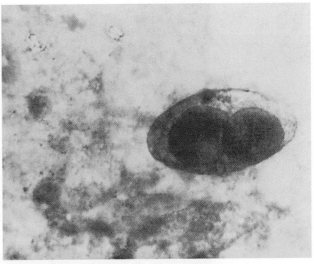

Figure 64.3 The coccidian protozoan *Isospora belli* causes a mild, self-limited diarrheal illness among immunocompetent persons but prolonged diarrhea among immunosuppressed persons. Infection with *I. belli* is diagnosed by identification of large (20–30 μm by 10–19 μm), oval, acid-fast oocysts that contain two sporoblasts in a fresh stool specimen (modified Kinyoun stain; magnification ×630). Source: Smith PD, Saini SS, Raffeld M, Manischewitz JF, Wahl SM. Cytomegalovirus induction of tumor necrosis facor-α by human monocytes and mucosal macrophages. J Clin Invest 1992;90: 1642. Reproduced with permission of Elsevier.

Figure 64.2 *Microsporida* protozoa in the small intestine of persons with HIV-1 infection is associated with a chronic diarrheal illness that clinically resembles cryptosporidiosis. **(a)** The intensity of infection is greatest in the jejunum, where densely stained elliptical spores are detected in the epithelial cell cytoplasm by light microscopic examination (semithin plastic section, methylene blue-azure II, basic fuchsin stain; original magnification ×630). **(b)** Electron micrograph shows a necrotic intestinal enterocyte in the final stage of being sloughed into the lumen; the enterocyte contains six microsporidian spores (magnification ×10 000). Source: Reproduced with permission of Dr. Jan M. Orenstein.

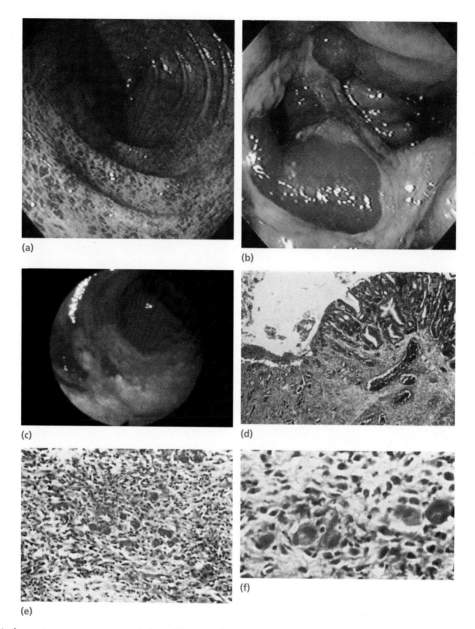

Figure 64.4 Colitis is the most common gastrointestinal manifestation of cytomegalovirus disease in AIDS. **(a)** Endoscopic view of diffuse colitis with prominent subepithelial hemorrhage in a patient with cytomegalovirus colitis. **(b)** Endoscopic visualization of a large well-circumscribed ulcer involving the ileocecal valve in a patient with cytomegalovirus colitis. **(c)** Endoscopic view of mucosal inflammation, ulceration, and bleeding in a patient with cytomegalovirus colitis. **(d)** Light microscopic examination of a colon biopsy specimen from the patient in **(c)** shows ulceration and hemorrhage, **(e)** infiltration by large numbers of inflammatory cells, and **(f)** numerous cytomegalic inclusion cells, which are pathognomonic of the infection. **(d, e, f)** hematoxylin and eosin; **(d)** magnification ×30; **(e)** magnification ×62; **(f)** magnification ×125.

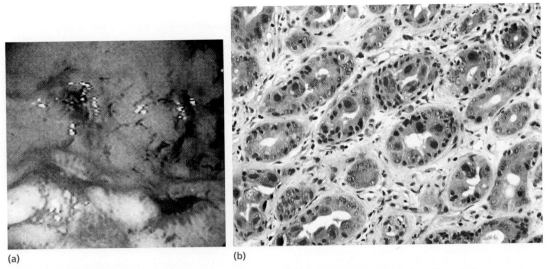

(a)   (b)

Figure 64.5 Cytomegalovirus infection may cause inflammation and ulceration in any organ of the gastrointestinal tract in immunosuppressed persons. **(a)** Endoscopic view of an antral ulcer in the gastric antrum in a woman with AIDS, who presented with nausea, vomiting, and weight loss. **(b)** Biopsy of the ulcer shows both nuclear and cytoplasmic inclusions, which are characteristic of cytomegalovirus infection, in cells of the glands, lamina propria, and vascular endothelium. Source: Smith PD, Saini SS, Raffeld M, Manischewitz JF, Wahl SM. Cytomegalovirus induction of tumor necrosis factor-α by human monocytes and mucosal macrophages. J Clin Invest 1992;90:1642. Reproduced with permission of Elsevier.

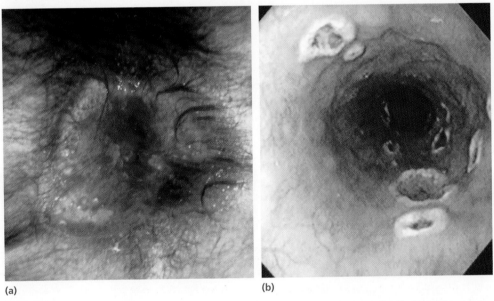

(a)   (b)

Figure 64.6 Herpes simplex virus is a latent infection among immunocompetent persons, but in persons infected with HIV-1, the virus can cause severe inflammation and ulceration of the anus, perianal region, and esophagus (esophagitis). **(a)** The perianal ulceration of this severely immunosuppressed patient with HIV-1 infection caused pain, tenesmus, and bleeding. Culture of a biopsy of the ulcer bed revealed herpes simplex virus. **(b)** Multiple small, well-circumscribed, shallow ulcers are typical for herpes simplex virus esophagitis.

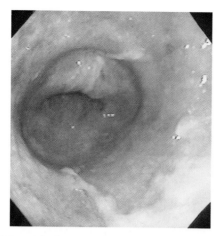

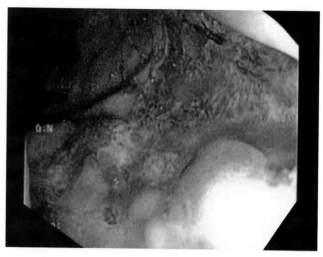

Figure 64.7 Bacterial infections with *Salmonella* spp., *Shigella flexneri*, and *Campylobacter jejuni* cause a similar clinical illness in persons infected with human immunodeficiency virus-1. This is characterized by recurrent or chronic diarrhea that is commonly associated with fever and abdominal cramps. Unlike infections with these pathogens in otherwise healthy persons, the infections in patients with HIV-1/AIDS are more often complicated by bacteremia. Endoscopic visualization of the colon of an HIV-1-infected patient shows superficial erosions, erythema, pus, and loss of the normal vascular pattern. A biopsy specimen of the area grew *C. jejuni*.

Figure 64.9 Lymphogranuloma venereum (LGV) is an invasive, sexually transmitted infection caused by *Chlamydia trachomatis*. LGV proctocolitis resulting in rectal bleeding, mucoid discharge, and tenesmus occurs with increased frequency in HIV-1-infected patients due to LGV serovar outer membrane A (OmpA). In an HIV-1-infected man with proctocolitis, colonoscopy showed erythema and friability in the distal colonic mucosa and, as shown here, shallow to deep ulcers, some measuring 20 mm in diameter. Histopathology of tissue obtained by biopsy of the rectal ulcer shown in the figure revealed ulceration with dense infiltration by chronic inflammatory cells and focal areas of acute inflammation. Strand displacement amplification of material obtained by rectal swab was positive for *C. trachomatis* and sequencing of the *C. trachomatis ompA* gene indicted OmpA type LGV 2b. In the absence of molecular testing, *C. trachomatis* can be diagnosed serologically by complement fixation (titer >1:64) or microimmunofluorescence (titer >1:256). The patient was cured of LGV with two 21-day courses of doxycycline 100 mg twice daily. Source: Geisler WM, Kapil R, Waites KB, Smith PD. Chronic rectal bleeding due to lymphogranuloma venereum proctocolitis. Am J Gastroenterol 2012;107:488.

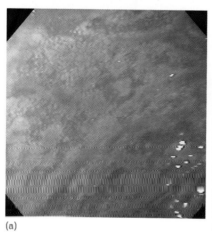

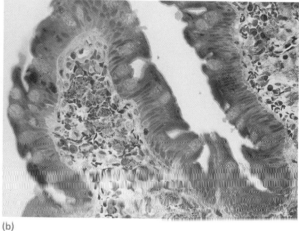

(a)   (b)

Figure 64.8 *Mycobacterium avium* complex is one of the most common bacterial pathogens identified in the gastrointestinal tracts of immunosuppressed patients with human immunodeficiency virus-1. Gastrointestinal involvement usually indicates disseminated infection and is associated with diarrhea, weight loss, fever, and a high bacterial burden in tissues. (a) Endoscopic image of the duodenum in a patient with AIDS and *M. avium* complex infection. The patient presented with diarrhea, abdominal pain, weight loss, and fever. The image shows multiple small yellow plaques, some of which have coalesced in the second portion of the duodenum. (b) Light micrograph of a biopsy section from the duodenum shows numerous lamina propria macrophages engorged with mycobacteria (methylene blue-azure II, basic fuchsin; magnification ×100).

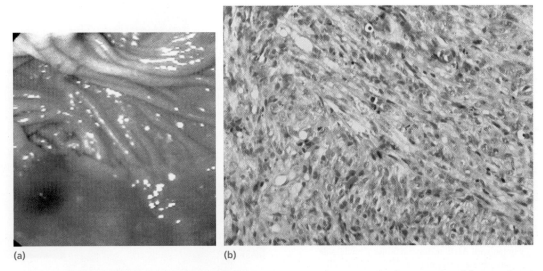

(a)   (b)

Figure 64.10 Kaposi sarcoma, a neoplasm associated with human herpes virus type 8 infection, may involve any region of the gastrointestinal tract. As a consequence of the widespread use of highly active antiretroviral therapy, Kaposi sarcoma has become uncommon in AIDS in the United States and Europe. **(a)** Endoscopic view of the stomach in a patient with AIDS shows a bleeding Kaposi sarcoma lesion; although the tumor is quite vascular, Kaposi sarcoma lesions bleed infrequently. **(b)** Biopsy of the stomach shows the characteristic proliferation of neoplastic spindle cells, some of which contain intracytoplasmic eosinophilic material (magnification ×40).

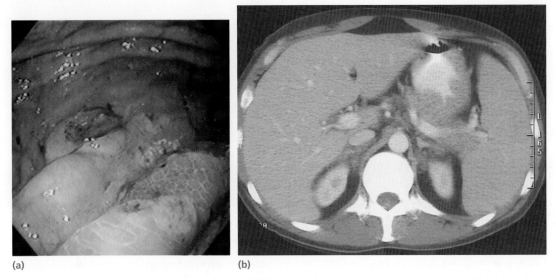

(a)   (b)

Figure 64.11 (a) Endoscopic view of the stomach from a patient with AIDS and non-Hodgkin gastric lymphoma shows thickened mucosal folds with superficial erosions and edema. **(b)** Abdominal computed tomography scan with contrast from the same patient shows markedly thickened gastric mucosa; gastric distention was limited owing to mucosal infiltration by tumor. Although the overall survival of patients with AIDS and non-Hodgkin lymphoma has increased since the introduction of highly active antiretroviral therapy, the incidence of this B-cell tumor among these patients has not decreased significantly as has that of many opportunistic infections.

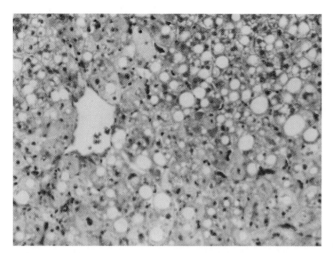

Figure 64.12 A woman with AIDS taking stavudine, a nucleoside analogue reverse transcriptase inhibitor (NRTI), presented with abdominal pain, nausea, vomiting, myalgias, hepatomegaly, elevated liver enzymes, and type B lactic acidosis. Liver biopsy shows macro- and microvesicular steatosis without cholestasis (magnification ×20). Fatty infiltration is the most common hepatic complication in patients with AIDS, particularly those taking NRTI antiretroviral drugs, such as zidovudine, didanosine, and stavudine. In addition to hepatic steatosis, these agents have been infrequently associated with myopathy, type B lactic acidosis, and fulminate hepatic failure.

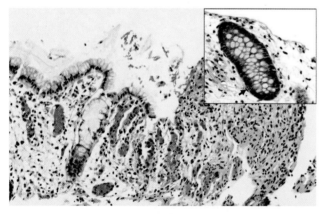

Figure 64.13 Acute graft-versus-host disease usually occurs within 3–4 weeks after stem cell transplantation and may involve the skin, liver, lung, and intestine. The clinical features of intestinal disease include watery diarrhea, anorexia, nausea, vomiting, abdominal pain, and bleeding. Intestinal biopsy from a patient with graft-versus-host disease shows flattening of crypts, crypt degeneration, edema, ulceration (magnification ×20) (top right) and typical epithelial cell apoptosis with (arrow) apoptotic bodies, necrotic epithelial cells, and minimal inflammatory cell infiltration (magnification ×40).

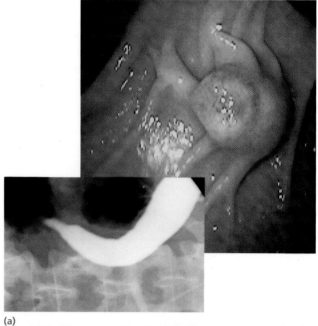

(a)

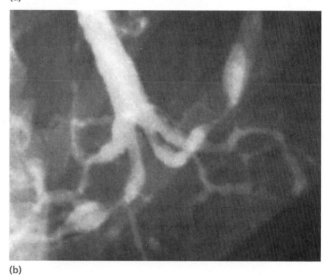

(b)

Figure 64.14 AIDS cholangiopathy is caused by inflammation of the biliary tract mucosa in patients infected with HIV-1 and is most commonly due to *Cryptosporidium*, cytomegalovirus, and microsporidia. **(a)** Endoscopic view of the ampulla of Vater in a patient with AIDS, abdominal pain and an elevated alkaline phosphatase shows an edematous, erythematous, and partially exudative papilla. Insert shows endoscopic retrograde cholangiogram of the patient's stenotic distal common bile duct. Biopsy of the ampulla of Vater revealed *Cryptosporidium*. **(b)** Endoscopic retrograde cholangiography in a patient with AIDS and cholangiopathy shows an irregular and distorted biliary tree with multiple areas of dilation and stricture.

CHAPTER 65

Gastrointestinal manifestations of immunological disorders

Paula O'Leary and Fergus Shanahan
University College Cork, Cork, Ireland

Immunodeficiency

Immunodeficiency disorders are a heterogeneous group of conditions that may be classified broadly into primary and secondary syndromes. Selective immunoglobulin A (IgA) deficiency and common variable immunodeficiency (CVID) (Figures 65.1 and 65.2) are the most common primary immunodeficiency syndromes among adults. Secondary immunodeficiencies are much more common than primary disorders. Causes include malnutrition, infection (HIV), protein-losing enteropathy such as intestinal lymphangiectasia (Figure 65.3), cancer, and iatrogenic immunosuppression.

The gastrointestinal tract is a primary target organ in both primary and secondary immunodeficiency disorders because of its large surface area and constant exposure to environmental

pathogens. The gut mucosa is composed of the single largest collection of lymphoid tissue in the body, primed to respond effectively to microbial challenge while at the same time regulated closely to avoid inappropriate and potentially harmful immune responses to the extensive and varied exposures experienced at this host–environment interface. The principal gastrointestinal consequence of immunodeficiency is increased susceptibility to infection. This includes infection with unusual agents, atypical manifestations of infection with commonly encountered pathogens, and bacterial overgrowth with organisms normally present in the gastrointestinal tract. There is also an increased prevalence of autoimmune disorders or chronic inflammatory conditions such as atrophic gastritis, inflammatory bowel disease, and celiac disease. In some immunodeficiency states there is an increased incidence of malignant tumors, particularly lymphoma. Benign diffuse nodular lymphoid hyperplasia may occur among some patients, whereas lymphoid atrophy may be a feature among others. Patients with severe immunodeficiency may have graft-versus-host disease caused by transplacentally acquired maternal lymphocytes or unintentional transfusion of nonirradiated blood products. However, patients with mild or selective forms of immunodeficiency, such as selective IgA deficiency, frequently are free of infections or other manifestations.

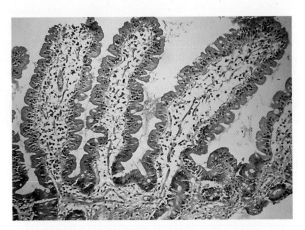

Figure 65.1 Small-bowel biopsy specimen from a patient with hypogammaglobulinemia shows a paucity of plasma cells in the lamina propria. Among patients with selective immunoglobulin A (IgA) deficiency, the absence or paucity of IgA-producing cells is compensated for by an increase in IgM-producing cells. Source: Courtesy of Dr. Klaus Lewin.

Nodular lymphoid hyperplasia

Diffuse nodular lymphoid hyperplasia occurs among approximately 20% of patients with CVID. The lymphoid nodules are in the lamina propria and submucosa and produce a nodularity that is visible on radiographic studies and at endoscopy (Figure 65.4). They are most prevalent in the small bowel, in some cases extend into the colon, and rarely extend into the stomach. At microscopic examination, the nodules consist of large lymphoid

Yamada's Atlas of Gastroenterology, Fifth Edition. Edited by Daniel K. Podolsky, Michael Camilleri, J. Gregory Fitz, Anthony N. Kalloo, Fergus Shanahan, and Timothy C. Wang.
© 2016 John Wiley & Sons, Ltd. Published 2016 by John Wiley & Sons, Ltd.
Companion website: www.yamadagastro.com/atlas

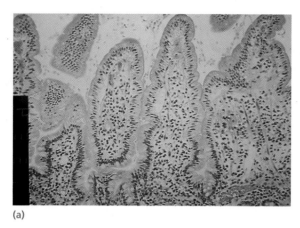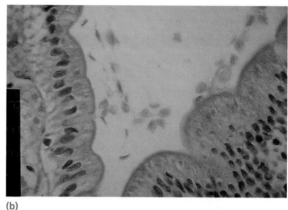

(a) (b)

Figure 65.2 (a, b) Giardiasis (*Giardia lamblia*) is the most common gastrointestinal parasitic infection in primary immunodeficiency syndromes. It occurs most frequently among patients with common variable hypogammaglobulinemia. Giardiasis usually does not distort the villous structure but may do so among patients with immunodeficiencies. Although the diagnosis of giardiasis can be made from inspection of histological sections of small bowel, finding the organism by means of this method is difficult and tedious when the infection burden is low. The diagnosis is made more conveniently by examination of the stools for cysts, or identification of the trophozoite form in intestinal fluid or smears of mucus adherent to the biopsy specimen.

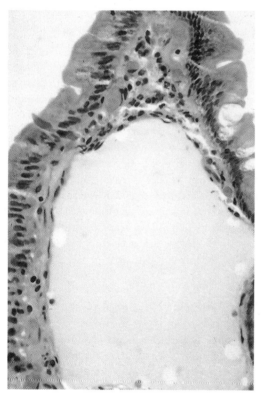

Figure 65.3 Secondary immunodeficiency: intestinal lymphangiectasia. Immunodeficiency caused by enteric protein loss may be a component of any severe inflammatory disorder of the gastrointestinal tract. The most severe cases of gastrointestinal protein loss occur with lymphangiectasia, which may be primary or secondary to lymphatic obstruction. Protein loss from the gastrointestinal tract is nonselective, and hypogammaglobulinemia is always accompanied by hypoalbuminemia. Among patients with lymphangiectasia there is also loss of lymphocytes, particularly T cells, and immunoglobulins. Source: Mitros FA. Atlas of Gastrointestinal Pathology. London: Gower, 1988. Copyright ©1988 Elsevier.

follicles with germinal centers (Figure 65.5). Plasma cells are usually absent. Lymphoid hyperplasia is believed to be caused by proliferation of B cells that are unable to undergo full differentiation to immunoglobulin secretion and therefore are unresponsive to feedback regulation of proliferation. Nodular lymphoid hyperplasia may be asymptomatic, but can be associated with bleeding, pain, diarrhea, and, when very large, obstructive symptoms. Potential for malignant transformation is possible but rare. Monitoring and surveillance guidelines are not defined. Unlike the situation with CVID, nodular lymphoid hyperplasia does not occur in X-linked hypogammaglobulinemia, probably because there is defective pre-B-cell to B-cell differentiation with hypoplasia of peripheral lymphoid tissue and a paucity of mature B cells. It is important to recognize that localized forms of nodular lymphoid hyperplasia, particularly in the large bowel, may occur among apparently healthy immunocompetent persons. Small nodules of lymphoid tissue on a background of normal folds of small bowel are normal and are a common finding among children and young adults. Infections may be a trigger.

Other gastrointestinal manifestations of common variable immunodeficiency

In addition to nodular lymphoid hyperplasia, a number of other gastrointestinal manifestations arise in patients with CVID. Celiac-like sprue lesions are commonly found in small intestinal biopsy. The lesion in CVID is characteristic for the paucity of antibody-producing plasma cells in the lamina propria (Figure 65.6). This can also be a feature in IgA deficiency. However, the sprue associated with CVID is not usually responsive clinically to gluten withdrawal whereas exclusion diet may be of benefit in affected patients with selective IgA deficiency. Inflammatory

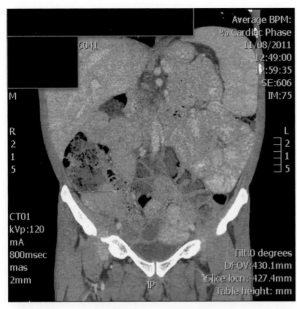
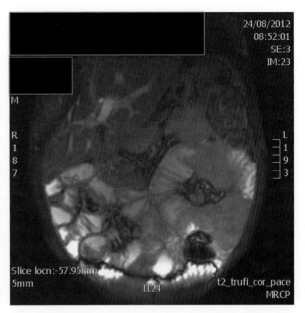

Figure 65.4 (a) Computed tomography (CT) abdomen coronal view and **(b)** magnetic resonance cholangiopancreatography (MRCP) axial view in a patient with common variable immunodeficiency (CVID) and chronic gastrointestinal symptoms of diarrhea and impaired absorption of vitamin B-12 and folate. One of the prominent features of both the CT and MRI images is the thickening and nodularity of the gut mucosa caused by diffuse nodular lymphoid hyperplasia, also noted at endoscopic examination in this patient. Moderate splenomegaly and intraabdominal lymphadenopathy, both features of the immune dysregulation seen in some patients with CVID, are also features. Source: Courtesy of Professor Michael Maher.

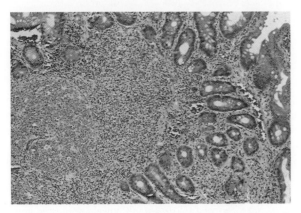

Figure 65.5 Histological features of diffuse nodular lymphoid hyperplasia in a patient with immunodeficiency. This jejunal biopsy specimen contains lymphoid tissue with germinal centers. Plasma cells were not identified. Radiographic evidence of nodular lymphoid hyperplasia was present. A cluster of *Giardia* organisms is present (top right). Source: Mitros FA. Atlas of Gastrointestinal Pathology. London: Gower, 1988. Copyright ©1988 Elsevier.

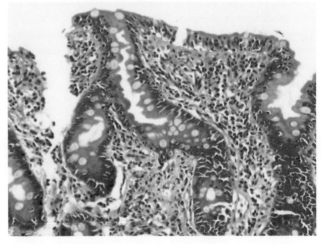

Figure 65.6 A duodenal biopsy section H&E stained, at ×200 magnification, from a patient with common variable immunodeficiency and diarrhea, showing intraepithelial lymphocytic infiltration, a feature also seen in celiac disease. The absence of plasma cells in the lamina propria is notable here and is a feature suggestive of primary immunodeficiency. Source: Courtesy of Dr. Louise Burke.

bowel disease-like lesions also occur in CVID. Histological features are similar to features in immunocompetent affected individuals, but subtle differences, such as diminishment in plasma cell numbers in the lamina propria, may occur. Therapy is similar to that used in immunocompetent patients. A number of different hepatic manifestations occur in patients with CVID, including cholestasis, autoimmune hepatitis, and primary biliary cirrhosis. Hepatic granulomatous disease may be part of a more generalized dysregulatory granulomatous process involving spleen, lymph nodes, bone marrow, and lungs characteristically (Figure 65.7). Antiinflammatory and immunosuppressive therapy may be required to control the process in some patients.

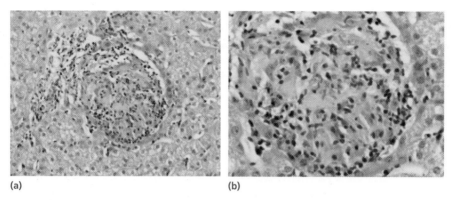

(a)   (b)

Figure 65.7 Two magnifications ((**a**) ×200, (**b**) ×400) of H&E stained liver sections from a patient with common variable immunodeficiency, altered liver biochemistry (raised alkaline phosphatase), and hepatomegaly, showing nonnecrotizing, well-formed epithelioid granulomata. These were distributed throughout the liver parenchyma. Zeill–Neilsen staining was negative. Source: Courtesy of Dr. Louise Burke.

Graft-versus-host disease

Gastrointestinal complications occur among virtually all patients at some stage during recovery from bone marrow transplantation. In addition to graft-versus-host disease, causes of gastrointestinal symptoms after bone marrow transplantation include the effects of chemotherapy and chemoradiation therapy given before bone marrow grafting and opportunistic infections that may be caused by the immunosuppressive protocol or the immunodeficiency associated with graft-versus-host disease. The gastrointestinal and liver damage associated with chemoradiation therapy usually resolves within 20–30 days after transplantation. Opportunistic infections may occur at any stage after bone marrow transplantation; bacterial and fungal infections tend to be more common during the first month and viral infections more common thereafter.

The clinical severity and extent of gastrointestinal involvement with acute and chronic graft-versus-host disease are highly variable. Acute graft-versus-host disease usually occurs 20–60 days after transplantation and primarily affects the skin, liver, and gastrointestinal tract. Chronic graft-versus-host disease is a multisystem disorder with clinical features resembling those of sicca syndrome and systemic sclerosis. Gastrointestinal involvement is particularly common in the oral mucosa (mucositis), esophagus, and small bowel. Chronic graft-versus-host disease usually occurs 80–400 days after transplantation.

The earliest morphological feature of acute intestinal graft versus host disease at light microscopic examination is apoptosis of individual cells in the intestinal crypts (Figure 65.8). This characteristic finding is diagnostic if obtained from normal-appearing mucosa at least 20 days after transplantation (when the effects of chemoradiation therapy have resolved). Inflammatory cells or microorganisms are not present in adjacent mucosa. Later, the histopathology can progress to total denudation of the mucosa; the apoptotic lesion is no longer evident, and changes are not specific.

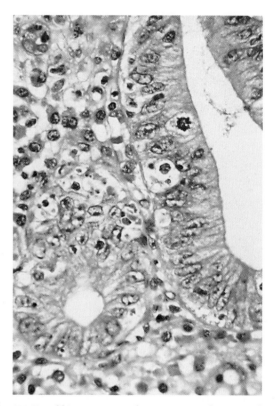

Figure 65.8 Rectal biopsy specimen from a patient with acute graft-versus-host disease after bone marrow transplantation. The individual crypt cell apoptosis (karyolytic debris in vacuoles near crypt base) is characteristic if found after day 20, when damage from chemoradiation therapy has resolved. Source: Courtesy of Dr. Klaus Lewin.

The radiographic appearance of graft-versus-host disease also varies with the severity and with the stage of the disease. During the acute phase there is mucosal and submucosal edema, particularly in the distal small bowel. In addition to thickening of the bowel wall there may be mucosal ulceration, sloughing, and

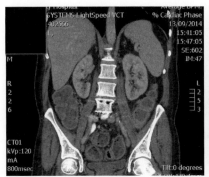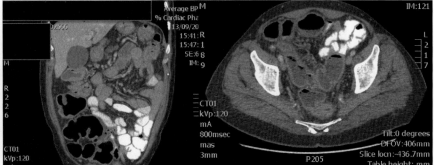

Figure 65.9 Computed tomography (CT) abdomen images from a patient with acute graft-versus-host disease presenting with florid watery diarrhea and abdominal pain. The notable features are the diffuse bowel wall thickening, luminal excess fluid, and mucosal hyperenhancement following contrast. While these features are not specific to graft-versus-host disease, in the appropriate clinical situation, they support this diagnosis. Source: Courtesy of Professor Michael Maher.

pneumatosis cystoides intestinalis. The changes are not specific and may be mimicked by coexisting cytomegalovirus (CMV) infection (Figure 65.9).

The endoscopic appearance of acute graft-versus-host disease may be normal, show patchy erythema, or show extensive mucosal sloughing, particularly in the ileum, cecum, and ascending colon, with relative sparing of the rectal and gastric mucosa. In contrast, esophageal involvement is particularly common in chronic graft-versus-host disease. Lesions include desquamation of the upper esophagus and upper esophageal webs; the distal esophagus usually is spared.

Cytomegalovirus infection

Gastrointestinal infection with CMV is found in several clinical settings. It may be associated with primary or secondary immunodeficiency states, particularly when there is defective cell-mediated immunity. CMV infection is seen increasingly among patients with iatrogenic immunosuppression associated with cancer therapy, transplantation, or chronic inflammatory disorders such as lupus or inflammatory bowel disease. Infection with CMV occurs in as many as one-third of patients undergoing transplantation. After oroesophageal candidiasis it is probably the most common gastrointestinal infection among patients with AIDS. CMV infection has also been described

among apparently immunocompetent persons with a variety of disorders including hypertrophic gastropathy, self-limited colitis, and ulcerative colitis, particularly when complicated by development of toxic megacolon. Although the manifestations of gastrointestinal CMV infection are highly variable, severity tends to correlate with the degree of immunosuppression. Inflammation with ulceration may be focal or diffuse (Figure 65.10a), superficial or deep (Figure 65.10b), and may lead to bleeding and perforation. Any part of the esophagus and small or large intestine may be involved. Multifocal involvement with CMV is usual among patients with AIDS, whereas CMV is often limited to the cecum (typhlitis) and ascending colon after transplantation.

Endothelial cells are the most frequent cell types infected (Figure 65.10c,d). Smooth muscle cells and the myenteric plexus occasionally are involved. Infected macrophages also may be seen in the lamina propria, whereas epithelial cells are seldom involved. CMV-infected cells are large with a granular cytoplasm and nuclei that are filled with intranuclear (Cowdry type A) inclusions, often with a periinclusion halo. Unlike cells infected with herpes simplex virus, which tend to be superficial, characteristic CMV-infected cells usually are found in the deeper layers of resected or biopsy specimens (Figure 65.10e). Identification of CMV infection may be facilitated by in situ hybridization or immunocytochemical analysis with virus-specific antibodies (Figure 65.10d,e).

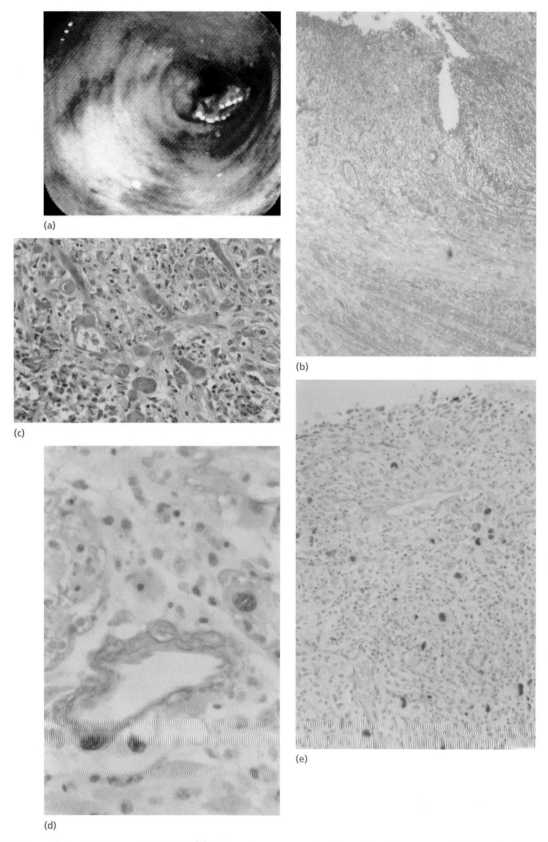

Figure 65.10 Cytomegalovirus (CMV)-associated colitis. **(a)** Endoscopic appearance of patchy erythematous mucosa with linear streaks. **(b)** Histopathological section of surgically resected colonic tissue shows penetrating ulceration with transmural inflammation in an immunodeficient patient with bloody diarrhea, abdominal pain, and peritoneal signs. **(c)** High-power light microscopic image of resected colonic tissue shown in **(b)** shows CMV-infected cells with characteristic nuclear inclusions within the lamina propria and submucosa. CMV has a propensity to infect endothelial cells, although smooth muscle cells, macrophages, and the myenteric plexus may be involved. **(d)** Immunocytochemical analysis with CMV-specific monoclonal antibody shows CMV within endothelial cells. **(e)** Full-thickness resected tissue stained immunocytochemically with viral-specific antibody shows that CMV-infected cells are usually found in the deeper layers of gastrointestinal specimens.

CHAPTER 66

Parasitic diseases: protozoa

Ellen Li and Samuel L. Stanley Jr.

Stony Brook University Hospital, Stony Brook, NY, USA

The intestinal parasitic protozoa are being increasingly recognized as important causes of diarrheal illness worldwide. Infestation with *Entamoeba histolytica*, the causative agent of amebic dysentery and amebic liver abscess, is primarily a disease of developing countries. Infestation with *Giardia lamblia, Cryptosporidium parvum*, and *Cyclospora cayetanensis*, however, poses serious threats to public health in the United States and the rest of the world. Physicians (gastroenterologists in particular) must consider these pathogens in the differential diagnosis of acute and chronic diarrhea and should be familiar with the optimal diagnostic (Table 66.1) and therapeutic approaches to these diseases. Because conventional microscopic examination of the stool for ova and parasites is time consuming and expensive, special requests for microscopic examinations may need to be made to the laboratory. In some hospitals, only fecal immunoassay(s) directed against *Giardia* and *Cryptosporidium* species may be performed when stool ova and parasite testing is requested.

Amebiasis

Improved sanitation conditions have greatly reduced the number of cases of amebiasis in the United States. Disease in the United States is probably most commonly detected among immigrants and should be considered for all persons with dysentery and an appropriate travel or exposure history. *E. histolytica* trophozoites can be seen in wet mounts of stool, ulcer scrapings, or intestinal aspirates obtained during endoscopy and in fixed specimens stained with trichrome (Figure 66.1). An important diagnostic problem is that *E. histolytica* is morphologically identical to the genetically distinct nonpathogenic *Entamoeba dispar* species. New antigen detection enzyme-linked immunosorbent assays (ELISA) that specifically recognize *E. histolytica* and not *E. dispar* in stool may replace microscopic examination as the test of choice for the diagnosis of intestinal amebiasis.

E. histolytica trophozoites invade the colonic mucosa and cause discrete ulcers covered with yellowish-white exudate (Figure 66.2a), multiple well-defined ulcers (Figure 66.2c), diffuse erythema and ulceration (Figure 66.2d), and, rarely, heaped-up inflammatory and granulation tissue that forms an ameboma (Figure 66.2b). Pseudomembrane formation can be seen.

The most frequent extraintestinal manifestation of *E. histolytica* infestation is amebic liver abscess. Patients usually have the triad of fever, right upper quadrant pain and tenderness, and a space-occupying lesion in the liver. As illustrated in Figure 66.3, an initial clue to the presence of amebic liver abscess may be an abnormal chest radiograph showing elevation of the right hemidiaphragm, right pleural effusion, and possibly a right basilar infiltrate. Amebic liver abscesses are often visible on computed tomographic (CT) scans as large, generally homogenous, low-attenuation lesions (Figure 66.4). However, multiple abscesses can develop.

Blastocystis hominis

Blastocystis hominis is one of the protozoan organisms frequently detected in stools (Figure 66.5). The pathogenicity of this organism continues to be controversial.

Giardiasis

G. lamblia has been the most common intestinal parasitic cause of diarrhea in the United States in recent years. Groups at high risk for giardiasis include children in day-care facilities and their adult contacts, travelers, and those who consume contaminated water. Abundant *Giardia* trophozoites may be seen in biopsy samples from the small intestine of these persons (Figure 66.6). The diagnosis of *G. lamblia* infestation is based primarily on detection of trophozoites and cysts in the stool by means of microscopic analysis of stained stool specimens (Figure 66.7).

Yamada's Atlas of Gastroenterology, Fifth Edition. Edited by Daniel K. Podolsky, Michael Camilleri, J. Gregory Fitz, Anthony N. Kalloo, Fergus Shanahan, and Timothy C. Wang.
© 2016 John Wiley & Sons, Ltd. Published 2016 by John Wiley & Sons, Ltd.
Companion website: www.yamadagastro.com/atlas

Table 66.1 Morphological features of human gastrointestinal protozoan parasites.

Type of parasite	Stool	Intestinal biopsy
Extracellular ameboid		
Entamoeba histolytica	Trophozoite 10–20 μm with pale, round nucleus with small central karyosome; cyst 9–25 μm with four nuclei Morphologically indistinguishable from Entamoeba dispar; immunoassays for detection of trophozoite antigen can differentiate E. histolytica from E. dispar; serological testing may be a useful adjunct	Trophozoites but not cysts seen invading colonic mucosa causing colonic ulcerations
Blastocystis hominis (pathogenicity is controversial)	Organisms 6–40 μm, round with large central body or vacuole	
Flagellates		
Giardia lamblia	Trophozoite pear shaped, 10–20 μm long, characteristic face-like image because of two nuclei, each with prominent karyosome Cyst oval, 7–10 μm long; direct fluorescence antibody test available in many laboratories for detection of cysts Fecal immunoassays are routinely used to detect Giardia in many US hospitals	Trophozoites seen most commonly on duodenal mucosal surface, but also on jejunal and ileal biopsy specimens Histological features usually normal, but villous atrophy seen in severe infections
Dientamoeba fragilis	Appears ameboid in shape, 10–15 μm, with flagella not visible, one or two nuclei No known cyst form	
Ciliate		
Balantidium coli (rare)	Trophozoite 50–200 μm in length, motile Cysts are rarely seen in stool and are 50–75 μm in diameter	Trophozoites can invade into colonic mucosa causing ulceration
Intracellular coccidia		
Cryptosporidium parvum	Modified acid-fast stain: oocysts stain uniformly, are round, 4–6 μm, contain four sporozoites that may or may not be visible Direct fluorescence assay may be helpful in detecting cysts Fecal immunoassays are used for detection of Cryptosporidium in many hospitals	Intracellular forms seen as 4-μm extracytoplasmic dots on the apical surface of enterocytes; distribution may be patchy
Isospora belli	May be observed on wet preparation May need to submit special request to laboratory Modified acid-fast stain: oocysts stain uniformly, appear oval, 20–30 μm, with two sporocysts, each containing four sporozoites	Intracellular forms seen as 20-μm intracytoplasmic inclusions within the enterocyte on light microscopic examination; distribution may be patchy
Cyclospora cayetanensis	May be observed on wet preparation May need to submit special request to laboratory Modified acid-fast stain: oocysts stain variably, resemble Cryptosporidium oocysts but are larger (8–10 μm), contain two sporocysts, each with two sporozoites Oocysts autofluoresce under ultraviolet light (365 nm)	Intracellular forms difficult to see on light microscopic examination but have been seen on electron microscopic examination as intracytoplasmic inclusions

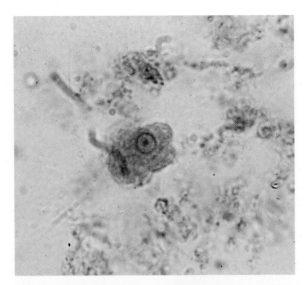

Figure 66.1 *Entamoeba histolytica* trophozoite in stool. This trophozoite is approximately 20 μm in diameter and has the characteristic round nucleus with a small, centrally placed karyosome. Source: Courtesy of Patrick Murray, PhD.

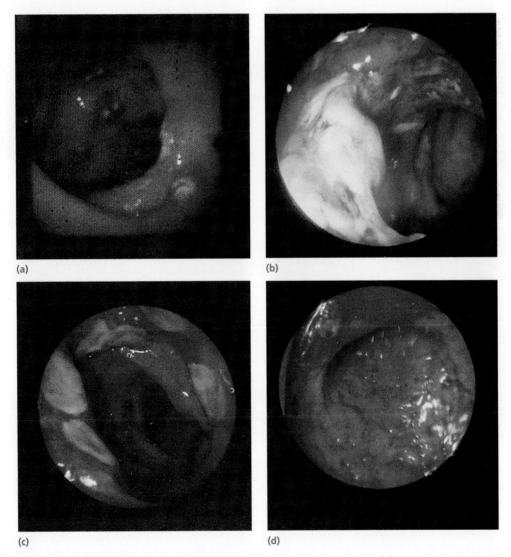

Figure 66.2 Rectosigmoidoscopic images show part of the pathological spectrum of intestinal amebiasis. **(a)** Ulcers covered with yellowish-white secretion. **(b)** Heaped-up granulation tissue forming an ameboma. **(c)** Multiple well-defined ulcers. **(d)** Diffuse erythema and ulceration. Source: Sepulveda B, Manzo N. Clinical manifestations and diagnosis of amebiasis. In: Martinez-Palomo A (ed.). Amebiasis. Amsterdam: Elsevier, 1986. Reproduced with permission of Elsevier.

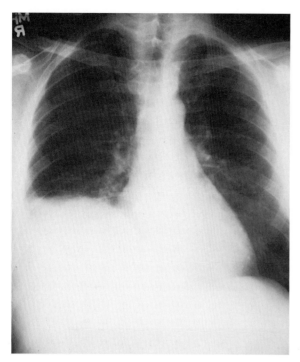

Figure 66.3 Chest radiograph of a patient with amebic liver abscess that has ruptured into the right pleural space. Elevated right hemidiaphragm, pleural effusion, and basilar infiltrate are depicted. This patient was initially thought to have bacterial pneumonia and empyema.

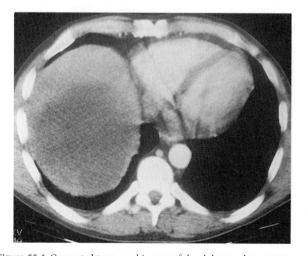

Figure 66.4 Computed tomographic scan of the abdomen demonstrates a large amebic liver abscess in the right lobe of the liver.

Antigen detection tests are available that permit detection of *G. lamblia*, as well as *E. histolytica* and *C. parvum*; these tests may be valuable as initial screening tests for individuals with diarrhea. Immunofluorescence assays (MeriFluor, Meridian Bioscience, Cincinnati, OH) can be used to detect both *G. lamblia* cysts and *C. parvum* oocysts (Figure 66.8).

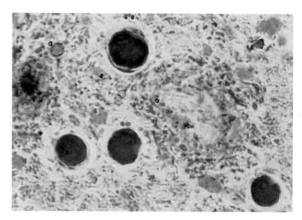

Figure 66.5 Trichrome stain of *Blastocystis hominis*. Source: Healy GR, Garcia LS. Intestinal and urogenital protozoa. In: Murray PR (ed.). Manual of Clinical Microbiology. Washington, DC: ASM Press, 1995. Reproduced with permission of ASM Press.

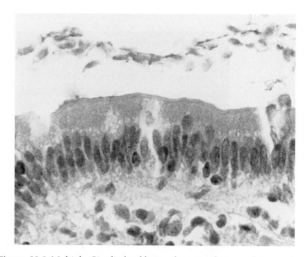

Figure 66.6 Multiple *Giardia lamblia* trophozoites that were lying on the surface of the duodenal mucosa. Source: Case records of the Massachusetts General Hospital. Weekly clinicopathological exercises. Case 8-1997. A 65-year-old man with recurrent abdominal pain for five years. N Engl J Med 1997;336:786. Reproduced with permission of the Massachusetts Medical Society.

Dientamoeba fragilis

Dientamoeba fragilis, a species of flagellated protozoa, is ameboid in shape and ranges in size from 5 to 15 μm; the flagella are not visible (Figure 66.9). There is no known cyst form. Symptoms ascribed to this organism include mild diarrhea, abdominal pain, anorexia, and fatigue.

Balantidiasis

Balantidium coli is a ciliate parasite that can invade the colonic mucosa (Figure 66.10) and cause colonic ulceration. Diagnosis

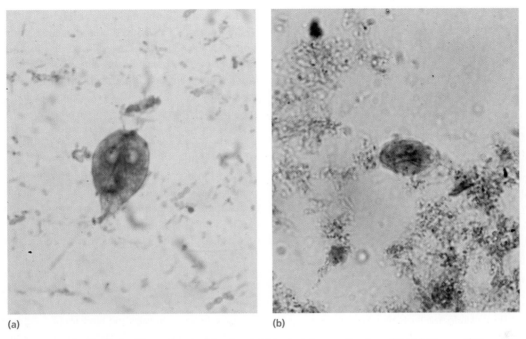

(a)   (b)

Figure 66.7 Trichrome stain of a *Giardia lamblia* trophozoite **(a)** and cyst **(b)** in stool. Source: Courtesy of Patrick Murray, PhD.

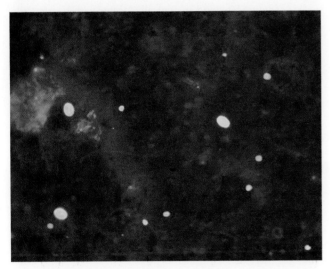

Figure 66.8 *Giardia lamblia* cysts (larger, ellipsoid, with some internal detail present) and *Cryptosporidium parvum* oocysts (smaller, spherical) in a stool sample are revealed by direct fluorescence assay. Source: Courtesy of Meridian Diagnostics.

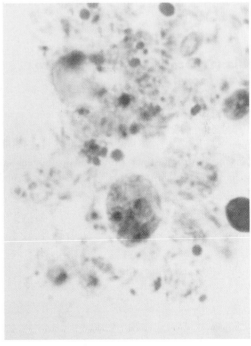

Figure 66.9 Trichrome stain of *Dientamoeba fragilis*. Although this organism is a flagellate, its appearance mimics that of amebas. Source: Healy GR, Garcia LS. Intestinal and urogenital protozoa. In: Murray PR (ed.). Manual of Clinical Microbiology. Washington, DC: ASM Press, 1995. Reproduced with permission of ASM Press.

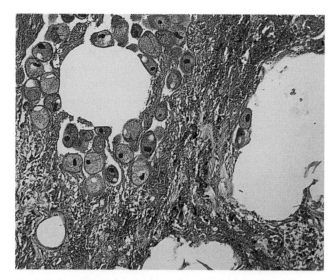

Figure 66.10 Balantidiasis. Numerous large trophozoites in the wall of the intestine in a patient with acquired immunodeficiency syndrome. Source: Farar WE, Wood MJ, Innes JA, et al. Infectious Diseases: Text and Color Atlas. St Louis: Mosby-Year Book, 1992. Reproduced with permission of Elsevier.

is made by observation of the large motile trophozoites in saline mounts of stool.

Coccidia (*Cryptosporidium, Isospora, and Cyclospora*)

Since the onset of the acquired immunodeficiency syndrome (AIDS) epidemic, coccidial organisms from the genera *Cryptosporidium, Cyclospora,* and *Isospora* have emerged not only as important gastrointestinal protozoan pathogens among immunocompromised hosts but also as causative agents of

diarrhea among immunocompetent hosts. *C. parvum* is a common cause of diarrhea among patients with AIDS in the United States and is one of the leading causative agents of waterborne disease outbreaks in the United States. *Cyclospora* and *Isospora* are seen less commonly in the United States but are prevalent in developing countries and should be suspected among travelers returning from endemic areas.

These organisms are intracellular pathogens with similar life cycles (Figure 66.11), which may account for their similar clinical manifestations.

The diagnosis of these parasitic diseases generally is made by examination of the stool. The acid-fast stain may be the most useful stain for detecting these organisms (Figures 66.12 and 66.13). Some laboratories may not routinely search for these organisms, and the physician may need to submit special requests to the laboratory. The organisms differ in size and shape (see Figures 66.12 and 66.13; Table 66.1). *Cryptosporidium* and *Cyclospora* are particularly difficult to differentiate from each other, and measurements must be made to confirm the size difference. Smears and biopsies of small intestinal aspirates may be useful for the diagnosis of infestation with these organisms (Figures 66.14, 66.15, and 66.16; see Table 66.1). Cryptosporidia can be easily detected on routine light microscopic examination as 4-μm basophilic dots on the apical surface of enterocytes and are typically located within crypt cells (see Figure 66.14). The organism is intracellular but extracytoplasmic (see Figure 66.15). A direct fluorescence assay allows screening by fluorescent microscopic examination, which can provide rapid and accurate results (see Figure 66.8). *Isospora* organisms can be detected on light microscopic examination as 20-μm inclusions within the enterocyte and are typically located within villous enterocytes (see Figure 66.16). With a heavy organism burden, *Cyclospora* organisms have been identified on light microscopic examination of duodenal biopsy specimens, but transmission electron microscopic examination may be a more sensitive approach.

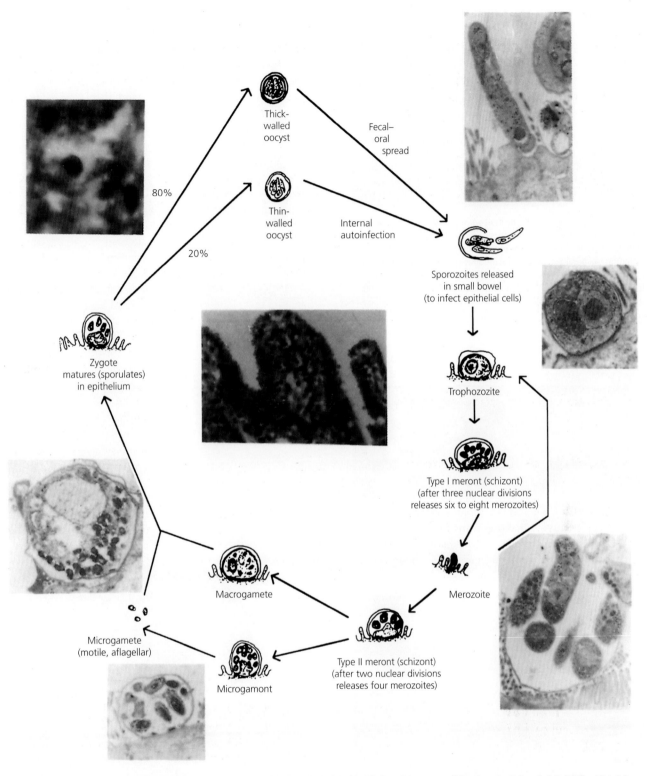

Figure 66.11 Life cycle of *Cryptosporidium*. Source: Guerrant RL, Petri WA, Wanke CS. Parasitic causes of diarrhea. In: Lebenthal E, Duffey M (eds). Paraphysiology of Secretory Diarrhea. Boston: Raven Press, 1990. Reproduced with permission of Elsevier.

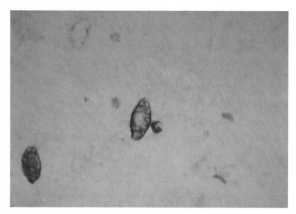

Figure 66.12 Acid-fast stain of an *Isospora belli* oocyst (large oocyst) and a *Cryptosporidium* oocyst (small oocyst) in a patient from Haiti. Source: Soave R, Weikel CS. Cryptosporidium and other protozoa including Isospora, Sarcocystis, Balantidum coli, and Blastocystis. In: Mandell GL, Douglas RG Jr, Bennett JE (eds). Principles and Practice of Infectious Diseases, 3rd edn. New York: Churchill Livingstone, 1990. Reproduced with permission of Elsevier; Courtesy of Dr. Madeline Boncy and Dr. Rosemary Soave.

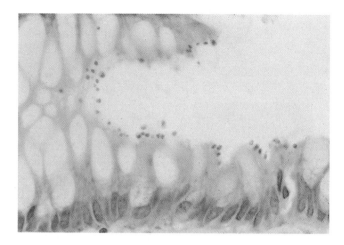

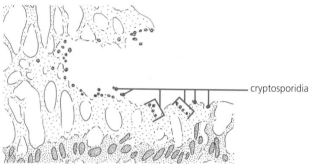

Figure 66.14 Cryptosporidia are seen as 4-μm dots on the apical surface of enterocytes.

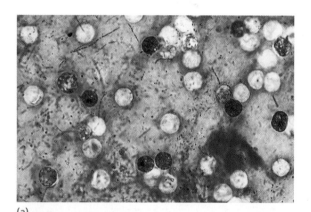

(a)

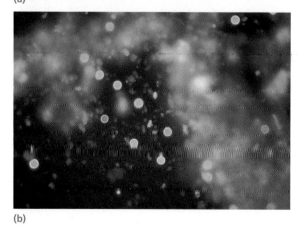

(b)

Figure 66.13 *Cyclospora cayetanensis.* **(a)** Modified acid-fast stain of *Cyclospora* oocysts shows multiple well-stained, poorly stained, and unstained oocysts within the same field. **(b)** Autofluorescence of *Cyclospora* oocysts. Source: Courtesy of Earl G. Long.

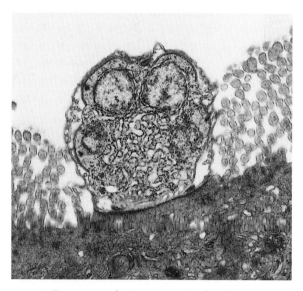

Figure 66.15 Transmission electron micrograph of a schizont stage of *Cryptosporidium parvum* attached to the intestinal epithelium. The organism is surrounded by the enterocyte plasma membrane but is separated from the cytoplasm by the membrane of a parasitophorous vacuole. Source: Courtesy of Dr. Paul Swanson.

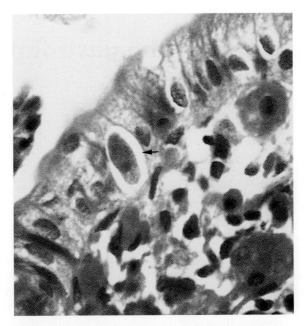

Figure 66.16 A single *Isospora belli* organism (arrow) appears as a 20-μm inclusion within an enterocyte.

CHAPTER 67

Helminthic infections of the gastrointestinal tract and liver

Thormika Keo, John Leung, and Joel V. Weinstock
Tufts Medical Center, Boston, MA, USA

Introduction

Helminths are multicellular eukaryotic organisms that are common parasites of the human gastrointestinal tract. Throughout human history, infestation with intestinal helminths has been a normal part of the human condition (Figures 67.1–67.23). Helminths are categorized into three major groups: nematodes, trematodes, and cestodes. Nematodes are round worms with a tubular gut, including both mouth and anus. There are two groups of flatworms: trematodes and cestodes. Trematodes, or flukes, are flat leaf-shaped organisms with a blind gut. All trematodes require an obligate freshwater snail host. The cestodes, or tapeworms, typically have two distinct forms. The adult stage is a tapeworm in the gut of the definitive host with an attachment organ, the scolex, and segments, termed proglottids. The external cestode surface tegument performs many of the same functions of the mammalian digestive tract. The proglottids are hermaphroditic, containing both ovaries and testes. The larval stage develops into cystic lesions in the tissues of the intermediate host. Some species have a second intermediate host. As members of the animal kingdom, helminths are multicellular organisms with their own organs and are large enough to be visible to the human eye during their life cycle. Thus, it is not uncommon to encounter these organisms during endoscopic procedures performed on high-risk populations.

Acknowledgment

This work was supported by NIH grants DK38327 and DK058755.

Yamada's Atlas of Gastroenterology, Fifth Edition. Edited by Daniel K. Podolsky, Michael Camilleri, J. Gregory Fitz, Anthony N. Kalloo, Fergus Shanahan, and Timothy C. Wang.

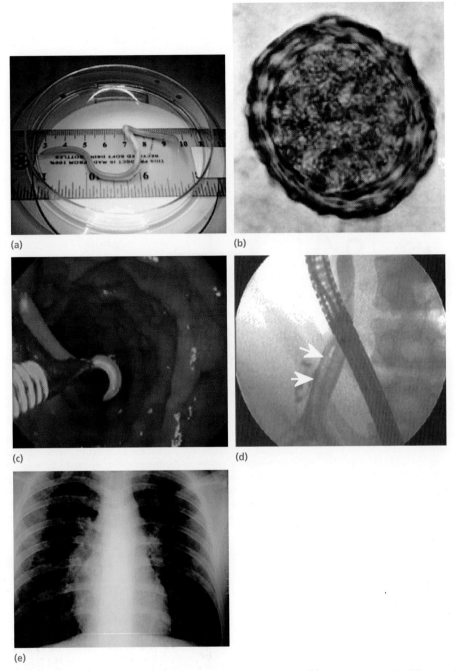

Figure 67.1 *Ascaris lumbricoides.* **(a)** The adult female worm measures up to 40 cm in length. **(b)** *Ascaris* ova are often bile-stained and demonstrate a thick mammillated shell. **(c)** Endoscopic extraction of an *Ascaris* located at the papilla. **(d)** Visualization of *Ascaris* in the common bile duct during endoscopic retrograde cholangio pancreatography (ERCP). **(e)** Loeffler's syndrome (or pneumonia) develops in some individuals during the acute stage of infection with *A. lumbricoides*. Chest x-ray may reveal unilateral or bilateral abnormalities ranging from diffuse interstitial pneumonitis to nodular densities. Sources: **(a)** Centers for Disease Control and Prevention (http://www.dpd.cdc.gov/DpDx/HTML/ImageLibrary/Ascariasis_il.htm). **(b)** http://en.wikipedia.org/wiki/File:Ascaris_lumbricoides.jpg. **(d)** Astudillo et al. Journal of the American College of Surgeons 2008;207:527–532. Reproduced by permission of Elsevier. **(e)** Lau et al. Journal of Clinical Pathology 2007, 60 (2) 202–3. Reproduced with permission from BMJ Publishing Group Ltd.

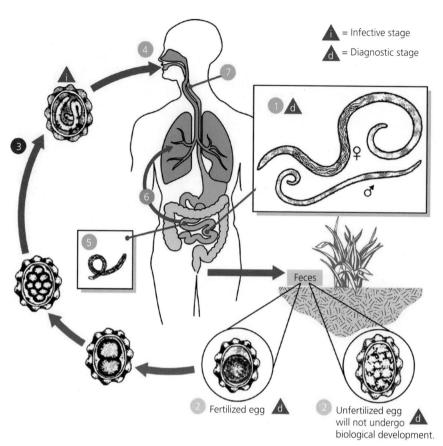

Figure 67.2 The life cycle of *Ascaris lumbricoides*. Adult worms (1) live in the lumen of the small intestine. A female may produce approximately 200 000 eggs per day, which are passed with the feces (2). Unfertilized eggs may be ingested but are not infective. Fertile eggs embryonate and become infective after 18 days to several weeks (3), depending on the environmental conditions (optimum: moist, warm, shaded soil). After infective eggs are swallowed (4), the larvae hatch (5), invade the intestinal mucosa, and are carried via the portal, then systemic circulation to the lungs (6). The larvae mature further in the lungs (10 to 14 days), penetrate the alveolar walls, ascend the bronchial tree to the throat, and are swallowed (7). Upon reaching the small intestine, they develop into adult worms (1). Between 2 and 3 months are required from ingestion of the infective eggs to oviposition by the adult female. Adult worms can live 1 to 2 years. Source: Centers for Disease Control and Prevention (http://www.dpd.cdc.gov/DpDx).

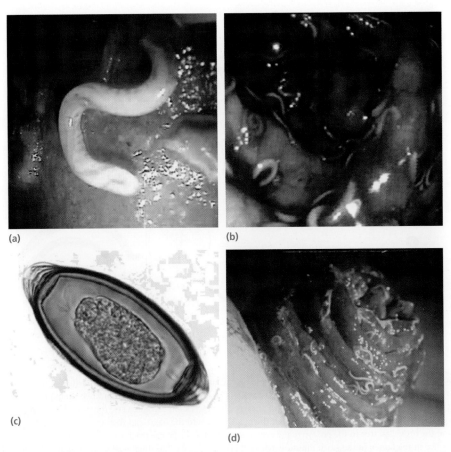

Figure 67.3 **(a)** Adult *Trichuris trichiura* inhabit the colon and can be visualized during colonoscopy. **(b)** Massive infection can be associated with diarrhea, colonic bleeding, or **(d)** rectal prolapse. *T. trichiura* **(c)** ova are characterized by polar plugs at both ends. Sources: **(a)** Courtesy of Richard Goodgame **(c)** Centers for Disease Control and Prevention (http://www.dpd.cdc.gov/DpDx).

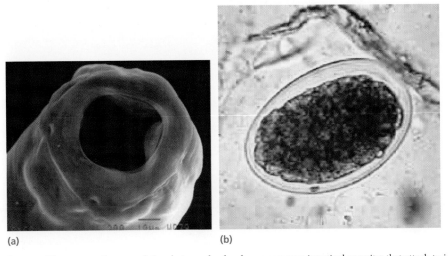

Figure 67.4 Human hookworms, *Necator americanus* and *Ancylostoma duodenale*, are common intestinal parasites that attach to intestinal villi and feed on blood. Low burden infections are typically asymptomatic, but heavy infection may cause iron-deficiency anemia. **(a)** Electron microscopy of *N. americanus* reveals two pairs of teeth for adhesion to bowel mucosa. **(b)** Hookworm ova typically display segmented larvae within a thin clear shell. Sources: **(a)** Jian et al. Experimental Parasitology 2003; 105 (3–4) 192–200. Reproduced by permission of Elsevier. **(b)** Centers for Disease Control and Prevention (http://www.dpd.cdc.gov/healthypets/diseases/hookworm.htm).

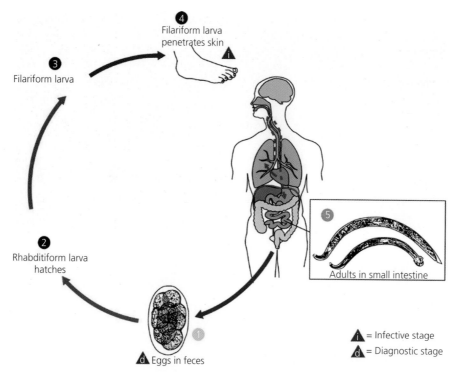

Figure 67.5 Human hookworm life cycle. Eggs are passed in the stool (1), and under favorable conditions (moisture, warmth, shade), larvae hatch in 1 to 2 days. The released rhabditiform larvae grow in the feces and/or the soil (2), and after 5 to 10 days (and two molts) they become filariform (third-stage) larvae that are infective (3). These infective larvae can survive 3 to 4 weeks in favorable environmental conditions. On contact with the human host, the larvae penetrate the skin and are carried through the blood vessels to the heart and then to the lungs. They penetrate into the pulmonary alveoli, ascend the bronchial tree to the pharynx, and are swallowed (4). The larvae reach the small intestine, where they reside and mature into adults. Adult worms live in the lumen of the small intestine, where they attach to the intestinal wall with resultant blood loss by the host (5). Most adult worms are eliminated in 1 to 2 years, but the longevity may reach several years. Some *A. duodenale* larvae, following penetration of the host skin, can become dormant (in the intestine or muscle). In addition, infection by *A. duodenale* may probably also occur by the oral and transmammary route. *N. americanus*, however, requires a transpulmonary migration phase. Source: Centers for Disease Control and Prevention (http://www.dpd.cdc.gov/DpDx).

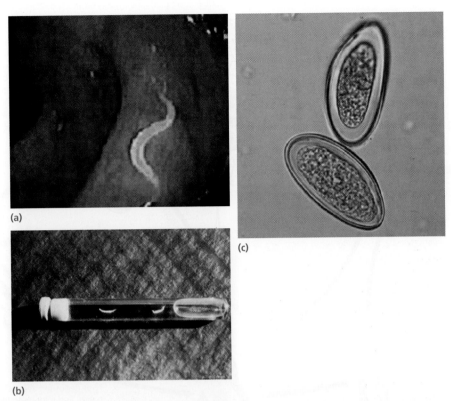

Figure 67.6 (a) An adult pinworm, *Enterobius vermicularis*, alive in the colon as seen through a colonoscope. **(b)** At night, the adult worms emerge and lay ova on the perianal skin. **(c)** The ova, which are found on the perianal skin, are flattened on one side. Sources: **(a)** Courtesy of Richard Goodgame. **(b)** From Zaiman H/ASTMH, "A pictoral presentation of parasites."

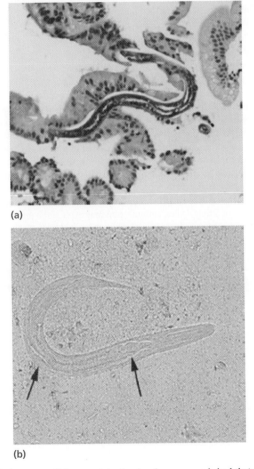

Figure 67.7 (a) The adult females of *Strongyloides stercoralis* burrow into duodenal mucosa and shed their ova, that hatch in the gastrointestinal tract, and **(b)** rhabditiform larvae are later voided into stool.

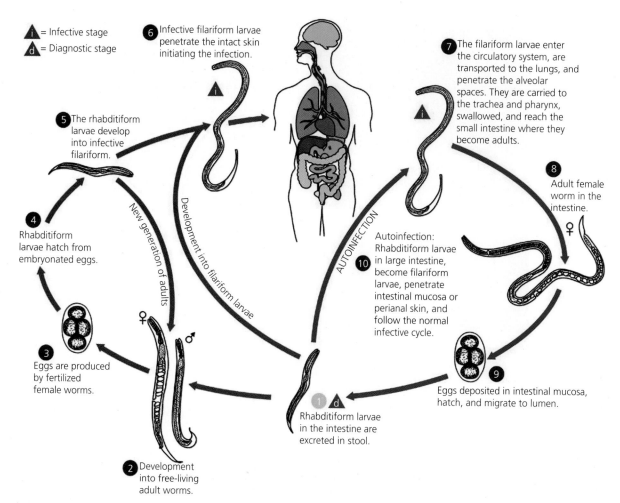

Figure 67.8 *Strongyloides* **Free-living cycle:** The rhabditiform larvae passed in the stool (1) (see "Parasitic cycle" further on) can either molt twice and become infective filariform larvae (direct development), (6) or molt four times and become free living adult males and females (2) that mate and produce eggs (3) from which rhabditiform larvae hatch (4). The latter in turn can either develop (5) into a new generation of free-living adults (as represented in [2]), or into infective filariform larvae (6). The filariform larvae penetrate the human host skin to initiate the parasitic cycle (see further on) (6). **Parasitic cycle:** Filariform larvae in contaminated soil penetrate the human skin (6), and are transported to the lungs where they penetrate the alveolar spaces; they are carried through the bronchial tree to the pharynx, are swallowed and then reach the small intestine (7). In the small intestine they molt twice and become adult female worms (8). The females live threaded in the epithelium of the small intestine and by parthenogenesis produce eggs (9), which yield rhabditiform larvae. The rhabditiform larvae can either be passed in the stool (1) (see "Free-living cycle" previously), or can cause autoinfection (10). In autoinfection, the rhabditiform larvae become infective filariform larvae, which can penetrate either the intestinal mucosa (internal autoinfection) or the skin of the perianal area (external autoinfection); in either case, the filariform larvae may follow the previously described route, being carried successively to the lungs, the bronchial tree, the pharynx, and the small intestine where they mature into adults; or they may disseminate widely in the body. To date, occurrence of autoinfection in humans with helminthic infections is recognized only in *Strongyloides stercoralis* and *Capillaria philippinensis* infections. In the case of *Strongyloides*, autoinfection may explain the possibility of persistent infections for many years in persons who have not been in an endemic area and of hyperinfection in immunosuppressed individuals. Source: Centers for Disease Control and Prevention (http://www.dpd.cdc.gov/DpDx).

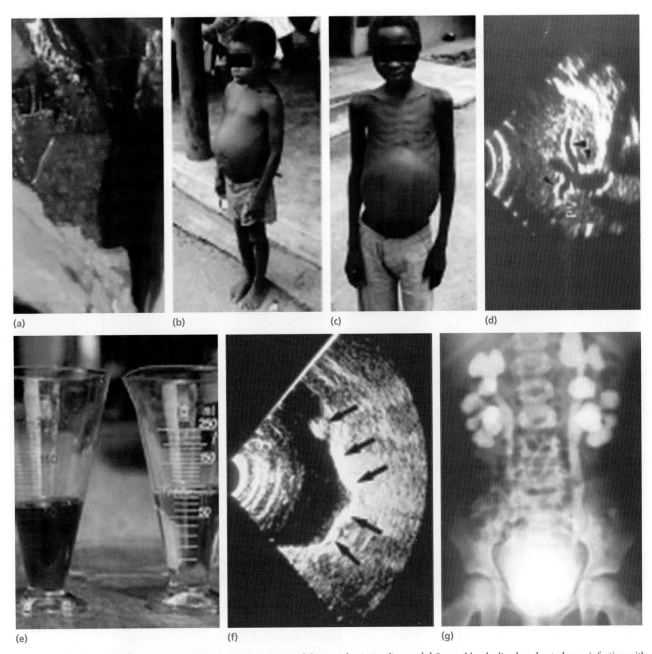

Figure 67.9 The blood flukes of the genus *Schistosoma* cause intestinal, liver, and urinary disease. **(a)** Severe bloody diarrhea due to heavy infection with *S. mansoni*. **(b)** 6-year-old boy with gross reactive hepatosplenomegaly. **(c)** 19-year-old man with symptoms of chronic fibrotic hepatic schistosomiasis: splenomegaly, external varices, ascites and growth retardation. Ultrasonography in chronic hepatic schistosomiasis may reveal **(d)** portal venodilatation secondary to advanced periportal fibrosis. Urinary involvement with *S. haematobium* can lead to **(e)** hematuria. Ultrasound detection of **(f)** bladder polyps, and **(g)** bilateral hydronephrosis complicating urinary schistosomiasis. Source: Gryseels et al. Lancet 2006;368(9541):1106. Reproduced by permission of Elsevier.

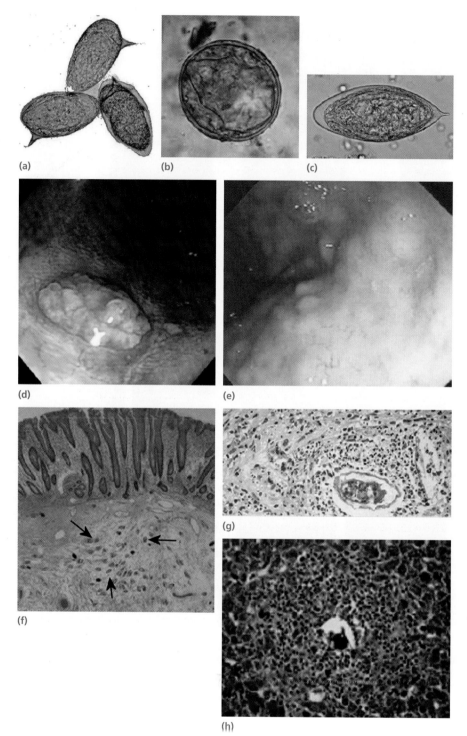

Figure 67.10 (a) Ova of *S. mansoni* have a characteristic lateral spin. (b) Ova of *S. japonicum* are more rounded and have only a vestigial spine. (c) The ova of *S. haematobium* have a solitary polar spine. *Schistosoma* ova incite granulomatous inflammation that may occur in the colon as a (d) single polyp (identified during colonoscopy after indigo carmine application), or (e) intestinal polyposis during colonoscopy. (f) Histologic examination of a colonic polyp revealing a closter of schistosome ova (arrows). (g) *S. mansoni* ovum surrounded by eosinophilic granulomatous inflammation in the colonic mucosa. (h) A schistosome ovum lodged in the liver inducing a granuloma. Sources: (d), (f) Abe et al. Journal of Gastroenterology and Hepatology 2006;21:1216. Reproduced by permission of John Wiley & Sons. (e), (g) Mesquita et al. Gastrointestinal Endoscopy 2003;58:910–911. Reproduced by permission of Elsevier. (h) Gryseels et al. Lancet 2006;368(9541):1106–1118. Reproduced by permission of Elsevier.

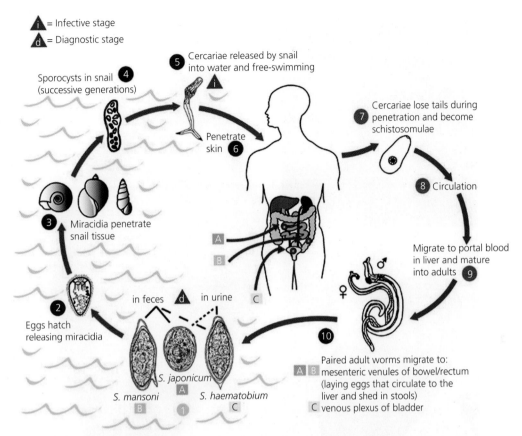

i = Infective stage

d = Diagnostic stage

Sporocysts in snail 4 (successive generations)

Cercariae released by snail 5 into water and free-swimming

3 Miracidia penetrate snail tissue

Penetrate skin 6

Cercariae lose tails during 7 penetration and become schistosomulae

8 Circulation

Migrate to portal blood in liver and mature into adults 9

2 Eggs hatch releasing miracidia

in feces d in urine

S. japonicum

A

S. mansoni

B

S. haematobium

C

1

10

Paired adult worms migrate to:
A B mesenteric venules of bowel/rectum (laying eggs that circulate to the liver and shed in stools)
C venous plexus of bladder

Figure 67.11 Schistosome life cycle. Eggs are eliminated with feces or urine (1). Under optimal conditions the eggs hatch and release miracidia (2), which swim and penetrate specific snail intermediate hosts (3). The stages in the snail include two generations of sporocysts (4), and the production of cercariae (5). Upon release from the snail, the infective cercariae swim, penetrate the skin of the human host (6), and shed their forked tail, becoming schistosomulae (7). The schistosomulae migrate through several tissues and stages to their residence in the veins (8), (9). Adult worms in humans reside in the mesenteric venules in various locations, which at times seem to be specific for each species (10). For instance, *S. japonicum* is more frequently found in the superior mesenteric veins draining the small intestine (A), and *S. mansoni* occurs more often in the superior mesenteric veins draining the large intestine (B). However, both species can occupy either location, and they are capable of moving between sites, so it is not possible to state unequivocally that one species only occurs in one location. *S. haematobium* most often occurs in the venous plexus of bladder (C), but it can also be found in the rectal venules. The females (size 7 mm to 20 mm; males slightly smaller) deposit eggs in the small venules of the portal and perivesical systems. The eggs are moved progressively toward the lumen of the intestine (*S. mansoni* and *S. japonicum*), and of the bladder and ureters (*S. haematobium*), and are eliminated with feces or urine, respectively (1). Pathology of *S. mansoni* and *S. japonicum* schistosomiasis includes: Katayama fever, hepatic perisinusoidal egg granulomas, Symmers' pipe stem periportal fibrosis, portal hypertension, and occasional embolic egg granulomas in brain, or spinal cord. Pathology of *S. haematobium* schistosomiasis includes: hematuria, scarring, calcification, squamous cell carcinoma, and occasional embolic egg granulomas in brain, or spinal cord. Human contact with water is thus necessary for infection by schistosomes. Various animals, such as dogs, cats, rodents, pigs, hourse and goats, serve as reservoirs for *S. japonicum*, and dogs for *S. mekongi*. Source: Centers for Disease Control and Prevention (http://www.dpd.cdc.gov/DpDx).

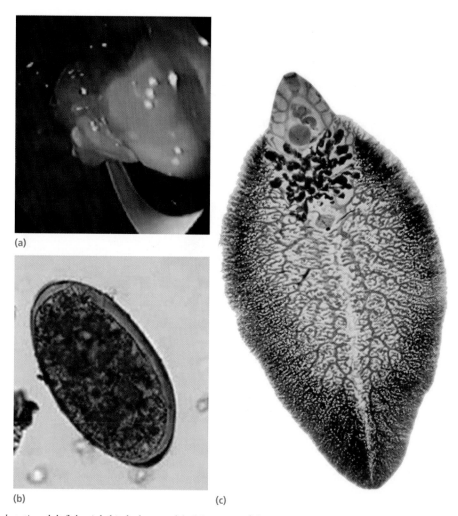

(a)

(b)   (c)

Figure 67.12 *Fasciola hepatica* adult flukes inhabit the lumen of the biliary tract. **(a)** Removal of *F. hepatica* from the common bile duct during endoscopic retrograde cholangio pancreatography (ERCP). **(b)** The ova are stained with bile, oval and have an indistinct operculum at one pole. **(c)** Adult *Fasciola hepatica* isolated from the peritoneal cavity of a patient during surgery. The patient had chronic abdominal pain associated with peripheral eosinophilia. Source: **(c)** Courtesy of Joel V. Weinstock, MD, Tufts Medical Center.

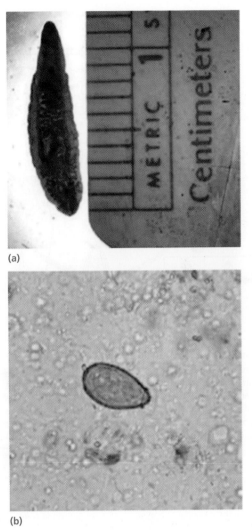

(a)

(b)

Figure 67.13 Liver flukes, *Clonorchis sienensis* and *Opisthorchis* species.
(a) Adult *C. sienensis* are flat trematodes and release (b) ova, oval-shaped
with a single polar operculum, into the bile duct.

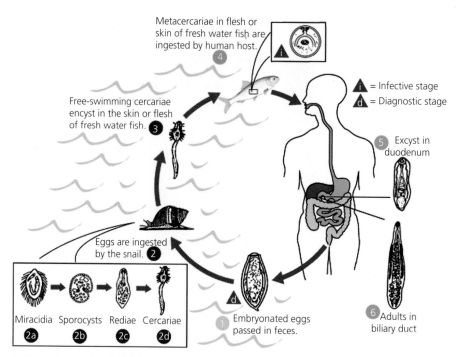

Figure 67.14 Life cycle of *Clonorchis sinensis* and *Opisthorchis* species. Embryonated eggs are discharged in the biliary ducts, and in the stool (1). Eggs are ingested by a suitable snail intermediate host (2). Each egg releases a miracidia (2a), which go through several developmental stages: sporocysts (2b), rediae (2c), and cercariae (2d). The cercariae are released from the snail and after a short period of free-swimming time in water, they come in contact and penetrate the flesh of freshwater fish, where they encyst as metacercariae (3). Infection of humans occurs by ingestion of undercooked, salted, pickled, or smoked freshwater fish (4). After ingestion, the metacercariae excyst in the duodenum (5), and ascend the biliary tract through the ampulla of Vater (6). Maturation takes approximately 1 month. The adult flukes (measuring 10 mm to 25 mm × 3 mm to 5 mm) reside in small and medium sized biliary ducts. In addition to humans, carnivorous animals can serve as reservoir hosts. Source: Centers for Disease Control and Prevention (http://www.dpd.cdc.gov/DpDx).

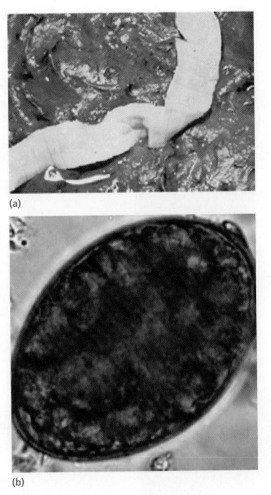

(a)

(b)

Figure 67.15 *Diphyllobothrium latum.* **(a)** The proglottids are broad and off-white in color readily visible in freshly passed stool. **(b)** The ova have an indistinct monopolar operculum and characteristic "knob" on the opposite pole.

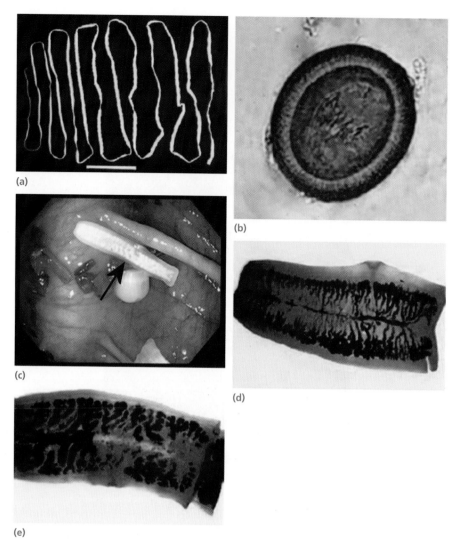

Figure 67.16 *Taenia saginata* and *Taenia solium* are the major human tapeworms acquired from beef and pork. **(a)** The adult worms form ribbon-like chains of proglottids that can reach lengths of up to 30 feet. **(b)** The ova for these two species have identical morphology. **(c)** *T. saginata* proglottids are motile and can be incidental findings during colonoscopy. **(d)** *T. saginata*, with 12–30 main lateral uterine branches compared with **(e)** *T. solium* has 8–13 branches. Source: **(c)** Courtesy of Dr. Moises Guelrud and Dr. Suraj Gupta, Division of Gastroenterology, Tufts Medical Center.

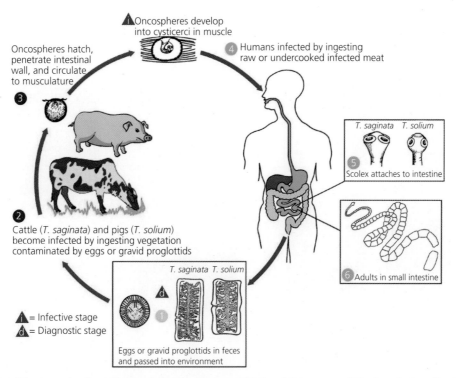

Figure 67.17 Life cycle of *Taenia* species. Taeniasis is the infection of humans with the adult tapeworm of *Taenia saginata* or *Taenia solium*. Humans are the only definitive hosts for *T. saginata* and *T. solium*. Eggs or gravid proglottids are passed with feces (1); the eggs can survive for days to months in the environment. Cattle (*T. saginata*), and pigs (*T. solium*) become infected by ingesting vegetation contaminated with eggs, or gravid proglottids (2). In the animal's intestine, the oncospheres hatch (3), invade the intestinal wall, and migrate to the striated muscles, where they develop into cysticerci. A cysticercus can survive for several years in the animal. Humans become infected by ingesting raw or undercooked infected meat (4). In the human intestine, the cysticercus develops over 2 months into an adult tapeworm, which can survive for years. The adult tapeworms attach to the small intestine by their scolex (5) and reside in the small intestine (6). Length of adult worms is usually 5 meters (m) or less for *T. saginata* (however it may reach up to 25 m), and 2 m to 7 m for *T. solium*. The adults produce proglottids which mature, become gravid, detach from the tapeworm, and migrate to the anus, or are passed in the stool (approximately 6 per day). *T. saginata* adults usually have 1000 to 2000 proglottids, while *T. solium* adults have an average of 1000 proglottids. The eggs contained in the gravid proglottids are released after the proglottids are passed with the feces. *T. saginata* may produce up to 100 000 and *T. solium* may produce 50 000 eggs per proglottid respectively. Source: Centers for Disease Control and Prevention (http://www.dpd.cdc.gov/dpdx/HTML/Taeniasis.htm).

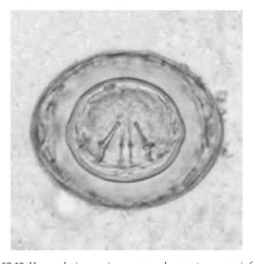

Figure 67.18 *Hymenolepis nana* is a common human tapeworm infection, but is usually asymptomatic. Ova are surrounded by a striated outer membrane separated by a clear space from the internal membrane containing the larvae, which have six hooks.

Type of cyst

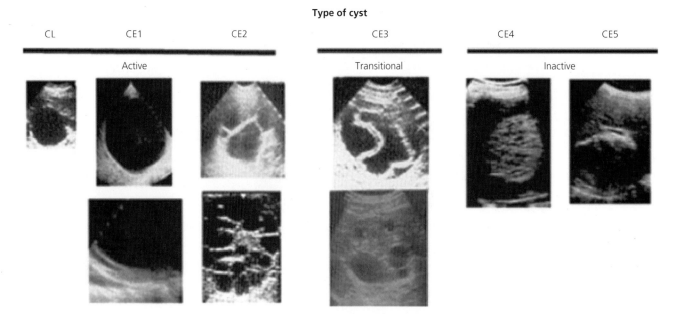

Figure 67.19 *Echinococcus granulosus* and related organisms cause cystic hydatid disease. Ultrasound staging of hydatid cysts. Source: WHO Informal Working Group on Echinococcosis 2003. Reproduced by permission of Elsevier.

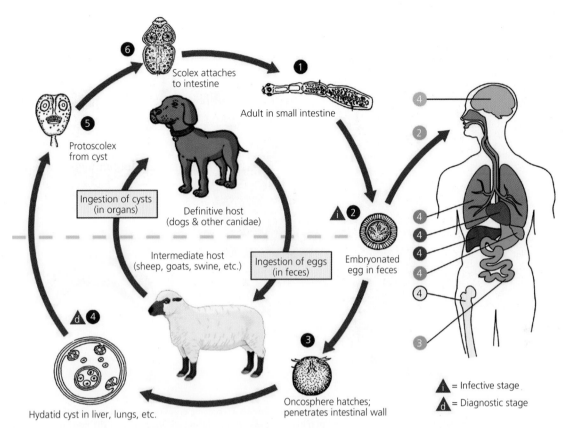

Figure 67.20 Life cycle of *Echinococcus granulosus*. The adult *Echinococcus granulosus* (3 mm to 6 mm long) (1), resides in the small bowel of the definitive hosts, dogs or other canids. Gravid proglottids release eggs (2) that are passed in the feces. After ingestion by a suitable intermediate host (under natural conditions: sheep, goat, swine, cattle, horses, camel), the egg hatches in the small bowel and releases an oncosphere (3) that penetrates the intestinal wall and migrates through the circulatory system into various organs, especially the liver and lungs. In these organs, the oncosphere develops into a cyst (4) that enlarges gradually, producing protoscolices, and daughter cysts that fill the cyst interior. The definitive host becomes infected by ingesting the cyst-containing organs of the infected intermediate host. After ingestion, the protoscolices (5) evaginate, attach to the intestinal mucosa (6), and develop into adult stages (1) in 32 to 80 days. The same life cycle occurs with *E. multilocularis* (1.2 mm to 3.7 mm), with the following differences: the definitive hosts are foxes, and to a lesser extent dogs, cats, coyotes, and wolves; the intermediate host are small rodents; and larval growth (in the liver) remains indefinitely in the proliferative stage, resulting in invasion of the surrounding tissues. With *E. vogeli* (up to 5.6 mm long), the definitive hosts are bush dogs and dogs; the intermediate hosts are rodents; and the larval stage (in the liver, lungs and other organs) develops both externally and internally, resulting in multiple vesicles. *E. oligarthrus* (up to 2.9 mm long) has a life cycle that involves wild felids as definitive hosts and rodents as intermediate hosts. Humans become infected by ingesting eggs (2), with resulting release of oncospheres (3) in the intestine and the development of cysts (all the 4's) in various organs. Source: Centers for Disease Control and Prevention (http://www.dpd.cdc.gov/DpDx).

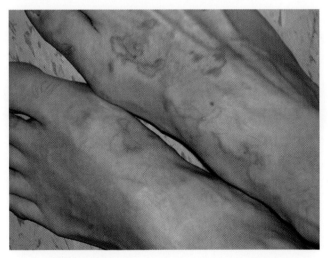

Figure 67.21 Photograph of cutaneous larvae migrans caused by *Toxocara* species. Source: Lemery J. Annals of Emergency Medicine. 2008 Jul;52(1):82. Reproduced by permission of Elsevier.

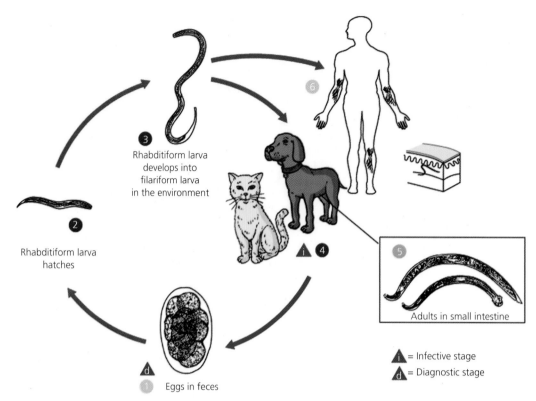

3
Rhabditiform larva
develops into
filariform larva
in the environment

2
Rhabditiform larva
hatches

Adults in small intestine

= Infective stage

= Diagnostic stage

Eggs in feces

Figure 67.22 Dog and cat hookworm life cycle. Cutaneous larval migrans (also known as creeping eruption) is a zoonotic infection with hookworm species that do not use humans as a definitive host, the most common being *Ascaris* braziliense and *Ascaris caninum*. The normal definitive hosts for these species are dogs and cats. The cycle in the definitive host is very similar to the cycle for the human species. Eggs are passed in the stool (1), and under favorable conditions (moisture, warmth, shade), larvae hatch in 1 to 2 days. The released rhabditiform larvae grow in the feces and/or the soil (2), and after 5 to 10 days (and two molts) they become filariform (third-stage) larvae that are infective (3). These infective larvae can survive 3 to 4 weeks in favorable environmental conditions. On contact with the animal host (4), the larvae penetrate the skin and are carried through the blood vessels to the heart and then to the lungs. They penetrate into the pulmonary alveoli, ascend the bronchial tree to the pharynx, and are swallowed. The larvae reach the small intestine, where they reside and mature into adults. Adult worms live in the lumen of the small intestine, where they attach to the intestinal wall. Some larvae become arrested in the tissues, and serve as source of infection for pups via transmammary (and possibly transplacental) routes (5). Humans may also become infected when filariform larvae penetrate the skin (6). With most species, the larvae cannot mature further in the human host, and migrate aimlessly within the epidermis, sometimes as much as several centimeters a day. Some larvae may persist in deeper tissue after finishing their skin migration. Source: Centers for Disease Control and Prevention (http://www.dpd.cdc.gov/DpDx).

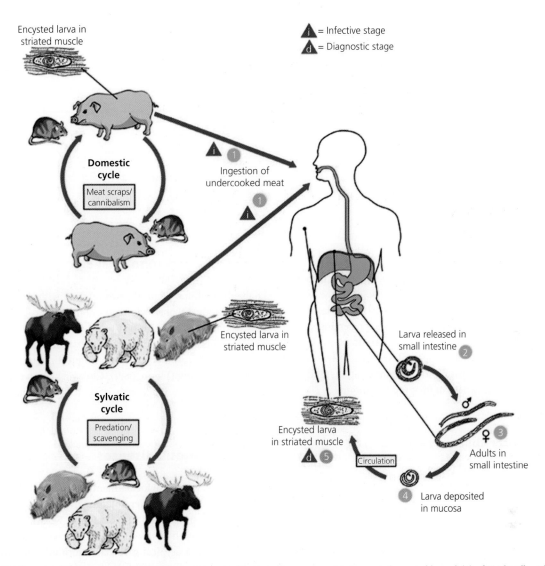

Figure 67.23 Life cycle of *Trichinella spiralis*. Trichinosis is acquired by ingesting meat containing cysts (encysted larvae) (1) of *Trichinella*. After exposure to gastric acid and pepsin, the larvae are released (2) from the cysts and invade the small bowel mucosa where they develop into adult worms (3) (female 2.2 mm in length, males 1.2 mm; life span in the small bowel: 4 weeks). After 1 week, the females release larvae (4) that migrate to the striated muscles where they encyst (5). *Trichinella pseudospiralis*, however, does not encyst. Encystment is completed in 4 to 5 weeks and the encysted larvae may remain viable for several years. Ingestion of the encysted larvae perpetuates the cycle. Rats and rodents are primarily responsible for maintaining the endemicity of this infection. Carnivorous/omnivorous animals, such as pigs or bears, feed on infected rodents or meat from other animals. Different animal hosts are implicated in the life cycle of the different species of *Trichinella*. Humans are accidentally infected when eating improperly processed meat of these carnivorous animals (or eating food contaminated with such meat). Source: Centers for Disease Control and Prevention (http://www.dpd.cdc.gov//parasites/trichinosis/biology.html).

CHAPTER 68

Gastrointestinal manifestations of systemic diseases

Eran Israeli[1] and Charles N. Bernstein[2]

[1] Hadassah–Hebrew University Medical Center, Jerusalem, Israel
[2] University of Manitoba, Winnipeg, Canada

Many systemic diseases are commonly manifest by gastrointestinal signs or symptoms. The liver or gut may be the principal targets of the disease process or indirectly affected by the disease or by a side-effect of treatment for the disease. In some instances, the gastrointestinal manifestation may be the presenting sign of the disease and a cause for seeking medical attention. In this chapter we present selected images of systemic diseases that have well-recognized gastrointestinal manifestations and that can be identified by a variety of imaging techniques.

Cardiovascular diseases

Aortic stenosis has been associated with an increased risk of gastrointestinal bleeding secondary to vascular ectasia of the gut (Figure 68.1). Severe abdominal pain can be a presentation of cocaine toxicity due to dissection of the celiac axis (Figure 68.2).

Genetic disease

Adults with type 1 Gaucher disease present with hepatosplenomegaly and pathological bone fractures (Figure 68.3).

Connective tissue diseases

Connective tissue diseases commonly affect the gastrointestinal tract directly, as in the case of scleroderma (Figure 68.4), or as a side-effect of immunosuppressive treatment, for example esophageal candidiasis in a patient treated with corticosteroids (Figure 68.5).

Endocrine and renal diseases

Diabetes mellitus commonly presents with gastrointestinal complications secondary to autonomic neuropathy such as gastric dilatation (Figure 68.6) and colonic dilatation (Figure 68.7) or atherosclerosis of mesenteric vasculature (Figure 68.8). Endometriosis can involve the gastrointestinal tract due to anatomical proximity (Figure 68.9). Chronic kidney disease is also associated with vascular ectasia of the gastrointestinal tract (Figures 68.10 and 68.11).

Granulomatous diseases

Granulomas, which are focal inflammatory processes composed of macrophages and other inflammatory cell types, form in the gastrointestinal tract in association with many noninfectious diseases, such as sarcoidosis (Figure 68.12), and infectious diseases, such as atypical mycobacterium infection in an HIV-positive patient (Figure 68.13).

Hematological diseases

Gastrointestinal bleeding can occur in patients with an inherited or acquired deficiency in coagulation factors. Figure 68.14 depicts an uncommon complication of warfarin ingestion presenting with an intramural hematoma of the esophagus. Eosinophilic infiltration and thickening of the gastrointestinal tract wall, as well as infiltration of other organs, can be seen in hypereosinophilic syndrome (Figure 68.15). Hypercoagulability is an important cause of gastrointestinal morbidity. Spontaneous thrombosis of the mesenteric veins can cause intestinal ischemia and infarction (Figure 68.16).

Yamada's Atlas of Gastroenterology, Fifth Edition. Edited by Daniel K. Podolsky, Michael Camilleri, J. Gregory Fitz, Anthony N. Kalloo, Fergus Shanahan, and Timothy C. Wang.
© 2016 John Wiley & Sons, Ltd. Published 2016 by John Wiley & Sons, Ltd.
Companion website: www.yamadagastro.com/atlas

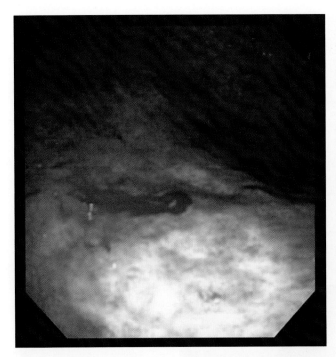

Figure 68.1 Actively bleeding gastric vascular ectasia in a patient with aortic stenosis.

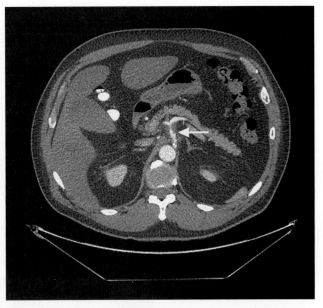

Figure 68.2 Computed tomography angiogram showing irregular narrowing of the true lumen of the celiac axis (arrow) secondary to a cocaine-induced dissection. Source: Courtesy of Iain Kirkpatrick, MD, Department of Radiology, University of Manitoba.

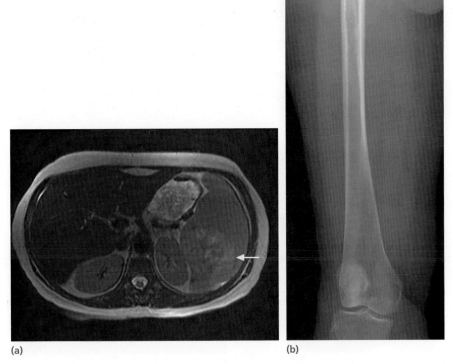

(a)   (b)

Figure 68.3 A patient with Gaucher disease developed left upper quadrant pain, and a computed tomograph **(a)** showed a heterogeneous mass in the enlarged spleen (arrow), which on splenectomy was found to be lymphoma. A radiograph of the femur in the same patient shows the characteristic "Erlenmeyer flask deformity" **(b)**, in which the diaphysis is narrow and the metaphysis is flared outwards. Source: Courtesy of Iain Kirkpatrick, MD, Department of Radiology, University of Manitoba.

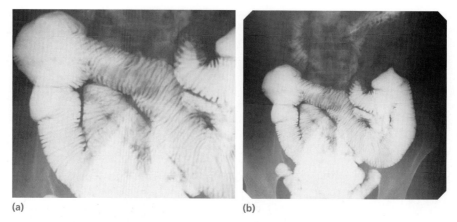

Figure 68.4 (a, b) Scleroderma affecting the small bowel manifest as a "hidebound appearance" seen on small bowel barium enteroclysis. Source: Courtesy of Jacob Sosna, MD, Department of Radiology, Hadassah–Hebrew University Medical Center.

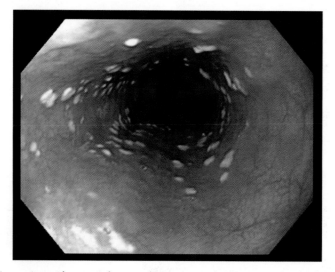

Figure 68.5 Esophageal candidiasis in a patient with systemic lupus erythematosus on chronic corticosteroids.

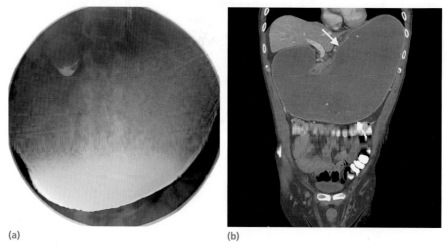

Figure 68.6 Spot image from an upper gastrointestinal barium study **(a)** and a coronal computed tomography image **(b)** in a patient with gross gastric dilatation (arrows) and fluid retention secondary to diabetic neuropathy. Source: Courtesy of Iain Kirkpatrick, MD, Department of Radiology, University of Manitoba.

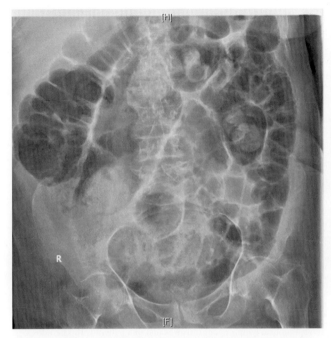

Figure 68.7 Colonic dilation from autonomic neuropathy secondary to diabetes. Source: Courtesy of Yaacov Bar-Ziv, MD, Department of Radiology, Hadassah–Hebrew University Medical Center.

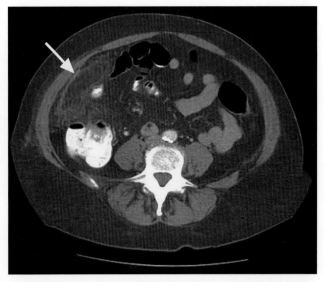

Figure 68.8 Transverse computed tomography image of a diabetic patient with omental inflammation related to spontaneous omental infarction (arrow). Source: Courtesy of Iain Kirkpatrick, MD, Department of Radiology, University of Manitoba.

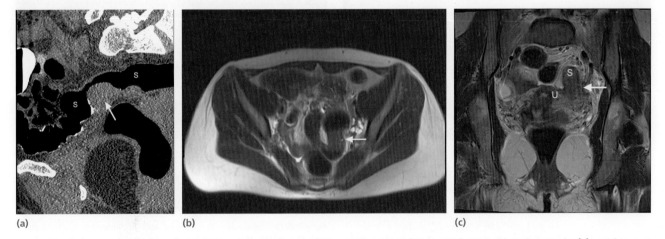

(a) (b) (c)

Figure 68.9 Endometriosis involving the gastrointestinal tract. A curved planar reformation of a computed tomography colonography **(a)** stretching out the lumen of the sigmoid colon (S) shows luminal narrowing related to an eccentric extrinsic mass (arrow). Transverse **(b)** and coronal **(c)** T2-weighted magnetic resonance images show the mass stuck down to the left of the uterus (U), involving the adnexa and broad ligament (arrow). Laparoscopy showed fibrotic endometriosis. Source: Courtesy of Iain Kirkpatrick, MD, Department of Radiology, University of Manitoba.

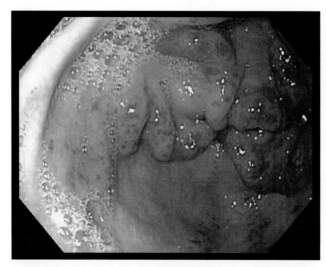

Figure 68.10 Gastric antral vascular ectasia (GAVE) in a patient with chronic kidney disease secondary to diabetes.

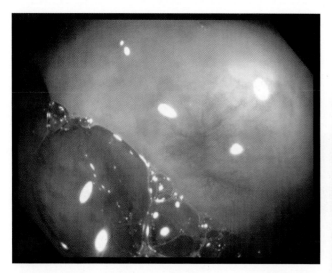

Figure 68.11 Cecal vascular ectasia in a patient with chronic kidney disease secondary to diabetes that leads to obscure gastrointestinal bleeding.

Vasculitis

Figure 68.17 shows considerable narrowing of the lumen of the abdominal aorta in a patient with chronic Takayasu arteritis.

Cancer

Intestinal metastasis from tumors originating in locations outside the gastrointestinal system can produce significant symptoms (Figures 68.18 and 68.19). Non-Hodgkin lymphoma can originate primarily in the gastrointestinal tract, for example gastric lymphoma (Figure 68.20). As many as 10% of patients with non-Hodgkin lymphoma originating from a nongastrointestinal site develop secondary involvement of the gastrointestinal

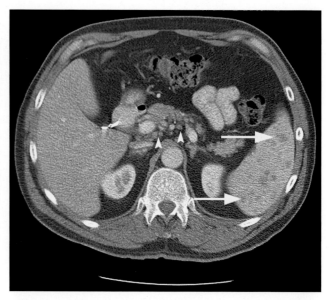

Figure 68.12 Transverse computed tomography image shows multiple hypodense splenic granulomas (arrows) and numerous small but excessive retroperitoneal lymph nodes (arrowheads) in a patient with sarcoidosis. Source: Courtesy of Iain Kirkpatrick, MD, Department of Radiology, University of Manitoba.

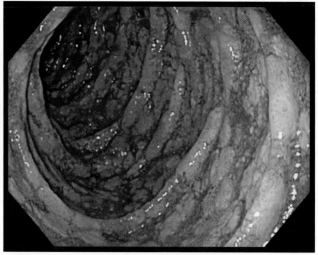

Figure 68.13 *Mycobacterium avium intracellulare* infection in a patients with HIV/AIDS. This is an endoscopic photo of the duodenum with raised yellow plaques.

tract (Figure 68.21). Neutropenic enterocolitis is a well-known complication following chemotherapy-induced neutropenia, most often in patients with leukemia (Figures 68.22 and 68.23). Neutropenia can also be complicated with hepatosplenic candidiasis (Figure 68.24). Other gastrointestinal complications of cancer treatment include graft-versus-host disease following stem cell transplantation (Figure 68.25), *Clostridium difficile* pseudomembranous colitis induced by broad-spectrum antibiotic therapy (Figure 68.26), and postirradiation proctitis (Figure 68.27).

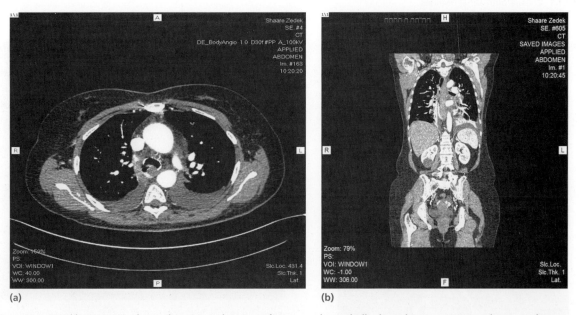

Figure 68.14 Intramural hematoma in the esophagus secondary to warfarin use and a markedly elevated INR on a computed tomography scan axial image **(a)** and on coronal image **(b)**. Source: Courtesy of Yaacov Bar-Ziv, MD, Department of Radiology, Hadassah–Hebrew University Medical Center.

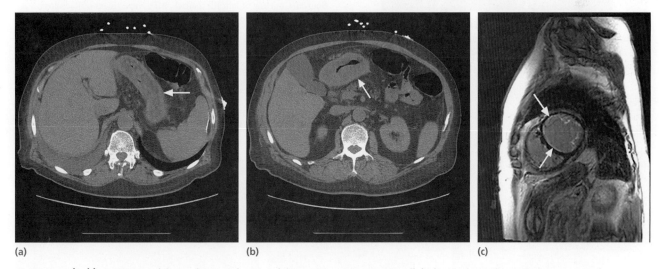

Figure 68.15 (a, b) Hypereosinophilic syndrome with eosinophilic gastritis causing gastric wall thickening (arrows) on transverse computed tomography images. **(c)** The same patient shows diffuse circumferential subendocardial delayed enhancement (arrows) on an inversion recovery-prepared T1-weighted gradient echo image of the heart, consistent with eosinophilic myocarditis. Source: Courtesy of Iain Kirkpatrick, MD, Department of Radiology, University of Manitoba.

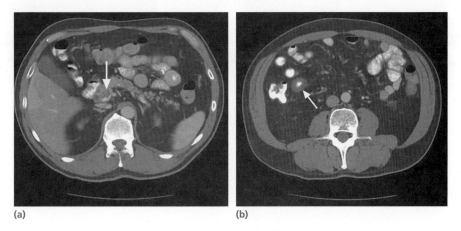

Figure 68.16 (a) Superior mesenteric venous thrombus (arrow) resulting in considerable small bowel wall thickening from congestion and **(b)** venous ischemia (arrow) in a patient with protein C deficiency as seen in transverse computed tomography images. Source: Courtesy of Iain Kirkpatrick, MD, Department of Radiology, University of Manitoba.

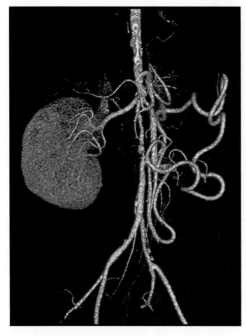

Figure 68.17 Chronic Takayasu arteritis has resulted in a considerable narrowing of the lumen of the abdominal aorta as recorded by a three-dimensional volume-rendered computed tomography angiogram. Source: Courtesy of Iain Kirkpatrick, MD, Department of Radiology, University of Manitoba.

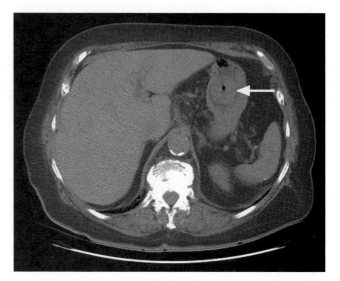

Figure 68.18 Transverse computed tomography image in a patient with longstanding human immunodeficiency virus and Kaposi sarcoma shows an ulcerated metastasis end-on in the gastric wall (arrow). Source: Courtesy of Iain Kirkpatrick, MD, Department of Radiology, University of Manitoba.

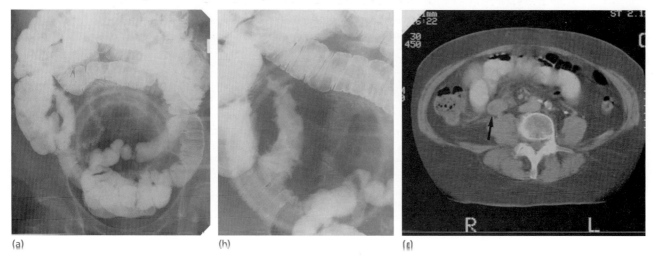

(a) (b) (c)

Figure 68.19 This patient has breast cancer metastasis to the ileum **(a, b)** as seen on small bowel barium enteroclysis. A computed tomography scan axial image **(c)** demonstrates neocecum (arrow) and adjacent nodes with necrosis. Source: Courtesy of Jacob Sosna, MD, Department of Radiology, Hadassah–Hebrew University Medical Center

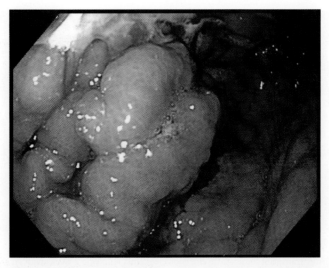

Figure 68.20 Gastric non-Hodgkin lymphoma manifest as prominent folds in the proximal stomach and bleeding from an ulcerated lesion more distally in the stomach.

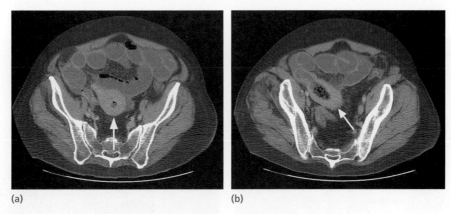

(a)   (b)

Figure 68.21 (a, b) Transverse computed tomography images of segmental small bowel wall thickening (arrows) secondary to non-Hodgkin lymphoma. Source: Courtesy of Iain Kirkpatrick, MD, Department of Radiology, University of Manitoba.

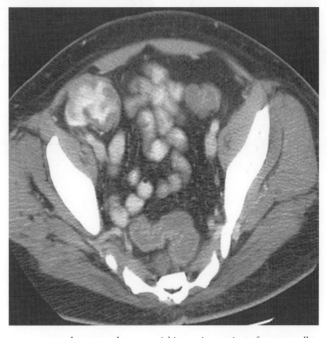

Figure 68.22 Neutropenic cecitis as seen on computed tomography scan axial image in a patient after stem cell transplant for non-Hodgkin lymphoma. Source: Courtesy of Jacob Sosna, MD, Department of Radiology, Hadassah–Hebrew University Medical Center.

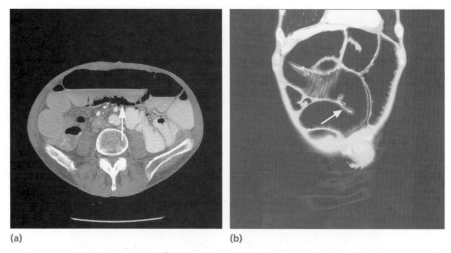

(a)   (b)

Figure 68.23 A patient after bone marrow transplant for acute myelogenous leukemia following 2 weeks with an absolute neutrophil count of 0. Transverse soft tissue window **(a)** and coronal lung window **(b)** images show extensive pneumatosis (arrows). Widespread neutropenic enterocolitis was found at autopsy. Source: Courtesy of Iain Kirkpatrick, MD, Department of Radiology, University of Manitoba.

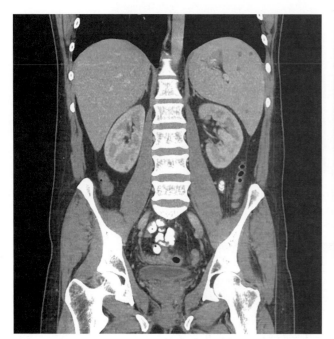

Figure 68.24 Splenic candidiasis seen as multiple hypodense splenic lesions on computed tomography in a patient who developed febrile neutropenia and candidemia. Source: Courtesy of Iain Kirkpatrick, MD, Department of Radiology, University of Manitoba.

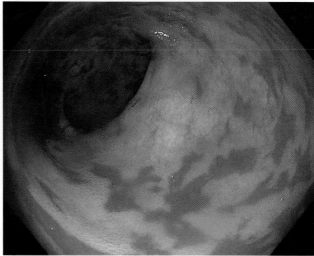

Figure 68.25 Chronic colonic graft-versus-host disease seen at colonoscopy in a patient after stem cell transplant for acute myelogenous leukemia.

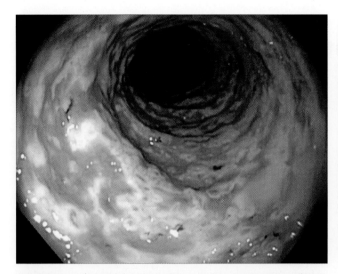

Figure 68.26 Pseudomembranous colitis secondary to *Clostridium difficile* infection visualized by colonoscopy in a patient being treated with chemotherapy for acute lymphoblastic leukemia who received broad-spectrum antibiotics.

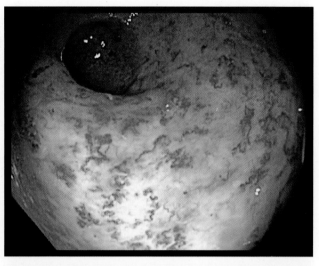

Figure 68.27 Radiation proctitis seen at lower endoscopy in a patient who received external beam radiotherapy for treatment of prostate cancer.

CHAPTER 69

Skin lesions associated with gastrointestinal and liver diseases

Kim B. Yancey and Travis W. Vandergriff
University of Texas Southwestern Medical Center, Dallas, TX, USA

Many diseases of the gastrointestinal tract have characteristic dermatological manifestations. Such manifestations may develop before, concomitantly with, or after the onset of gastrointestinal diseases. Recognition of the cutaneous manifestations of gastrointestinal diseases may be of significance for purposes of diagnosis and management. In addition, primary skin diseases may affect the gastrointestinal tract, display characteristic alterations, and/or produce specific complications.

In this chapter, the cutaneous manifestations of diseases with the following overall characteristics are illustrated:

- Inherited disorders with an increased risk of gastrointestinal malignancy (Figures 69.1, 69.2, 69.3, 69.4, 69.5, and 69.6)
- Genodermatoses (i.e., inherited skin disorders) with characteristic gastrointestinal manifestations (Figures 69.7–69.15)
- Paraneoplastic and related syndromes with gastrointestinal and cutaneous manifestations (Figures 69.16, 69.17, 69.18, 69.19, 69.20, and 69.21).

- The cutaneous manifestations of inflammatory bowel disease (Figures 69.22–69.35)
- Immunologically mediated diseases with gastrointestinal manifestations (Figures 69.36–69.56)
- The cutaneous manifestations of liver disease (Figures 69.57–69.77)
- The mucocutaneous manifestations of nutritional deficiencies (Figures 69.78, 69.79, and 69.80)
- Cutaneous alterations arising during treatment of hepatitis C virus infection (Figure 69.81)
- Miscellaneous disorders associated with cutaneous and gastrointestinal manifestations (Figures 69.82, 69.83, 69.84, and 69.85).

Yamada's Atlas of Gastroenterology, Fifth Edition. Edited by Daniel K. Podolsky, Michael Camilleri, J. Gregory Fitz, Anthony N. Kalloo, Fergus Shanahan, and Timothy C. Wang.
© 2016 John Wiley & Sons, Ltd. Published 2016 by John Wiley & Sons, Ltd.
Companion website: www.yamadagastro.com/atlas

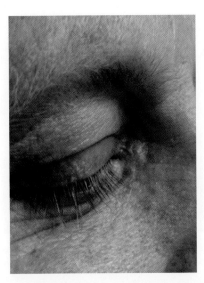

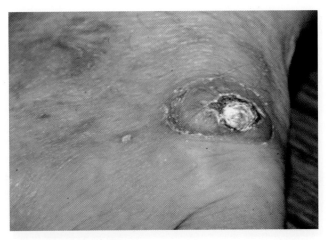

Figure 69.3 Keratoacanthoma.

Figure 69.1 Sebaceous carcinoma. Sebaceous carcinoma is commonly located on or near the eyelids; it is seen in patients with Muir–Torre syndrome. Source: Courtesy of Joseph Nezgoda, MD, MBA and Atif Collins, MD.

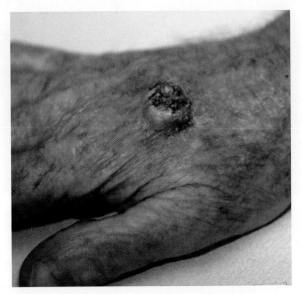

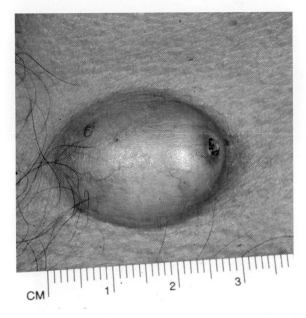

Figure 69.2 Keratoacanthoma. In Muir–Torre syndrome, sebaceous tumors and keratoacanthomas occur in association with internal malignancies (e.g., colonic adenocarcinomas, neoplasms of the genitourinary tract).

Figure 69.4 Epidermal inclusion cyst. In Gardner syndrome, epidermal inclusion cysts, pilomatricomas, lipomas, fibromas, and desmoid tumors are seen in association with colonic adenocarcinomas.

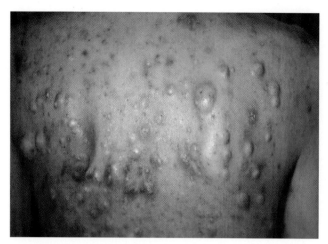

Figure 69.5 Multiple epidermal inclusion cysts.

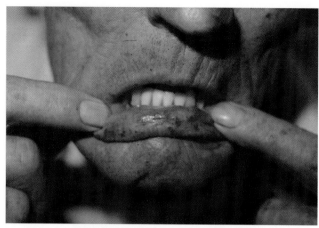

Figure 69.8 Hereditary hemorrhagic telangiectasia is characterized by diffuse mucocutaneous telangiectases and visceral arteriovenous malformations.

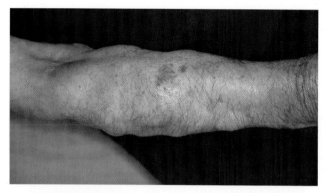

Figure 69.6 Lipomas.

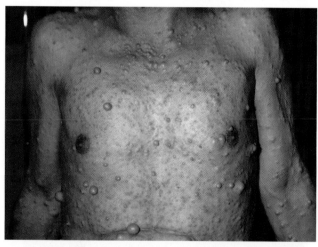

Figure 69.9 Neurofibromatosis type 1 (NF1, von Recklinghausen disease). Cutaneous manifestations of NF1 include café-au-lait macules, axillary or inguinal freckling, and neurofibromas.

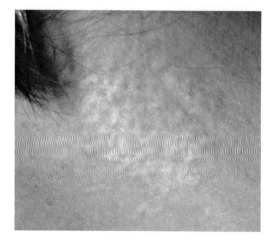

Figure 69.7 Pseudoxanthoma elasticum (PXE). PXE is an inherited connective tissue disease characterized by abnormalities in elastin fibers. Skin lesions dominate in flexural areas and display a cobblestone appearance. Vascular involvement commonly results in hemorrhage (e.g., gastric hemorrhage).

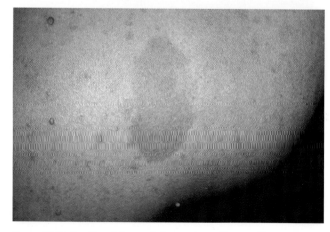

Figure 69.10 A café-au-lait macule in a patient with neurofibromatosis type 1.

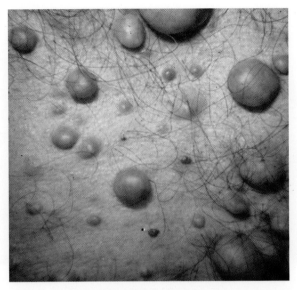

Figure 69.11 Dermal neurofibromas in a patient with neurofibromatosis type 1.

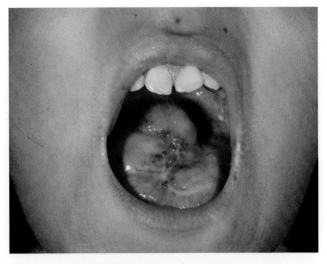

Figure 69.13 Blue rubber bleb nevus syndrome.

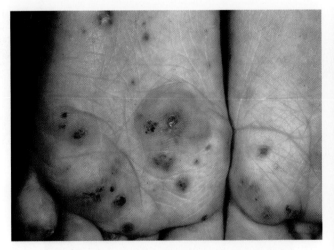

Figure 69.12 Blue rubber bleb nevus syndrome is a systemic disease characterized by cutaneous and gastrointestinal venous malformations; its most significant gastrointestinal complication is hemorrhage.

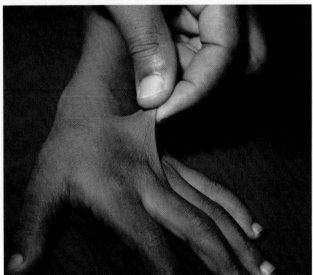

Figure 69.14 Ehlers–Danlos syndrome (EDS). Patients with most subtypes of EDS display skin hyperextensibility and joint hypermobility.

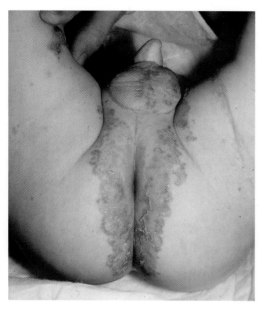

Figure 69.15 Acrodermatitis enteropathica, a rare disorder of zinc uptake and metabolism, typically features pink, scaly, psoriasiform plaques in an acral and/or periorificial distribution.

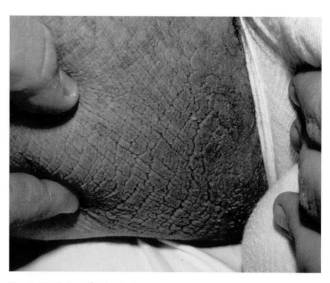

Figure 69.17 Acanthosis nigricans.

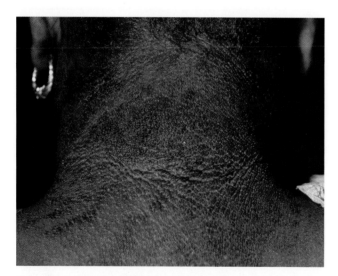

Figure 69.16 Acanthosis nigricans (AN) is characterized by hyperpigmented velvety lesions that typically affect skin on the neck, axillae, groin, or other sites. In rare instances, AN signifies a paraneoplastic phenomenon.

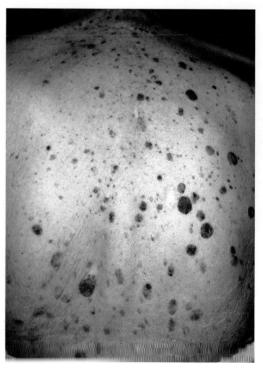

Figure 69.18 Seborrheic keratoses (SKs) are benign skin neoplasms that are quite common and usually multiple. The sign of Leser–Trelat, a rare cutaneous manifestation of internal malignancy (e.g., gastric adenocarcinomas, colon adenocarcinomas, breast carcinoma, lymphoma), represents an abrupt and striking increase in the number and/or size of SKs.

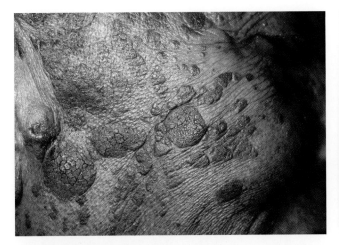

Figure 69.19 Seborrheic keratoses.

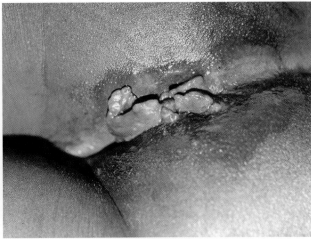

Figure 69.22 Alterations of the perianal mucosa signify a manifestation of cutaneous Crohn's disease.

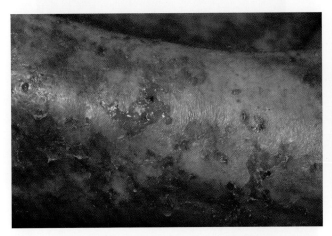

Figure 69.20 Necrolytic migratory erythema, an erosive, painful, pruritic, and typically periorificial eruption that develops in patients with elevated glucagon levels (e.g., patients with pancreatic islet cell tumors or pseudoglucagonoma syndrome).

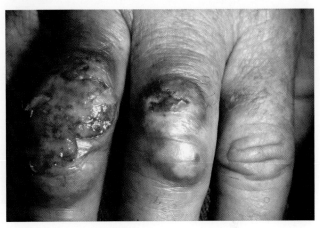

Figure 69.23 Pyoderma gangrenosum.

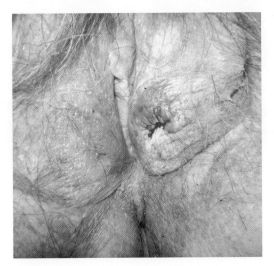

Figure 69.21 Extramammary Paget disease, a rare cutaneous adenocarcinoma that may be unifocal or associated with an underlying adnexal, genitourinary, or gastrointestinal neoplasm.

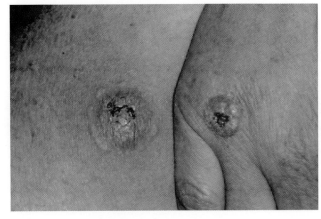

Figure 69.24 Early lesions of pyoderma gangrenosum.

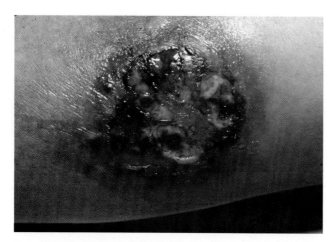

Figure 69.25 Pyoderma gangrenosum.

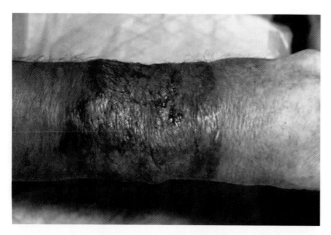

Figure 69.26 A partially healed lesion of pyoderma gangrenosum.

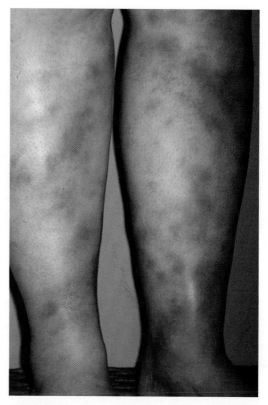

Figure 69.27 Erythema nodosum. Source: Courtesy of William D. James, MD.

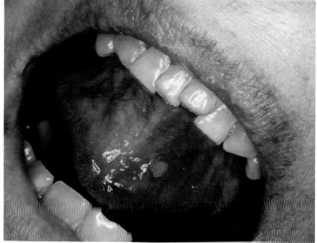

Figure 69.28 A small, round, white ulcer surrounded by a rim of erythema displays morphological features characteristic of an aphthae.

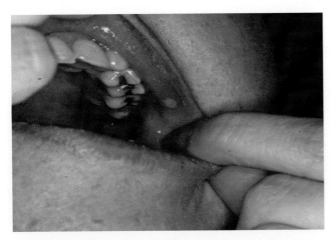

Figure 69.29 An aphthous ulcer on the upper lip.

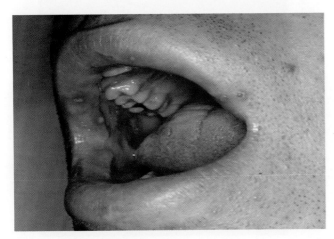

Figure 69.30 Multiple aphthous ulcers.

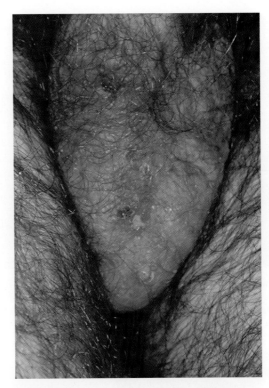

Figure 69.31 Scrotal ulcers in a patient with Behçet disease.

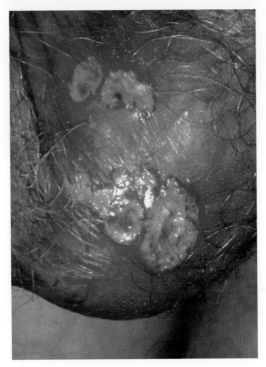

Figure 69.32 Scrotal ulcers in a patient with Behçet disease.

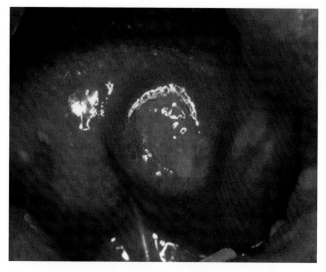

Figure 69.33 Sutton disease (periadenitis mucosa necrotica recurrens) is characterized by "major aphthae", deep, painful ulcerative lesions that are greater than 10 mm in diameter. Source: Courtesy of Jacqueline Plemons, DDS, MS.

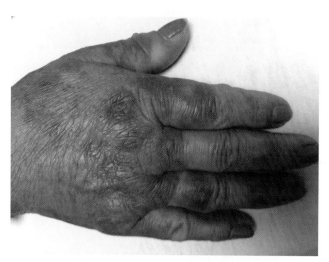

Figure 69.34 Sweet syndrome (acute febrile neutrophilic dermatosis) is characterized by the abrupt onset of red, edematous papulonodules, fever, and neutrophilia.

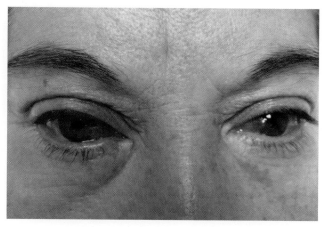

Figure 69.35 Conjunctivitis in a patient with Sweet syndrome.

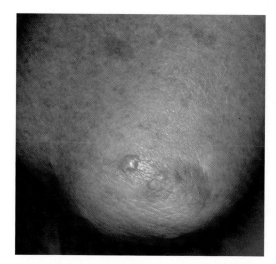

Figure 69.36 Dermatitis herpetiformis.

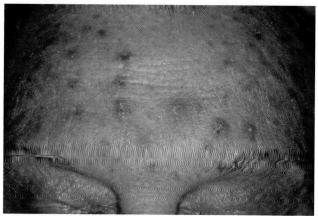

Figure 69.37 Inflammatory papulovesicles on the forehead of a patient with dermatitis herpetiformis.

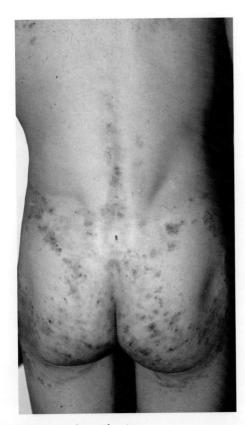

Figure 69.38 Dermatitis herpetiformis.

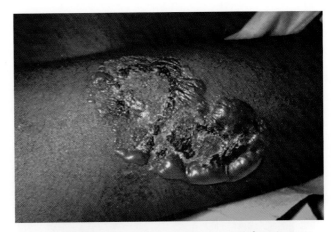

Figure 69.40 Epidermolysis bullosa acquisita, an acquired autoimmune blistering disease caused by IgG autoantibodies to type VII collagen in epidermal basement membrane, may present as an inflammatory blistering disorder that resembles bullous pemphigoid (shown here) or as a "dermolytic", mechanobullous process characterized by skin fragility and scarring.

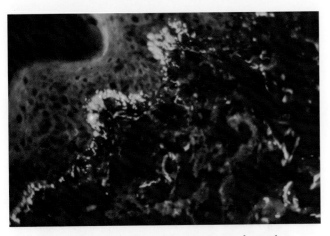

Figure 69.39 Direct immunofluorescence microscopy of normal-appearing perilesional skin from a patient with dermatitis herpetiformis shows in situ granular deposits of IgA in dermal papillae and the epidermal basement membrane.

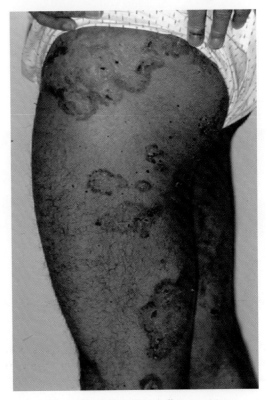

Figure 69.41 Inflammatory epidermolysis bullosa acquisita.

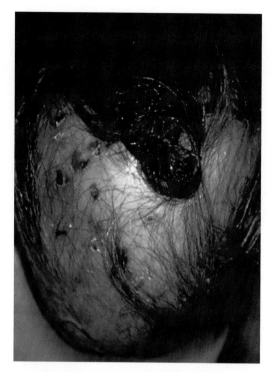

Figure 69.42 Crusted erosions on a scarred scalp typify lesions that can develop in patients with dermolytic epidermolysis bullosa acquisita.

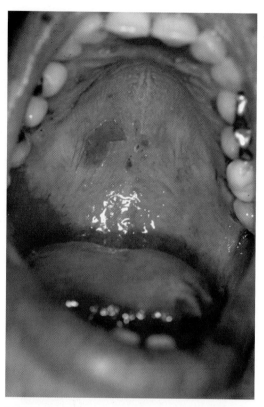

Figure 69.44 Erosive lesions on the palate in a patient with epidermolysis bullosa acquisita.

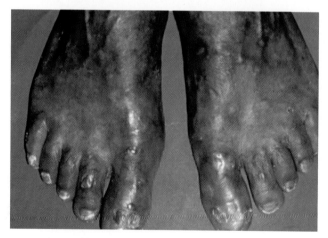

Figure 69.43 Nail loss and round sites of postinflammatory change and scarring typify lesions of dermolytic epidermolysis bullosa acquisita.

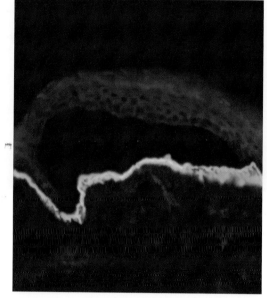

Figure 69.45 Circulating IgG autoantibodies from patients with epidermolysis bullosa acquisita bind the dermal side of 1 M NaCl split skin by indirect immunofluorescence microscopy.

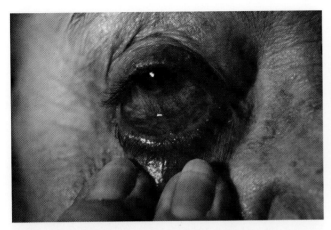

Figure 69.46 Mucous membrane pemphigoid, an autoimmune subepidermal blistering disease, affecting the eye.

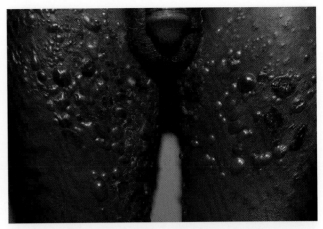

Figure 69.49 Bullous pemphigoid, an autoimmune subepidermal blistering disease.

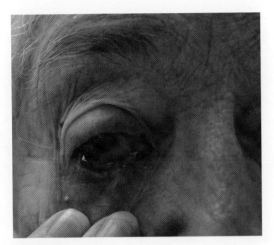

Figure 69.47 Inflammation and symblephara signify advanced ocular mucous membrane pemphigoid.

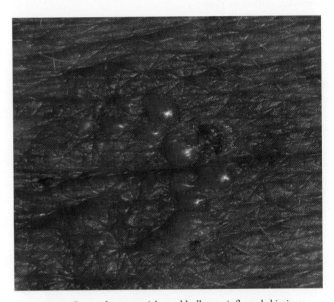

Figure 69.50 Grouped tense vesicles and bullae on inflamed skin in a patient with bullous pemphigoid.

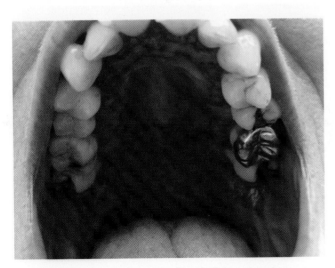

Figure 69.48 Mucous membrane pemphigoid affecting the palate.

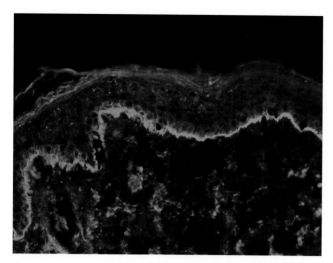

Figure 69.51 Patients with bullous pemphigoid have in situ deposits of IgG (and C3) in the epidermal basement membrane of their normal-appearing, perilesional skin.

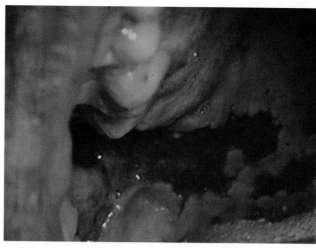

Figure 69.53 Pemphigus vulgaris affecting the palate. Source: Courtesy of Jacqueline Plemons, DDS, MS.

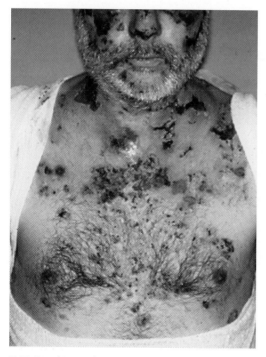

Figure 69.52 Pemphigus vulgaris, a rare, potentially life threatening mucocutaneous blistering disease, develops as a consequence of autoimmunity to desmosomal cadherins.

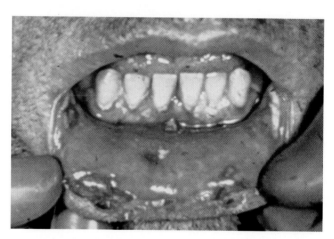

Figure 69.54 Pemphigus vulgaris affecting the lips and gingivae.

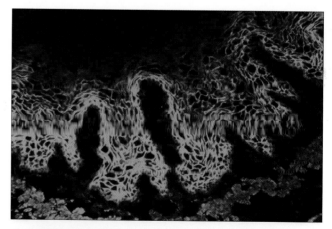

Figure 69.55 Circulating IgG autoantibodies from patients with pemphigus vulgaris bind to desmosomal cadherins on the plasma membranes of keratinocytes in stratified squamous epithelia by indirect immunofluorescence microscopy.

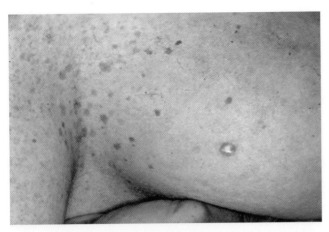

Figure 69.56 Degos disease (malignant atrophic papulosis) characteristically displays focal, porcelain-white lesions surrounded by erythema.

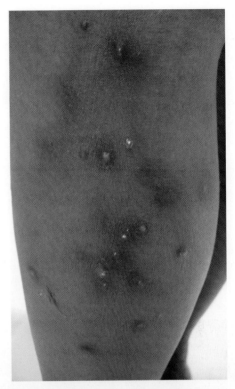

Figure 69.58 Prurigo nodules and sites of postinflammatory hyperpigmentation due to excessive scratching and rubbing of skin.

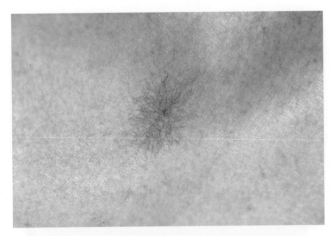

Figure 69.57 Spider angioma (vascular spider, spider nevus, nevus araneus) represent vascular anomalies commonly seen in young children, pregnancy, and patients with liver disease.

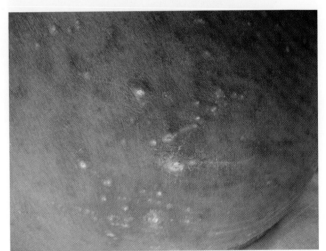

Figure 69.59 Prurigo nodules, lichenification, and sites of postinflammatory hyperpigmentation at sites of scratching.

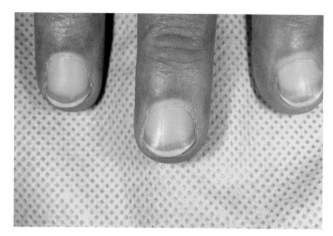

Figure 69.60 Terry nails. In Terry nails, the distal nail bed shows a normal pink color while the proximal nail bed is white. Terry nails are seen in patients with cirrhosis, chronic congestive heart failure, or diabetes mellitus; they are also sometimes seen in normal individuals.

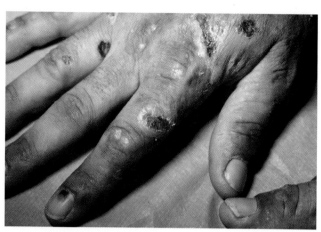

Figure 69.62 Porphyria cutanea tarda.

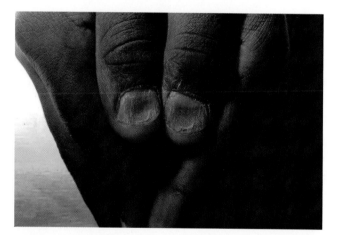

Figure 69.61 Koilonychia (spoon nails) represents a nail abnormality characterized by thinned, concave nails. Koilonychia is seen in individuals with iron deficiency, Plummer–Vinson syndrome, or hemachromatosis. It is also considered physiological in the toenails of children, a common finding in the nails of adults with thermal exposure, and idiopathic or familial in other cases.

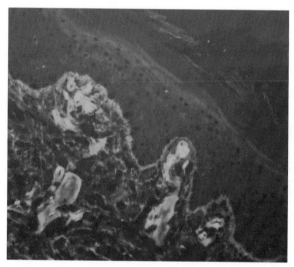

Figure 69.63 Direct immunofluorescence microscopy of affected skin from patients with porphyria cutanea tarda often displays in situ deposits of IgG and C3 in the epidermal basement membrane and the walls of blood vessels in the papillary dermis.

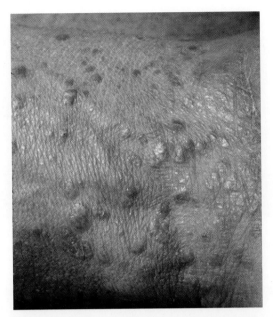

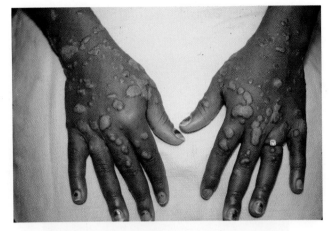

Figure 69.66 Hypertrophic lichen planus.

Figure 69.64 Lichen planus. Hepatic disorders associated with the development of lichen planus include hepatitis C virus infection, hepatitis B immunization, and primary biliary cirrhosis.

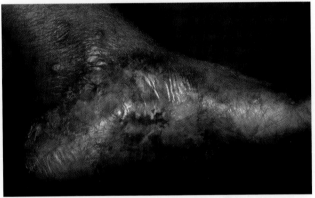

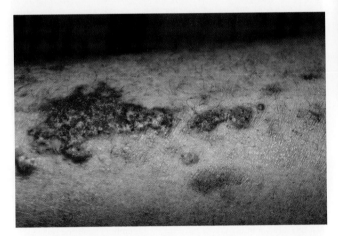

Figure 69.67 Inflammatory lesions of lichen planus on the palms and soles may be characterized by erosions, ulcers, and severe pain.

Figure 69.65 Hypertrophic lichen planus may develop as a consequence of the rubbing and scratching that this pruritic disease sometimes elicits.

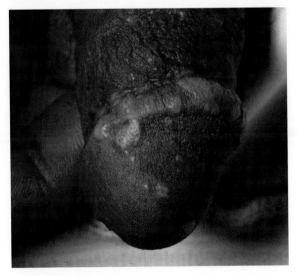

Figure 69.68 Lichen planus on the penis.

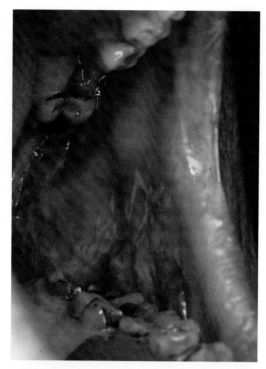

Figure 69.69 Reticulate white lesions on the buccal mucosa signify an oral manifestation of lichen planus.

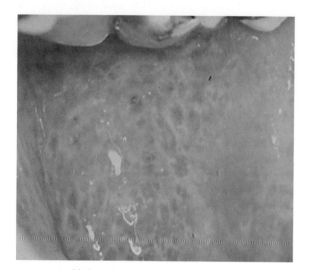

Figure 69.70 Oral lichen planus. Source: Courtesy of Jacqueline Plemons, DDS, MS.

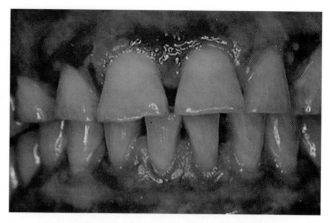

Figure 69.71 Lichen planus affecting the gingiva. Source: Courtesy of Jacqueline Plemons, DDS, MS.

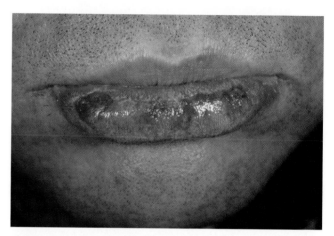

Figure 69.72 Erosive lichen planus on the lips.

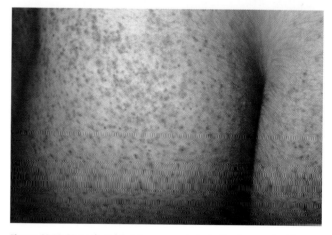

Figure 69.73 Henoch–Schönlein purpura is typically characterized by an eruptive cutaneous vasculitis that is often associated with arthralgias, abdominal pain, and/or renal disease.

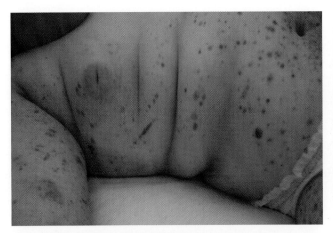

Figure 69.74 A child with Henoch–Schönlein purpura displays numerous sites of palpable purpura in the same phase of evolution.

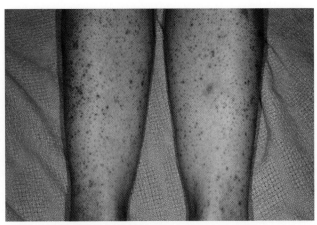

Figure 69.76 Leukocytoclastic vasculitis.

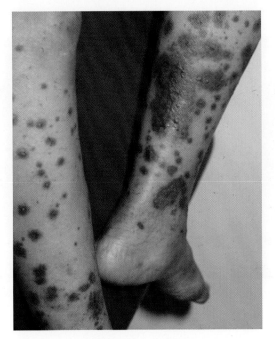

Figure 69.75 Leukocytoclastic vasculitis (LCV). LCV tends to predominate on the lower extremities and display sites of palpable purpura. On occasion, lesions become so inflamed that superficial vesicles and/or erosions develop.

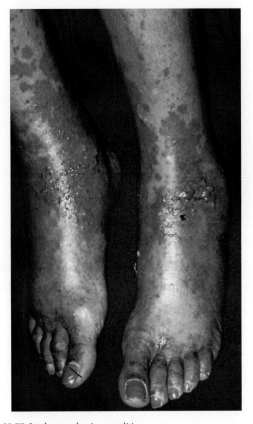

Figure 69.77 Leukocytoclastic vasculitis.

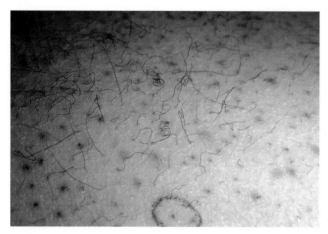

Figure 69.78 Scurvy or vitamin C deficiency displays perifollicular hemorrhages and cork-screw hairs (i.e., hair shafts curled within follicles capped by keratotic plugs).

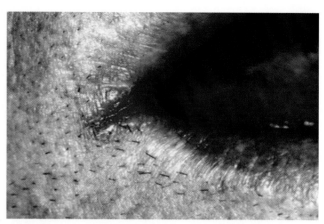

Figure 69.80 Angular cheilitis (perleche) is seen in patients with ill-fitting dentures, intraoral candidiasis, diabetes mellitus, Down syndrome, Sjögren syndrome, or riboflavin deficiency. Source: Courtesy of Jacqueline Plemons, DDS, MS.

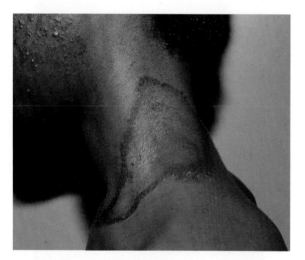

Figure 69.79 Pellagra. The most characteristic cutaneous manifestation of pellagra is a photosensitive eruption that is often seen on the face, neck, upper chest, and upper extremities. Pellagra usually results from a deficiency of niacin (vitamin B-3) or its precursor amino acid tryptophan. Pellagra can also be induced by medications (e.g., isoniazid, azathioprine, 5-fluorouracil).

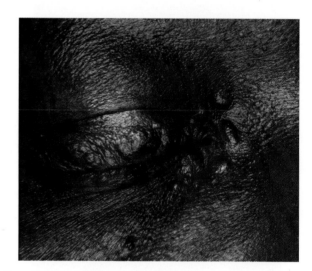

Figure 69.81 Sarcoidosis.

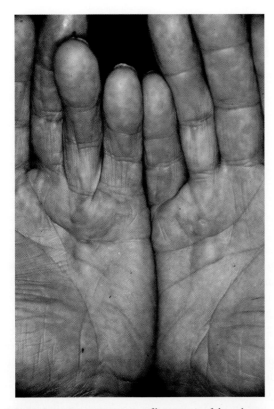

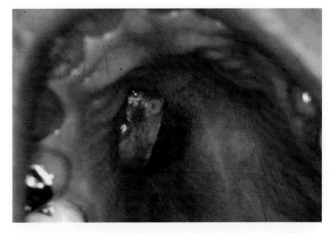

Figure 69.84 Kaposi sarcoma in a patient with human immunodeficiency virus infection. Source: Courtesy of Jacqueline Plemons, DDS, MS.

Figure 69.82 Dupuytren contracture, a fibromatosis of the palmar aponeurosis that is most common in men aged 30–50 years. Dupuytren contracture is associated with Peyronie disease, plantar fibromatosis, and knuckle pads; a familial predisposition for this problem exists. It occurs at times with cirrhosis, diabetes mellitus, and chronic epilepsy.

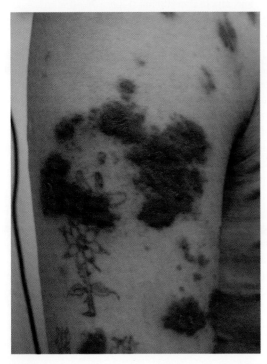

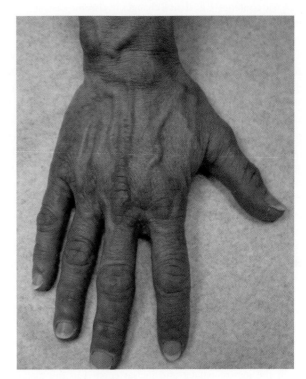

Figure 69.85 An adult with dermatomyositis displays Gottron papules and tendon streaking.

Figure 69.83 Kaposi sarcoma in a patient with human immunodeficiency virus infection.

CHAPTER 70

Oral manifestation of gastrointestinal diseases

Vidyasagar Ramappa and Yashwant R. Mahida

University of Nottingham and Nottingham University Hospitals NHS Trust, Nottingham, UK

Lesions in the oral cavity and adjacent tissues may occur due to a variety of mechanisms. These include disease processes that are similar to those occurring in the rest of the gastrointestinal tract (e.g., inflammation in oral manifestations of Crohn's disease), nutritional deficiencies (e.g., glossitis and angular cheilitis secondary to malabsorption), and persistent exposure to gastric contents (e.g., dental changes in chronic gastroesophageal reflux). In some uncommon gastrointestinal disorders features in the oropharynx may provide important diagnostic clues, such as venous malformation in blue rubber bleb nevus syndrome and characteristic mucocutaneous lesions in Peutz–Jeghers syndrome and hereditary hemorrhagic telangiectasias. Recurrent aphthous stomatitis is more common and can be associated with the gastrointestinal conditions celiac disease and inflammatory bowel disease. Involvement of the oral cavity is frequent in chronic graft-versus-host disease and may lead to significant symptoms and difficulties in chewing and swallowing food. The figures in this chapter illustrate lesions in the oral cavity (and adjacent tissues) that occurred in association with specific disease processes affecting other parts of the gastrointestinal tract.

Figure 70.1 illustrates oral manifestations of gastroesophageal reflux disease. In Figure 70.1a broad shallow erosion with thinning of the enamel has resulted in an increased translucency of the incisal region of the anterior maxillary central incisors, associated with increased grayness. Figure 70.1b shows that the thinner enamel in the cervical regions (around the neck) of the teeth has been eroded to varying degrees, accentuating the yellow appearance of the underlying dentin. Erosion resulting in the loss of palatal and incisal enamel of the maxillary incisors is shown in Figure 70.1c. In Figure 70.1d long-standing erosion has caused severe loss of occlusal enamel and dentin of lower molar teeth resulting in cupping of these teeth. For example, there is a severe cupping of the occlusal surface of the mandibular first molar tooth adjacent to the resin composite restoration.

Oral manifestations of Crohn's disease in children are shown in Figure 70.2. They include lip swelling with fissures (Figure 70.2a), cobblestone appearance of the buccal mucosa (Figure 70.2b), linear ulceration deep in the mandibular vestibule (Figure 70.2c), mucosal tag on the buccal aspect of the gingiva (Figure 70.2d), and mucogingivitis in relation to the maxillary permanent incisors (Figure 70.2e).

Figure 70.3 shows features of pyostomatitis vegetans in patients with ulcerative colitis. Multiple confluent pustules on the palate and tongue are shown in Figure 70.3a,b, vegetating pyoderma gangrenosum in Figure 70.3c, and pustules assuming a figurate pattern in Figure 70.3d. Other features shown are confluent pustules and erosions assuming a "snail track" pattern (Figure 70.3e) and gingival edema and pustules (Figure 70.3f).

In the oral cavity, chronic graft-versus-host-disease may lead to mucoceles (Figure 70.4a), atrophy, and perioral fibrosis (Figure 70.4b); mucosal edema and lichenoid lesions (Figure 70.4c); and mucosal erythema (Figure 70.4d).

Figure 70.5 shows characteristic lip telangiectasias in a patient with hereditary hemorrhagic telangiectasia.

A venous malformation lesion in the oral cavity of a patient with blue rubber bleb nevus syndrome is shown in Figure 70.6. Endoscopic appearance of venous malformations in the colon in blue rubber bleb nevus syndrome can be seen in Figure 70.7.

Figure 70.8a shows multiple osteomas arising from the mandible of a patient with Gardner syndrome. The corresponding radiograph (Figure 70.8b) shows homogenous radiopaque masses over the right and left inferior aspect of the mandible, which are suggestive of osteomas. Also, multiple small, homogeneous radiopaque masses surrounded by a radiolucent halo can be seen throughout the maxilla and mandible suggestive of complex odontomas. These sclerotic masses are present throughout the body of mandible giving it a mottled appearance.

Perioral pigmentation (Figure 70.9) may provide an important clue regarding the diagnosis of Peutz–Jeghers syndrome.

Yamada's Atlas of Gastroenterology, Fifth Edition. Edited by Daniel K. Podolsky, Michael Camilleri, J. Gregory Fitz, Anthony N. Kalloo, Fergus Shanahan, and Timothy C. Wang.

© 2016 John Wiley & Sons, Ltd. Published 2016 by John Wiley & Sons, Ltd.

Companion website: www.yamadagastro.com/atlas

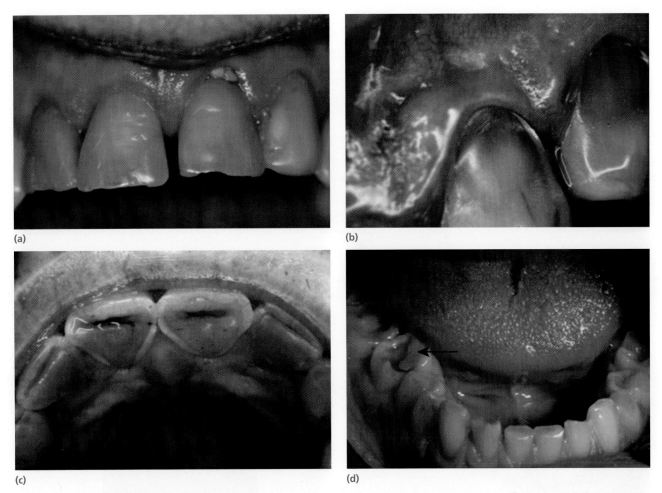

Figure 70.1 Oral manifestations of gastroesophageal reflux disease. **(a)** Broad shallow erosion with thinning of the enamel has resulted in an increased translucency of the incisal region of the anterior maxillary central incisors, associated with increased grayness. **(b)** The thinner enamel in the cervical regions (around the neck) of the teeth has been eroded to varying degrees, accentuating the yellow appearance of the underlying dentin. **(c)** Erosion has resulted in the loss of palatal and incisal enamel of the maxillary incisors. **(d)** Long-standing erosion has caused severe loss of occlusal enamel and dentin of lower molar teeth, resulting in cupping of these teeth. For example there is a severe cupping of the occlusal surface of the mandibular first molar tooth adjacent to the resin composite restoration (black arrow). Source: Ranjitkar S, Smales RJ, Kaidonis JA. Oral manifestations of gastroesophageal reflux disease. J Gastroenterol Hepatol 2012;27:21. Reproduced with permission of John Wiley & Sons. Source: **(a)** Courtesy Dr. A. Dickson.

In angular cheilitis (Figure 70.10) inflammation occurs at the angles of the mouth and is commonly associated with deficiencies of B vitamins such as riboflavin (B-2), niacin (B-3), and pyridoxine (B-6). Secondary infection with *Candida* or staphylococci may occur.

Glossitis (Figure 70.11) is an inflammatory condition that leads to atrophy of the filiform papillae on the dorsal surface of the tongue, resulting in a smooth, featureless, and erythematous appearance. Fissuring may also occur. Glossitis is often due nutritional deficiency arising from an underlying gastrointestinal condition.

Figure 70.12 shows an aphthous ulcer. Aphthae appear as small, shallow white ulcers distributed along mucous membranes. Although observed in normal individuals, multiple or persistent lesions can be associated with underlying conditions, such as inflammatory bowel disease or Behçet disease.

Macroglossia due to infiltration of the tongue in a patient with primary amyloidosis is shown in Figure 70.13. There is evidence of repeated tongue-biting in this photograph.

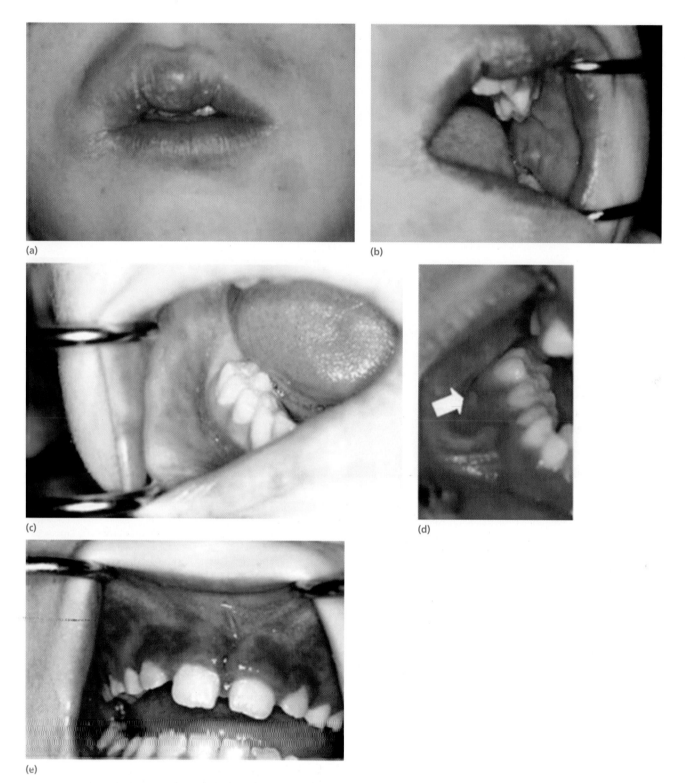

Figure 70.2 Oral manifestations of Crohn's disease in children. **(a)** Lip swelling with fissures. **(b)** Cobblestone appearance of the buccal mucosa. **(c)** Linear ulceration deep in the mandibular vestibule. **(d)** Mucosal tag (arrow) on the buccal aspect of the gingiva. **(e)** Mucogingivitis in relation to the maxillary permanent incisors. Source: Harty S, Fleming P, Rowland M, et al. A prospective study of the oral manifestations of Crohn's disease. Clin Gastroenterol Hepatol 2005;3:886. Reproduced with permission of Elsevier.

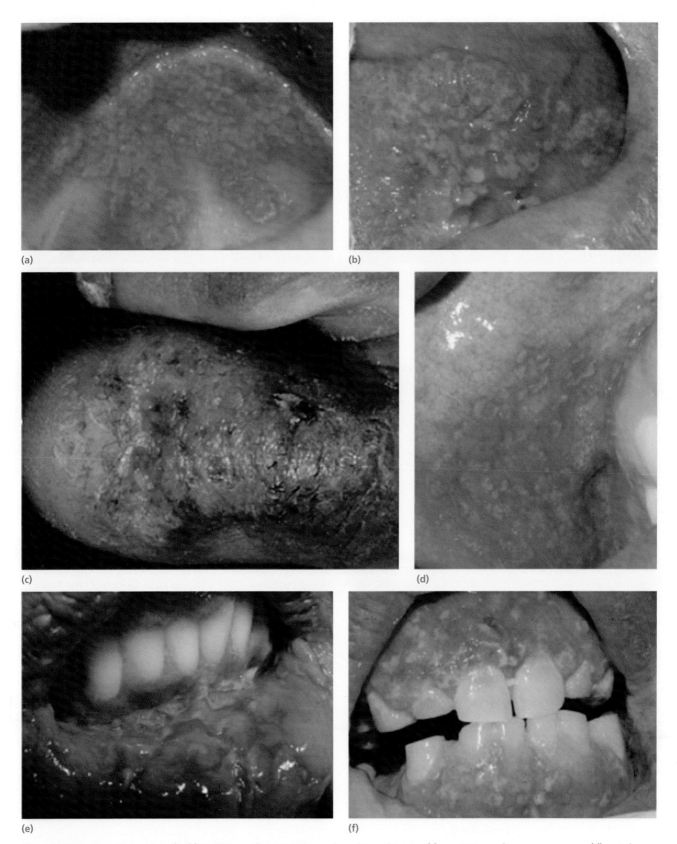

Figure 70.3 Pyostomatitis vegetans: **(a, b)** multiple confluent pustules on the palate and tongue; **(c)** vegetating pyoderma gangrenosum; **(d)** pustules assuming a figurate pattern; **(e)** confluent pustules and erosions assuming a "snail track" pattern; **(f)** gingival edema and pustules. Source: Nico MM, Hussein TP, Aoki V, et al. Pyostomatitis vegetans and its relation to inflammatory bowel disease, pyoderma gangrenosum, pyodermatitis vegetans, and pemphigus. J Oral Pathol Med 2012;4:584. Reproduced with permission of John Wiley & Sons.

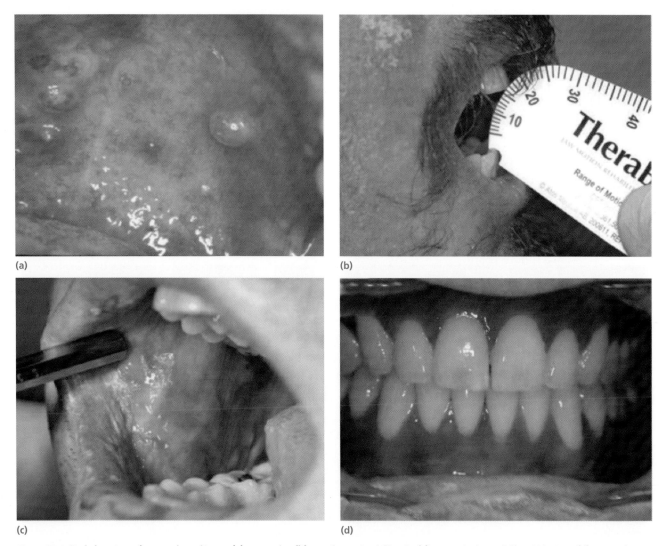

(a)

(b)

(c)

(d)

Figure 70.4 Oral chronic graft-versus-host-disease: **(a)** mucoceles; **(b)** atrophy, perioral fibrosis; **(c)** mucosal edema, lichenoid lesions; **(d)** mucosal erythema. Source: Mays JW, Sarmadi M, Moutsopoulos NM. Oral manifestations of systemic autoimmune and inflammatory diseases: diagnosis and clinical management. J Evid Based Dent Pract 2012;12(3 Suppl):265. Reproduced with permission of Elsevier. Source (a, b): Courtesy of Carol Bassim, DMD, MS, and Dean Edwards, DDS.

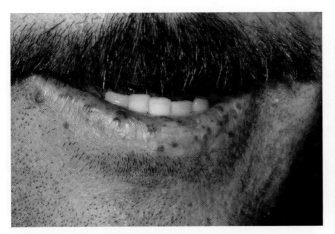

Figure 70.5 Lip telangiectasias in hereditary hemorrhagic telangiectasia. Source: van Dijk HA, Fred HL. Images of Memorable Cases: Cases 115 & 116, OpenStax CNX, 2008. Available at: http://cnx.org/content/m15016/1.3/, accessed 5 October 2013.

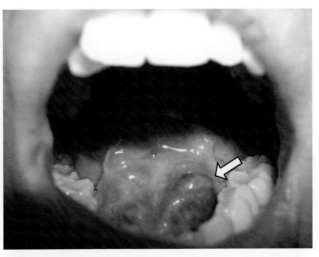

Figure 70.6 Oral cavity showing a venous malformation lesion (arrow) in a patient with blue rubber bleb nevus syndrome. Source: Ochiai D, Miyakoshi K, Yakubo K, et al. Familial blue rubber bleb nevus syndrome in pregnancy with spinal epidural involvement. Case Rep Obstet Gynecol 2013;2013:141506.

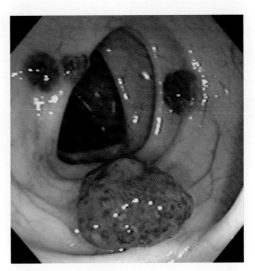

Figure 70.7 Endoscopic appearance of venous malformations in blue rubber bleb nevus syndrome. Source: Fishman SJ, Smithers CJ, Folkman J, et al. Blue rubber bleb nevus syndrome: surgical eradication of gastrointestinal bleeding. Ann Surg 2005;241:523. Reproduced with permission of Wolters Kluwer Health.

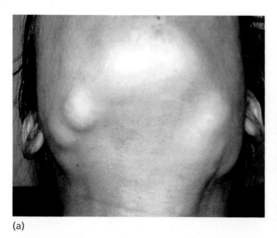

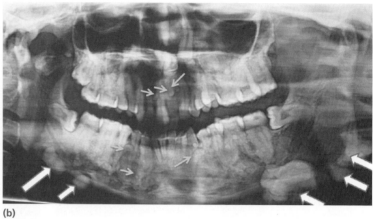

(a)

(b)

Figure 70.8 Gardner syndrome. **(a)** Multiple osteomas arising from the mandible. **(b)** Corresponding radiograph showing homogenous radiopaque masses over the right and left inferior aspect of the mandible (large arrows) suggestive of osteomas. Also, multiple small, homogenous radiopaque masses surrounded by a radiolucent halo can be seen throughout the maxilla and mandible suggestive of complex odontomes (small arrows). Diffuse sclerotic masses are present throughout the body of mandible giving it a mottled appearance. Source: Panjwani S, Bagewadi A, Keluskar V, et al. Gardner's syndrome. J Clin Imag Sci 2011;1:65.

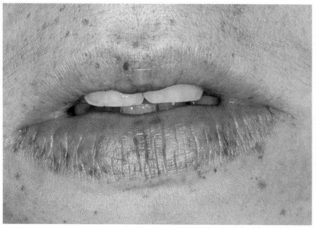

Figure 70.9 Perioral pigmentation in Peutz–Jeghers syndrome. Source: Meleti M, Vescovi P, Mooi WJ, et al. Pigmented lesions of the oral mucosa and perioral tissues: a flow-chart for the diagnosis and some recommendations for the management. Oral Surg Oral Med Oral Pathol Oral Radiol Endod 2008;105:606. Reproduced with permission of Elsevier.

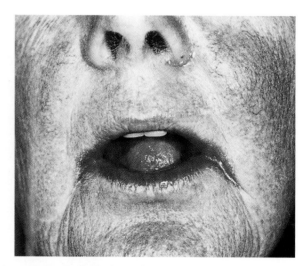

Figure 70.10 Angular cheilitis. Inflammation at the angles of the mouth is commonly associated with deficiencies of B vitamins such as riboflavin (B-2), niacin (B-3), and pyridoxine (B-6). Secondary infection with *Candida* or staphylococci may occur. Source: Habif TP. In: Baxter S, ed. Clinical Dermatology, 3rd edn. St. Louis: Mosby, 1996. Reproduced with permission of Elsevier.

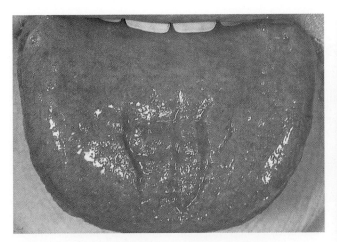

Figure 70.11 A raw, fissured tongue, especially in the setting of peripheral neuropathy, should raise the suspicion of vitamin B-12 deficiency. In later stages, the tongue may appear more atrophic with a bald, glistening surface. Source: Allison MC. Diagnostic Picture Tests in Gastroenterology. London: Mosby,1991. Reproduced with permission of Elsevier.

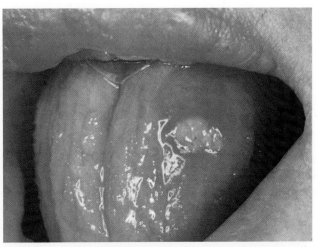

Figure 70.12 Aphthous ulcer. Aphthae appear as minute, shallow white ulcers distributed along mucous membranes. Although observed in normal individuals, multiple or persistent lesions mandate exclusion of an underlying disease process, such as inflammatory bowel disease or Behçet disease. Source: Allison MC. Diagnostic Picture Tests in Gastroenterology. London: Mosby, 1991. Reproduced with permission of Elsevier.

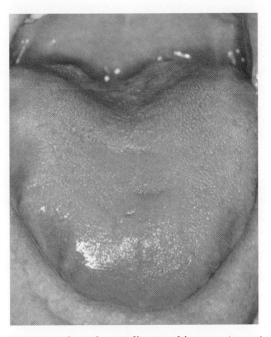

Figure 70.13 Macroglossia due to infiltration of the tongue in a patient with primary amyloidosis. Evidence of repeated tongue-biting is illustrated in this photograph. Source: Allison MC. Diagnostic Picture Tests in Gastroenterology. London: Mosby, 1991. Reproduced with permission of Elsevier.

CHAPTER 71

Intestinal ischemia and vasculitides

Juan-Ramón Malagelada and Carolina Malagelada

Hospital Universitari Vall d'Hebron, Autonomous University of Barcelona, Spain

Intestinal ischemia comprises a variety of disorders that develop as a result of inadequate blood supply to some portion of the gastrointestinal tract. The gastrointestinal tract is supplied by three major branches of the aorta: the celiac axis (CA), the superior mesenteric artery (SMA), and the inferior mesenteric artery (IMA). The first provides blood to the stomach and proximal duodenum, as well as to liver and pancreas. The second, supplies the distal duodenum, small bowel, and proximal colon, and the third the distal colon. There are key collaterals that link these territories, chiefly, the arc of Riolan (which connects the proximal middle colic artery with a branch of the left colic artery) and the marginal artery of Drummond (which connects the SMA with the IMA).

Acute mesenteric ischemia is a consequence of an abrupt interruption of blood flow to the small bowel. Five subgroups are defined on the basis of causation: SMA embolus, SMA thrombosis, focal segmental ischemia, nonocclusive mesenteric ischemia (NOMI), and acute mesenteric venous thrombosis. Among the various causes of acute mesenteric ischemia, SMA embolism is the most common (50%), followed by SMA thrombosis and NOMI (15%–30% for each). Superior mesenteric vein thrombosis is the least common (5%) cause of acute mesenteric ischemia. Chronic mesenteric ischemia develops as a result of chronically impaired blood flow to the stomach and/or small bowel. There are two major categories of chronic mesenteric ischemia. One form, most common in young individuals, results from extrinsic compression of aortic branches due to anatomic or inflammatory defects. A second form, which affects mostly elderly individuals, results from chronic arteriosclerotic occlusion of mesenteric vessels.

The diagnosis of mesenteric ischemia rests upon the combination of clinical suspicion and imaging findings. The key features of CT imaging in acute mesenteric ischemia involve vessel abnormalities, morphological changes in the bowel wall, and indirect signs that may be present in the mesentery and peritoneum (Figures 71.1, 71.2, 71.3, 71.4, and 71.5). Mesenteric angiography is another key diagnostic procedure that doubles as a therapeutic tool with a major impact on reducing mortality from mesenteric ischemia. Angiographic procedures include the therapeutic option of intraarterial infusion of vasodilators or thrombolytic agents. In the setting of underlying arteriosclerotic disease, endovascular stenting has increasingly been used to provide adequate revascularization and to reduce the need for surgery (Figures 71.6, 71.7, 71.8, 71.9, 71.10, and 71.11).

Ischemic colitis is a condition that develops when the blood supply to the colon is insufficient to sustain tissue needs. Small vessel disease and/or vasomotor dysfunction appear to be the main underlying mechanism. There are four main forms of ischemic colitis: transient ulcerating ischemic colitis (Figures 71.12, 71.13, 71.14, 71.15, 71,16, and 71.17), reversible ischemic colopathy (Figure 71.18), segmental ulcerating colitis with stricture (Figures 71.19, 71.20, 71.21, and 71.22), and fulminant universal ischemic colitis (Figures 71.23 and 71.24). Irrespective of the presentation, definitive diagnosis of ischemic colitis requires appropriate imaging and histological confirmation (Figures 71.25 and 71.26). Diagnostic means include barium enema, colonoscopy, and computed tomography.

Yamada's Atlas of Gastroenterology, Fifth Edition. Edited by Daniel K. Podolsky, Michael Camilleri, J. Gregory Fitz, Anthony N. Kalloo, Fergus Shanahan, and Timothy C. Wang.

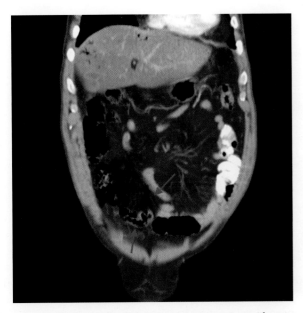

Figure 71.1 Computed tomography appearance in a patient with acute mesenteric ischemia. Note marked pneumatosis along the portal and mesenteric venous branches as well as intramurally (arrows).
Source: Courtesy of Dr. Sergi Quiroga, Radiology Unit, Hospital Universitari Vall d'Hebron, Barcelona.

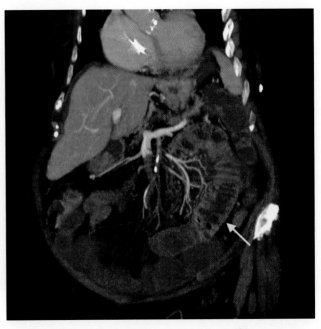

Figure 71.2 Computed tomography appearance in acute mesenteric ischemia secondary to superior mesenteric artery embolus. Pictures show embolus lodged near the origin of the superior mesenteric artery (red arrow) as well as ischemic loops of bowel. Note poor contrast penetration inside the intestinal wall with reduced blood flow and dilatation of the small bowel loops (yellow arrow). Source: Courtesy of Dr. Sergi Quiroga, Radiology Unit, Hospital Universitari Vall d'Hebron, Barcelona.

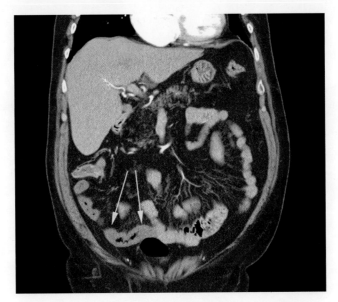

Figure 71.3 Computed tomography appearance of acute ileal ischemia. Note the marked thickening of the wall of affected ileal loops with narrowing of the intestinal lumen (arrows). Source: Courtesy of Dr. Sergi Quiroga, Radiology Unit, Hospital Universitari Vall d'Hebron, Barcelona.

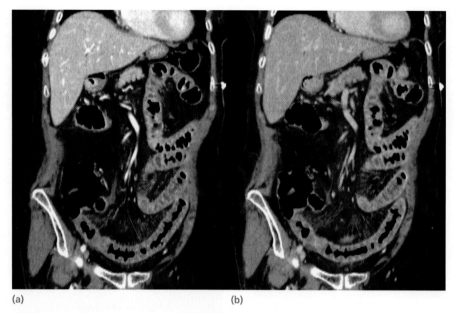

(a)   (b)

Figure 71.4 (a, b) Computed tomography appearance in subacute mesenteric ischemia. Note the extensive thickening of the wall of the small bowel loops with smooth serosal surfaces and appearance of rigidity caused by wall infiltration and organized edema and hemorrhage (arrows). Source: Courtesy of Dr. Sergi Quiroga, Radiology Unit, Hospital Universitari Vall d'Hebron, Barcelona.

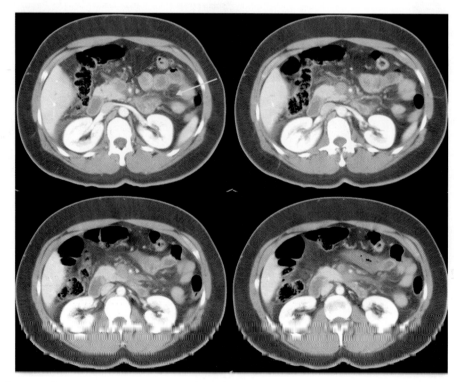

Figure 71.5 Computed tomography appearance in acute superior mesenteric vein thrombosis. Note the thrombus inside the mesenteric vein (red arrow). There is marked edema of the mesentery (yellow arrow) in addition to the less specific thickening of the small bowel wall. Source: Courtesy of Dr. Sergi Quiroga, Radiology Unit, Hospital Universitari Vall d'Hebron, Barcelona.

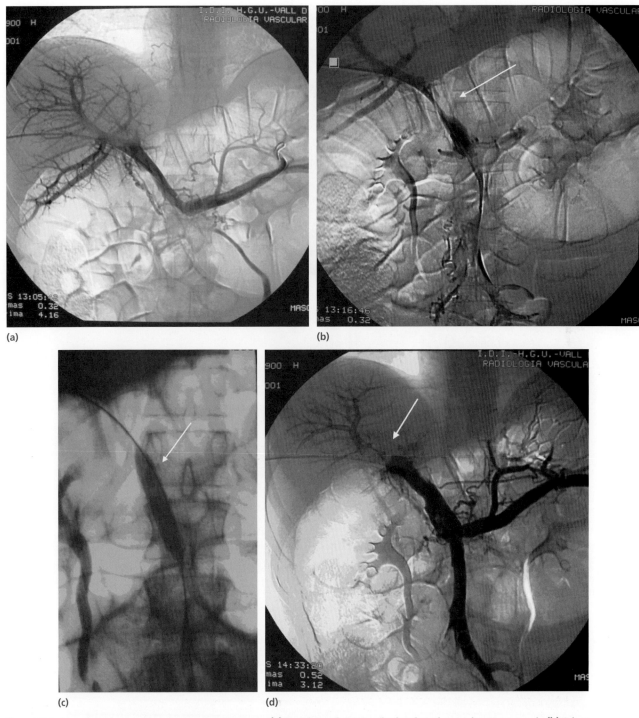

(a)

(b)

(c)

(d)

Figure 71.6 Acute thrombosis of the superior mesenteric vein. **(a)** Portal vascularization displayed via the transhepatic approach. **(b)** Selective catheterization of the mesenteric vein revealing extensive thrombosis. **(c)** Mechanical fragmentation of the thrombus (urokinase was contraindicated in this patient). **(d)** Repermeabilization by displacement of thrombus into the intrahepatic branches of the portal vein. Source: Courtesy of Dr. Mercedes Perez and Dr. Antoni Segarra, Interventional Radiology Unit, Hospital Universitari Vall d'Hebron, Barcelona.

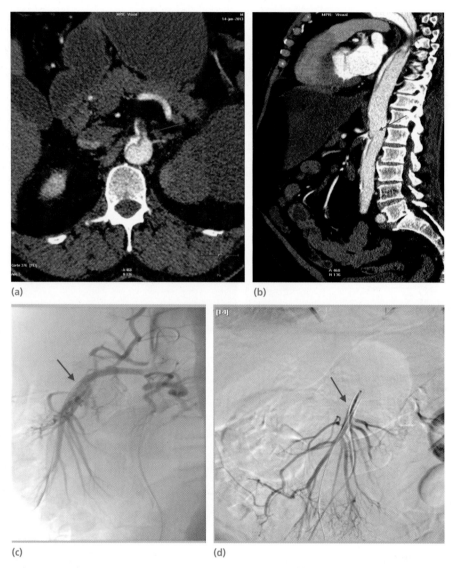

Figure 71.7 (a, b) Aortic dissection with superior mesenteric artery blockage by aortic flap. **(c)** Control after self-expanding prosthesis placement. **(d)** Repermeabilization of the superior mesenteric artery. Source: Courtesy of Dr. Mercedes Perez and Dr. Antoni Segarra, Interventional Radiology Unit, Hospital Universitari Vall d'Hebron, Barcelona.

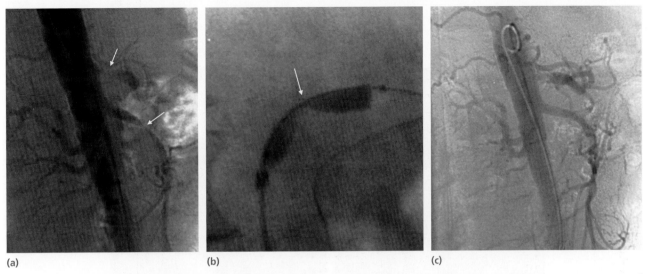

(a)   (b)   (c)

Figure 71.8 Double stenosis (celiac and superior mesenteric artery) treated with balloon dilation. **(a)** Abdominal aortogram demonstrating a stenosis of both the celiac axis and the superior mesenteric artery. **(b)** Balloon angioplasty. **(c)** Control after treatment. Source: Courtesy of Dr. Mercedes Perez and Dr. Antoni Segarra, Interventional Radiology Unit, Hospital Universitari Vall d'Hebron, Barcelona.

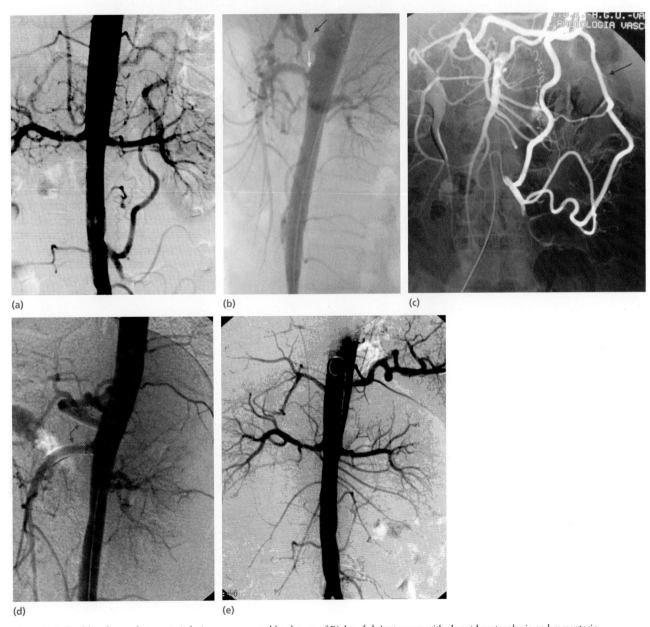

(a)   (b)   (c)

(d)   (e)

Figure 71.9 Double celiac and mesenteric lesion compensated by the arc of Riolan. **(a)** Aortogram with absent hepatosplenic and mesenteric vascularization. **(b)** Side view showing absence of the celiac axis (CA; red arrow) and stenosis of the superior mesenteric artery (SMA; yellow arrow). **(c)** Supraselective catheterization of the inferior mesenteric artery revealing compensation of the SMA and CA by the arc of Riolan and the gastroduodenal artery, respectively. **(d)** Double stenting of the SMA and CA. **(e)** The compensating collaterals disappear after stenting.
Source: Courtesy of Dr. Mercedes Perez and Dr. Antoni Segarra, Interventional Radiology Unit, Hospital Universitari Vall d'Hebron, Barcelona.

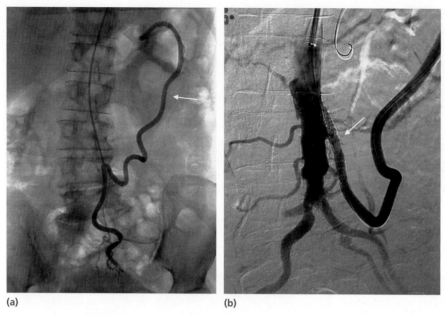

(a) (b)

Figure 71.10 Inferior mesenteric artery (IMA) stenosis pre- and poststent. **(a)** Percutaneous approach to the IMA via the axillar artery and a prominent compensating arc of Riolan (arrow). **(b)** Poststent control. Source: Courtesy of Dr. Mercedes Perez and Dr. Antoni Segarra, Interventional Radiology Unit, Hospital Universitari Vall d'Hebron, Barcelona.

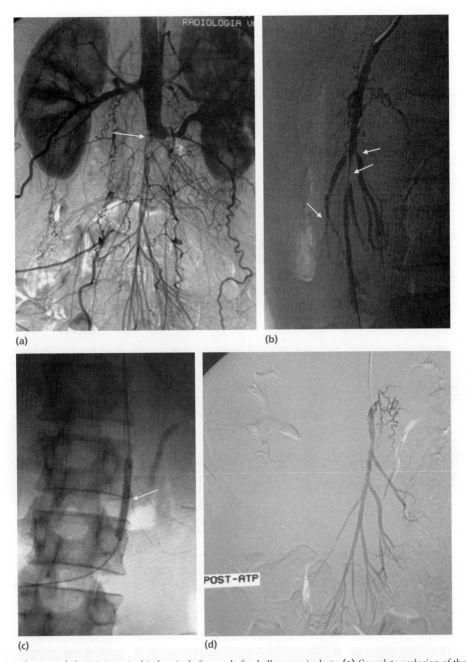

Figure 71.11 Leriche syndrome and chronic intestinal ischemia, before and after balloon angioplasty. **(a)** Complete occlusion of the infrarenal aorta.
(b) Extensive stenotic lesions of the superior mesenteric artery. **(c)** Balloon angioplasty. **(d)** Control showing resolution of the stenosis.
Source: Courtesy of Dr. Mercedes Perez and Dr. Antoni Segarra, Interventional Radiology Unit, Hospital Universitari Vall d'Hebron, Barcelona.

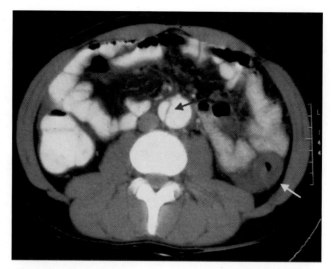

Figure 71.12 Computed tomography scan appearance of ischemic colitis in a patient with aortic dissection (red arrow). Note concentric thickening of the affected ascending colon (yellow arrow). Source: Courtesy of Lawrence J. Brandt, Montefiore Medical Center, New York.

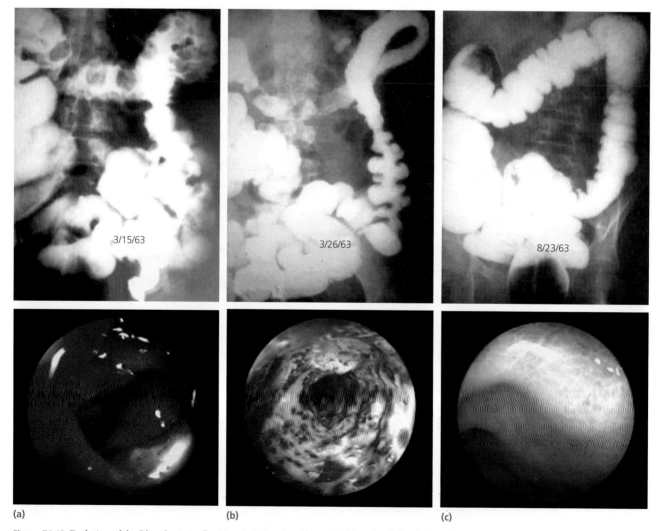

Figure 71.13 Evolution of the "thumbprinting" pattern in ischemic colitis at 24, 48, and 72 h (a–c) after clinical onset. Thumbprinting is most characteristic in the early stages but bulging tends to disappear later and turn into a flatter mucosal lesion. Source: Courtesy of Lawrence J. Brandt, Montefiore Medical Center, New York.

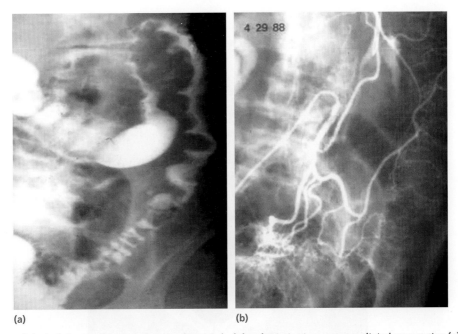

Figure 71.14 Transient radiological abnormalities in ischemic colitis. Marked thumbprinting is apparent at clinical presentation **(a)** but angiography **(b)** is unrevealing because of transient arterial blockage or small vessel ischemia. Source: Courtesy of Lawrence J. Brandt, Montefiore Medical Center, New York.

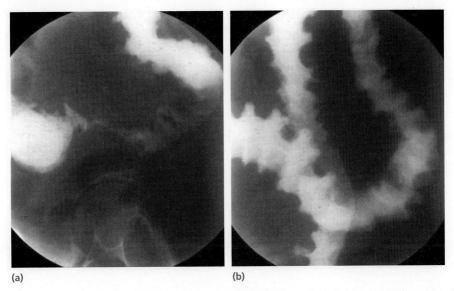

Figure 71.15 Ischemic colitis and acute diverticulitis may present concomitantly producing a mixed clinical picture. The more typical radiographic features of each of these two conditions may help identify the respectively affected segments, as illustrated by the barium enema pictures shown here: diverticulitis **(a)** and ischemic colitis **(b)**. Source: Courtesy of Lawrence J. Brandt, Montefiore Medical Center, New York.

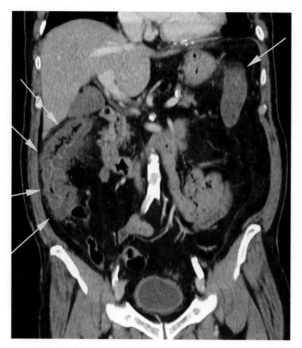

Figure 71.16 Computed tomography scan appearance of ischemic colitis affecting the right colon and splenic flexure. Note the markedly thickened bowel wall with some air remaining in the lumen (arrows).
Source: Courtesy of Dr. Sergi Quiroga, Radiology Unit, Hospital Universitari Vall d'Hebron, Barcelona.

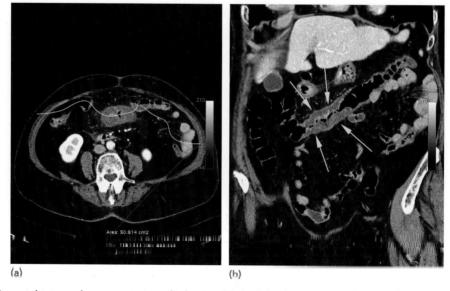

(a)   (b)

Figure 71.17 (a, b) Computed tomography scan appearance of ischemic colitis involving the transverse colon. Note the sharply different wall thickness between the affected transverse segment and the spared ascending colon and hepatic flexure (arrows). Source: courtesy of Dr. Sergi Quiroga, Radiology Unit, Hospital Universitari Vall d'Hebron, Barcelona.

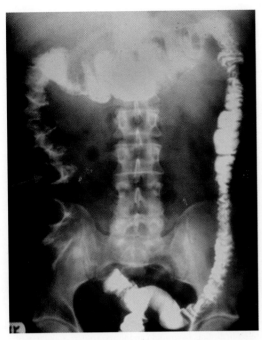

Figure 71.18 Barium enema appearance of acute right-sided ischemic colitis in a patient with hepatitis B virus-induced polyarteritis. Note the marked thumbprinting pattern in the ascending colon. Source: Courtesy of Lawrence J. Brandt, Montefiore Medical Center, New York.

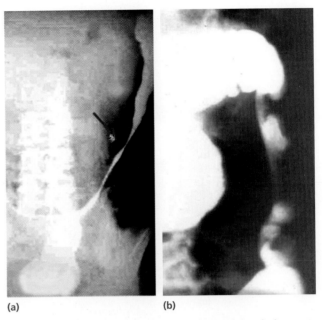

(a)   (b)

Figure 71.19 Irreversible ischemic strictures may develop at the later stages of ischemic colitis. Radiographically they may be long, with tapered edges **(a)** and usually distinct from the sharper-edged neoplastic strictures **(b)**. Source: Courtesy of Lawrence J. Brandt, Montefiore Medical Center, New York.

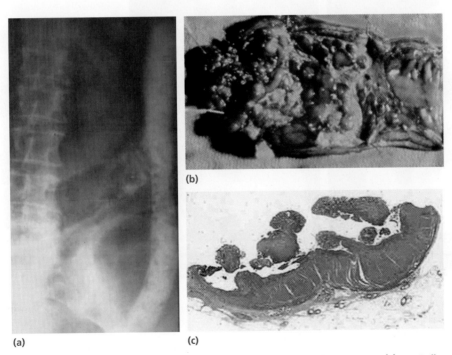

(a)   (c)

Figure 71.20 Pseudopolyps in chronic ischemic colitis as observed in the descending colon in the barium enema **(a)**, surgically resected specimen **(b)**, and microscopically **(c)**. The pseudopolyps may potentially lead to confusion with late-stage inflammatory bowel disease. Source: Courtesy of Lawrence J. Brandt, Montefiore Medical Center, New York.

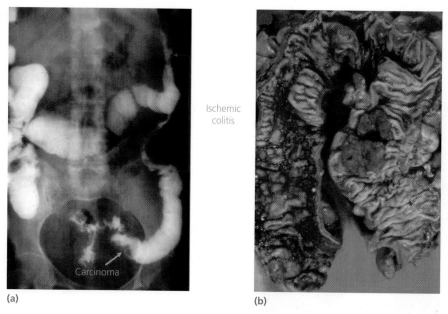

(a)   (b)

Figure 71.21 Ischemic colitis associated with sigmoid carcinoma. Note, on the barium enema picture **(a)**, the characteristic long thumbprinting and narrowing of a segment of the descending colon and **(b)** the surgically resected specimen including a sigmoid carcinoma. Source: Courtesy of Lawrence J. Brandt, Montefiore Medical Center, New York.

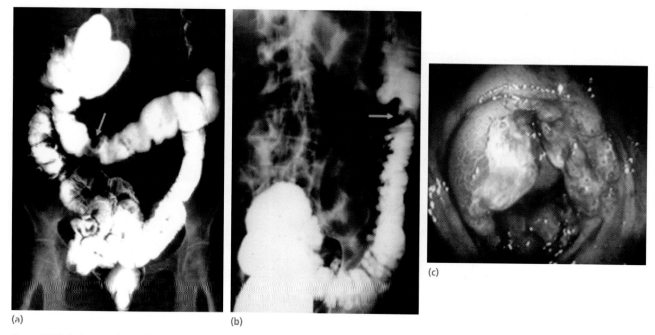

(a)   (b)   (c)

Figure 71.22 Ischemic colitis with a radiographic **(a, b)** and colonoscopic **(c)** appearance susceptible to confusion with colonic adenocarcinoma. There is luminal narrowing by a lobulated mass effect caused by edema and ulceration in the ischemic segment. Source: Courtesy of Lawrence J. Brandt, Montefiore Medical Center, New York.

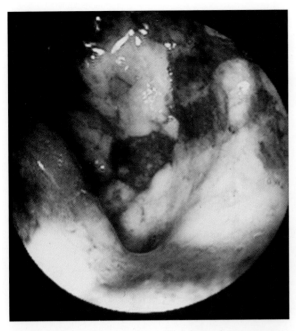

Figure 71.23 Colonoscopic appearance of ischemic colonic gangrene. Source: Courtesy of Lawrence J. Brandt, Montefiore Medical Center, New York.

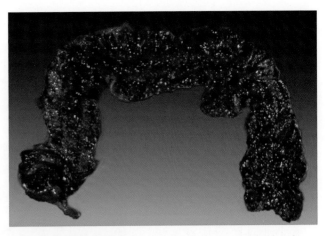

Figure 71.24 Surgically resected colon from a patient who developed fulminant universal ischemic colitis and who required emergency intervention. Source: Courtesy of Lawrence J. Brandt, Montefiore Medical Center, New York.

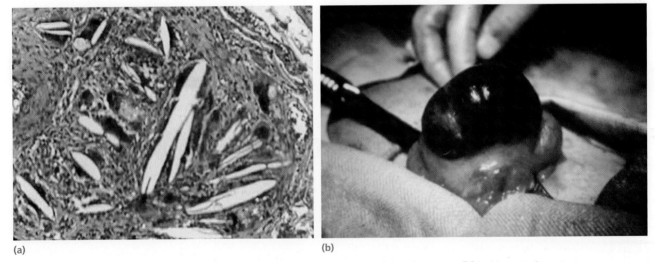

(a)   (b)

Figure 71.25 Cholesterol emboli (a) may lead to bowel ischemia and cecal necrosis, as observed at surgery (b) in this particular patient. Source: Courtesy of Lawrence J. Brandt, Montefiore Medical Center, New York.

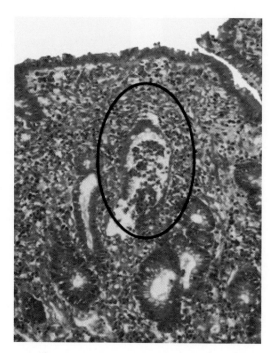

Figure 71.26 The microscopic appearance of ischemic bowel may incorporate features more characteristic of inflammatory bowel disease such as crypt abscesses, as in the present specimen. However, distinction may be usually established by the pathologist through multiple morphological features. Source: Courtesy of Lawrence J. Brandt, Montefiore Medical Center, New York.

CHAPTER 72

Radiation injury in the gastrointestinal tract

Steven M. Cohn[1] and Stephen J. Bickston[2]
[1] University of Viginia School of Medicine, Charlottesville, VA, USA
[2] Virginia Commonwealth University and McGuire VA Medical Center, Richmond, VA, USA

The gastroenterologist will continue to encounter and treat patients with gastrointestinal or hepatic complications resulting from the therapeutic use of ionizing radiation. The histopathological analysis of tissue specimens can often aid in establishing the diagnosis and excluding other etiologies for a patient's symptoms. The histological appearance of lesions observed in tissue specimens is often characteristic of acute or delayed radiation injury. However, no individual histological feature is pathognomonic for radiation-induced damage. Therefore, histological findings may mimic other pathological conditions and must be interpreted carefully within the appropriate clinical context for a given patient. Patients may present with acute symptoms days or weeks after radiation therapy is initiated or with delayed clinical syndromes that may occur years after therapy. The early effects primarily involve the mucosa, which is lined by rapidly proliferating epithelial cells that are sensitive to the acute effects of radiation injury. Clinical symptoms include odynophagia, diarrhea, nausea, vomiting, or gastrointestinal bleeding; the symptoms depend on the location of the radiation field, the dose of irradiation, and the fractionation schedule. The delayed effects of therapeutic irradiation are more likely to present with chronic diarrhea, fibrosis, ulcer formation, or bleeding, and are thought to be secondary to damage to the vasculature of the organs involved. The figures that follow (Figures 72.1–72.13) illustrate selected histopathological features of acute and chronic radiation injury in the gastrointestinal tract and liver.

The histopathological features of acute radiation injury are dominated by evidence of acute injury to the mucosa. Apoptosis of lamina propria lymphocytes and epithelial cells and the cessation of epithelial cell replication occur within hours of a radiation dose. Mature, differentiated epithelial cells continue to be lost in the absence of replacement by replication of the progenitor cells within these epithelia, resulting in the subsequent loss of mucosal function. Acute diarrhea may result under these circumstances. Mucosal and submucosal edema may also be observed within the radiation field as a result of endothelial dysfunction.

Specimens from patients with acute hepatic injury secondary to therapeutic irradiation for solid neoplasms are rarely obtained. However, venoocclusive disease is not uncommon in bone marrow transplant patients following cytoreductive therapy with combined chemotherapy and irradiation. Onset of venoocclusive disease in this setting usually occurs before 5 weeks posttransplant. Changes in hepatic histology include vascular congestion that is most prominent in centrilobular areas, subendothelial edema, endothelial destruction, sinusoidal dilation, and centrizonal hepatocyte necrosis with attenuation of the hepatocellular cords.

Evidence of vascular injury and regeneration is a hallmark of chronic radiation injury and is often observed in pathological specimens. Myointimal proliferation in medium-sized muscular arteries may lead to chronic ischemic injury and ulceration caused by the marked decrease in the luminal diameter of these vessels. The presence of lipophages or foamy macrophages in the intima of small arterioles is also a characteristic finding of delayed radiation injury, although these lesions may also result from other etiologies. Telangiectatic vessels in the lamina propria or submucosa are another frequent finding and account for the diffuse bleeding sometimes observed in radiation enteritis. Sclerosis or medial fibrosis indicative of healing vasculitic lesions may also be observed.

Changes in the mucosa and submucosa are also frequently observed in chronic radiation injury and are thought to be secondary to the chronic vascular changes described above. Cellular atypia may be observed in the epithelium lining any region of the alimentary tract that was within the radiation field. Mucosal atrophy resulting in impaired mucosal function is also sometimes observed. Fibrosis may be confined to the submucosa or extend through the muscularis propria and accounts for luminal strictures seen in chronic radiation injury. These strictures may occur within any irradiated region of the alimentary tract. The appearance of these fibrotic lesions in the small intestine may resemble that of Crohn's disease both on gross inspection and on radiological examination, although fistulae and creeping fat are rarely observed.

Yamada's Atlas of Gastroenterology, Fifth Edition. Edited by Daniel K. Podolsky, Michael Camilleri, J. Gregory Fitz, Anthony N. Kalloo, Fergus Shanahan, and Timothy C. Wang.
© 2016 John Wiley & Sons, Ltd. Published 2016 by John Wiley & Sons, Ltd.
Companion website: www.yamadagastro.com/atlas

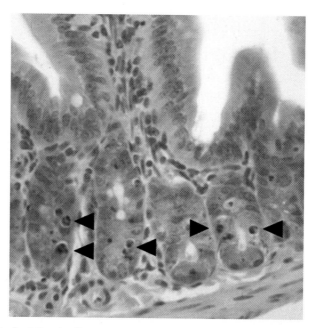

Figure 72.1 Acute radiation injury 6 h after 8 Gy γ-irradiation. Apoptotic cells (programmed cell death; arrowheads) appear within the small intestinal crypt epithelium by 3–6 h after irradiation (FVB/N inbred mouse strain; H & E stain; original magnification ×200). The remaining crypt epithelial cells undergo cell cycle arrest and migrate onto the villi, depleting the crypt of cells over the next 24 h. This experimental sample is from the laboratory mouse because tissue is rarely obtained during this time frame after irradiation in humans.

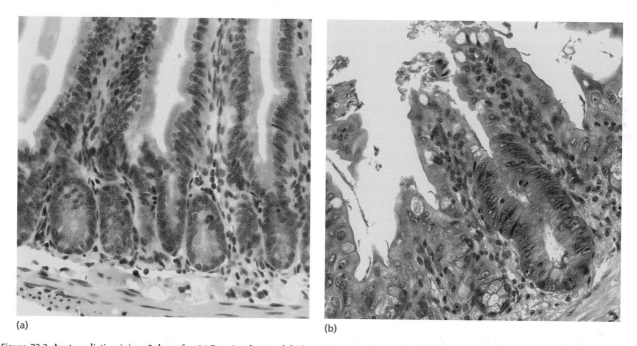

(a)   (b)

Figure 72.2 Acute radiation injury 3 days after 14 Gy γ-irradiation. **(a)** The architecture of normal epithelium in the adult mouse small intestine. **(b)** The histological features found in the small intestine 3 days after irradiation. Note the marked shortening of the intestinal villi, which results from cessation of crypt epithelial replication and lack of replacement of villous epithelial cells after irradiation. The loss of differentiated epithelial cells associated with villous blunting can result in impaired mucosal absorptive function. Expanded regenerative crypts first appear at this time and are composed of rapidly proliferating basophilic cells that are somewhat larger than those found in normal uninjured crypts (H & E stain, original magnification ×400). As in Figure 72.1, this experimental sample was obtained from the laboratory mouse to illustrate the regenerative process after irradiation because tissue is rarely obtained during this time frame after irradiation in humans.

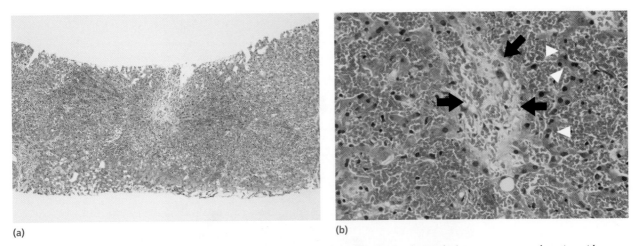

(a) (b)

Figure 72.3 Hepatic venoocclusive disease occurring in a 24-year-old woman after cytoreductive therapy for bone marrow transplantation with combined chemotherapy and irradiation. **(a)** A low-power view of a core biopsy that shows sinusoidal congestion with increased numbers of red blood cells in the centrolobar region (H & E stain; original magnification ×40). **(b)** A higher-power view of the same biopsy that demonstrates fibrinous deposits in a central vein (arrows), atrophy of the hepatic cords (arrowheads), and congestion of the sinusoids, which are packed with red blood cells (H & E stain; original magnification ×200). Source: Courtesy of Dr. Christopher Moskaluk.

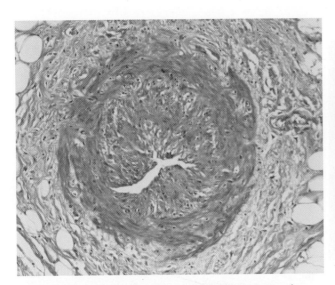

Figure 72.4 Myointimal proliferation nearly occludes the lumen of a moderate-sized mesenteric artery. This process usually occurs over several years after radiation injury and may lead to chronic ischemic injury caused by the marked decrease in the lumenal diameter of these vessels. Ulceration of the overlying mucosa can occur in areas of localized ischemia (H & E stain; original magnification ×100). Source: Courtesy of Dr. Christopher Moskaluk.

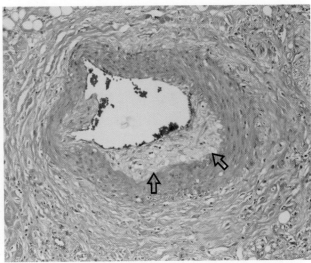

Figure 72.5 Intimal lipophage accumulation in intestinal arteriole following irradiation. These foam cells (arrows) may be seen in the intima of small arteries and arterioles of the intestine several years after irradiation, and may contribute to lumenal narrowing of these vessels and subsequent ischemic injury to the mucosa (H & E stain; original magnification ×100). Source: Courtesy of Dr. Christopher Moskaluk.

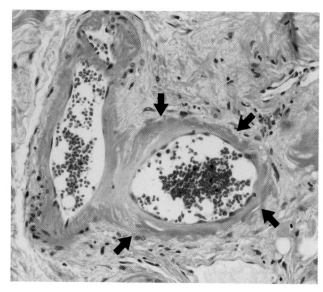

Figure 72.6 Radiation-induced sclerosis of small- to medium-sized blood vessels in the mesenteric vasculature. Sclerosis or medial fibrosis is a histological feature associated with healing vasculitic lesions. Note the hyalinization of the vessel walls (arrows) with prominent vascular ectasia (H & E stain; original magnification ×200). Source: Courtesy of Dr. Christopher Moskaluk.

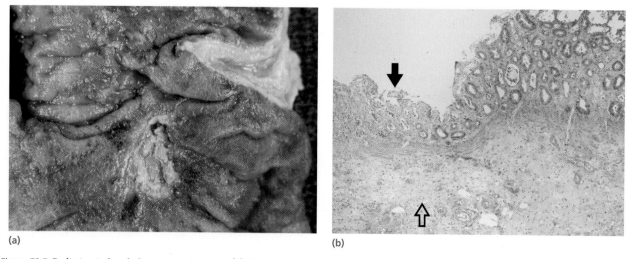

(a)   (b)

Figure 72.7 Radiation-induced ulceration in the colon. **(a)** The gross appearance of a well-demarcated ulcer present in the rectum years after external radiation for an adjacent neoplasm. **(b)** The histological appearance with chronic ulceration, mucosal necrosis similar to that seen in ischemic injury (closed arrow), and dense submucosal fibrosis (open arrow). The fibrosis may be confined to the submucosa or extend through the muscularis propria, and accounts for the thickening or strictures noted on gross examination. These strictures may occur within any irradiated region of the alimentary tract. The lesion is notable because of the absence of a prominent inflammatory infiltrate (H & E stain; original magnification ×20). Source: Courtesy of Dr. Christopher Moskaluk.

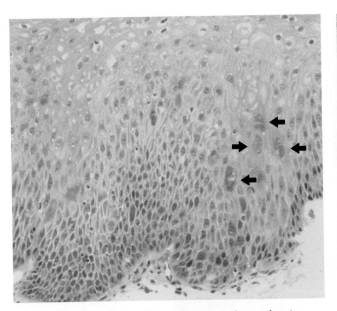

Figure 72.8 Epithelial atypia in the esophagus secondary to chronic radiation injury. Note the presence of enlarged atypical nuclei with irregular nuclear contours (arrows). Hyperchromasia of these atypical cells is rare in contrast to the cellular atypia that is characteristic of neoplastic processes and is an important histological feature distinguishing these two processes (H & E stain; original magnification ×800). Source: Courtesy of Dr. Christopher Moskaluk.

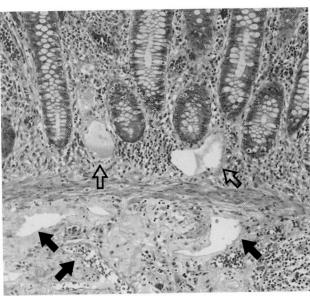

Figure 72.10 Telangiectasias are frequently observed in delayed radiation injury. Dilated venules and lymphatic channels may be seen in the lamina propria (open arrows) or in the submucosa (solid arrows) underlying relatively normal appearing colonic epithelium. These lesions likely account for the diffuse bleeding sometimes observed in chronic radiation enteritis (H & E stain; original magnification ×40). Source: Courtesy of Dr. Christopher Moskaluk.

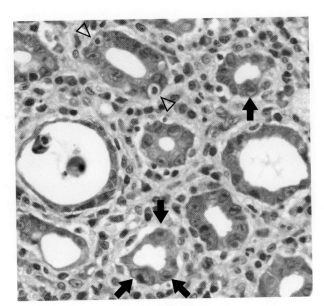

Figure 72.9 Epithelial alterations in the colon secondary to chronic radiation injury. Note the cells with enlarged irregular nuclei with prominent nucleoli (arrows). As in the esophagus in Figure 72.8, the epithelial cellular atypia characteristic of chronic radiation injury is not associated with the nuclear hyperchromasia that is commonly observed in atypia associated with neoplastic processes. Apoptotic cells are noted in some glands (arrowheads). Atrophic glands with flattened and sloughing epithelial cells are also prominent (H & E stain; original magnification ×400). Source: Courtesy of Dr. Christopher Moskaluk.

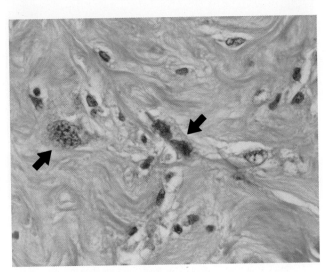

Figure 72.11 Atypical fibroblasts in radiation injury. Bizarre appearing fibroblasts with large pyknotic nuclei (arrows) are frequently seen in delayed phase of radiation injury in the alimentary tract. Although these atypical fibroblasts are frequently observed, their presence is not specific for radiation injury (H & E stain; original magnification ×400). Source: Courtesy of Dr. Christopher Moskaluk.

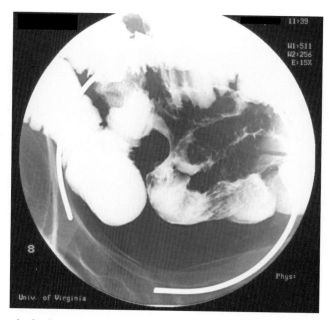

Figure 72.12 Small bowel spot radiograph of radiation enteritis. String-like stricturing and separation of bowel loops seen may give an appearance of Crohn's disease. Source: Courtesy of Dr. H. Shaffer.

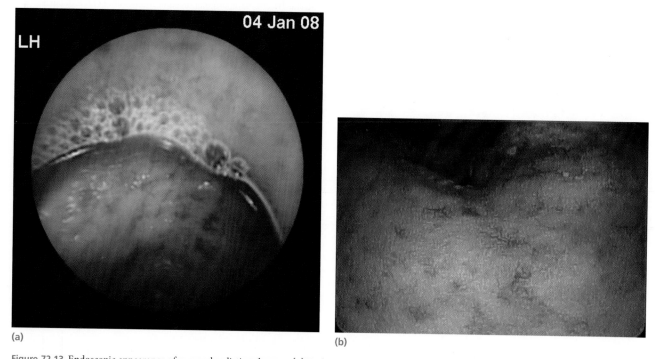

Figure 72.13 Endoscopic appearance of mucosal radiation damage. (a) Endoscopic image of radiation proctitis. Note the mucosal telangiectasias. (b) Capsule endoscopic image of the small intestine showing telangiectasia. Source: Courtesy of Dr. G.S. Raju, Galveston, TX.

PART 3

Diagnostic and therapeutic modalities in gastroenterology

CHAPTER 73

Upper gastrointestinal endoscopy

Ebubekir S. Daglilar,[1] Abdurrahman Kadayifci,[1,2] and William R. Brugge[1]

[1] Massachusetts General Hospital, Boston, MA, USA
[2] University of Gaziantep, Gaziantep, Turkey

The father of modern endoscopy is Rudolf Schindler. He pioneered the use of gastroscopy through the use and development of a semirigid gastroscope. The first endoscope, of a kind, was developed in 1806 by Philip Bozzini with his introduction of a "Lichtleiter" (light conductor) "for the examinations of the canals and cavities of the human body." However, the Vienna Medical Society disapproved of such curiosity. Apparently, an endoscope was first introduced into a human in 1853. The use of electric light was a major step in the improvement of endoscopy. The first such lights were external. Later, smaller bulbs became available, making internal light possible. Jacobeus has been given credit for early endoscopic explorations of the abdomen and the thorax with laparoscopy (1912) and thoracoscopy (1910). For diagnostic endoscopy, Basil Hirschowitz invented a superior glass fiber for flexible endoscopes. The technology resulted in not only the first useful medical endoscope, but the invention revolutionized other endoscopic uses and led to practical fiberoptics.

Technical considerations

Upper gastrointestinal endoscopy is a highly technical procedure that requires a close cooperative arrangement between physicians and nurses. A well-organized facility will optimize patient safety and the ability to provide the appropriate techniques. With only a few exceptions, upper GI endoscopy will be performed in a hospital or a medical care facility that can provide a reliable set of highly trained personnel and specialized equipment. In addition to a wide array of endoscopes and processors, the procedure unit should be equipped with an organized set of accessories used during endoscopy.

In addition to procedure rooms, it is critical to have a travel cart that will enable endoscopists to provide endoscopic procedures at sites remote from an endoscopy unit. Well-maintained, controlled access storage is essential for the endoscopic accessories. There must be a well-designed area for endoscope disinfection and preparation of accessories for sterilization. It is also critical to have preparation and recovery areas for the evaluation and monitoring of patients.

Electrocautery devices are critical to the performance of many endoscopic procedures. In many units, the devices are not installed in each procedure room. Because these devices are frequently used, it is critical that they be readily available during procedures and properly maintained by qualified personnel.

Videoendoscopes

Videoendoscopy, introduced in the mid-1980s, has dramatically improved and expanded the field of endoscopy. Videoendoscopy is now used almost universally. The endoscopic image is generated electronically using a charge-coupled device (CCD) located in the tip of the endoscope. Endoscope processors manage the images and display them on video monitors. Prior to video endoscopy, fiberoptics generated the images on small hand-held eye pieces.

The first videoendoscopes used black and white CCDs that required a color wheel. Green, red, or blue light was sequentially sent down the illumination bundle of the endoscope and activated the CCD at the tip. A color image was reconstructed using the three sets of images generated by the colored lights. The videoprocessor displayed a full-color image of the gastrointestinal tract lining, although with apparent image flickering during rapid movement. Most current videoendoscopes use a color CCD that obtains the image in color on the tip of the endoscope. These devices provide 30 000–850 000 pixels of resolution. By incorporating high-pixel density charged-coupled

Yamada's Atlas of Gastroenterology, Fifth Edition. Edited by Daniel K. Podolsky, Michael Camilleri, J. Gregory Fitz, Anthony N. Kalloo, Fergus Shanahan, and Timothy C. Wang.

devices, high-resolution endoscopes provide images that display vivid mucosal detail. High-resolution endoscopes are capable of discriminating objects 10–70 microns in diameter, compared to the naked eye, which is capable of discriminating objects 125–165 microns in diameter. The videoendoscope has controls for air, water, and suction; plus knobs for up-and-down and right-and-left bending of the tip. The instrument channel is shared for the passage of accessories and suction. There are also buttons on the videoendoscope control handle to activate digital video recording, image capture, and recording video images.

Video endoscopy has greatly expanded the viewing capabilities of procedures. Multiple monitors in the procedure room provide bright vivid images that enable many procedure personnel to participate in procedures. The live video images can also be distributed remotely to sites within an institution or to remote sites for teaching, research, and demonstration. The teaching, instruction, and training of endoscopy has improved dramatically with the use of video endoscopy. Documentation of procedures is provided by the saving, retrieval, and reviewing of stored digital images. Stored images can be recalled from a central image storage system and sent to any location in the endoscopy service. The storage drives can be used for image processing and management as well as a reliable storage of endoscopic images and information on PACS (picture archiving and communication system). The hardware and software are now available for the capture, editing, and storage of video clips. This type of material will further improve teaching and patient care.

Introducing the endoscope

Most small-diameter videoendoscopes can be easily passed under direct vision through the upper esophageal sphincter. The tip of the instrument is advanced in the midline into the direction of the closed cricopharyngeal sphincter. The patient is asked to swallow, and under direct vision the tip of the instrument is passed from the epiglottis and larynx into the proximal esophagus. In the past, endoscopes were passed blindly aided by the swallowing action. The direct vision technique allows an inspection of the pharynx, epiglottis, and vocal cords prior to insertion. Furthermore, direct imaging may decrease the risk of the inadvertent passage of the endoscope into a proximal esophageal diverticulum. Small-diameter videoendoscopes can also be passed transnasally and may provide the opportunity to perform unsedated endoscopy.

Endoscopes are designed with the endoscopic controls (e.g., air, water, and suction valves; tip direction wheels) to be controlled with the left hand. The right hand is used to advance the instrument and use the tip control knob. Torque of the endoscope is accomplished by rotating the instrument control handle with the right hand, which results in rotation of the entire shaft and tip of the endoscope. A central instrument channel is used for a wide variety of devices and accessories. The instrument channel is variable in diameter and there may be two instrument channels in some instruments.

Upper gastrointestinal endoscopy is the basis for many of the diagnostic and therapeutic procedures offered by endoscopists and gastroenterologists. Identification of normal mucosa and normal endoscopic anatomy is critical for determining what is abnormal. This chapter demonstrates normal and pathological endoscopic findings in the esophagus, stomach, and duodenum (Figures 73.1–73.80).

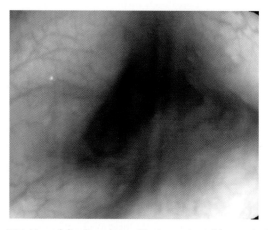

Figure 73.1 Normal distal esophagus. The impression of the vertebral column can be seen in the inferior aspect.

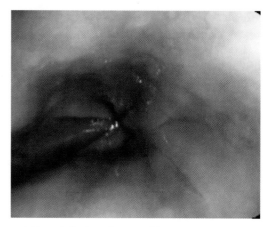

Figure 73.2 Normal distal esophagus and lower esophageal sphincter.

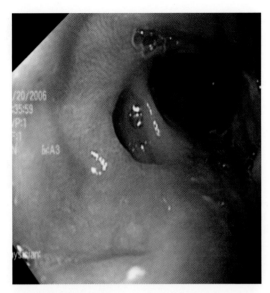

Figure 73.3 Esophageal diverticulum. A small diverticulum can be seen on the left in the distal esophagus.

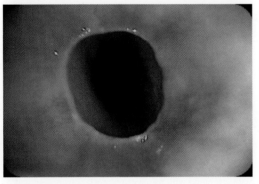

Figure 73.4 Schatzki ring. A Schatzki ring can be appreciated here in the distal esophagus. The junction between the squamous mucosa of the esophagus and the columnar mucosa of the stomach occurs in the vicinity of the ring.

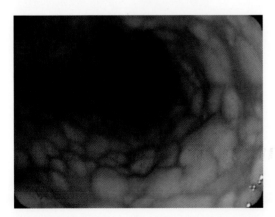

Figure 73.5 Diffuse glycogenic acanthosis. These white nodules represent esophageal glycogenic acanthosis, which is usually sparse and of little clinical significance. This patient has Cowden syndrome, with a marked diffuse presentation.

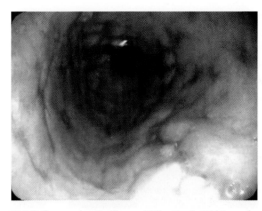

Figure 73.6 Reflux esophagitis. Savary–Miller Grade III (circumferential lesion, erosive, or exudative) reflux type esophagitis can be seen in this image. Multiple erosions in the lower third of the esophagus can be seen in this image.

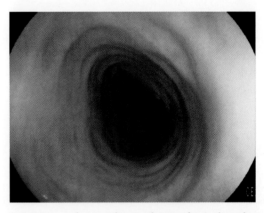

Figure 73.7 Feline esophagus. Feline esophagus refers to the endoscopic finding of a fine stacked concentric ring appearance in the esophagus. Feline esophagus is suggestive of eosinophilic esophagitis, which was proven by biopsy in this 36-year-old man.

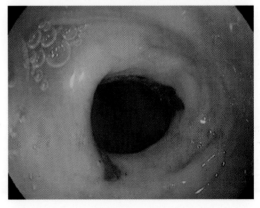

Figure 73.8 Benign intrinsic esophageal stenosis. Endoscopic view of a benign-appearing intrinsic stenosis in the esophagus in a patient with a history of photodynamic therapy for Barrett esophagus.

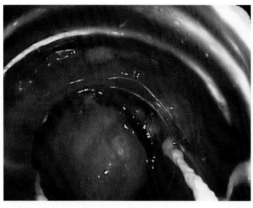

Figure 73.9 Endoscopic mucosal resection. In a region of Barrett esophagus with known high-grade dysplasia, a nodule was found. The nodule is being removed here with an endoscopic mucosal resection. Pathological examination revealed intramucosal adenocarcinoma.

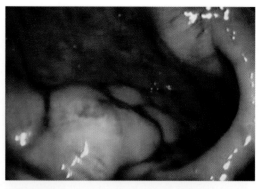

Figure 73.12 Esophageal varices. Large esophageal varices can be seen here in the distal esophagus. At approximately 7 o'clock, a fibrin cap overlies the varix and may have been the source of the bleeding.

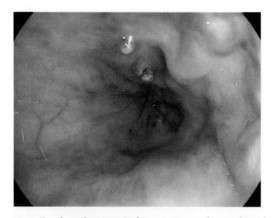

Figure 73.10 Esophageal varices. Endoscopic image of an eradicated varix with a visible vessel overlying it. It had stigmata of recent bleeding. The varices had no red wale signs. One band was successfully placed with complete eradication, resulting in hemostasis.

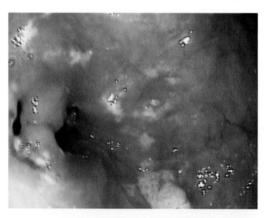

Figure 73.13 Esophageal perforation and fistula. In this image, an esophageal perforation with fistula can be seen. This patient had squamous cell carcinoma of the lung invasive to the esophagus.

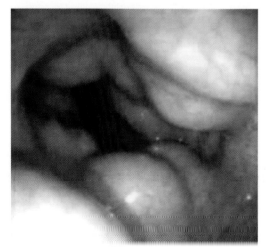

Figure 73.11 Esophageal leiomyoma. In a patient presenting with dysphagia, multiple submucosal masses were discovered on endoscopy. The masses proved to be esophageal leiomyomata.

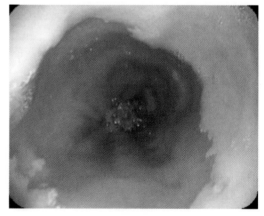

Figure 73.14 Barrett esophagus. This image demonstrates the characteristic salmon-pink mucosa of Barrett esophagus extending proximally from the gastroesophageal junction. The normal esophageal squamous mucosa is pearly white and can be seen here in the proximal portion of the esophagus.

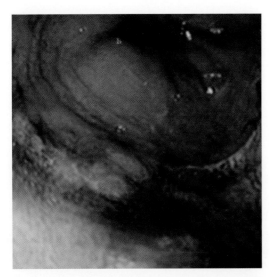

Figure 73.15 Chromoendoscopy. Chromoendoscopy involves staining the gastrointestinal mucosa for better endoscopic visualization, usually for the detection of malignant or premalignant lesions. In this image, Lugol solution has been used to stain the distal esophagus. Negative staining of nodular mucosa can be seen, and biopsy confirmed Barrett esophagus with mild dysplasia. Source: Courtesy of Dr. Moises Guelrud.

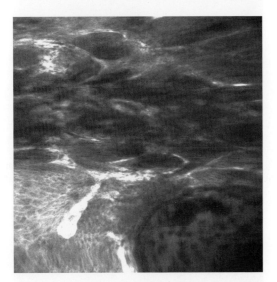

Figure 73.16 Confocal laser endomicroscopy (CLE), Barrett esophagus with high grade dysplasia. CLE is a high resolution endoscopic technique that may enhance the visualization of the fine vasculature and mucosal morphology and may increase diagnostic accuracy. In this patient with Barrett esophagus, high-grade dysplasia, and squamous overgrowth, CLE demonstrates black dysmorphic glands and (in the left corner) squamous epithelium.

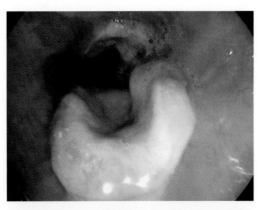

Figure 73.17 Esophageal adenocarcinoma. Endoscopic appearance of a large, malignant-appearing mass in the distal esophagus from 35 to 42 cm, which revealed undifferentiated esophageal adenocarcinoma on biopsy. Left upper corner, the mass appeared to be arising in the background of Barrett esophagus. The mass occupied approximately 30%–40% of the lumen of the esophagus.

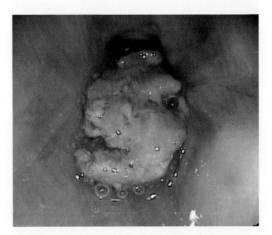

Figure 73.18 Food impaction. Food bolus in the distal esophagus proximal to an esophageal stricture in a patient with Barrett esophagus.

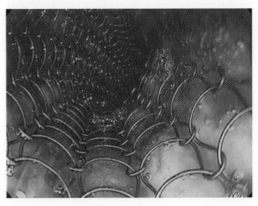

Figure 73.19 Esophageal stent. Metal stent placement for palliation of obstructing gastroesophageal junction adenocarcinoma. The wire mesh of the stent can be seen in this image overlying and compressing a fungating and ulcerated mass.

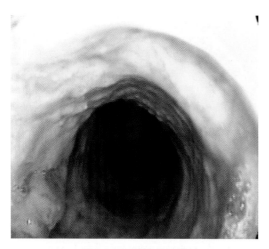

Figure 73.20 Squamous cell cancer of the esophagus. In the mid-esophagus, an irregular nodular plaque was observed in a patient with a history of alcohol and tobacco use. Biopsies revealed moderately differentiated squamous cell cancer of the esophagus.

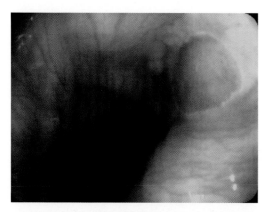

Figure 73.21 Esophageal inlet patch. This lesion in the right superior aspect of the image has the typical appearance of an inlet patch. An inlet patch is an area of heterotopic gastric mucosa characteristically found in the cervical esophagus.

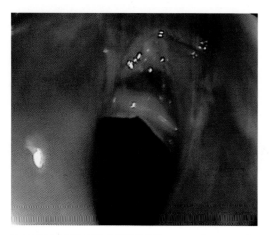

Figure 73.22 Esophageal web. A thin membrane can be seen in the superior aspect of the image. This patient had a cervical esophageal web, which was dilated with passage of the endoscope.

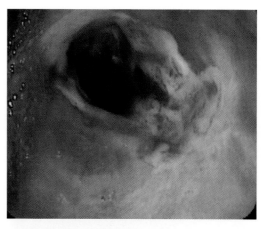

Figure 73.23 Radiation esophagitis. Distal esophageal circumferential ulceration and esophagitis in a patient who had received full-dose radiation therapy for regionally advanced adenocarcinoma.

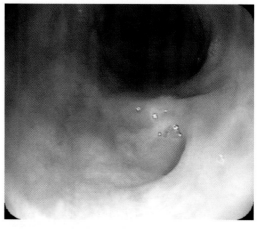

Figure 73.24 Cytomegalovirus esophageal ulcer. Upper endoscopy in a patient with AIDS and dysphagia revealed a distal esophageal ulceration. An immunohistochemical stain for CMV was positive.

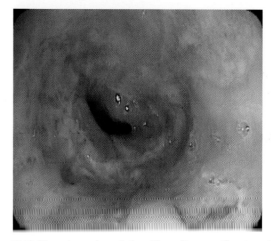

Figure 73.25 Herpetic esophageal ulcer. The earliest manifestation of herpes simplex esophagitis may be vesicular, though this is rarely seen. The herpetic lesions may coalesce. On endoscopy, a well-circumscribed, volcano-appearance has been described. In this case, HSV-1 was cultured from esophageal biopsies.

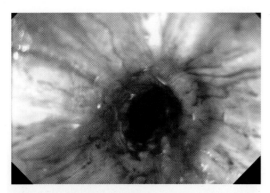

Figure 73.26 Caustic esophagitis. Severe caustic injury to the entire esophagitis in a patient with a history of a suicide attempt by alkaline ingestion.

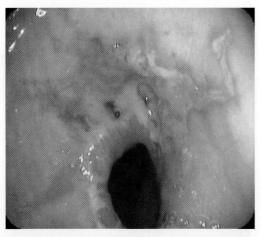

Figure 73.27 Esophagogastric anastomosis. Endoscopic appearance of the esophagogastric anastomosis in a patient who had had an Ivor–Lewis esophagectomy for high-grade dysplasia with intramucosal carcinoma arising in an area of Barrett esophagus.

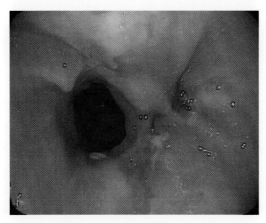

Figure 73.28 Esophagojejunal anastomosis. This patient had an esophagojejunal anastomosis after gastrectomy for gastric cancer. He presented with dysphagia, and a stricture at the anastomosis can be seen here.

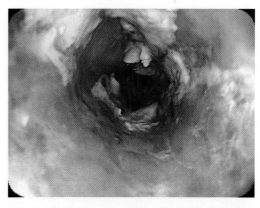

Figure 73.29 Candidal esophagitis. Inflammation with thick white adherent plaques in a patient with AIDS and candidal esophagitis. Fluconazole-sensitive *Candida albicans* was cultured from the esophageal brushing.

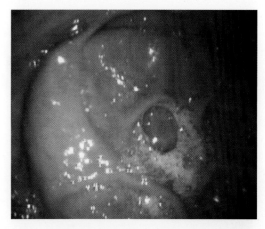

Figure 73.30 Normal gastric body. The appearance of the normal stomach with a prominent splenic impression. A prominent splenic impression may be noted in patients with a low body mass index.

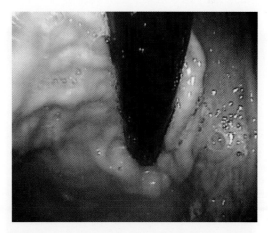

Figure 73.31 Normal gastric cardia. This is the endoscopic view in retroflexion of the normal gastric cardia. The proximal portion of the scope is seen exiting from the gastroesophageal junction.

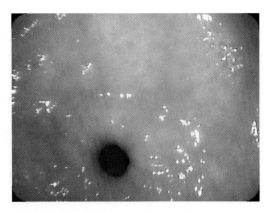

Figure 73.32 Normal gastric antrum. The muscular pylorus is in the lower mid portion of the image.

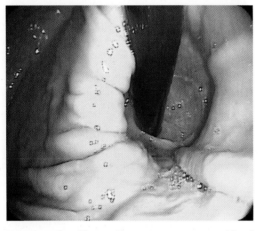

Figure 73.33 Large hiatal hernia. This patient was 86 years old and, on retroflexed view, a large hiatal hernia can be appreciated.

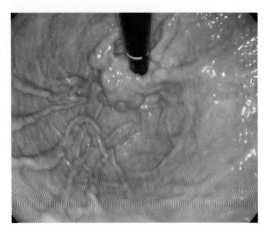

Figure 73.34 Gastric varices without bleeding. Portal hypertensive gastropathy was seen in gastric fundus.

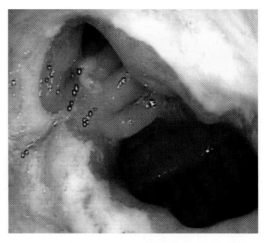

Figure 73.35 Anastomotic ulcer. Circumferential ulceration with overlying fibrinous material at the anastomosis in a patient status-post Roux-en-Y gastric bypass surgery. This patient ultimately underwent a redo gastrojejunostomy with ulcer excision.

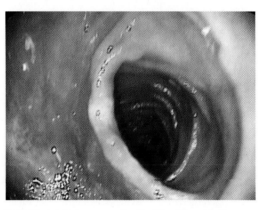

Figure 73.36 Gastric bypass anastomosis. A healthy appearing gastrojejunal anastomosis can be seen here in a woman who underwent a Roux-en-Y gastric bypass for obesity with multiple comorbid conditions.

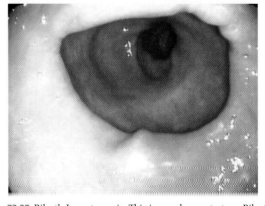

Figure 73.37 Bilroth I anastomosis. This image demonstrates a Bilroth type I anastomosis, where, following antrectomy, the duodenum is anastomosed to the proximal stomach. Antrectomy was common in the years prior to antisecretory therapy for peptic ulcer disease.

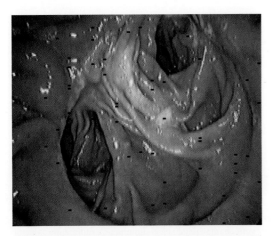

Figure 73.38 Bilroth II anastomosis. This image demonstrates a Bilroth type II anastomosis. In a Bilroth II procedure, a gastrojejunostomy is created. Both the afferent limb (which drains upstream pancreatobiliary secretions) and efferent limb (which allows food and secretions to flow downstream) are visible here.

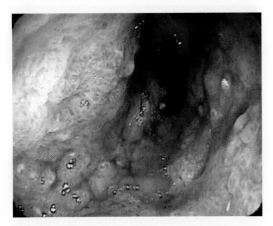

Figure 73.39 Menetrier disease. This patient with hypoalbuminemia presented with markedly enlarged gastric folds. Biopsies revealed edematous gastric mucosa with foveolar hyperplasia and no evidence of malignancy confirming Menetrier disease; however, years later he developed gastric leiomyosarcoma.

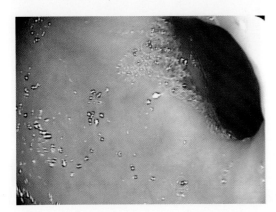

Figure 73.40 Atrophic gastritis. This patient had diffuse atrophic gastritis. The image of the antrum reveals thin mucosa with visible submucosal vessels. Biopsy confirmed chronic antral gastritis with marked intestinal metaplasia consistent with atrophic gastritis.

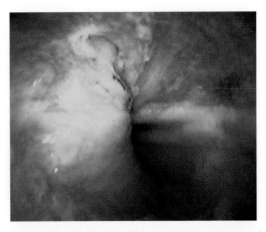

Figure 73.41 Mallory-Weiss tear. Mallory–Weiss tear in a 27-year-old man who presented with emesis followed by hematemesis. Mallory–Weiss tears are longitudinal intramural mucosal lacerations occurring in the distal esophagus and proximal stomach. They are usually associated with forceful retching.

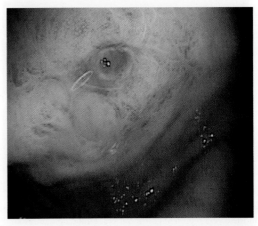

Figure 73.42 Dieulafoy lesion. A Dieulafoy lesion is an uncommon cause of upper gastrointestinal bleeding, resulting from an aberrant dilated submucosal artery eroding through the mucosa in the absence of a primary ulcer. A large Dieulafoy lesion can be seen here in the gastric body.

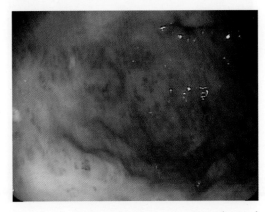

Figure 73.43 Gastric antral vascular ectasia presenting with typical erythematous lesions in the antrum of the stomach. These lesions may require repeated treatments with argon plasma coagulation or electrocautery to prevent recurrent gastrointestinal bleeding.

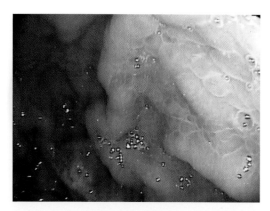

Figure 73.44 Portal hypertensive gastropathy. Endoscopic appearance of portal hypertensive gastropathy in a 55-year-old man with cirrhosis. Note the characteristic snakeskin appearance of the gastric mucosa.

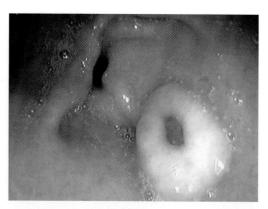

Figure 73.47 Pancreatic rest. Ectopic pancreatic tissue in the gastric antrum with characteristic apical dimpling. A rudimentary ductal system may empty into this depression.

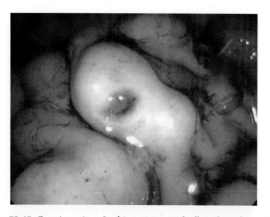

Figure 73.45 Gastric varices. In this patient, markedly enlarged gastric folds in the cardia represent gastric varices. Endoscopic ultrasound can confirm the presence of varices if the diagnosis is in question.

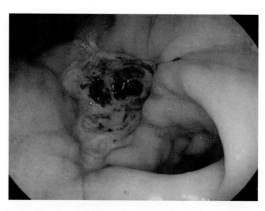

Figure 73.48 Gastric peptic ulcer. Antral gastric ulcer in a patient with a history of heavy nonsteroidal antiinflammatory drug (NSAID) exposure. The patient discontinued her NSAID use and on repeat upper endoscopy, the ulcer had resolved.

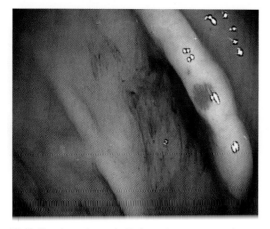

Figure 73.46 Gastric angioectasia. Endoscopic appearance of a gastric angioectasia on a rugal fold in the stomach. This patient presented with bleeding, and hematin (altered blood) can be seen adjacent to the angioectasia.

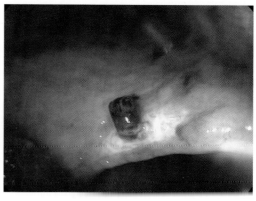

Figure 73.49 Gastric ulcer with adherent clot. This gastric ulcer was located on the incisura. The adherent clot is an endoscopic finding associated with an increased risk of rebleeding.

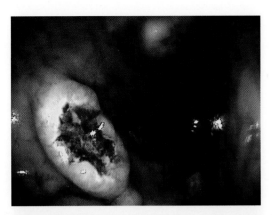

Figure 73.50 Malignant gastric ulcer. This large cratered gastric ulcer had heaped margins and a chronic appearance. Biopsies from this ulcer revealed a signet ring cell adenocarcinoma with ulceration and candidal overgrowth.

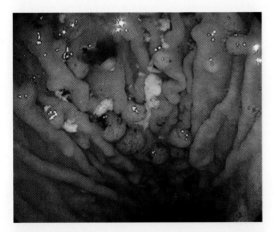

Figure 73.51 Gastric polyps. Multiple 3-mm to 15-mm sessile fundic gland-type polyps were found in the gastric body. Some of these had a hemorrhagic appearance on the surface. The largest and the hemorrhagic-appearing polyps were removed with a hotsnare. Many of the smaller polyps were snared with a cold snare. At least 20 polyps were removed. Pathology confirmed the polyps were consistent of proton pump inhibitor therapy. No polyps were seen after a year follow-up with use of an H_2 receptor blocker for gastroesophageal reflux disease symptoms.

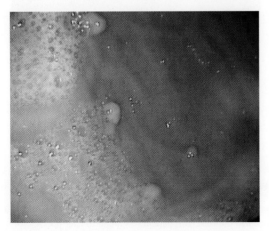

Figure 73.52 Fundic gland polyps. These small sessile polyps distributed in the body and fundus in a patient with a history of proton pump inhibitor therapy are characteristic of fundic gland polyps.

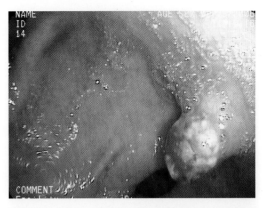

Figure 73.53 Hyperplastic polyp. An inflamed hyperplastic polyp is seen here in the antrum of the stomach. Hyperplastic polyps are the most common type of gastric polyp and, while they have a low malignant potential, should be removed at the time of endoscopy.

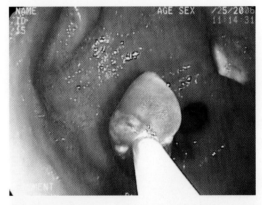

Figure 73.54 Endoscopic appearance of polyp tissue being removed after snare polypectomy in the gastric antrum.

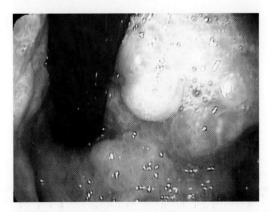

Figure 73.55 Gastric carcinoid tumor. A large fungating and submucosal noncircumferential mass was found in the cardia in this patient with multiple endocrine neoplasia type 1. Biopsies confirmed a low-grade carcinoid tumor.

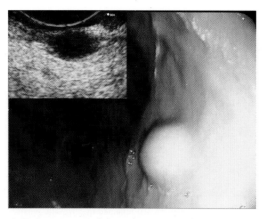

Figure 73.56 Gastrointestinal stromal tumor (GIST). Endoscopic appearance of a 1.3-cm GIST in the stomach. The lesion appeared to originate from within the submucosa (layer 3).

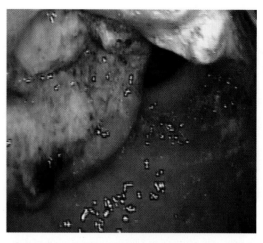

Figure 73.59 Moderately differentiated invasive gastric adenocarcinoma. An ulcerated mass in the antrum of the stomach seen here in an 84-year-old Korean woman with iron deficiency anemia. Stomach cancer is the most prevalent malignant neoplasm in Korea.

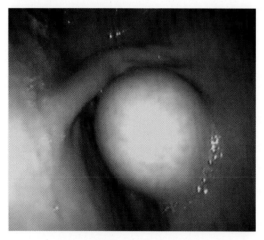

Figure 73.57 Gastric antral lipoma. A submucosal mass is seen here in the antrum. After resection, the pathological examination revealed a lipoma.

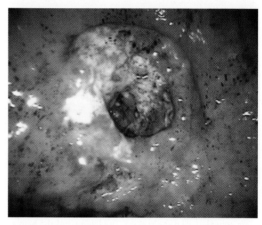

Figure 73.60 Gastric adenocarcinoma. Irregular fungating ulcerated pyloric channel mass. The mass was an invasive poorly differentiated adenocarcinoma on biopsy.

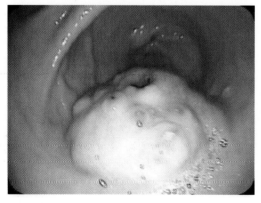

Figure 73.58 Glomus tumor. Endoscopic image of a glomus tumor in the antrum of the stomach. Glomus tumors are benign lesions originating from the modified smooth muscle cells of the glomus body and are rarely seen in the stomach. These submucosal lesions may present with overlying mucosal ulceration, as seen here.

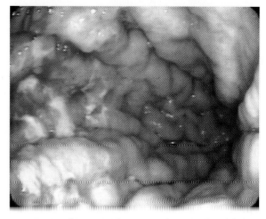

Figure 73.61 Linitis plastica. In this image, the rugal folds of the stomach are thickened diffusely. This patient was found to have poorly differentiated metastatic adenocarcinoma of the breast.

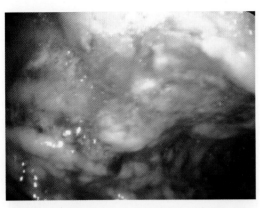

Figure 73.62 Gastric mucosa-associated lymphoid tissue (MALT) lymphoma. Friable ulcerated mucosa on the lesser curvature on the stomach. Biopsies revealed a dense lymphoid infiltrate with focal ulceration consistent with low-grade marginal zone (MALT) B-cell lymphoma.

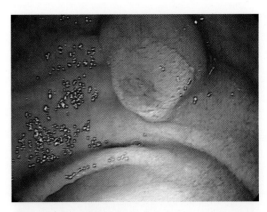

Figure 73.65 Normal ampulla. Using a side viewing endoscope, the papilla can usually be easily seen. The ampulla was normal in this patient.

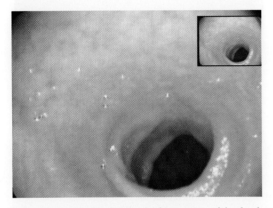

Figure 73.63 Normal duodenal bulb. The first portion of the duodenum, just after the pylorus, is referred to as the duodenal bulb.

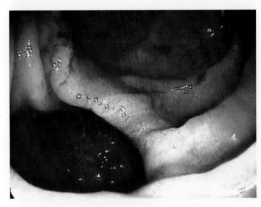

Figure 73.66 Large duodenal diverticulum. A large duodenal diverticular cavity can be seen in the lower left aspect of the image.

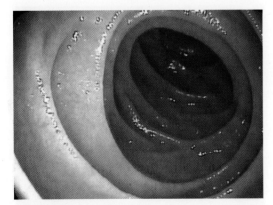

Figure 73.64 Normal duodenum. Normal appearance of the second portion of the duodenum.

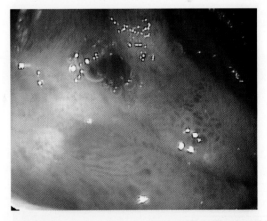

Figure 73.67 Duodenal ulcer. A duodenal ulcer with a pulsatile visible vessel was found in the duodenal bulb in a patient who presented with melena. The presence of a visible vessel is an endoscopic feature that is associated with an increased risk of recurrent bleeding.

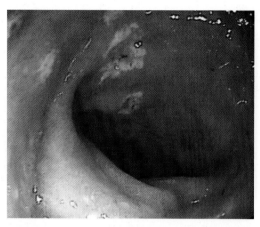

Figure 73.68 Duodenal erosions. White patches in the distal duodenal bulb. Erosions are differentiated from ulcers by the depth of penetration. In contrast to ulcers, erosions remain superficial to muscularis mucosa.

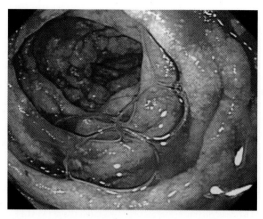

Figure 73.71 Intestinal lymphangiectasia. Endoscopic appearance of diffuse intestinal lymphangiectasia. The white papules arising from the duodenal mucosa represent lymph in dilated lacteals in the mucosa.

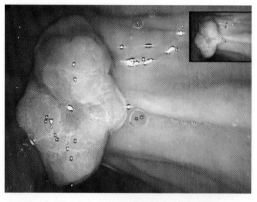

Figure 73.69 Periampullary mass. Endoscopic view of a large periampullary mass with clear yellow bile draining from the central portion of the lesion. After resection, this mass was found to be a tubular adenoma.

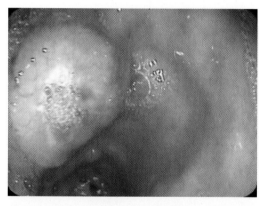

Figure 73.72 Duodenal metastatic tumor. A mass was found in the duodenal bulb in a patient with hepatocellular carcinoma. Biopsies confirmed metastatic hepatocellular carcinoma.

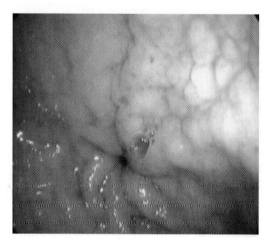

Figure 73.70 Celiac disease. Duodenal mucosa in the bulb with a scalloped mosaic appearance in a patient with celiac disease. This patient had a high titer of antiendomysial and tissue transglutaminase antibodies. Small bowel biopsies confirmed villous blunting, crypt hyperplasia, and markedly increased intraepithelial lymphocytes.

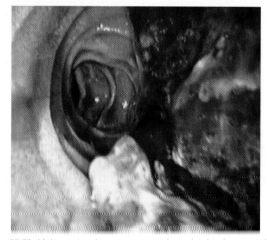

Figure 73.73 Malignant melanoma, metastatic to the duodenum. A large fungating pigmented mass with minimal bleeding can be seen here involving the second portion of the duodenum. The ampulla was not involved.

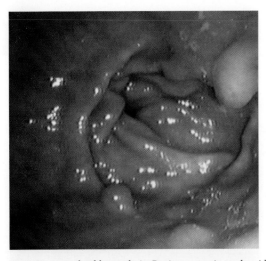

Figure 73.74 Brunner gland hyperplasia. Benign-appearing polypoid lesions can be seen here in the bulb of the duodenum. These are consistent with Brunner gland hyperplasia.

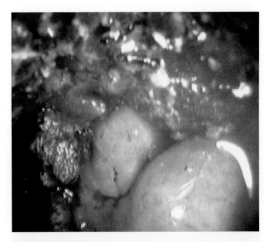

Figure 73.77 Duodenal lymphoma. A firm mass can be seen here in the fourth portion of the duodenum. This patient had a history of kidney transplant and biopsies confirmed a diffuse large B-cell lymphoma.

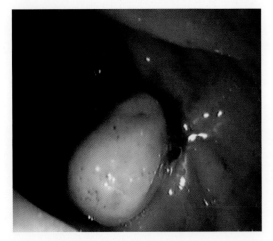

Figure 73.75 Duodenal lipoma. A submucosal mass can be seen in the second portion of the duodenum. Pathological examination confirmed the clinical impression of a lipoma.

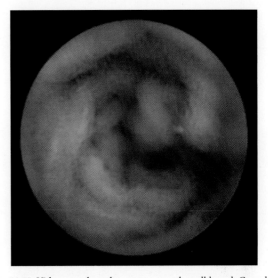

Figure 73.78 Video capsule endoscopy – normal small bowel. Capsule endoscopy involves ingestion of a capsule-sized device that obtains images of the gastrointestinal tract and transmits data to a recorder worn by patients during the study. This image reveals the typical appearance of the normal small bowel folds and villi. Source: Courtesy of Dr. Myles D. Keroack.

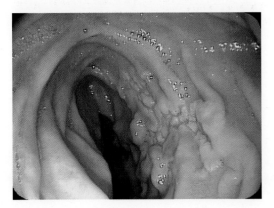

Figure 73.76 Duodenal adenoma. A mass can be appreciated in the second portion of the duodenum. Biopsies confirmed that the mass was a tubulovillous adenoma.

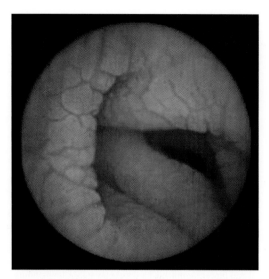

Figure 73.79 Video capsule endoscopy – celiac disease. Capsule endoscopy in a patient with celiac disease reveals scalloping of the small intestinal mucosa. Source: Courtesy of Dr. Myles D. Keroack.

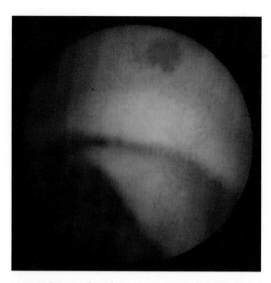

Figure 73.80 Video capsule endoscopy – angioectasia. Capsule endoscopy may be indicated in some patients with obscure gastrointestinal bleeding. This image reveals an angioectasia in the small intestine. Source: Courtesy of Dr. Myles D. Keroack.

CHAPTER 74

Capsule and small bowel endoscopy

Jonathan A. Leighton and Shabana F. Pasha
Mayo Clinic, Scottsdale, AZ, USA

The small bowel is a tortuous tubular organ 600–800 cm in length. Anatomically, it lies between the pylorus and the ileocecal valve. It comprises three segments: the duodenum, the jejunum, and the ileum. The duodenum is the most proximal and shortest segment of the small bowel, with a mean length of 25 cm. It is shaped like a C-loop. This is the only segment located in the retroperitoneal space, and it is therefore relatively fixed. It includes the duodenal bulb and the second, third, and fourth portions, and it extends up to the ligament of Treitz. The ampulla of Vater lies in the second portion of the duodenum. The remainder of the small bowel is suspended in the peritoneal cavity by a broad-based mesentery, and it is freely mobile. The proximal 40% of this portion is the jejunum and the remaining distal 60% is the ileum. The luminal surface of the small bowel has numerous folds called the plicae circulares. The plicae are most prominent in the proximal small bowel, and decrease in number distally.

Historically, suspected small bowel disease was classified as proximal and distal to the ligament of Treitz. Since the introduction of capsule endoscopy and deep enteroscopy, the small bowel is now divided into three segments: the upper tract proximal to the ligament of Treitz, the lower tract distal to the ileocecal valve, and the midgut, which refers to the portion of the small bowel located between the ampulla and the ileocecal valve that can be identified more definitively using these new imaging techniques.

These advances in small-bowel endoscopy have led to a significant improvement in the endoscopic evaluation and management of small bowel disorders, including obscure gastrointestinal bleeding, Crohn's disease, and small bowel tumors (Figures 74.1, 74.2, and 74.3). The entire small bowel can now be visualized in a noninvasive manner using capsule endoscopy. The patency capsule is useful to confirm patency of the gastrointestinal tract prior to administration of the capsule in patients with a suspected obstruction or stricture (Figure 74.4). Therapeutic management of small bowel lesions is now possible with deep enteroscopy techniques, including balloon-assisted and spiral enteroscopy. Each of these devices has unique advantages and disadvantages that should be taken into consideration during selection of the appropriate modality. As a result, capsule endoscopy and deep enteroscopy techniques are often complementary and utilized together in the evaluation of suspected small bowel disorders.

The images in this chapter illustrate the clinical usefulness of these new small bowel modalities in the evaluation of patients with vascular lesions (Figure 74.5), inflammatory lesions (Figure 74.6), celiac sprue (Figure 74.7), polyps (Figure 74.8), and tumors (Figures 74.9, 74.10, and 74.11).

Yamada's Atlas of Gastroenterology, Fifth Edition. Edited by Daniel K. Podolsky, Michael Camilleri, J. Gregory Fitz, Anthony N. Kalloo, Fergus Shanahan, and Timothy C. Wang.
© 2016 John Wiley & Sons, Ltd. Published 2016 by John Wiley & Sons, Ltd.
Companion website: www.yamadagastro.com/atlas

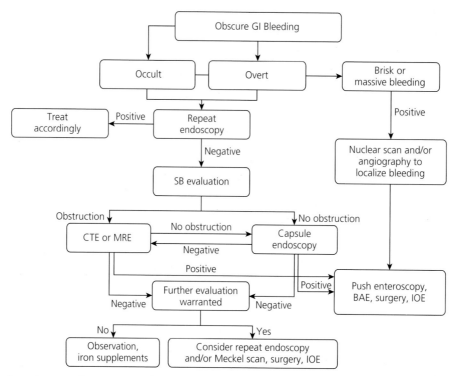

Figure 74.1 Algorithm for evaluation and management of patients with obscure gastrointestinal bleeding. BAE, balloon-assisted enteroscopy; CTE, computed tomography enterography; GI, gastrointestinal; IOE, intraoperative enteroscopy; MRE, magnetic resonance enterography; SB, small bowel. Source: Adapted from Leighton JA. The role of endoscopic imaging of the small bowel in clinical practice. Am J Gastroenterol 2011;106:27. Reproduced with permission.

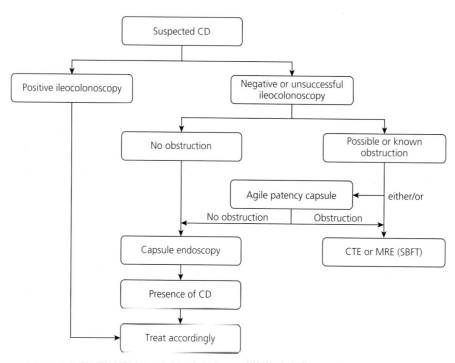

Figure 74.2 Algorithm for evaluation of patients with suspected Crohn's disease (CD). Crohn's disease; CTE, computed tomography enterography; MRE, magnetic resonance enterography; SBFT, small bowel follow through. Source: Mergener K, Ponchon T, Gralnek I, et al. Literature review and recommendations for clinical application of small-bowel capsule endoscopy, based on a panel discussion by international experts: consensus statements for small-bowel capsule endoscopy, 2006/2007. Endoscopy 2007;39:895. Erratum In: Endoscopy 2007;39:1105. Reproduced with permission of Thieme Publishing Group.

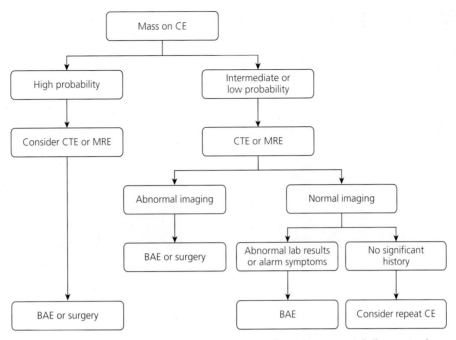

Figure 74.3 Algorithm for evaluation and management of patients with suspected small bowel tumor. BAE, balloon-assisted enteroscopy; CE, capsule endoscopy; CTE, computed tomography enterography; lab, laboratory; MRE, magnetic resonance enterography. Source: Adapted from Leighton JA. The role of endoscopic imaging of the small bowel in clinical practice. Am J Gastroenterol 2011;106:27. Reproduced with permission.

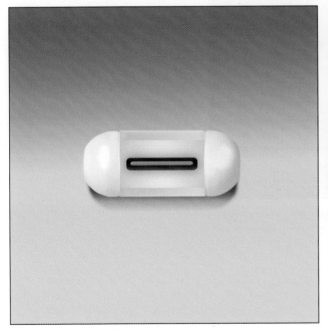

Figure 74.4 Patency capsule. The Agile Patency System (Given Imaging Ltd, Yoqneam, Israel) contains a radiofrequency identification tag covered with a dissolvable body of lactose and barium with a timer plug at either end. Image reproduced with permission.

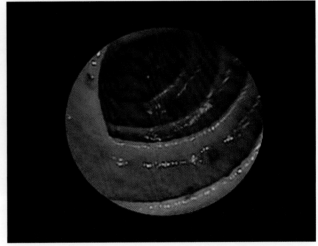

Figure 74.5 Antegrade double-balloon enteroscopy showing angiectasias. This 64-year-old woman presented with melena and iron-deficiency anemia.

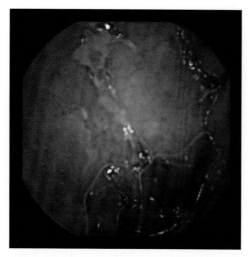

Figure 74.6 Capsule endoscopy showing mucosal ulcerations in the distal ileum. This 45-year-old man presented with abdominal pain and diarrhea. Ileocolonoscopy and computed tomography enterography were both negative. The diagnosis of Crohn's disease was confirmed with retrograde double-balloon enteroscopy and biopsies.

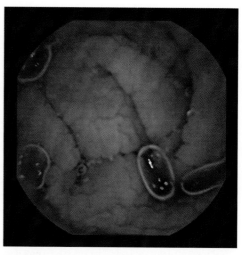

Figure 74.7 Capsule endoscopy showing mucosal nodularity and fissuring in the proximal small bowel. This 54-year-old woman had an elevated immunoglobin A tissue transglutaminase antibody titer of 75 U/mL. The diagnosis of celiac sprue was confirmed with push enteroscopy and biopsies.

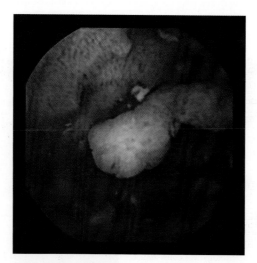

Figure 74.8 Capsule endoscopy view of a hamartomatous polyp in the small bowel of a 25-year-old woman with Peutz–Jeghers syndrome.

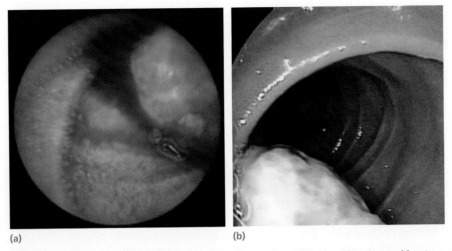

(a)   (b)

Figure 74.9 **(a)** Capsule endoscopy showing a polypoid lesion with active bleeding in the midjejunum. This 61-year-old patient presented with hematochezia. **(b)** Double-balloon enteroscopy showing a polypoid hemangioma. A polypoid hemangioma was also found in the 61-year-old patient with hematochezia in whom capsule endoscopy previously showed a polypoid lesion with active bleeding in the midjejunum.

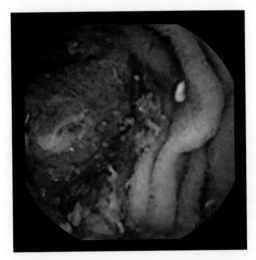

Figure 74.10 Capsule endoscopy showing a small bowel tumor in the proximal midjejunum. The capsule was retained proximal to the tumor. Surgical resection of the tumor was performed. Pathology was consistent with a melanoma.

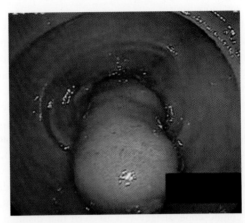

Figure 74.11 Large hamartomatous polyp in the ileum diagnosed on retrograde double-balloon enteroscopy. This 72-year-old man had intermittent hematochezia. Two prior capsule endoscopies had been negative.

To access the videos for this chapter, please go to

www.yamadagastro.com/atlas

Video 74.1 Deep enteroscopy performed for ablation of angioectasias with argon plasma coagulation. This 62-year-old man presented with recurrent iron-deficiency anemia. Upper endoscopy and colonoscopy were normal, but capsule endoscopy showed multiple angioectasias in the proximal small bowel.

Video 74.2 (a) Retrograde deep enteroscopy shows a jejunal varix with an adherent clot. This 72-year-old woman with a history of alcoholic cirrhosis presented with maroon stools. Push enteroscopy did not reveal an upper gastrointestinal source for the bleeding. Colonoscopy findings were also negative, although blood could be seen coming from the small bowel.

Video 74.2 (b) Injection of cyanoacrylate glue to control bleeding in the jejunal varix.

CHAPTER 75

Colonoscopy and flexible sigmoidoscopy

Peter H. Rubin, Steven Naymagon, Christopher B. Williams, and Jerome D. Waye

Icahn School of Medicine at Mount Sinai, New York, NY, USA

Colonoscopy is the most direct and effective modality for diagnosing diseases affecting the colonic and distal ileal mucosa. Various pathological findings can be readily identified, including polyps, cancers, inflammation, and vascular lesions. In addition, colonoscopy allows for interventions, including biopsy, polypectomy, hemostasis, and stricture dilation. While the list of pathologies that may affect the colon is quite expansive, the potential endoscopic findings resulting from these diseases is more limited.

As the endoscopist advances the colonoscope from the rectum to the cecum several key anatomical landmarks are encountered. The folds of rectum (or Houston's valves) are semilunar transverse folds that protrude into the lumen. Transition from rectum to colon is noted by the more circular haustra in the sigmoid and descending colon. Once the splenic flexure is traversed, the triangular folds of the transverse colon can be seen. The hepatic flexure is identified by the bluish shadow of the liver, which abuts the serosal surface of the colon. Upon reaching the cecum the appendiceal orifice appears as a semilunar slit and the ileocecal valve as a notched fold just distal to the caput cecum (Figure 75.1). If the terminal ileum is intubated by the colonoscope, shaggy villi are seen that distinguish the small bowel from the colonic mucosa, which is smooth and glassy with interlacing delicate vascularity visible through the transparent epithelial surface.

Diverticulosis is a common colonoscopic finding, especially in the left colon of patients older than 50 (Figure 75.2). The number and size of colonic diverticula can vary. In severe cases, innumerable large diverticular openings can be seen, sometimes challenging the endoscopist to identify the true lumen of the colon. In addition, diverticulosis may be associated with muscular hypertrophy causing the lumen to become even narrower with spasm and marked tortuosity. While most patients with diverticulosis are asymptomatic, some patients will develop diverticular bleeding. Colonoscopy can help diagnose active or recent diverticular hemorrhage, although the exact site of bleeding is rarely identified. If the culprit diverticulum is found, it

can be treated with bipolar cautery, epinephrine injection, or clipping. Another sequel of diverticulosis that may be identified colonoscopically is diverticular colitis, an inflammatory process of the interdiverticular mucosa. Findings include erythema, edema, friability, and ulceration in the colonic segment affected by diverticulosis but sparing the diverticular orifices themselves. Diverticular colitis may be difficult to distinguish from inflammatory bowel disease.

The most common reason for performing colonoscopy is screening and surveillance for colonic polyps. A polyp is a protuberance of mucosal origin above the normally flat colonic surface (Figures 75.3 and 75.4). These mucosal-based lesions are distinct from submucosal lesions, such as lipomas and carcinoid tumors, which may also cause protrusion into the colonic lumen (Figure 75.5). While most polyps arise sporadically, certain inherited conditions and a family history of colon polyps increases the risk. An extreme example is familial adenomatous polyposis, which is a genetic condition that may lead to the development of hundreds of polyps and typically requires colectomy (Figure 75.6).

Colonic polyps vary in their endoscopic appearance. Pedunculated polyps grow on a stalk of normal mucosa or fibrous tissue (Figure 75.7), while sessile polyps have a broad base without a discrete stalk (Figures 75.4 and 75.8). Histologically, polyps may be classified as adenomatous or hyperplastic. Adenomatous polyps, which may be either pedunculated or sessile, are dysplastic and have malignant potential. Upon close inspection, they often have a cerebriform mucosal pit pattern and obliteration of the normal mucosal vascular pattern (Figures 75.7 and 75.8). Hyperplastic polyps appear as pale, translucent, sessile lesions (Figure 75.3). They are usually seen in the left colon and are composed of nondysplastic cells. In recent years much attention has been paid to a class of polyps called serrated adenomas, which are typically sessile lesions arising in the right colon and may be identified by a mucus covering (Figure 75.4). It has been hypothesized that these lesions give rise to carcinoma through a distinct, accelerated mechanism.

Yamada's Atlas of Gastroenterology, Fifth Edition. Edited by Daniel K. Podolsky, Michael Camilleri, J. Gregory Fitz, Anthony N. Kalloo, Fergus Shanahan, and Timothy C. Wang.

© 2016 John Wiley & Sons, Ltd. Published 2016 by John Wiley & Sons, Ltd.

Companion website: www.yamadagastro.com/atlas

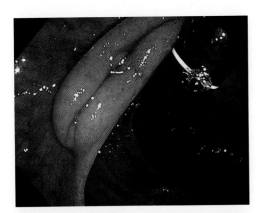

Figure 75.1 Ileocecal valve. The ileocecal valve is typically viewed in profile during colonoscopy such that only one side of the valve is visible. If retroflexion is performed in the cecum, a head-on view of the valve can be obtained as shown in this image. This affords a clear view of both lips of the valve and allows for closer inspection for polyps, inflammation, and ulcers. Retroflexion in the cecum and right colon is also a valuable technique for detecting polyps, which may be hidden behind colonic folds and may otherwise be missed.

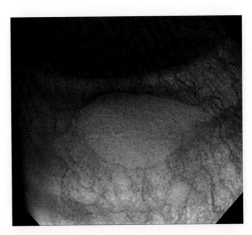

Figure 75.3 Hyperplastic polyp. These are typically found in the rectosigmoid region and can be identified by their sessile nature, pale coloration, and relatively normal pit pattern. These lesions are not dysplastic and have no malignant potential. However, because it may be difficult to definitively distinguish them from adenomas, hyperplastic polyps are often resected during colonoscopy.

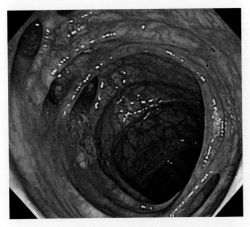

Figure 75.2 Diverticulosis. This is a common endoscopic finding typically seen in the sigmoid colon. Diverticula are out-pouchings of the colonic mucosa and submucosa at areas of weakness in the colonic wall. Dense diverticulosis can make colonoscopy challenging by creating numerous openings, which may be mistaken for the colonic lumen. In addition, severe diverticulosis has been associated with hypertrophy of colonic folds and segmental inflammation known as diverticular colitis.

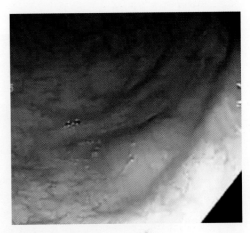

Figure 75.4 Sessile serrated adenoma. Sessile serrated adenomas/polyps pose a challenge for endoscopists. As shown in this image, the lesion may be very subtle. It is very flat and pale with an altered mucosal vascular pattern and a mucus cap. Sessile serrated polyps are often found in the right colon and may progress more rapidly through the adenoma–carcinoma sequence than traditional adenomas.

When a polyp is encountered the endoscopist has various management options. Ideally, the lesion can be completely removed via biopsy forceps in the case of small polyps or snare polypectomy for larger polyps (Figure 75.9). Cautery can be applied to the biopsy forceps or the snare in order to cauterize mucosal vessels and minimize bleeding. If needed, a submucosal injection of saline can be made at the base of the polyp to elevate it and create a "cushion" in order to decrease the risk of transmural burn or perforation. Large polyps can be removed using this technique called endoscopic mucosal resec-

tion (Figure 75.10). The specimen can then be retrieved and sent for histopathological analysis (Figure 75.11). If the lesion is deemed endoscopically unresectable, mucosal biopsies are taken to help with diagnosis and a carbon "tattoo" can be applied to permit localization of the lesion at future endoscopic sessions or surgery. Polypectomy is a safe procedure with a low risk of bleeding and perforation. If immediate or delayed bleeding occurs it can often be managed endoscopically with epinephrine injection, bipolar cautery, or application of clips to the polypectomy site. Perforations may occasionally be managed

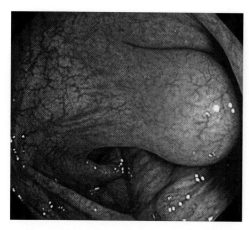

Figure 75.5 Lipoma. In contrast to colorectal polyps, which are of mucosal origin, lipomas are submucosal. Therefore, the mucosal surface of these lesions appears normal except for a yellow discoloration resulting from the underlying fat. If probed, lipomas are soft and demonstrate the "pillow sign." These lesions are benign and need not be removed.

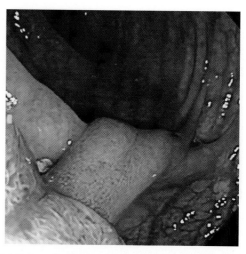

Figure 75.7 Pedunculated polyp. Adenomatous polyps may grow on a long stalk, or pedicle, which is created by chronic traction on the polyp by colonic peristalsis. In this image, the head of the polyp is in the lower left with a long stalk extending from the colonic mucosa. Note the difference in pit pattern between the head of the polyp and the stalk. The presence of the stalk often makes snare polypectomy simpler by allowing the endoscopist to capture the stalk and perform a clean en bloc resection.

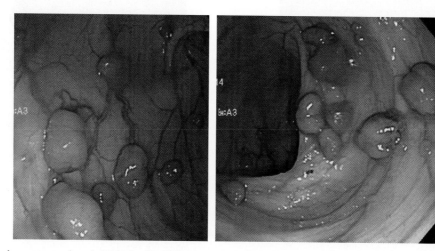

Figure 75.6 Familial adenomatous polyposis. Multiple colon polyps occur in familial adenomatous polyposis (FAP). Patients with FAP may develop innumerable colonic adenomas at a young age. The development of colorectal cancer is universal and early colectomy is usually recommended prophylactically.

endoscopically by applying clips to close the mucosal defect. However, even if endoscopic therapy is performed, surgical consultation is always prudent.

Unfortunately, some colonic lesions are identified only after progression to carcinoma. Malignant tumors of the colon grow in a haphazard manner. Ulceration is a frequent finding, as is sloughing of a portion of the surface (Figure 75.12). The endoscopic appearance may vary from an apparent indentation on the top of a polyp to an obvious, fungating tumor (Figure 75.13). The cancer may be bulky or may ulcerate and become relatively flat in configuration (Figure 75.14). The role of the endoscopist in these cases is to take adequate biopsies, mark the lesion so

that it can be readily identified in the operating room, and rule out synchronous polyps or cancers.

Inflammation or colitis is another common finding encountered by the endoscopist. Many diseases can cause colitis, including viral, bacterial, and parasitic infections, inflammatory bowel disease, transient or prolonged colonic ischemia, numerous medications including nonsteroidal antiinflammatory drugs, and various systemic diseases such as Behçet syndrome and graft-versus-host disease. Despite the broad differential diagnosis of colonic inflammation, the mucosal findings are fairly uniform. In mild colitis, mucosal erythema, edema, and friability are noted. This causes the mucosa to become opaque

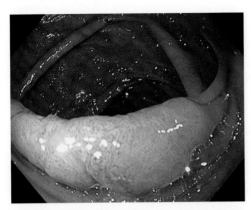

Figure 75.8 Sessile polyp. In contrast to pedunculated polyps, sessile polyps do not have a stalk but rather a broad flat base. This polyp morphology is more commonly found in the right colon where colonic contractions lack the vigor necessary to cause traction leading to formation of a stalk. This image shows a large sessile lesion occupying much of the surface area of a colonic fold. Due to the flat nature of these lesions polypectomy may be very challenging.

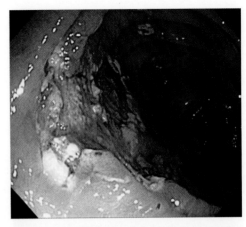

Figure 75.10 Postpolypectomy mucosal defect. This image shows a large mucosal defect following endoscopic mucosal resection of a broad-based sessile polyp. The blue tint in the defect is a result of injecting fluid containing blue dye into the submucosa under the polyp to lift it away from deeper layers of the colon wall and facilitate polypectomy. Demonstrated here is the use of argon plasma coagulation to destroy any residual adenomatous tissue at the edges of a polypectomy site.

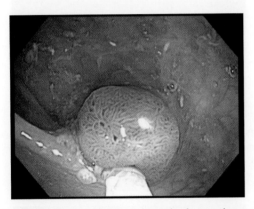

Figure 75.9 Snare polypectomy. Most colorectal polyps can be removed via snare polypectomy. In this image a lesion is being encircled by a polypectomy snare just prior to resection. "Cold snare" is often used for smaller polyps while larger lesions may require the use of electrocautery to provide better hemostasis. Note the polyp's cerebriform pit pattern, which is typical of an adenoma.

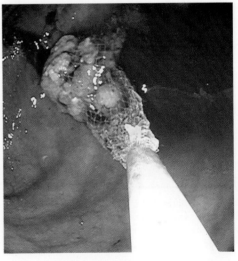

Figure 75.11 Basket retrieval. After polypectomy is completed the specimen must be retrieved for histopathological analysis. One technique for doing so employs a basket that is passed through the colonoscope and allows for several fragments to be collected at once.

and obscures the normal branching vascular pattern. In more severe cases, the inflammatory process can lead to frank ulceration, exudates, and spontaneous bleeding (Figure 75.15). Colitis can be diffuse, affecting most or all of the colonic surface area, or segmental, with sparing of some colonic segments.

In cases of chronic colitis, the inflammation may permanently damage the colonic mucosa. Mild cases may manifest as linear, pale scarring in the background of normal healed mucosa (Figure 75.16). In more extreme cases, ulcerations can become deeper and may interlink; with healing, the intervening islands of inflamed but not ulcerated mucosa exhibit a different growth

pattern than the thin, reepithelialized mucosa that regenerates over ulcerated segments (Figures 75.17 and 75.18). This difference in growth pattern may cause the development of mucosal protrusions known as postinflammatory polyps or "pseudopolyps." These lesions are typically small, shiny, worm-like, and may contain a white cap (Figure 75.19). Pseudopolyps have no malignant potential but if they become large and numerous they may cause obstruction, bleeding, or impede surveillance of the colon.

Another potential consequence of chronic colitis is the development of colorectal dysplasia and cancer. Patients with

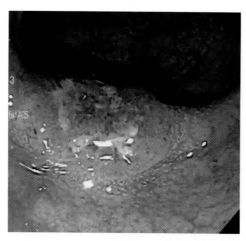

Figure 75.12 Malignant polyp. A sessile polyp with a central ulceration. If an endoscopist attempted to inject this lesion prior to performing polypectomy, it would likely demonstrate the "nonlifting sign," which results from tethering and invasion of the lesion into the submucosa consistent with malignancy. In such cases the role of the endoscopist is to obtain adequate biopsies for analysis and to mark the site of the lesion to facilitate intraoperative identification.

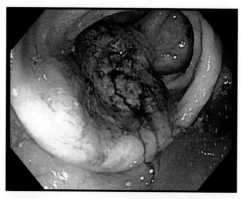

Figure 75.13 Colon cancer. This is a large adenocarcinoma in the sigmoid colon. The lesion occupies approximately half of the circumference of the colonic lumen. It has an area of central ulceration and necrosis, is very friable, and bleeds spontaneously.

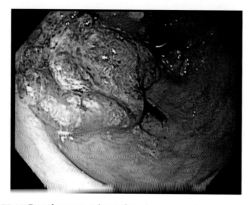

Figure 75.14 Rectal cancer. A large, fungating cancer is seen on retroflexion in the rectum. The lesion has a necrotic area in the center and bleeds spontaneously. Retroflexion of the colonoscope provides more complete inspection of the rectum.

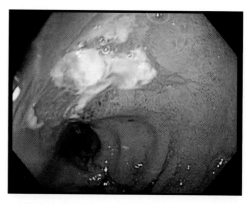

Figure 75.15 Ileal Crohn's disease. Crohn's disease most commonly involves the terminal ileum. This image demonstrates a large ulcer, friability, mucosal edema, and bleeding in the terminal ileum of a patient with Crohn's disease.

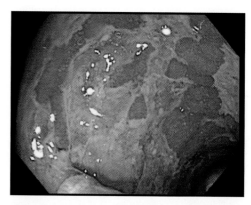

Figure 75.16 Colonic ulcers in Crohn's disease. Crohn's disease may cause serpiginous, coalescing ulcers to form on the mucosa. In such cases the adjacent areas of mucosa can appear edematous.

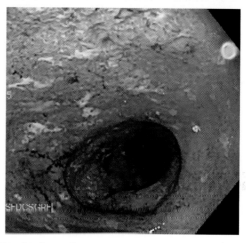

Figure 75.17 Moderate ulcerative colitis. Ulcerative colitis is a disease that is limited to the colonic mucosa. As such, it leads to characteristic mucosal findings, which are mucosal edema, erythema, friability, exudates, and bleeding. Note also the complete loss of the normal colonic vascular pattern, which can no longer be seen through an edematous, boggy mucosa.

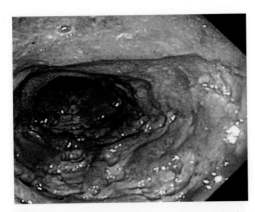

Figure 75.18 Severe ulcerative colitis. In severe disease, the inflammation in ulcerative colitis may spread beyond the mucosa. This image shows not only edema, friability, and loss of vascularity but also deep ulcers reminiscent of Crohn's disease.

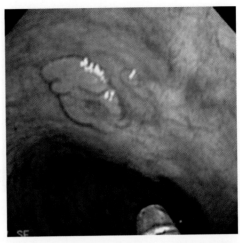

Figure 75.20 Chromoendoscopy. Chromoendoscopy, the application of a topical dye to the colonic surface, is a valuable technique for the detection and characterization of mucosal lesions. This image demonstrates the blue tint on the colonic mucosa created by dye spraying. A sessile polyp is clearly demarcated by chromoendoscopy thus facilitating polypectomy.

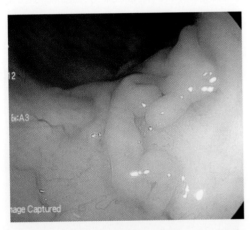

Figure 75.19 Pseudopolyps. Inflammatory polyps, or pseudopolyps, arise in areas of prior colitis as a result of mucosal regeneration after an insult. They are characterized by their pale coloration, smooth texture, and worm-like appearance. These lesions have no malignant potential and need not be removed. However, if they grow very large they may cause obstructive symptoms and make colonoscopy challenging.

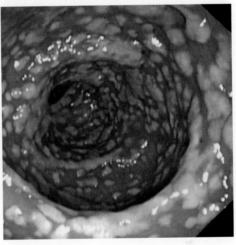

Figure 75.21 Pseudomembranous colitis. Pseudomembranes are yellow-white exudates that arise on the colonic mucosa. This finding is most common with *Clostridium difficile* infection but may occur with other infections as well.

long-standing, extensive ulcerative colitis and Crohn's colitis are at greatest risk and require periodic endoscopic surveillance. If the dysplasia is localized to a polypoid lesion it can be eradicated by colonoscopic polypectomy, just like polyps in noncolitic colons. However, some dysplasia may be subtle and undetectable in a field of colitis except by random circumferential biopsies throughout the colon. Chromoendoscopy, which involves the real-time application of a topical dye to the colonic mucosa, has been shown to highlight the mucosal pit pattern and help in the detection of dysplasia in inflammatory bowel disease (Figure 75.20).

While it is often difficult to diagnose the underlying etiology of colitis based solely on endoscopic appearance, some diseases have very characteristic findings at colonoscopy. Pseudomem-

branous colitis caused by *Clostridium difficile* infection may cause patchy clumps of creamy plaques on the mucosal surface (Figure 75.21). Ischemic colitis may be suspected based on its predilection for the "water-shed" segments of the colon. It may present with a wide array of mucosal appearances depending on the elapsed time from the ischemic episode to endoscopic examination. The ischemic segment may be friable and purplish-black in the initial phase of mucosal vascular insufficiency. In less severe cases, erythema alone may be encountered in the area of the descending colon or splenic flexure (Figure 75.22). Subsequent sloughing of the edematous mucosa may be associated with local or widespread ulceration. Another potential

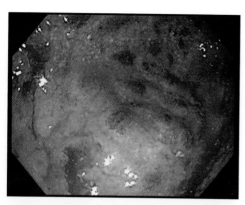

Figure 75.22 Ischemic colitis. The findings in mild to moderate ischemic colitis include mucosal edema, erythema, friability, ulceration, and exudates not unlike those seen in idiopathic ulcerative colitis. However, ischemic colitis may be suspected by its sudden onset and segmental distribution in the "watershed" areas of the colon. In more severe cases, the mucosa becomes purple and cyanotic.

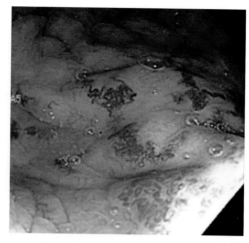

Figure 75.24 Radiation proctopathy. Pelvic radiation therapy may lead to damage to the colorectum. In the acute setting this may cause ulceration and edema. Chronic radiation proctopathy causes multiple ectatic blood vessels in a background of a pale mucosa. The area may bleed requiring endoscopic therapy.

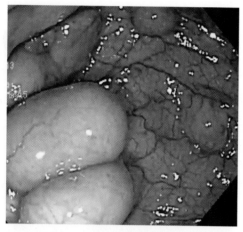

Figure 75.23 Pneumatosis cystoides intestinalis. Pneumatosis cystoides intestinalis, or pneumatosis cystoides coli when it is limited to the colon, is a condition in which air is present in the submucosa leading to the formation of multiple submucosal gas-filled cysts. The etiology is not clear but may be related to mechanical trauma to the mucosa or to bacterial infection. Pneumatosis cystoides coli has been associated with numerous inflammatory conditions of the colon, certain pulmonary diseases, and various medications. This condition may resolve spontaneously but complicated cases may require surgery.

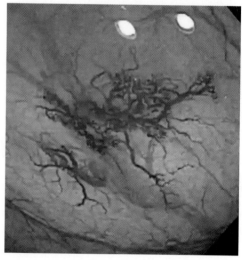

Figure 75.25 Angioectasia. These are characterized by their deep red color and ectatic, arborized blood vessels with an accompanying draining vein. They are most commonly found in the right colon in older patients and may cause bleeding and anemia. Endoscopic therapies including argon plasma coagulation and electrocautery can be used to ablate these lesions.

consequence of colonic inflammation is pneumatosis cystoides coli, a condition in which air is trapped beneath the mucosa (Figure 75.23).

Vascular abnormalities of the mucosa tend to be present at opposite ends of the large bowel, with radiation changes in the rectum and vascular ectasia in the right colon. Telangiectasia caused by radiation is more frequently encountered in the rectosigmoid area after pelvic radiation therapy for gynecological malignancy or in the distal rectum for prostate cancer. The postradiation proctopathy typically presents with rectal bleed-

ing. The endoscopic findings are confined to the area of radiation therapy and typically reveal multiple, small, interlacing blood vessels, friability, and mucosal pallor (Figure 75.24). Persistent bleeding may be treated with argon plasma coagulation of the affected area. Angiodysplasia or focal vascular ectasia, probably of degenerative origin, may develop in the proximal colon of elderly patients (Figure 75.25). These may be single or multiple and may cause bleeding or anemia. A draining vein is often visible at endoscopic examination and represents the hallmark angiographic descriptor of this vascular malformation. Endoscopic treatment options for vascular ectasias include argon plasma coagulation and bipolar cautery.

The terminal ileum can be intubated in most patients undergoing colonoscopy. This is often critical in assessing patients with colitis. Patients with ulcerative colitis typically have a normal-appearing terminal ileum or mild "backwash" ileitis. On the other hand, the terminal ileum is the most common site of Crohn's disease manifesting as aphthous erosions, deep ulcers,

exudates, friability, and bleeding (Figure 75.15). Other common findings in the terminal ileum include inflammatory polyps and lymphoid hyperplasia, which are benign conditions but may sometimes raise concern for malignancy or Crohn's disease.

Over the past several decades colonoscopy has revolutionized the diagnosis and management of gastrointestinal disorders. Colonoscopic technologies and techniques continue to rapidly evolve and it can be anticipated that endoscopists will become even more effective and efficient at identifying and treating a growing list of pathologies.

To access the videos for this chapter, please go to

www.yamadagastro.com/atlas

Video 75.1 Resection of a pedunculated polyp. A patient was referred for resection of a 4-cm polyp that filled the lumen of the sigmoid colon. Upon careful inspection, the polyp was found to have a broad pedicle. Polypectomy was performed by ensnaring the stalk of the polyp and applying pure coagulation current. Bleeding at the polypectomy site was controlled with the application of endoscopic clips.

Video 75.2 Endoscopic mucosal resection of a sessile polyp. A patient was referred for resection of a clam-shaped sessile polyp that encompassed both sides of a colonic fold. A submucosal injection was used to raise the lesion. A snare was then used to resect the lesion in piecemeal fashion. Argon plasma coagulation was used to ablate fragments of residual tissue at the resection margins.

Video 75.3 Six-month follow-up after polypectomy. Six months after the piecemeal resection of a clam-shaped sessile polyp (Video 75.2) there was no evidence of residual adenoma. A mucosal defect was noted at the polypectomy site.

CHAPTER 76

Endoscopic retrograde cholangiopancreatography: diagnostic and therapeutic

Mustafa A. Arain and Martin L. Freeman
University of Minnesota, Minneapolis, MN, USA

Endoscopic retrograde cholangiopancreatography (ERCP) is a specialized procedure for the management of biliary and pancreatic diseases using a combination of endoscopic and fluoroscopic guidance. Although initially used both as a diagnostic and therapeutic modality, in the modern era it is primarily a therapeutic procedure. Following the advances in noninvasive cross-sectional imaging modalities (magnetic resonance imaging [MRI] and computed tomography [CT]) as well as improvements in endoscopic ultrasound, which allows high-resolution endosonographic evaluation of the pancreatobiliary system and, if necessary, simultaneous tissue acquisition by fine-needle aspiration, the role of diagnostic ERCP is now primarily reserved for conditions in which the diagnosis remains elusive despite evaluation using noninvasive imaging and endoscopic ultrasound (EUS).

Diagnostic and therapeutic ERCP can be associated with a variety of complications, including pancreatitis, hemorrhage, and perforation, with pancreatitis being the most common. The risk of complications, and specifically pancreatitis, can be reduced by practicing the four "Ps" of complication prophylaxis, which are: (1) recognition of patient-related risk factors; (2) recognition and modification of procedure-related risk factors; (3) placement of prophylactic pancreatic stents in appropriately high-risk patients; and (4) pharmacological prevention, for example the use of rectal indomethacin to reduce the risk of pancreatitis (Figure 76.1).

The primary role of ERCP is to reestablish drainage of the biliary and pancreatic ductal systems in the setting of stones, strictures, and leaks, to remove localized tumors of the papillary orifices, and, increasingly, as an adjunct to EUS-guided access and drainage using a minimally invasive endoscopic approach for the management of complications of pancreatitis, specifically pancreatic pseudocysts and walled off pancreatic and peripancreatic necrosis. The most common indication for ERCP is for the removal of bile duct stones (Figure 76.2). Several techniques, including stone extraction with balloon catheters and baskets, mechanical lithotripsy, large balloon dilation of the papillary orifice, and intraductal lithotripsy techniques such as electrohydraulic and laser lithotripsy, can be used to achieve complete stone removal (Figure 76.3). Biliary strictures may be benign (e.g., in the setting of surgery) or malignant (e.g., due to pancreatic or hilar tumors), and are treated with balloon dilation of the stricture and placement of plastic or metal biliary stents (Figure 76.4). Biliary system leaks are treated with a biliary sphincterotomy to reduce the resistance of biliary flow across the major papilla and transpapillary stent placement. Papillary tumors that are not cancerous and do not extend into the bile duct or pancreas can be removed endoscopically. However, the risk of complications, including bleeding, pancreatitis, and retroperitoneal perforation, is increased in this setting (Figure 76.5).

Improvements in endoscopic technologies and techniques enable ERCP to play an increasingly safe and effective role in the management of pancreatic diseases. ERCP for pancreatic diseases are technically more demanding and riskier than ERCP for most biliary conditions, and therefore should ideally be performed by dedicated endoscopists with advanced endoscopic expertise in a multidisciplinary context, with appropriate understanding of the disease processes and involvement of specialized surgeons and interventional radiologists, as appropriate. Complications of chronic pancreatitis, including pancreatic duct stones, strictures, or leaks, are the main indications for ERCP (Figures 76.6, 76.7, and 76.8). A small pancreatic orifice, the presence of a concomitant pancreatic stricture, and the hard, calcific nature of pancreatic stones make stone removal by ERCP technically more difficult. Extracorporeal shock wave lithotripsy (ESWL) may be used alone or as an adjunct to ERCP for pancreatic stone removal. The principles of ERCP-guided pancreatic stone removal include pancreatic sphincterotomy, careful dilation of the pancreatic orifice, and use of baskets

Yamada's Atlas of Gastroenterology, Fifth Edition. Edited by Daniel K. Podolsky, Michael Camilleri, J. Gregory Fitz, Anthony N. Kalloo, Fergus Shanahan, and Timothy C. Wang.
© 2016 John Wiley & Sons, Ltd. Published 2016 by John Wiley & Sons, Ltd.
Companion website: www.yamadagastro.com/atlas

rather than balloons. Difficult pancreatic stones may require pancreatic stent placement to aid pancreatic orifice or stricture dilation and stone fragmentation and ESWL or surgery. The role of ERCP for the management of recurrent acute pancreatitis is often debated due to the risks of the procedure, primarily worsening of pancreatitis and uncertain benefits. ERCP is often offered in the hope of alleviating pain and breaking the cycle of recurrent attacks by optimizing drainage from the pancreatic orifice through pancreatic sphincterotomy and/or stent placement (Figures 76.9 and 76.10).

Surgical procedures that result in alterations of the gastric, duodenal, and/or biliary anatomy may result in anatomic changes that make ERCP access to the major papilla/biliary tree technically difficult or impossible. Depending on the surgical anatomy, options include enteroscopy-assisted ERCP, which is limited by the number of accessories available to perform the procedure, or if feasible a surgical approach, for example in the setting of a Roux-en-Y gastric bypass. The latter approach is more invasive but allows placement of a dedicated duodenoscope to perform ERCP utilizing the full spectrum of ERCP accessories and devices (Figures 76.11 and 76.12).

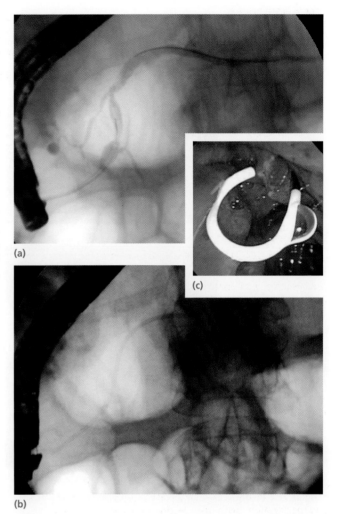

(a)

(c)

(b)

Figure 76.1 (a, b) Fluoroscopic and **(c)** endoscopic views of placement of a long (9 cm), unflanged 4 French soft material pancreatic stent to the midbody of a normal configuration pancreatic duct for prevention of postendoscopic retrograde cholangiopancreatography pancreatitis.

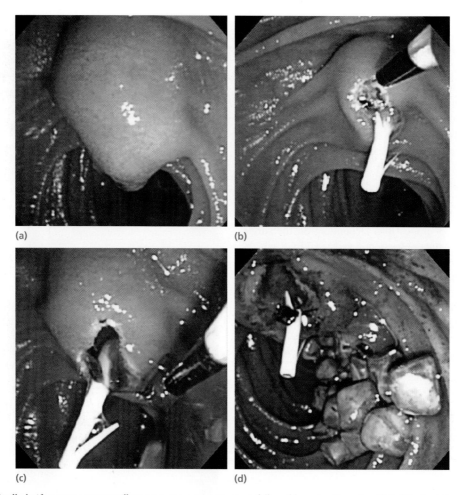

Figure 76.2 (a–d) Needle-knife precut access papillotomy over a pancreatic stent, followed by extraction of multiple bile duct stones.

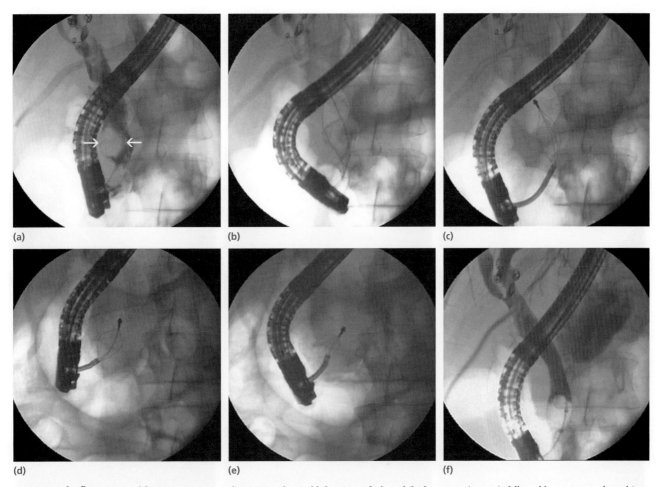

(a)   (b)   (c)

(d)   (e)   (f)

Figure 76.3 (a–f) Sequence of fluoroscopic images showing mechanical lithotripsy of a large bile duct stone (arrows), followed by capture and crushing of the stone, with final clearance of the duct.

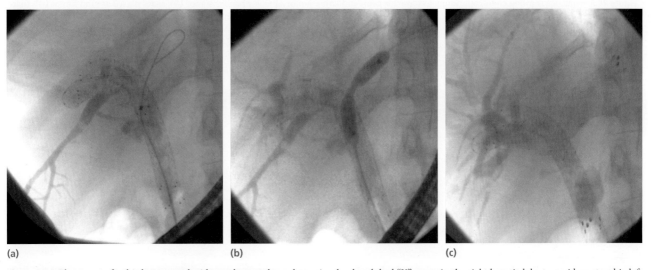

(a)   (b)   (c)

Figure 76.4 Placement of a third uncovered wide-mesh stent through previously placed dual "Y" stents in the right hepatic lobe to avoid an atrophic left hepatic lobe, after delayed presentation with cholangitis 3 months after initial stent insertion. **(a)** Dual stents in "Y" configuration in right anterior and posterior sectoral ducts. **(b)** Dilating balloon and guidewire passed through stents into the left hepatic duct. **(c)** Third metallic stent placed into the left duct, resulting in drainage of all three sectors.

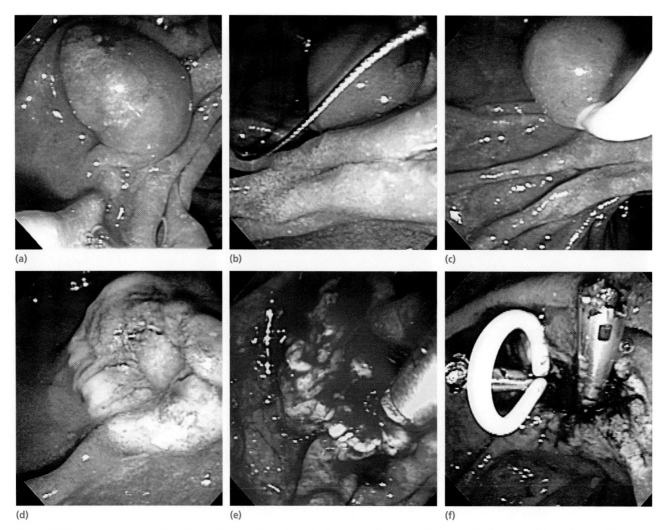

(a)   (b)   (c)

(d)   (e)   (f)

Figure 76.5 Sequence showing endoscopic ampullectomy for neuroendocrine tumor of major papilla: tumor **(a)**, snare passed around tumor **(b)**, snare closed **(c)**, postampullectomy **(d)**, bleeding **(e)**, controlled after placement of a pancreatic stent (white) with injection of adrenaline and placement of clips **(f)**.

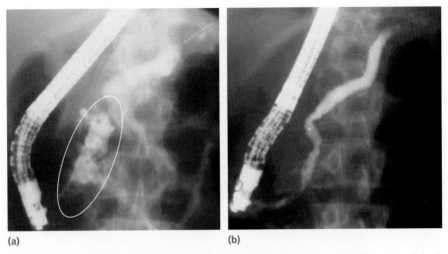

Figure 76.6 Endoscopic retrograde cholangiopancreatography showing very large pancreatic stone prior to extracorporeal shock wave lithotripsy (ESWL) (circle) **(a)**, and after ESWL **(b)**, with complete stone fragmentation and clearance.

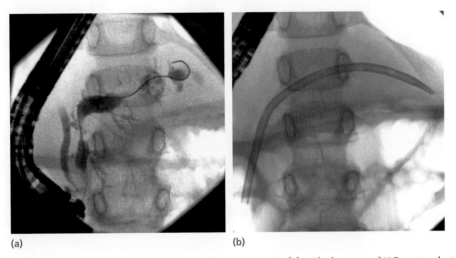

Figure 76.7 Complex multiple strictures in a 7-year-old child with hereditary pancreatitis **(a)**, with placement of 10 F stent to the tail of the pancreatic duct **(b)**.

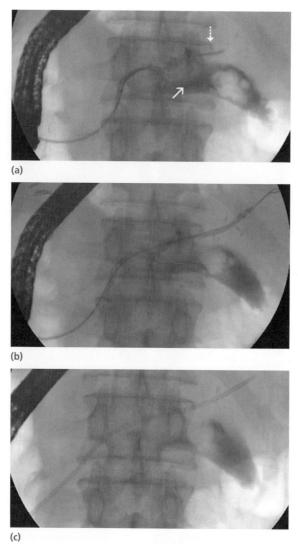

(a)

(b)

(c)

Figure 76.8 Pancreatic duct leak. Disrupted duct **(a)**(solid arrow shows leak, dashed arrow shows upstream disconnected duct); passage of guidewire to the tail beyond disruption **(b)**; placement of 5 F stent to the tail bridging the leak **(c)**.

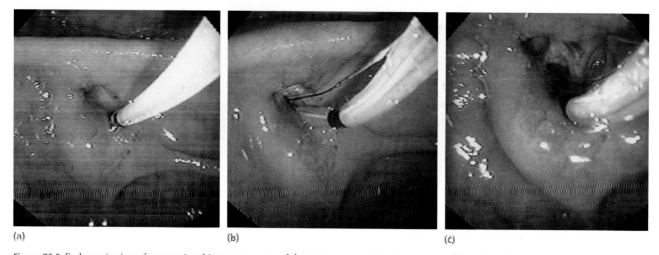

(a)   (b)   (c)

Figure 76.9 Endoscopic view of pancreatic sphincter manometry **(a)**, traction pancreatic sphincterotomy **(b)**, and patulous pancreatic sphincterotomy **(c)** for acute recurrent pancreatitis.

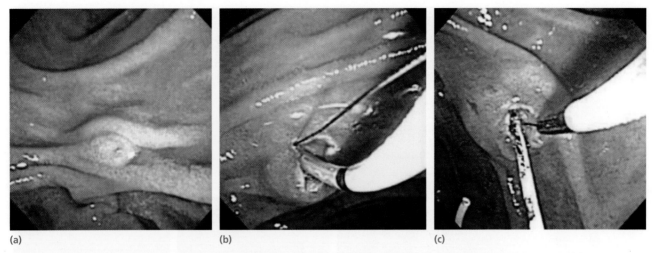

(a) (b) (c)

Figure 76.10 Minor papillotomy for pancreas divisum with acute recurrent pancreatitis, using two different techniques. Minor papilla **(a)**, traction papillotomy **(b)**, and needle-knife papillotomy over a dorsal pancreatic duct stent **(c)**.

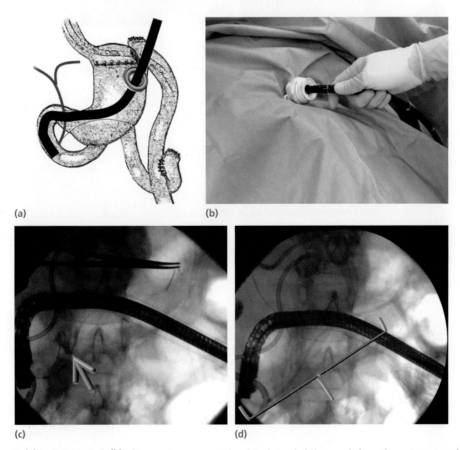

(a) (b)

(c) (d)

Figure 76.11 A schematic **(a)** and photograph **(b)** of a percutaneous port placed in the excluded stomach for endoscopic retrograde cholangiopancreatography (ERCP) access in the setting of a Roux-en-Y gastric bypass. ERCP **(c)** using a duodenoscope through a percutaneous port in a gastric bypass patient who presented with necrotizing pancreatitis, retroperitoneal fat necrosis, and a pancreatic leak (arrow), which was treated with a pancreatic stent **(d)**. Two percutaneous drains placed for peripancreatic necrosis are seen in the background.

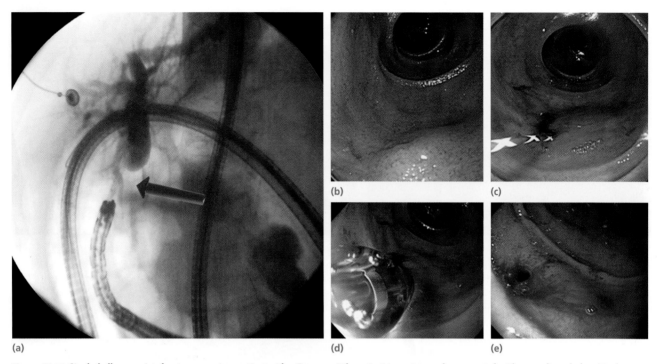

(a)   (b)   (c)   (d)   (e)

Figure 76.12 Single-balloon-assisted enteroscopy in a patient with a Roux-en-Y hepaticojejunostomy who presented with ascending cholangitis due to stenosis of the biliary anastomosis **(a, b)**. After wire placement **(c)**, the stricture was balloon dilated **(d)** resulting in widening of the anastomotic orifice **(e)**.

CHAPTER 77

Gastrointestinal dilation and stent placement

Shayan Irani and Richard A. Kozarek
Virginia Mason Medical Center, Seattle, WA, USA

Although dilation of gastrointestinal strictures was traditionally limited to the esophagus and the anorectum, the development of polyethylene balloons has expanded the endoscopist's therapeutic horizons. Advanced over a guidewire or directly through an endoscope, such balloons allow access to stenotic lesions of the stomach, small intestine, colon, and pancreaticobiliary tract. Exemplifying the ability to dilate previously inaccessible stenoses has been the development of newer dilating systems for use in the esophagus. For bougienage, polyvinyl dilators have virtually supplanted the Eder–Puestow metal olives (Pauldrach Medical, Garben, Germany), and lesions previously considered "undilatable" have been recategorized (Figures 77.1 and 77.2). More recent modifications, such as over-the-scope bougies or balloons with a controllable expansion radius, may further improve the safety and efficacy of dilation (Figure 77.3, 77.4, 77.5, and 77.6).

Consequently, these expanded capabilities have led endoscopists into widespread dilation therapy for a variety of stenoses, despite the absence of data or contradictory results from studies assessing risks and benefits of dilation compared with more conventional therapy such as surgery. Similarly, as pharmacological and radiation therapies evolve, it is unclear whether dilation provides a desirable alternative or adjuvant to these treatments. For example, stenoses with deep ulcerations caused by Crohn's disease, which would have historically necessitated surgery, are increasingly being dilated by endoscopists. Whether these dilations may be made more successful, or even obviated, by new immunomodulatory treatments for inflammatory bowel disease remains unknown.

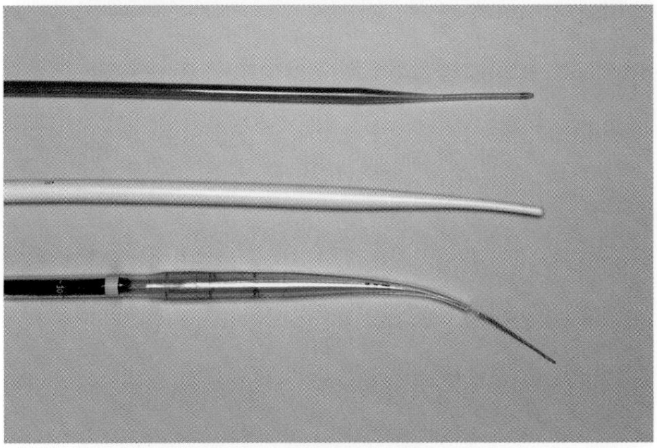

As with dilation, technological advances have driven the increased use of, and indications for, endoluminal stents in the alimentary canal. Expandable stent therapy has virtually supplanted conventional prosthesis placement in the esophagus, due to the relative ease of placement and improved safety profile during insertion (Figure 77.7). Nevertheless, critical evaluation of this technology suggests that the need for intervention actually may increase after placement of expandable esophageal stents. This reintervention is a direct consequence of stent design: uncovered stents elicit granulation tissue and allow tumor ingrowth, and completely covered prostheses have a penchant for migration. All prostheses have the capability to cause erosion with fistulization, gastrointestinal bleeding, or occlusion by food bolus (Figures 77.8, 77.9, 77.10, and 77.11).

Expandable stent technology allows at least the potential to open obstructed luminal orifices for patients at high risk and patients with widespread metastases, and to open nonesophageal locations. Some uncertainty exists in choosing between stents and other modalities, reflecting the paucity of controlled studies regarding placement of these stents into locations other than the esophagus or biliary tract (Figures 77.12, 77.13, 77.14, 77.15, 77.16, and 77.17). The ongoing evolution of the various stents themselves and their respective delivery systems is also a reason for uncertainty in management choices. Finally, the cost of this technology – US$1000 to US$3000 per device depending on stent design and length – raises uncertainty as to the potential cost effectiveness in some circumstances. It is hoped that in the future, the various stent types can be better placed into perspective with regard to each other and with other potential therapies in the future.

Figure 77.1 Dilating systems. Savary–Gilliard (top), American (middle), and Optical (bottom) dilators. All are wire-guided, with the optical dilator also admitting an endoscope for direct visualization.

Yamada's Atlas of Gastroenterology, Fifth Edition. Edited by Daniel K. Podolsky, Michael Camilleri, J. Gregory Fitz, Anthony N. Kalloo, Fergus Shanahan, and Timothy C. Wang.
© 2016 John Wiley & Sons, Ltd. Published 2016 by John Wiley & Sons, Ltd.
Companion website: www.yamadagastro.com/atlas

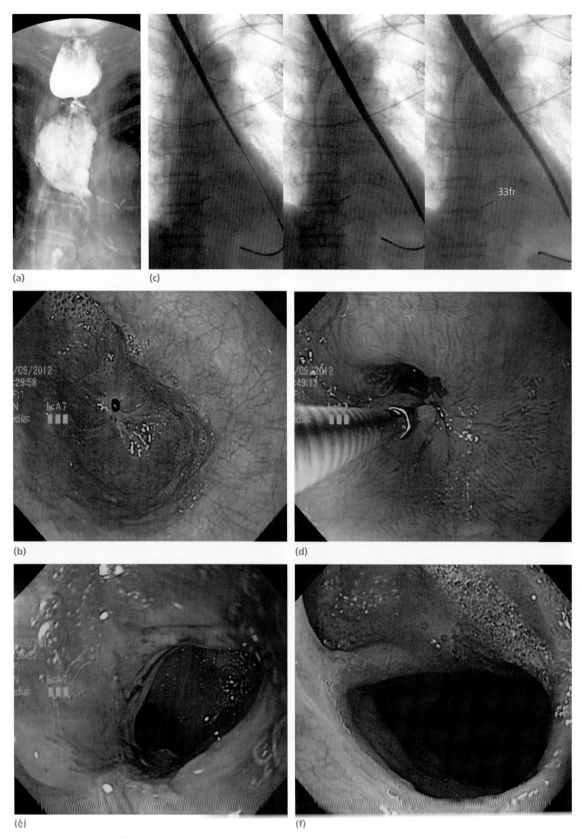

Figure 77.2 (a) Esophogram and (b) endoscopy demonstrating a high-grade, benign, esophagogastric anastomotic stenosis. (c) Barium-impregnated Savary-type dilator (American Dilator; Cook Medical, Winston-Salem, NC) passed over a guidewire (distal portion of free guidewire in stomach) across stricture. (d) Four-quadrant injection of steroid into the same refractory stenosis. (e) Endoscopic view immediately after dilation of stenosis and (f) 2 months later.

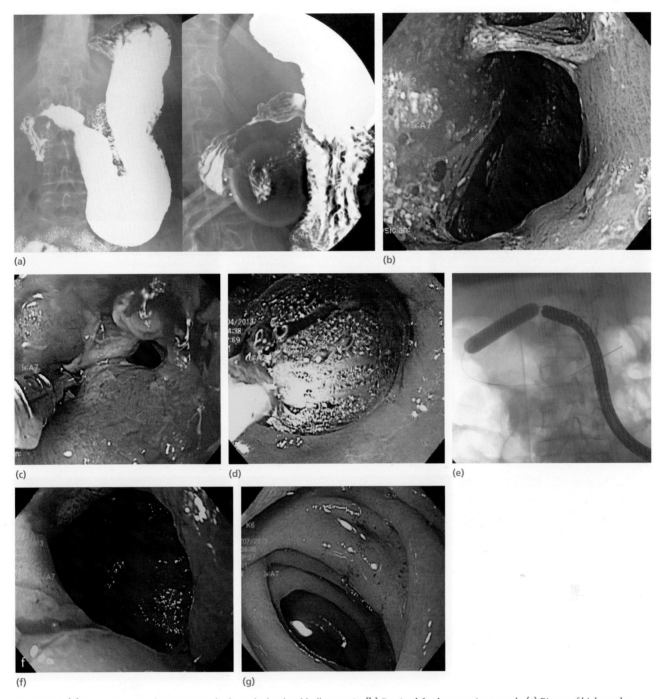

Figure 77.3 (a) Upper GI series demonstrating high-grade duodenal bulb stenosis. **(b)** Retained food present in stomach. **(c)** Biopsy of high-grade duodenal stenosis. **(d, e)** Dilation of stricture using a 10–12-mm controlled radial expansion balloon (Boston Scientific, Natick, MA) under endoscopic and fluoroscopic guidance. **(f, g)** Endoscopic inspection of stenosis and postbulbar duodenum after balloon dilation.

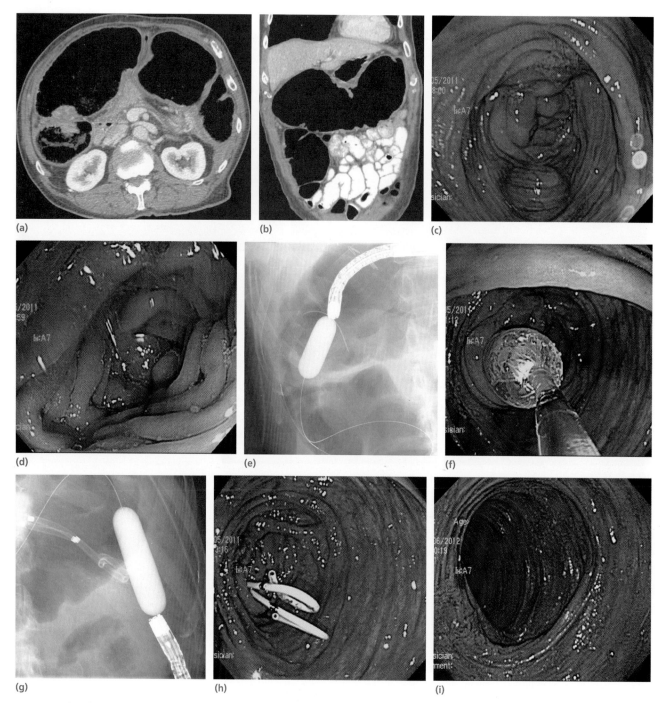

Figure 77.4 (a, b) Computed tomography scan demonstrating a markedly dilated transverse colon due to benign strictures of the ascending and descending colon secondary to a prior episode of severe pancreatitis. **(c, d)** Endoscopic view of ascending and descending colon strictures. **(e–g)** Through-the-scope, 15-mm controlled radial expansion balloon dilation (Boston Scientific, Natick Ma) of ascending and descending colon strictures. **(h)** Two double pigtail plastic biliary stents placed to allow decompression of the **(i)** markedly distended transverse colon.

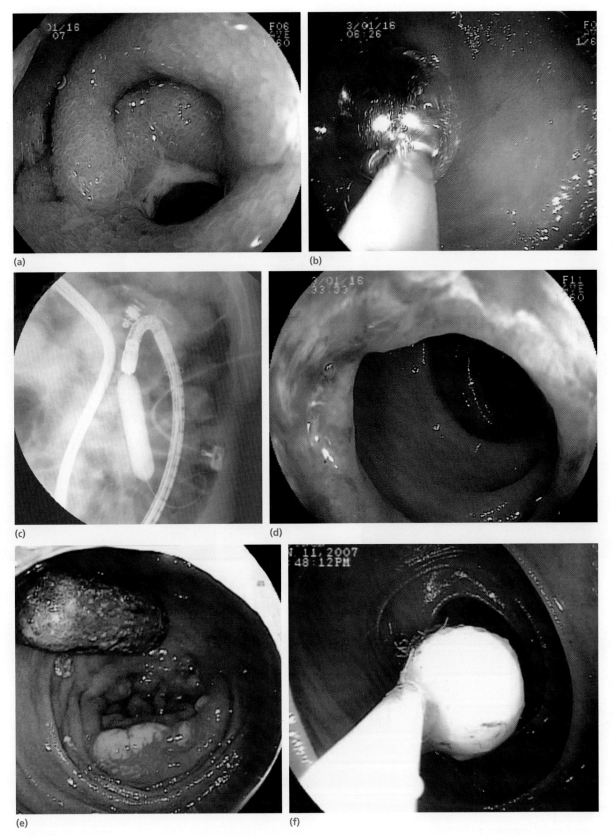

Figure 77.5 (a) Endoscopic view of benign midileal stricture discovered at retrograde double-balloon enteroscopy performed for a retained video capsule. **(b, c)** Controlled radial expansion balloon dilation (Boston Scientific, Natick, MA) to 10 mm under endoscopic and fluoroscopic control. **(d)** Postdilation inspection of stricture and small bowel upstream to the stenosis. **(e, f)** Retained video capsule reached and retrieved with a Roth Net (US Endoscopy, Mentor, OH).

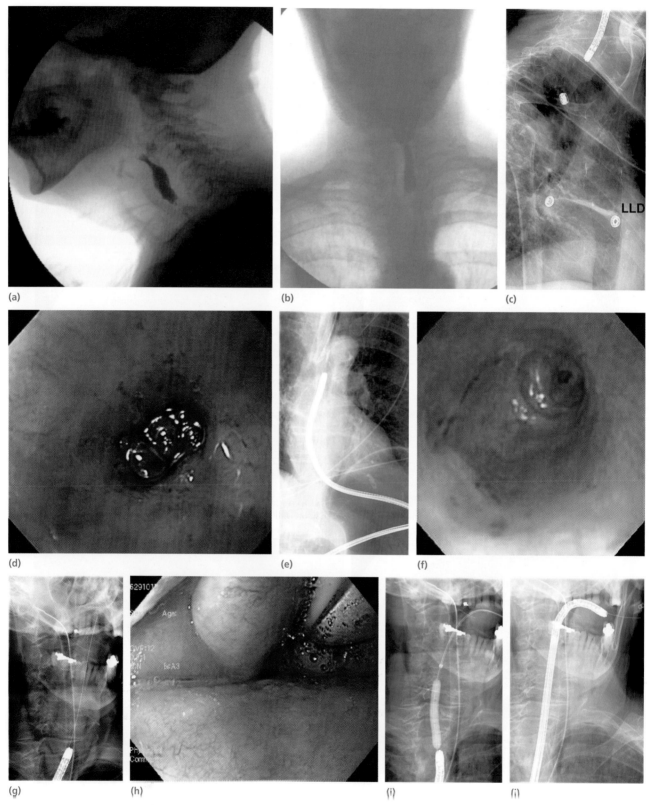

Figure 77.6 **(a, b)** Esophogram demonstrating complete cut off in the proximal esophagus in a patient secondary to radiation injury for a previously treated squamous cell pharyngeal cancer. Fluoroscopic and endoscopic view demonstrating a complete occlusion of the proximal esophageal lumen, both **(c, d)** antegrade (through mouth) and **(e, f)** retrograde (through gastrostomy). **(g, h)** Stiff end of a 0.035 inch (0.89 mm) guidewire (arrow) used to dissect through the membranous occlusion in the proximal esophagus under fluoroscopic and endoscopic guidance, until the wire emerges through the mouth. **(i, j)** Controlled radial expansion balloon dilation (Boston Scientific, Natick, MA) to 8 mm under endoscopic and fluoroscopic control, followed by advancement of the endoscope in retrograde fashion to the mouth.

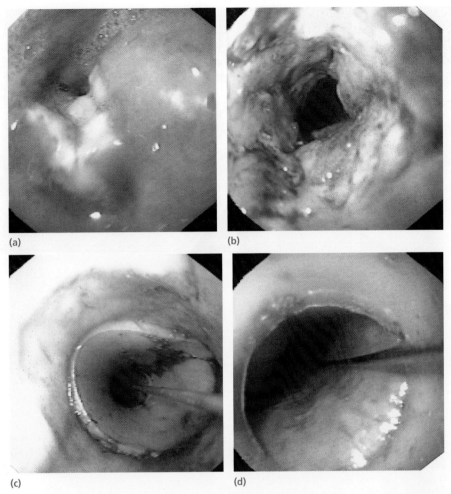

(a) (b) (c) (d)

Figure 77.7 Conventional esophageal prosthesis placement. A stricture caused by midesophageal squamous cell carcinoma was managed with a conventional prosthesis (Wilson-Cook, Winston-Salem, NC) pushed into position with a Dumon introducer. Endoscopic photographs show original neoplasm **(a)**, appearance after dilation **(b)**, and proximal **(c)** and distal **(d)** stent margin.

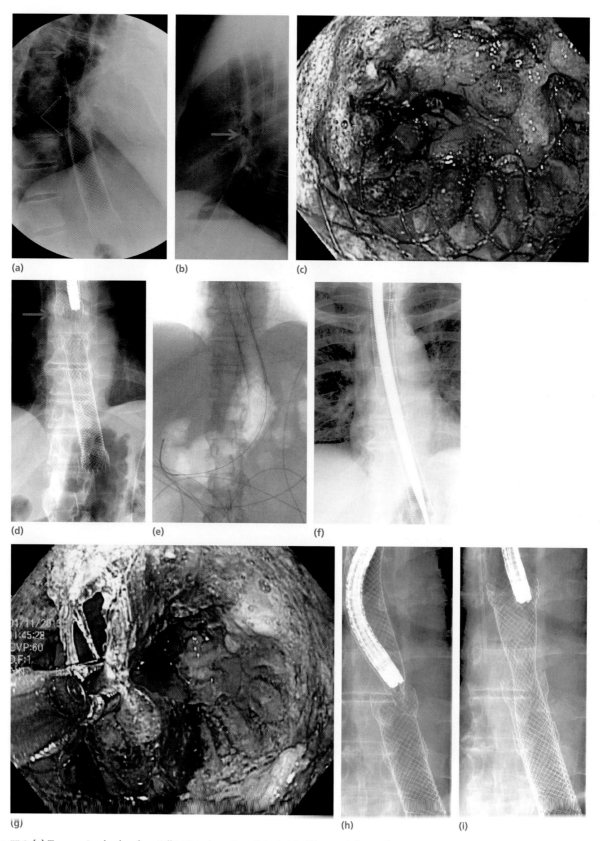

Figure 77.8 (a) Two previously placed partially covered esophageal stents (double arrow) for esophageal adenocarcinoma with granulation ingrowth and stenosis at the proximal end, treated with a fully covered esophageal stent (large arrow). **(b)** Proximal migration of a fully covered esophageal stent (arrow) 1 month later with associated recurrent dysphagia. **(c, d)** Distal end of a fully covered esophageal stent (arrow) lying above the stenosis at the proximal end of the previously placed partially covered stent. **(e, f)** Spring-tipped guidewire passed into stomach, followed by dilation with a 36 Fr American Dilator (Cook Medical, Winston-Salem, NC) to facilitate **(g–i)** repositioning of migrated fully covered stent, to bridge the stenosis.

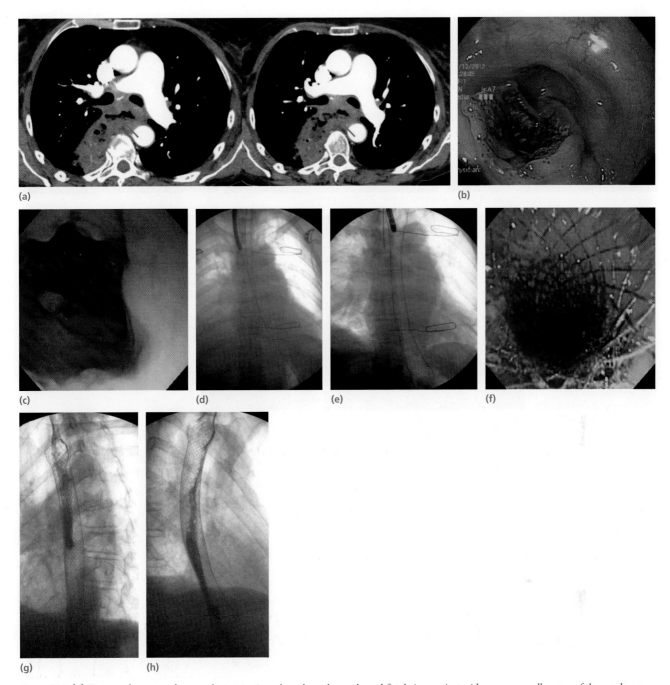

Figure 77.9 (a) Computed tomography scan demonstrating a large bronchoesophageal fistula in a patient with squamous cell cancer of the esophagus. **(b)** Endoscopic view of bronchoesophageal fistula and associated **(c)** lung abscess. **(d–f)** External markers taped to chest wall to aid fluoroscopic deployment in addition to endoscopic visualization with a pediatric gastroscope for precise placement. **(g, h)** Esophogram the following day confirms closure of bronchoesophageal fistula.

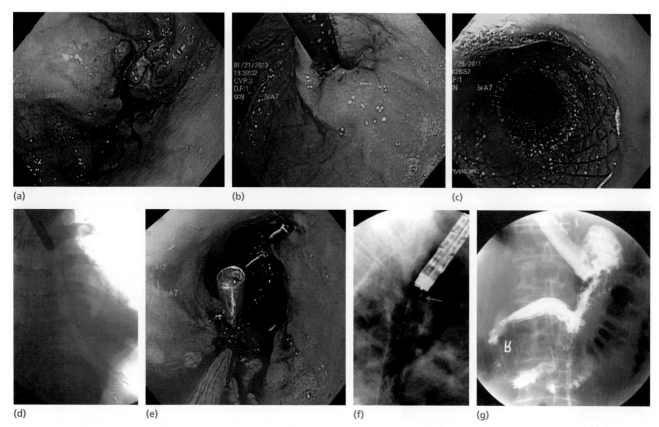

(a)   (b)   (c)

(d)   (e)   (f)   (g)

Figure 77.10 (a, b) Endoscopic view of esophageal adenocarcinoma extending into the gastric cardia and fundus. **(c, d)** Fully covered esophageal stent placed across stricture. **(e, f)** Hemostatic clips used to secure the proximal end of the stent to reduce the chance of migration. **(g)** Esophogram the following day confirms the stable position and patency of the stent.

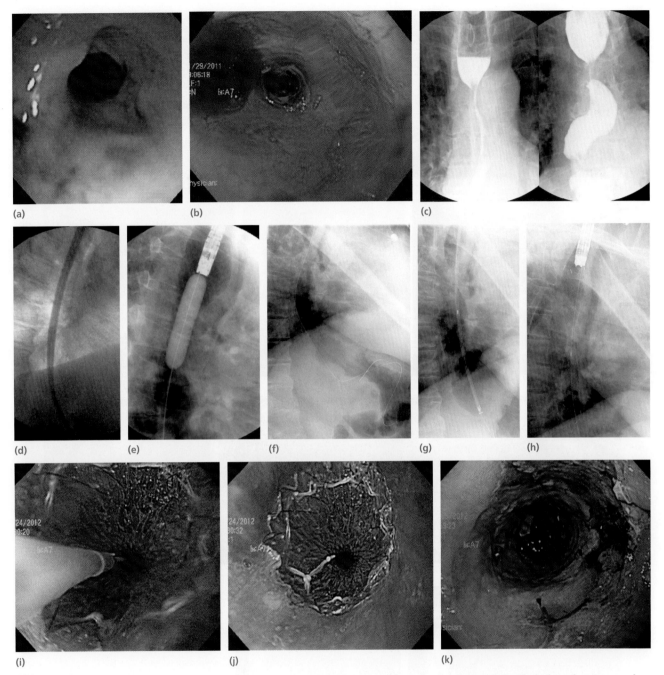

Figure 77.11 (a, b) Endoscopic views of high-grade, benign peptic esophageal stricture. **(c)** Esophogram demonstrating the high-grade stricture and an associated hiatal hernia. Despite repeated dilations with **(d)** American (Cook Medical, Winston-Salem, NC) and **(e)** controlled radial expansion balloon dilators (Boston Scientific, Natick, MA), a refractory stricture persisted. **(f–j)** A through-the-scope fully covered metal stent is deployed over a 0.035-inch (0.89-mm) guidewire. **(k)** Endoscopic appearance at removal of the fully covered stent 3 months later demonstrating resolution of the stricture.

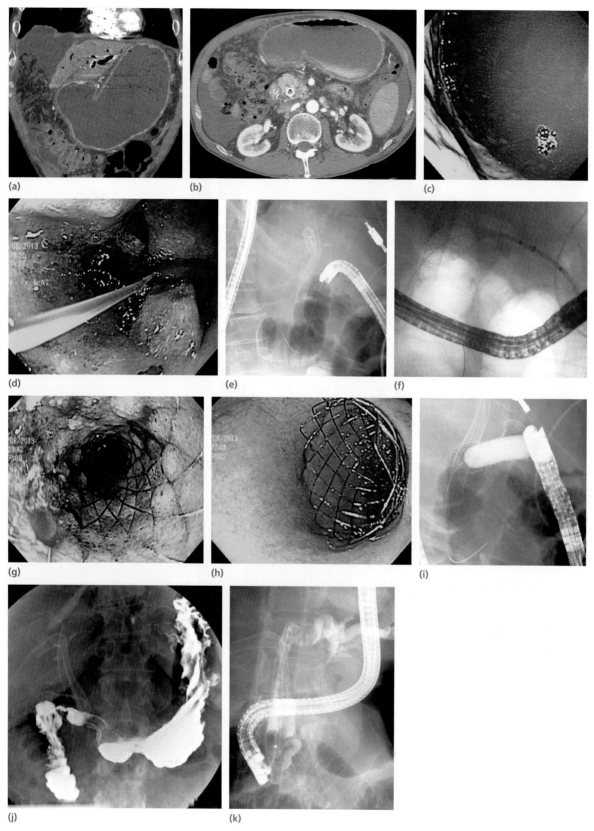

Figure 77.12 **(a, b)** Computed tomography scan demonstrating gastric outlet obstruction secondary to gallbladder cancer. **(c)** Endoscopic view of a large amount of retained gastric contents with **(d)** guidewire advanced through a high-grade duodenal bulb stricture. Deployment of a 6-cm Duodenal WallFlex stent (Boston Scientific, Natick, MA) under **(e, f)** fluoroscopic and **(g, h)** endoscopic control. **(i)** Despite controlled radial expansion balloon dilation (Boston Scientific, Natick, MA) to 15 mm, at the time of stent deployment, it was not possible to advance the duodenoscope into the second part of duodenum to perform a cholangiogram. **(j)** Upper GI series the next day demonstrating a patent and fully expanded duodenal stent, **(k)** followed by the ability to perform endoscopic retrograde cholangiopancreatography (ERCP).

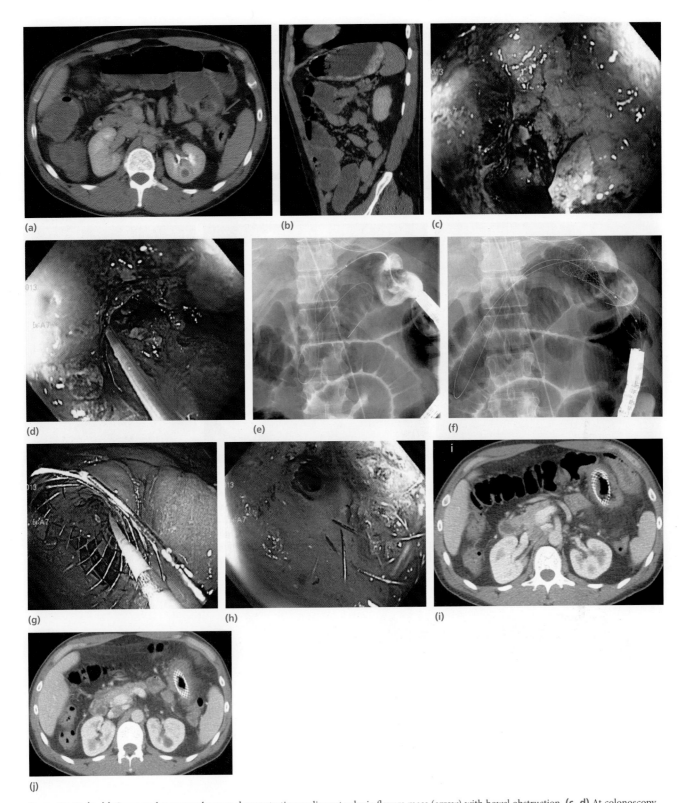

Figure 77.13 (a, b) Computed tomography scan demonstrating malignant splenic flexure mass (arrow) with bowel obstruction. **(c, d)** At colonoscopy, a high-grade malignant obstruction was encountered, which is traversed with a 0.035-inch (0.89-mm) guidewire. **(e, f)** Under fluoroscopic and **(g, h)** endoscopic guidance, a 9-cm Colonic WallFlex stent (Boston Scientific, Natick, MA) is deployed. **(i, j)** Computed tomography scan 2 days later demonstrated good stent position with resolution of bowel obstruction.

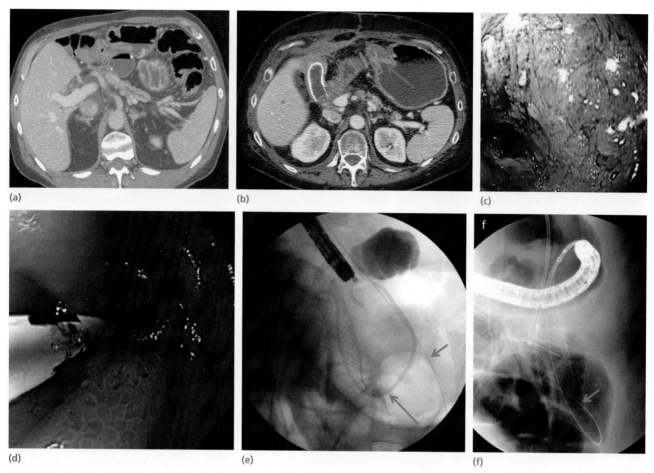

Figure 77.14 (a, b) Computed tomography scan demonstrating recurrent gastric outlet obstruction at the level of gastrojejunostomy (large arrow) in a patient with locally advanced pancreatic cancer and previous placed duodenal stent (small arrow). Obstruction of **(c)** efferent and **(d)** afferent limbs. A double pigtail stent is placed into the afferent limb to identify later for placement of a second metal stent. **(e, f)** Double pigtail stent (large arrow) in the afferent limb and 0.035 inch (0.89-mm) guidewire (small arrow) in efferent limb over which a 6-cm Duodenal WallFlex stent (Boston Scientific, Natick, MA) is deployed. **(g–j)** Through the tines of the efferent limb stent, a partially covered biliary WallFlex stent (small arrow) is deployed alongside the pigtail stent. **(k)** Upper GI series the following day and **(l)** computed tomography scan 6 weeks later demonstrate patency of both metal stents.

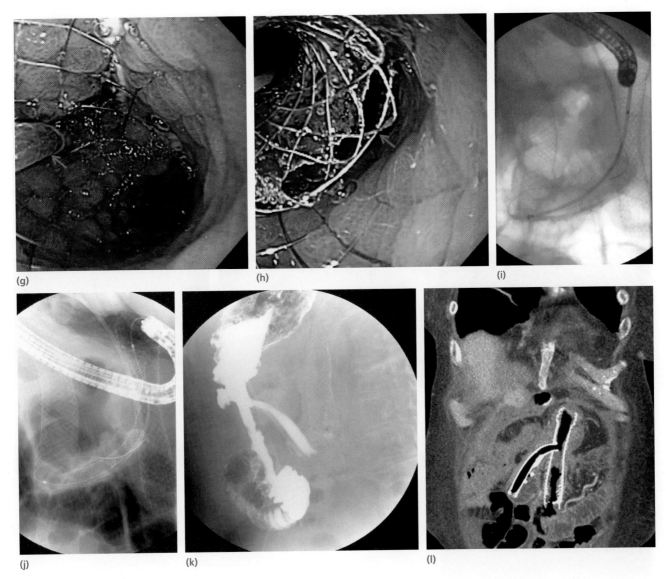

(g) (h) (i)

(j) (k) (l)

Figure 77.14 (*Continued*)

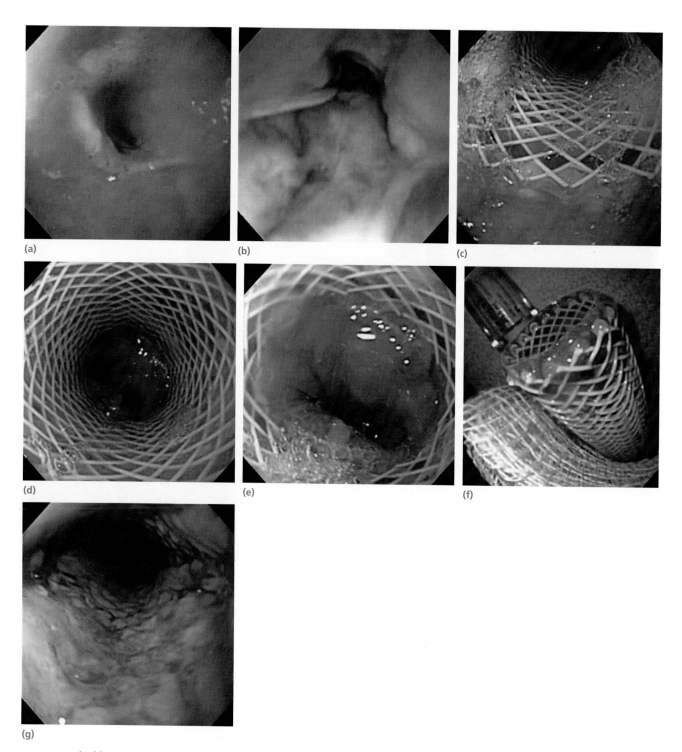

Figure 77.15 (a, b) High-grade radiation-induced proximal esophageal stricture. **(c)** Proximal, **(d)** mid, and **(e)** distal portion of self-expandable plastic stent (SEPS) (Polyflex stent, Boston Scientific, Natick, MA) placed above the level of the esophagogastric junction. **(f)** After removal of the SEPS, **(g)** endoscopic resolution of the stricture is noted.

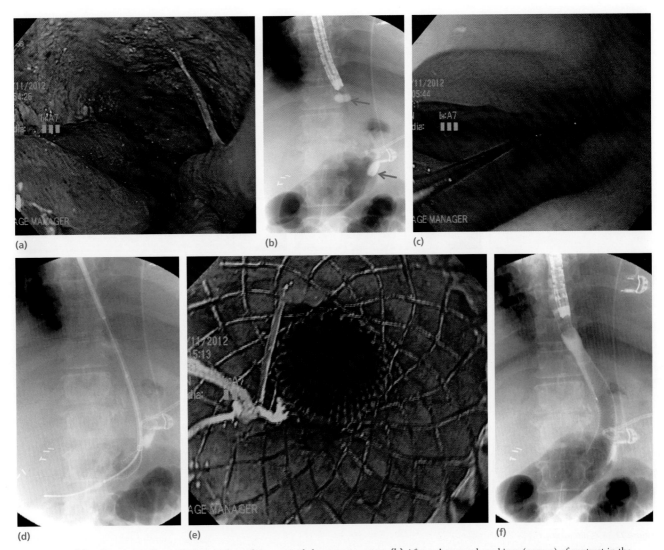

(a)　　　　　　　　　　(b)　　　　　　　　　　(c)

(d)　　　　　　　　　　(e)　　　　　　　　　　(f)

Figure 77.16 **(a)** Dehiscence at the staple line 10 days after a vertical sleeve gastrectomy. **(b)** After submucosal markings (arrows) of contrast in the stomach and esophagus, **(c–f)** a partially covered esophageal stent is placed across the dehiscence to provide a "water-tight" seal. **(g, h)** Upper GI series confirms closure of the leak. **(i)** Two months later, significant granulation ingrowth at the proximal end (arrow), prevents stent removal. **(j)** A fully covered stent of the same diameter is placed to facilitate "stent-in-stent" removal. **(k, l)** Two weeks later, both stents are fairly easily removed and endoscopy demonstrates closure of dehiscence.

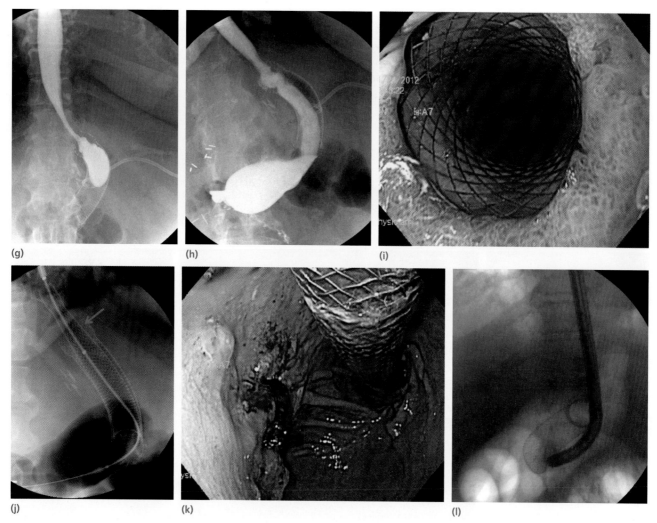

(g)   (h)   (i)

(j)   (k)   (l)

Figure 77.16 (*Continued*)

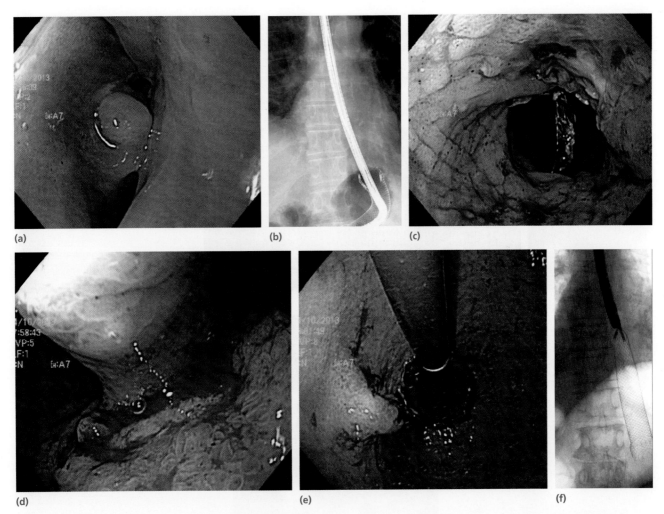

(a)

(b)

(c)

(d)

(e)

(f)

Figure 77.17 (a) Migrated fully-covered esophageal stent, despite previously placed hemostatic clips, in a patient with a midesophageal stenosis due to metastatic breast cancer, presenting with hematemesis and recurrent dysphagia. **(b, c)** Proximal end of the stent at the esophagogastric junction, with **(d, e)** the distal end impacted in the lesser curvature of the stomach causing a pseudopolyp and ulceration. **(f–h)** The same fully-covered stent withdrawn proximally above the midesophageal stenosis, and secured to the esophageal wall with an over-the-scope-clip (arrow). **(i, j)** Esophogram the following day confirms the stable position of the stent, and failure of migration for the ensuing 3 months.

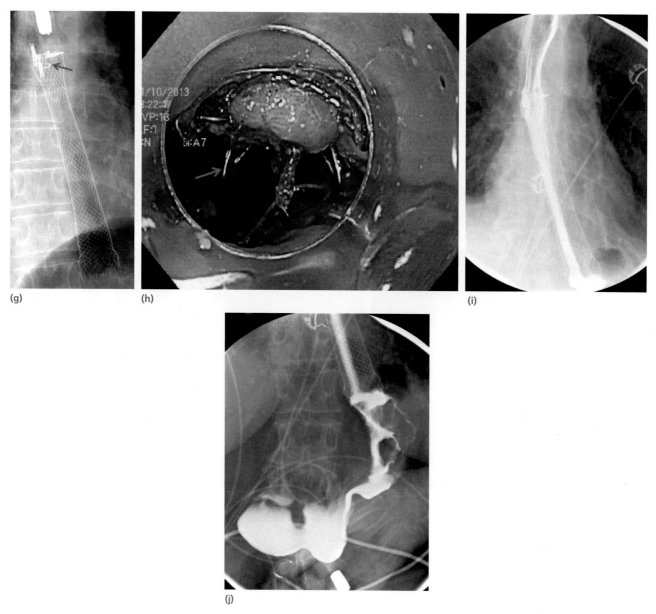

(g)

(h)

(i)

(j)

Figure 77.17 (*Continued*)

To access the videos for this chapter, please go to
www.yamadagastro.com/atlas

Video 77.1 Bearclaw self-expandable metal stent. Treatment of a high-grade, benign, esophagogastric anastomotic stricture with dilation, steroid injection, and a fully covered esophageal self-expandable metal stent secured to the esophageal wall with an over-the-scope clip.

Video 77.2 Rendezvous esophageal reconnection and self-expandable metal stent insertion. This 54-year-old man had a total laryngectomy and irradiation for laryngeal cancer 4 years prior and has had total aphagia requiring enteral feeding for the past 3 years. Per os endoscopy demonstrated a tiny, non-patent esophageal inlet. Endoscopy through the patient's gastrostomy orifice demonstrated complete obstruction, and attempts to pass an endoscopic ultrasound (EUS) needle into the hypopharynx from the esophagus were unsuccessful. Ultimately, an endoscopic retrograde cholangiopancreatography (ERCP) catheter and guidewire passed through a per os endoscope could reestablish continuity with the aid of biopsy forceps. Following guidewire insertion into the esophagus, the neolumen was dilated with an 8-mm balloon followed by placement of a 10-mm partially covered self-expandable metal stent. The latter was subsequently clipped in place distally using the endoscope placed through the gastrostomy. Four weeks later, the stent was retrieved and the patient dilated to 42 Fr. Following several additional dilations, he has remained dysphagia free.

CHAPTER 78

Management of upper gastrointestinal hemorrhage related to portal hypertension

Tinsay A. Woreta and Zhiping Li
Johns Hopkins University, Baltimore, MD, USA

The anatomy of the portal venous system is shown in Figure 78.1. Portal hypertension is defined as the pathological increase in portal venous pressure, in which the pressure gradient between the portal vein and inferior vena cava is increased above the normal value of 5 mmHg. Cirrhosis is the most common cause of portal hypertension. When the portal venous pressure gradient exceeds a certain threshold, collaterals develop at sites of communication between the portal and systemic circulations (Figure 78.2).

Three-dimensional computed tomography (CT) (Figure 78.3) and magnetic resonance imaging (MRI) (Figure 78.4) are very useful modalities to image the portal vein and assess for the presence of portosystemic collaterals. The most commonly used method to measure portal venous pressure is an indirect approach in which the hepatic venous pressure gradient (HVPG) is determined (Figure 78.5).

Portal venous pressure is directly related to vascular resistance and portal venous blood flow. Increased intrahepatic vascular resistance occurs in cirrhosis due to both structural changes and endothelial dysfunction, which results in intrahepatic vasoconstriction (Figure 78.6). In splanchnic and systemic circulations, endothelial dysfunction leads to arterial vasodilation, which increases splanchnic flow and worsens portal hypertension (Figure 78.7).

Gastroesophageal collaterals are of important clinical significance due to the risk of rupture and variceal hemorrhage (Figure 78.8). Esophageal varices are graded according to their size as follows: F0, no varices; F1, small; F2, medium; and F3, large (Figure 78.9). The size of varices and the presence of red signs (Figure 78.10) are important predictors of the risk of hemorrhage. Gastric varices are classified according to whether they are in continuity with esophageal varices and their location

(Figure 78.11). Fundal varices have the highest risk of bleeding (Figure 78.12).

Acute variceal hemorrhage (Figure 78.13) is a medical emergency that requires optimal management to prevent mortality. The first-line treatment is the combination of vasoactive drugs and emergency endoscopic therapy. The endoscopic therapy of choice for esophageal varices is variceal ligation, as it is more effective than sclerotherapy with fewer side-effects (Figures 78.14 and 78.15). The treatment of choice for gastric varices is endoscopic variceal obturation with the tissue adhesive N-butyl-2-cyanoacrylate. Endoscopic ultrasound-guided therapy with combined coiling and cyanoacrylate injection is a promising new strategy to increase efficacy and minimize the risk of embolization (Video 78.1). Targeting perforating veins that feed gastric varices is another innovative approach (Figure 78.16). Transjugular intrahepatic portosystemic shunt (TIPS) is also an effective therapy (Figure 78.17). Surgical shunt therapy may also be considered in patients with Child–Pugh A cirrhosis (Figure 78.18).

Portal hypertensive gastropathy (Figure 78.19) is another possible source of bleeding in patients with portal hypertension and should be distinguished from gastric antral vascular ectasia (GAVE) (Figure 78.20), as they require different treatment approaches.

Acknowledgment

We sincerely thank Dr. Payal Saxena, Dr. Marcia Canto, and Dr. Mouen Khashab in the Division of Gastroenterology/Hepatology at Johns Hopkins Hospital for providing multiple images and the video clip for this chapter.

Yamada's Atlas of Gastroenterology, Fifth Edition. Edited by Daniel K. Podolsky, Michael Camilleri, J. Gregory Fitz, Anthony N. Kalloo, Fergus Shanahan, and Timothy C. Wang.
© 2016 John Wiley & Sons, Ltd. Published 2016 by John Wiley & Sons, Ltd.
Companion website: www.yamadagastro.com/atlas

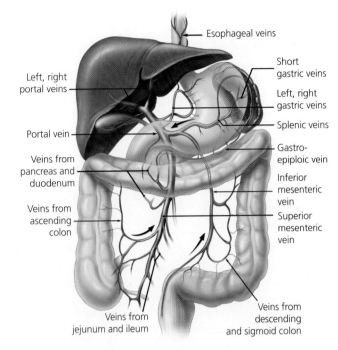

Figure 78.1 Anatomy of the portal venous system.

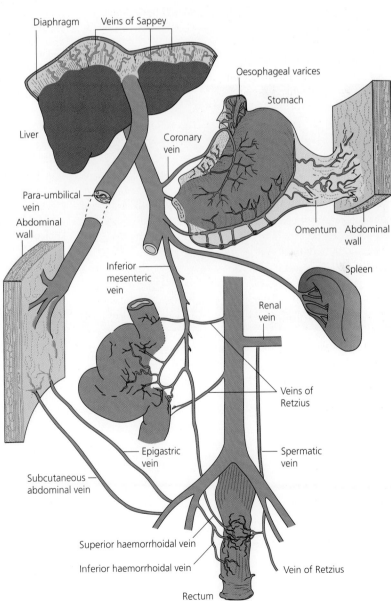

Figure 78.2 Sites of portosystemic collateral circulation in portal hypertension and cirrhosis. Source: Dooley J, Sherlock S. Sherlock's Diseases of the Liver and Biliary System, 12th edn, 2011. Reproduced with permission of John Wiley & Sons.

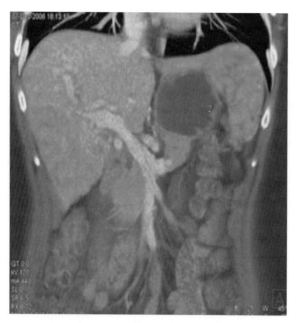

Figure 78.3 Three-dimensional computed tomography scan is a sensitive method to assess portal venous anatomy.

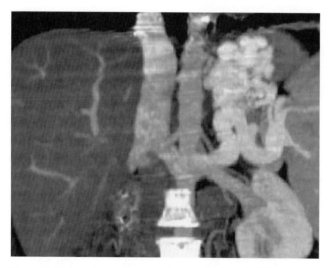

Figure 78.4 Magnetic resonance imaging showing large fundal varices.

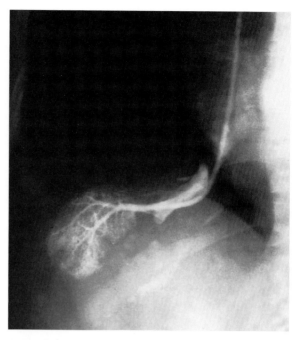

Figure 78.5 Indirect measurement of portal venous pressure via hepatic vein catheterization. A catheter is inserted into the internal jugular vein and wedged into the hepatic vein. The wedged position is confirmed by injecting a small amount of contrast, which enters the hepatic sinusoids. Source: Dooley J, Sherlock S. Sherlock's Diseases of the Liver and Biliary System, 12th edn, 2011. Reproduced with permission of John Wiley & Sons.

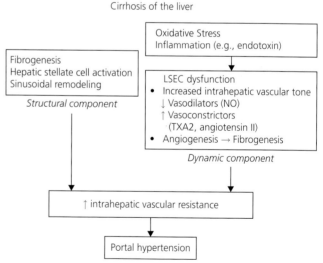

Figure 78.6 Summary of the changes that occur in the intrahepatic circulation in cirrhosis that lead to increased intrahepatic vascular resistance and subsequent development of portal hypertension. LSEC, liver sinusoidal endothelial cell; NO, nitric oxide; TXA2, thromboxane A2.

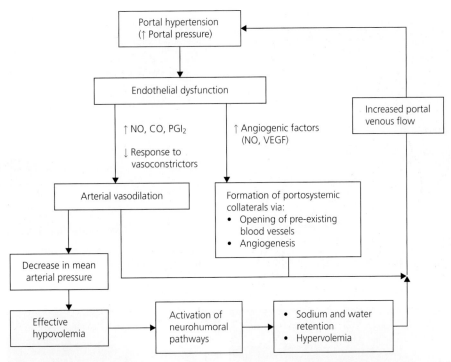

Figure 78.7 Summary of the changes that occur in splanchnic and systemic circulation in cirrhosis that lead to increased portal flow and exacerbate portal hypertension. NO, nitric oxide; CO, carbon monoxide; PGI$_2$, prostacyclin; VEGF, vascular endothelial growth factor.

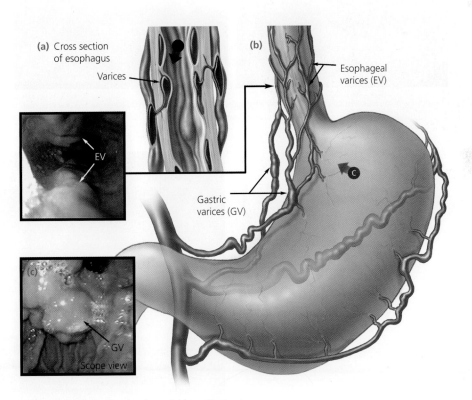

Figure 78.8 Development of gastroesophageal varices in portal hypertension.

F1   F2   F3

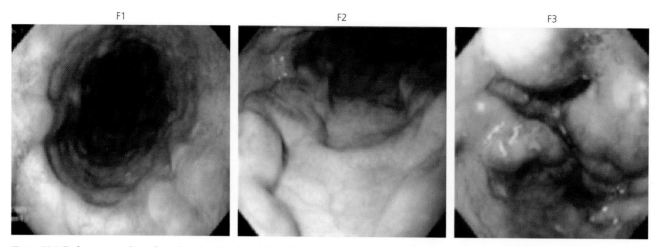

Figure 78.9 Endoscopic grading of esophageal varices from F1 to F3 based on size. Source: Maruyama HS, Arun J. Portal hypertension: nonsurgical and surgical management. In: Schiff's Diseases of the Liver, 11th edn. Schiff ER, Maddrey WC Sorrell MF (eds), 2012. Reproduced with permission of John Wiley & Sons.

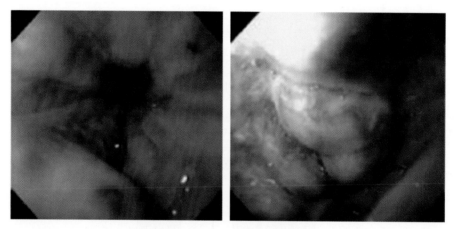

Figure 78.10 Red signs of esophageal varices, which predict the risk of variceal hemorrhage. Cherry red spots are discrete, flat, red spots that overlie varices. Red wale marks are longitudinal dilated venules on the surface of varices.

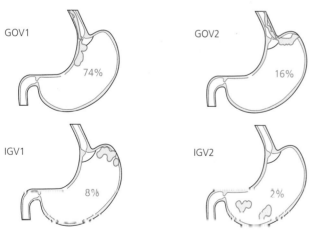

Figure 78.11 Sarin's classification of gastric varices.

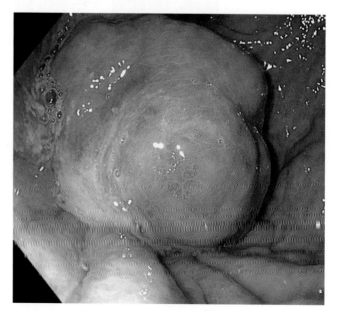

Figure 78.12 Endoscopic appearance of large IGV1 varix upon retroflexed view. Source: Courtesy of Dr. Payal Saxena and Dr. Marcia Canto.

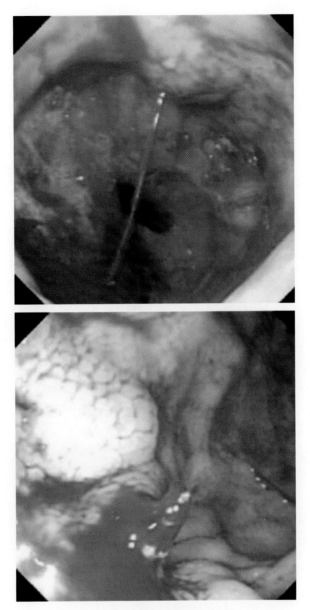

Figure 78.13 Actively spurting esophageal and gastric varices.

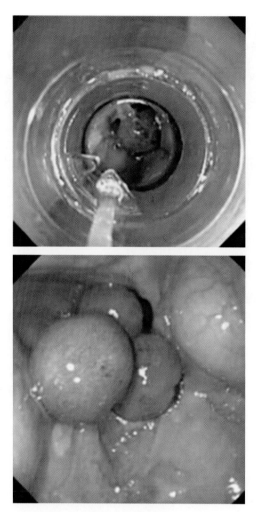

Figure 78.14 Multiple bands applied to esophageal varices.

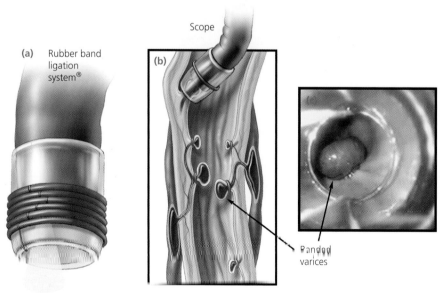

Figure 78.15 (a–c) Schematic depiction of esophageal variceal banding.

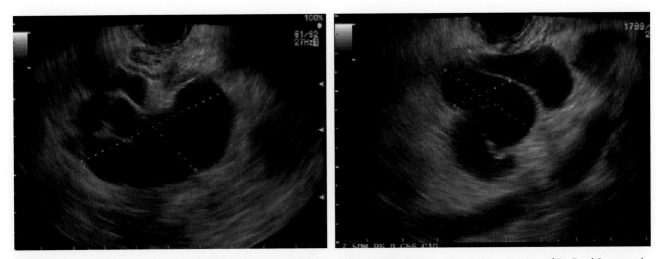

Figure 78.16 Endoscopic ultrasound revealing large gastric varix and perforating veins feeding gastric varix. Source: Courtesy of Dr. Payal Saxena and Dr. Mouen Khashab.

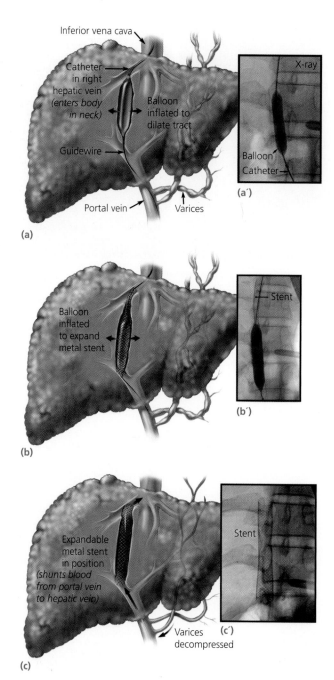

Figure 78.17 (a–c) Schematic showing the technique of transjugular intrahepatic portosystemic shunt (TIPS). Source: Reproduced with permission of Division of Gastroenterology, Johns Hopkins University www.hopkins-gi.org.

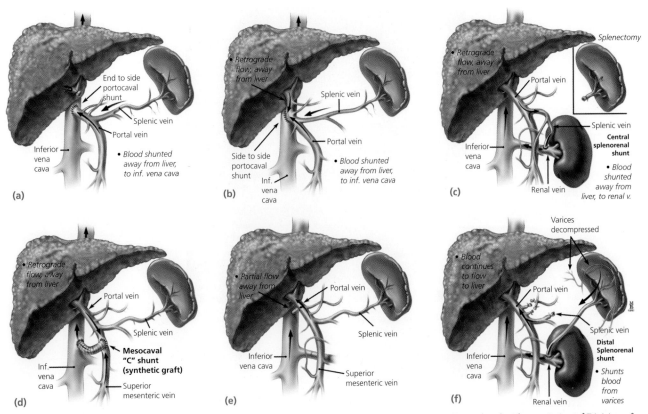

Figure 78.18 (a–f) Various types of shunt surgeries used for management of portal hypertension. Source: Reproduced with permission of Division of Gastroenterology, Johns Hopkins University www.hopkins-gi.org.

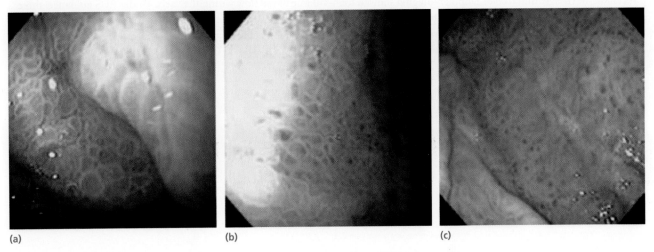

Figure 78.19 Endoscopic appearance of portal hypertensive gastropathy, ranging from mild (a) to severe (c).

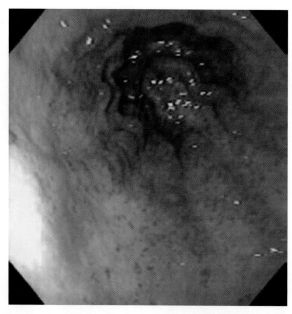

Figure 78.20 Endoscopic appearance of gastric antral vascular ectasia (GAVE).

To access the video for this chapter, please go to
www.yamadagastro.com/atlas

Video 78.1 Endoscopic ultrasound (EUS)-guided coiling and cyanoacrylate injection of large IGV1 varix with stigmata of recent hemorrhage. Initial color Doppler imaging showed high-volume blood flow within the varix. Under EUS guidance, three embolization coils were deployed into the varix followed by cyanoacrylate injection. Repeat color Doppler after treatment showed no significant flow within the varix. Probing of the varix with an injection catheter tip revealed firm consistency, confirming complete obliteration. Source: Courtesy of Dr. Payal Saxena and Dr. Marcia Canto.

CHAPTER 79

Endoscopic diagnosis and treatment of nonvariceal upper gastrointestinal hemorrhage

David J. Bjorkman

Florida Atlantic University, Boca Raton, FL, USA

Upper gastrointestinal (UGI) bleeding from peptic ulcer disease and other nonvariceal causes is a frequent cause of hospitalization (250 000–300 000 hospital admissions per year in the United States). Advances in endoscopic diagnosis and therapy have not substantially affected the overall mortality rate of this disorder, which remains in the range of 5%–15% depending on age and comorbid medical conditions.

Initial treatment should focus on vigorous volume resuscitation. A combination of clinical characteristics and endoscopic findings can predict the risk for rebleeding and mortality. This allows the level of care to be tailored to the risk for the individual patient. In the setting of bleeding peptic ulcers the best predictor of persistent or recurrent bleeding, the need for surgical intervention, and mortality is the endoscopic appearance of the ulcer. Lesions with active bleeding or a visible vessel have a high likelihood of rebleeding (40%–55%) and a mortality rate that exceeds 10%. On the other hand, lesions with a clean base have a very low risk of rebleeding (<5%) and a mortality rate that approaches 0%. Early endoscopic evaluation can, therefore, determine the optimal treatment approach for each patient.

Endoscopic therapy is indicated for all lesions that are considered to have a high risk of rebleeding (active bleeding or visible vessel). Ulcers with adherent clots that obscure the underlying lesions may benefit from careful endoscopic therapy.

Endoscopic therapies can be thermal (electrocoagulation, direct heat application, or laser therapy), involve injection with various agents, or employ mechanical compression of the bleeding site (hemostatic clips or bands). All of these methods have a high rate (90%) of success in stopping active bleeding, and significantly reduce the risk of rebleeding. Endoscopic therapy also reduces morbidity, mortality, transfusion requirements,

and the costs of care. The technique of choice for a specific patient depends on the clinical situation, the location of the lesion, and the skill of the endoscopist.

This chapter demonstrates some of the endoscopic findings predictive of the outcome of a bleeding lesion, some of the devices used to treat the lesions, and the results of therapy (Figures 79.1–79.14).

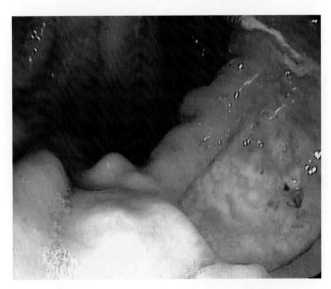

Figure 79.1 Deep gastric ulcer with flat pigmented spots in the base. This lesion, despite its depth, has a low (<10%) risk of rebleeding and a mortality rate of less than 5%. Endoscopic therapy is not indicated for this lesion.

Yamada's Atlas of Gastroenterology, Fifth Edition. Edited by Daniel K. Podolsky, Michael Camilleri, J. Gregory Fitz, Anthony N. Kalloo, Fergus Shanahan, and Timothy C. Wang.

© 2016 John Wiley & Sons, Ltd. Published 2016 by John Wiley & Sons, Ltd.

Companion website: www.yamadagastro.com/atlas

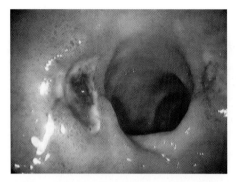

Figure 79.2 A duodenal ulcer with a central smooth-surfaced protuberance indicating a visible vessel. Despite the absence of active bleeding, the risk of rebleeding in this lesion is greater than 40% and the mortality rate is greater than 10%. Both of these figures can be considerably reduced by appropriate endoscopic therapy. Source: Dooley J, Sherlock S. Sherlock's Diseases of the Liver and Biliary System, 12th edn. Oxford: Wiley-Blackwell, 2011. Reproduced with permission of John Wiley & Sons.

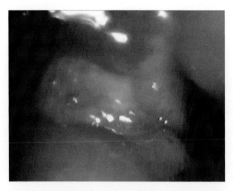

Figure 79.3 A large, deep duodenal ulcer with a visible vessel with bleeding is seen in the center of the base of the ulcer. The position of this lesion is ideal for direct application of thermal therapy to coagulate the vessel.

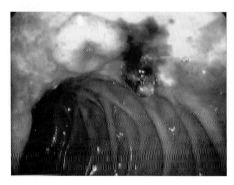

Figure 79.4 This large ulcer at the apex of the duodenal bulb shows a visible vessel extending into the lumen. The risk of rebleeding from this lesion is very high without endoscopic therapy.

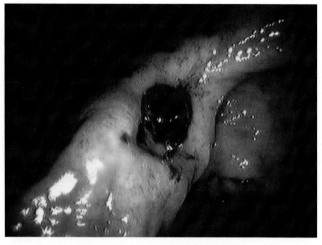

Figure 79.5 This deep ulcer on the gastric angularis has an adherent clot (remains after vigorous washing) that obscures the ulcer base. The risk of rebleeding in this setting depends on the underlying lesion. Removal of the clot may precipitate active bleeding. Optimal treatment of this lesion remains controversial. If the clot is removed to evaluate the underlying lesion, injection therapy with epinephrine (adrenaline) should be performed before clot manipulation to limit or prevent active bleeding. Source: Dooley J, Sherlock S. Sherlock's Diseases of the Liver and Biliary System, 12th edn. Oxford: Wiley-Blackwell, 2011. Reproduced with permission of John Wiley & Sons.

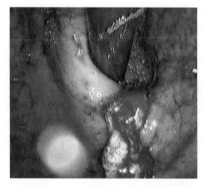

Figure 79.6 This clot extending from the gastroesophageal junction into the cardia of the stomach overlies and obscures a Mallory–Weiss tear. There is oozing at the superior aspect of the clot from the Mallory–Weiss tear. The endoscope is retroflexed with the proximal part of the scope seen entering the stomach from the esophagus. Although Mallory–Weiss tears usually stop bleeding spontaneously, endoscopic therapy is indicated for actively bleeding lesions such as this.

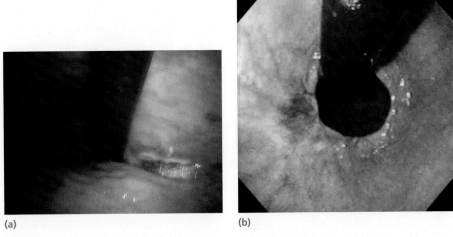

(a)   (b)

Figure 79.7 (a, b) Two Mallory–Weiss tears at the gastroesophageal junction are demonstrated in these images.

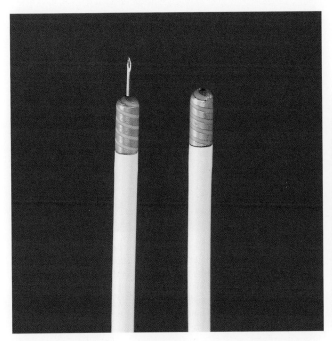

Figure 79.8 Multipolar electrocoagulation catheter with electrodes that circle the end of the catheter and a central channel for vigorous water irrigation. This catheter also has a retractable central injection needle to allow combined electrocoagulation and injection therapy. The probe is inserted through the working channel of the endoscope and applied directly to the bleeding lesion while electrical energy is repeatedly passed between the electrodes through the tissue. The resistance of the tissue results in heat that cauterizes the lesion and seals the walls of the bleeding vessel together in what is called coaptive coagulation. Control of energy delivery and water irrigation is achieved by foot pedals attached to the electrical generator and the probe.

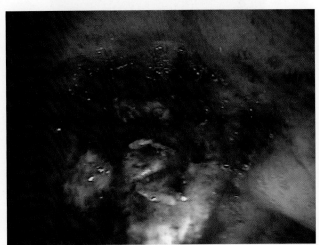

Figure 79.9 Active bleeding from a duodenal ulcer. Initial injection with saline or dilute epinephrine can control the bleeding. Subsequent thermal therapy can be applied to the specific bleeding site. Injection alone is not as effective as injection followed by thermal therapy. Source: Maruyama HS, Arun J. Portal hypertension: nonsurgical and surgical management. In: Schiff ER, Maddrey WC, Sorrell MF (eds). Schiff's Diseases of the Liver, 11th edn. Oxford: Wiley-Blackwell, 2011. Reproduced with permission of John Wiley & Sons.

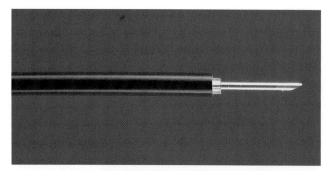

Figure 79.10 Endoscopic injection needle. This needle is attached to a syringe containing the desired solution for injection. The needle is retracted into the catheter and then passed through the working channel of the endoscope. The needle is then advanced out of the catheter and repeated injections are made around the bleeding lesion. When saline or dilute epinephrine is used, large volumes of injected fluid (10 mL or more) can be used to tamponade the bleeding lesion. Smaller volumes (0.1- to 0.2-mL aliquots) should be injected when absolute alcohol is used. Injection of saline or epinephrine is very helpful in slowing active bleeding in preparation for more definitive thermal or injection therapy. Data suggest that saline injection alone is not as effective as contact thermal methods in preventing rebleeding.

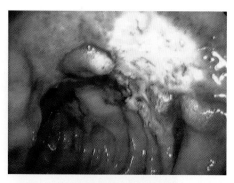

Figure 79.12 Appearance of a duodenal ulcer after successful thermal therapy. The bleeding site and the surrounding area have been successfully heated, leaving the white coagulated tissue behind with no evidence of a persistent visible vessel or bleeding. The surrounding edema is the result of thermal therapy and may also help reduce blood flow to the area.

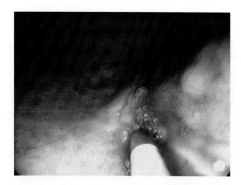

Figure 79.11 Direct application of a multipolar probe to a visible vessel in the base of a gastric ulcer. The central injection needle can be used to inject saline or dilute epinephrine around the vessel. The definitive thermal therapy can then be applied with firm pressure of the probe using long bursts of low energy.

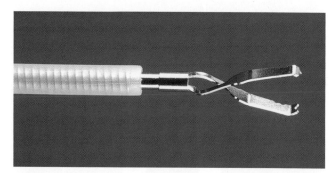

Figure 79.13 A hemostatic clip attached to the delivery catheter. The clip is similar to that used in surgery and is applied to a bleeding vessel to close it. After several days, the clip sloughs into the lumen and is passed. The clip can be rotated to provide a better position for application. The clip is then closed via the handle on the delivery catheter and released from the delivery device. Because the bleeding vessel is not always visible or accessible, multiple clips are often required to achieve the appropriate hemostatic effect.

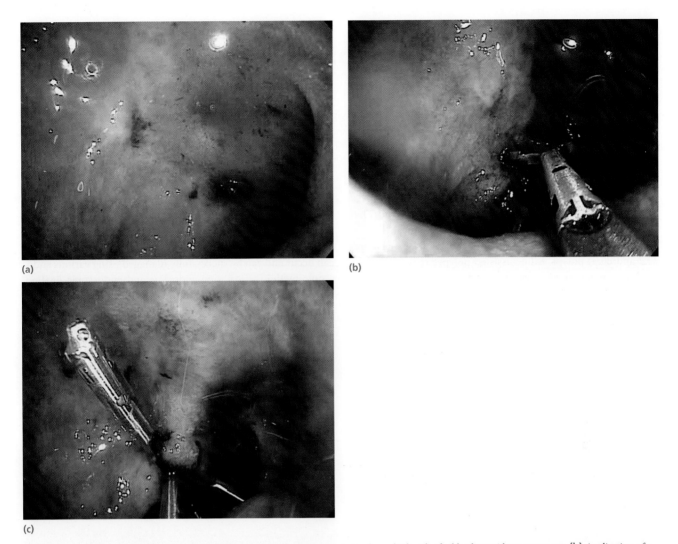

Figure 79.14 (a) Deep duodenal ulcer with a visible vessel in the base. This lesion has a high risk of rebleeding without treatment. **(b)** Application of a hemostatic clip to the ulcer seen in (a). The position of the ulcer facilitates the placement of the clip. Clips may be difficult to place in ulcers that are behind folds or when the ulcer base is extremely fibrotic. Manipulation of the visible vessel may precipitate active bleeding, as seen here. **(c)** Appearance of the same ulcer after successful placement of multiple hemostatic clips. The bleeding has been controlled.

CHAPTER 80

Endoscopic therapy for polyps and tumors

Mouen A. Khashab,[1] Sergey V. Kantsevoy,[1] and Heiko Pohl[2]
[1] Johns Hopkins University School of Medicine Baltimore, MD, USA
[2] Dartmouth-Hitchcock Medical Center and VA White River Junction, White River Junction, VT, USA

Endoscopic resection of gastrointestinal polyps and tumors has become an important addition to traditional surgical therapy. This includes resection of small (Figure 80.1) and large (Figures 80.2 and 80.3) polyps. Saline-assisted polypectomy is typically used for resection of larger flat and sessile gastrointestinal polyps (Figures 80.4 and 80.5). Older data suggested that use of argon plasma coagulation to ablate margins of polypectomy sites may result in a decrease in polyp recurrence during follow-up (Figure 80.6). Detachable snares can be placed around thick stalks of larger pedunculated polyps to prevent post-polypectomy bleeding (Figure 80.7). Closing large polypectomy sites with endoclips may also play a role in the prevention of delayed postpolypectomy bleeding (Figure 80.8). Both immediate bleeding (Figure 80.9) and delayed bleeding (Figure 80.10) can occur and can be successfully managed using various endoscopic methods, including endoclips and endoscopic ligation. Endoscopic submucosal dissection can also be employed for en bloc resection of large gastrointestinal lesions (Figures 80.11 and 80.12). Perforations can occur during resection and can be closed using standard endoclips (Figure 80.13) or over-the-scope clips (Figure 80.14).

Yamada's Atlas of Gastroenterology, Fifth Edition. Edited by Daniel K. Podolsky, Michael Camilleri, J. Gregory Fitz, Anthony N. Kalloo, Fergus Shanahan, and Timothy C. Wang.
© 2016 John Wiley & Sons, Ltd. Published 2016 by John Wiley & Sons, Ltd.
Companion website: www.yamadagastro.com/atlas

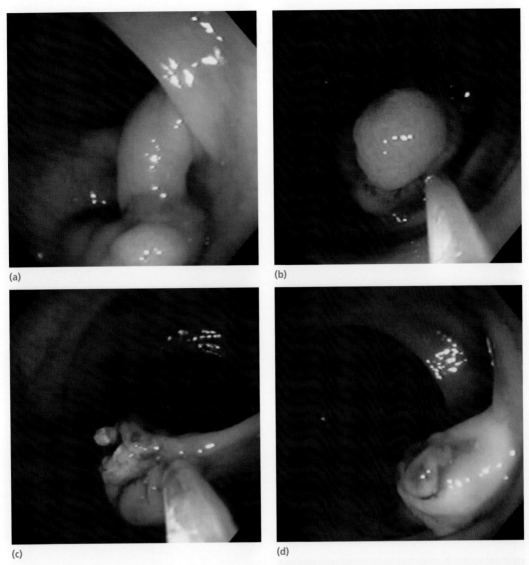

Figure 80.1 Endoscopic removal of small pedunculated colonic polyp. **(a)** Colonic polyp on a long, thin stalk. **(b)** A polypectomy snare applied to the stalk below the head of the polyp. **(c)** The polyp pulled away from the colonic wall to prevent electrical damage to the bowel wall when electrocautery was applied. **(d)** The stalk is transected by the snare without any bleeding from the remaining portion of the stalk. It is very important to leave at least a small portion of the stalk, which can be used for ligation or cautery if postpolypectomy bleeding occurs (as illustrated later in Figure 80.10).

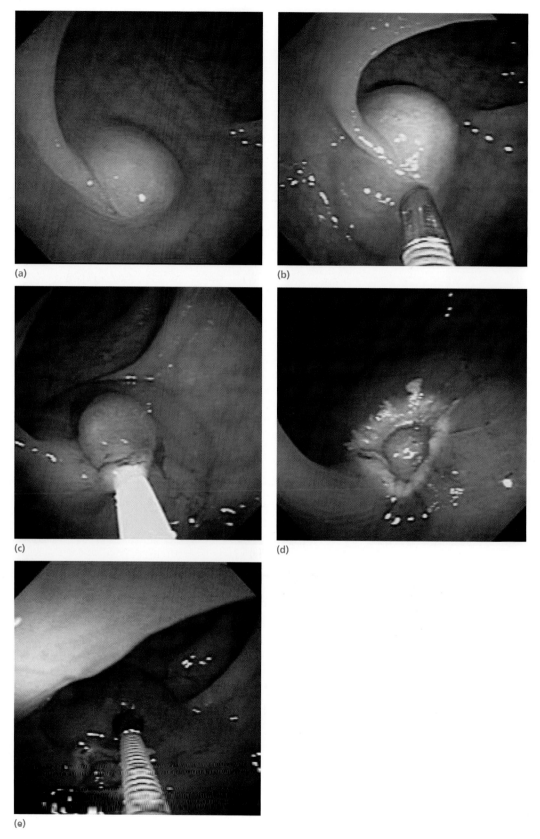

Figure 80.2 Saline-assisted polypectomy of a sessile polyp. **(a)** Flat sessile polyp, 1 cm in diameter, located in the ascending colon. **(b)** Normal saline (5 mL) is injected into the submucosal layer of the colon to elevate the polyp. **(c)** The polyp is raised on the submucosal cushion made by injection of normal saline. A polypectomy snare is tightened around the polyp. **(d)** The polyp is excised by the endoscopic snare and removed. The submucosal cushion is still present following the polypectomy. **(e)** The polypectomy site is tattooed using a submucosal injection of Spot® (GI Supply, Camp Mill, PA).

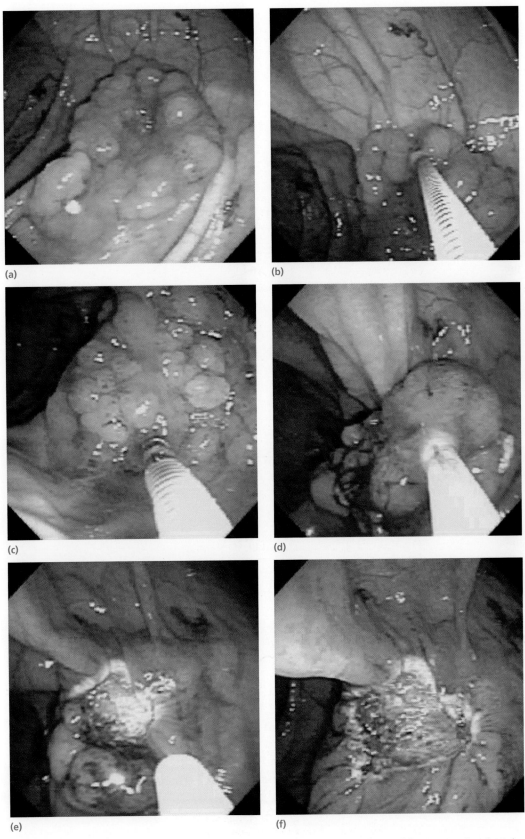

Figure 80.3 Piecemeal removal of a large, flat, sessile colonic polyp with saline-assisted injection technique. **(a)** A large sessile polyp is located in the proximal ascending colon. **(b)** Submucosal injection of normal saline performed in the most proximal portion of the polyp. **(c)** Submucosal injection into the most distal portion of the polyp completes creation of the submucosal cushion under the polyp. **(d)** The polypectomy snare is applied around the proximal portion of the polyp. **(e)** The proximal half of the polyp is removed. **(f)** The polypectomy is completed without technical problems or complications. **(g)** The polypectomy site is tattooed using submucosal injection of Spot® (GI Supply, Camp Mill, PA). **(h, i)** The resected polyp is removed for pathological examination with a Roth Net® (US Endoscopy, Mentor, OH) retrieval net. **(j)** A repeat colonoscopy 3 months following initial removal demonstrates complete healing of the polypectomy site without any residual polypoid tissue.

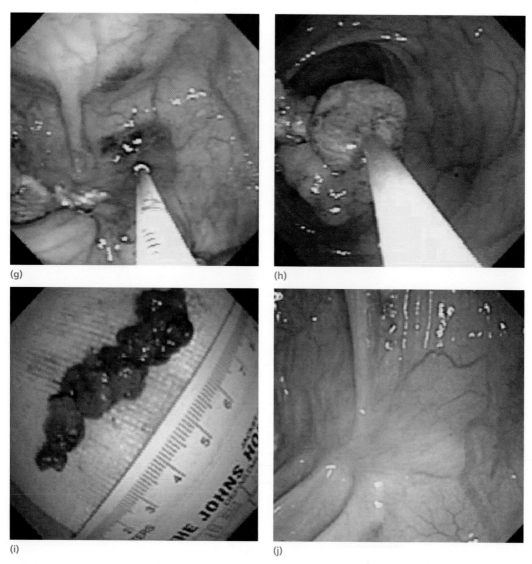

(g)

(h)

(i)

(j)

Figure 80.3 (*Continued*)

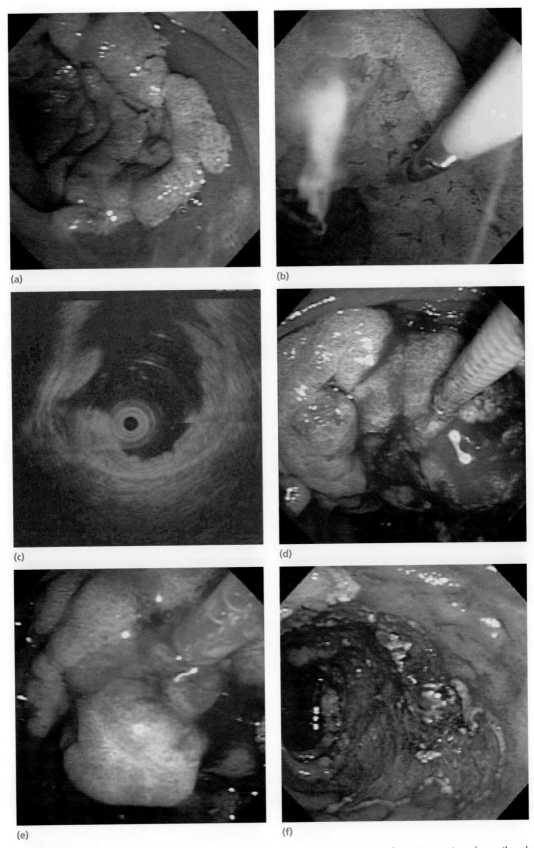

Figure 80.4 Endoscopic ultrasound for detection of the depth of the bowel wall involvement prior to endoscopic resection of a sessile polypoid lesion. **(a)** A large flat sessile polypoid lesion is seen in the second portion of the duodenum. **(b)** The duodenum is filled with water (to create acoustic interface for endoscopic ultrasound) and a 20-MHz endoscopic ultrasound probe (Olympus Optical Ltd, Tokyo, Japan) is advanced toward the lesion. **(c)** Endoscopic ultrasound demonstrates polypoid thickening of the mucosal layer with intact submucosal layer of the duodenum. **(d)** Normal saline is injected into the submucosal layer to facilitate polypectomy. **(e)** The polypectomy snare is applied to the polyp. The polyp is excised by the piecemeal technique. **(f)** Final endoscopic view demonstrating the polypectomy site after complete resection of the polyp.

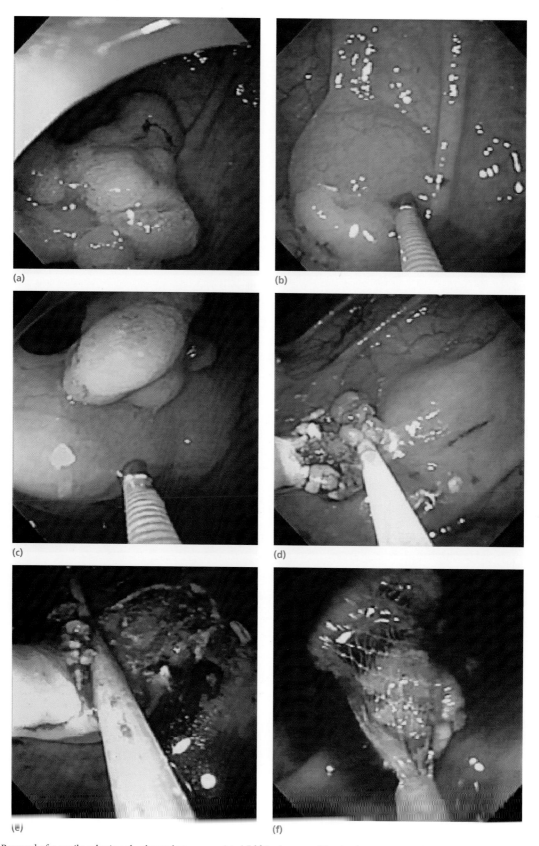

Figure 80.5 Removal of a sessile colonic polyp located on an angulated fold in the area of fixed colonic turns can be technically difficult and cause perforation of the colonic wall. Submucosal injection prior to polypectomy facilitates removal of the lesion and decreases the risk of perforation. (a) Large fungating polyp with a broad base located in the hepatic flexure on top of the colonic fold. (b) Submucosal injection of normal saline solution started with the most proximal portion of the polyp. (c) Submucosal injection is completed when the polyp is elevated above the colonic fold. (d) The polyp is excised using the piecemeal technique with a polypectomy snare. (e) Polypectomy is completed without perforation or bleeding from the polypectomy site. (f) All resected parts of the polyp are collected with a Roth Net® (US Endoscopy, Mentor, OH) retrieval net.

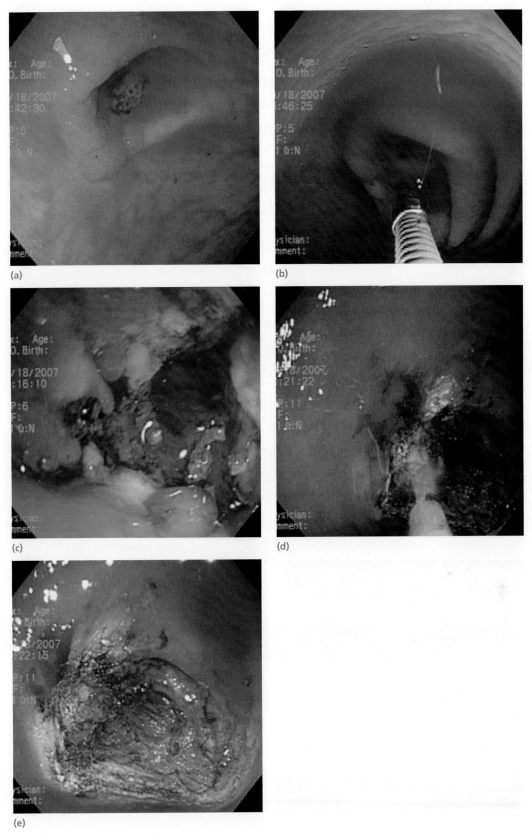

Figure 80.6 Argon plasma coagulation is frequently used to eliminate residual polypoid tissue at the margins and the base of the polypectomy site in order to prevent recurrence of the polyp after polypectomy. **(a)** Endoscopic view of the sessile polyp located inside the appendicular orifice. **(b)** The polyp is elevated with submucosal injection of normal saline solution. **(c)** The polyp is excised with an endoscopic polypectomy snare. **(d)** The base and margins of the polypectomy site are treated with the argon plasma coagulator to remove residual polypoid tissue at the margins and the base of the polypectomy site. **(e)** Final view of the polypectomy site with no visible residual polypoid tissue.

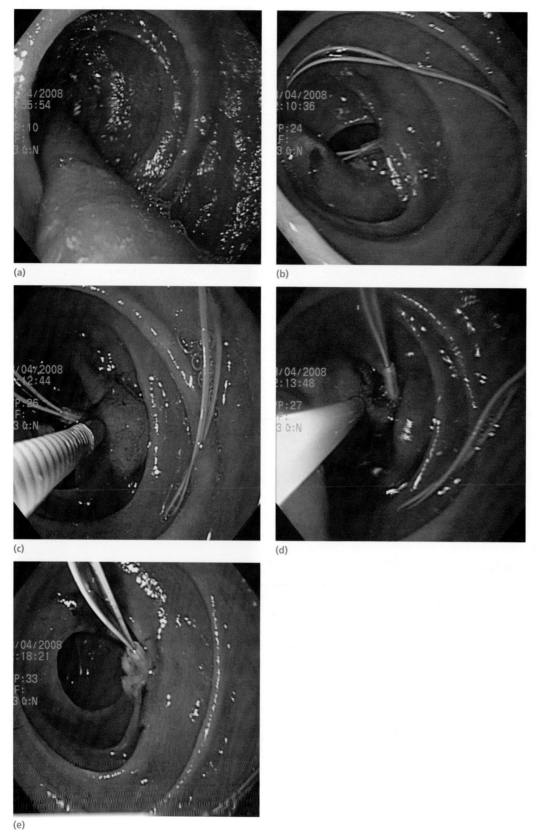

Figure 80.7 Use of detachable snare to prevent postpolypectomy bleeding following removal of a pedunculated polyp with a large (thick) stalk. **(a)** Pedunculated polyp with a large stalk (>1 cm in diameter) located in the second portion of the duodenum. **(b)** Detachable loop (PolyLoop® HX-400U-30, Olympus Optical Inc, Tokyo, Japan) is applied to the base of the stalk at the point of its attachment to the duodenal wall. **(c)** The future polypectomy site is tattooed using a submucosal injection of Spot® (GI Supply, Camp Mill, PA). **(d)** An endoscopic snare is applied to the stalk of the polyp above the previously deployed detachable loop. **(e)** The polyp is excised and removed. The detachable loop is clearly seen at the site of its application. There is no bleeding from the remnant of the stalk.

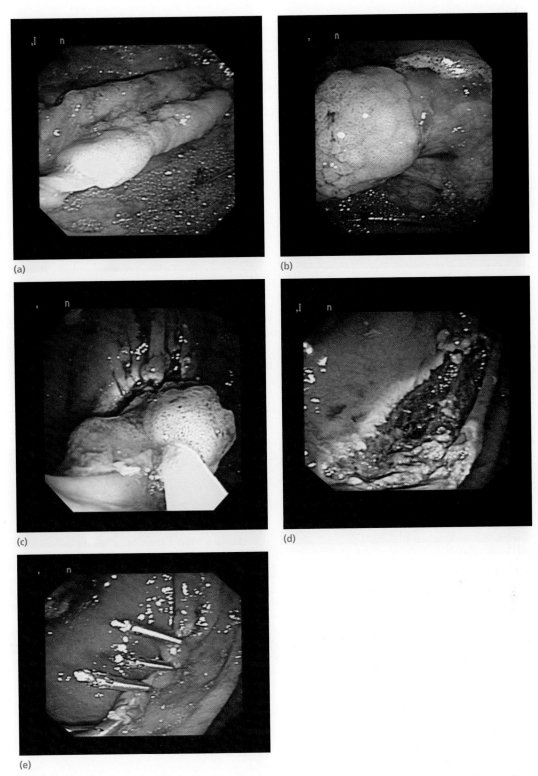

Figure 80.8 Endoscopic resection of a large sessile polyp in an anticoagulated patient. (a) A flat 25-mm polyp was seen in the ascending colon. (b) The polyp was lifted with a mixture of saline and 0.25% indigo carmine. (c) Piecemeal resection was then performed using a 33-mm snare. (d) The edges of the polypectomy site were then treated with argon plasma coagulation to decrease chance of residual/recurrent polyp during follow-up. (e) The polypectomy site was closed with multiple hemoclips to prevent postpolypectomy bleeding.

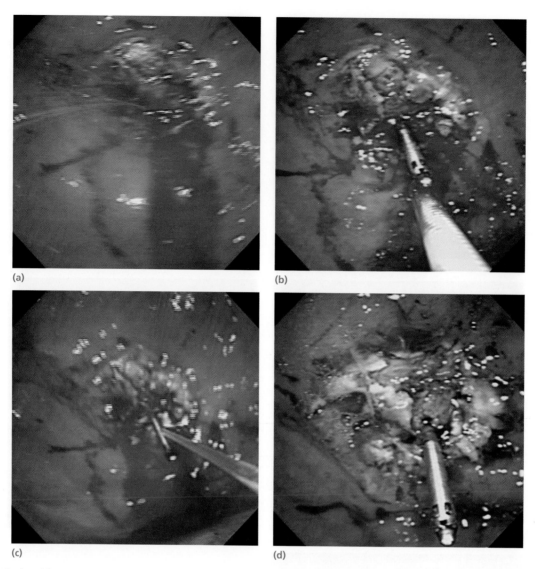

(a)

(b)

(c)

(d)

Figure 80.9 Bleeding following endoscopic polyp removal. Endoscopic hemostasis is usually successful in controlling the bleeding. **(a)** Active arterial bleeding from a polypectomy site. **(b)** Endoscopic clip (Resolution® Boston Scientific Microvasive, Natick, MA) is applied to the bleeding vessel. **(c)** The blood from the polypectomy site is washed away. **(d)** Final view of the polypectomy site demonstrating successful hemostasis without any active bleeding.

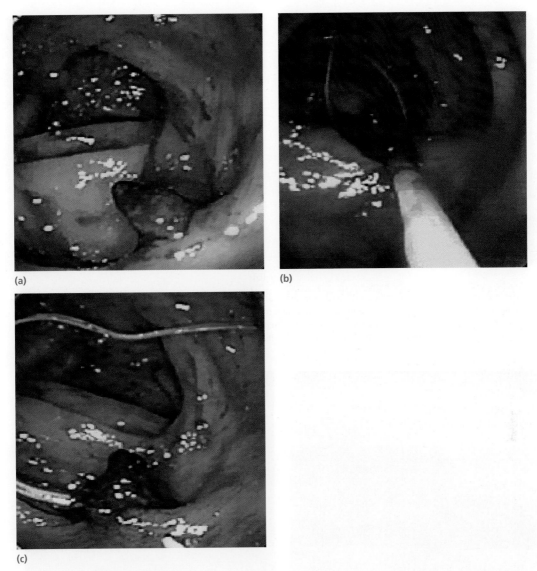

Figure 80.10 Delayed bleeding postpolypectomy controlled with endoscopic ligation. **(a)** The patient presented with rectal bleeding 24 h postpolypectomy. Colonoscopy demonstrates active bleeding from the remnant of the polyp's stalk post previous polypectomy. **(b)** Endoscopic detachable loop (PolyLoop® HX-400U-30, Olympus Optical Inc., Tokyo, Japan) is positioned around the remnant of the polyp's stalk. **(c)** Full deployment of the detachable loop with successful endoscopic hemostasis.

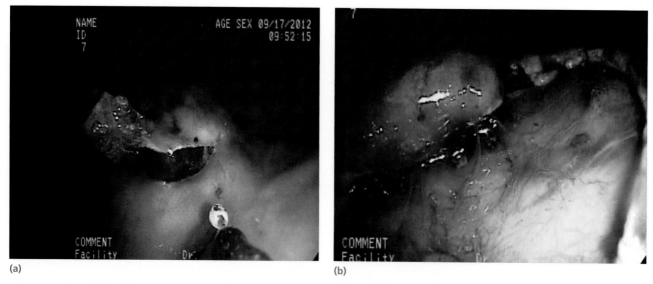

(a)

(b)

Figure 80.11 Gastric endoscopic submucosal dissection (ESD) performed in an animal model using a new endoscopic gel (Cook Medical Inc, Winston-Salem, NC) with submucosal dissecting properties. **(a)** Submucosal injection of the viscous gel is performed to lift the lesion. Circumferential incision is then performed using an ESD knife. The gel is seen extruding through the incision. **(b)** Gel has dissecting properties and submucosal dissection is, therefore, not required. Complete resection is achieved by circumferential incision using an ESD knife and submucosal dissection by the gel.

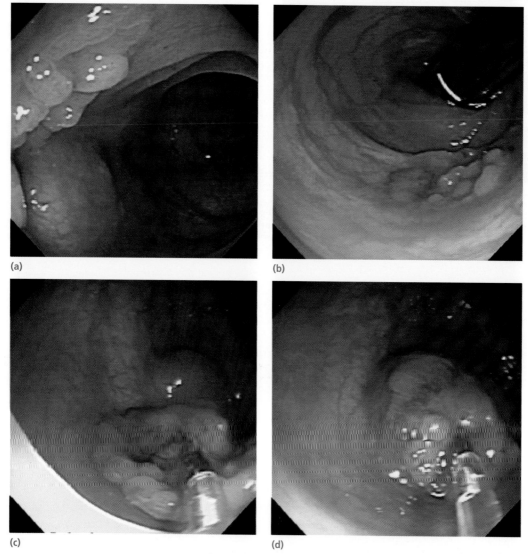

(a)

(b)

(c)

(d)

Figure 80.12

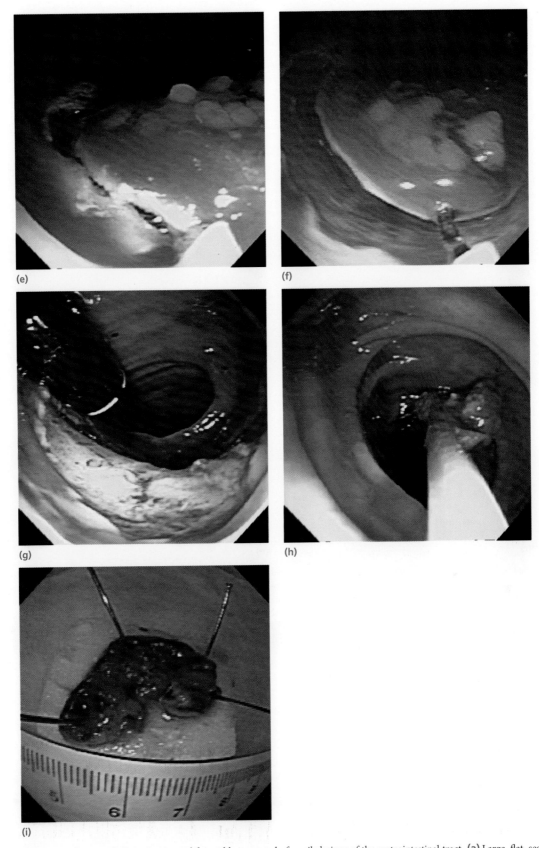

Figure 80.12 Endoscopic submucosal dissection is used for en bloc removal of sessile lesions of the gastrointestinal tract. **(a)** Large, flat, sessile polyp located in descending colon. Please note suboptimal visualization of the polyp on forward view due to its location behind the colonic fold. **(b)** Retroflex position of the colonoscope significantly improves visualization of the polyp. **(c)** Submucosal injection of normal saline solution lifting the most distal portion of the polyp. **(d)** The entire polyp is lifted with the submucosal injection of normal saline. **(e)** A circumferential incision is made around the polyp using the tip of a polypectomy snare. **(f)** The polyp is dissected from underlining muscularis layer using the tip of the polypectomy snare. **(g)** Appearance of the polypectomy site after completion of the endoscopic submucosal dissection without any evidence of bleeding or perforation. **(h)** Resected polyp is removed using a Roth Net® (US Endoscopy, Mentor, OH) retrieval net. **(i)** Pathological specimen demonstrating en bloc removal of the large (3 cm in diameter) polyp within the healthy tissues.

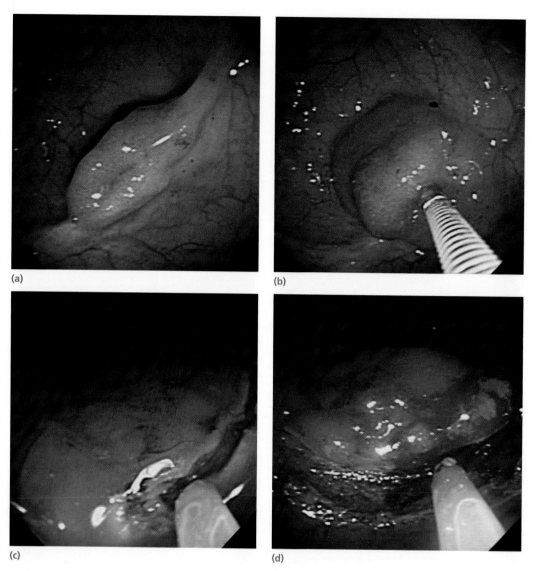

Figure 80.13 Small perforations after endoscopic submucosal dissection repaired with application of endoscopic clips. **(a)** A sessile polyp located on a colonic fold in the descending colon. **(b)** The polyp is raised with a submucosal injection of normal saline solution. **(c)** A circumferential incision around the polyp performed with the tip of an endoscopic polypectomy snare. **(d)** Endoscopic submucosal dissection is performed with the tip of an endoscopic polypectomy snare. **(e)** The polyp is removed en bloc with endoscopic submucosal dissection; however, the small perforation is clearly visible in the muscularis layer of the colon. **(f)** Endoscopic clip (Resolution® Boston Scientific Microvasive, Natick, MA) is ready for application to close the perforation. **(g)** Application of two endoscopic clips to completely close the colonic perforation.

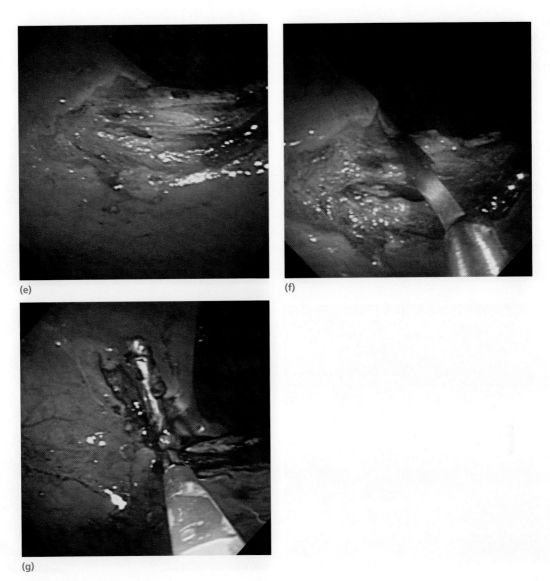

(e)

(f)

(g)

Figure 80.13 (*Continued*)

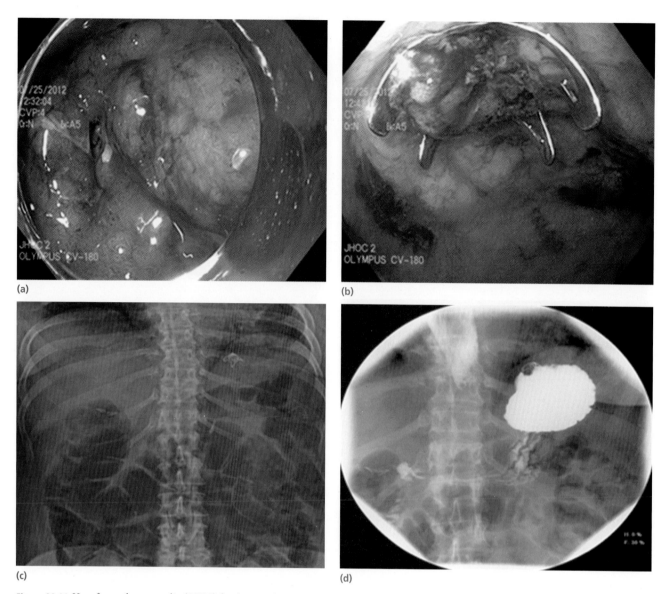

(a)

(b)

(c)

(d)

Figure 80.14 Use of over-the-scope clip (OTSC) for closure of gastric perforation due to penetrating foreign body. **(a)** Full-thickness defect was noted in gastric fundus after removal of the foreign body. **(b)** One OTSC clip was placed and resulted in complete closure of gastric defect. **(c)** An abdominal radiograph was obtained and showed the clip in the left upper quadrant. **(d)** An upper gastrointestinal series demonstrated no evidence of leak.

To access the videos for this chapter, please go to
www.yamadagastro.com/atlas

Video 80.1 Video clip demonstrating endoscopic resection of a giant duodenal bulb polyp in retroflexion. Resection on forward viewing was not possible. The gastroscope was retroflexed in the bulb and then the polyp was lifted with saline/indigo carmine. The polyp was then resected in a piecemeal fashion using a 33-mm snare. The edges of the polypectomy site were treated with argon plasma coagulation.

Video 80.2 Video clip demonstrating endoscopic resection of a dysplastic flat polyp in a patient with ulcerative colitis. The polyp margins were marked with argon plasma coagulation. Subsequently, the polyp was lifted and then resected en bloc with a large snare. The edges were treated with argon plasma coagulation.

Video 80.3 Video clip demonstrating ligation-assisted endoscopic mucosal resection (EMR) of a duodenal bulb carcinoid in a cirrhotic patient. One band was placed around the tumor using a gastroscope. The resection angle was not optimal using a forward-viewing endoscope. This was replaced with a side-viewing duodenoscope and the tumor was then resected en bloc using a hot snare. The EMR site was completely closed with placement of multiple hemoclips as the patient was at high risk for post-EMR bleeding.

CHAPTER 81

Laparoscopy and laparotomy

Ricardo Zorron[1] and Gustavo Carvalho[2]

[1] Klinikum Bremerhaven Reikenheide, Bremerhaven, Germany
[2] Universidade Federal de Pernambuco, Recife, Brazil

Indications for diagnostic laparoscopy and laparotomy

Staging laparoscopy for intraabdominal malignancies

Gastrointestinal (gastric, pancreatic) staging and laparoscopic evaluation of pelvic masses is useful because of the relative inability of computed tomography (CT) to detect small (<5 mm) peritoneal and superficial liver metastases, saving some patients with unsuspected local unresectability from a nontherapeutic laparotomy.

It is performed with a single trocar in cases where only the peritoneal surface and liver will be evaluated (usually a 10-min procedure). Three trocars are used when retroperitoneal exploration with opening of the bursa omentalis and laparoscopic ultrasound are performed. When a locally advanced tumor is found to be unresectable, laparoscopic palliative therapy may be performed.

Acute abdomen

The majority of patients with an acute abdomen will benefit from therapeutic laparoscopy (Figure 81.1), with the exception of intestinal obstruction, where the procedure is compromised by excessive bowel distension and inadequate visualization, and in cases of intestinal ischemia. Generally, contraindications for diagnostic laparoscopy are similar to those for exploratory laparotomy. Unique contraindications in the case of laparoscopy are patients unable to tolerate pneumoperitoneum, and those with clinical abdomen compartment syndrome (when laparotomic decompression is also desired), hypercapnia, and coagulopathy.

Diagnostic laparoscopy in the intensive care unit

Early diagnosis of catastrophic, acute life-threatening intraabdominal conditions, such as mesenteric ischemia, acute intestinal perforation, cholecystitis, and sepsis among critically ill patients, remains a diagnostic challenge. The sensitivity, specificity, and diagnostic accuracy of diagnostic laparoscopy are high (75%–100%), and dependent on several factors, such as patients habitus, experience of the surgeon, abdominal bowel distension, and previous abdominal surgery with adhesions.

Performing bed-side laparoscopy in the intensive care unit may improve outcomes, as the risks of interruption of medicine, transport, and morbidity of open exploration can be avoided.

Diagnostic and therapeutic laparoscopy for trauma

Stable patients with blunt abdominal trauma may undergo diagnostic laparoscopy to assess potential injury. In patients with penetrating trauma, it is very effective in detecting peritoneal penetration and to potentially treat organ injuries. Laparoscopy for abdominal trauma is appropriate in patients demonstrating: (1) hemodynamic stability upon arrival or after initial resuscitation, (2) normality in the Glasgow scale, (3) limitation on associated nonabdominal trauma, and (4) technical and staff availability. Current data recognize diagnostic laparoscopy is effective in selecting patients who will benefit from open surgery.

Technique for diagnostic laparoscopy

For bedside laparoscopy, pulse oximetry, electrocardiogram, and blood pressure should be monitored. Patients who are not intubated receive sedation with midazolam and/or propofol as needed. Patients not requiring mechanical ventilation prior to laparoscopy usually do not need to be intubated for the procedure. A monitor, insufflator, light source, camera, and pertinent instruments must be available.

The patient is positioned supine on an ICU bed. The abdomen is prepped with betadine solution and then sterile drapes

Yamada's Atlas of Gastroenterology, Fifth Edition. Edited by Daniel K. Podolsky, Michael Camilleri, J. Gregory Fitz, Anthony N. Kalloo, Fergus Shanahan, and Timothy C. Wang.
© 2016 John Wiley & Sons, Ltd. Published 2016 by John Wiley & Sons, Ltd
Companion website: www.yamadagastro.com/atlas

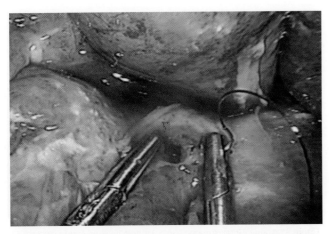

Figure 81.1 Diagnostic laparoscopy. A perforated duodenal ulcer with diffuse peritonitis was identified and treated (suture and omentoplastic of the ulcer) laparoscopically.

arranged as in the operating room. Local anesthesia using a mix of 1% lidocaine with 1% ropivacaine (50%–50%) is used to anesthetize the trocar sites. An incision is made intraumbilical or supraumbilical and a 5- or 10-mm trocar and camera inserted using an open Hasson technique. After insufflation with CO_2 to a pressure of 10–14 mmHg, additional trocars are placed under direct laparoscopic view as needed to manipulate the bowel and complete the exploration. The presence and character of intraperitoneal fluid are noted, and fluid collected for microbiological examinations. The viability and integrity of the bowel can be assessed, and the condition of the liver and gallbladder evaluated. Additional maneuvers are performed as needed. Evaluation of the retroperitoneum is limited. Diagnostic evaluation for morbidly obese patients and those with intestinal obstruction may be impaired.

Technique for explorative laparotomy

Under general anesthesia, the patient is positioned in the supine position, unless there is a high likelihood of rectal anastomosis, in which case the Lloyd–Davies position is preferable. Full abdominal wall relaxation is required, as a very good overview is needed, especially in the very obese patient. Clinical history and image methods should guide the location of the incision for infraumbilical (diseases of colon and rectum, appendix, gynecological) or supraumbilical (stomach, pancreas, gallbladder) incision. A median laparotomy is chosen for explorative laparotomy because of easy access to all abdominal and retroperitoneal organs. After skin, subcutaneous, and fascial incision, dissection of adhesions is usually necessary in patients who have undergone previous surgery. Dissection of very dense adhesions may result in small bowel injury, and the need for suture repair. Exploration includes visualization and palpation of liver, stomach, spleen, major omentum, and pelvic organs. Hernias of

the abdominal wall are investigated but if not the primary cause of the acute abdomen they should only rarely be treated in the same procedure. Intestinal exploration starts with the appendix, through ascending, transverse, descending, and sigmoid colon to rectum. Small bowel evaluation starts from the Treitz ligament in the direction of the terminal ileum. Retroperitoneal masses, lymph nodes, and peritoneal lesions may be observed and can be biopsied. Intraoperative ultrasound enhances the identification of deep hepatic and pancreas lesions and is mainly used for staging cancer.

Abdominal closure is now preferentially performed using a strong, absorbable or nonabsorbable running suture as a one-layer closure for the aponeurosis. Some transverse incisions may require a double-layer suture, and many surgeons prefer single sutures instead of running ones. The closure of subcutaneous tissue is not always performed, and skin closure is accomplished with intradermal running suture, skin staplers, or biological glue. Subcutaneous drains may be placed to reduce hematoma when there is a large dissection surface, in contaminated operations, or in obese patients.

Complications of laparoscopy and laparotomy

Intraoperative complications for diagnostic laparoscopy include:
- Bowel perforation
- Laceration of solid organs
- Subcutaneous or retroperitoneal emphysema
- Vascular injury
- Tension pneumothorax
- Port site infection.

Single-port surgery

Laparoscopic surgery through a single-site incision can be obtained by the insertion of an adapted platform (single port) (Figures 81.2 and 81.3), or using multiple trocars inserted in different fascial orifices, but through the same umbilical skin incision (multiport, single-site surgery).

Advantages of the single-port technique include: (1) similar technique to traditional laparoscopic surgery, (2) minimization of the skin incision, (3) superior cosmesis due to occult intraumbilical incision, and (4) opportunity for the surgeon to "convert" the procedure to multiport laparoscopy. Compared with natural orifice translumenal endoscopic surgery (NOTES) techniques, single-port surgery is simpler and possibly safer, and uses rigid instruments for retraction and conventional laparoscopic instruments and clips.

Novel applications of single-port surgery includes transrectal NOTES using a single port, transvaginal insertion, or direct percutaneous intragastric insertion to perform submucosal excision or stapled sleeve resections of large gastric

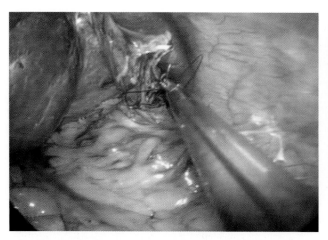

Figure 81.2 Single-port surgery. Splenectomy for splenomegaly can be performed using a single intraumbilical incision. Operative view of ligation of the splenic hilum with unabsorbable suture.

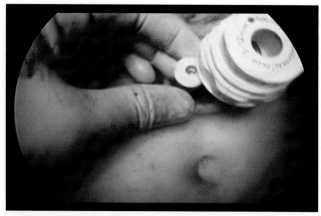

Figure 81.4 Single-port surgery. Using a single incision and inserting a single-port system (SILS, Covidien, New Haven, USA) directly in the gastric lumen, intragastric surgical resection of a large gastrointestinal stromal tumor (GIST) is performed with laparoscopy instruments.

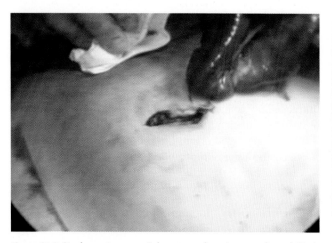

Figure 81.3 Single-port surgery. Splenectomy for splenomegaly, umbilical extraction of the specimen.

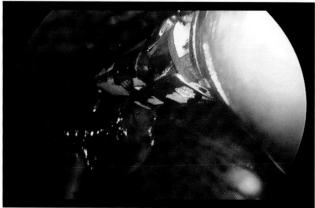

Figure 81.5 Intragastric resection of a gastrointestinal stromal tumor (GIST) using single-port surgery. After direct access of the single-port system inside the stomach, intragastric stapling is performed to achieve entire resection with clear margins. The tumor is extracted through the single port or transorally through a gastroscope.

adenomas or gastrointestinal stromal tumors (GIST) (Figures 81.4 and 81.5).

Minilaparoscopy

The advent of NOTES and subsequently single-port surgery has prompted efforts to develop even less invasive approaches to surgical access. Minilaparoscopy (MINI) is a natural advance, which may diminish surgical trauma by reducing the diameter of the standard laparoscopic instruments, without losing range of motion in triangulation, a significant concern in NOTES and single-port surgery.

To access the videos for this chapter, please go to
www.yamadagastro.com/atlas

Video 81.1 Single-port extragastric and intragastric resection for submucosal tumors. Intragastric surgery performed by direct percutaneous single-port insertion inside the stomach. Sleeve resection of the anterior wall was performed intragastrically through consecutive application of the stapling device. These indications of large gastric tumors not suitable for endoscopic resection were previously treated by formal laparoscopy or laparotomy. A formal single-port gastric resection is also shown for comparison.

Video 81.2 Left lateral liver segmentectomy using single-port and radiofrequency coagulation. The new technology for hepatic resections using radiofrequency and single-port access is an innovative way to perform safe laparoscopic major hepatic resections. We show a clinical case of a 37-year-old female patient with a large (9.2 cm) hemangioma at liver segments II and III, with indication for liver resection and cholecystectomy. After insertion of an umbilical single-port device, resection margins were marked and deeply delimitated with monopolar radiofrequency (Cool-tipTM, Covidien, USA). Intrahepatic section was performed without clips or sutures, and major pedicles were transected with an endostapler. The specimen was extracted with an extraction bag through the umbilical single port. Liver resections can nowadays have broader indications for primary laparoscopic and single-port resection. The concurrent use of radiofrequency technology to perform the intrahepatic resection can potentially minimize blood loss and reduce operative time, with better cosmesis.

Video 81.3 Single-port splenectomy for splenomegaly and wandering cystic spleen. In a young female patient with Wolf-Hirschhorn syndrome, with abdominal pain and the diagnosis of wandering spleen with splenomegaly (25 cm diameter), led to indication of elective splenectomy. In the supine position, single-port umbilical splenectomy was performed without laparoscopic assistance, splenic vessels were ligated by sutures, and the specimen was transumbilically extracted.

Video 81.4 Flexible natural orifice translumenal endoscopic surgery (NOTES) transvaginal cholecystectomy. Using a hybrid technique with umbilical laparoscopy, dissection of the gallbladder was performed using a transvaginal colonoscope through a transvaginal surgical platform.

Video 81.5 Revisional bariatric surgery: one-step transforming failed gastric band (LGB), vertical banded gastroplasty (Mason, VBG), and sleeve gastrectomy (LSG) to Roux-en-Y gastric bypass (LRYGB). Revision from failed bariatric restrictive procedures to LRYGB produces an effective result in achieving excess weight loss and reducing comorbidities. The video shows fundamental surgical steps in transforming LGBs, VGBs, and LSGs to LRYGB, in morbidly obese patients (BMI 45.3 to 57 kg/m^2) submitted to restrictive procedure more than 2 years before and with inadequate weight loss. Technical steps included: (1) full adhesiolysis and dissection of the small curvature including hiatus; (2) liberation of the hiatus and upper greater curvature with ultrasonic energy; (3) resection of the band and fibrous tissue and creating a small stapled gastric pouch over a 32 Fr bougie; (4) hand-sewn gastrojejunal anastomosis, PDS 3.0, at 70 cm from the Treitz ligament, stapled jejunojejunal anastomosis at 150 cm; and (5) leak testing with methylene blue and drainage. Careful identification of the altered anatomy and hand-sewing skills are important preconditions for the surgeon in performing advanced revisional procedures in bariatric surgery.

CHAPTER 82

Natural orifice translumenal endoscopic surgery (NOTES)

Vivek Kumbhari and Anthony N. Kalloo

Johns Hopkins University School of Medicine, Baltimore, MD, USA

Natural orifice translumenal endoscopic surgery (NOTES) is heralded as a paradigm shift in minimally invasive surgery. NOTES potentially offers a less invasive, safer, and more cost-effective alternative to laparoscopic surgery. Although originally designed for transgastric access to peritoneal structures, the transvaginal approach rapidly disseminated because of greater familiarity with the technique by surgeons and its ability to provide better orientation to organs of the upper gastrointestinal tract. This limited the clinical experience to women and led to decreased participation by the gastroenterologist. However, the development of new closure devices has also allowed the approach for NOTES to shift from transvaginal to transrectal, which will overcome the aforementioned obstacles. Transrectal NOTES allows preservation of spatial orientation, intuitive movements, and a large port for the introduction of instruments and removal of large specimens.

Although the original concept was designed around targeting organs in the gastrointestinal tract, preclinical experiments have demonstrated the feasibility and safety of NOTES for gynecological, fetal, and even orthopedic (spinal) interventions. The true value of NOTES may emerge from shifting the focus of competing directly with currently satisfactory procedures, toward providing novel approaches to difficult problems where an ideal solution is currently lacking. This is evidenced by the worldwide dissemination of submucosal endoscopy (an offshoot of NOTES). Peroral endoscopic myotomy (POEM) and submucosal tunneling endoscopic resection (STER) are two such examples that have the potential to supplant current surgical methods. This chapter chronologically portrays the evolution of NOTES in the 21st century (Figures 82.1–82.22), and reminds the reader that despite ongoing advances, its maximal potential has not been reached.

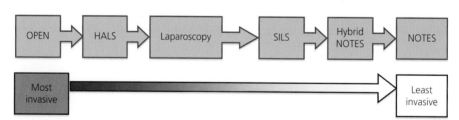

Figure 82.1 The concept of natural orifice translumenal endoscopic surgery (NOTES) includes the evolution of surgery to the goal of less invasive procedures. Minimally invasive techniques have considerably reduced the morbidity associated with abdominal incisions. Efforts to achieve so-called "scarless" surgery have taken this a step further. NOTES avoids percutaneous incisions and instead creates a visceral incision to gain access to the thoracic or peritoneal cavity. Hybrid NOTES involves procedures that require a percutaneous port for assistance. Potential advantages over conventional laparoscopic surgery and single-incision laparoscopic surgery (SILS) include the abolishment of incision-related complications such as wound infections, incisional hernia, postoperative pain, and adhesions. Additional benefits include reduced recovery time and improved cosmesis. HALS, hand-assisted laparoscopic surgery.

Yamada's Atlas of Gastroenterology, Fifth Edition. Edited by Daniel K. Podolsky, Michael Camilleri, J. Gregory Fitz, Anthony N. Kalloo, Fergus Shanahan, and Timothy C. Wang.
© 2016 John Wiley & Sons, Ltd. Published 2016 by John Wiley & Sons, Ltd.
Companion website: www.yamadagastro.com/atlas

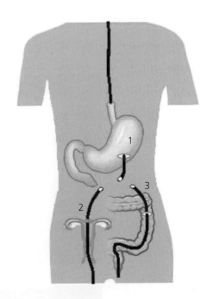

Figure 82.2 Several access routes for natural orifice translumenal endoscopic surgery (NOTES) have been proposed, including the transesophageal, transgastric, transvaginal, transcolonic, and transurethral approaches. The transesophageal approach involves the endoscope being inserted orally and then being advanced through the mediastinal cavity by penetration of the esophageal wall to perform mediastinal or thoracic surgery. Similarly, with the transgastric approach (1), the endoscope is inserted orally and advanced into the peritoneal cavity by incision in the gastric wall to perform peritoneal or retroperitoneal surgery. The transvaginal approach (2) has been performed for decades in gynecological practice with closure of the vaginal wall being performed manually. The disadvantage with this approach is that it is only applicable to women. The transcolonic approach (3) involves the endoscope being inserted through the anus and being advanced through the rectal or colonic wall into the peritoneal cavity. The widespread application of this approach is hampered by the need for a reliable closure method and need for infection control. The transurethral approach involves the endoscope being inserted into the urethra and through the bladder into the peritoneum. The advantage of this technique is that this conduit is sterile but the disadvantage is that instruments to perform a surgery must be of limited size. Source: Tomikawa M, Xu H, Hashizume M. Current status and prerequisites for natural orifice translumenal endoscopic surgery (NOTES). Surg Today 2010;20:909. Reproduced with permission of Springer Science and Business Media.

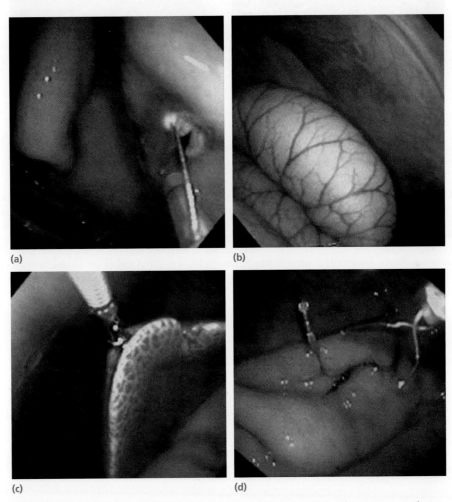

(a)

(b)

(c)

(d)

Figure 82.3 Natural orifice translumenal endoscopic surgery (NOTES) has gained worldwide attention from gastroenterologists and surgeons since it was first described in 2000. Transgastric peritoneoscopy and liver biopsy was performed in survival porcine study. This was the first study to show that the peroral transgastric approach to the peritoneal cavity might serve as an alternative to laparoscopy or laparotomy. **(a)** Endoscopic view of gastric wall incision being made with a sphincterotome. **(b)** Endoscopic view of the peritoneal cavity showing small bowel. **(c)** Endoscopic view of peroral transgastric liver biopsy. **(d)** Endoscopic view showing closure of the gastric incision with standard endoclips. Source: Kalloo AN, Singh VK, Jagannath SB, et al. Flexible transgastric peritoneoscopy: a novel approach to diagnostic and therapeutic interventions in the peritoneal cavity. Gastrointest Endosc 2004;60:114. Reproduced with permission of Elsevier.

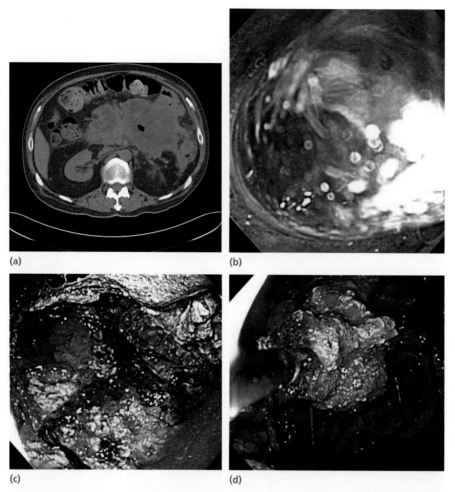

Figure 82.4 Endoscopic drainage of walled-off pancreatic necrosis has been in practice for over a decade and was one of the earliest endoscopic procedures that purposely breached the gastric lumen. These collections are often found in the retrogastric position. Once the necrotic cavity is cleared, the gastrotomy is left to close by secondary intention. **(a)** Representative computed tomography (CT) image demonstrating walled-off pancreatic necrosis in a 62-year-old woman who had acute pancreatitis 57 days previously. **(b)** Dilatation of the gastrostomy tract using a through-the-endoscope balloon. **(c)** Intracavitary image demonstrating necrotic debris attached to the wall of the cavity. **(d)** Intracavitary debridement of the cavity using standard endoscopic accessories. Source: Gardner TB, Coelho-Prabhu N, Gordon SR, et al. Direct endoscopic necrosectomy for the treatment of walled-off pancreatic necrosis: results from a multicenter U.S series. Gastrointest Endosc 2011;4:718. Reproduced with permission of Elsevier.

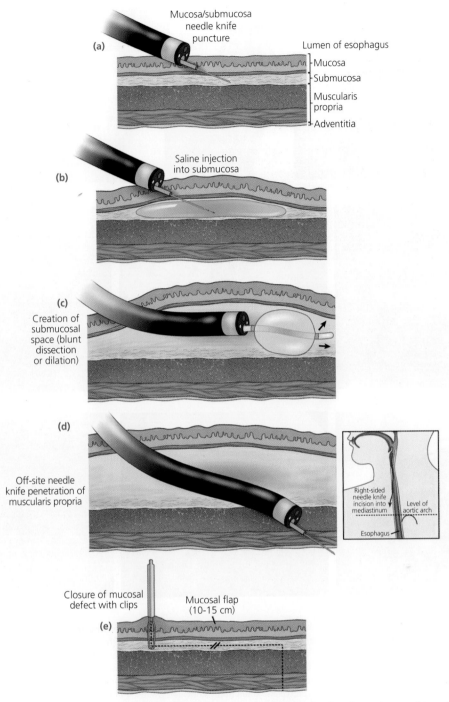

Figure 82.5 Most transesophageal natural orifice translumenal endoscopic surgery (NOTES) studies describe a submucosal tunneling technique for mediastinal access. The submucosal tunnel creates a flap that acts as a seal to prevent mediastinal contamination and can be subsequently closed with tissue-approximating devices at the end of the procedure. **(a)** Saline/methylene blue solution is injected into the submucosa. **(b)** Needle knife mucosal/submucosal puncture. **(c)** Creation of submucosal space by blunt dissection and/or balloon dilation. **(d)** Off-site needle knife penetration of the muscularis propria with subsequent entry into the mediastinum (see inset). **(e)** Offset closure of muscular defect with overlying mucosal flap.
Source: Khashab MA, Kalloo AN. NOTES: current status and new horizons. Gastroenterology 2012;142:704. Reproduced with permission of Elsevier.

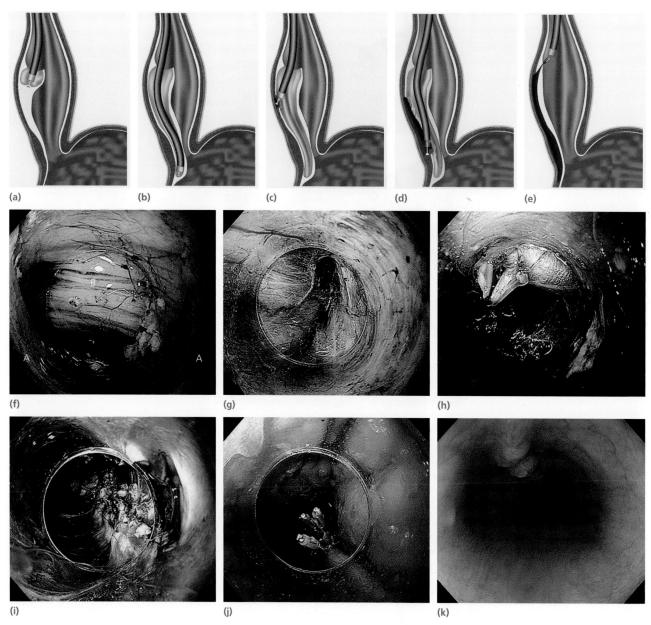

Figure 82.6 (a–e) These schematic diagrams illustrate the technical steps in performing a peroral endoscopic myotomy (POEM). POEM is the first routine clinical application of the natural orifice translumenal endoscopic surgery (NOTES) paradigm. **(a)** Entry to submucosal space. After submucosal injection, a 2-cm longitudinal mucosal incision is made at approximately 13 cm proximal to the gastroesophageal junction (GEJ). **(b)** Submucosal tunneling. A long submucosal tunnel is created to 3 cm distal to the GEJ. **(c)** Endoscopic myotomy is begun at 3 cm distal to the mucosal entry point, and is carried out in a proximal to distal direction to a total length of 10 cm. **(d)** Long endoscopic myotomy of inner circular muscle bundles is done, leaving the outer longitudinal muscle layer intact. The expected end point of myotomy is 2 cm distal to the GEJ. **(e)** Closure of mucosal entry: the mucosal incision is closed using endoclips. **(f–k)** These endoscopic images correspond to the steps illustrated in **(a–e)**. **(f)** The tip of the cap-fitted endoscope has been introduced into the submucosal space. The white bundles demonstrate the thickened inner circular muscle layer. A, mucosal layer; B, inner circular muscle bundle. **(g)** Submucosal tunnel created with the left half of the image revealing the mucosal flap. **(h)** Endoscopic myotomy was begun at 3 cm distal to the mucosal entry. **(i)** Completion of endoscopic myotomy. Circular muscle bundles were dissected and the 10 cm myotomy was completed. **(j)** The mucosal entry incision was tightly closed using an endoclip. **(k)** Follow-up endoscopy at 7 days showed only a small scar at the mucosal entry site. Source: Inoue H, Minami H, Kobayashi Y, et al. Peroral endoscopic myotomy (POEM) for esophageal achalasia. Endoscopy 2010;42:265. Reproduced with permission of Thieme Publishing Group.

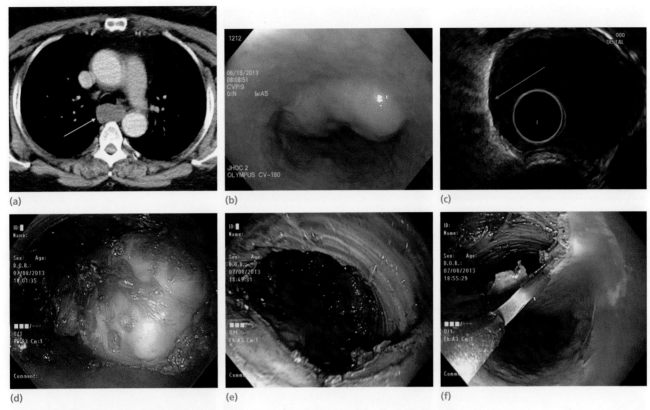

Figure 82.7 These images depict the diagnosis and management of a mediastinal mass, which was subsequently found to be a leiomyoma. This patient underwent a submucosal tunneling endoscopic resection (STER), which is an extension of transesophageal natural orifice translumenal endoscopic surgery (NOTES). Forty-eight hours after her procedure she was discharged to home and able to consume oral intake. (**a**) Axial computed tomography (CT) revealing a slice of a 2 × 6 cm mass (yellow arrow) adjacent to the aorta. (**b**) Upper endoscopy showed indentation of the esophageal lumen by the mass. (**c**) Endoscopic ultrasound suggested a hypoechoic mass originating from the muscular layer (red arrow) of the esophagus. (**d**) Submucosal fibers were dissected resulting in a tunnel with the mucosa on one side, mass in the middle, and normal muscle on the other side. (**e**) Complete endoscopic resection and retrieval of the leiomyoma was performed resulting in an empty tunnel. (**f**) Commencement of closure of the mucosal opening at the top of the tunnel with endoclips.

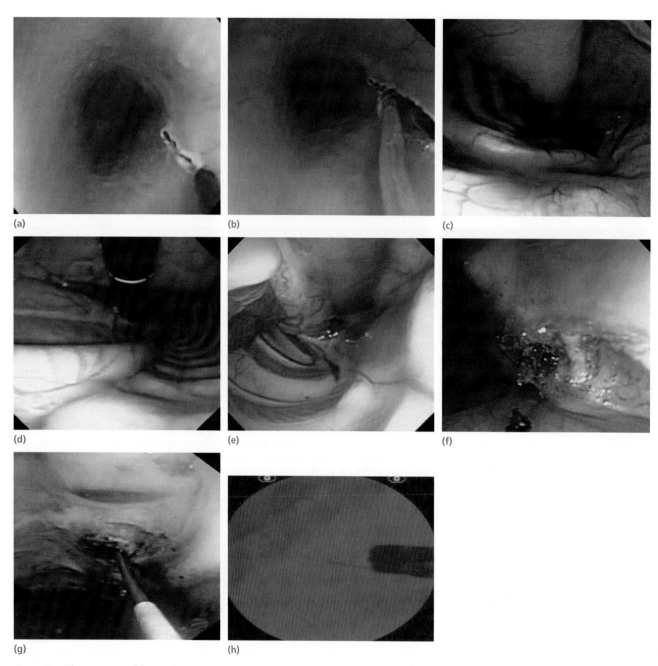

Figure 82.8 The proximity of the esophagus to the vertebral column provides close and direct access to the thoracic spine. This may open the doors for multilevel anterior spinal procedures using natural orifice translumenal endoscopic surgery (NOTES) techniques. These images depict a nonsurvival porcine experiment to demonstrate the feasibility of transesophageal biopsy of thoracic vertebrae. **(a)** Esophageal wall incision. **(b)** Submucosal tunnel. **(c)** Visualization of the lung, pleura, aorta, thoracic spine, and esophagus in the forward scope position. **(d)** Retroflexed endoscopic views at the distal thoracic spine. **(e)** Retroflexed endoscopic views at the proximal thoracic spine. **(f)** Incision over the anterior longitudinal ligament and exposure of the intravertebral space and vertebral bone. **(g)** Insertion of a 19-gauge needle into the thoracic vertebrae. **(h)** Fluoroscopic view of vertebral bone biopsy. Source: Magno P, Khashab MA, Mas M, et al. Natural orifice translumenal endoscopic surgery for anterior spinal procedures. Minim Invasive Surg 2012;2012:365814. Reproduced with permission.

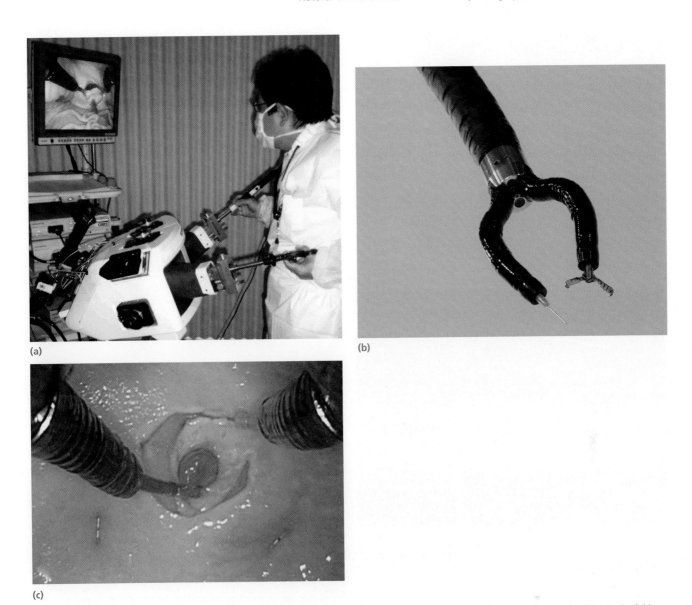

(a)

(b)

(c)

Figure 82.9 The advent of natural orifice translumenal endoscopic surgery (NOTES) has accelerated the development of new technology in the field or gastrointestinal endoscopy. Traditional endoscopes are not ideal for intraabdominal surgery. New multitasking platforms have been developed to facilitate NOTES interventions. The EndoSAMURAI (Olympus Corporation, Tokyo, Japan) is an example of one such platform. **(a)** The EndoSAMURAI is a single-operator system with both hands required for manipulation of the device. **(b)** The two arms are preloaded with accessories. **(c)** Endoscopic image during a full-thickness gastric resection of a simulated lesion in an ex vivo model. Note that with this platform counter-traction can be applied whilst the second arm carries out the dissection. Source: Ikeda K, Sumiyama K, Tajiri K, et al. Evaluation of a new multitasking platform for endoscopic full thickness resection. Gastrointest Endosc 2011;73:117. Reproduced with permission of Elsevier.

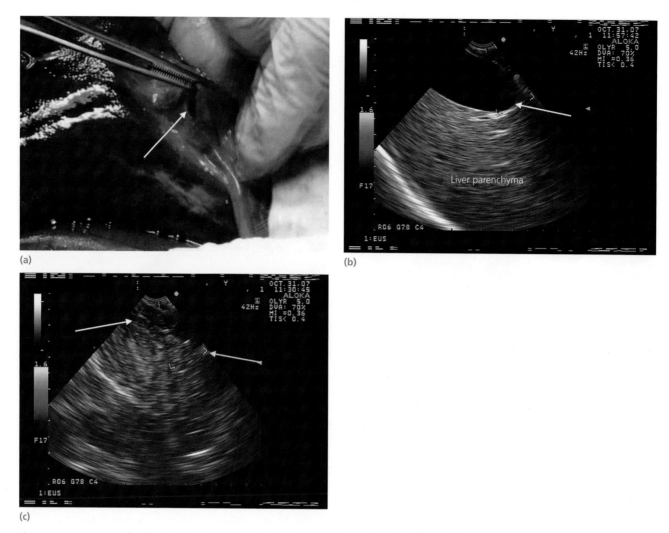

(a)

(b)

(c)

Figure 82.10 Many natural orifice translumenal endoscopic surgery (NOTES) procedures have been performed through the anterior stomach wall. In a porcine model, blind NOTES access through the stomach wall resulted in major complications. Endoscopic ultrasonography (EUS)-guided access reduced but did not eliminate the risk of complications. **(a)** Inadvertent gallbladder puncture (arrow) from access through a gastric antral access site. **(b)** EUS performed at the site of blind puncture revealing the gallbladder (arrow) within hepatic parenchyma abutting the serosa of the stomach. **(c)** An example of an EUS image of a safe access site. Note the nonspecific echogenicity that is present in the absence of any identifiable structures (white arrow). Also note the absence of a Doppler signal in the intended trajectory of the initial NOTES puncture (yellow arrow). Source: Elmunzer BJ, Schomish SJ, Trunzo JA, et al. EUS in localizing safe alternate access sites for natural orifice translumenal endoscopic surgery: initial experience in a porcine model. Gastrointest Endosc 2009;69:108. Reproduced with permission of Elsevier.

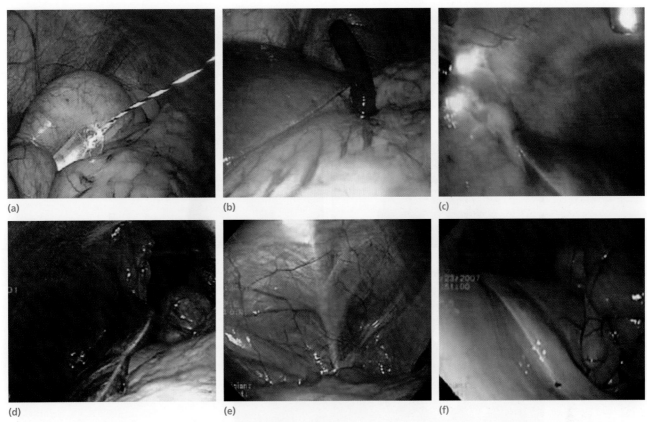

(a)   (b)   (c)

(d)   (e)   (f)

Figure 82.11 Natural orifice translumenal endoscopic surgery (NOTES) peritoneoscopy using a hybrid technique. NOTES peritoneoscopy through an anterior gastrotomy by using a standard endoscope permits adequate visualization of organs in the peritoneum. The accuracy of NOTES compared with laparoscopy in identifying intraabdominal pathology remains to be determined. These images demonstrate hybrid NOTES diagnostic peritoneoscopy in humans. **(a)** NOTES gastrotomy performed with balloon dilation over a guidewire. **(b)** Endoscope passed into the peritoneal cavity for assessment. **(c)** Laparoscopic view of flexible endoscope positioned to visualize the liver. **(d)** The view of the right upper quadrant and liver seen through the flexible endoscope. **(e)** NOTES visualization of the right inguinal region clearly demonstrating the inferior epigastric vessels. **(f)** View of the appendix and right paracolic gutter through the flexible endoscope after retroflexion in the pelvis. Source: Nikfarjam M, McGee MF, Trunzo JA , et al. Transgastric natural-orifice transluminal endoscopic surgery peritoneoscopy in humans: a pilot study in efficacy and gastrotomy site selection by using a hybrid technique. Gastrointest Endosc 2010;72:279. Reproduced with permission of Elsevier.

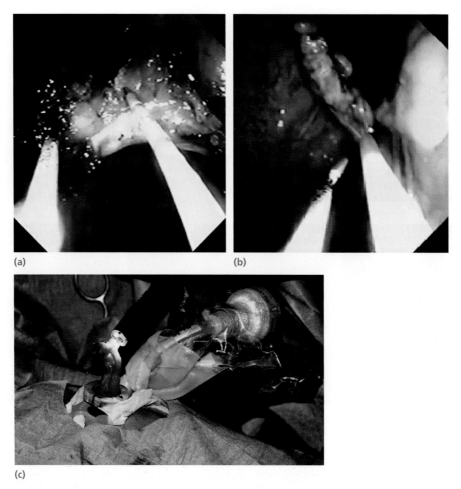

Figure 82.12 The first translumenal organ resection was a transgastric appendectomy in 2004. Natural orifice translumenal endoscopic surgery (NOTES) appendectomy is technically demanding with current instrumentation and lack of triangulation. These images were taken during a human NOTES appendectomy and demonstrate some of the steps involved in the procedure. **(a)** Dissection of mesoappendix at the base of the appendix using a needle-knife. **(b)** An endoloop was applied at the base of the dissected appendix. **(c)** The appendix was removed through an oral overtube.
Source: Park PO, Bergstrom M. Transgastric peritoneoscopy and appendectomy: thoughts on our first experience in humans. Endoscopy 2010;42:81. Reproduced with permission of Thieme Publishing Group.

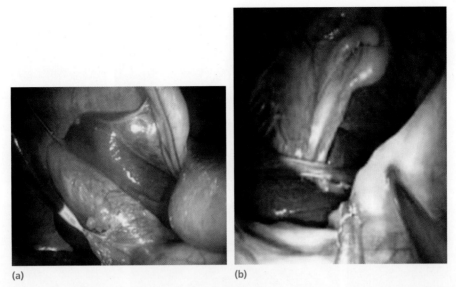

Figure 82.13 Although most experts believe that the transgastric route will dominate natural orifice translumenal endoscopic surgery (NOTES) in the future, the current lack of instrumentation for triangulation and hence the ability to retract organs for dissection are limiting its broad acceptance. Whilst a transvaginal grasper can be used in a transvaginal cholecystectomy to provide retraction, this is not possible in the transgastric route and transparietal assistance is obligatory. These images depict a hybrid transgastric cholecystectomy in a human. **(a)** Retraction of the gallbladder with a laparoscopic instrument introduced in the right hypochondrium. **(b)** Dissection of the cystic pedicle with a flexible endoscope. Source: Dallemagne B, Perretta S, Allemann P, et al. Transgastric cholecystectomy: From the laboratory to clinical implementation. World J Gastrointest Surg 2010;7:187. Reproduced with permission.

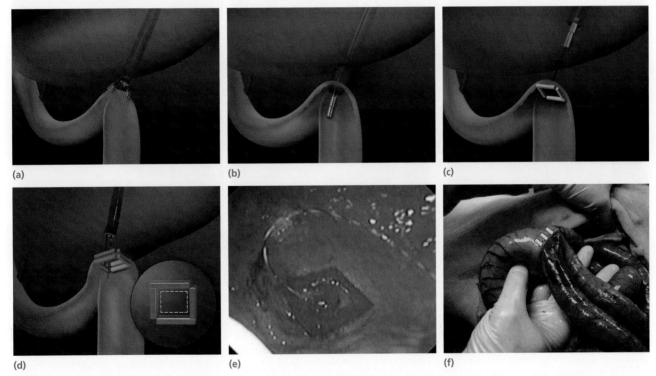

Figure 82.14 Gastrojejunostomy is important for palliation of malignant gastric outlet obstruction and surgical obesity procedures. A less invasive endoscopic technique for gastrojejunostomy creation is attractive. A novel device for compression anastomosis that uses self-assembling magnets allows for transoral creation of immediate and large-caliber gastrojejunostomy in a porcine model. The steps for transoral delivery of the self-assembling magnets for endoscopy (SAMSEN) magnets are: **(a)** natural orifice translumenal endoscopic surgery (NOTES) gastrotomy is followed by small bowel mobilization and enterotomy creation by using a custom grasping overtube; **(b)** injection of the small-bowel magnet; **(c)** opening of the small-bowel magnet followed by deployment of the gastric magnet; **(d)** mating of magnets followed by immediate gastrojejunostomy access. **(e)** Endoscopic view of the gastric magnet. **(f)** External view at necropsy of the gastrojejunal interface with robust coupling of magnets (yellow arrows). Source: Ryou M, Cantillon-Murphy P, Azagury D, et al. Smart self-assembling magnets for endoscopy (SAMSEN) for transoral endoscopic creation of immediate gastrojejunostomy (with video). Gastrointest Endosc 2011;73:353. Reproduced with permission of Elsevier.

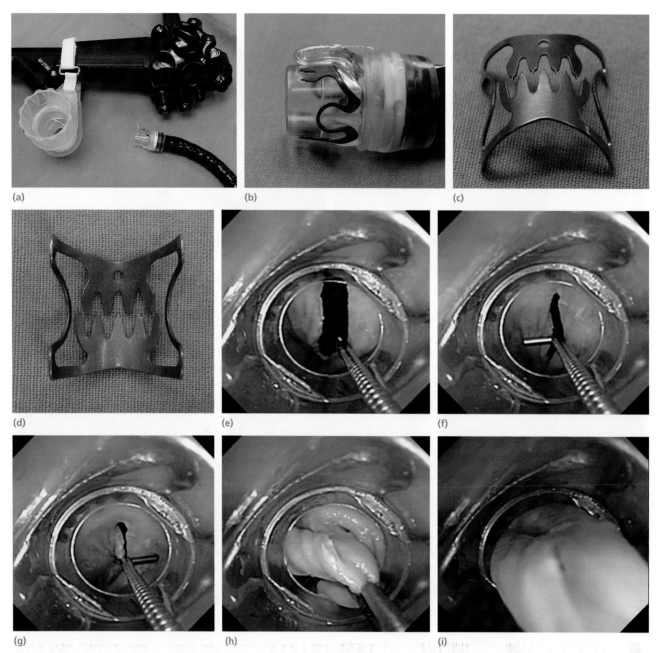

Figure 82.15 Over-the-scope clip (OTSC) system has been shown to be superior to standard endoclips for visceral wall closure. This is related to the ability of the OTSC to incorporate the entire thickness of the visceral wall, as opposed to just the mucosa or a partial-thickness closure. Deployment of the clip takes simply a matter of minutes. **(a)** Endoscope with mounted hand wheel and applicator cap. **(b)** A 12-mm transparent cap with OTSC mounted onto the tip of the endoscope. **(c, d)** OTSC once deployed. Endoscopic view of the OTSC closure procedure: **(e)** the edges were endoscopically aligned in a 6 to 12 o'clock direction; **(f)** left lateral edge of the perforation was grasped with the twin grasper; **(g)** right lateral edge of the perforation was grasped with the twin grasper; **(h)** the re-apposed tissue was pulled into the OTSC cap; **(i)** sufficient suction was maintained to aspirate the tissue surrounding the perforation into the cap before application of the OTSC; **(j)** endoscopic inspection and insufflation following OTSC application. Assisting instruments to gather a GI wall defect into the applicator cap: **(k, l)** the twin grasper has two jaws that can open and close separately to approximate wound edges; **(m, n)** the anchor has three needle pins that can be deployed into tissue for secure grasping and manipulation. Source: (a–d) von Renteln D, Rudolph HU, Schmidt A, et al. Endoscopic closure of duodenal perforations by using an over-the-scope clip: a randomized, controlled porcine study. Gastrointest Endosc 2010;71:131. Reproduced with permission of Elsevier. (e–j) von Renteln D, Denzer UW et al. Endoscopic closure of GI fistulae by using an over-the-scope clip (with videos). Gastrointest Endosc 2010;72:1289. Reproduced with permission of Elsevier. (k–n) Matthes K, Jung Y, Kato M, et al. Efficacy of full-thickness GI perforation closure with a novel over-the-scope clip application device: an animal study. Gastrointest Endosc 2011;74:1369. Reproduced with permission of Elsevier.

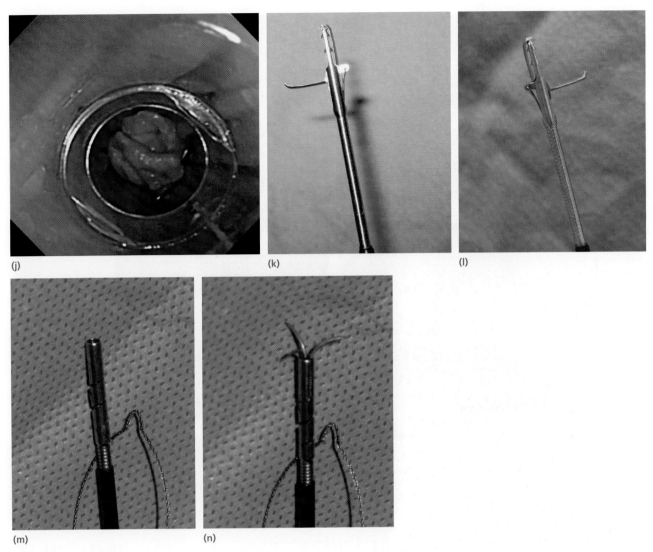

(j)

(k)

(l)

(m)

(n)

Figure 82.15 (*Continued*)

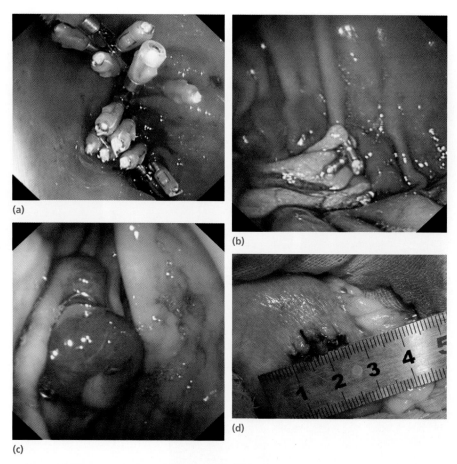

Figure 82.16 Gastrotomy closures of different approaches in a canine model: **(a)** standard endoclip closure where two mucosal surfaces are approximated and healing is without seromuscular apposition; **(b)** omentoplasty closure where omentum was pulled into the gastric lumen and fixed endoscopically with endoclips; **(c)** over-the-scope clip (OTSC) closure; and **(d)** surgical hand-suturing closure. Source: Sun G, Yang Y, Zhang X, et al. Comparison of gastrotomy closure modalities for natural orifice translumenal surgery: a canine study. Gastrointest Endosc 2013;77:774. Reproduced with permission of Elsevier.

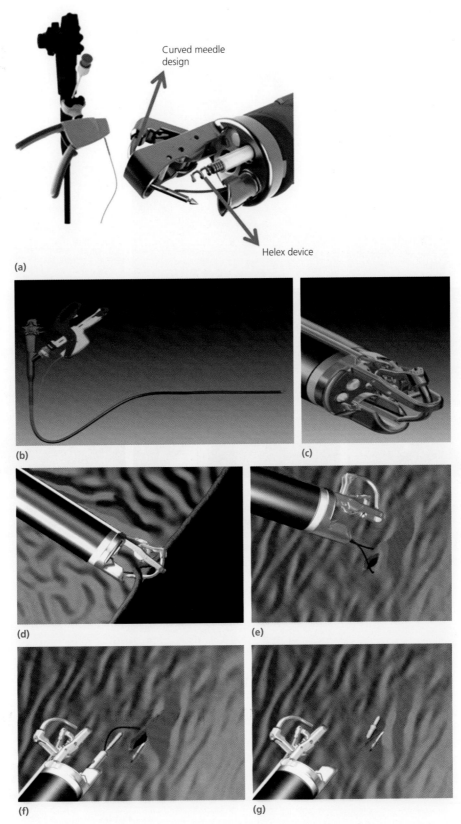

Figure 82.17 The pursuit of a reliable technique for closure of visceral translumenal defects has led to endoscopic suturing devices. **(a)** One such device depicted here (Overstitch; Apollo Endosurgery, Austin, TX, USA) has been developed to allow full-thickness suturing to mimic surgical suturing. This device is capable of the placement of interrupted or running sutures without tying a knot. The diagrams demonstrate the suturing technique: **(b)** OverStitch suturing device is mounted on the double-channel endoscope; **(c)** magnified view of the working portion of the suturing device frontloaded to the tip of the endoscope; **(d)** needle puncturing the gastric wall above the fistula; **(e)** a needle and thread are passed through the gastric wall above and below the fistula; **(f)** the needle is released out of the suturing device to serve as a tissue anchor, and a cinching mechanism is advanced into the stomach; **(g)** the thread is tightened, closing the fistula, then the cinching mechanism is deployed completing the stitch. Source: Abu Dayyeh BK, Ranjan E, Gostout CJ. Endoscopic sleeve gastroplasty: a potential endoscopic alternative to surgical sleeve gastrectomy for treatment of obesity. Gastrointest Endosc 2013;78:530. Reproduced with permission of Elsevier.

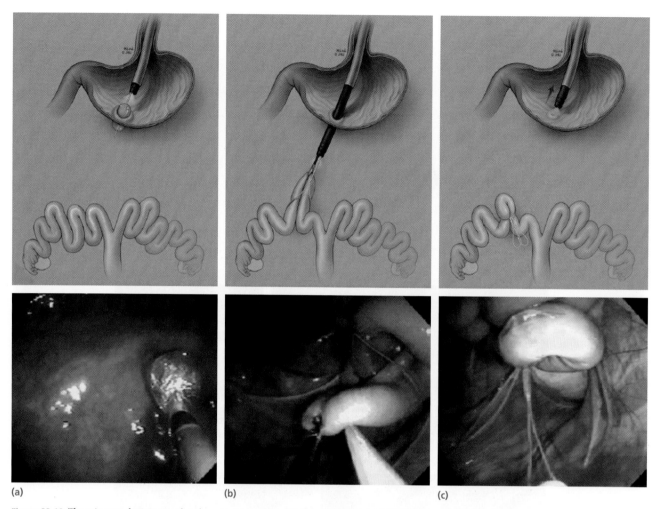

(a) (b) (c)

Figure 82.18 These images depict peroral endoscopic transgastric ligation of a unilateral fallopian tube in a long-term survival porcine model.
(a) Schematic drawing and endoscopic view of balloon dilation of the gastric wall. **(b)** Schematic drawing and endoscopic view of unilateral ligation of the fallopian tube with an endoloop. **(c)** Schematic drawing and endoscopic view of the fallopian tube postligation with two endoloops.
Source: Jagannath SB, Kantsevoy SV, Vaughn CA, et al. Peroral transgastric endoscopic ligation of fallopian tubes with long-term survival in a porcine model. Gastrointest Endosc 2005;51: 449. Reproduced with permission of Elsevier.

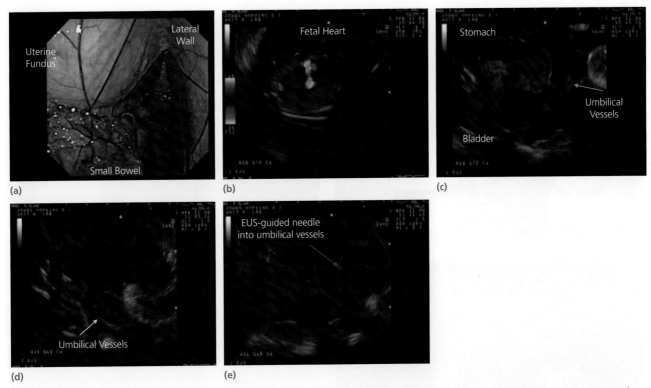

Figure 82.19 Despite advances in fetal surgery, morbidity and mortality are not insignificant. A nonsurvival study was performed in two pregnant sheep and a third sheep was survived. Both transgastric and transvaginal access approaches were utilized. The study showed that intraperitoneal endoscopic ultrasonography (EUS) via a natural orifice translumenal endoscopic surgery (NOTES) approach provides excellent access and visualization of the intrauterine cavity and fetal parts. **(a)** Transgastric view of the peritoneum with a flexible endoscope. **(b)** Intraperitoneal EUS revealing excellent visualization of the four chambers of the fetal heart. **(c)** Sonographic visualization of the fetal stomach, bladder, and umbilical vessels (blue arrow). **(d)** Sonographic view of the umbilical vessels in cross-section (yellow arrow). **(e)** EUS-guided saline injection into the umbilical vein (red arrow). Source: Giday SA, Buscaglia JM, Althaus J, et al. Successful diagnostic and therapeutic intrauterine fetal interventions by natural orifice translumenal endoscopic surgery (with videos). Gastrointest Endosc 2009;70:377. Reproduced with permission of Elsevier.

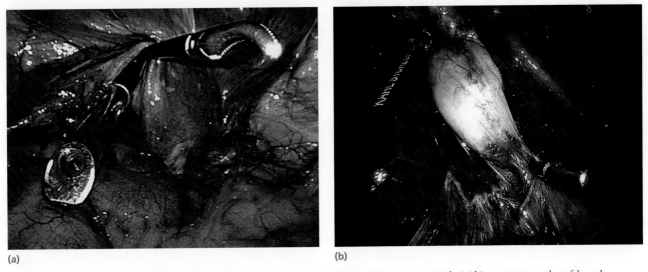

Figure 82.20 Transvaginal natural orifice translumenal endoscopic surgery (NOTES) cholecystectomy with rigid instruments can be safely and effectively performed in humans. Most transvaginal NOTES procedures are performed using a hybrid technique although expert centers are becoming proficient using a pure NOTES technique. These images are taken at different stages of NOTES transvaginal cholecystectomy in humans. **(a)** Inserting the dissector and the optic through the posterior fornix of the vagina (uterus on the right side). **(b)** Retracting the gallbladder with the vaginal dissector and dissecting the triangle of Calot with the instrument inserted through the umbilicus. Source: Zornig Z, Mofid H, Siemssen L, et al. Transvaginal NOTES hybrid cholecystectomy: feasibility results in 68 cases with mid-term follow-up. Endoscopy 2009;41:391. Reproduced with permission of Elsevier.

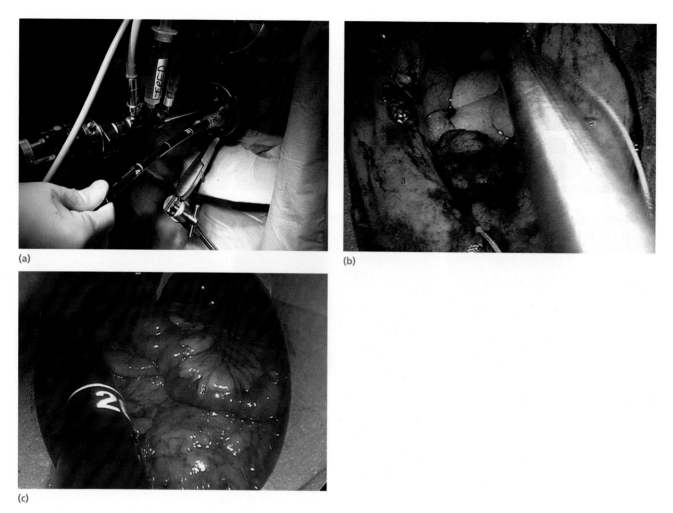

Figure 82.21 Transanal endoscopic microsurgery (TEM) is a minimally invasive technique for full-thickness resection of rectal tumors, followed by suture closure of the resultant defect. Entry into the peritoneal cavity during a resection of rectosigmoid lesions has been described with safe closure obtained. These images are from a preclinical study where standard TEM instrumentation and a flexible endoscope demonstrated the feasibility of transrectal natural orifice translumenal endoscopic surgery (NOTES) in peritoneal access, peritoneoscopy, liver biopsy, and colorectal resections. **(a)** Close-up view of gastroscope inserted through one 10-mm silastic seal in the TEM faceplate. **(b)** TEM peritoneal access with rectal mucosa labeled and bowel visible through a rectotomy. **(c)** Endoscope, examining the upper abdomen. Source: Denk PM, Swanstrom LL, Whiteford MH. Transanal endoscopic microsurgical platform for natural orifice surgery. Gastrointest Endosc 2008;68:954. Reproduced with permission of Elsevier.

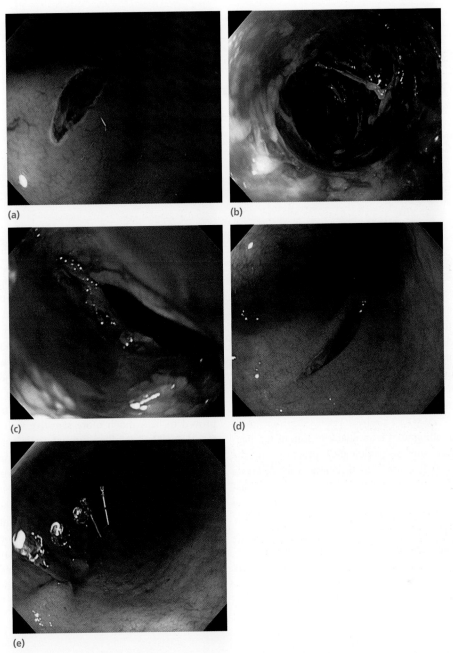

Figure 82.22 Although most natural orifice translumenal endoscopic surgery (NOTES) procedures have been performed via a transgastric or transvaginal approach, the transcolonic approach has several theoretical advantages. The major benefit is more direct access to upper abdominal structures. Additionally, a transcolonic approach is can be used in both sexes. A major concern in any transcolonic approach is the risk of infectious adverse events. To decrease these risks, a submucosal endoscopic approach with a mucosal flap can be utilized. Herein are endoscopic pictures of transcolonic peritoneoscopy with submucosal endoscopy with mucosal flap in a porcine survival model. **(a)** Mucosal incision on the submucosal fluid cushion. **(b)** Submucosal tunnel created by balloon dissection. **(c)** Seromuscular incision at the end of submucosal tunnel. **(d)** Mucosal incision site after peritoneoscopy before closure. **(e)** Complete closure of the mucosal incision site with endoclips. Source: Takizawa K, Brahmbhatt R, Knipschield, et al. Transcolonic peritoneoscopy by using submucosal endoscopy with mucosal flap for the detection of peritoneal bead targeting in the porcine survival model: a feasibility and effectiveness study. Gastrointest Endosc 2014;79:127. Reproduced with permission of Elsevier.

CHAPTER 83

Plain and contrast radiology

Marc S. Levine[1] and Stephen E. Rubesin[2]
[1] University of Pennsylvania Medical Center, Philadelphia, PA, USA
[2] Hospital of the University of Pennsylvania, Philadelphia, PA, USA

Plain radiographs of the abdomen are useful for evaluating abdominal pain or distention, obstructive symptoms, or clinical signs of an acute abdomen. The combination of supine and upright or decubitus horizontal beam radiographs allows the diagnosis of adynamic ileus or obstruction of the small bowel or colon, free intraperitoneal air (pneumoperitoneum) (Figure 83.1), ischemic or necrotic bowel with air in the bowel wall (pneumatosis) (Figure 83.2), air in the bile ducts (pneumobilia), and portal venous gas (Figure 83.3). Nevertheless, computed tomographic (CT) scanning is a more sensitive modality for evaluating acute abdominal symptoms (see Chapter 86).

Double-contrast radiography is a valuable technique for diagnosing a wide spectrum of pathological processes in the gastrointestinal tract. Because this technique can delineate normal mucosal surface patterns in the pharynx, upper gastrointestinal tract, small bowel, and colon, it is particularly helpful in detecting a variety of inflammatory or neoplastic diseases involving the mucosa. In some cases, barium studies may demonstrate abnormalities that are missed or misinterpreted at endoscopic examination. Double-contrast radiography and endoscopy should be considered as complementary procedures for evaluating suspected gastrointestinal disease.

Double-contrast radiography can delineate in detail the normal anatomic features of the pharynx (Figure 83.4). As a result, inflammatory (Figure 83.5) or neoplastic (Figures 83.6 and 83.7) lesions that disrupt or obliterate the normal anatomic landmarks can be demonstrated readily. In the upper gastrointestinal tract, double-contrast techniques allow detection of esophagitis caused by plaques or ulcers (Figure 83.8), esophageal cancer (Figure 83.9), benign gastric ulcer (Figure 83.10), early gastric cancer (Figure 83.11), duodenal ulcer (Figure 83.12), erosive gastritis or duodenitis, and other inflammatory or neoplastic lesions. The small bowel enema (enteroclysis) has proved to be a much more sensitive technique than conventional small bowel follow-through examination for determining the site and cause of small bowel obstruction (Figure 83.13) and a variety of other abnormalities in the small bowel (Figures 83.14–83.16). Double-contrast barium enema examination is a valuable technique for detecting colonic polyps or carcinoma (Figure 83.17) and for diagnosing inflammatory bowel disease (granulomatous and ulcerative colitis) or its complications (Figure 83.18). Double-contrast studies may also be performed to evaluate the colon after a surgical procedure (Figure 83.19). Although rare, complications of these studies may be encountered (Figure 83.20).

Yamada's Atlas of Gastroenterology, Fifth Edition. Edited by Daniel K. Podolsky, Michael Camilleri, J. Gregory Fitz, Anthony N. Kalloo, Fergus Shanahan, and Timothy C. Wang.
© 2016 John Wiley & Sons, Ltd. Published 2016 by John Wiley & Sons, Ltd.
Companion website: www.yamadagastro.com/atlas

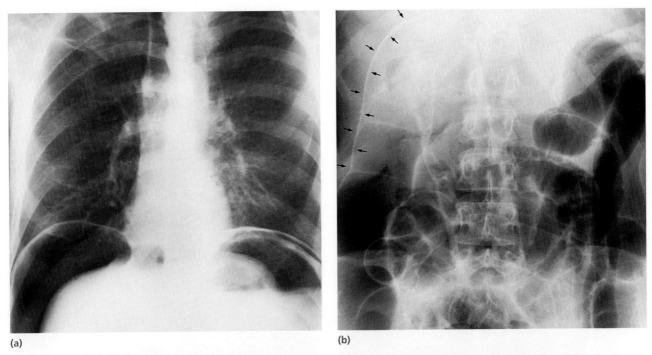

(a)

(b)

Figure 83.1 Pneumoperitoneum. **(a)** Upright chest radiograph shows large amounts of free intraperitoneal air beneath both sides of the diaphragm of this patient with a perforated duodenal ulcer. **(b)** Supine plain radiograph of the abdomen of another patient shows an indirect sign of pneumoperitoneum, air on both sides of the bowel wall (Rigler sign; arrows) after perforation at colonoscopy. Source: Levine MS. Plain radiograph diagnosis of the acute abdomen. Emerg Med Clin North Am 1985;3:541. Reproduced with permission of Elsevier.

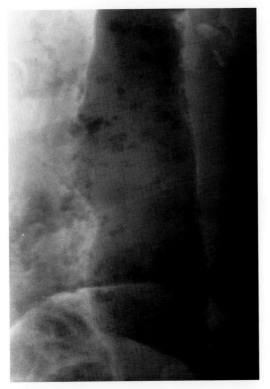

Figure 83.2 Pneumatosis caused by infarction of the left colon after a surgical procedure. Close-up view of supine plain radiograph of the abdomen shows tiny, mottled and linear collections of gas in the wall of the descending colon.

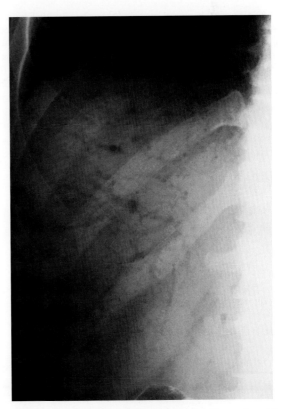

Figure 83.3 Close-up view of the right upper quadrant on supine plain radiograph of the abdomen shows linear, branching collections of gas in the portal venous system caused by intestinal infarction. Gas shadows extend to the periphery of the liver. This appearance is characteristic of portal venous gas. Source: Levine MS. Plain radiograph diagnosis of the acute abdomen. Emerg Med Clin North Am 1985;3:541. Reproduced with permission of Elsevier.

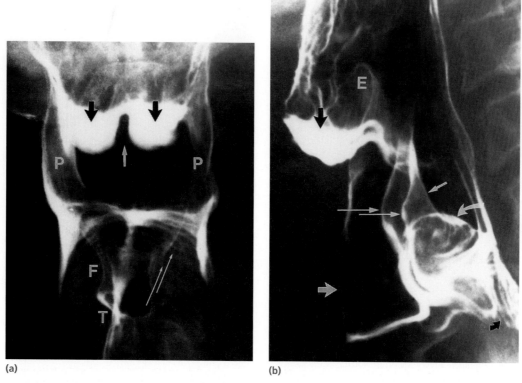

(a)   (b)

Figure 83.4 Normal pharyngeal anatomy. **(a)** Frontal view of pharynx shows cup-shaped valleculae (black arrows) separated by the median glossoepiglottic fold (short white arrow). More inferiorly, pyriform sinuses (P) form the anterior portion of lateral food channels. The arcuate line (long white arrows) is caused by normal laryngeal impression on the collapsed hypopharynx. In this case, both true (T) and false (F) vocal cords are outlined with aspirated barium in the larynx. **(b)** Lateral view during phonation shows the epiglottic tip (E), valleculae (short black arrow), aryepiglottic folds (medium-length white arrow), and anterior walls of pyriform sinuses (long white arrows). Redundant mucosal folds overlie the muscular process of the arytenoid (curved white arrow) and cricoid (curved black arrow) cartilages. Aspirated barium outlines the laryngeal vestibule (short white arrow) and ventricle. Source: Rubesin SE, Glick SN. The tailored double-contrast pharyngogram. CRC Crit Rev Diagn Imaging 1988;28:133. Reproduced with permission of Taylor and Francis Informa UK Ltd.

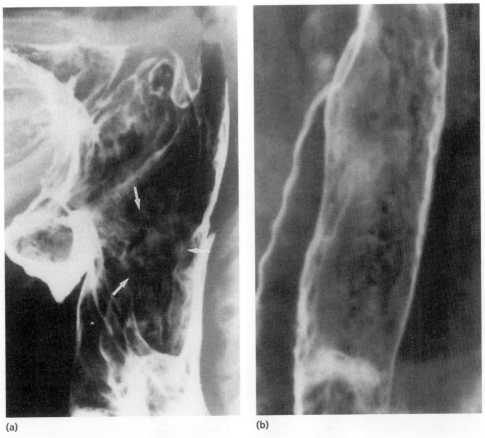

(a)   **(b)**

Figure 83.5 *Candida* pharyngitis and esophagitis in an immunosuppressed patient undergoing chemotherapy for metastatic breast cancer. **(a)** Lateral view of the pharynx shows small, sharply circumscribed plaques (arrows) in the hypopharynx. **(b)** Double-contrast esophagogram also shows multiple plaque-like lesions in the esophagus caused by concomitant *Candida* esophagitis.

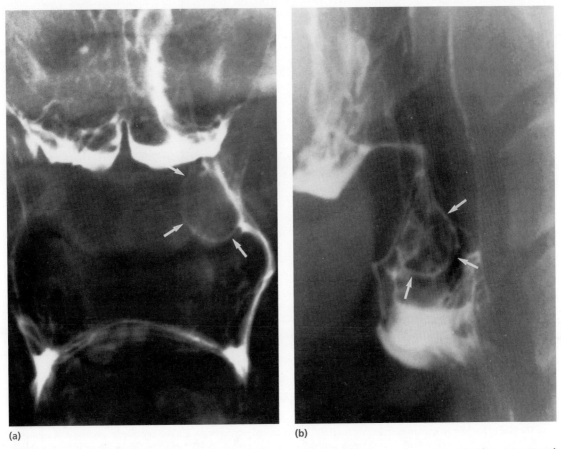

(a)   **(b)**

Figure 83.6 Aryepiglottic fold cyst. **(a)** Frontal view of the pharynx shows the cyst as a smooth submucosal mass (arrows) with an approximately 90° angle between the border of the mass and the adjacent pharyngeal wall. **(b)** Lateral view shows the lesion as a round, sharply circumscribed mass (arrows).

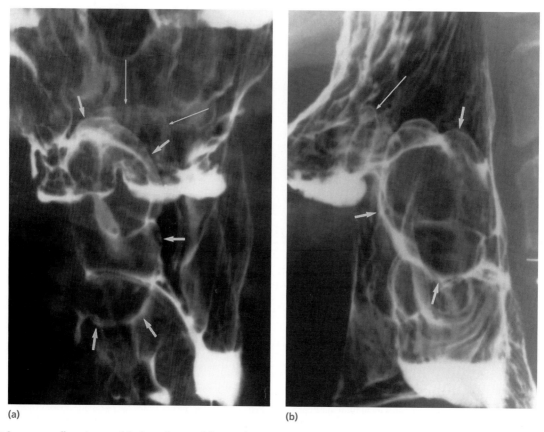

(a)   (b)

Figure 83.7 Squamous cell carcinoma of the hypopharynx. **(a)** Frontal view of the pharynx shows a large polypoid mass (short arrows) obliterating the right lateral wall of the hypopharynx. The tumor extends across the midline. Valleculae and the tip of the epiglottis (long arrows) are preserved. **(b)** Lateral view demonstrates a lobulated mass (short arrows) in the hypopharynx. The epiglottic tip (long arrow) is preserved. Source: Rubesin SE, Glick SN. The tailored double-contrast pharyngogram. CRC Crit Rev Diagn Imaging 1988;28:133. Reproduced with permission of Taylor and Francis Informa UK Ltd.

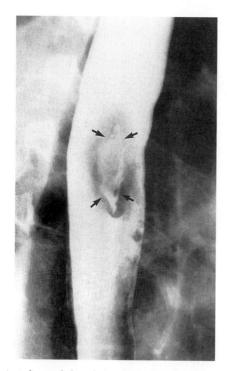

Figure 83.8 Single-contrast esophagram shows a giant, diamond-shaped ulcer (arrows) with a surrounding radiolucent rim of edema in the midesophagus. The patient has human immunodeficiency virus (HIV) infection and odynophagia. Endoscopic biopsy specimens, brushings, and cultures revealed no evidence of cytomegalovirus infection, so the ulcer probably was caused directly by HIV infection (idiopathic or HIV-related ulcer).

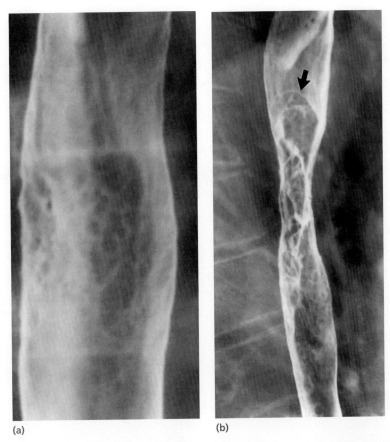

(a)   (b)

Figure 83.9 Esophageal carcinoma. **(a)** Superficial spreading carcinoma with focal nodularity of the midesophagus caused by tiny, coalescent nodules and plaques. **(b)** Advanced infiltrating esophageal carcinoma with irregular narrowing of the lumen. The tumor has an abrupt shelf-like proximal border (arrow). Source: Levine MS, Rubesin SE, Herlinger H, et al. Double contrast upper gastrointestinal examination: technique and interpretation. Radiology 1988;168:584. Reproduced with permission of the Radiological Society of North America.

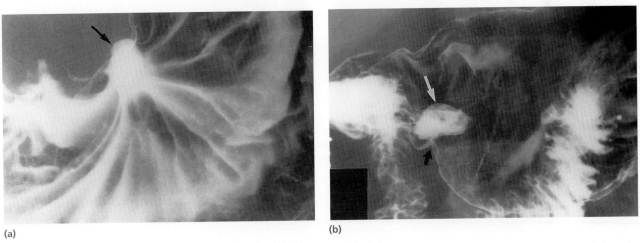

(a)   (b)

Figure 83.10 Benign gastric ulcers. **(a)** Lesser curvature ulcer (arrow). Smooth folds radiate to the edge of the crater. This lesion fulfils the radiological criteria for a benign gastric ulcer. **(b)** Greater curvature ulcer (white arrow) caused by aspirin ingestion. Deformity of the greater curvature (black arrow) is depicted adjacent to the ulcer.

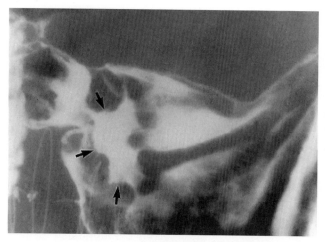

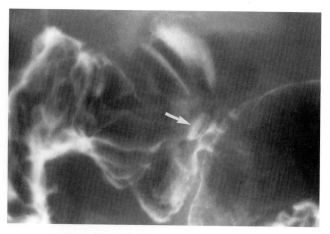

Figure 83.11 Early gastric cancer manifested by an irregular ulcer (arrows) on the posterior wall of the antrum with scalloped borders and nodular, clubbed folds surrounding the ulcer. Source: Levine MS, Creteur V, Kressel HY, et al. Benign gastric ulcers: diagnosis and follow-up with double contrast radiography. Radiology 1987;164:9. Reproduced with permission of the Radiological Society of North America.

Figure 83.12 Linear duodenal ulcer (arrow) at the base of the bulb. Thickened folds are present above the ulcer.

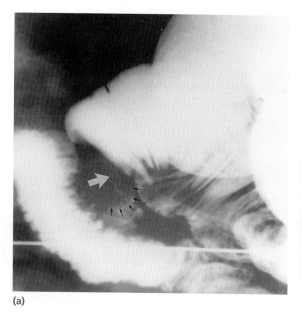

(a)

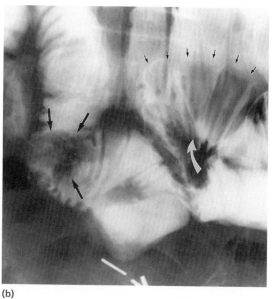

(b)

Figure 83.13 Small bowel metastases causing obstruction. **(a)** High-grade small bowel obstruction caused by annular metastasis from gastric carcinoma. Tight, constricted segment (white arrow) and distal mass effect (black arrows) are visible. **(b)** Partially obstructing metastases from sigmoid carcinoma. One metastasis causes spiculation and fixation of the small bowel wall (white arrow) with normal distensibility of the opposite wall (small black arrows). Another metastasis appears en face as a filling defect (large black arrows) causing distortion of folds.

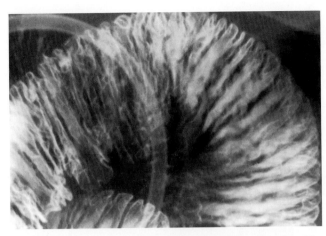

Figure 83.14 Intestinal lymphangiectasia manifested by thickened, mildly irregular folds and tiny nodules representing engorged villi.

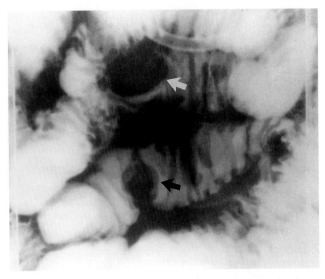

Figure 83.15 Carcinoid tumors in the ileum. The smaller, more distal lesion appears as a smooth submucosal mass (black arrow). However, a larger lesion (white arrow) is associated with outward extension into the mesentery.

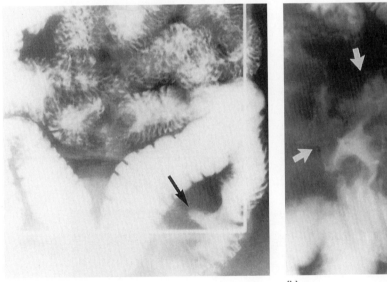

(a)

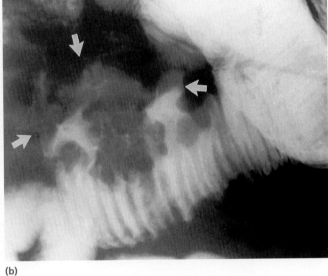

(b)

Figure 83.16 Non-Hodgkin lymphoma of the small bowel. **(a)** Radiograph from small-bowel follow-through study shows focal obliteration of folds of the small bowel with associated ulcer (arrow) on the mesenteric border of the bowel. Because of a history of systemic lupus erythematosus, these findings were attributed to lupus-related vasculitis. **(b)** Spot radiograph from small bowel enema examination performed during later hospital admission shows exoenteric excavation (arrows) from previously ulcerated area. This finding is characteristic of non-Hodgkin lymphoma involving the small bowel.

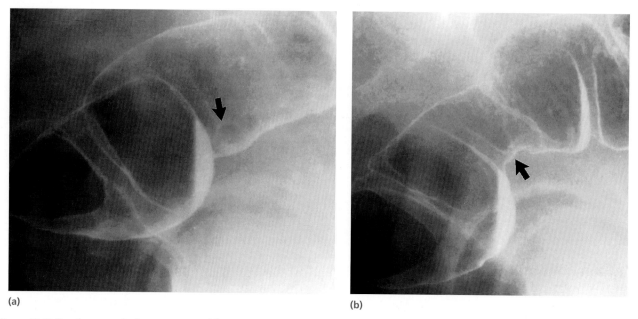

(a)

(b)

Figure 83.17 Development of colonic carcinoma. **(a)** Initial radiograph shows a small polypoid lesion (arrow) on the anterior wall of the distal sigmoid colon. **(b)** Repeat radiograph from double-contrast barium enema examination several years later shows how the polyp has developed into an infiltrating carcinoma (arrow).

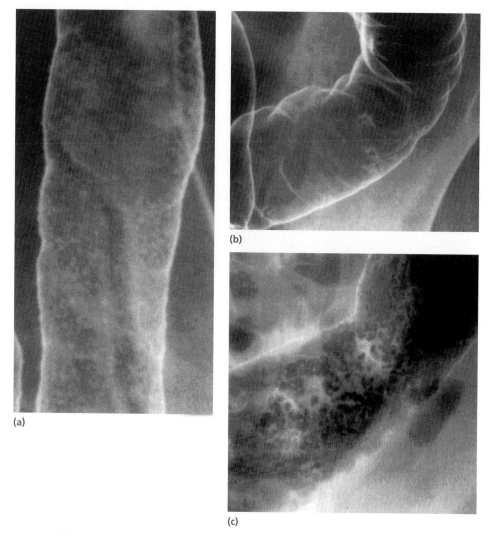

(a)

(b)

(c)

Figure 83.18 Ulcerative colitis. **(a)** Stippling of colonic mucosa caused by innumerable superficial erosions in acute ulcerative colitis. **(b)** Postinflammatory (filiform) polyposis in a patient with quiescent colitis. **(c)** Epithelial dysplasia (precancerous) in a patient with chronic ulcerative colitis. Faceted, angular filling defects are characteristic of "macroscopic" dysplasia. Source: (c) Courtesy of Dr. FM Kelvin.

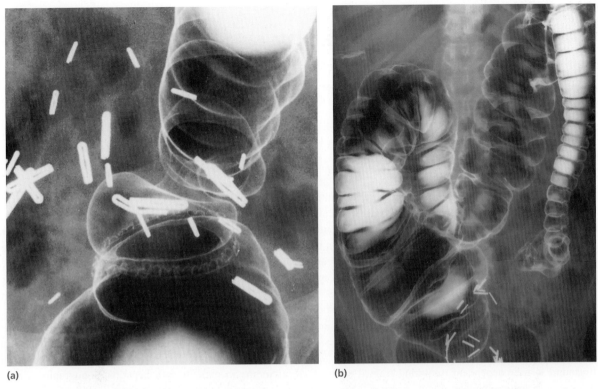

(a)

(b)

Figure 83.19 Postoperative colons of two patients. **(a)** Normal double-contrast appearance of colorectal anastomosis. The site of anastomosis is indicated by the staple line. **(b)** Radiograph from double-contrast colostomy enema examination shows a normal postoperative colon. This examination is important for detecting recurrent or metachronous carcinoma.

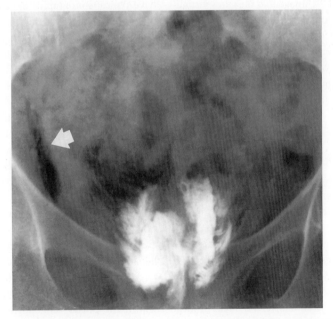

Figure 83.20 Complication of barium enema caused by laceration of the rectum by inflated rectal balloon. Radiograph shows extravasation of barium into perirectal tissue. Retroperitoneal air (arrow) is visible along the right lateral wall of the pelvis.

CHAPTER 84

Transabdominal sonography

Stephanie F. Coquia, Linda C. Chu, and Ulrike M. Hamper
Johns Hopkins University School of Medicine, Baltimore, MD, USA

Ultrasound (US) is one of the diagnostic imaging modalities that can be used to image the intraabdominal organs. In comparison to other available imaging modalities, such as computed tomography (CT) and magnetic resonance imaging (MRI), US is nonionizing, portable, and less expensive. Unlike CT and MRI, US in the United States currently does not have the capability of intravenous contrast agents to evaluate masses or patency of vasculature. However, with the use of color and spectral Doppler sonography, direction and speed of flow within a vessel may be determined, parameters that cannot be assessed by CT or MRI.

Ultrasound is user dependent, requiring trained sonographers and sonologists to obtain pertinent images of the patient's anatomy. The images obtained are also affected by the patient's body habitus, respiratory motion, and artifacts, which need to be compensated for during the examination by the performing imager. For example, air, such as that within the gastrointestinal tract, creates shadowing within the image that obscures visualization of organs deep to it (Figure 84.1). To work around this, the imager may have to use a different approach (sonographic window) or have the patient change position. Therefore, unlike CT and MRI, the performance of each exam may be quite variable as the sonographer or sonologist may use a variety of techniques and positions to obtain the same set of images across all patients.

Liver

Primary indications for liver sonography include evaluation of diffuse parenchymal disease, focal liver mass, vascular disease, trauma, and transplantation.

Parenchymal diseases such as fatty liver and cirrhosis have typical sonographic appearances that are useful in confirming the clinical diagnosis. Hepatic steatosis commonly appears as a diffusely echogenic liver, but fatty infiltration may also appear geographic and focal within the liver. Conversely, areas of focal fatty sparing appear hypoechoic and appear in typical locations such as the gallbladder fossa (Figure 84.2) or dorsal left hepatic lobe. Cirrhosis presents with a nodular liver contour and coarsened liver echotexture. If advanced, the liver is small in size and may be accompanied by ascites. Hepatitis has a nonspecific appearance on US, and the liver can appear normal. One presentation that has been described is the "starry sky" appearance related to edema within the portal triads (Figure 84.3).

Although sonography is less sensitive than CT or MRI in detecting focal liver masses, it remains a good initial screening modality. As such it is used in surveillance of hepatocellular carcinoma in patients with hepatitis. Sonography is also frequently used to characterize abnormalities found on other imaging modalities such as CT or MRI, primarily by characterizing lesions as either cystic or solid. Common benign liver masses such as liver cysts (Figure 84.4, in a patient with autosomal dominant polycystic kidney disease) and hemangiomas have typical sonographic appearances that allow for confident diagnoses. Other masses, however, are indeterminate and require further imaging or biopsy for diagnosis. One such indeterminate appearing but histologically benign mass is focal nodular hyperplasia (FNH), the second most common benign solid mass in the liver after hemangioma. An example of an FNH is seen in Figure 84.5. When multiple solid lesions are present, especially in the setting of a known primary malignancy, metastatic disease should be considered (Figure 84.6). Hepatocellular carcinoma may have associated vascular involvement of the portal and hepatic veins, and US can be used to evaluate for extension of tumor thrombus into these vessels (Figure 84.7).

Doppler sonography is the first-line modality in evaluation of hepatic vascular disease. A dedicated liver duplex evaluates the hepatic arteries (Figure 84.8), portal veins, hepatic veins, and inferior vena cava. It is a noninvasive method to detect the sequela of cirrhosis and the alterations of hemodynamics seen in portal hypertension, such as slow flow within the portal vein, portal vein thrombosis, development

Yamada's Atlas of Gastroenterology, Fifth Edition. Edited by Daniel K. Podolsky, Michael Camilleri, J. Gregory Fitz, Anthony N. Kalloo, Fergus Shanahan, and Timothy C. Wang.
© 2016 John Wiley & Sons, Ltd. Published 2016 by John Wiley & Sons, Ltd.
Companion website: www.yamadagastro.com/atlas

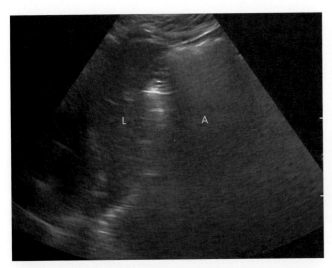

Figure 84.1 Sagittal image of the left hepatic lobe (L) showing extensive shadowing related to air (A) within the stomach, obscuring structures deep to the stomach such as the pancreas and aorta.

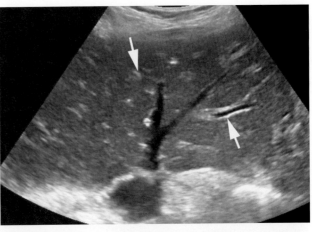

Figure 84.3 Hepatitis. Transverse sonogram of the liver shows brightly echogenic portal triads (arrows) that are sharply defined against the background of relatively hypoechoic liver. This pattern has been referred to as the "starry sky" pattern, and can be seen in hepatitis.

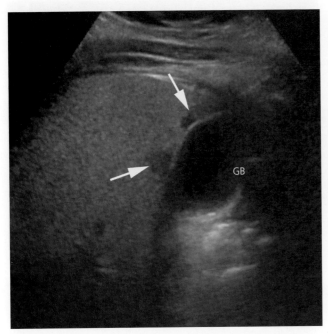

Figure 84.2 Focal fatty sparing. Sagittal sonogram of the right hepatic lobe shows echogenic liver with coarsened echotexture in the setting of hepatic steatosis. Two small hypoechoic structures (arrows) along the gallbladder fossa represent focal fatty sparing. Focal fatty infiltration and focal fatty sparing tend to occur in characteristic locations: the falciform ligament, porta hepatis, and gallbladder (GB) fossa.

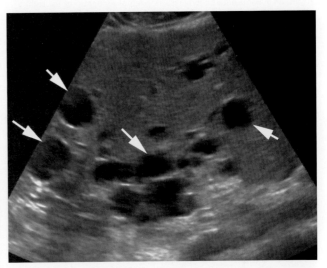

Figure 84.4 Polycystic liver disease. Sagittal sonogram of the right hepatic lobe shows innumerable well-circumscribed anechoic cystic masses in the liver (arrows) in a patient with polycystic liver disease. Some of these cysts demonstrate increased through transmission typical of cysts.

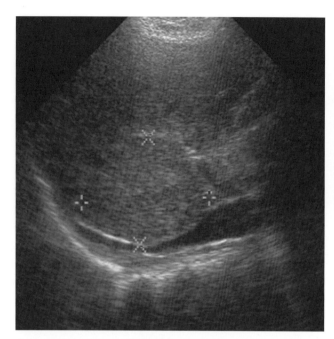

Figure 84.5 Focal nodular hyperplasia. Sagittal sonogram of the right hepatic lobe shows a subtle isoechoic mass (between calipers). Sonographic appearance of focal nodular hyperplasia can be variable and usually requires further evaluation with computed tomography (CT), magnetic resonance imaging (MRI), and/or biopsy.

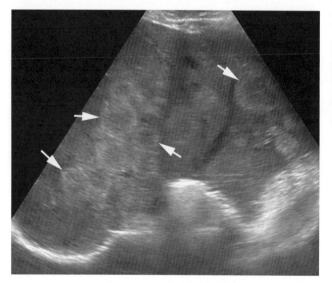

Figure 84.6 Diffuse metastatic disease. Transverse sonogram of the right hepatic lobe shows innumerable masses with isoechoic centers and thick peripheral hyperechoic halos (arrows), compatible with metastatic disease.

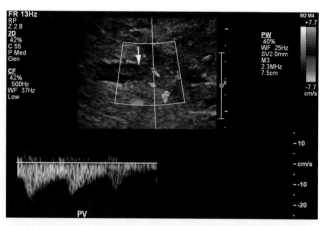

Figure 84.7 Sonogram of the main portal vein demonstrates nonocclusive thrombus (arrow) within the main portal vein. Spectral Doppler interrogation of the thrombus demonstrates an arterial waveform within the thrombus. The presence of internal vascularity and arterial waveform differentiates tumor thrombus from bland thrombus.

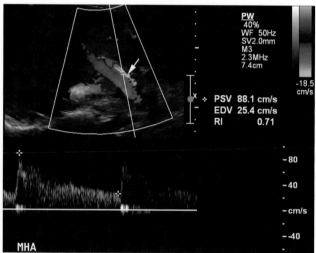

Figure 84.8 Normal hepatic artery duplex. Color and spectral Doppler of the main hepatic artery (arrow) show a normal low resistance arterial waveform with normal resistive index of 0.71.

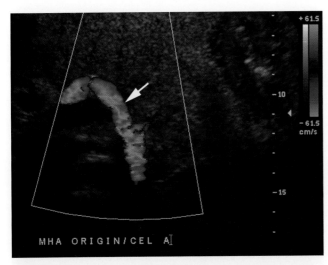

Figure 84.9 Corkscrew hepatic artery. Color Doppler image of the main hepatic artery (arrow) shows an enlarged and tortuous main hepatic artery to supply blood flow to the liver in the setting of portal vein thrombosis. The large tortuous main hepatic artery is also referred to as a "corkscrew" hepatic artery.

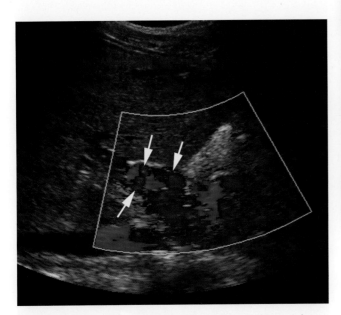

Figure 84.10 Cavernous transformation of the main portal vein. Color Doppler image of the porta hepatis shows numerous collateral vessels in the region of the porta hepatis (arrows) supplying the liver. The normal main portal vein is chronically occluded and is not visualized.

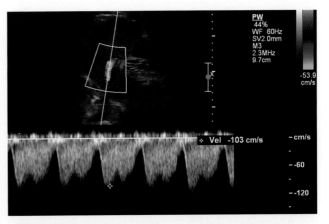

Figure 84.11 Normal transjugular intrahepatic portosystemic shunt (TIPSS). Color and spectral Doppler interrogation of the TIPSS shows blood flow from the right portal vein to the right hepatic vein. The direction of blood flow is appropriately away from the transducer with peak velocity of 103 cm/s, which is within normal limits for TIPSS.

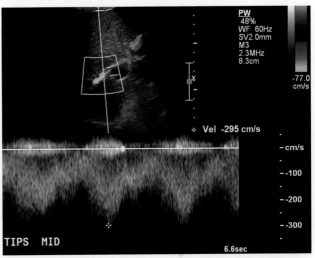

Figure 84.12 Transjugular intrahepatic portosystemic shunt (TIPSS) stenosis. Spectral Doppler waveform in midportion of TIPSS shows abnormally elevated peak velocity of 295 cm/s, compatible with TIPSS stenosis. Hepatopetal flow within left portal vein (not shown) is also an important sign of TIPSS malfunction.

of corkscrew hepatic arteries (Figure 84.9) in response to the diminished flow in the portal vein, and cavernous transformation after long-standing portal vein thrombosis (Figure 84.10). In patients with transjugular intrahepatic portosystemic shunts (TIPSS), sonography can readily detect complications such as TIPSS stenosis or occlusion. A normal TIPSS is seen in Figure 84.11; a stenosed TIPSS is seen in Figure 84.12. Sonography is also an important screening tool for posttransplant vascu-

lar complications and is helpful in detecting signs of vascular compromise before catastrophic loss of the transplant allograft (Figures 84.13, 84.14, 84.15, and 84.16). Hepatic vein occlusion may be seen in the setting of Budd–Chiari syndrome (Figure 84.17).

Ultrasound can be used to perform image-guided interventions, such as abscess drainage, biopsy, and tumor ablation. In experienced hands, ultrasound-guided percutaneous procedures are quicker and easier to perform than CT-guided procedures. Sonography can directly depict the needle tip as it is placed in the lesion in order to ensure accurate tissue sampling.

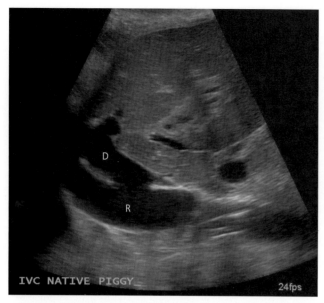

Figure 84.13 Orthotopic liver transplant with donor inferior vena cava (IVC) to recipient IVC "piggyback" anastomosis. Sonogram of the IVC anastomosis shows end-to-side donor IVC (D) to recipient IVC (R) anastomosis.

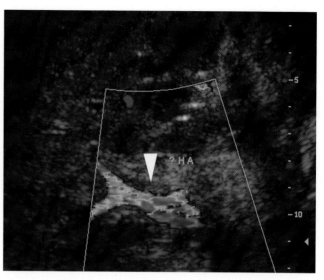

Figure 84.15 Transplant liver with occlusion of main hepatic artery. Color Doppler image of the porta hepatis shows patent main portal vein with absence of flow in the main hepatic artery (arrowhead).

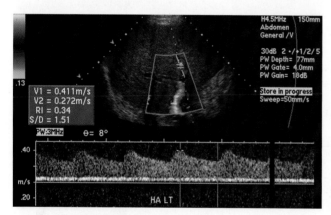

Figure 84.14 Transplant liver with stenosis of the main hepatic artery anastomosis. Color and spectral Doppler of the left hepatic artery branch shows a parvus et tardus waveforms with abnormally low resistive index of 0.34, concerning for upstream stenosis of the hepatic artery anastomosis.

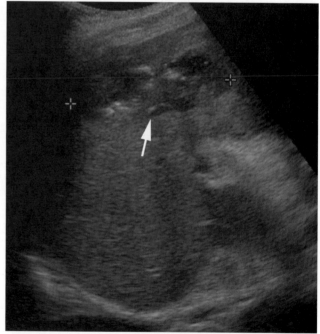

Figure 84.16 Hepatic artery occlusion in transplant liver with liver infarction. Transverse sonogram of the transplant liver shows a heterogeneous collection within the right hepatic lobe from liver infarction (arrow).

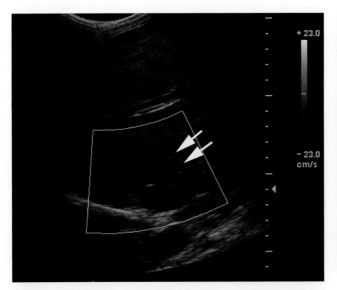

Figure 84.17 Budd–Chiari syndrome. Grayscale sonogram of the hepatic vein confluence shows multiple thin webs (arrows) within the main hepatic vein, compatible with Budd–Chiari syndrome. Flow in the hepatic vein is present on color Doppler images (not shown).

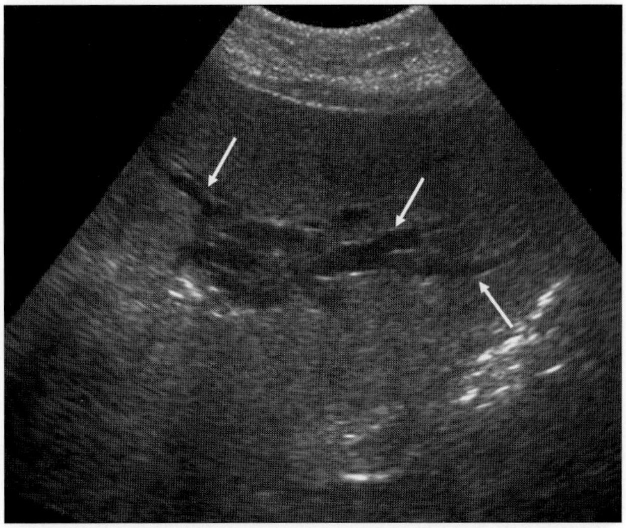

Figure 84.18 Intrahepatic biliary ductal dilation. Multiple tubular structures are seen within the left hepatic lobe (arrows). Interrogation with color Doppler showed that some of these structures did not fill in with color, confirming the presence of dilated ducts.

Gallbladder and biliary tract

Ultrasound is the imaging modality of choice in the evaluation of the gallbladder and the biliary tree. Common indications for a right upper quadrant ultrasound include evaluation for gallstones, cholecystitis, biliary ductal dilation, or choledocholithiasis to explain a patient's elevated liver function tests.

Ultrasound can be used to evaluate for the presence of both intrahepatic (Figure 84.18) and extrahepatic biliary ductal dilation. If present, US can also be used to evaluate for a specific cause such as stone in the biliary tree or a pancreatic head mass causing upstream biliary obstruction. If the exam is unrevealing as to a cause for the dilation, further imaging could be pursued with magnetic resonance cholangiopancreatography (MRCP) or endoscopic retrograde cholangiopancreatography (ERCP). After ERCP and sphincterotomy, air may be present in the biliary tree, which can be visualized on US (Figure 84.19).

Gallstones appear as echogenic, mobile masses that demonstrate posterior acoustic shadowing, an artifact related to the lack of echoes able to penetrate the stone resulting in a "black sound void" deep to the stone. Sometimes stones may be large or numerous and occupy the entire gallbladder lumen, leaving only the anterior wall visible, a sonographic sign known as the WES sign, or wall-echo-shadow sign (Figure 84.20). Calcification in the gallbladder wall is known as a porcelain gallbladder (Figure 84.21). The calcification in the anterior wall causes posterior acoustic shadowing that obscures the gallbladder lumen, and so a porcelain gallbladder may be confused with a gallbladder full of stones. The WES sign helps to make this distinction. Porcelain gallbladder has been associated with gallbladder carcinoma.

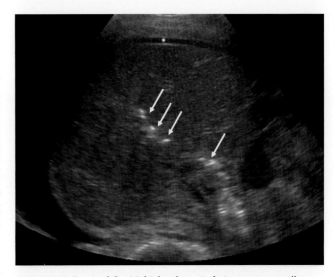

Figure 84.19 Pneumobilia. Multiple echogenic foci are seen centrally within the liver in a linear configuration (arrows). None of the foci were seen in the portal vein, confirming the presence of the air within the biliary tree. Note that perihepatic ascites is also present (*).

Gallstones may become impacted in the cystic duct leading to biliary colic and acute cholecystitis. Sonographic findings present in acute cholecystitis include gallbladder wall thickening, wall hyperemia, pericholecystic fluid, and a sonographic Murphy sign (marked tenderness over the gallbladder when the transducer is pressed over the gallbladder). Complications of acute cholecystitis include gangrenous cholecystitis (Figure 84.22), emphysematous cholecystitis (Figure 84.23), and gallbladder perforation, which may result in abscess formation within the adjacent liver.

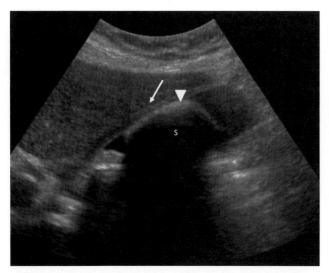

Figure 84.20 "Wall-echo-shadow" sign. A large gallstone is seen within the gallbladder, nearly occupying the entire gallbladder lumen and causing posterior acoustic shadowing (S). However, a discrete gallbladder wall (arrow) is seen separate to the echogenic rim of the gallstone (arrowhead), confirming that the calcification is within the gallbladder, not within the wall.

In addition to stones, sludge may be present in the gallbladder lumen (Figure 84.24). Sludge is also mobile but does not shadow like a stone. It may appear mass-like, commonly referred to as tumefactive sludge. Sludge does not show flow on color Doppler US, enabling adherent sludge to be distinguished from gallbladder neoplasms.

Pancreas

The pancreas is usually imaged as part of the routine evaluation of the right upper quadrant. It is usually of similar echogenicity to the liver or slightly hyperechoic to the liver. Commonly it may become fatty replaced, such as in older patients (Figure 84.25) or in patients with cystic fibrosis. In the setting of acute pancreatitis, it can become hypoechoic and enlarged due to edema. Peripancreatic fluid may also be present. Ultrasound is not commonly ordered in the diagnosis of acute pancreatitis, but it is ordered to evaluate for gallstones as a cause of pancreatitis. In chronic pancreatitis, parenchymal calcifications and ductal dilation can be seen.

While US is not the imaging modality of choice in the evaluation for pancreatic masses, these may be seen in the work-up for biliary ductal dilation or abnormal liver function tests. Masses may present with upstream pancreatic ductal dilation or atrophy (Figure 84.26). When visualized it is important to evaluate for adjacent vessel involvement or evidence of metastatic disease within the liver, as the presence of either has important implications in regard to management of the pancreatic mass.

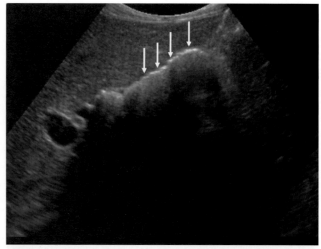

(a)

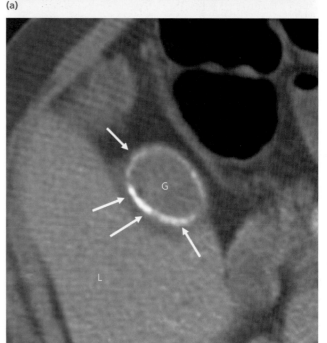

(b)

Figure 84.21 Porcelain gallbladder. **(a)** Curvilinear echogenicity (arrows) in the region of the gallbladder, causing significant posterior acoustic shadowing. A discrete gallbladder wall is not seen separate to the echogenicity and there was no change in the appearance of the echogenicity when the patient changed position. **(b)** The patient had a computed tomography (CT) scan, which confirmed the presence of calcification (arrows) within the gallbladder wall (G), consistent with a porcelain gallbladder. The liver is also depicted (L).

Gastrointestinal tract

Sonography is used in a limited number of indications to evaluate the gastrointestinal tract. In children it is used to evaluate for appendicitis and intussusception so as to avoid radiation from abdominal radiography, CT, or air reduction enema. An

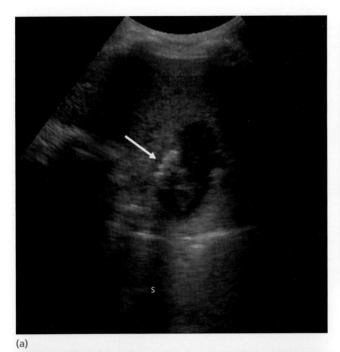

(a)

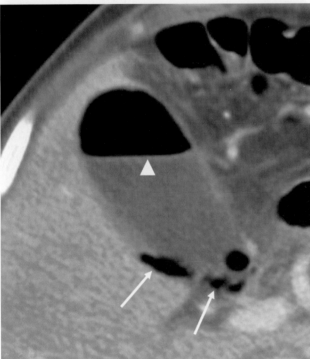

(b)

Figure 84.22 Emphysematous cholecystitis. **(a)** Echogenic foci are seen within the nondependent wall of the gallbladder (arrow), causing dirty posterior acoustic shadowing (S), suggesting emphysematous cholecystitis. **(b)** Subsequent computed tomography (CT) confirms the presence of air in the gallbladder wall (arrows). An air–bile level is seen within the gallbladder lumen (arrowhead).

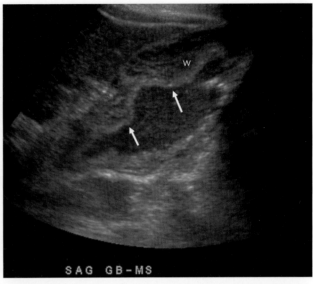

Figure 84.23 Gangrenous cholecystitis. The wall of the gallbladder (W) is markedly thickened with a striated, multilaminar appearance. The mucosal layer (arrows) is irregular in contour. A sonographic Murphy sign may be absent in gangrenous cholecystitis due to denervation.

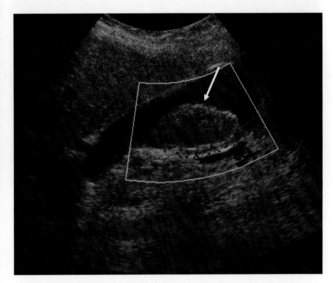

Figure 84.24 Tumefactive sludge. Focal nonvascular, nonshadowing mobile hypoechoic mass (arrow) within the gallbladder. It does not show internal vascularity on color Doppler as would be expected for a neoplasm of that size and it does not show posterior acoustic shadowing as seen in gallstones. The mass moved with a change in patient positioning, confirming its mobility.

example of an ileocolic intussusception is seen in Figure 84.27. Diagnosis of acute appendicitis requires visualization of a non-compressible, dilated (diameter 7 mm or larger), blind-ending tubular structure compatible with an obstructed appendix. As with identifying pancreatic masses, bowel pathology may be

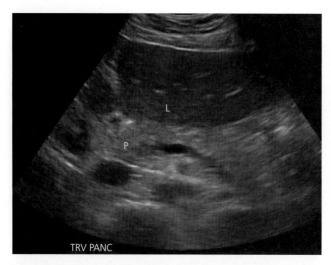

Figure 84.25 Fatty infiltration of the pancreas. The pancreas (P) is hyperechoic to the liver (L) and similar in echotexture to the retroperitoneal fat.

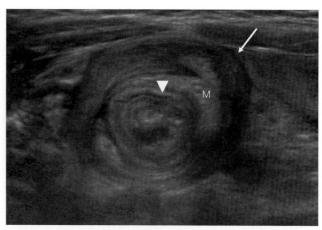

Figure 84.27 Ileocolic intussusception in the transverse plane. Two hypoechoic eccentric rings are seen, denoting the bowel wall of the intussusceptum (arrowhead) and the intussuscipiens (arrow). The echogenic area between the two rings is the mesenteric fat (M) accompanying the intussusceptum into the intussuscipiens.

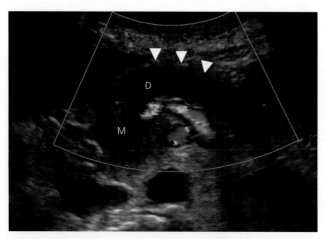

Figure 84.26 Pancreatic adenocarcinoma. Transverse image of the pancreas shows pancreatic ductal dilation (D), abruptly terminating in the pancreatic head secondary to an ill-defined hypoechoic mass (M). There is associated pancreatic atrophy as minimal parenchyma is seen surrounding the dilated pancreatic duct (arrowheads).

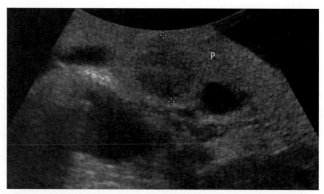

Figure 84.28 Hypoechoic mass (calipers) in the body of the pancreas (P) seen with intraoperative ultrasound. Note that the superior part of the image does not show the usual anterior abdominal wall musculature, as the transducer was placed immediately over the pancreas. This mass was excised with pathology of islet cell tumor.

identified during the evaluation of the other intraabdominal organs for causes of abdominal pain, for example evaluation of the other intraabdominal organs, for example bowel obstruction (dilated bowel) or inflammatory bowel disease or diverticulitis (hyperemic and thickened bowel walls).

Peritoneal cavity

Common indications to evaluate the peritoneal cavity with ultrasound include evaluation for ascites and abdominal fluid collections. Ultrasound guidance can also be used during paracentesis and the percutaneous drainage of visualized fluid collections.

Intraoperative ultrasound

Ultrasound can be used within the operating room to detect tumors for biopsy and resection. With an open abdomen, the probe can be placed on the organ of interest, improving resolution and detection of focal masses (Figure 84.28) as compared to conventional transabdominal ultrasound.

CHAPTER 85

Endoscopic ultrasonography

Marcia Irene Canto and Mouen A. Khashab
Johns Hopkins University, Baltimore, MD, USA

Introduction

Endoscopic ultrasonography (EUS) is an established diagnostic and therapeutic modality in gastroenterology. Although most gastroenterologists are not trained in the practice of EUS, it is important that they understand the principles of the technique and the indications for EUS in order to offer optimal patient care.

This chapter provides case vignettes with selected images that illustrate common diagnostic and therapeutic indications for EUS. A brief overview of the role of EUS in such indications is included. As a complete representation of images encountered in endosonography could not be provided here, the authors recommend that anyone interested in learning EUS should review textbooks dedicated to the practice of EUS and seek out an established EUS training program.

Types of echoendoscopes

There are two major types of echoendoscopes: radial imaging and linear imaging. Radial echoendoscopes provide cross-sectional anatomical imaging. Newer generations of the radial echoendoscope include electronic array, which allows for the addition of Doppler to the radial echoendoscope (Figure 85.1a). Linear echoendoscopes transmit ultrasound waves in the same axis as the long shaft of the transducer, which allows for real-time therapeutic intervention, most commonly fine-needle aspiration (Figure 85.1b). Figures 85.2, 85.3, 85.4, 85.5, and 85.6 depict selected images of normal histology or anatomy as visualized by EUS. Case examples showing the use of EUS follow.

Case 1 A 57-year-old man with a history of reflux presents with 2 months of progressive dysphagia for solids more than liquids. He reports a 15 lb weight loss. A computed tomography (CT) scan of the thorax reveals thickening of the distal esophagus. Upper endoscopy reveals a narrowed esophageal stricture

(Figure 85.7a). The EUS (Figure 85.7b) shows an asymmetric hypoechoic image of the stricture region that reflects the mass at 40 cm from the incisors. The mass extends beyond the esophageal muscularis propria and invades the adjacent left pleura. A malignant periesophageal lymph node is identified that was not seen on the CT scan (Figure 85.7c). EUS stage is T4N1Mx.

Case 2 A 43-year-old man with history of cystic fibrosis presents with hemoccult positive stools and mild anemia. Upper endoscopy reveals a polypoid mass in the distal esophagus (Figure 85.8a). Biopsy confirms adenocarcinoma. EUS shows an asymmetric, hypoechoic mass with submucosal invasion (Figure 85.8b). Endoscopic mucosal resection was performed as ablative therapy (Figure 85.8c).

Case 3 A 65-year-old woman with weight loss undergoes CT of the abdomen. The CT scan shows a left adrenal mass. Upper endoscopy reveals a large gastric ulcer in the fundus (Figure 85.9a). Radial EUS demonstrates a mass in the left adrenal (Figure 85.9b), and a mass in the left upper lobe of the lung. The results of a fine needle aspiration confirmed the diagnosis of stage IV nonsmall cell lung cancer (Figure 85.9c).

Case 4 A 47-year-old man with a history of gastroesophageal reflux undergoes upper endoscopy. A submucosal mass of about 3 cm is identified (Figure 85.10a). Radial EUS demonstrates a well-circumscribed, hypoechoic mass originating from the muscularis layer of the stomach (Figure 85.10b). Fine-needle aspiration demonstrates spindle-shaped cells that stain positive for C-kit protein. A gastrointestinal stromal cell tumor (GIST) was diagnosed.

Case 5 A 57-year-old woman undergoes upper endoscopy for epigastric pain. An ulcerated mucosa was identified from a biopsy, confirming adenocarcinoma (Figure 85.11a). EUS revealed mucosal and submucosal infiltration (Figure 85.11b). Curative subtotal gastrectomy was performed.

Case 6 A 68-year-old man presents with epigastric pain and weight loss. A CT scan shows pancreatic head enlargement

Yamada's Atlas of Gastroenterology, Fifth Edition. Edited by Daniel K. Podolsky, Michael Camilleri, J. Gregory Fitz, Anthony N. Kalloo, Fergus Shanahan, and Timothy C. Wang.
© 2016 John Wiley & Sons, Ltd. Published 2016 by John Wiley & Sons, Ltd.
Companion website: www.yamadagastro.com/atlas

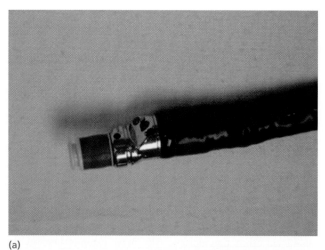

(a)

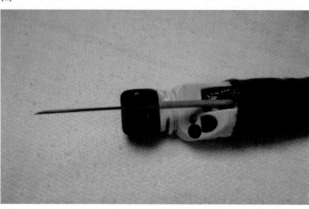

(b)

Figure 85.1 **(a)** Electronic radial echoendoscope (Olympus). **(b)** Linear echoendoscope with a protruding needle used for a fine-needle aspiration (Olympus).

without a discrete mass. EUS shows a hypoechoic mass (Figure 85.12a), which is confirmed to be adenocarcinoma by EUS-guided fine-needle aspiration (Figure 85.12b).

Case 7 A 49-year-old woman suffers from episodes of hypoglycemia. Prior imaging studies failed to identify a clinically suspected insulinoma. EUS reveals a 5-mm well-circumscribed hypoechoic lesion in the pancreatic tail (Figure 85.13). Distal pancreatectomy was performed and symptoms were resolved.

Case 8 A 48-year-old man presents with steatorrhea and persistent abdominal pain. EUS demonstrates hyperechoic foci and strands, pseudolobulations and lobularity of the pancreatic gland (Figure 85.14). Other features (not shown) included calcifications and an echogenic pancreatic duct. These EUS features are most consistent with chronic pancreatitis.

Case 9 An asymptomatic 65-year-old man has a 2.5 cm pancreatic cyst. EUS reveals a multiseptated, well-circumscribed, anechoic lesion with posterior acoustic enhancement. Echogenic debris is noted within the cyst (Figure 85.15). The results of a fine-needle aspiration confirm a mucinous tumor.

Case 10 A 29-year-old man with a history of rectal pain and bleeding. Colonoscopy reveals multiple polyps and an anorectal stricture that is nearly causing obstruction (Figure 85.16a). EUS reveals an irregular hypoechoic mass with infiltration into adjacent soft tissue (EUS stage T4NxMx) (Figure 85.16b).

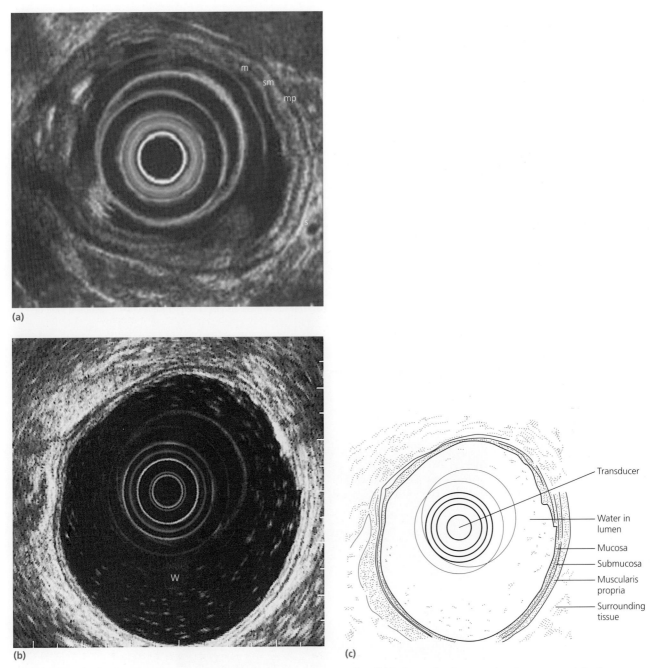

Figure 85.2 (a) Endoscopic ultrasonography showing the five layers of the stomach wall. The image showing normal anatomy was created using a 5.0 MHz radial scanning endoscope. **(b)** A healthy stomach imaged with a 7.5 MHz radial scanning endoscope. Water (W) in the gastric lumen facilitates imaging of the wall layers that correspond to mucosa, submucosa, muscularis propria, and surrounding tissue. **(c)** Diagrammatic image showing labels. m, mucosa; sm, submucosa; mp, muscularis propria; s, serosa; w, water.

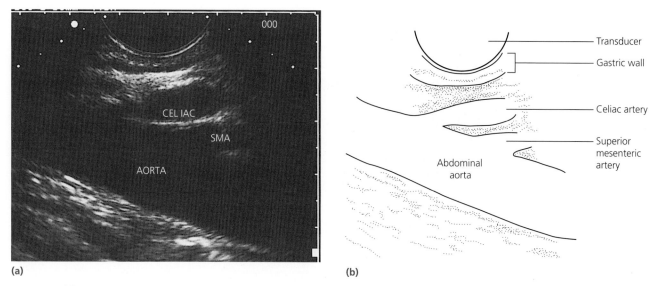

Figure 85.3 (a) The abdominal aorta and the origins of the celiac and superior mesenteric arteries (SMA) imaged through the gastric wall with an electronic curvilinear-array ultrasound endoscope, with diagrammatic image **(b)**. This instrument also has Doppler capability for demonstration of blood flow in these vessels.

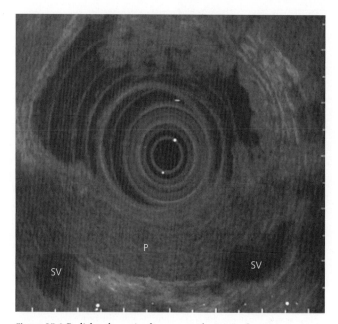

Figure 85.4 Radial endoscopic ultrasonography image showing characteristic normal "salt-and-pepper pattern" of the pancreas. P, body of the pancreas; SV, splenic vein.

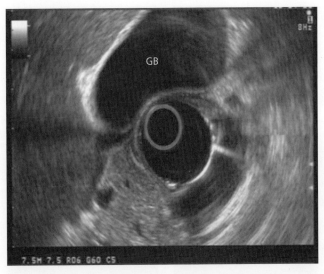

Figure 85.5 Radial endoscopic ultrasonography image showing image of a healthy gallbladder. GB, gallbladder.

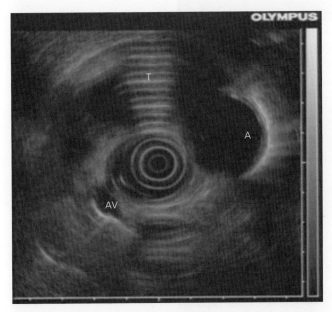

Figure 85.6 Radial endoscopic ultrasonography image showing normal mediastinal anatomy. A, aorta; AV, azygos vein; T, trachea.

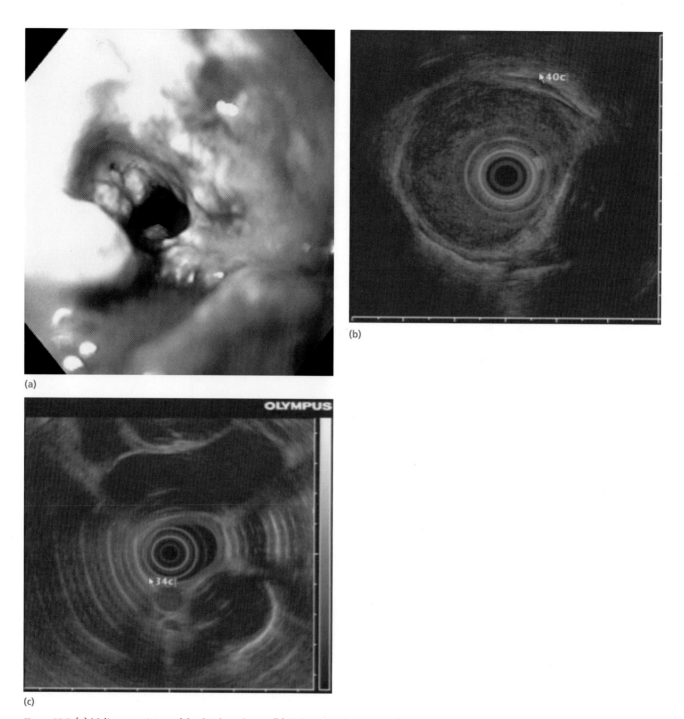

Figure 85.7 (a) Malignant stricture of the distal esophagus. **(b)** Endoscopic ultrasonography image of esophageal carcinoma (T4) with pleural invasion. **(c)** EUS reveals a hypoechoic, sharply defined periesophageal lymph node suspicious for malignancy. EUS-guided fine-needle aspiration confirms malignant status of the lymph node.

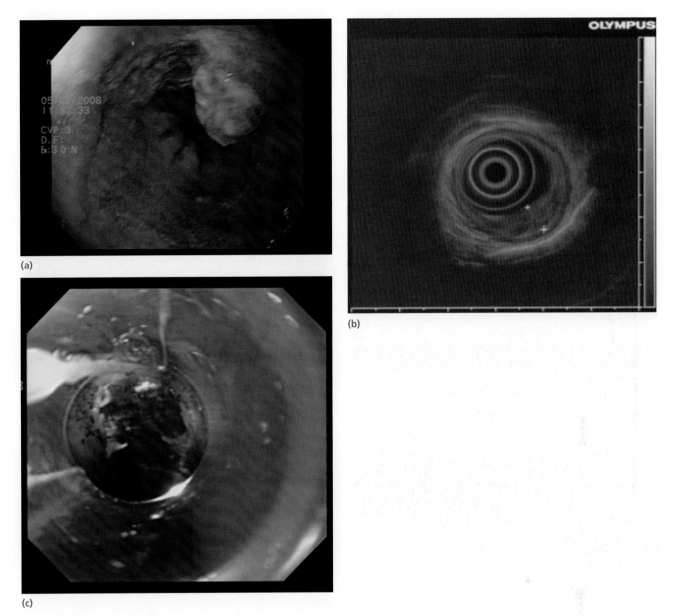

Figure 85.8 (a) Upper endoscopy image showing a polypoid lesion in the distal esophagus. The results of the biopsies confirmed adenocarcinoma.
(b) Endoscopic ultrasonography image showing esophageal cancer. **(c)** Patient was treated with endoscopic mucosal resection.

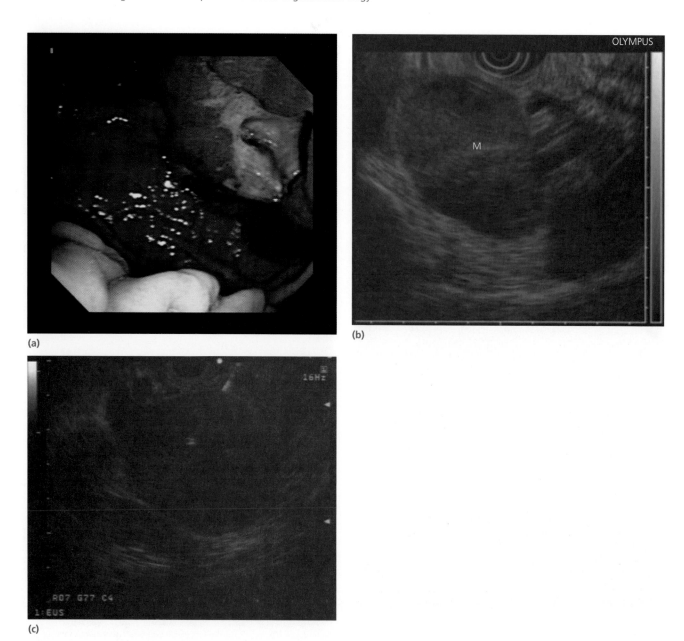

Figure 85.9 **(a)** Upper endoscopy image showing ulcerated gastric mass in fundus. **(b)** Radial endoscopic ultrasonography demonstrates a hypoechoic mass (M) of the left adrenal gland. **(c)** Fine-needle aspiration of the mass in **(b)**.

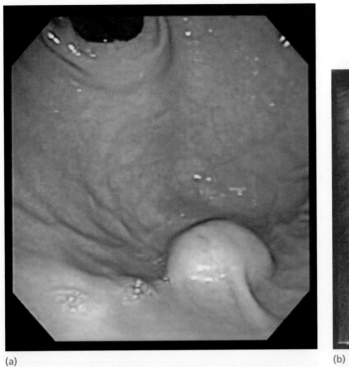

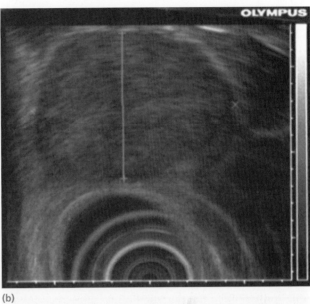

(a)

(b)

Figure 85.10 (a) An upper gastrointestinal endoscopy image of the stomach showing a submucosal mass. (b) Endoscopic ultrasonography demonstrates a hypoechoic mass originating from the gastric muscularis propria.

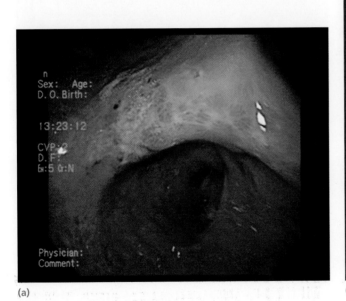

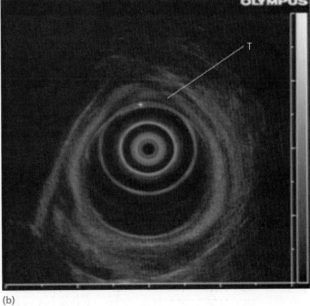

(a)

(b)

Figure 85.11 (a) Endoscopy revealing an ulcerated mucosa along the gastric incisura. (b) Endoscopic ultrasonography shows mucosal and submucosal thickening, which suggests T1N0 gastric malignancy. T, tumor.

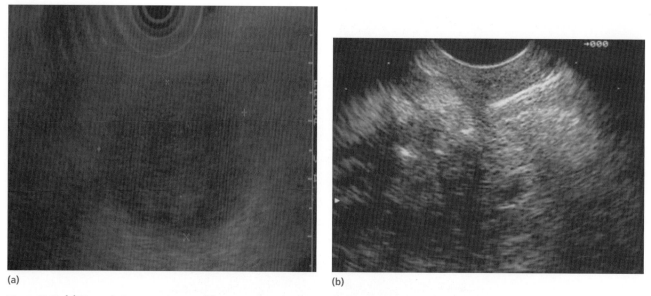

(a)   (b)

Figure 85.12 (a) Hypoechoic pancreatic mass. **(b)** Fine-needle aspiration needle entering pancreatic mass. The biopsy results confirmed adenocarcinoma.

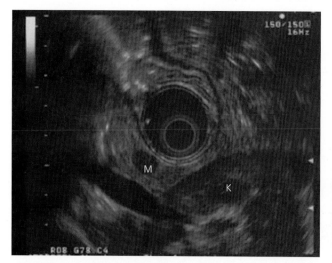

Figure 85.13 Endoscopic ultrasonography reveals 5 mm well-circumscribed hypoechoic lesion (M) in the pancreatic tail. K, left kidney.

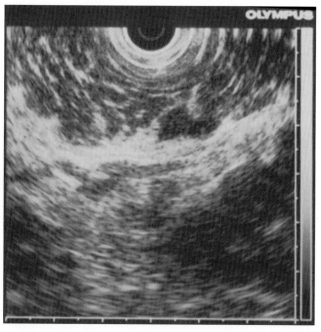

Figure 85.14 Endoscopic ultrasonography image of chronic pancreatitis.

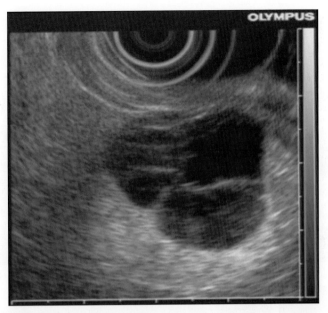

Figure 85.15 Endoscopic ultrasonography image showing a multiseptated, well-circumscribed, anechoic lesion with posterior acoustic enhancement. Echogenic debris is evident within the cyst.

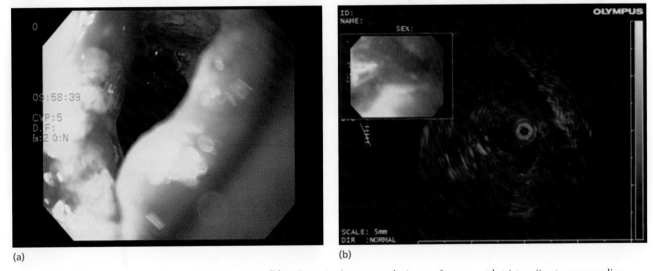

(a)   (b)

Figure 85.16 **(a)** Endoscopic image of an anorectal stricture. **(b)** Endoscopic ultrasonography image of an anorectal stricture (inset: corresponding endoscopic image).

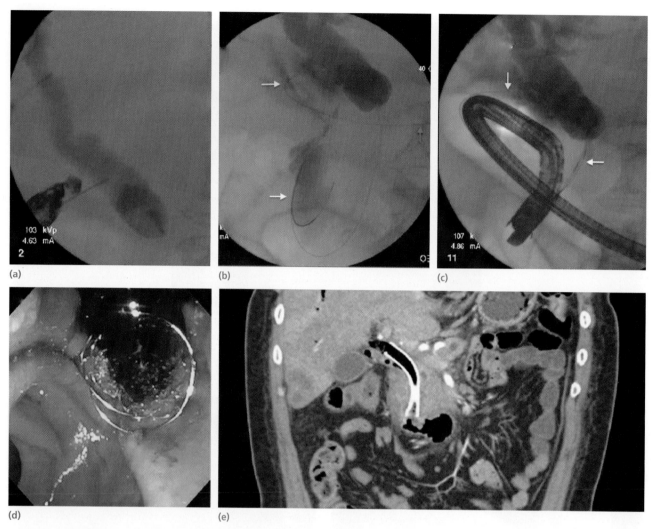

Figure 85.17 EUS-guided biliary drainage using the rendezvous technique. **(a)** The common bile duct (CBD) was punctured with a 19-gauge needle under endosonographic guidance and antegrade cholangiography revealed dilated CBD with distal obstruction. **(b)** Antegrade passage of guidewire can be seen passing via the stomach (red arrow), duodenal bulb (yellow arrow), through the papilla and coiled in the distal duodenum (white arrow). **(c)** The wire was grasped through a duodenoscope and a sphincterotome was passed over the wire (white arrow). The wire was withdrawn from the duodenal bulb (yellow) and re-advanced in a retrograde fashion to facilitate transpapillary stent placement. **(d)** Dark bile flowing through transpapillary self-expandable metallic biliary stent. **(e)** Coronal CT showing self-expandable metallic stent placed across distal biliary stricture due to pancreatic mass.

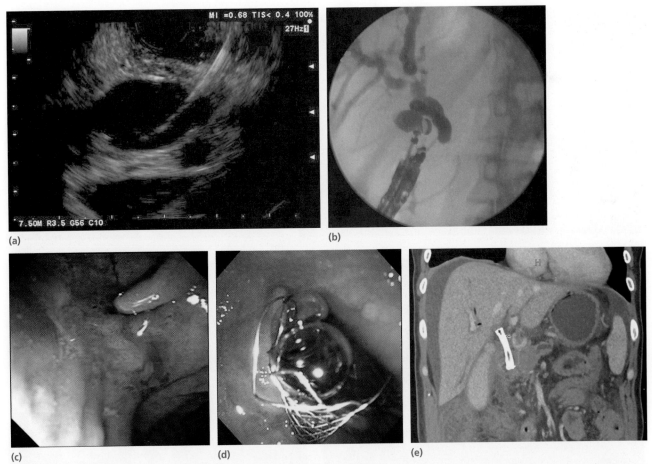

(a)

(b)

(c)

(d)

(e)

Figure 85.18 EUS-guided biliary drainage using direct transluminal technique. **(a)** Endosonographic demonstrating needle and guide wire within the common bile duct (CBD). **(b)** Antegrade cholangiography demonstrating intra- and extra-hepatic biliary dilation with an abrupt cut off in the mid CBD. Prophylactic pancreatic stent placed at failed ERCP remains *in situ*. **(c)** The choledochoduodenostomy (CDS) was dilated with a dilating bougie catheter (4–7 Fr). **(d)** Large volume of bile flowing through the fully covered self-expanding metallic biliary stent that was placed across the CDS. **(e)** Coronal CT 4 weeks post EUS-BD reveals optimal stent position and absence of biliary ductal dilatation

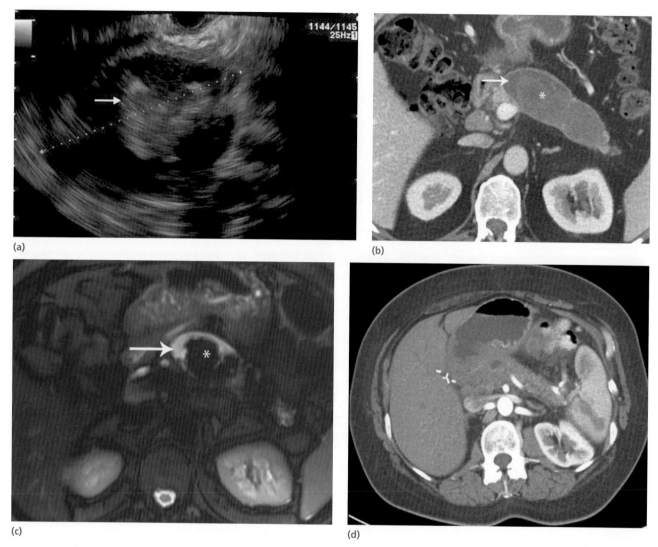

Figure 85.19 EUS-guided drainage of walled-off pancreatic necrosis (WOPN). **(a)** EUS image of WOPN prior to EUS guided drainage. Hyperechoic solid material (yellow arrow) is seen within the cyst. **(b)** Axial contrast enhanced CT shows a large intrapancreatic collection with near complete replacement of the pancreatic parenchyma measuring 11.7 cm. The collection has a large amount of debris (asterisk) with a thin sliver of fluid (arrow). **(c)** Axial T2 weighted MRI of abdomen demonstrates the presence of a collection measuring 11.6 cm that contains predominantly solid debris (asterisk) with small amount of fluid (arrow). **(d)** Axial contrast enhanced CT performed 2 months after stent placement demonstrates marked decrease in the size of the collection.

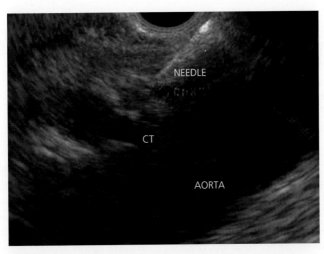

Figure 85.20 EUS-guided celiac plexus neurolysis (CPN) using single central injection technique. The celiac trunk (CT) is easily identified as the first take-off from the aortal. An FNA needle is advanced and CPN is carried under EUS guidance.

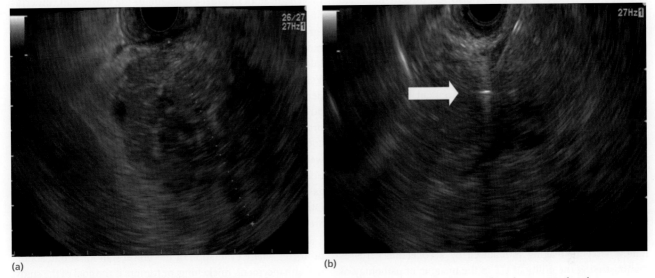

(a)   (b)

Figure 85.21 EUS-guided fiducial placement. **(a)** EUS image of a mass in the head of the pancreas. EUS-FNA confirmed pancreatic ductal adenocarcinoma. **(b)** EUS image showing FNA needle and a deployed hyperechoic fiducial (arrow).

CHAPTER 86

Computed tomography of the gastrointestinal tract

Siva P. Raman, Karen M. Horton, Pamela T. Johnson, and Elliot K. Fishman

Johns Hopkins University, Baltimore, MD, USA

Introduction

Since the introduction of computed tomography (CT) in the late 1970s, there have been remarkable technical advancements in terms of both scanner hardware and software. Today's multidetector CT (MDCT) scanners allow submillimeter collimation (0.6 mm) and fast scanning speeds (0.33 s per rotation), resulting in dramatic improvements in both temporal and spatial resolution that have greatly improved our ability to image the body. For example, the latest dual-source MDCT scanners can now image the entire abdomen and pelvis in less than 1 second. In addition to dramatically reducing motion and respiratory artifacts, this narrow temporal window has directly impacted protocol design, enabling the consistent acquisition of images at peak enhancement. This has proven particularly valuable in the imaging of traditionally hypervascular tumors such as hepatocellular carcinoma, pancreatic neuroendocrine tumor, and renal cell carcinoma, all of which are much better visualized when imaged during peak arterial enhancement. Following data acquisition, easy-to-use three-dimensional (3D) postprocessing software is now widely available and routinely utilized in practices across the country, allowing the radiologist to view the scan data in any imaging plane and utilize 3D techniques that can accentuate sites of pathology. Beyond improved image quality and diagnostic efficacy for existing applications, these advancements have facilitated the development of new CT applications, including so-called virtual colonoscopy and coronary CT angiography. In this chapter, a discussion of CT techniques for hollow visceral imaging is followed by a collection of cases demonstrating the utility of CT in the imaging of pathology of the hollow viscera, solid organs, and peritoneal cavity.

The hollow viscera of the gastrointestinal tract

Techniques
Oral contrast

Identifying abnormalities of the luminal gastrointestinal tract, whether neoplastic or inflammatory, relies on the ability to adequately visualize the bowel wall and gauge abnormalities in either bowel wall thickness or enhancement. In general, a complete evaluation of the bowel wall requires optimal distension of the bowel lumen with an enteric contrast agent. There are a variety of CT enteric contrast agents that can be administered either orally or rectally, and these agents are broadly categorized as positive agents, neutral agents, or negative agents.

Positive agents appear "white" on CT and usually consist of diluted (1.5%–2%) iodinated water-soluble contrast or diluted (2%) barium suspensions. These are the agents traditionally used for routine CT scans of the abdomen. While quite useful in differentiating loops of bowel from adjacent structures, they are often associated with "beam-hardening" or streak artifacts that might limit optimal evaluation of the bowel wall (in terms of enhancement or thickening). Neutral contrast agents appear "gray" on CT and usually have a density similar to water. The most commonly used neutral agents include water, methylcellulose agents, and commercially available products such as Volumen (E-Z-Em; Lake Success, New York), which has a density value slightly greater than water. Given that these agents do not result in beam hardening or streak artifact, while still producing very good distension of the bowel lumen, they are considered the best contrast agents for evaluating the bowel wall. "Negative" agents are not widely utilized in clinical practice, but include gas granules administered orally or insufflated gas (especially during CT colonoscopy) which appear "black." Other negative agents such as oil-based products (peanut oil) are not used routinely.

Neutral agents are most commonly utilized in enterography protocols where evaluation of the bowel wall for subtle abnormal enhancement, thickening, or tumors is the goal of the study, as these agents allow excellent visualization of the enhancing wall that may otherwise be obscured by positive agents. In addition, when 3D postprocessing is performed, it is beneficial to use neutral contrast agents, as they allow 3D reconstructions of the vasculature without the need for extensive postprocessing to segment the bowel loops. Alternatively, when positive oral agents are used these "white" loops need to be manually removed using postprocessing, as they will otherwise obscure the adjacent contrast enhanced vessels, particularly when maximum intensity projection reconstruction techniques are utilized. Positive oral contrast agents help delineate loops of bowel

Yamada's Atlas of Gastroenterology, Fifth Edition. Edited by Daniel K. Podolsky, Michael Camilleri, J. Gregory Fitz, Anthony N. Kalloo, Fergus Shanahan, and Timothy C. Wang.

© 2016 John Wiley & Sons, Ltd. Published 2016 by John Wiley & Sons, Ltd.

Companion website: www.yamadagastro.com/atlas

studies where the enteric contrast agent is utilized merely to distinguish bowel loops from other adjacent structures, such as studies performed for nonspecific abdominal pain.

Intravenous contrast

Intravenous (i.v.) contrast-enhanced images expand the diagnostic range of CT and have now become essential for most clinical indications. With a few rare exceptions (such as CT scans performed for the identification of renal calculi), intravenous contrast is an essential component of most scan protocols. Intravenous contrast enhancement dramatically increases the conspicuity of pathological processes throughout the gastrointestinal tract, which in many cases may not be visible on studies performed without intravenous contrast. Even the basic assessment of whether a particular loop of bowel is truly thickened may be difficult without i.v. contrast, and identifying abnormal bowel wall enhancement or the presence of a bowel tumor may be impossible on noncontrast studies. Similarly, a complete evaluation of the solid organs of the abdomen is often impossible without intravenous contrast, as many liver or pancreatic tumors may be invisible to the radiologist on noncontrast studies. Even if a pathological entity can be recognized on a noncontrast study, contrast may be necessary to narrow a differential diagnosis or provide a specific diagnosis, as the degree of enhancement and vascularity associated with a pathologic process can be a vital clue as to the correct diagnosis. For example, while the distinction between a benign liver hemangioma and a malignant hepatoma may be quite obvious on a contrast-enhanced CT, liver lesions cannot be properly characterized as benign or malignant without i.v. contrast.

Nonionic iodinated contrast agents are typically utilized, and the specific protocol for contrast administration will vary depending on the clinical indication. While some indications may require only the acquisition of venous-phase images, other indications may require more complex protocols with acquisition in multiple different "phases" of contrast enhancement. For example, in patients with suspected mesenteric ischemia, it is important to acquire images in both the arterial and venous phases in order to ensure adequate visualization of both the mesenteric arteries and veins, in addition to assessment of bowel wall enhancement. The radiologist will tailor the scan protocol based on the clinical question, and it is therefore essential that appropriate clinical information is provided by the ordering physician in order for scans to be performed correctly.

Scanning protocol

In general, a CT scan performed on the latest generation of CT scanners entails the acquisition of high-resolution volumetric datasets, including images with extremely thin collimation (as small as 0.5–0.75 mm). These datasets are now usually "isotropic" (identical resolutions in the x, y, and z axes), allowing the creation of detailed multiplanar and 3D reconstructions from the source data set. Images can be reconstructed in multiple different ways from the source data, including 3–5 mm slices for "routine" review of the axial images, multiplanar

reconstructions in the coronal and sagittal plane that are usually created directly at the CT scanner console, and additional 3D reconstructions created at an independent workstation. While older generations of scanners often required the technologist to manually select individual scan parameters, such as tube voltage and tube current, this process has largely been automated on the latest generation of scanners, which include "automated exposure control" or "automated tube potential selection" software, which select the best scan parameters depending on the patient's size, the type of study being performed, and the part of the body being scanned.

Three-dimensional imaging

Traditionally, evaluation of a CT dataset entailed only reviewing the axial images in order to make a diagnosis. However, it is now clear that properly evaluating any pathological process requires viewing the dataset from multiple different perspectives and planes, as the axial images alone may not be sufficient to make an accurate diagnosis. As a result, 3D postprocessing has now become a standard part of CT interpretation, including multiplanar reconstruction (MPR), volume rendering, and maximum intensity projection (MIP).

Multiplanar reconstructions are the most basic form of 3D imaging, allowing the radiologist to scroll through the dataset in any plane. These reconstructions are quite simple to create, and are often automatically created at the CT console following the completion of the scan. "Volume rendering" (VR) and maximum intensity projection (MIP) are more robust and computationally intensive methods that require the radiologist to interactively manipulate the dataset using advanced reconstruction software, most often at an independent workstation. Volume rendering is a technique that allows the brightness, opacity, window width, and window level to be adjusted in real time in order to accentuate certain tissue types or to permit selective viewing of the vasculature. Manipulating trapezoidal transfer functions interactively modifies the image contrast and the related pixel attenuations in the final image. This function allows unique color and opacity assignments to each voxel and can be adjusted to alter the display. Although initial volume rendering software was somewhat labor intensive, modern software packages are relatively easy to use and can be adjusted in real time. Moreover, the process can be simplified by creating automatic presets that can be applied quickly, following which only minor adjustments are needed. MIP reconstructions display the brightest voxel along a ray, and are most often utilized for a detailed evaluation of the vasculature (including small branch vessels). The radiologist often utilizes a combination of these different 3D tools to optimally display the relevant anatomy and pathology, and subsequently make a final diagnosis.

The images shown in this chapter relate to: the gastrointestinal tract (Figures 86.1–86.13); the liver (Figures 86.14, 86.15, 86.16, and 86.17); the pancreas (Figures 86.18, 86.19, 86.20, 86.21, and 86.22); the biliary tract (Figure 86.23); the peritoneum (Figure 86.24); and hernias (Figure 86.25).

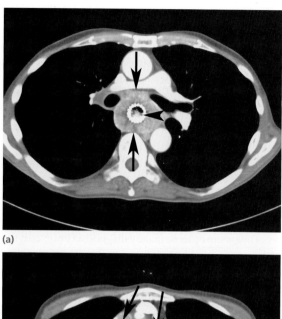

(a)

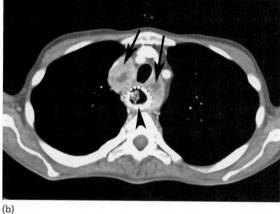

(b)

Figure 86.1 **(a)** Axial intravenous contrast-enhanced multidetector computed tomography (MDCT) image reveals a large circumferential esophageal mass (arrows). The mass splays the carina. An esophageal stent is in place (arrowhead). **(b)** Axial intravenous contrast-enhanced MDCT image demonstrates bulky mediastinal adenopathy (arrows). The esophageal stent is again noted (arrowhead).

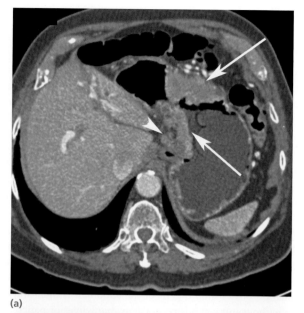

(a)

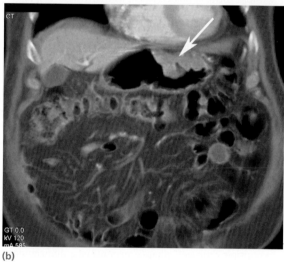

(b)

Figure 86.2 **(a)** Axial intravenous contrast-enhanced multidetector computed tomography (MDCT) image in a patient with gastric adenocarcinoma shows an infiltrating mass in the gastric body (arrows). There is extension into the gastrohepatic ligament (arrowhead). **(b)** Coronal volume-rendered image nicely demonstrates the bulky gastric mass (arrow).

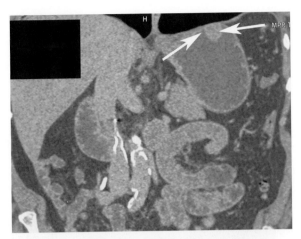

Figure 86.3 Intravenous contrast-enhanced coronal multiplanar reconstruction using water as oral contrast demonstrates a 1.3-cm intramural gastric mass (arrows) compatible with a gastrointestinal stromal tumor. This was an incidental finding.

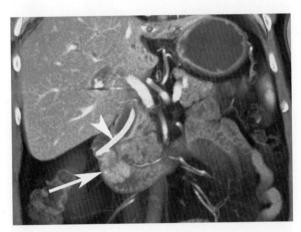

Figure 86.4 Intravenous contrast-enhanced coronal volume-rendered image using water as oral contrast demonstrates a 2-cm lobulated mass (arrow) in the second portion of the duodenum. A common bile duct stent is in place (arrowhead). The patient underwent Whipple surgery and pathology revealed adenocarcinoma arising in a tubular adenoma.

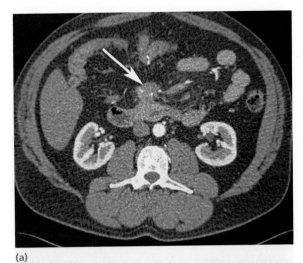

(a)

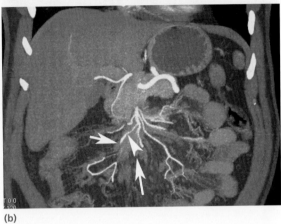

(b)

Figure 86.5 (a) Axial intravenous contrast-enhanced multidetector computed tomography (MDCT) image shows a 1.5-cm infiltrating mass (arrow) in the root of the mesentery, compatible with carcinoid. **(b)** Coronal maximum intensity projection nicely demonstrates encasement of the superior mesenteric artery branches (arrowhead) by the infiltrating tumor (arrows).

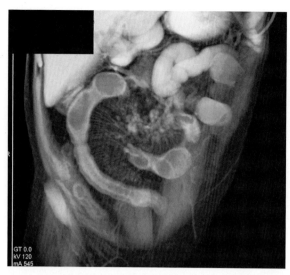

Figure 86.6 Coronal volume-rendered image from an intravenous and oral contrast-enhanced computed tomography (CT) in a patient with Crohn's disease demonstrates small bowel wall thickening, mucosal hyperemia, and engorgement of the vasa recta. This is an example of the comb sign, indicating active disease.

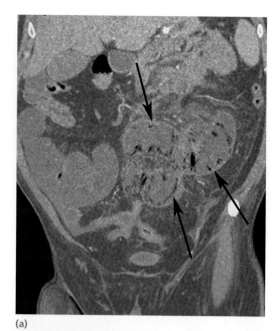

(a)

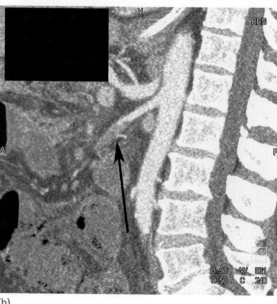

(b)

Figure 86.7 (a) Coronal multiplanar reconstruction (MPR) from intravenous contrast-enhanced computed tomography (CT) demonstrates dilated small bowel with pneumatosis (arrows). **(b)** Sagittal MPR demonstrates thrombosis in the superior mesenteric artery (arrow).

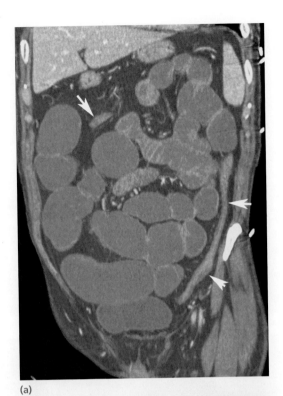

(a)

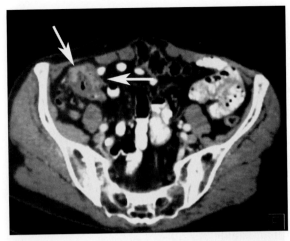

Figure 86.9 Axial intravenous and oral contrast-enhanced multidetector computed tomography (MDCT) image demonstrates a subtle mass (arrows) in the right colon. Colonoscopy and biopsy revealed adenocarcinoma.

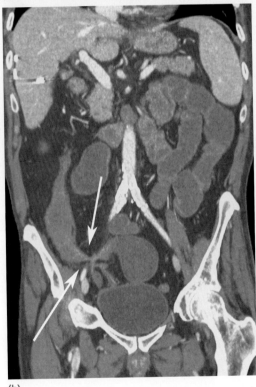

(b)

Figure 86.8 **(a)** Intravenous contrast-enhanced coronal multiplanar reconstruction (MPR) using water as oral contrast demonstrates moderate small bowel dilatation. The colon is decompressed (arrows). **(b)** Intravenous contrast-enhanced coronal MPR using water as oral contrast demonstrates multiple fistulae (arrows) in the distal small bowel and colon. This was the source of the small bowel obstruction in this patient with Crohn's disease.

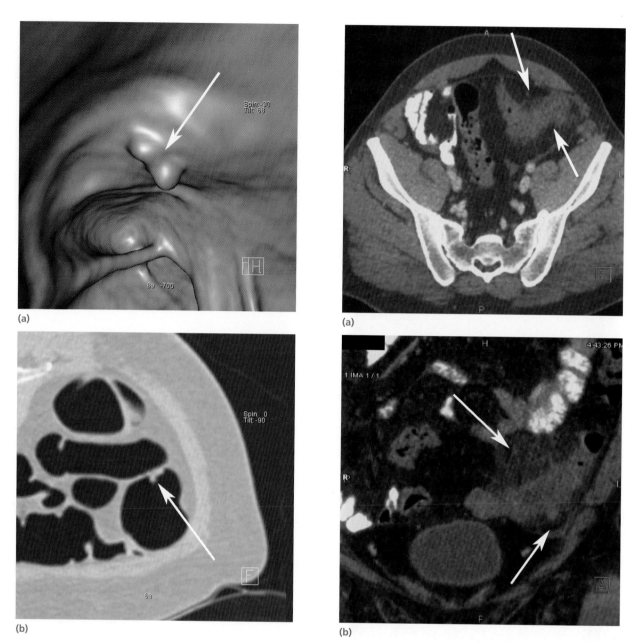

Figure 86.10 (a) Endolumenal fly-through view from virtual colonoscopy shows 8-mm polyp (arrow). **(b)** Axial prone image from virtual colonoscopy demonstrates an 8-mm polyp (arrow) in the right colon.

Figure 86.11 (a) Axial oral and intravenous contrast-enhanced multidetector computed tomography (MDCT) image reveals thickening of the sigmoid colon with pericolonic stranding (arrows) compatible with diverticulitis. **(b)** Coronal multiplanar reconstruction shows extensive inflammation and minimal fluid in the pericolonic fat (arrows) typical of diverticulitis.

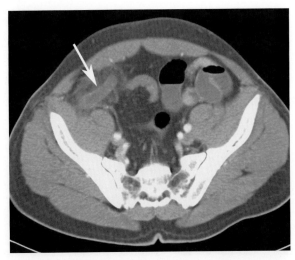

Figure 86.12 Axial intravenous contrast-enhanced multidetector computed tomography (MDCT) in a patient with right lower quadrant pain demonstrates an enlarged fluid-filled appendix (arrow) with moderate periappendiceal inflammation, compatible with acute appendicitis.

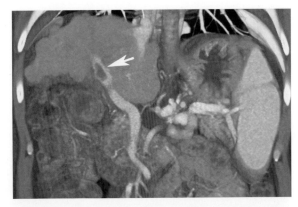

Figure 86.14 Coronal volume-rendered image from intravenous contrast-enhanced computed tomography (CT) demonstrates a small shrunken nodular liver compatible with cirrhosis. Splenomegaly reflects portal hypertension. Thrombus is present in the intrahepatic portal vein (arrow).

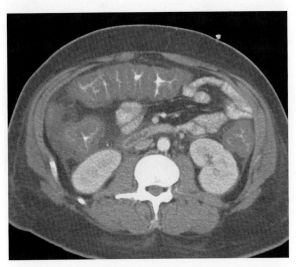

Figure 86.13 Axial intravenous and oral contrast-enhanced multidetector computed tomography (MDCT) demonstrates marked diffuse colonic thickening compatible with pseudomembranous colitis.

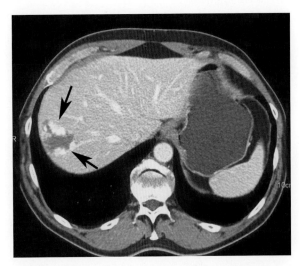

Figure 86.15 Intravenous contrast-enhanced axial multidetector computed tomography (MDCT) demonstrates a 2.5-cm mass (arrows) in the right lobe of the liver with peripheral nodular enhancement characteristic of a hemangioma.

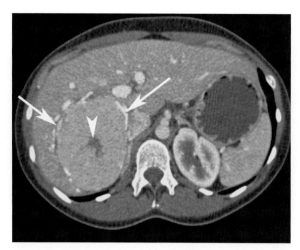

Figure 86.16 Axial intravenous contrast-enhanced multidetector computed tomography (MDCT) during portal venous phase of enhancement demonstrates a large mass in the right lobe of the liver (arrows), with a central scar (arrowhead). This is a typical CT appearance of focal nodular hyperplasia.

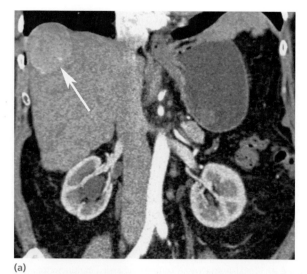

(a)

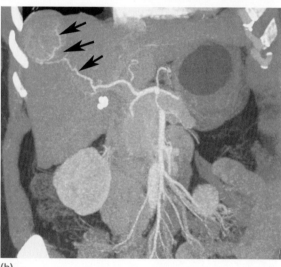

(b)

Figure 86.17 (a) Coronal intravenous contrast-enhanced multiplanar reconstruction from an arterial phase acquisition demonstrates a 4-cm enhancing hepatoma (arrow) in the dome of the liver. The liver is shrunken, compatible with cirrhosis. (b) Coronal maximum intensity projection demonstrates the arterial vessel (arrows) feeding the hepatoma.

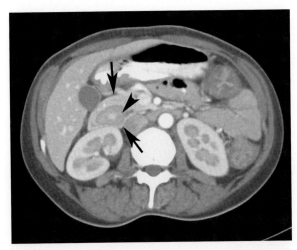

Figure 86.18 Oral and intravenous contrast-enhanced axial computed tomography (CT) demonstrates pancreatic tissue (arrows) surrounding the second portion of the duodenum (arrowhead), compatible with annular pancreas.

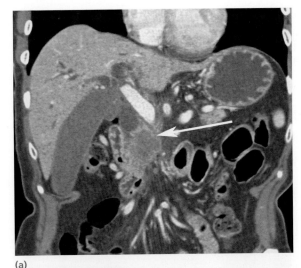

(a)

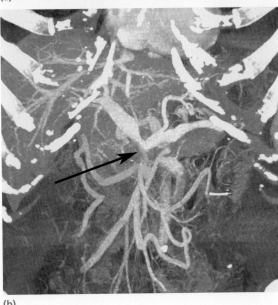

(b)

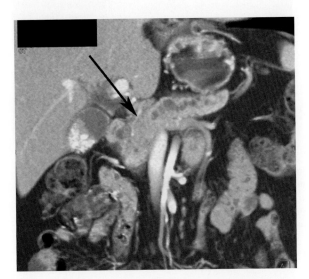

Figure 86.19 Intravenous contrast-enhanced coronal multiplanar reconstruction image demonstrates 1.5-cm pancreatic mass (arrow) with distal pancreatic ductal obstruction. At surgery this was an adenocarcinoma.

Figure 86.20 (a) Intravenous contrast-enhanced coronal multiplanar reconstruction image demonstrates a 4-cm mass (arrow) in the head of the pancreas causing common bile duct obstruction. The gallbladder is also distended. Biopsy revealed pancreatic adenocarcinoma. (b) Coronal maximum intensity projection demonstrates encasement of the superior mesenteric vein (arrow) with resulting collaterals. The patient was deemed unresectable.

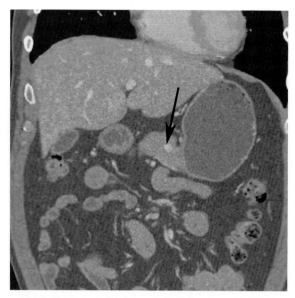

Figure 86.21 Coronal intravenous contrast-enhanced multiplanar reconstruction demonstrates a 5-mm enhancing lesion (arrow) in the body of the pancreas. This was an insulinoma.

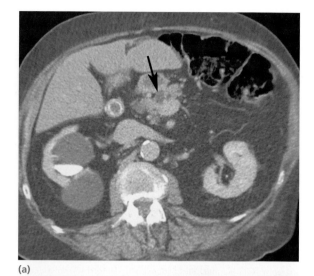

(a)

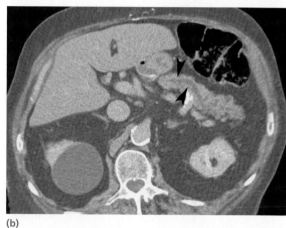

(b)

Figure 86.22 **(a)** Axial intravenous contrast-enhanced multidetector computed tomography (MDCT) demonstrates a 1-cm cystic lesion (arrow) in the pancreatic neck. **(b)** Axial image also demonstrates pancreatic ductal dilatation (arrowheads). These findings are very suspicious for intraductal pancreatic mucinous neoplasm.

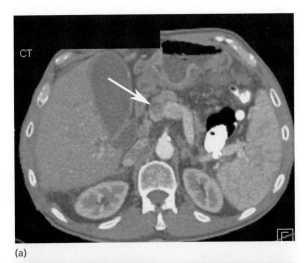

(a)

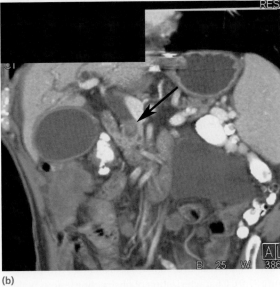

(b)

Figure 86.23 **(a)** Axial intravenous contrast-enhanced multidetector computed tomography (MDCT) in a patient with obstructive jaundice shows a subtle filling defect in the common duct (arrow). **(b)** Coronal multiplanar reconstruction better demonstrates the stone (arrow) in the distal common bile duct.

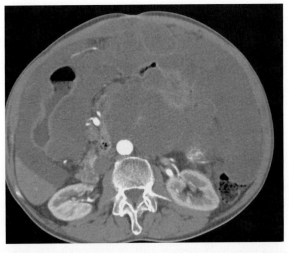

Figure 86.24 Intravenous contrast-enhanced axial computed tomography (CT) in a patient with pseudomyxoma peritonei demonstrates extensive low-density implants filling the peritoneal cavity.

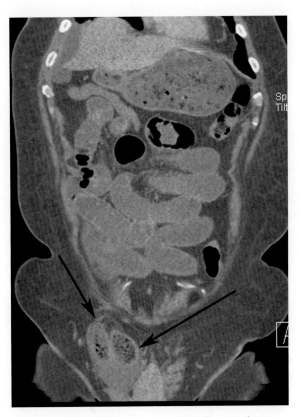

Figure 86.25 Coronal multiplanar reconstruction shows moderate dilatation of small bowel loops due to an obstructing right inguinal hernia (arrows).

CHAPTER 87

Magnetic resonance imaging

Diane Bergin
University Hospital Galway, Galway, Ireland

Magnetic resonance imaging (MRI) allows a comprehensive evaluation of the intraabdominal solid organs including the liver, pancreas, and spleen, and is the most sensitive noninvasive imaging modality for evaluating the biliary system.

Since the development of MRI, its applications for imaging the gastrointestinal tract have expanded rapidly. MRI of the abdomen was initially hampered because of artifacts associated with respiratory and bowel motion. The development of fast imaging techniques has overcome these effects of motion, enabling examination of structures and organs that were previously not reliably imaged.

MRI utilizes several parameters to characterize tissues including T1, T2, lipid content, and magnetic susceptibility. The generation of MR images involves the spatial localization of radiofrequency signals elicited from water- or fat-containing tissue in the body. The variation in grayscale on the image from white to black represents the strength of these signals and is called the signal intensity. Tissues and structures that are bright on the MR image are described as being of high signal intensity, and tissues and structures that are black on the image are of low signal intensity. When the specific technical parameters are changed on the MR magnet system, images can be generated that evaluate different tissue properties. Two tissue properties, T1 and T2, are examined on T1- and T2-weighted sequences respectively. The presence of lipid within tissue is identified using chemical shift images. Other properties, such as vascularity, biliary secretion, or macrophage activity, are imaged using a wide array of different contrast agents. Blood flow in vessels is selectively visualized with gradient-echo sequences called magnetic resonance angiography.

One of the most frequent applications of MRI of the abdomen is characterization of a liver lesion. The most common benign liver lesions are hepatic cysts (Figure 87.1) and hepatic hemangiomas (Figure 87.2), which have very high signal on T2-weighted sequences. Hemangiomas enhance from the periphery with a discontinuous nodular pattern. Hepatic cysts do not enhance. Arterial enhancing lesions that are commonly seen in women are focal nodular hyperplasia (Figure 87.2). Hepatic lesions that are of moderately high signal intensity on T2-weighted images are malignant lesions, including hepatocellular carcinoma (Figure 87.3), and hepatic metastases (Figures 87.4 and 87.5).

MRI can be used to diagnose diffuse liver disease such as cirrhosis, fatty infiltration, and hemochromatosis. Fatty infiltration is diagnosed using chemical shift imaging (Figure 87.6). Iron deposition is characterized by marked low signal on T2 and gradient-echo sequences (Figure 87.7). Cirrhosis is accurately diagnosed on MRI by visualization of the regenerating nodules, which are separated from each other by the fibrovascular septae. Larger regenerating nodules can be differentiated from small hepatocellular carcinomas on the basis of their arterial phase enhancement during dynamic scanning (Figure 87.8).

MR cholangiography (MRC) and MR cholangiopancreatography (MRCP) are used for evaluating the biliary tract and pancreatic duct. They selectively image fluid in the abdomen, including bile and secretions in the biliary tract and pancreatic duct. Using these sequences and displaying them in a format similar to conventional endoscopic retrograde cholangiopancreatography or cholangiography, one can identify obstruction of the biliary duct and pancreatic duct. Filling defects such as calculi appear as low-signal abnormalities within the duct (Figure 87.9). Characterization of obstructing lesions is aided by dynamic gadolinium-enhanced images. Cholangiocarcinoma typically demonstrates delayed enhancement (Figure 87.10).

The normal pancreatic parenchyma is high signal on T1-weighted images (Figure 87.11). Chronic pancreatitis is characterized by loss of this high T1 signal as well as irregular dilation of the pancreatic duct (Figure 87.12). Pancreatic adenocarcinoma typically is hypoenhancing relative to the normal pancreas and depending on its location may cause secondary ductal dilation (Figure 87.13).

The potential of MRI for evaluating the bowel has been explored. Bowel motion can be reduced by the intravenous injection of antiperistaltic agents such as glucagon. These techniques can differentiate bowel from pathological processes. Intrinsic intestinal wall abnormalities such as inflammatory bowel disease can be characterized (Figure 87.14).

Yamada's Atlas of Gastroenterology, Fifth Edition. Edited by Daniel K. Podolsky, Michael Camilleri, J. Gregory Fitz, Anthony N. Kalloo, Fergus Shanahan, and Timothy C. Wang.

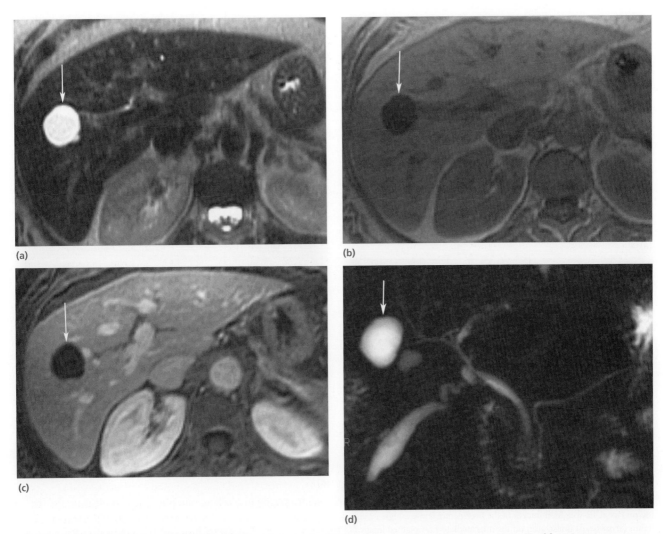

Figure 87.1 Simple hepatic cyst. Axial T2-weighted **(a)**, axial T1-weighted **(b)**, postcontrast three-dimensional gradient-echo **(c)**, and magnetic resonance cholangiopancreatography (MRCP) **(d)**. Images demonstrate a high T2 signal lesion (arrow) and a low T1 signal nonenhancing lesion (arrow), consistent with a simple hepatic cyst.

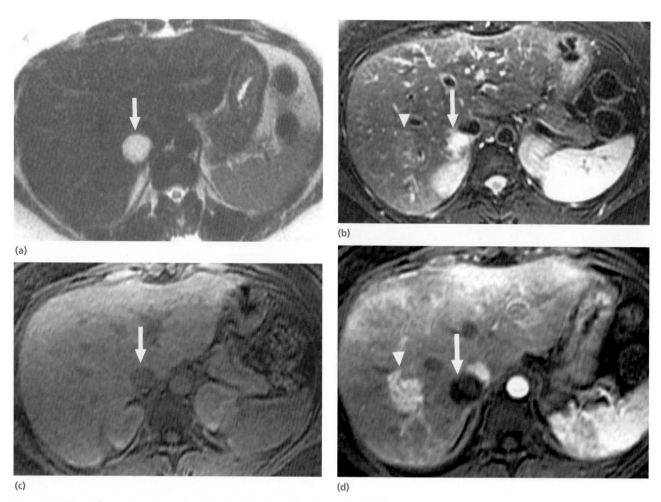

Figure 87.2 Hepatic hemangioma (arrow) and focal nodular hyperplasia (arrowhead). **(a)** Long time to echo (TE) (180 ms), and **(b)** intermediate TE (80 ms) axial T2-weighted images of the liver demonstrate a high T2 signal lesion (arrow) adjacent to the inferior vena cava (IVC). Of note, a second lesion (arrowhead) is also seen on the intermediate T2-weighted image **(b)** but not on the long T2-weighted image **(a)**. **(c)** Three-dimensional gradient echo image before contrast; **(d)** during arterial phase. Following contrast administration, the paracaval lesion (arrow) demonstrates discontinuous peripheral enhancement with progressive delayed enhancement consistent with a hemangioma. The second lesion (arrowhead) enhances avidly in the arterial phase and becomes isointense to hepatic parenchyma on subsequent imaging consistent with focal nodular hyperplasia.

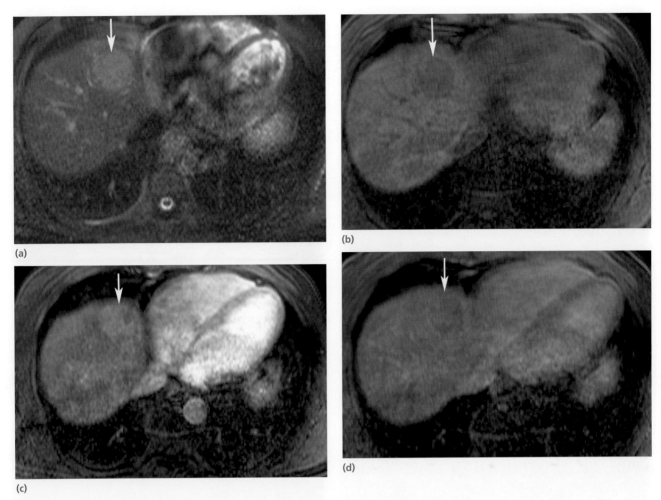

(a)

(b)

(c)

(d)

Figure 87.3 Hepatocellular carcinoma. Intermediate time to echo (TE) axial T2-weighted **(a)**, precontrast three-dimensional gradient-echo **(b)**, arterial phase **(c)**, and delayed postcontrast three-dimensional gradient-echo **(d)**. Images demonstrate a high T2 signal lesion with arterial hyperenhancement and "washout" on delayed images following contrast administration (arrows).

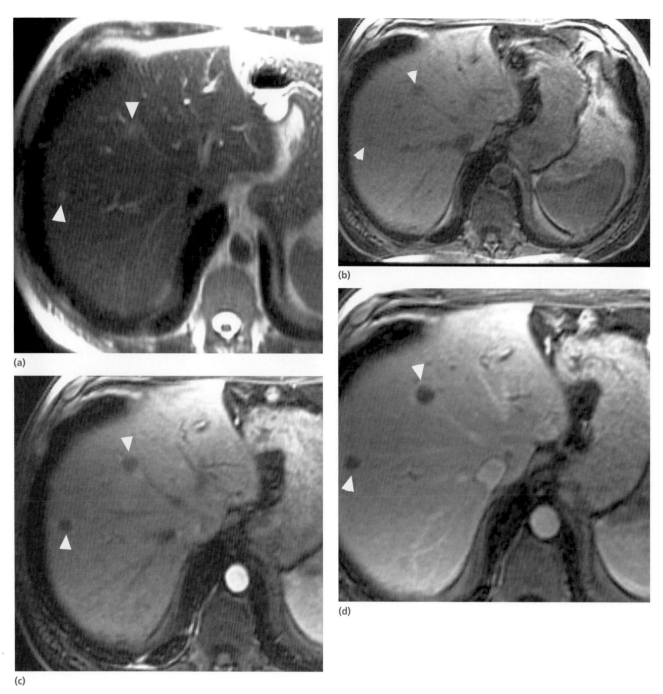

Figure 87.4 Hypovascular hepatic metastases. Axial T2-weighted **(a)**, precontrast three-dimensional gradient-echo **(b)**, arterial phase **(c)**, and postcontrast three-dimensional gradient-echo enhanced **(d)**. Images demonstrate hypoenhancing metastatic lesions (arrowheads) with rim enhancement in a patient with metastatic pancreatic carcinoma.

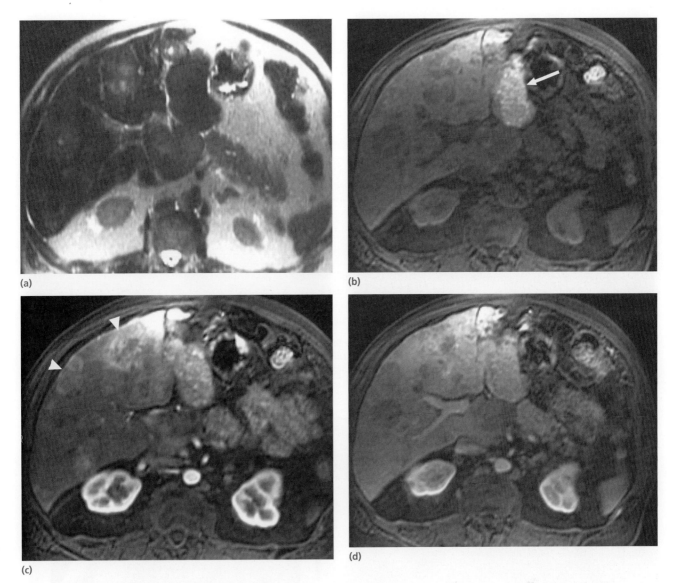

(a)

(b)

(c)

(d)

Figure 87.5 Hypervascular hepatic metastases. Axial T2-weighted **(a)**, precontrast **(b)**, arterial phase **(c)**, portal venous phase postcontrast three-dimensional gradient-echo **(d)**. Images demonstrate multiple arterial enhancing lesions (arrowheads) in this patient with melanoma metastases **(c)**. Note the increased signal on precontrast T1-weighted images in the lesion in the lateral segment of the left lobe of the liver (arrow) secondary to melanin or hemorrhage **(b)**.

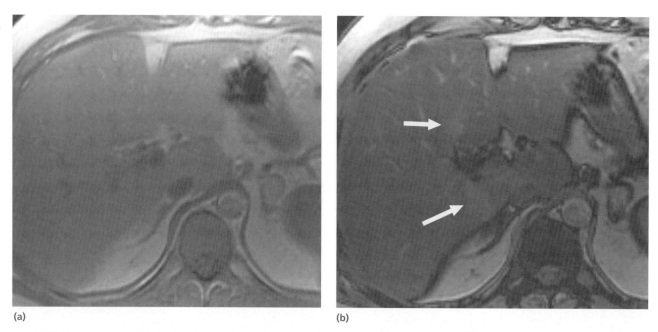

(a)   (b)

Figure 87.6 Hepatic steatosis. **(a)** Axial in-phase gradient-echo image with time to echo (TE) of 4.6 ms and **(b)** opposed-phase gradient-echo image with TE of 2.2 ms of the liver demonstrate a drop in signal of the liver parenchyma on opposed-phase images consistent with hepatic steatosis. There is a relative lack of a drop in signal near the gallbladder fossa (arrows) consistent with focal fatty sparing.

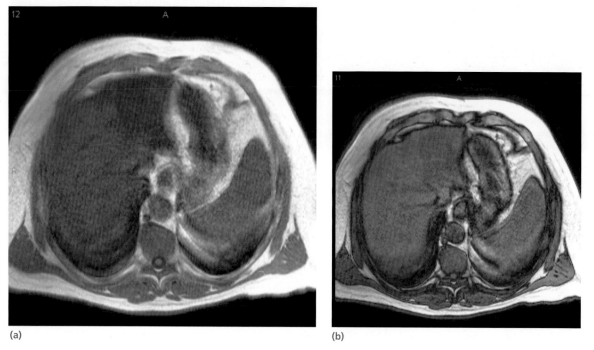

(a)   (b)

Figure 87.7 Secondary hepatic hemosiderosis. Axial in-phase **(a)**, and opposed-phase **(b)** gradient-echo images with time to echo (TE) of 4.6 ms and 2.2 ms, respectively, demonstrate a relatively decreased signal on the in-phase images of the hepatic and splenic parenchyma consistent with secondary hemosiderosis.

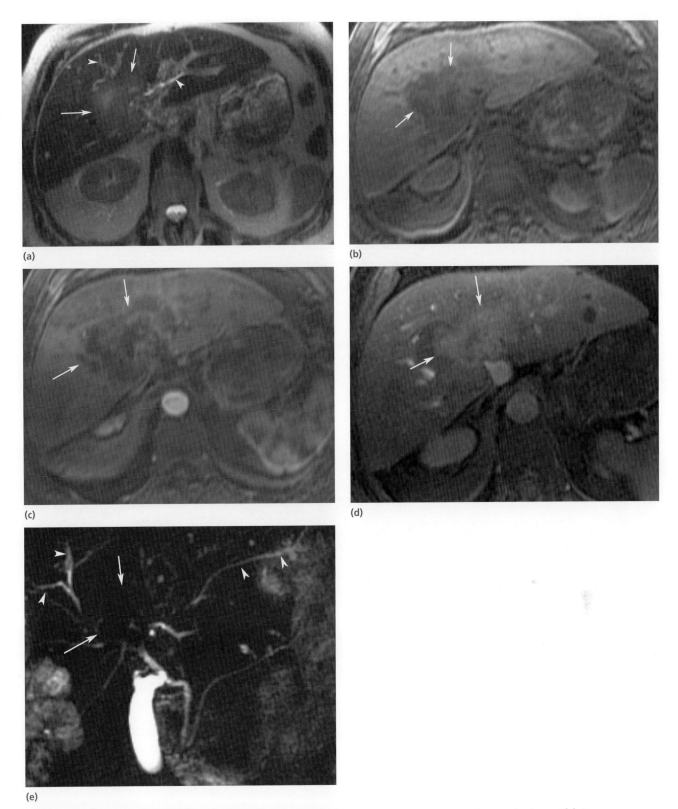

Figure 87.8 Hepatic cirrhosis with iron-containing regenerative nodules and hepatocellular carcinoma. Axial T2-weighted image **(a)** demonstrates cirrhotic liver with nodular contour (arrowheads). There is an arterial enhancing lesion (arrow) in the left lobe of the liver seen on precontrast **(b)**, and arterial phase **(c)** three-dimensional gradient-echo images that demonstrates "washout" on portal venous phase imaging **(d)**. Two-dimensional gradient-echo in-phase image **(e)** demonstrates scattered subcentimeter low T1 signal lesions throughout the liver parenchyma consistent with iron-containing regenerative nodules.

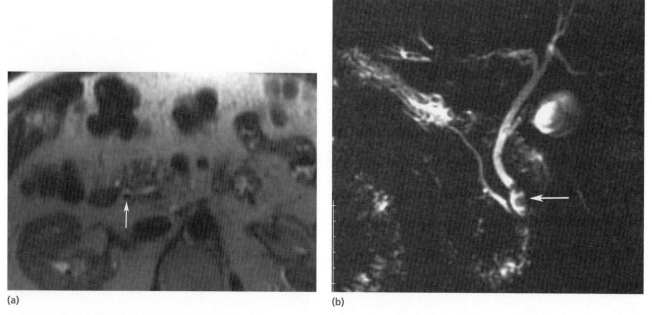

(a)

(b)

Figure 87.9 Choledocholithiasis. Axial T2-weighted **(a)** and magnetic resonance cholangiopancreatography (MRCP) **(b)** images show a low signal void (arrow) consistent with common bile duct calculi.

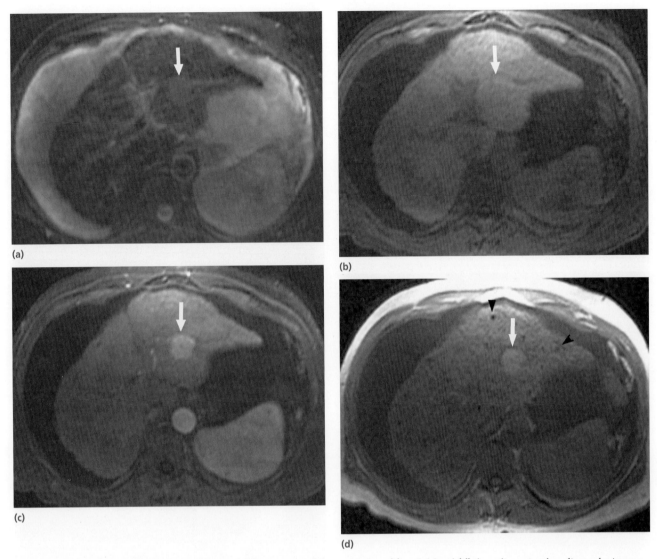

(a)

(b)

(c)

(d)

Figure 87.10 Cholangiocarcinoma. Axial T2-weighted **(a)**, precontrast **(b)**, arterial phase **(c)**, and delayed **(d)** three-dimensional gradient-echo images show a large central mass (arrow) that demonstrates delayed enhancement following contrast administration. There is mild peripheral intrahepatic biliary dilation (arrowheads) secondary to obstruction.

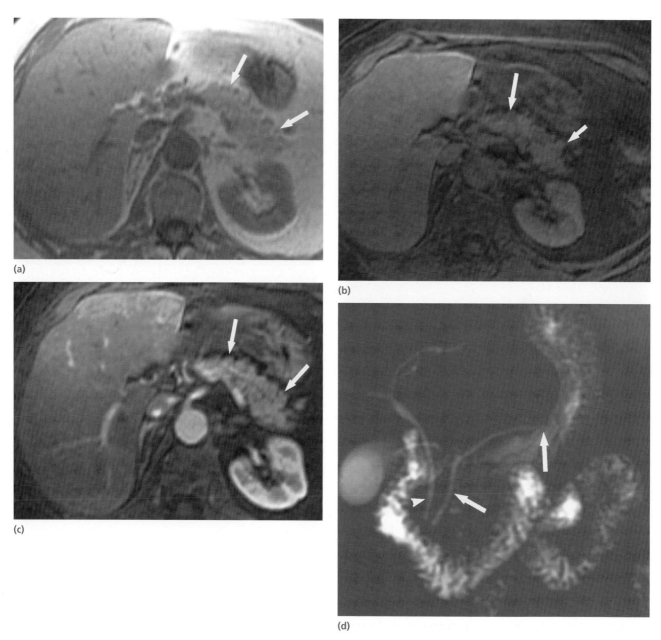

Figure 87.11 Normal pancreas. Axial two-dimensional gradient-echo **(a)**, and precontrast three-dimensional gradient-echo fat-suppressed T1-weighted **(b)** images demonstrate a normal magnetic resonance imaging signal of the pancreatic parenchyma of the body and tail of pancreas, which is isointense or higher in signal than liver parenchyma. Axial three-dimensional gradient-echo arterial phase images **(c)** demonstrate normal peak enhancement of the pancreatic parenchyma in the arterial phase. Magnetic resonance cholangiopancreatography (MRCP) **(d)** demonstrates normal relative anatomy of the common bile duct (arrowhead) and the pancreatic duct (arrows).

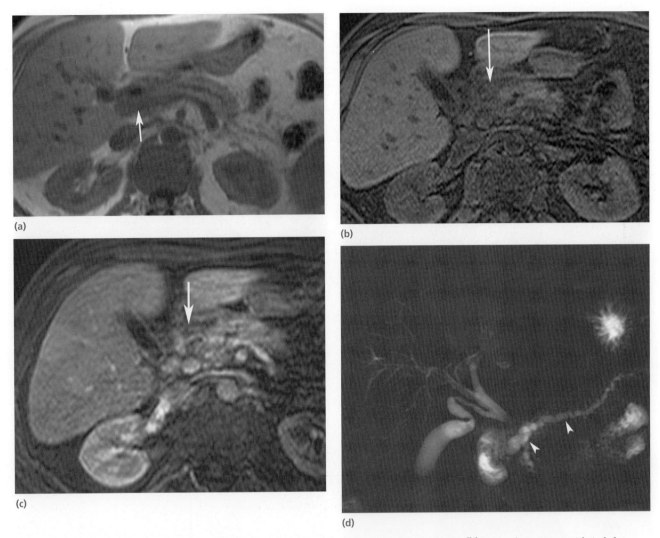

Figure 87.12 Chronic pancreatitis. Axial T1-weighted **(a)** and precontrast three-dimensional gradient-echo **(b)** images demonstrate a relatively low signal (arrow) in the region of the head of the pancreas with relative hypoenhancement following contrast administration on postcontrast images **(c)**. Magnetic resonance cholangiopancreatography (MRCP) **(d)** demonstrates associated diffuse dilation of the pancreatic duct (arrowheads).

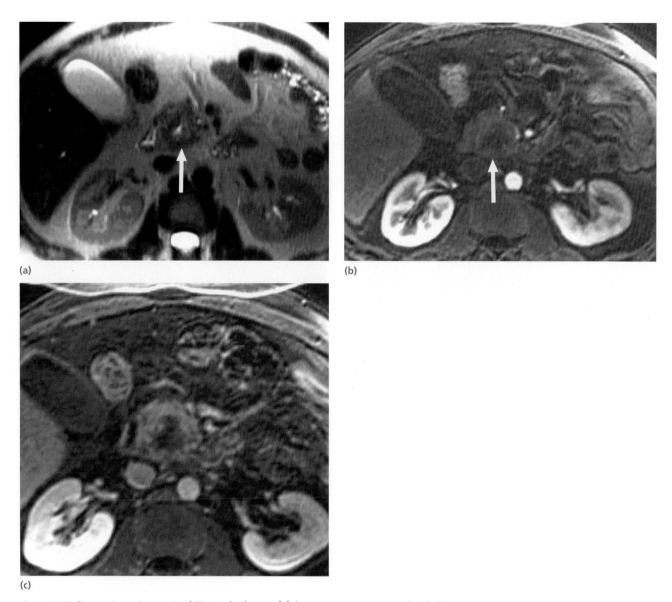

(a)

(b)

(c)

Figure 87.13 Pancreatic carcinoma. Axial T2-weighted image (a) demonstrates a mass in the head of the pancreas (arrow) with some central necrosis that hypoenhances relative to the remainder of the pancreas on postcontrast arterial three-dimensional gradient-echo (b) and portal venous (c) images.

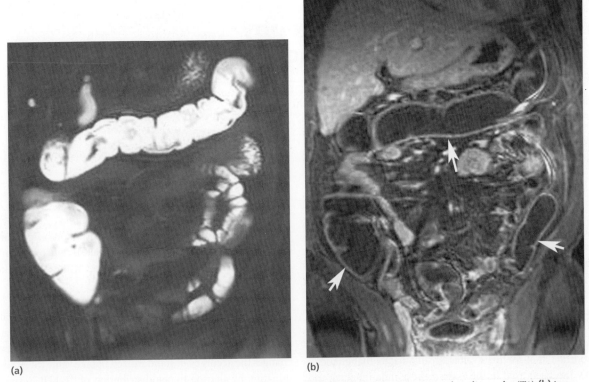

(a)   (b)

Figure 87.14 Magnetic resonance colonography (MRC). Coronal T2-weighted **(a)** and coronal three-dimensional gradient-echo (T1) **(b)** images demonstrate a fluid-distended normal colon (arrows). Source: Courtesy of Thomas Lauenstein MD, Atlanta, GA.

CHAPTER 88

Positron emission tomography in the gastrointestinal tract

Manuela Matesan,[1] Jonathan Sham,[1] James Park,[1] and Satoshi Minoshima[2]

[1] University of Washington, Seattle, WA, USA
[2] University of Utah, Salt Lake City, UT, USA

Positron emission tomography (PET) is an imaging technique that provides both structural and functional information, in contrast to other imaging modalities which provide mostly structural information such as computed tomography (CT) and magnetic resonance imaging (MRI).

Currently, the most common radiotracer used clinically for PET images is the glucose analogue 2-deoxy-2-[^{18}F]fluoro-D-glucose (^{18}F-fluorodeoxyglucose or ^{18}F-FDG), which has become an important tool for the evaluation of various malignancies and has also been used in the assessment of inflammatory and infectious disease.

The radiotracer has a half-life of approximately 110 min, enabling its production at regional facilities which then manage distribution to clinical sites.

Patient preparation is critical to the quality of ^{18}F-FDG PET. Patients should avoid strenuous exercise for 24 h before the ^{18}F-FDG PET study to minimize uptake of the radiotracer in muscles. Patients should, as much as possible, be on a low-carbohydrate diet for 24 h before the study. Fasting is required for at least 4–6 h (based on Society of Nuclear Medicine and Molecular Imaging procedure standard for tumor imaging with ^{18}F-FDG PET/CT) prior to the study. A longer period of fasting (of approximately 12 h) and low-carbohydrate diet for 24 h may decrease ^{18}F-FDG accumulation by the myocardium and improve detection of mediastinal metastases. A high-fat, low-carbohydrate, protein-preferred meal the day before the scan more effectively suppresses cardiac activity by increasing free fatty acid (FFA) availability, which promotes FFA oxidation and inhibits glucose use. Fasting is also important in order to minimize competitive inhibition of FDG uptake by glucose in tumors (most institutions reschedule the patient if the blood glucose level is greater than 150–200 mg/dL).

While fasting, patients should consume at least two to three 355-mL (12-oz) glasses of water to ensure adequate hydration. Insulin should not be used to adjust the blood glucose at the time of the imaging procedure; recent insulin administration changes the accuracy of standardized uptake value (SUV) determination by altering the biodistribution of ^{18}F-FDG, especially in insulin-sensitive tissue such as muscle, myocardium, and fat. Recent insulin administration also causes low hepatic ^{18}F-FDG uptake.

Because ^{18}F-FDG is mainly eliminated by urinary excretion, additional preparation can be performed for specific imaging of the pelvic region. This includes i.v. hydration, Lasix administration during the study, Foley catheter in the bladder, and retrograde filling of the bladder with sterile saline solution.

A collection of ^{18}F-FDG PET images in malignant and inflammatory/infectious diseases are presented in this chapter (Figures 88.1–88.24). Two examples of other more specific PET radiotracers currently not approved for clinical use in the USA, one 3,4-dihydroxy-6-^{8}F-fluoro-L-phenylalanine (^{18}F-FDOPA), an amino acid that resembles natural L-DOPA, the precursor of the neurotransmitter dopamine (Figure 88.25), and another one ^{68}Ga-OTA-D-Phe(1)-Tyr(3)-octreotide (^{68}Ga-DOTA-TOC), which is a somatostatin receptor analog labeled at the positron emitter ^{68}Ga (Figure 88.26), are also included in this chapter.

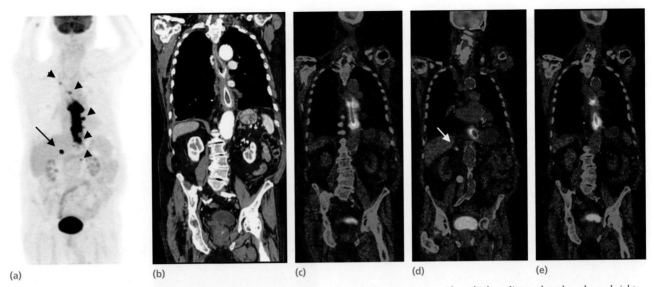

Figure 88.1 A 80-year-old male with poorly differentiated mid and distal esophageal adenocarcinoma with multiple malignant lymph nodes and right adrenal gland metastasis. An ^{18}F-fluorodeoxyglucose positron emission tomography (^{18}F-FDG PET) scan was performed for initial staging. ^{18}F-FDG PET maximum intensity projection (MIP) images (a), coronal image of a contrast computed tomography (CT) (b), and multiple fused images (c–e) show a primary esophageal mass and malignant lymph nodes (in a marked by arrowheads localized periesophageal, anterior mediastinal, left gastric, celiac, left paraaortic next to the left renal vein) and right adrenal metastasis (arrow in a, d). Involvement of left paraaortic lymph nodes at the level of the renal vessels is not uncommon in advanced esophageal cancer. ^{18}F-FDG PET is often able to detect distant metastases not clearly visualized on anatomic imaging, significantly changing management.

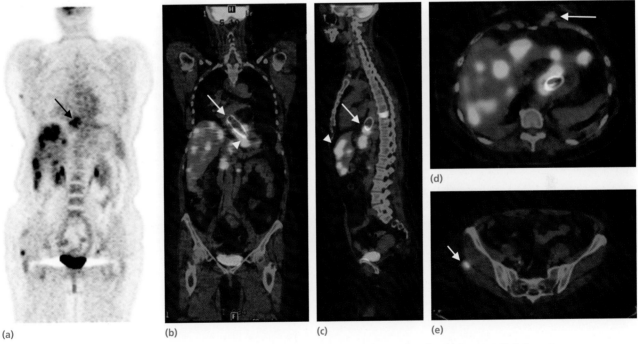

Figure 88.2 A 62-year-old female with adenocarcinoma of the distal esophagus/proximal stomach and multiple metastatic lesions. An ^{18}F-fluorodeoxyglucose positron emission tomography (^{18}F-FDG PET) scan was performed for initial staging. ^{18}F-FDG PET scan coronal image (a) and fused images (b, c) show a hypermetabolic lesion at the distal esophagus and proximal stomach (arrow in a, b, c), multiple hypermetabolic lymph nodes in the upper abdomen (arrowhead in b), multiple hepatic metastases, and bony lesions. There are also subcutaneous (arrow in axial fused image d) and intramuscular (arrow in axial fused image e) metastatic lesions. Metastatic lesions from esophageal cancer commonly include lungs, liver, bones, and adrenal glands; uncommon sites of metastatic lesions include the brain, skeletal muscle, subcutaneous tissues, thyroid gland, and pancreas.

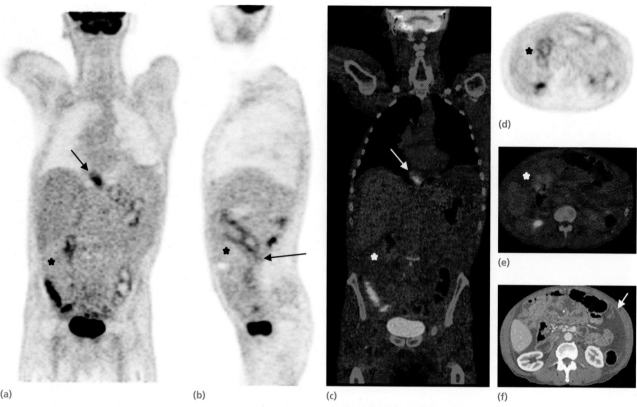

(a) (b) (c) (f)

Figure 88.3 A 58-year-old male with recently diagnosed adenocarcinoma of the esophagus. An ^{18}F-fluorodeoxyglucose positron emission tomography (^{18}F-FDG PET) scan was performed for initial staging. ^{18}F-FDG PET scan coronal image **(a)** and fused PET/computed tomography (CT) image **(c)** show radiotracer uptake associated with distal esophageal lesion (arrow in a, c). There is also diffuse uptake associated with the peritoneum consistent with peritoneal carcinomatosis seen in all PET images **(a, b, d)** and fused PET/CT images **(c, e)** (marked by star). Axial contrast CT image **(f)** performed after the PET scan at the time of staging shows distortion and retraction of the small bowel mesentery and abnormal increased attenuation throughout the omentum (arrow in **f**). U-shaped hypermetabolic peritoneal activity, straight-line sign demarcating involved peritoneum from uninvolved retroperitoneum (arrow in **b**), and diffuse, low-grade glucose hypermetabolism throughout the abdomen and pelvis obscuring visceral outlines has been reported in diffuse peritoneal carcinomatosis. However, the aspect is nonspecific and can be seen also in infectious or inflammatory etiology of peritonitis. Malignant ascites has been reported in 4.0% of patients with esophageal cancer.

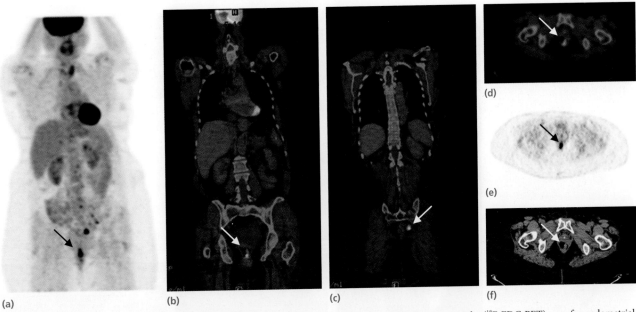

(a)   (b)   (c)   (f)

(d)

(e)

Figure 88.4 A 56-year-old female who underwent a staging ^{18}F-fluorodeoxyglucose positron emission tomography (^{18}F-FDG PET) scan for endometrial adenocarcinoma with incidental finding of anorectal squamous cell carcinoma. Special preparation ("bladder protocol") was used in order to increase the sensitivity of the study for detection of abnormalities in the pelvic region. ^{18}F-FDG PET maximum intensity projection (MIP) image **(a)** and axial image **(e)**, and fused PET/computed tomography (CT) images **(b, d)** show a hypermetabolic focus in the rectal region consistent with incidentally discovered anorectal squamous cell carcinoma (arrow in **a, b, d, e**). There were hypermetabolic pelvic lymph nodes, including one left perirectal lymph node (arrow on coronal fused image **c**). **(f)** The rectal lesion (arrow) is difficult to characterize on attenuation correction noncontrast CT. On ^{18}F-FDG PET, the presence of intense uptake in the pelvis due to radioactive urine in the bladder can cause artifacts or may obscure hypermetabolic lesions in the vicinity. In order to evaluate the pelvic region for primary or metastatic lesions, special preparation (bladder protocol) is helpful. Protocols include intravenous hydration, administration of furosemide, catheterization to remove excreted radiotracer, and retrograde filling of the bladder with saline solution.

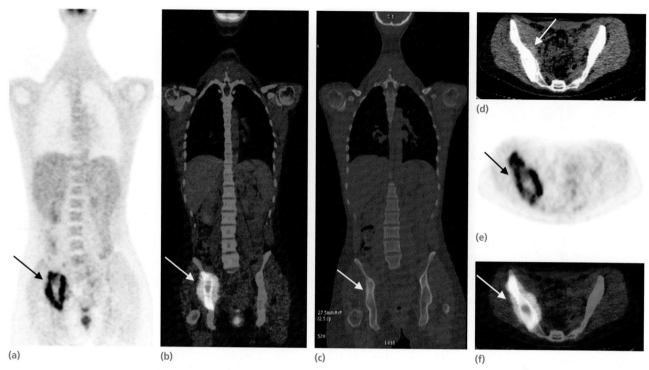

(a)   (b)   (c)   (d)

(e)

(f)

Figure 88.5 A 26-year-old women with history of stage 1 rectal adenocarcinoma (pT2, N0) surgically resected who presented 2 years later with mildly elevated carcinoembryonic antigen (CEA) level (5.7 ng/mL) and right hip pain. ^{18}F-fluorodeoxyglucose positron emission tomography (^{18}F-FDG PET) scan images **(a, e)** and fused images **(b, f)** showed hypermetabolic focus in the right pelvic region, including acetabulum, right ilium, and sacrum (arrow in **a, b, e, f**). The coronal computed tomography (CT) image **(c)** shows minimal sclerotic right pelvic bones with a soft tissue component in the iliacus muscle (arrow in axial CT image **d**) consistent with skeletal metastasis. Pulmonary metastases were diagnosed later at short time interval (not on this PET scan). Colorectal cancer metastasizes mainly to liver, lung, and peritoneum; skeletal metastasis occur less frequently in primary colorectal carcinomas.

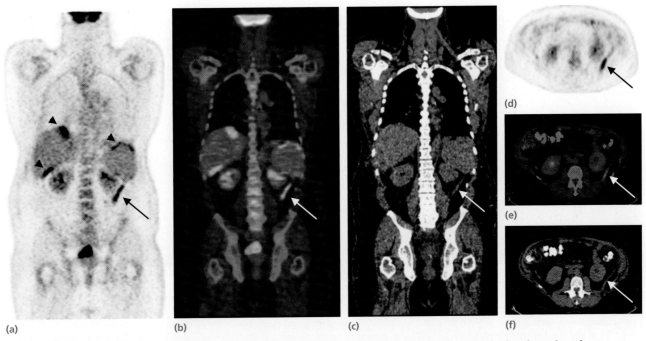

Figure 88.6 A 60-year-old male with a history of rectosigmoid junction adenocarcinoma who, 1 week postsurgery, developed complicated intraabdominal sepsis secondary to a disrupted low anterior anastomosis. An ^{18}F-fluorodeoxyglucose positron emission tomography (^{18}F-FDG PET) scan was performed 6 weeks later. ^{18}F-FDG PET images **(a, d)** and fused images **(b, e)** show hypermetabolic foci localized peritoneal around the liver and spleen (arrowhead in a) and retroperitoneal at the posterior renal fascia, also called the fascia of Zuckerkandl (arrow in **b, d, e**), due to prior episode of fecal peritonitis with residual inflammation/granulomatous reaction. Thickening of the posterior renal fascia is seen in attenuation correction computed tomography (CT) scan **(c, f)**. Benign conditions like inflammation and infection can have ^{18}F-FDG uptake with similar intensity per unit volume compared to malignant lesions (for example peritoneal metastases) and history and the pattern of distribution of hypermetabolic foci (in this case involvement also of the posterior renal fascia) are important factors to be taken into consideration. Source: Courtesy of Hubert Vesselle PhD, MD, University of Washington.

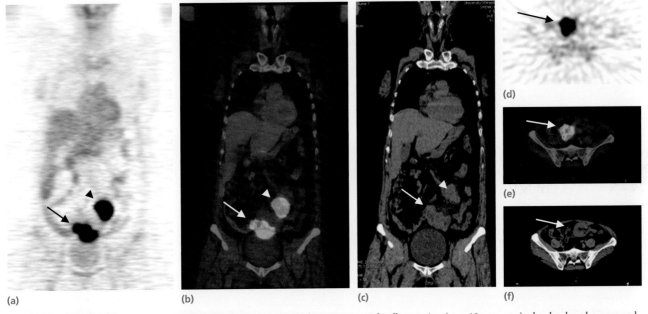

Figure 88.7 A 56-year-old women with history of melanoma in situ in the cutaneous right elbow region (over 10 years ago) who developed nausea and vomiting. A computed tomography (CT) abdomen showed a mesenteric mass and small bowel wall thickening; ^{18}F-fluorodeoxyglucose positron emission tomography (^{18}F-FDG PET) was performed for further characterization. ^{18}F-FDG PET images **(a, d)** and fused PET/CT images **(b, e)** show intense radiotracer uptake associated with a small bowel loop (arrow in **a, b, d, e**) and a large mesenteric nodal mass (arrowhead in **a, b**) consistent with metastatic melanoma. Segmental thickening of the small bowel wall is seen on noncontrast CT images **(c, f)**. Secondary tumors of the small intestine are 2.5 times more common than primary small bowel carcinoma. Melanoma is the most common malignancy to metastasize to the small intestine, although testis, lung, breast, and ovarian cancers also frequently involve the small intestine by metastatic spread.

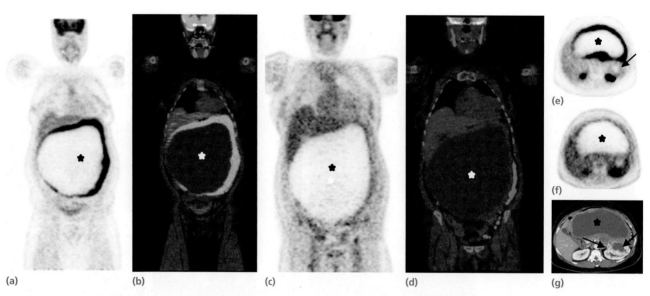

Figure 88.8 A 59-year-old female with gastrointestinal stromal cell tumor (GIST) of gastric origin (with greater than 99% necrosis and cystic changes) and left kidney clear cell renal carcinoma. An ^{18}F-fluorodeoxyglucose positron emission tomography (^{18}F-FDG PET) scan pre- and posttreatment with imatinib mesylate (5 weeks interval between the scans) was performed for staging and assessment of the preoperative treatment response. ^{18}F-FDG PET images **(a, e)** and fused image **(b)** showed a large abdominal mass with central necrosis corresponding to gastric GIST. A PET scan performed 5 weeks later **(c, d, f)** showed good response to treatment with no significant residual ^{18}F-FDG uptake. No abnormal increased uptake in left renal mass (arrow in **e**) was seen on the contrast computed tomography (CT) axial image (arrow in **g**) consistent with renal cell carcinoma. ^{18}F-FDG PET/CT has a role in initial staging, response to therapy, and detection of recurrence of GISTs. ^{18}F-FDG PET can detect response to imatinib mesylate treatment in patients with malignant GISTs as early as 1 week after starting therapy.

A metaanalysis of the diagnostic performance of ^{18}F-FDG PET and PET/CT in renal cell carcinoma showed a sensitivity and specificity of 62% and 88%, respectively.

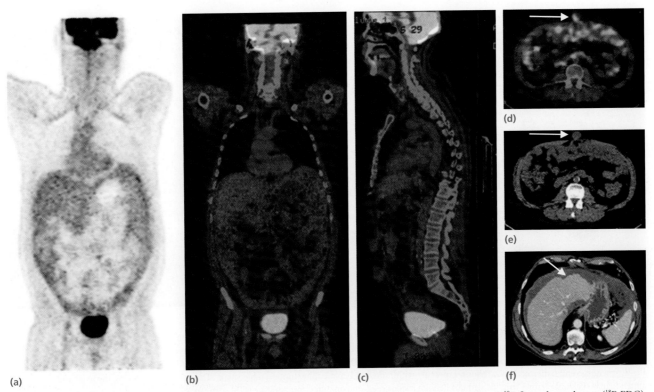

(a)   (b)   (c)   (d)   (e)   (f)

Figure 88.9 A 68-year-old male with appendiceal mucinous adenocarcinoma and resulting pseudomyxoma peritonei. ^{18}F-fluorodeoxyglucose (^{18}F-FDG) images (a) and fused images (b, c, d) show diffuse minimal low-level FDG uptake in the peritoneal cavity and greater omentum associated with extensive low-density material throughout the abdominal cavity surrounding the liver, spleen, anteriorly in the location of the greater omentum, and in the ventral and umbilical hernia (arrow in d, e), consistent with pseudomyxoma peritonei. Axial contrast-enhanced computed tomography (CT) images of the abdomen and pelvis demonstrate lobulated, low-attenuation masses scalloping the border of the liver (arrow in f). Some metastatic peritoneal deposits are cystic or mucinous in nature and thus may be low in attenuation on CT and do not have or have only faint FDG avidity, mimicking loculated fluid.

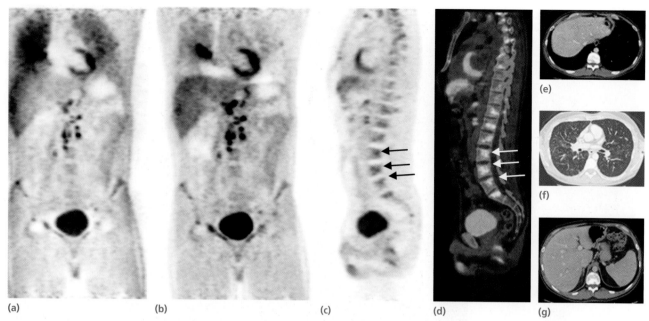

(a) (b) (c) (d) (e) (f) (g)

Figure 88.10 A 41-year-old male with sarcoidosis involving the lungs, liver, spleen, skeleton, and multiple lymph nodes localized supra and infradiaphragmatic. ^{18}F-fluorodeoxyglucose positron emission tomography (^{18}F-FDG PET) nonattenuation-corrected coronal (NAC) images **(a)**, attenuation correction (AC) images **(b, c)**, and fused sagittal image **(d)** show diffuse hypermetabolic foci in the lungs and heterogeneous uptake within the liver with several hypermetabolic lesions, especially within the left hepatic lobe. Innumerable small FDG-avid foci involving the axial and appendicular skeleton (arrows in **c, d**) without definite lesions seen on computed tomography (CT) scan, are most likely related to sarcoidosis. Hypermetabolic infradiaphragmatic lymph nodes are also seen. Axial contrast-enhanced CT images show multiple hypodense lesions in the liver **(e)** and spleen **(g)** consistent with sarcoidosis (biopsy proven for liver and spleen). The axial chest CT image **(f)** shows multiple pulmonary nodules in a perilymphatic distribution. The patient is status postsplenectomy on PET images. ^{18}F-FDG PET scan has been increasingly used for the assessment of infectious and inflammatory diseases, including sarcoidosis. Liver and spleen are involved in 5%–15% of cases, whereas other gastrointestinal localizations are rare (1%–3%).

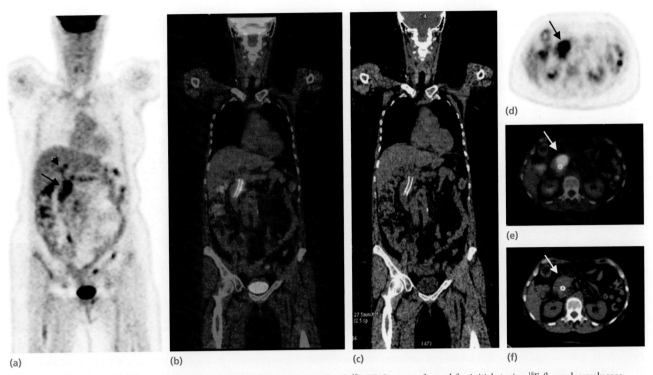

(a)   (b)   (c)   (d)   (e)   (f)

Figure 88.11 A 59-year-old woman with adenocarcinoma of the pancreatic head. ^{18}F-FDG was performed for initial staging. ^{18}F-fluorodeoxyglucose positron emission tomography (^{18}F-FDG PET) scan images (**a, c**) and fused images (**b, e**) show a hypermetabolic pancreatic head mass consistent with known malignancy (arrow in **a**) and mild uptake in the rest of the pancreas representing inflammation secondary to pancreatic duct obstruction. Minimal uptake along the right and left hepatic ducts and common hepatic/biliary duct probably represent mild inflammation (arrowhead in **a**). In solid pancreatic lesions ^{18}F-FDG PET/computed tomography (CT) is most helpful, and superior to contrast-enhanced CT, for the identification of unsuspected distal metastases. On PET scan, mild biliary tract FDG uptake has been previously described after stent placement.

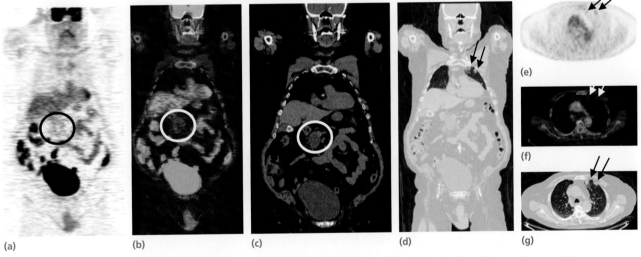

(a)   (b)   (c)   (d)   (e)   (f)   (g)

Figure 88.12 A 77-year-old male referred for evaluation of multiple bilateral pulmonary nodules and one indeterminate cystic pancreatic mass. ^{18}F-fluorodeoxyglucose positron emission tomography (^{18}F-FDG PET) coronal images (**a**) and fused images (**b**) showed no abnormal ^{18}F-FDG uptake associated with the cystic pancreatic head lesion (circle in **a, b**), which was described as multilobulated with thickened walls and septations on magnetic resonance imaging (MRI) (not shown); noncontrast computed tomography (CT) shows cystic pancreatic mass (circle in **c**). Only minimal uptake is seen in the lungs associated with multicentric bilateral lung consolidations (arrows in **d, e, f, g**). Findings were consistent with pulmonary low-grade mucinous multifocal adenocarcinoma (biopsy proven). Pancreatic fluid cytology (post fine-needle aspiration) was negative for malignancy and was mucin positive. False-negative results on ^{18}F-FDG PET have been described associated with mucinous tumors. Overall sensitivity on ^{18}F-FDG PET scan is low for mucinous tumors, possibly due to low cellularity of the lesion. In this case the lung lesions had faint FDG uptake and were consistent (based on the pathology report) with adenocarcinoma in situ (low-grade mucinous neoplasm with bronchioloalveolar pattern of spread and no definite invasive carcinoma, 1 cm greatest dimension). The absence of ^{18}F-FDG uptake on PET associated with pancreatic cystic and/or mucin-producing tumors does not exclude malignancy given the limited sensitivity of ^{18}F-FDG PET for this type of lesion.

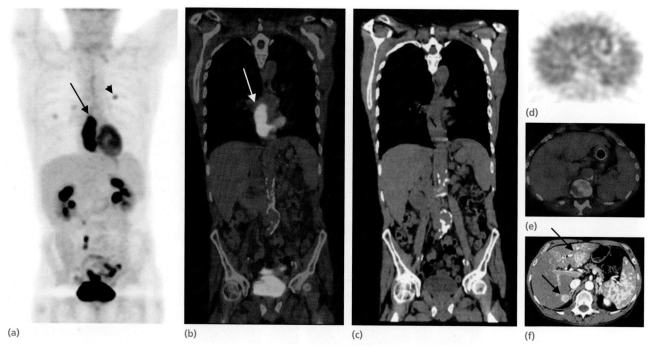

Figure 88.13 A 60-year-old man with squamous cell carcinoma of the esophagus; positron emission tomography (PET) scan was performed for staging of the disease. The patient also has cirrhosis with multifocal hepatocellular carcinoma.[18]F-fluorodeoxyglucose (^{18}F-FDG) PET images **(a, d)** and fused images **(b, e)** do not show any increased uptake associated with multiple hepatocellular carcinoma lesions seen on contrast-enhanced computed tomography (CT) scan (arrows in **f**). There is uptake associated with the esophageal adenocarcinoma (arrow in **a**); the left supraclavicular lymph node and pulmonary nodule are suspicious for being metastatic from esophageal cancer (arrowhead in **a**). Minimal uptake associated with asymmetric gynecomastia is seen in the right chest. Varying accumulation of ^{18}F-FDG has been described in hepatocellular carcinomas (HCC) depending on the degree of tumor differentiation, which leads to variable levels of glucose-6-phosphatase activity (glucose-6-phosphatase dephosphorylates intracellular ^{18}F-FDG-6-phosphate, which can then leave the hepatocyte). Well-differentiated HCC can have uptake similar to normal liver and may not be detected on FDG PET examinations.

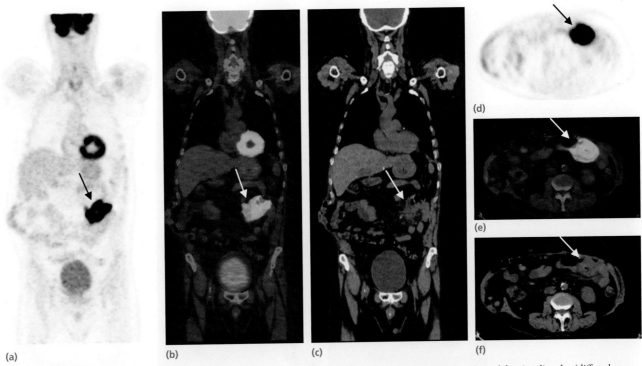

(a)   (b)   (c)   (d)   (e)   (f)

Figure 88.14 A 64-year-old male with a history of orthotopic liver transplant and recurrent posttransplant lymphoproliferative disorder (diffuse large B-cell lymphoma, Epstein–Barr virus [EBV] negative). ^{18}F-fluorodeoxyglucose positron emission tomography (^{18}F-FDG PET) images **(a, d)** and fused images **(b, e)** show segmental circumferential bowel wall thickening of the proximal jejunum, which has high ^{18}F-FDG uptake (arrows in **a, b, d, e**) consistent with diffuse large B-cell lymphoma. Thickened bowel wall is seen on noncontrast computed tomography (CT) (arrow in **c, f**). Posttransplant lymphoproliferative disease (PTLD) is a well-recognized complication of both solid organ transplantation and allogeneic hematopoietic stem cell transplantation. In most cases, PTLD is associated with EBV infection of B cells, either as a consequence of reactivation of the virus posttransplantation or from primary EBV infection. The incidence of PTLD is thought to be bimodal; cases in the first year after solid-organ transplantation are typically related to EBV. A second incidence occurs more than 1 year following transplantation and is typically not related to EBV. FDG PET has a high sensitivity of 89% for detection of PTLD.

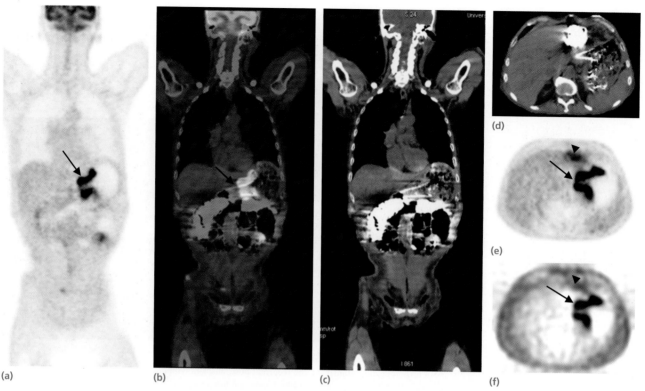

(a)   (b)   (c)   (d)   (e)   (f)

Figure 88.15 A 73-year-old male with invasive gastric adenocarcinoma involving the antrum and body of the stomach. ^{18}F-fluorodeoxyglucose positron emission tomography (^{18}F-FDG PET) images **(a)** and fused images **(b)** show a circumferential intense hypermetabolic area involving the antrum and body of the stomach with gastric wall thickening consistent with known malignancy (arrows in **a, b, e, f**). An additional focus of increased radiotracer uptake in the transverse colon is seen on attenuation correction axial images (arrowhead in e), which is not visualized in the same area on nonattenuation-correction images (arrowhead in f), and this represents an artifact due to the presence of barium in the bowel. In this patient on pathological specimen, carcinoma penetrated to the surface of the visceral peritoneum (serosa) and directly invaded adjacent structures (retroperitoneal fibroadipose tissue). As with many malignancies, tumor stage (T) is poorly assessed with PET/computed tomography (CT) because of the limited spatial resolution on PET and the blooming artifact. When reviewing PET/CT images it is important to examine not only the attenuation correction images but also the nonattenuation corrected images. Scatter and attenuation correction require an accurate attenuation map, which is difficult to perform for high-density materials (high-Z materials) like metal implants and dense CT contrast agents (iodine, barium).

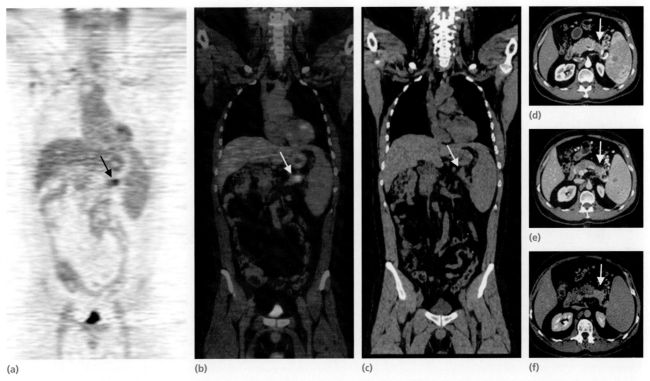

(a) (b) (c) (d) (e) (f)

Figure 88.16 A 47-year-old male who underwent work-up for thrombocytopenia and splenomegaly secondary to splenic vein thrombosis, diagnosed with nonsecretory pancreatic neuroendocrine tumor. ^{18}F-fluorodeoxyglucose positron emission tomography (^{18}F-FDG PET) coronal images (a) and fused images (b) show increased radiotracer uptake associated with the pancreatic tail mass. A malignant peripancreatic lymph node found at surgery was not hypermetabolic on PET scan. Attenuation correction noncontrast computed tomography (CT) scan (c) shows splenomegaly. Multiphase contrast-enhanced CT images show a pancreatic tail mass that is hypovascular on arterial phase (d), iso- to hypervascular on portal venous phase (e), and hyperdense on delayed phase (f). The CT features are suspicious for an adenocarcinoma with a desmoplastic stromal component and are atypical for pancreatic neuroendocrine tumors, which usually are hypervascular on arterial phase; however, this tumor was a biopsy-proven pancreatic neuroendocrine tumor. Well-differentiated neuroendocrine tumors are best assessed with ^{111}In-Octreoscan or ^{68}Ga-DOTA-peptides and are usually false negative on ^{18}F-FDG PET. Tumors that are negative on somatostatin receptor analog study but positive on ^{18}F-FDG PET scan carry a worse prognosis.

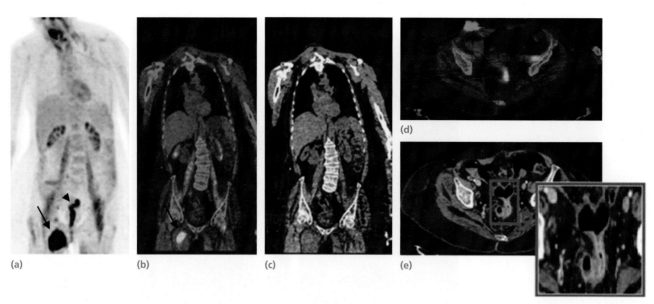

Figure 88.17 A 56-year-old female with an anal polyp representing invasive squamous cell carcinoma with large right inguinal necrotic lymph node. There is concurrent proctitis. ¹⁸F-fluorodeoxyglucose positron emission tomography (¹⁸F-FDG PET) image **(a)** and fused image **(b)** show a hypermetabolic right inguinal large necrotic metastatic lymph node (arrow in a, b) and diffuse uptake in the rectal and rectosigmoid region (arrowhead in a). The axial image of contrast-enhanced computed tomography (CT) scan **(e)** shows bowel wall thickening in the rectal and rectosigmoid region with mucosal enhancement at this level (without discontinuities of mucosal enhancement along the thickened segment, no perirectal lymph nodes, and a long segment of the bowel wall which is thickened); findings are compatible with the patient's known proctitis. In addition, on ¹⁸F-FDG PET there is diffuse increased uptake associated with the musculature (psoas and iliopsoas muscles), which is physiological (positional). ¹⁸F-FDG PET uptake is nonspecific and hypermetabolic lesions do not always indicate malignancy. Correlation with CT images, as in this case, can often allow detection of the responsible nonneoplastic hypermetabolic conditions (e.g., infection or inflammation), thereby preventing false-positive interpretation.

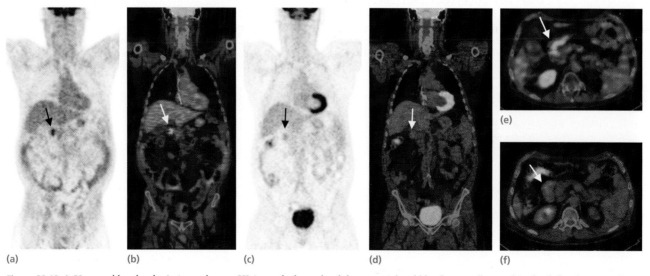

Figure 88.18 A 58-year-old male who is 4 months post HLA-matched, unrelated donor, peripheral blood stem cell transplant for diffuse large B-cell non-Hodgkin lymphoma; 8 weeks posttransplant the patient was diagnosed with graft-versus-host disease. ¹⁸F-fluorodeoxyglucose positron emission tomography (¹⁸F-FDG PET) images coronal **(a)** and fused **(b, e)** obtained 4 months posttransplant show increased radiotracer uptake in the duodenum (arrows in a, b, e), which was not seen on a prior PET scan performed before the stem cell transplant **(c, d, f)**. Biopsy results showed graft-versus-host disease. The patients with an allogeneic bone marrow transplant may develop an immune response against the body, producing graft-versus-host disease, which can be acute (typically occurs within the first few months after transplant) or chronic (occurs more than 3 months after transplant). Data show that in the bowel ¹⁸F-FDG PET has a good sensitivity for detecting sites of bowel affected by graft-versus-host disease. Source: Courtesy of Cheng Han Shih MD, University of Washington.

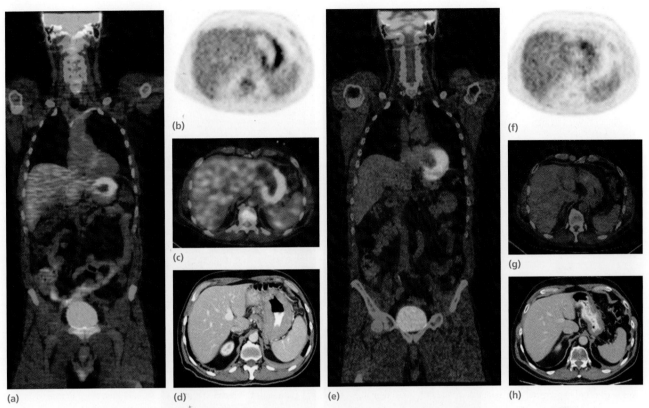

(a)   (b)   (c)   (d)   (e)   (f)   (g)   (h)

Figure 88.19 A 64-year-old male with prior history of right upper lobe pulmonary mucosa-associated lymphoid tissue (MALT) lymphoma, and now with biopsy-proven gastric MALT lymphoma. ^{18}F-fluorodeoxyglucose positron emission tomography (^{18}F-FDG PET) scan was performed pre- and posttreatment. Pretreatment ^{18}F-FDG PET image **(b)** and fused images **(a, c)** show increased FDG uptake associated with diffuse gastric wall thickening. Axial contrast computed tomography (CT) image **(d)** shows a mildly enhancing thickened gastric wall. Posttreatment ^{18}F-FDG PET image **(f)** and fused images **(e, g)** show interval resolution of the previously seen increased FDG uptake associated with the gastric wall. Axial contrast CT image **(h)** shows interval resolution of the previously seen gastric wall thickening. The intense uptake in the lower thoracic region seen on posttreatment PET scan **(e)** is due to physiological uptake in the heart, which can be variable from one scan to another depending on the length of the fasting time and 24-h diet before the scan. MALT is an indolent form of lymphoma (a type of marginal zone lymphoma) and the sensitivity of detection by FDG PET scan depends on the location of the involvement, sensitivity being high in pulmonary MALT lymphoma but significantly lower in gastric MALT, due to the fact that the gastric uptake may be increased both physiologically and due to inflammation. However, higher-grade lymphoma and associated ulceration increased the rate of detection of gastric MALT lymphoma.

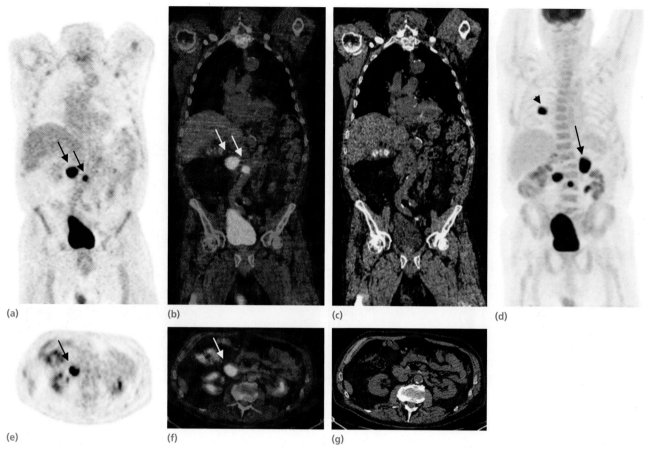

(a)   (b)   (c)   (d)

(e)   (f)   (g)

Figure 88.20 A 75-year-old male underwent ^{18}F-fluorodeoxyglucose positron emission tomography (^{18}F-FDG PET) staging for duodenal epithelioid angiosarcoma. ^{18}F-FDG PET images coronal and axial **(a, e)** and maximum intensity projection (MIP) **(d)**, and also fused images **(b, f)**, show hypermetabolic lesions within the third portion of the duodenum consistent with known duodenal epithelioid angiosarcoma (arrows in **a, b, e, f**). Adrenal metastasis (arrow in **d**) and one rib metastasis (arrowhead in **d**) are also visualized. Epithelioid angiosarcoma is a highly aggressive endothelial cell malignancy, most commonly arising in the deep soft tissues, but a variety of primary sites, including the adrenals, thyroid, skin, bone, and breast, are encountered; the gastrointestinal tract is rarely involved. ^{18}F-FDG PET is often able to detect lesions that are difficult to visualize on anatomic imaging (for example small bowel lesions), potentially drastically altering management.

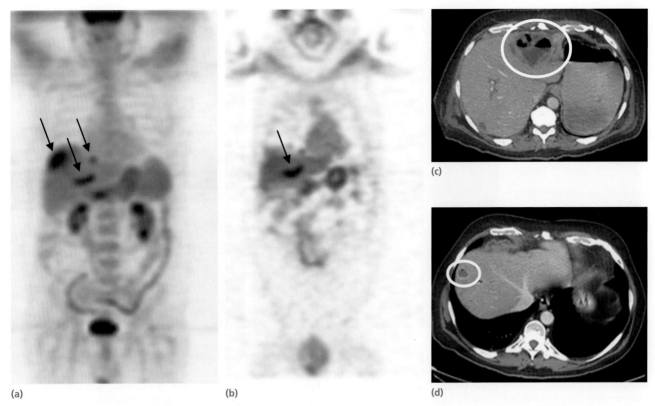

(a)   (b)   (c)
                                                                  (d)

Figure 88.21 A 64-year-old male with pancreatic cancer status post Whipple procedure complicated by injury to the hepatic artery, hepatic necrosis, and development of multiple liver abscesses. ^{18}F-fluorodeoxyglucose positron emission tomography (^{18}F-FDG PET) images maximum intensity projection (MIP) **(a)** and coronal **(b)** show multiple foci of increased radiotracer uptake in the liver consistent with the patient's known polymicrobial liver abscesses. Axial images of contrast-enhanced computed tomography (CT) scan show wedge-shaped areas of hypodensities in the left and right lobes of the liver (one wedge-shaped hypodense area, which is gas containing, is shown in **c**). One of the lesions presents rim enhancement on contrast-enhanced CT **(d)**. Knowledge of the benign pathological causes of increased ^{18}F-FDG uptake is necessary for the accurate interpretation of ^{18}F-FDG PET images. ^{18}F-FDG PET is not a specific marker for malignancy and correlation with clinical information and other imaging modalities is very important.

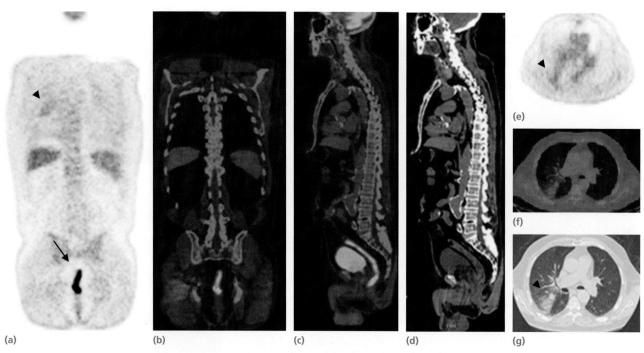

(a)   (b)   (c)   (d)   (g)

Figure 88.22 A 76-year-old male with lung adenocarcinoma and ulcerative colitis involving the rectum and rectosigmoid region. ^{18}F-fluorodeoxyglucose positron emission tomography (^{18}F-FDG PET) coronal **(a)**, axial **(e)**, fused image **(f)**, and one computed tomography (CT) axial image **(g)** show minimal uptake (max standardized uptake value [SUV] 2.4) in the right upper lung corresponding to ground-glass opacity with 1.5 cm solid component consistent with (invasive) adenocarcinoma with a peripheral lepidic growth pattern (growth of neoplastic cells along preexisting structures and alveolar septa) (arrowheads in **a, e, f, g**). ^{18}F-FDG PET coronal **(a)** and fused images **(b, c)** also show intense uptake seen in the rectum and rectosigmoid region corresponding to thickening of the bowel wall seen on the CT image consistent with patient's known ulcerative colitis (arrow in **a**). SUV values cannot differentiate between benign and malignant lung lesions, given that slow-growing malignant pulmonary lesions can have only minimal ^{18}F-FDG uptake. In this case, FDG uptake in the lung lesion was not significantly higher than the mediastinal blood pool. Regarding inflammatory bowel disease (IBD), ^{18}F-FDG PET was used in differentiation between a flare of inflammatory bowel disease versus the onset of a noninflammatory process causing similar symptoms in patients with known IBD. Many unanswered questions remain, but PET appears to be a promising tool in the noninvasive evaluation of IBD.

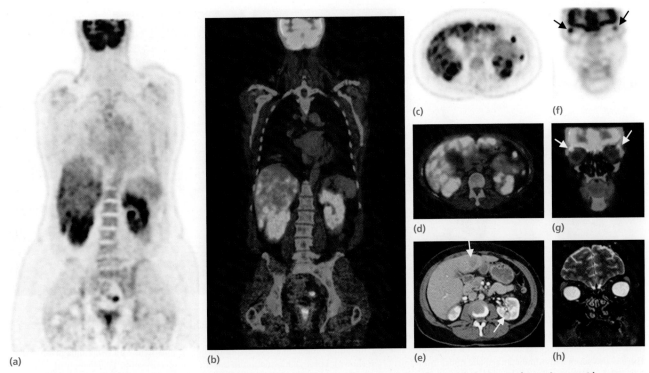

(a)   (b)   (c)   (d)   (e)   (f)   (g)   (h)

Figure 88.23 A 58-year-old woman with history of breast cancer and hepatitis C (treated with interferon and ribavirin in the past), now with a new diagnosis of Burkitt lymphoma with central nervous system involvement and also lymph nodes, liver, kidneys, and lacrimal glands involvement. ^{18}F-fluorodeoxyglucose positron emission tomography/computed tomography (^{18}F-FDG PET/CT) images (**a, c**) and fused images (**b, d**) show multiple hypermetabolic foci in the liver and kidneys. Prominent lacrimal glands seen on T2 magnetic resonance coronal images (**h**) with increased ^{18}F-FDG uptake on PET scan (arrows in **f, g**) likely are consistent with lymphoma involvement also. Hypodense lesions are seen on contrast-enhanced CT scan in the liver and kidneys (arrows in **e**). The hypermetabolic foci seen on PET scan (including the lacrimal gland uptake) have resolved on follow-up posttreatment scan (not shown). Burkitt lymphoma is a highly aggressive B-cell neoplasm with very high mitotic rate (high Ki67) and can be divided in endemic, sporadic, and immunodeficiency related. This type of lymphoma frequently involves extranodal sites, including abdominal organs and central nervous system, and can also involve ovaries, testicles, breast, kidneys, and peripheral blood. Endemic cases frequently involve facial bones and HIV-related cases often involve lymph nodes and bone marrow.

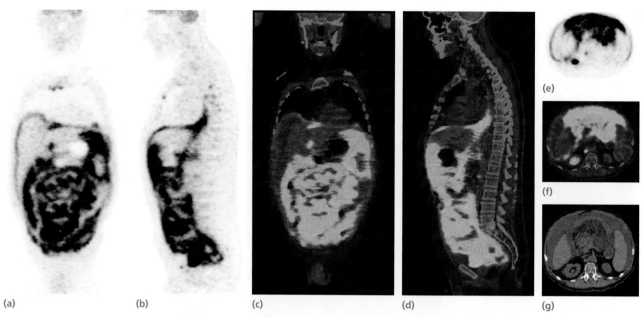

(a) (b) (c) (d) (e) (f) (g)

Figure 88.24 A 63-year-old male with diffuse large B-cell lymphoma demonstrating a large volume of ascites and hypermetabolic peritoneal lining consistent with lymphoma involvement. ^{18}F-fluorodeoxyglucose positron emission tomography (^{18}F-FDG PET) **(a, b, e)** and fused images **(c, d, f)** show intense uptake associated with the peritoneal lining, including omentum and serosa of the bowel, consistent with lymphoma involvement. There is also supra and infradiaphragmatic nodal involvement (not shown). Limited information in the attenuation correction axial computed tomography (CT) noncontrast images **(g)** show significant amount of ascites. Normal ^{18}F-FDG biodistribution includes intense brain uptake and mild radiotracer uptake in the liver and spleen (with splenic ^{18}F-FDG uptake similar or slightly lower compared to the liver). In this case there is altered ^{18}F-FDG biodistribution with very low radiotracer uptake in the brain, liver, and spleen. Decreased ^{18}F-FDG uptake in the brain has been described in patients with hyperglycemia; however, in this case the glucose level is within normal limits (116 g/dL). There is also no visualization of the myocardium; however, the myocardium uptake is highly variable depending mostly on the patient's diet the day before the study and the length of fasting. In this case, the most likely explanation for the altered biodistribution is intense metabolic activity associated with peritoneal involvement with less radiotracer available for uptake at the usual sites of FDG metabolism.

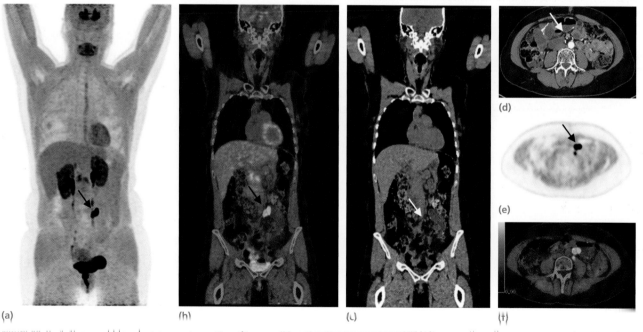

(a) (b) (c) (d) (e) (f)

Figure 88.25 A 46-year-old female status post resection of two small bowel neuroendocrine carcinoids now with malignant mesenteric lymph nodes. 3,4-dihydroxy-6-^{18}F-fluoro-L-phenylalanine (^{18}F-FDOPA) images **(a, e)** and fused images **(b, f)** show uptake in mesenteric lymph nodes consistent with malignant lymph nodes. Small subcentimeter mesenteric lymph nodes are seen in the attenuation correction computed tomography (CT) images (arrow in **c, d**). ^{18}F-FDOPA (an analog of L-DOPA) is an agent being explored for imaging of neuroendocrine tumors. Normal tracer uptake can be seen in the striatum and pancreas, and there is elimination via the biliary path (resulting in gallbladder visualization), digestive, and urinary tracts (kidneys and urinary bladder are seen). Liver and myocardial uptake is generally mild.

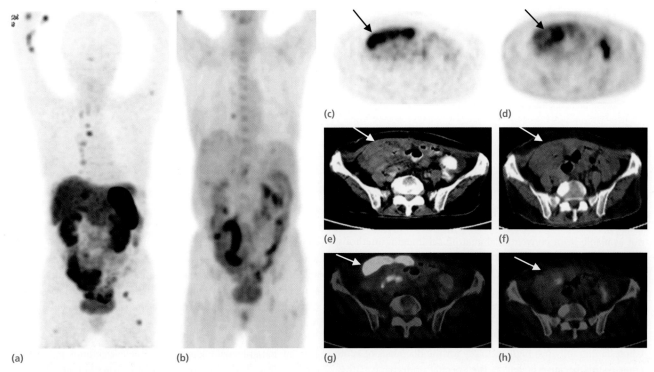

(a)   (b)   (c)   (d)   (e)   (f)   (g)   (h)

Figure 88.26 A 68-year-old female with terminal ileum carcinoid with diffuse metastatic disease. ^{68}Ga-OTA-D-Phe(1)-Tyr(3)-octreotide (^{68}Ga-DOTA-TOC) images show a higher number of metastatic lesions than ^{18}F-fluorodeoxyglucose positron emission tomography (^{18}F-FDG PET) images. ^{68}Ga-DOTA-TOC coronal **(a)**, axial **(c)**, and fused images **(g)** shows hypermetabolic foci in the skeleton (left acetabulum, left and right femurs, left humerus, and right sternal manubrium) liver, right internal mammary lymph nodes, multiple mesenteric, and peritoneal hypermetabolic soft tissue deposits. ^{18}F-FDG PET coronal **(b)**, axial **(d)**, and fused images **(h)** show fewer metastatic lesions (skeletal lesions in the left acetabulum and left femur are less conspicuous and other lesions like left humeral lesion, some of the mediastinal lymph nodes, and liver metastatic lesions are not seen). The hypermetabolic soft tissue omental deposit seen on axial ^{68}Ga-DOTA-TOC study (arrow in **c, e, g**) shows significantly higher uptake compared to the ^{18}F-FDG PET study (arrow in **d, f, h**). Normal biodistribution on ^{68}Ga-DOTA-peptides PET includes, spleen, kidneys, pituitary, adrenals, thyroid, salivary glands, and bowel. Prominent physiological pancreatic uncinate process activity has also been described.

CHAPTER 89

Radionuclide imaging of the gastrointestinal tract

Harvey A. Ziessman
Johns Hopkins University, Baltimore, MD, USA

Nuclear medicine image interpretation is based on physiology and function, as well as diagnostic information, which is often not available from conventional anatomical imaging methods, for example ultrasonography, computed tomography (CT), and magnetic resonance imaging (MRI).

Acute cholecystitis

Cholescintigraphy has high accuracy for the diagnosis of acute cholecystitis because it detects the specific underlying pathophysiology, that is obstruction of the cystic duct, seen as nonfilling of the gallbladder. Sensitivity for the diagnosis is greater than 95% and specificity 90%.

Nonvisualization of the gallbladder 60 min after injection of technetium 99m (Tc-99m) dimethyl iminodiacetic acid (HIDA) is abnormal. However, delayed imaging is required to diagnose or exclude acute cholecystitis. If the gallbladder does not fill by 3–4 h, acute cholecystitis is diagnosed; if it fills, acute cholecystitis is excluded. An alternative to 3–4 h delayed imaging is to administer morphine sulfate, 0.04 mg/kg intravenously, if the gallbladder is not seen at 60 min. The diagnosis can be confirmed or excluded within 30 min. Morphine contracts the sphincter of Oddi, increases intrabiliary pressure, and produces preferential bile flow towards and through the cystic duct, if it is patent (Figure 89.1).

The scintigraphic "rim sign" is seen in 25%–35% of patients with acute cholecystitis (Figure 89.2). This sign is very specific for acute cholecystitis and, importantly, is associated with severe advanced cholecystitis with an increased potential for complications, for example gangrene and perforation. The sign is seen as increased uptake in the liver adjacent to the gallbladder fossa, due to inflammatory spread from the gallbladder to the adjacent liver, causing increased blood flow and extraction of the Tc-99m HIDA in that region.

Chronic cholecystitis

Chronic calculous cholecystitis is often diagnosed in a patient with recurrent biliary colic-like pain who has cholelithiasis on anatomical imaging. These patients are usually directed to surgery for cholecystectomy. Their histopathology shows chronic inflammatory and fibrotic changes in the gallbladder, as well as stones.

Chronic acalculous gallbladder disease is seen in more than 10% of patients who have had cholecystectomy for chronic cholecystitis. They are clinically and histopathologically indistinguishable, except for the presence or absence of gallstones. Symptoms resolve with cholecystectomy.

The challenge is to make the diagnosis of chronic acalculous gallbladder disease noninvasively and preoperatively. Cholecystokinin (CKK, sincalide) cholescintigraphy with calculation of a gallbladder ejection fraction (GBEF) has proven valuable for preoperative diagnosis and predicting response to cholecystectomy. Diseased gallbladders do not contract well and have a low GBEF. Greater than 90% of patients with symptoms suggestive of chronic acalculous gallbladder disease and a low GBEF are cured of their symptoms with cholecystectomy (Figure 89.3).

Biliary obstruction

The diagnosis of *acute biliary obstruction* is commonly made with anatomical imaging, for example ultrasonography, which demonstrates dilated biliary ducts. However, it may take 24–72 h after the onset of acute obstruction for the bile ducts to dilate. Tc-99m HIDA imaging can confirm the diagnosis immediately after obstruction by demonstrating the underlying pathophysiology, that is reduced bile flow. Typically, with high-grade biliary obstruction, cholescintigraphy shows good hepatic extraction

Yamada's Atlas of Gastroenterology, Fifth Edition. Edited by Daniel K. Podolsky, Michael Camilleri, J. Gregory Fitz, Anthony N. Kalloo, Fergus Shanahan, and Timothy C. Wang.
© 2016 John Wiley & Sons, Ltd. Published 2016 by John Wiley & Sons, Ltd.
Companion website: www.yamadagastro.com/atlas

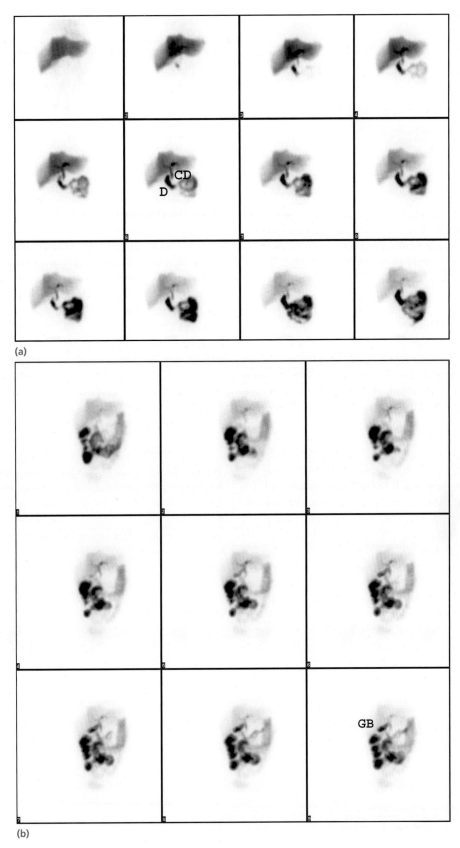

(a)

(b)

Figure 89.1 Cholescintigraphy with morphine sulfate. **(a)** Sequential images over 60 min. The right lobe has an abnormal appearance due to a loculated pleural effusion. There is normal hepatic uptake and biliary clearance into the common duct (CD) and duodenum (D) and more distal small bowel. However, no filling of the gallbladder is seen. **(b)** After morphine injection, imaging is continued for 30 min. The gallbladder (GB) fills progressively, ruling out acute cholecystitis.

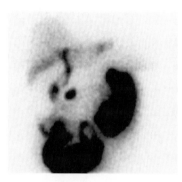

Figure 89.2 Rim sign in acute cholescystitis. A 40-year-old female was referred for suspected acute cholecystitis. The technetium 99m-labeled hepatic iminodiacetic acid (Tc-99m HIDA) study showed nonfilling of the gallbladder at 1 h (not shown). Further delayed images were obtained at 3 h. The image shows no gallbladder filling and a "rim" sign, that is increased uptake in the liver adjacent to the gallbladder fossa. There is normal transit to the small intestines. The rim sign is specific for acute cholecystitis and suggests severe disease with an increased likelihood of complications such as gangrene and perforation.

but no biliary or intestinal clearance, that is a persistent hepatogram (Figure 89.4).

Partial low-grade biliary obstruction has a somewhat different imaging pattern. Bile ducts often do not become dilated because of the lower intraductal pressure compared to high-grade obstruction. Cholescintigraphic images show good hepatic function, prompt secretion into biliary ducts, but retention of radiotracer in biliary ducts and delayed transit into the small intestines.

Cholescintigraphy can provide diagnostic information in patients with the *postcholecystectomy syndrome*. Common biliary causes for recurrent pain after cholecystectomy are residual or recurrent biliary duct stones, biliary stricture, and sphincter of Oddi dysfunction. All have a scintigraphic picture of partial biliary obstruction. Image analysis and quantification can be diagnostic. If stones, tumor, and stricture are eliminated by endoscopic retrograde cholangiopancreatography (ERCP), sphincter of Oddi dysfunction is likely (Figure 89.5).

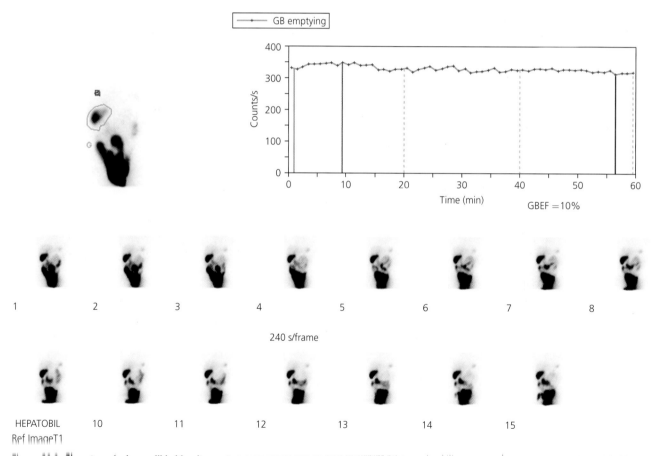

Figure 89.3 Chronic acalculous gallbladder disease in a 44-year-old female with recurrent biliary colic. Ultrasonography was negative. The gallbladder filled during the first 60 min of the study (not shown). Shown are sequential 2-min images made during the 60 min infusion of sincalide (cholecystokinin, CCK). A region of interest was drawn on the computer around the gallbladder and a time–activity curve generated. Very poor gallbladder contraction is seen. The calculated gallbladder ejection fraction (GBEF) was 10% (normal ≥38%). Histopathology showed a chronically inflamed gallbladder without stones.

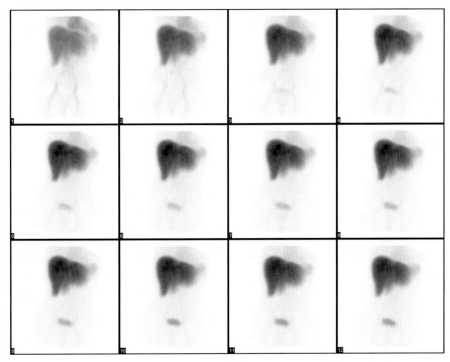

Figure 89.4 Acute biliary obstruction. The patient had acute onset of upper abdominal pain and presented in the emergency room. Ultrasonography showed normal-size biliary ducts. Sequential 5-min images over 1.5 h show good hepatic function but no biliary excretion into biliary ducts, consistent with a high-grade acute biliary obstruction.

Biliary atresia

This neonatal disease presents as cholestatic jaundice. It is caused by a progressive inflammatory sclerosis that obliterates extahepatic and intrahepatic biliary ducts. Early diagnosis is critical and must be made within the first 60 days of life to prevent irreversible liver failure. Treatment requires a palliative hepatoportoenterostomy (Kasai procedure), but ultimately liver transplantation. The differential diagnosis includes neonatal hepatitis of various etiologies.

Patient preparation for cholescintigraphy requires 3–5 days of phenobarbital to activate liver excretory enzymes and increase bile flow. Cholescintigraphic images demonstrate a high-grade obstruction, with a persistent hepatogram and no biliary to bowel transit over 24 h. The negative predictive value of the study is very high, approaching 100%. The positive predictive value is somewhat lower. False-positive studies occur in some patients with severe parenchymal liver disease (Figure 89.6).

Biliary leak

Bile leaks usually occur as an acute complication of cholecystectomy or biliary tract surgery. Although ultrasonography and CT can detect fluid collections, the cause may be uncertain. Cholescintigraphy can determine if there is active biliary leakage, estimate the rate of leakage, and determine whether a fluid collection is of biliary origin, rather than caused by ascites, infection, etc. Slow bile leaks often resolve spontaneously with conservative therapy, whereas more rapid leaks usually require intervention.

Bile leakage is seen on cholescintigraphy as progressively increasing radiotracer collection in the region of the gallbladder fossa or hepatic hilum. It can move into the subdiaphragmatic space, over the dome of the liver, into the colonic gutters, or spread diffusely as free bile throughout the abdomen (Figure 89.7). Peritoneal tubing, drains, and collection bags may exhibit accumulation and at times be the only evidence of leakage.

F-18 FDG PET imaging of inflammatory bowel disease

[18]F-labeled fluorodeoxyglucose (18-F FDG) PET (positron emission tomography) is increasingly used for diagnosis and to evaluate patients with known inflammatory bowel disease. FDG is transported into cells proportional to their metabolic cell activity. Neutrophils and macrophages accumulate FDG. The PET study may be useful in patients with suspected disease where endoscopic evaluation is not feasible due to patient safety or patient fear of an endoscopic exam. In patients with a diagnosis, the study can provide evidence of disease activity and location, evaluate treatment efficacy, provide evidence of relapse, and suggest complications (Figure 89.8).

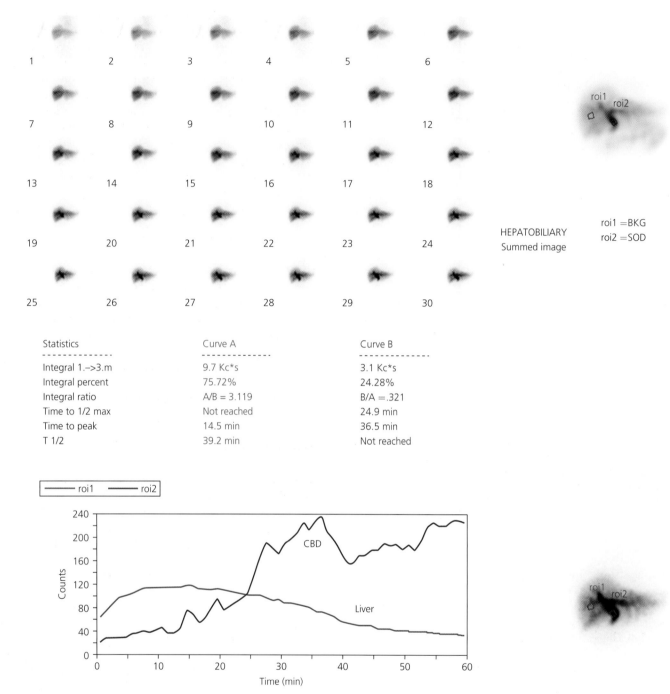

Statistics	Curve A	Curve B
Integral 1.–>3.m	9.7 Kc*s	3.1 Kc*s
Integral percent	75.72%	24.28%
Integral ratio	A/B = 3.119	B/A =.321
Time to 1/2 max	Not reached	24.9 min
Time to peak	14.5 min	36.5 min
T 1/2	39.2 min	Not reached

HEPATOBILIARY
Summed image

roi1 =BKG
roi2 =SOD

Figure 89.5 Sphincter of Oddi dysfunction. Postcholecystectomy pain in a 38-year-old female with chronic recurrent biliary colic beginning 5 months postsurgery. Sequential technetium 99m-labeled hepatic iminodiacetic acid (Tc-99m HIDA) 2-min images over 1 h show clearance into biliary ducts, but persistent prominent activity in biliary ducts and little bile transit to the intestines. The common bile duct (CBD) time–activity curve shows a progressive rise in activity. This is consistent with a partial biliary obstruction. No stones or biliary stricture were found on endoscopic retrograde cholangiopancreatography (ERCP). Sphincterotomy was performed with subsequent symptom resolution.

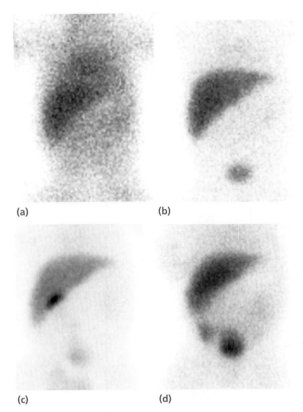

(a)   (b)

(c)   (d)

Figure 89.6 Biliary atresia. A 6-week-old child with persistent hyperbilirubinemia referred to rule out biliary atresia. The technetium 99m-labeled hepatic iminodiacetic acid (Tc-99m HIDA) study shows images immediately after injection **(a)**, 1 h **(b)**, 6 h **(c)**, and 24 h **(d)**. Hepatic function is good. Biliary clearance is seen at 6 h with filling of the gallbladder and at 24 h in the intestines. The study could have been stopped at 6 h because gallbladder filling excludes the diagnosis of biliary atresia.

Tc-99m sulfur colloid for liver and spleen scanning

Tc-99m sulfur colloid liver spleen scans are less commonly used today than in the past. However, for certain specific indications, it can be very useful, for example to diagnose *focal nodular hyperplasia*. Another important indication is to diagnose or confirm *splenosis* or *splenic remnants*. Planar imaging may be diagnostic; however, single photon emission computed tomography (SPECT) imaging can further increase detectability and interpretation confidence (Figure 89.9).

Tc-99m-labeled red blood cell scintigraphy to diagnose cavernous hemangioma of the liver

Tc-99m red blood cell (RBC) scintigraphy has been used for decades to confirm the diagnosis of cavernous hemangiomas in

the liver. Today, MRI is most commonly used for this purpose because of its superior anatomic resolution and high sensitivity for detecting small lesions and hemangiomas adjacent to vascular structures. However, MRI specificity is less than Tc-99m-labeled RBC, because some benign and malignant lesions can have findings similar to hemangioma. A false-positive Tc-99m RBC study is extremely rare. Using SPECT, sensitivity approaches 100% for hemangiomas greater than 1.4 cm in size. Sensitivity decreases for small-size hemangiomas, although hemangiomas as small as 0.5 cm may be detected (Figure 89.10). On scintigraphy, cavernous hemangiomas have increased activity compared to normal liver.

Esophageal motility

Images are acquired as the patient swallows liquids or semisolids with radiotracer. Dynamic image acquisition is performed. Qualitative image analysis with cinematic display is often sufficient to diagnose abnormal esophageal motility; however, a strength of the radionuclide method is quantification. Calculation of an esophageal transit time or the percent residual esophageal activity is performed. Although scintigraphy can serve as a screening test, it is most commonly performed today to evaluate response to therapy (Figure 89.11).

Gastroesophageal reflux

The radionuclide gastroesophageal reflux study is a very sensitive method for detecting reflux. The study's high sensitivity for reflux detection is due to the rapid framing rate used during acquisition (10-s frames for 1 h) (Figure 89.12). For children, formula or milk is mixed with Tc-99m sulfur colloid and ingested and images are acquired for 1 h. For adults, orange juice is commonly used. In addition to visual assessment, quantitative methods are used.

Gastric motility

The radionuclide gastric emptying study has been the standard test for the evaluation of gastric motility for decades. Various radiolabeled meals have been used. Some form of egg meal, often a sandwich, has been common. Collaboration between the American Motility Society and the Society of Nuclear Medicine has resulted in published Consensus Recommendations for solid gastric emptying. The Recommendations call for a specific standardized protocol (Tougas G, Eaker EY, Abell TL, et al. Assessment of gastric emptying using a low fate meal: establishment of international control values. Am J Gastoenterol 2000;95:1456–62), a simplified protocol, a study length of 4 h, 1-min images at 0, 1, 2, and 4 h, and validated normal values (Figure 89.13).

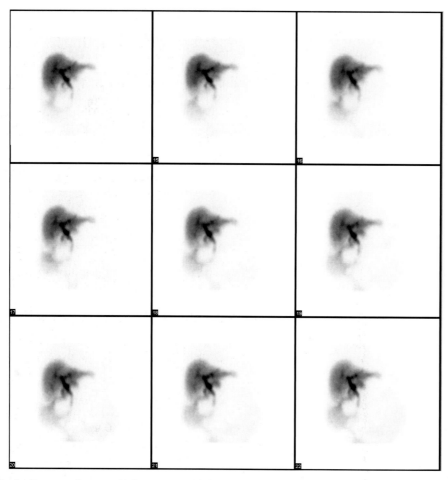

Figure 89.7 Biliary leak after liver transplantation. Technetium 99m-labeled hepatic iminodiacetic acid (Tc-99m HIDA) images show progressive biliary leakage, initially in the right upper quadrant, which increases in intensity and size with time. Bile dispersed throughout much of the abdominal cavity.

It had been standard teaching for years that liquid studies are less sensitive for detecting gastroparesis than solid studies, and thus should only be used when a patient cannot tolerate solids. However, studies have shown that more than 30% of patients with a normal solid study have delayed liquid emptying (Figure 89.14).

Tc-99m red blood cell labeling to detect gastrointestinal bleeding

The patient's RBCs are radiolabeled and imaging is performed initially for 60–90 min and acquired in a rapid framing rate of 0.5–1.0 min/frames. The bleeding study can determine if bleeding is active, the approximate site of the active bleed, and the rate of bleeding (Figure 89.15). Bleeding rates as low as 0.1 mL/min can be detected, which is 10 times more sensitive than contrast angiography. Thus angiographers often request a RBC study prior to angiography. If the RBC study is negative for active bleeding, angiography is very likely to be negative.

Meckel diverticulum and ectopic gastric mucosa

Tc-99m pertechnetate is secreted by gastric mucosa in the stomach and ectopic gastric mucosa, for example Meckel diverticulum. For decades, the Tc-99m pertechnetate *Meckel scan* has been an accurate and accepted methodology to preoperatively confirm the diagnosis. Cimetidine administered as 20 mg/kg orally in divided doses for 2 days prior to the study increases detection by inhibiting release of Tc-99m from the gastric mucosa.

Somatostatin receptor imaging (OctreoScan™)

Somatostatin receptor imaging has proven useful for imaging neuroendocrine tumors, for example gastroenteropancreatic and carcinoid tumors. *Gastroenteropancreatic tumors* are slow growing and often quite small. Most have high concentrations

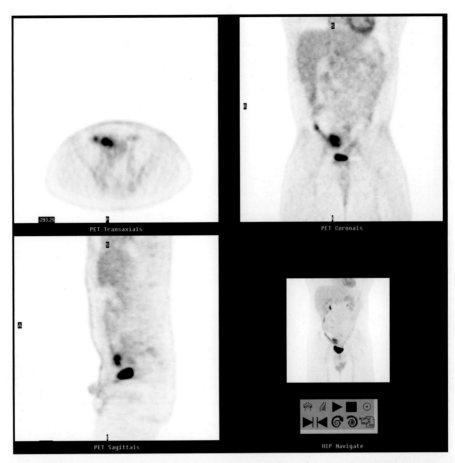

Figure 89.8 Crohn's disease and ^{18}F-labeled fluorodeoxyglucose positron emission tomography (F-18 FDG PET) study. A 33-year-old female presented with symptoms suggestive of intestinal obstruction and a history of Crohn's disease. Computed tomography showed markedly thickened distal ileum. The PET study shows intense increased uptake in the region of the distal ileum consistent with very active inflammation. The patient had an ileal resection for persistent high-grade obstruction.

of somatostatin receptors. Symptoms are secondary to the hormonal activity expressed, for example hypoglycemia, gastric ulcers, severe diarrhea, and flushing. Frequently, the tumors have metastasized by the time of diagnosis, to liver, lymph nodes, bone, lungs, and skin. *Gastrointestinal carcinoid tumors* are derived from the foregut, midgut, or hindgut. The midgut carcinoids with liver metastases cause the carcinoid syndrome with symptoms and signs of flushing, diarrhea, wheezing, and valvular right heart disease.

In-111 pentreotide (OctreoScan®) is a somatostatin receptor imaging radiopharmaceutical. Sensitivity for detection of carcinoid tumors and gastrinomas is high (80%–90%), lower for VIPomas and glucagonomas (75%), and poorest for insulinomas (50%) (Figures 89.16 and 89.17). Conventional imaging, for example ultrasonography, MRI, and CT, have lower tumor detection rates. Somatostatin receptor imaging is used at the time of initial diagnosis to detect metastatic disease, for staging, and evaluating response to therapy. It can help select patients likely to respond favorably to octreotide therapy. OctreoScan

imaging positively impacts patient management in 25%–45% of patients.

F-18 FDG PET imaging of gastrointestinal malignancies

F-18 FDG PET is a well-accepted method to diagnose, stage, restage, and monitor response to therapy for many gastrointestinal malignancies. F-18 FDG is a radiolabeled glucose analog. It is transported into the cell and phosphorylated by the same mechanism as glucose but is unable to be metabolized further and is therefore trapped intracellularly. Most malignant tumor cells exhibit increased glucose metabolism compared to normal tissue cells and have increased uptake of F-18 FDG. Whole-body cross-sectional imaging is routinely performed. Most PET scanners today are hybrid PET/CT cameras. The PET and CT images are obtained sequentially with the patient lying on a table that moves between the two adjacent scanners. Images are

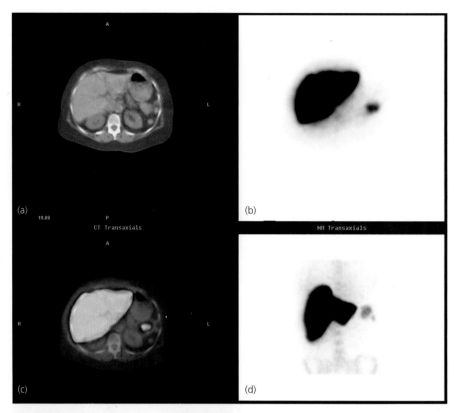

Figure 89.9 (a–d) Splenosis. This 68-year-old female had acute abdominal pain. A left-sided mass was seen on computed tomography (CT), thought possibly to be splenic tissue. The patient has a history of splenectomy secondary to trauma. A Tc-99m sulfur colloid liver–spleen single photon emission computed tomography (SPECT)/CT scan showed uptake in the mass consistent with splenic tissue. A second smaller adjacent mass is seen on the maximum intensity projection (MIP) image **(d)**.

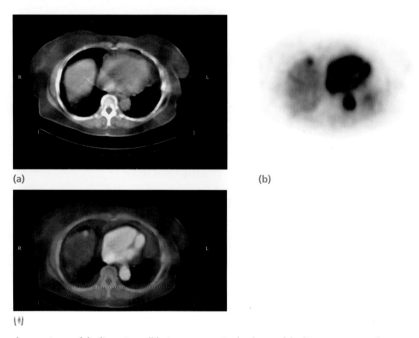

Figure 89.10 Cavernous hemangioma of the liver. A small lesion was seen in the dome of the liver on computed tomography (CT) in a patient with a history of colon cancer **(a)**. The CT report suggested a possible cavernous hemangioma, but could not exclude tumor. The Tc-99m radiolabeled red blood cell study shows increased uptake on the single photon emission computed tomography (SPECT) **(b)** and the fused SPECT/CT study **(c)**, confirming a hemangioma.

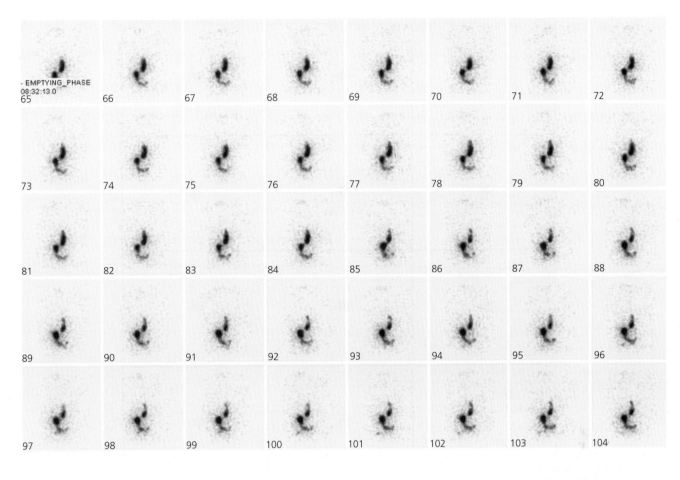

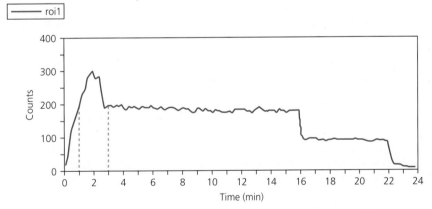

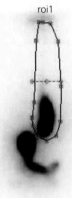

Figure 89.11 Achalasia. Esophageal swallow study. Sequential 15-s images (posterior view) (24 min acquisition) after ingestion of a corn flake and milk meal with Tc-99m sulfur colloid demonstrates very slow and delayed clearance from the esophagus. A region of interest (ROI) drawn around the esophagus generates a time–activity curve and allows for quantification of the delayed clearance. The drop in counts at 16 and 24 min is due to the ingestion of additional clear liquids.

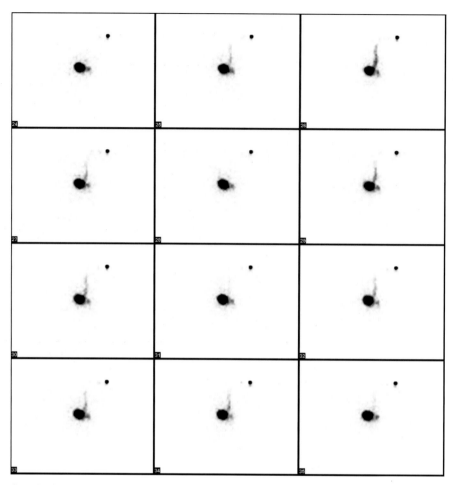

Figure 89.12 Gastroesophageal reflux. A neonate with failure to thrive ingested her usual formula meal with Tc-99m sulfur colloid. Ten-second sequential frames show frequent episodes of reflux of varying length, but mostly high level (above mid esophagus). The black dot in the left upper corner is a radioactive marker to show the level of the mouth.

registered and fused (overlayed) for functional and anatomical correlation (Figure 89.18).

F-18 FDG uptake is quite high in many gastrointestinal malignancies, including colorectal cancer, esophageal cancer, and pancreatic cancer. Although not routinely used for primary diagnosis in colorectal cancer, it can be helpful in patients at high risk for metastases. FDG PET can detect tumor recurrence when other imaging modalities are negative in patients with an elevated serum carcinoembryonic antigen level. It is used to evaluate patients with a single known liver metastasis that is potentially resectable. Preoperative detection of distant metastases is poor by conventional methods. This is a major strength of FDG PET. FDG PET frequently changes patient management, with a reported clinical impact on patient care in 30%–40% of patients. FDG PET can determine the effectiveness of chemotherapy and radiation therapy. It is commonly used for patients with esophageal and pancreatic cancer, for staging, restaging, and evaluating response to therapy.

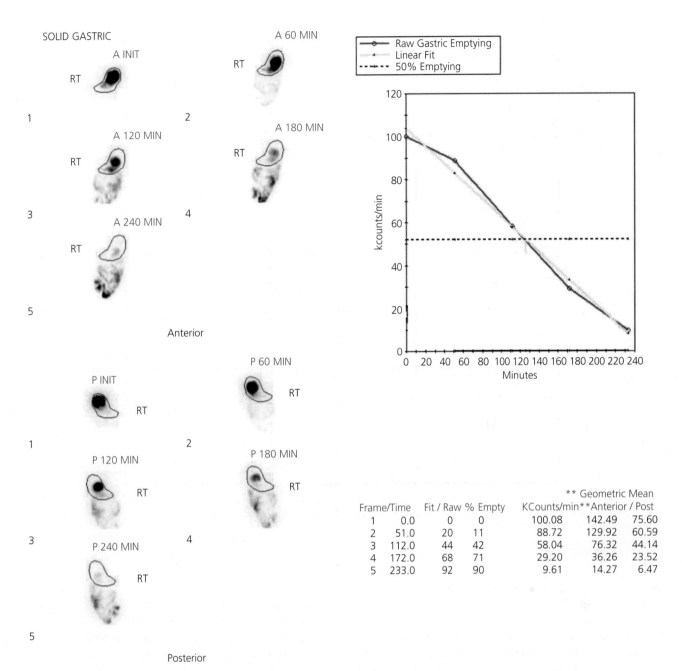

Frame/Time		Fit / Raw	% Empty	KCounts/min	** Geometric Mean Anterior / Post	
1	0.0	0	0	100.08	142.49	75.60
2	51.0	20	11	88.72	129.92	60.59
3	112.0	44	42	58.04	76.32	44.14
4	172.0	68	71	29.20	36.26	23.52
5	233.0	92	90	9.61	14.27	6.47

Figure 89.13 Normal solid gastric emptying. Anterior (A) and posterior (P) images were acquired each hour for 4 h. Regions of interest are drawn in the anterior and posterior view and attenuation correction performed. Emptying is normal (normal is >40% at 2 h and >90% at 4 h).

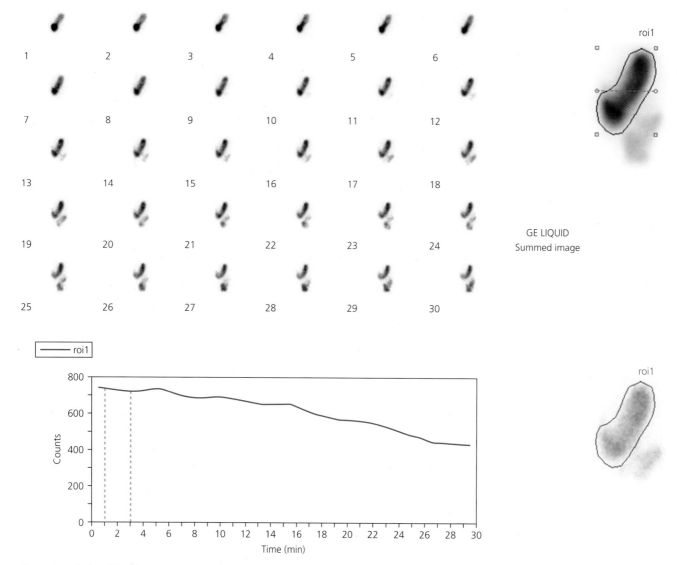

Figure 89.14 Delayed liquid gastric emptying. The patient had symptoms suspicious for gastroparesis. However, the solid emptying study was normal (Figure 89.13). The patient drank 300 mL water with Tc-99m sulfur colloid for the exam. Images were acquired every minute for 30 min. A region of interest (roi) was drawn around the stomach and the time–activity curve generated showed delayed emptying. The emptying half-time was determined to be 45 min (normal <23 min).

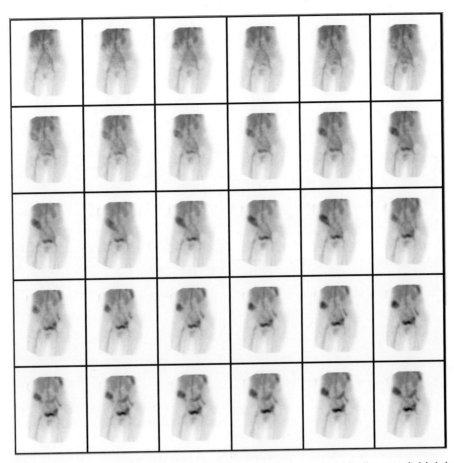

Figure 89.15 Gastrointestinal bleeding scan in patient referred for recent melena. The patient's red blood cells were radiolabeled and thus the images show the normal blood pool in the kidneys, spleen, great vessels, and in this case some increasing urinary activity in the bladder due to unlabeled Tc-99m pertechnetate. Sequential images were acquired for 90 min. Increasing radioactivity is seen over time in the right upper quadrant in the region of the hepatic flexure. With time it transited to the descending colon and rectosigmoid. This was consistent with an active, fairly rapid hepatic flexure colon bleed, confirmed by angiography, due to angiodysplasia.

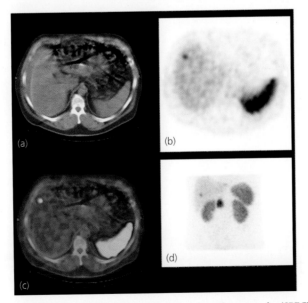

Figure 89.16 Somatostatin receptor imaging (OctreoScan) single photon emission computed tomography (SPECT)/CT of pancreatic islet cell tumor: CT slice **(a)**, SPECT transaxial slice **(b)**, fused SPECT/CT image **(c)**. The maximum intensity projection (MIP) image (anterior view), a three dimensional reconstructed abdominal image **(d)**, shows normal uptake in spleen and kidneys and focal hot uptake in a midline mass, the patient's islet cell tumor. In addition, a small focus of uptake is seen in the anterior inferior portion of the liver on the MIP view, the SPECT, and the fused images. This is a metastasis.

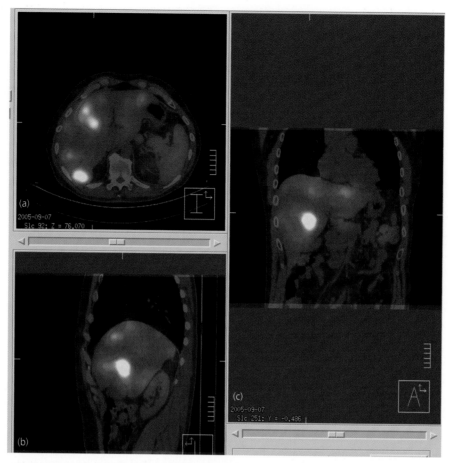

Figure 89.17 OctreoScan single photon emission computed tomography (SPECT)/CT of carcinoid tumor. Fused SPECT and CT images with transverse **(a)**, sagittal **(b)**, and coronal **(c)** slices. Intense uptake is seen in multiple large carcinoid tumors metastatic to the liver.

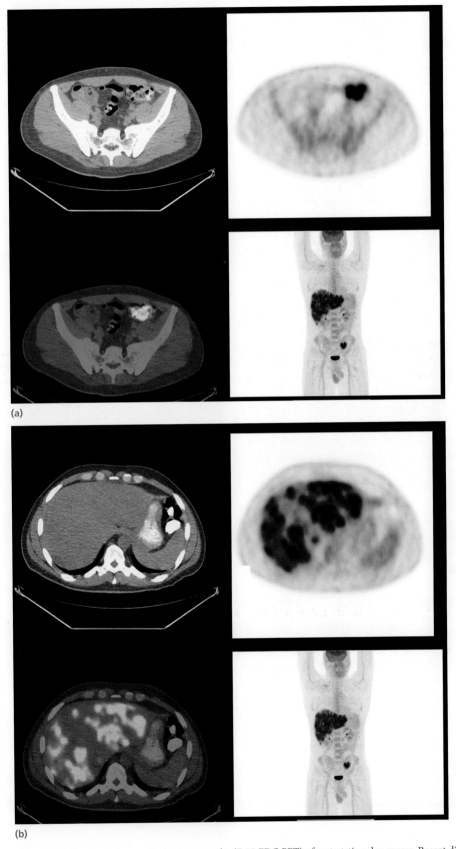

(a)

(b)

Figure 89.18 ¹⁸F-labeled fluorodeoxyglucose positron emission tomography (F-18 FDG PET) of metastatic colon cancer. Recent diagnosis of adenocarcinoma of sigmoid colon. **(a)** Transverse cuts through the primary tumor in the sigmoid colon. Whole-body maximum intensity projection (MIP) anterior view (right lower) shows the primary cancer in the left lower quadrant and extensive metastases to the liver. Multiple small regions of focal uptake are seen in renal calyces, which is normal urinary clearance, and bladder clearance. Transverse cross-sectional FDG PET slice (right upper) shows intense FDG uptake in the primary malignancy that corresponds to the CT lesion (left upper) and fused CT and FDG images (left lower). **(b)** Transverse cuts through the liver. Multiple regions of uptake in the liver consistent with metastases.

CHAPTER 90
Abdominal angiography

Kyung Jae Cho
University of Michigan Cardiovascular Center, Ann Arbor, MI, USA

Angiography is performed to establish a specific diagnosis of neoplasm and vascular lesions, to evaluate hepatoportal hemodynamics, and to obtain specific information about vascular anatomy and variation before radiological or surgical intervention. In this chapter the technique and use of angiography in the diagnosis and management of gastrointestinal, pancreatic, hepatic, and splenic lesions are illustrated.

General angiographic technique

Gastrointestinal angiography is performed by means of percutaneous retrograde femoral arterial catheterization (Seldinger technique). The common femoral artery usually is punctured with a 21-gauge (0.032 inch) single-wall puncture needle. The Seldinger technique using the micropuncture set and femoral artery access under ultrasound guidance is shown in Figure 90.1. When the femoral artery cannot be used because of its occlusion, the left axillary or brachial artery is used. The radial artery may also be used for access. Most visceral angiography is performed with 4F or 5F catheters with preshaped configurations. Three commonly used preshaped catheter configurations for visceral angiography are the shepherd's hook, cobra, and sidewinder catheters.

Intraarterial digital subtraction angiography (IA DSA) is currently used for visceral angiography. Conventional angiography using the cut-film technique is no longer used. Both iodinated contrast medium and carbon dioxide (CO_2) are used as a contrast agent. CO_2 is the preferred contrast agent for detection of gastrointestinal (GI) bleeding, wedged hepatic venography, bleeding from traumatic injury of the spleen and liver, and splenoportography (Figure 90.2). Because CO_2 causes no known allergic reactions and nephrotoxicity, the gas should be used as an alternative contrast agent in patients with hypersensitivity to iodinated contrast material or renal insufficiency.

The techniques used in visceral angiography are aortography, selective and superselective visceral angiography, indirect portography (arterial portography), direct portography (transhepatic, transjugular, transsplenic or transumbilical approach), hepatic venography, and wedged hepatic venography. The coaxial catheterization method using a 3F microcatheter is used for superselective catheterization for embolization of GI bleeding, tumors, and vascular lesions.

Gastrointestinal angiography

Visceral angiography often begins with lateral aortography to visualize the origins of the celiac and superior mesenteric arteries in patients suspected of having mesenteric ischemia (Figure 90.3). Visceral angiography includes the injection into the celiac and superior mesenteric arteries to demonstrate vascular anatomy (Figures 90.4–90.7). Visceral angiography is used for the diagnosis of arterial occlusive disease (Figure 90.8), collateral circulation (Figure 90.9), aneurysms (Figure 90.10), arteriovenous fistulae (Figure 90.11), and portal vein aneurysm (Figure 90.12).

Angiography plays an important role in the diagnosis of upper and lower gastrointestinal bleeding (Figures 90.13–90.16). Angiography is especially useful in identifying chronic gastrointestinal bleeding from tumors (Figure 90.17), vascular malformations (Figure 90.18), and colonic vascular ectasia (Figure 90.19). Visualization of the portal venous system is important in the evaluation of cirrhosis, portal hypertension, and pancreatic, biliary, and hepatic tumors. The portal vein can be evaluated by means of indirect portography (arterial portography) (Figures 90.20 and 90.21) or direct portography (Figures 90.22 and 90.23). Angiography is used to differentiate occlusive from nonocclusive mesenteric ischemia. It is also useful in the diagnosis of carcinoid tumor (Figure 90.24) and both pancreatic (Figure 90.25) and hepatic (Figure 90.26) metastases. Diagnostic angiography is performed prior to balloon angioplasty of superior mesenteric artery stenosis and transcatheter embolization for control of upper and lower GI bleeding, and

Yamada's Atlas of Gastroenterology, Fifth Edition. Edited by Daniel K. Podolsky, Michael Camilleri, J. Gregory Fitz, Anthony N. Kalloo, Fergus Shanahan, and Timothy C. Wang.
© 2016 John Wiley & Sons, Ltd. Published 2016 by John Wiley & Sons, Ltd.
Companion website: www.yamadagastro.com/atlas

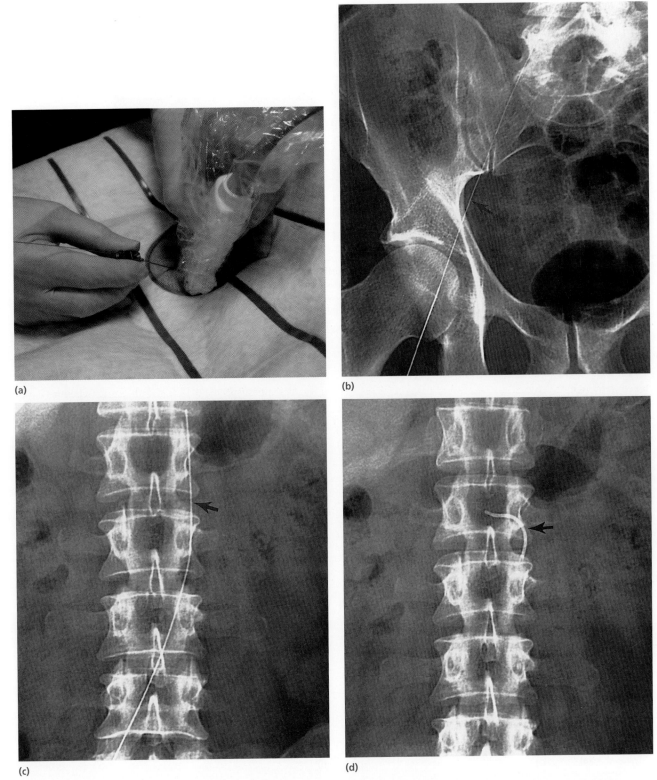

(a)

(b)

(c)

(d)

Figure 90.1 Seldinger technique for percutaneous angiography with micropuncture technique. **(a)** The common femoral artery is accessed with a 21-gauge needle under ultrasound guidance. **(b)** The 0.018-inch (0.46-mm) guidewire (arrow) is introduced through the iliac artery into the aorta. **(c)** The 0.035-inch guidewire (arrow) is introduced into the aorta through a 4F coaxial dilator, which was advanced over the 0.018-inch guidewire. **(d)** The 5F shepherd's hook catheter (arrow) has been placed in the abdominal aorta for catheterization of the branches of the aorta. A pigtail catheter should be used for abdominal aortography with contrast medium whereas an end-hole catheter is used for CO_2 aortography.

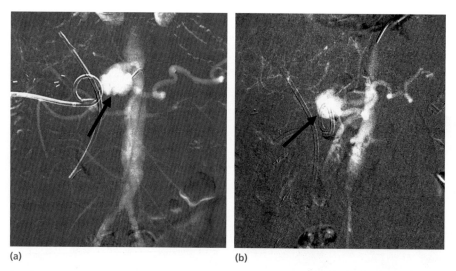

(a)   (b)

Figure 90.2 CO$_2$ celiac digital subtraction arteriogram in a 61-year-old woman with a history of gallbladder cancer presented with massive upper GI bleeding following wedge liver resection. **(a)** CO$_2$ injection into the celiac axis shows a pseudoaneurysm (arrow). CO$_2$ reflux visualizes the aorta and its branches. There are a biliary plastic stent and a percutaneous drainage catheter for bile leak. **(b)** Cross-table lateral projection with CO$_2$ shows the pseudoaneurysm (arrow) arising from the celiac artery. Coil embolization occluded the pseudoaneurysm, resulting in cessation of GI bleeding.

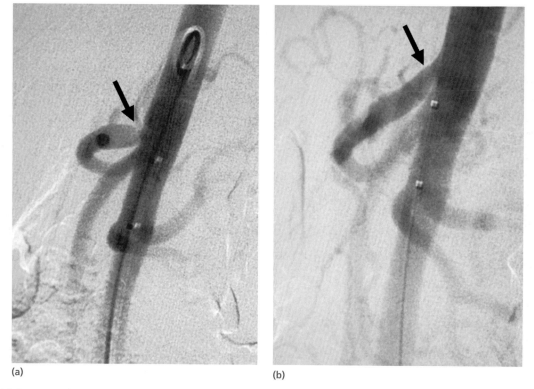

(a)   (b)

Figure 90.3 Median arcuate ligament compression of the celiac artery in a 28-year-old woman with postprandial abdominal pain. **(a)** Full expiration. The origin of the celiac axis has a 60% stenosis (arrow) caused by median arcuate ligament compression. **(b)** Full inspiration. The origin of the celiac axis shows no stenosis (arrow).

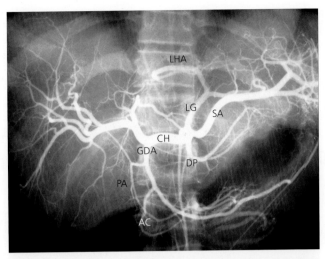

Figure 90.4 Celiac axis anatomy. The celiac axis gives off the splenic (SA), left gastric (LG), and common hepatic (CH) arteries. There is an aberrant left hepatic artery (LHA) originating from the left gastric artery. The common hepatic artery divides into the gastroduodenal artery (GDA) and proper hepatic arteries. The gastroduodenal artery gives rise to the posterior arcade (PA) and anterior arcade (AC) arteries, which join to form the inferior pancreaticoduodenal artery. The dorsal pancreatic (DP) artery originates from the celiac artery.

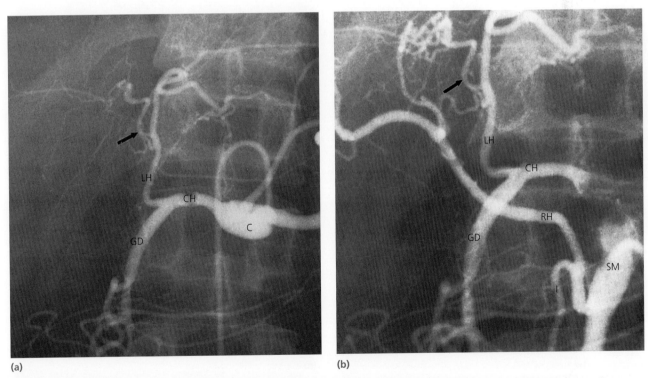

(a)   (b)

Figure 90.5 Aberrant right hepatic artery originating from the superior mesenteric artery. **(a)** The common hepatic artery (CH) divides into the gastroduodenal (GD) and left hepatic (LH) arteries. The middle hepatic artery (arrow) originates from the left hepatic artery (LH). **(b)** Arterial phase of superior mesenteric arteriogram of the same patient. The replaced right hepatic (RH) originates from the superior mesenteric artery (SM), and the inferior pancreaticoduodenal (I) artery originates from the aberrant right hepatic artery. The gastroduodenal (GD) and left hepatic (LH) arteries are filled from the superior mesenteric artery because of celiac stenosis.

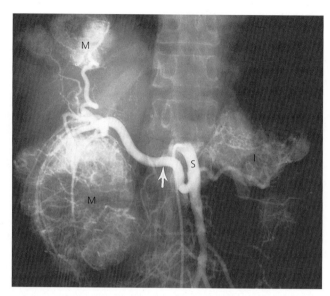

Figure 90.6 Hepatic artery variation. Superior mesenteric arteriogram in a patient with hepatic metastases (M) from nonfunctioning islet cell carcinoma of the pancreas (I). The right hepatic artery (arrow) is replaced from the superior mesenteric artery (S) and supplies hypervascular metastases (M) in the liver. The splenic, left gastric, and common hepatic arteries originate from the celiac axis (not shown).

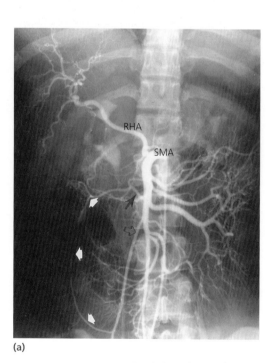
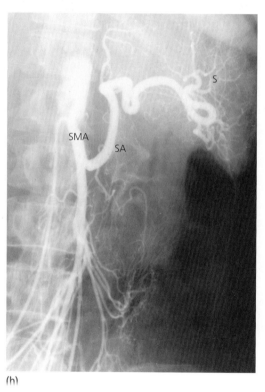

(a)   (b)

Figure 90.7 Celiac trunk variations. (a) Arterial phase of a superior mesenteric angiogram. The right hepatic artery (RHA) has a replaced origin from the superior mesenteric artery (SMA). The middle colic (black arrow) and right colic (black open arrow) arteries form the paracolic arcade (white arrows) along the ascending colon. The common hepatic and splenic arteries arise from the celiac trunk (not shown). (b) Arterial phase of a superior mesenteric angiogram. The splenic artery (SA) has a replaced origin from the superior mesenteric artery (SMA). In this patient, the celiac trunk gives off a left gastric artery and a common hepatic artery (not shown). S, spleen.

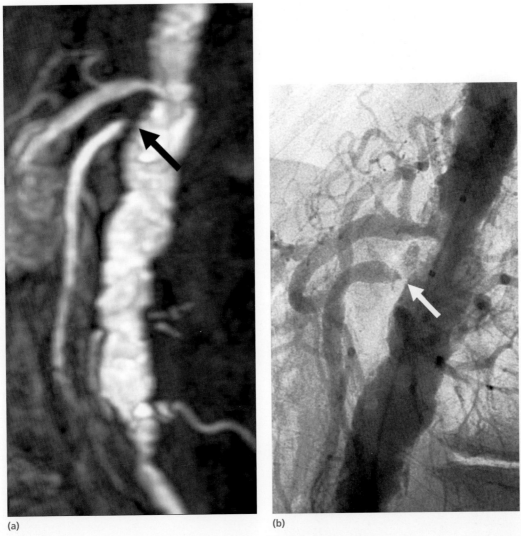

(a)

(b)

Figure 90.8 Superior mesenteric artery occlusion. **(a)** Magnetic resonance angiography (sagittal view) demonstrates mild celiac stenosis and occlusion of the superior mesenteric artery (arrow). **(b)** Lateral aortogram. The superior mesenteric artery is occluded (arrow).

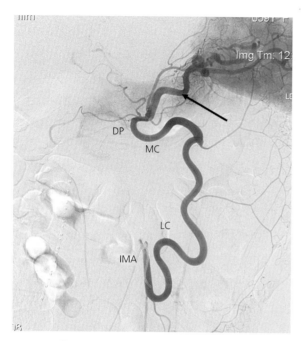

Figure 90.9 Collateral circulation from interior mesenteric artery in celiac artery occlusion. The left colic branch (LC) of the inferior mesenteric artery (IMA) is markedly dilated. Blood flows through this artery to the middle colic (MC), to the dorsal pancreatic (DP) and to the splenic artery (arrow).

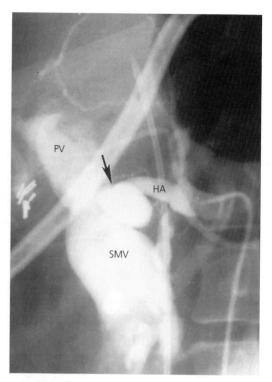

Figure 90.11 Arterioportal fistula that developed after a gunshot wound. Selective hepatic arteriogram (oblique view) demonstrates a large fistula (arrow) and aneurysm between the hepatic artery (HA) and portal vein (PV). SMV, superior mesenteric vein.

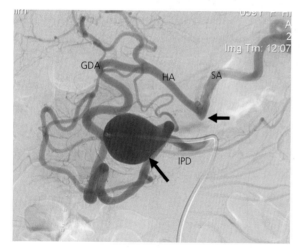

Figure 90.10 Pancreatic artery aneurysm. Arteriogram with the injection of contrast medium into the inferior pancreaticoduodenal artery (IPD). There is an aneurysm (arrow) on the posterior arcade artery. The celiac artery is occluded (shorter arrow). The posterior and anterior arcades are markedly dilated, and blood flows through these arteries to the gastroduodenal (GDA) and to the hepatic (HA) and splenic (SA) arteries.

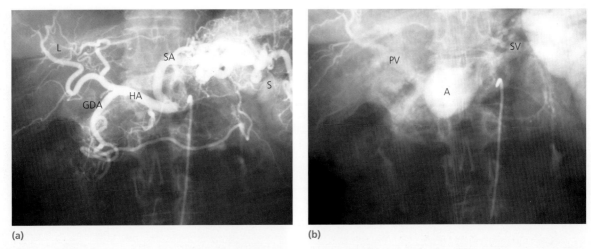

(a)

(b)

Figure 90.12 Portal venous aneurysm. **(a)** Celiac arteriogram shows tortuous splenic artery (SA), patent hepatic (HA) and gastroduodenal (GDA) artery. S, spleen, L, liver. **(b)** Venous phase of the celiac angiogram shows a portal vein aneurysm (A) arises from the junction of the splenic (SV) and portal (PV) veins. Venous aneurysms may occur in the splenic, superior mesenteric, and portal veins. Most portal vein aneurysms are found incidentally and cause no specific symptoms.

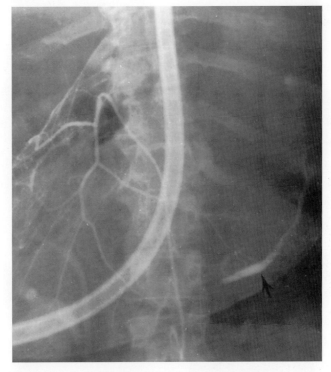

Figure 90.13 Arterial bleeding from a peptic ulcer. The catheter has been selectively placed into the left gastric artery. Angiogram shows extravasation of contrast medium in the body of the stomach near the greater curvature. The extravasated contrast medium gives the appearance of a vein ("pseudovein" sign) (arrow). The bleeding was successfully controlled by gelatin sponge (Gelfoam, Upjohn, Kalamazoo, MI) embolization.

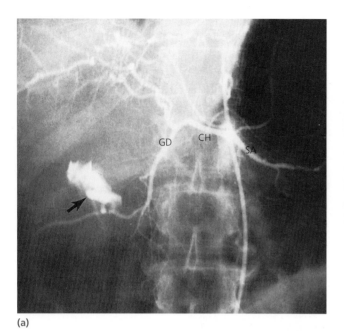

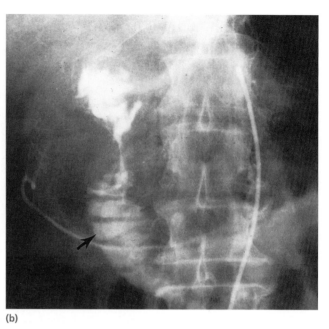

(a)

(b)

Figure 90.14 Massive arterial bleeding into the duodenum of a patient with peptic ulcer. **(a)** Celiac arteriogram (arterial phase) shows branches of the celiac artery with severe vasoconstriction caused by hypovolemic shock. Massive contrast extravasation is demonstrated in the duodenal bulb (arrow) from the proximal gastroepiploic artery. SA, splenic artery; CH, common hepatic artery; GD, gastroduodenal artery. **(b)** Venous phase of same angiogram shows extravasated contrast medium outlining the mucosal folds of the duodenum (arrow).

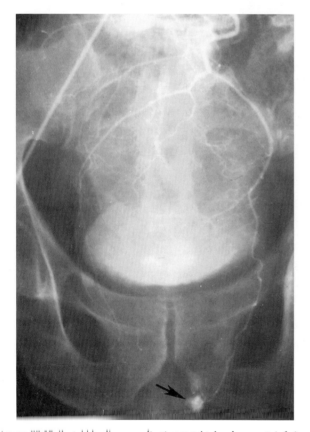

Figure 90.15 Rectal bleeding complicating rectal tube placement. Inferior mesenteric arteriogram shows active bleeding (arrow) into the distal rectum. Vasopressin infusion stopped the bleeding. Superselective embolization may also be used for control of the bleeding.

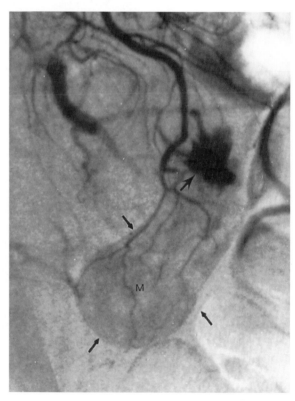

Figure 90.16 Intestinal bleeding from Meckel diverticulum. Superior mesenteric arteriogram of a 7 year old girl with lower gastrointestinal bleeding shows Meckel diverticulum (M, small arrows) and extravasation of the contrast medium (large arrow) near its attachment to the ileum.

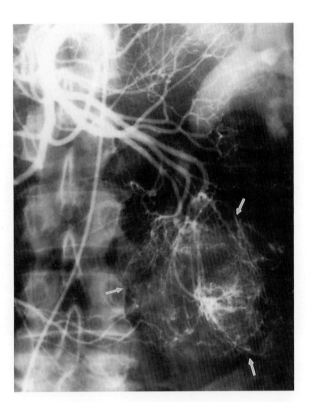

Figure 90.17 Intestinal leiomyosarcoma. Superior mesenteric arteriogram demonstrates a vascular tumor with dilated feeding arteries and tumor vessels (arrows). The inhomogeneous tumor blush and poor margin of the tumor suggest a malignant tumor.

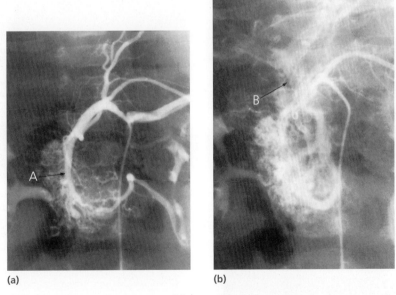

(a)

(b)

Figure 90.18 Pancreatic and duodenal arteriovenous malformations. **(a)** Arterial phase of a gastroduodenal angiogram of a 7-month-old boy with gastrointestinal hemorrhage demonstrates tortuous abnormal vascular channels in the duodenum and pancreas. The gastroduodenal artery (A) and its branches supply the malformations. **(b)** Parenchymal phase demonstrates mottled staining and early, dense venous opacification from the lesion. B, portal vein. Source: Chuang VP, Pulmano CM, Walter JF, et al. Angiography of pancreatic arteriovenous malformation. Am J Roentgenol 1977;129:1015. Reproduced with permission of the American Roentgen Ray Society.

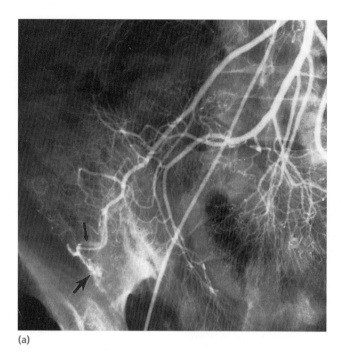

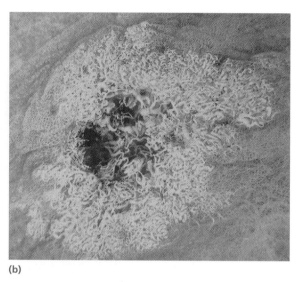

(a)

(b)

Figure 90.19 Vascular ectasia of the cecum. **(a)** Superior mesenteric arteriogram of a 70-year-old woman with recurrent lower gastrointestinal bleeding. Dilated cecal artery feeds a small mucosal vascular ectasia (large arrow). An early draining vein (small arrow) is beginning to fill. **(b)** The resected cecum has been injected with Microfil (Canton Bio-Medical Products, Inc., Boulder, CO) and has undergone the clearing process. Mucosal vascular ectasia is present.

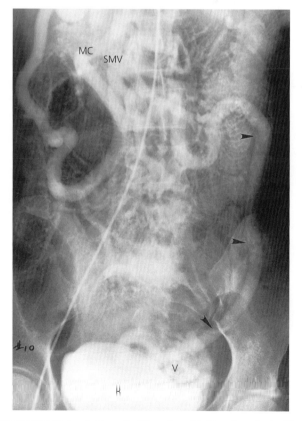

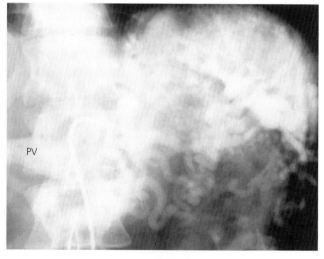

Figure 90.21 Isolated gastric varices of a patient with splenic vein occlusion associated with pancreatitis. Venous phase of splenic angiogram shows varices in the wall of the stomach and upper abdomen. Varices reconstitute the portal vein (PV). Splenectomy is curative for bleeding gastric varices. Partial splenic artery embolization is a safe, effective alternative to surgical treatment.

Figure 90.20 Varices in the wall of the urinary bladder of a patient with hematuria. Venous phase of superior mesenteric angiogram shows large varices (V) in the wall of the bladder (B) filled from the superior mesenteric vein (SMV) through the middle (MC) and left colic (arrowheads) veins.

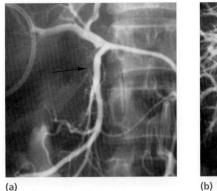
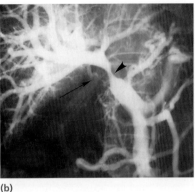

(a)　　　　　　　　　　　(b)

Figure 90.22 Invasion of common bile duct by gallbladder carcinoma. **(a)** Arterial phase of a hepatic angiogram demonstrates occlusion of the bile duct artery (arrow). **(b)** Portal venogram through the percutaneous transhepatic approach shows that vein of the bile duct (arrow) and portal vein (arrowhead) are encased, indicating unresectability of the tumor.

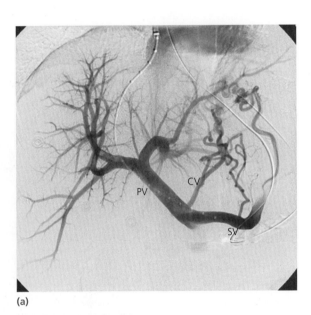
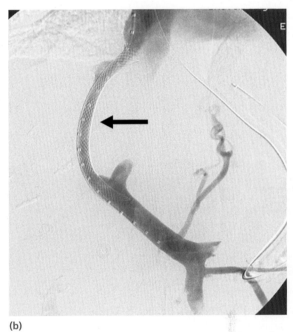

(a)　　　　　　　　　　　(b)

Figure 90.23 Transjugular portography in a patient with cirrhosis and portal hypertension. **(a)** Direct splenoportogram: the splenic and portal veins are patent, and portal blood flows toward the liver (hepatopetal). The coronary vein (CV) and gastric varices are filled. **(b)** After creation of a portosystemic shunt (TIPS), the TIPS stent (arrow) is patent, and blood flows through this TIPS stent and to the hepatic vein.

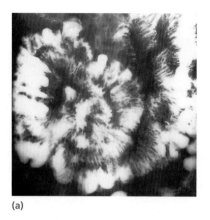

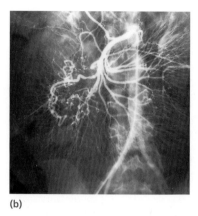

(a)   **(b)**

Figure 90.24 Ileal carcinoid tumor with mesenteric metastases. **(a)** Barium study of a 52-year-old woman with diarrhea and abdominal pain shows that loops of small bowel are retracted and their walls are thickened. **(b)** Superior mesenteric arteriogram shows that right colic and ileocolic arteries are encased and the mesenteric artery branches are retracted into a stellate pattern. Source: Reuter SR, Redman HC, Cho KJ. Gastrointestinal Angiography, 3rd edn, 1986. Reproduced with permission of Elsevier.

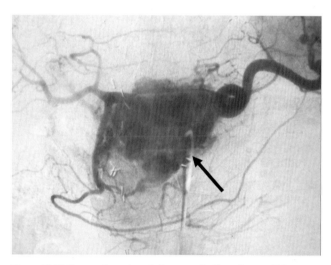

Figure 90.25 Pancreatic metastasis from renal cell carcinoma. Celiac angiogram shows a large hypervascular tumor (arrow) in the head and neck region of the pancreas.

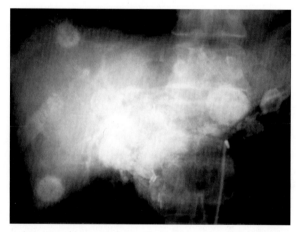

Figure 90.26 Liver metastases from renal cell carcinoma. Parenchymal phase of a hepatic angiogram shows multiple hypervascular metastases. Other vascular hepatic metastases are from pancreatic neuroendocrine tumors, carcinoid tumors, renal cell carcinoma, medullary thyroid carcinoma, and melanoma.

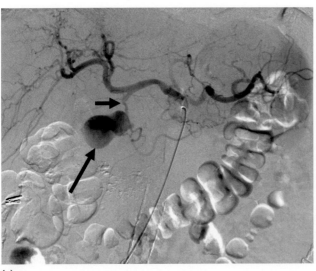

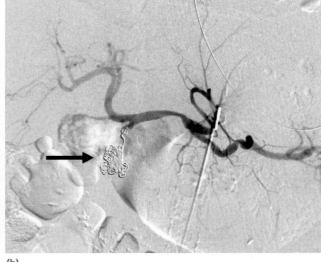

(a)   **(b)**

Figure 90.27 Gastroduodenal artery pseudoaneurysm in a 57-year-old man with chronic pancreatitis and hemtochezia. **(a)** Celiac arteriogram (arterial phase) demonstrates a 3-cm pseudoaneurysm (longer arrow) arising from the gastroduodenal artery (shorter arrow). **(b)** Celiac arteriogram following embolization of the gastroduodenal artery pseudoaneurysm with coils and Gelfoam pledgets demonstrates occlusion of the pseudoaneurysm and gastroduodenal artery (arrow). Hematochezia stopped following the embolization.

occlusion of splanchnic artery aneurysms and pseudoaneurysms (Figure 90.27).

Pancreatic angiography

Ultrasound, computed tomography (CT), and magnetic resonance imaging (MRI) are the initial diagnostic procedures for inflammatory and neoplastic pancreatic lesions. Endoscopic retrograde cholangiopancreatography with cytological examination is commonly performed for suspected pancreatic cancer. If endoscopy is unsuccessful in patients with a mass in the pancreatic head and obstructive jaundice, percutaneous transhepatic cholangiogram with biliary drainage is performed. Once pancreatic lesions have been demonstrated by other imaging modalities, angiography may be performed to obtain a specific diagnosis and to assess the vascular anatomy and resectability of the tumor before surgical intervention.

Endoscopic ultrasound scanning is commonly used to localize pancreatic islet cell tumors. When it reveals a pancreatic mass in a patient with hyperinsulinism, surgical therapy is possible without additional localization procedures. For occult insulinomas, selective arterial calcium stimulation localizes the source of hyperinsulinism through assay of insulin from the hepatic vein at 30 s and 60 s, following stimulation of the potential supplying arteries. Angiography localizes insulinoma in approximately 60% of cases (Figure 90.28). Angiography is often negative for gastrinomas because they are usually hypovascular. However, selective secretin injection regionalizes occult gastrinomas through blood sampling from the hepatic vein at 30 s

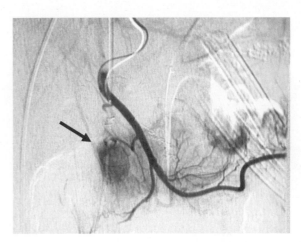

Figure 90.28 Insulinoma. Gastroduodenal arteriogram shows a vascular lesion in the head of the pancreas (arrow) representing an islet cell adenoma.

and 60 s following stimulation of the potential feeding artery. Angiography is usually positive for other neuroendocrine tumors, including vasoactive intestinal polypeptide-secreting tumor (VIPoma), pancreatic polypeptide-producing tumor (PPoma), somatostatinoma, and glucagonoma (Figure 90.29). Angiography is important in the diagnosis and management of gastrointestinal bleeding complicating pancreatitis and pseudocysts (Figure 90.30). In this setting, bleeding may originate from an aneurysm or varices associated with portal or splenic venous thrombosis.

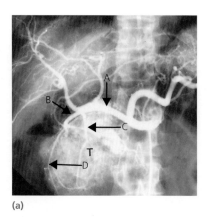
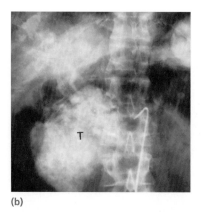

(a) **(b)**

Figure 90.29 Glucagonoma. **(a)** Arterial phase of a celiac angiogram of a 64-year-old man with dermatitis, diabetes mellitus, and anemia. Hypervascular tumor (T) in the head of the pancreas is supplied by the pancreatic arcade arteries. A, common hepatic artery; B, gastroduodenal artery; C, posterior arcade artery; D, anterior arcade artery. **(b)** Parenchymal phase shows tumor has homogeneous dense contrast accumulation characteristic of an islet cell tumor. Source: Cho, KJ, Wilcox CW, Reuter SR. Glucagon-producing islet cell tumor of the pancreas. Am J Roentgenol 1977;129:159. Reproduced with permission of the American Roentgen Ray Society.

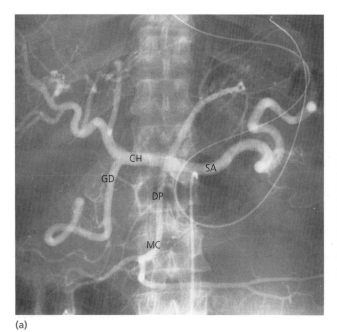
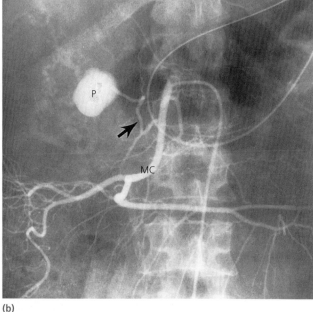

(a) **(b)**

Figure 90.30 Bleeding into a pancreatic pseudocyst. **(a)** Celiac angiogram (arterial phase) shows middle colic artery (MC) arising from the dorsal pancreatic (DP) artery that originates from the celiac axis. SA, splenic artery; CH, common hepatic artery; GD, gastroduodenal artery. **(b)** Selective injection into the dorsal pancreatic artery demonstrates a pseudoaneurysm (P) filled from a branch of the dorsal pancreatic artery (arrow).

Hepatic angiography

Ultrasound, CT (with and without contrast enhancement), and MRI are used for the diagnosis of hepatic mass lesions. Angiography is sensitive in detecting vascular tumors in the liver, including hepatoma, cavernous hemangioma (Figure 90.31), focal nodular hyperplasia (Figure 90.32), and bleeding associated with hepatic adenoma (Figure 90.33).

Hepatic angiography plays an important role in the preoperative evaluation for resectability of tumors; involvement of both lobes, regional lymph node metastases, and portal vein invasion indicate unresectability of the tumor (Figure 90.34). The portal venous phase of high-dose superior mesenteric angiography is used to evaluate the portal venous system. Angiography localizes lesions and can be used for treatment of patients with clinically significant hemobilia (Figure 90.35) or bleeding after

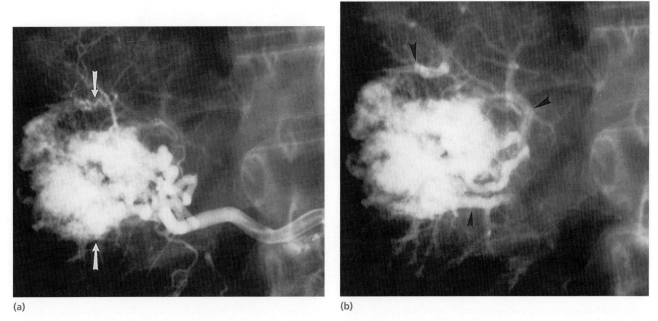

(a)   (b)

Figure 90.31 Cavernous hemangioma. **(a)** Hepatic angiogram (arterial phase) shows dilated hepatic artery and the vascular spaces of the hemangioma filled with contrast medium (arrows). **(b)** Vascular spaces have retained contrast medium through the venous phase, characteristic of hemangioma. Portal veins (arrowheads) are opacified, indicating arteriovenous shunting. Arteriovenous shunting is an unusual finding with hemangioma.

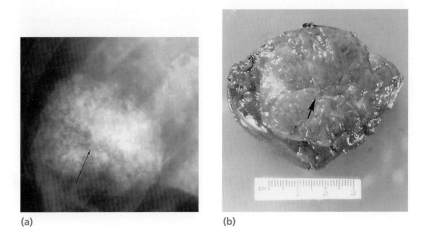

(a)   (b)

Figure 90.32 Focal nodular hyperplasia. **(a)** Parenchymal phase of a hepatic angiogram, magnification technique, of a 26-year-old woman demonstrates nodular accumulation of contrast medium with central scar formation (arrow) typical of focal nodular hyperplasia. **(b)** Section of the resected mass shows a nodular pattern, central scar (arrow), and radiating septa. Source: Reuter SR, Redman HC, Cho KJ. Gastrointestinal Angiography, 3rd edn, 1986. Reproduced with permission of Elsevier.

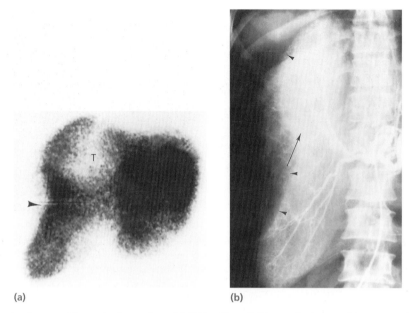

Figure 90.33 Ruptured hepatic adenoma with massive hemorrhage. (a) ⁹⁹ᵐTc sulfur colloid scan of a 30-year-old woman with a history of use of oral contraceptives demonstrates a photon-deficient area (T) and large subcapsular hematoma (arrowhead) in the right lobe of the liver. (b) Arterial phase of a hepatic angiogram demonstrates an avascular mass (arrow) associated with a large subcapsular hematoma (arrowheads). Liver is displaced from the lateral abdominal wall. Source: Reuter SR, Redman HC, Cho KJ. Gastrointestinal Angiography, 3rd edn, 1986. Reproduced with permission of Elsevier.

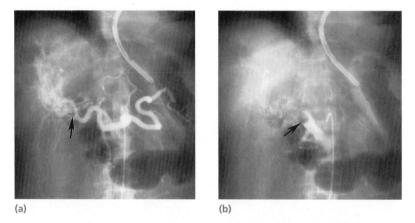

Figure 90.34 Invasion of the portal vein by hepatoma in a patient with esophageal variceal bleeding. (a) Arterial phase of a celiac angiogram shows linear abnormal vessels (arrow) running along the portal vein, known as the threads and streaks sign. (b) Venous phase of same angiogram demonstrates tumor thrombus (arrow) in the portal vein.

laparoscopic cholecystectomy (Figure 90.36). Selective arterial embolization is effective in controlling bleeding from intrahepatic sources and eliminates the need for major surgical intervention.

Panhepatic angiography, including both arterial and venous assessment with manometry, is an important preoperative procedure for portosystemic shunt operations and endovascular interventions. Angiography is essential in the diagnosis of Budd–Chiari syndrome (Figure 90.37). Hepatic venography

with injection of contrast medium into the occluded hepatic vein or patent accessory vein usually demonstrates typical spider web collaterals. Angiographic methods used for the management of Budd–Chiari syndrome include percutaneous transluminal angioplasty, placement of metallic stents, and transjugular intrahepatic portacaval shunt (TIPS). Wedged hepatic venography and manometry is important in the angiographic evaluation of patients with cirrhosis and portal hypertension. Wedged hepatic venography is performed to

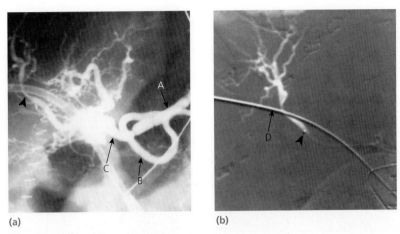

Figure 90.35 Superselective catheterization of a hepatic artery branch in a patient with hemobilia subsequent to percutaneous biliary drainage. **(a)** Celiac arteriogram shows biliary catheter has injured a right hepatic arterial branch (arrowhead). **(b)** Digital subtraction arteriogram through a 3F coaxial catheter (arrowhead) in the bleeding artery demonstrates arterial injury. Hemobilia was controlled by means of embolization. A, celiac artery; B, splenic artery; C, hepatic artery; D, transhepatic biliary catheter.

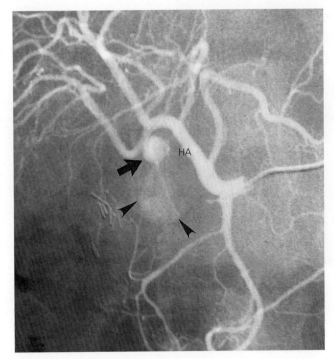

Figure 90.36 Massive bleeding complicating laparoscopic cholecystectomy. Hepatic angiogram (arterial phase) demonstrates bleeding (arrowheads) from pseudoaneurysm (arrow) of the right hepatic artery (HA).

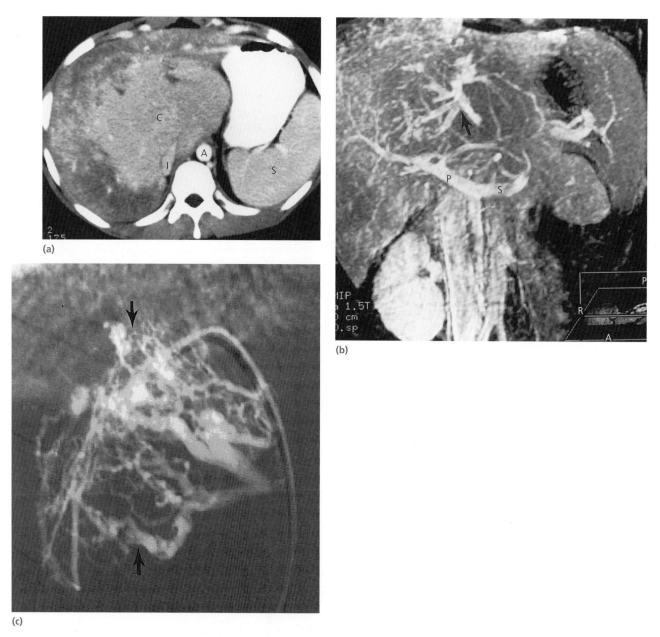

(a)

(b)

(c)

Figure 90.37 Budd–Chiari syndrome. **(a)** Computed tomographic scan of a 23-year-old woman with ascites and pulmonary embolism demonstrates an enlarged caudate lobe (C) and inhomogeneous perfusion in the periphery of the liver. A, aorta; I, inferior vena cava; S, spleen. **(b)** Three-dimensional contrast magnetic resonance angiogram demonstrates obliteration of the hepatic veins. The dilated accessory hepatic veins (arrow) drain from the caudate lobe into the inferior vena cava. The splenic (S) and portal (P) veins are patent. **(c)** Wedged hepatic venogram with injection of contrast medium through the occluded hepatic vein demonstrates typical spider web hepatic venous collateral vessels (arrows). The patient underwent orthotopic liver transplantation.

diagnose portal vein occlusion (Figure 90.38), facilitate transjugular liver biopsy (Figure 90.39), and to visualize the portal vein target for a TIPS procedure. In the absence of presinusoidal obstruction, wedged hepatic venous pressure reflects sinusoidal pressure.

Splenic angiography

The splenic artery is a branch of the celiac artery, but rarely originates from the superior mesenteric artery. The splenic artery gives rise to the dorsal pancreatic, pancreatica magna, caudal pancreatic, and left gastroepiploic arteries before branching into the segmental arteries of the spleen. Occasionally, it gives rise to accessory left gastric and superior polar splenic artery before entering the hilus of the spleen. The short gastric arteries arise from the splenic arterial branches in the upper pole of the spleen. All branches of the splenic artery provide collateral pathways in occlusion of the celiac, superior mesenteric, and splenic artery. The splenic artery is visualized with the injection of contrast medium into the celiac axis. Selective catheterization of the splenic artery can be performed by advancing a 4F or 5F catheter into the splenic artery over a guide wire. The coaxial catheterization method using a 3F microcatheter is useful for superselective catheterization of the splenic artery and its branches for transcatheter embolization. Splenic angiography is performed for the diagnosis of pancreatic tumor, aneurysm (Figures 90.40 and 90.41), and splenic vein occlusion. Indications for splenic artery embolization include: control of traumatic splenic hemorrhage (Figure 90.42), hypersplenism, using partial splenic artery embolization, gastric variceal bleeding from isolated splenic vein occlusion, prior to

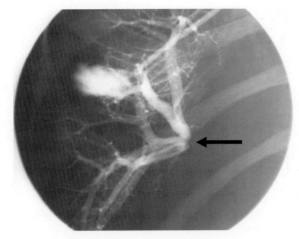

Figure 90.38 Portal vein occlusion. Wedged hepatic venogram with contrast medium shows occlusion of the portal vein (arrow) at the hilus.

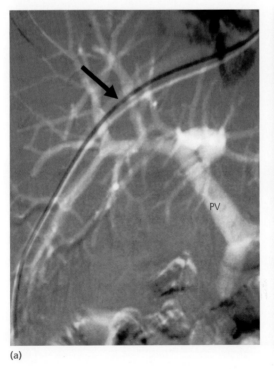

(a)

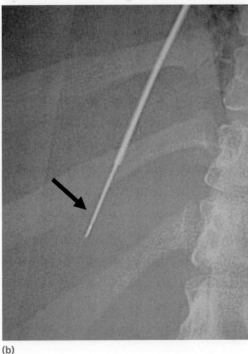

(b)

Figure 90.39 Transjugular liver biopsy. **(a)** CO_2 wedged hepatic venogram shows filling of the portal vein (PV). The right hepatic vein with the catheter in place (arrow) overlies the intrahepatic portal vein branches in the right hepatic lobe. **(b)** Digital image taken during liver biopsy shows a Quick-Core biopsy needle (arrow).

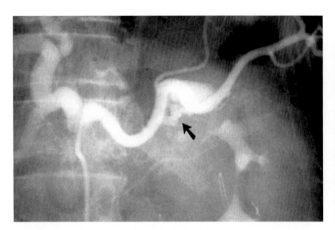

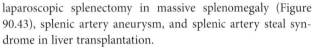

Figure 90.40 Splenic artery aneurysm bleeding into the pancreatic duct. Celiac angiogram shows an aneurysm in the mid part of the splenic artery from which contrast medium extravasates into the pancreatic duct (arrow).

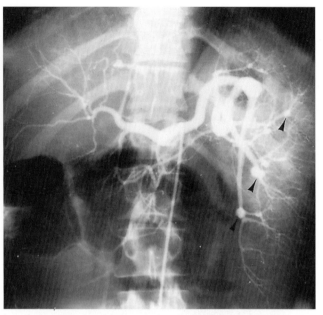

Figure 90.41 Splenic artery aneurysms associated with portal hypertension. Multiple aneurysms are present in the splenic artery branches (arrowheads). The spleen is enlarged because of portal hypertension.

laparoscopic splenectomy in massive splenomegaly (Figure 90.43), splenic artery aneurysm, and splenic artery steal syndrome in liver transplantation.

Percutaneous splenoportography is useful for evaluating the splenic and portal veins in patients with cirrhosis and portal hypertension, and splenic vein occlusion. Noninvasive imaging and indirect splenoportography with the injection of large volume of contrast medium into the splenic artery have largely replaced splenoportography. CO_2 splenoportography with a skinny needle (22- to 25-gauge needle) is a safe, useful technique in visualizing the splenic and portal veins, and portosystemic collaterals. Splenic arterial wedge injection with CO_2 using a microcatheter can visualize the splenic vein and facilitate the diagnosis of splenic vein occlusion.

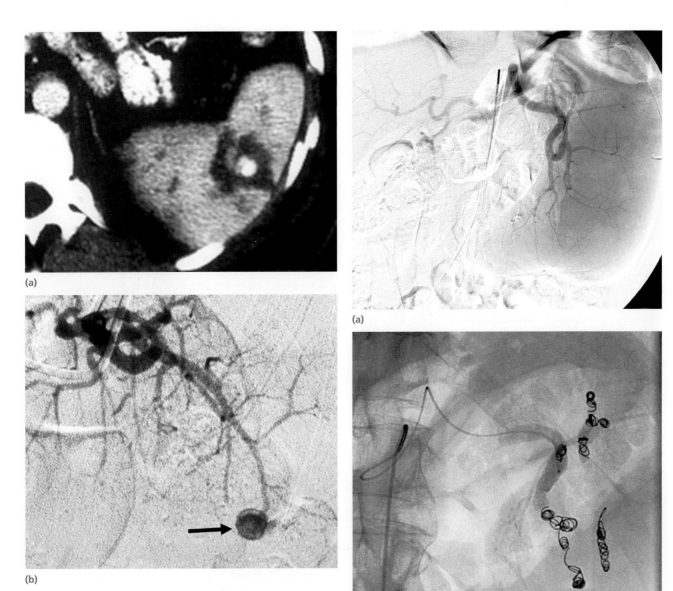

(a)

(b)

Figure 90.42 Traumatic splenic artery pseudoaneurysm. **(a)** Computed tomography taken after splenic injury shows a dense contrast collection within the spleen surrounded by a low-density area. **(b)** Splenic arteriogram shows a discrete pseudoaneurysm in the lower pole of the spleen (arrow). The aneurysm was treated with transcatheter embolization.

(a)

(b)

Figure 90.43 Splenic embolization prior to laparoscopic splenectomy in a 70-year-old man with chronic lymphocytic leukemia. **(a)** Splenic arteriogram shows massive splenomegaly. **(b)** After embolization of the segmental branches of the splenic artery and the distal main splenic artery with coils, an avascular segment is created in the splenic artery to facilitate laparoscopic splenectomy.

CHAPTER 91

Interventional radiology

Todd R. Schlachter, Julius Chapiro, Rafael Duran, Vania Tacher, Camila Zamboni, Luke Higgins, and Jean-Francois Henri Geschwind

Johns Hopkins University School of Medicine, Baltimore, MD, USA

Percutaneous therapies of liver tumors

Vascular and interventional radiology utilize minimally invasive, image-guided, targeted procedures to diagnose and treat diseases in nearly every organ system. In the past decade, advances in technology have combined with the skill set of interventional radiologists and resulted in significant changes in patient care. Interventional radiology procedures frequently offer less risk, less pain, and less recovery time compared to open surgery.

Treatment of primary and secondary liver cancer

Image-guided therapies for primary and secondary liver cancer include intraarterial therapies and percutaneous ablative techniques. With respect to the former, local drug delivery is facilitated by lipiodol emulsions (conventional transarterial chemoembolization, cTACE) or drug-eluting beads (DEB-TACE). Alternatively, radioembolization affords deposition of radiation via beta emitters following intraarterial local delivery, markedly reducing systemic radiation dose. In the context of the liver, ablative therapies utilize thermal heating (microwave or radiofrequency ablation) (Figures 91.1–91.7).

Vascular interventions

Vascular interventions of the gastrointestinal tract are directed at maintaining sufficient perfusion of the abdominal viscera, stopping bleeding, and equilibrating venous pressure. Angiography of the abdominal vasculature is employed both for diagnosis and treatment planning for stenotic vessels, aneurysm formation, and hemorrhagic source (Figures 91.8–91.13).

Transjugular intrahepatic portosystemic shunt and portal vein interventions

Portal hypertension is a common manifestation of chronic liver disease. In the appropriate patient populations, treatment of an increased portal pressure gradient can be achieved with placement of a transjugular intrahepatic portosystemic shunt (TIPS). For example, patients with Budd–Chiari syndrome can undergo TIPS placement or direct intrahepatic portocaval shunt (DIPS) in order to relieve liver congestion, thus obviating the immediate need for liver transplantation (Figures 91.14 and 91.15).

Biliary interventions in interventional radiology

There are innumerable strategies employed by interventionalists for the treatment and diagnosis of diseases affecting the biliary tract, including percutaneous transhepatic cholangiography, biliary drain placement, biliary stent placement, and cholecystostomy tube placement (Figures 91.16, 91.17, 91.18, and 91.19).

Percutaneous gastric, gastrojejunostomy, and jejunostomy feeding tubes

Abdominal interventions are readily used to achieve short or long-term enteric access for nutritional support or gastrointestinal decompression (Figures 91.20, 91.21, and 91.22).

Yamada's Atlas of Gastroenterology, Fifth Edition. Edited by Daniel K. Podolsky, Michael Camilleri, J. Gregory Fitz, Anthony N. Kalloo, Fergus Shanahan, and Timothy C. Wang.
© 2016 John Wiley & Sons, Ltd. Published 2016 by John Wiley & Sons, Ltd.
Companion website: www.yamadagastro.com/atlas

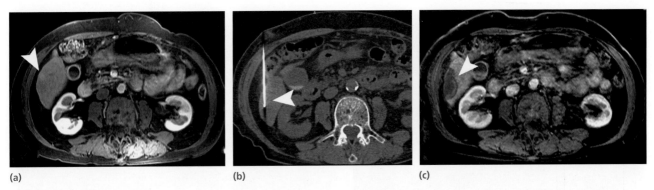

(a)   (b)   (c)

Figure 91.1 Radiofrequency ablation. A patient with a 2.5-cm hepatocellular carcinoma lesion in the left lobe of the liver. **(a)** Baseline magnetic resonance image (MRI) shows enhancement of the target lesion (arrowhead). **(b)** Radiofrequency ablation needle placed under computed tomography guidance (arrowhead). **(c)** Ablation zone in a follow-up MRI 1 month after treatment (arrowhead).

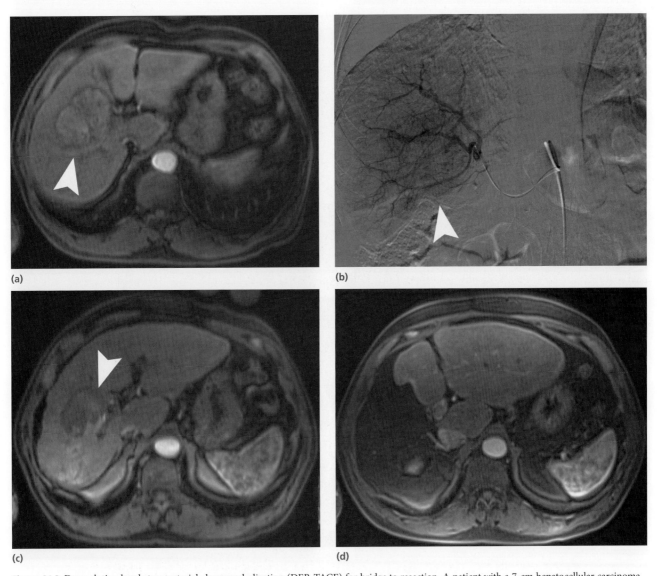

(a)   (b)

(c)   (d)

Figure 91.2 Drug-eluting beads transarterial chemoembolization (DEB-TACE) for bridge to resection. A patient with a 7-cm hepatocellular carcinoma lesion in the right lobe of the liver. **(a)** Baseline magnetic resonance image (MRI) shows homogenous enhancement of the target lesion (arrowhead). **(b)** Angiogram of the right hepatic artery shows a tumor blush (arrowhead). **(c)** Follow-up MRI 1 month after treatment shows a largely necrotic lesion (arrowhead). **(d)** MRI after surgical resection of the right lobe.

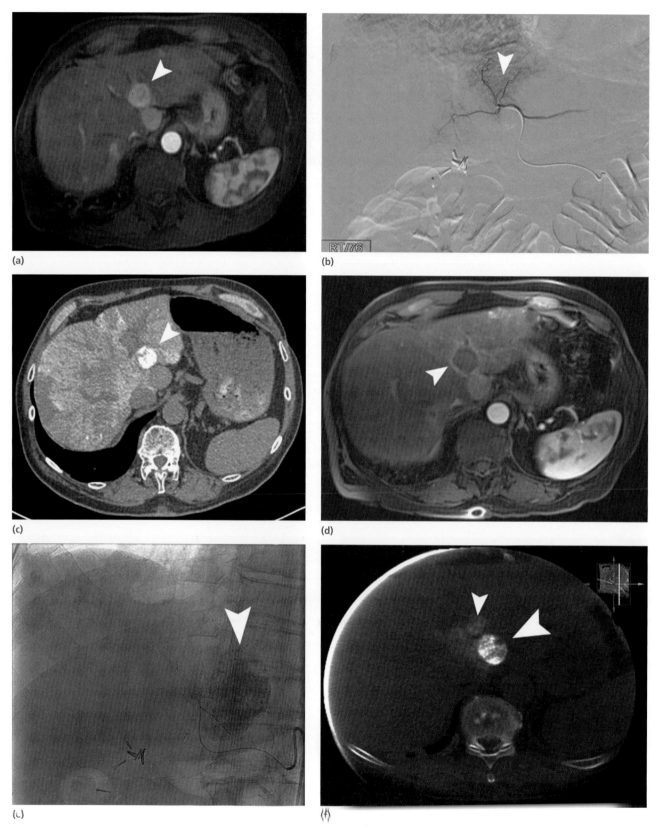

Figure 91.3 Conventional transarterial chemoembolization (cTACE). A patient diagnosed with hepatocellular carcinoma presented with two new 3-cm lesions in the left lobe. **(a)** Baseline magnetic resonance image (MRI) shows two enhancing lesions (arrowhead indicates the target lesion for the initial cTACE). **(b)** Angiogram of the arteries supplying the target lesion (tumor blush, arrowhead). **(c)** Postprocedural computed tomography (CT) scan shows successful deposition of embolic material (arrowhead). **(d)** Follow-up MRI shows necrotic target lesion (arrowhead) next to a viable nontarget lesion. **(e)** Second cTACE, angiogram of the viable lesion (tumor blush, arrowhead). **(f)** Intraprocedural cone-beam CT showing fresh embolic material within the target lesion (large arrowhead) and remaining material within the previously treated lesion (small arrowhead).

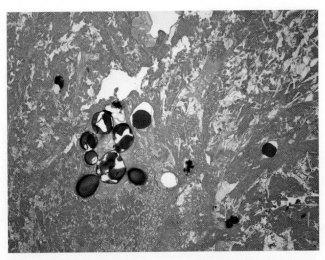

Figure 91.4 Drug-eluting beads and microparticles. H & E-stained slide of an hepatocellular carcinoma lesion, treated with conventional transarterial chemoembolization (cTACE) and drug-eluting beads transarterial chemoembolization (DEB-TACE), shows both microparticles (darker blue) and drug-eluting beads (damaged though cutting artefacts).

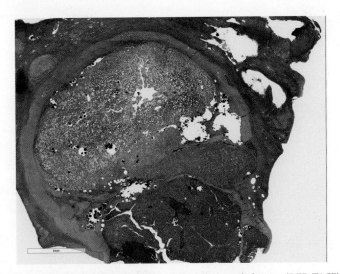

Figure 91.5 Histopathology of a target lesion after drug-eluting beads transarterial chemoembolization (DEB-TACE). H & E-stained slide of a tumor after surgical resection in a patient with hepatocellular carcinoma shows complete necrosis of the lesion and accumulation of drug-eluting beads within the tumor capsule.

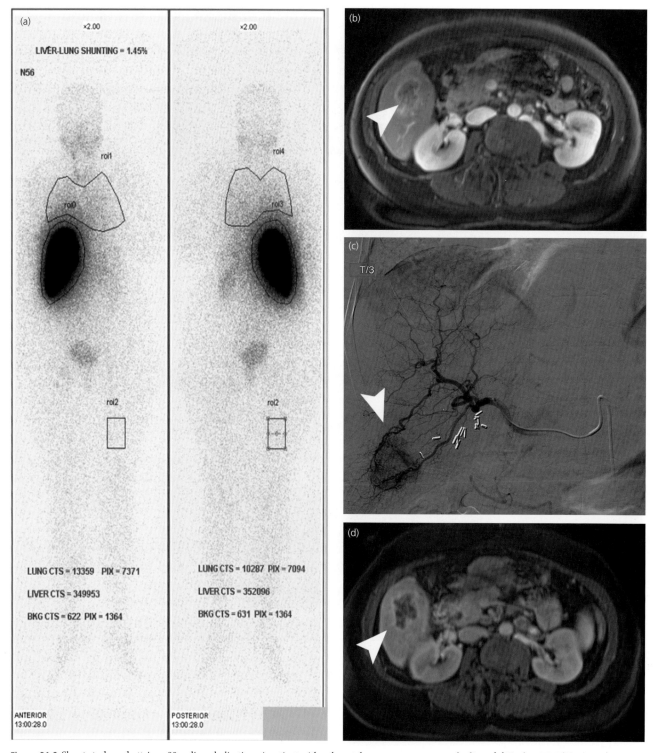

Figure 91.6 Shunt study and yttrium-90 radioembolization. A patient with colorectal cancer metastases to the liver. **(a)** Evaluation of the liver–lung shunting prior to the delivery of yttrium-90. **(b)** Baseline magnetic resonance image (MRI) shows a largely viable lesion within the liver (arrowhead). **(c)** Angiogram of the right hepatic artery prior to the delivery of the payload shows two tumor-feeding arteries and a tumor blush (arrowhead). **(d)** Follow-up MRI shows a largely necrotic lesion (arrowhead) 1 month after treatment.

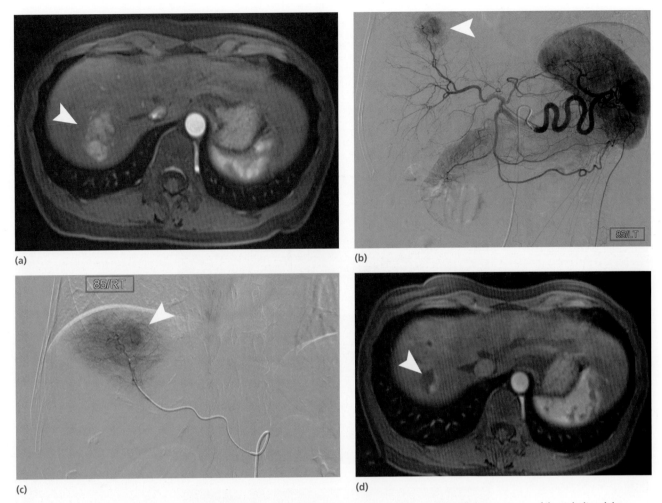

Figure 91.7 Drug-eluting beads transarterial chemoembolization (DEB-TACE). A patient with an hepatocellular carcinoma of the right liver lobe. **(a)** Baseline magnetic resonance image (MRI) shows a well-enhancing lesion (arrowhead) on arterial-phase images. **(b)** Angiogram of the coeliac trunk shows a tumor blush (arrowhead) of the target lesion with a well-contrasted tumor-feeding artery. **(c)** Super-selective angiogram of the tumor-feeding artery (arrowhead) prior to embolization. **(d)** Follow-up MRI shows good tumor response (arrowhead) after treatment.

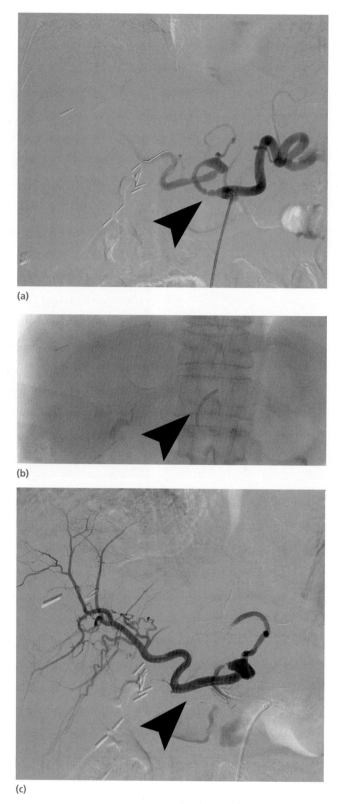

(a)

(b)

(c)

Figure 64.9 Hepatic artery stenosis. A case of a 39-year-old man with history of orthotropic liver transplant complicated with a hepatic artery stenosis at the anastomosis. (a) Celiac axis arteriogram though a catheter showed a high-grade narrowing of the hepatic artery anastomosis (arrowhead). (b) Angioplasty of hepatic artery anastomosis was carried out with a balloon (arrowhead). (c) Successful angioplasty of hepatic artery anastomoses (arrowhead) on the celiac axis arteriogram. Note the visualization of the hepatic arteriogram.

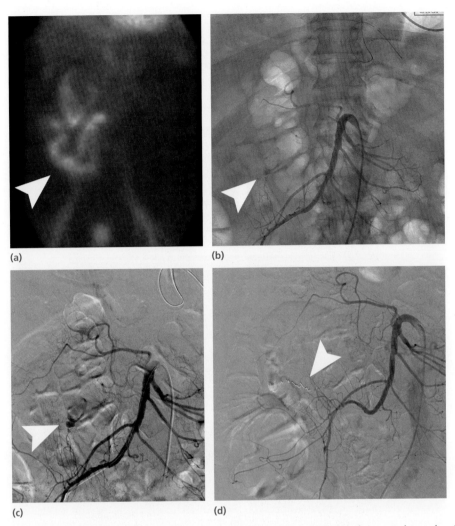

Figure 91.9 Upper gastrointestinal hemorrhage. A 68-year-old man with a lower gastrointestinal bleeding documented on technetium-99m red blood cell imaging in small bowel (arrowhead) **(a)**. The superior mesenteric artery (SMA) was selected by a catheter and an SMA angiography was performed. **(b)** A large pseudoaneurysm (arrowhead) was noted with rapid extravasation of contrast into the jejunum in the right upper quadrant on fluoroscopy images. **(c)** These finding were better visualized (arrowhead) on digital subtraction angiography (DSA) than on fluoroscopy. **(d)** A super-selective catheterization was performed with a microcatheter to a small jejunal branch vessel feeding the pseudoaneurysm. Coils (arrowhead) were used to occlude the feeding vessel. SMA angiographies were performed postcoiling and confirmed occlusion of the pseudoaneurysm and the absence of persistent bleeding.

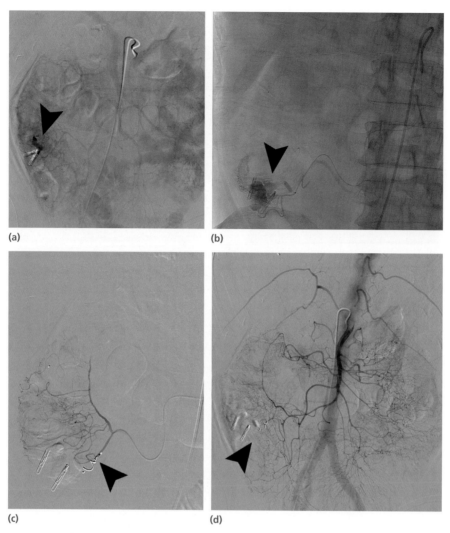

Figure 91.10 Cecal hemorrhage. An 80-year-old man with the history of episodic bleeding of the right colon requiring blood transfusion and with current rebleeding. The bleeding diverticulum was initially treated by clips placed endoscopically. **(a)** On a late phase of a superior mesenteric artery (SMA) angiography though a catheter, extravasation of contrast into the bowel (bowel folds outlined active bleeding, arrowhead) was seen in the region of the cecum, close to the clips. **(b)** A selective digital subtraction angiogram (DSA) of the terminal cecal branch of the ileocecal artery though a microcatheter inserted co-axially to the catheter confirmed the location of the bleed (arrowhead). **(c)** Coils (arrowhead) were deployed through the microcatheter to the terminal cecal branch. Selective angiography and then global DSA though the SMA **(d)** confirmed the absence of bleeding (arrowhead).

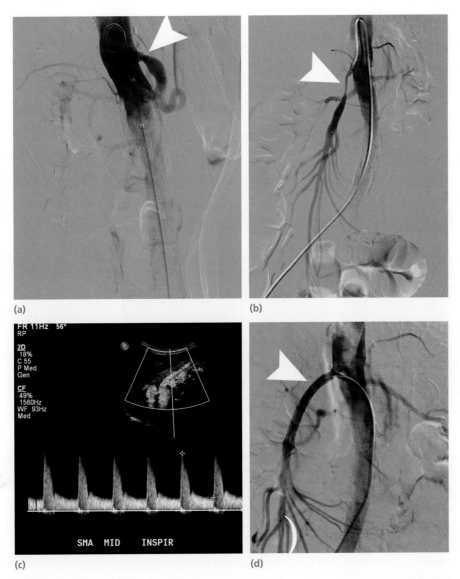

Figure 91.11 Chronic mesenteric ischemia. A case of a 79-year-old woman with a history of chronic epigastric pain and weight loss. Abdomen magnetic resonance angiography (MRA) demonstrated severe stenosis of the proximal superior mesenteric artery (SMA) and mild to moderate stenosis of the origin of the celiac trunk. **(a)** Abdominal aortic aortography (lateral position) was performed and evidenced a proximal narrowing of the celiac trunk (arrowhead). **(b)** The SMA was selected using a catheter and the arteriography was performed in lateral and oblique positions. A significant short-segment stenosis within the proximal SMA, approximately 1–2 cm distal to the SMA origin, was seen (arrowhead). **(c)** This finding was consistent with the duplex Doppler ultrasound, which demonstrated hemodynamically significant stenosis of the proximal SMA. **(d)** A percutaneous transluminal angioplasty was performed in the region of significant stenosis for predilatation. A bare metal stent was deployed across the stenosis and a balloon dilatation of the stent was performed. A final angiogram of the SMA demonstrated significantly improved flow through the superior mesenteric (arrowhead).

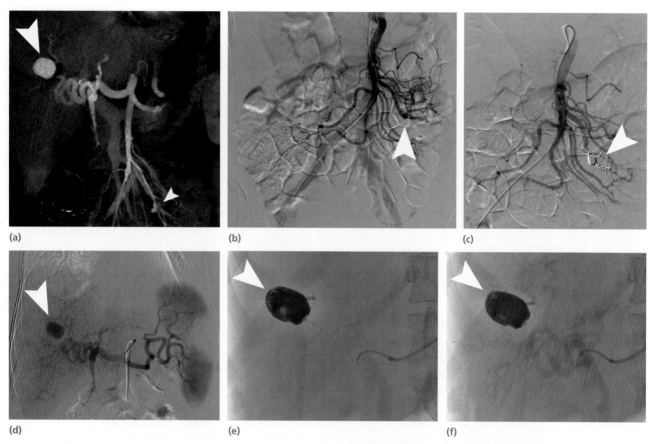

Figure 91.12 Visceral artery aneurysm. This was a case of a 29-year-old man with a history of intravenous drug abuse and endocarditis. **(a)** A coronal reconstructed computed tomography angiogram of the abdomen revealed large pseudoaneurysms within the liver (large arrowhead) and in the superior mesenteric artery (SMA) distribution (small arrowhead). **(b)** The patient was presented for angiography and potential embolization. An angiogram was performed though a catheter placed in the SMA and this showed the pseudoaneurysm. A microcatheter was used to select a proximal ileal branch of the left lower quadrant off the SMA and this confirmed the location of the pseudoaneurysm (arrowhead). The pseudoaneurysm was embolized with coils. **(c)** A nonselective angiogram of the SMA evidenced the occlusion of pseudoaneurysm (arrowhead). **(d)** The catheter was then placed into the celiac trunk and angiography was performed, which showed a pseudoaneurysm arising from the right hepatic artery (arrowhead). **(e)** A microcatheter was advanced to the pseudoaneurysm (arrowhead), which enabled its embolization with a liquid embolic agent (Onyx), until the absence of residual contrast filling of the pseudoaneurysm evidenced on the hepatic arteriography (arrowhead) **(f)**.

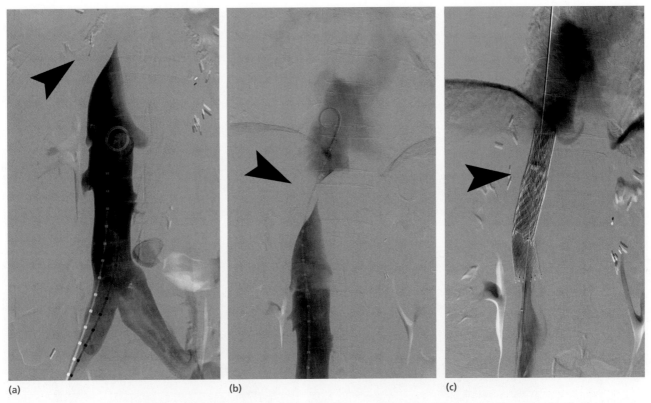

(a)   (b)   (c)

Figure 91.13 Inferior vena cava (IVC) stenosis. This was a case of a 56-year-old woman with advanced liposarcoma who presented with subcutaneous abdominal edema and lower extremity edema. **(a)** A venogram of the IVC was performed through a catheter and demonstrated a prominent IVC with abrupt narrowing at the level of the intrahepatic IVC (arrowhead). **(b)** A catheter was advanced into the right atrium. A concurrent superior vena cava (SVC)/IVC venogram through the catheter showed an approximately 4-cm near occlusion of the intrahepatic IVC (arrowhead). **(c)** Two consecutive stents were deployed successfully at the level of the intrahepatic IVC stenosis and were angioplastied by a balloon. A poststents angiogram was performed and showed a widely patent IVC (arrowhead) with prompt flow into the right atrium consistent with good technical success.

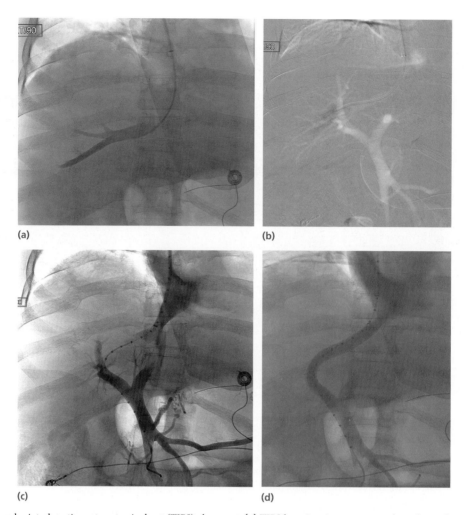

Figure 91.14 Transjugular intrahepatic portosystemic shunt (TIPS) placement. **(a)** TIPS hepatic vein access was achieved into the right internal jugular vein under ultrasound guidance, using a micropuncture set. A Bentson wire was advanced down into the inferior vena cava (IVC) and a 10 Fr 40-cm vascular sheath was advanced into the right atrium. The right hepatic vein was then accessed. **(b)** A CO_2 portovenogram was performed to target the portal vein for transhepatic puncture. **(c)** Stent mapping: after portal vein access was achieved, simultaneous hepatic and portal venograms were performed to delineate stent size and relative anatomy. **(d)** Post-TIPS stent placement veinogram: after stent deployment and angioplasty a portal venogram confirmed stent placement and decompression of gastric and esophageal varices.

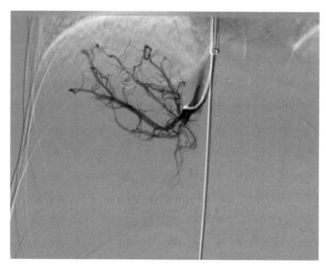

Figure 91.15 Budd–Chiari syndrome. Hepatic venogram showing the classic "cobweb" appearance of chronically occluded hepatic veins.

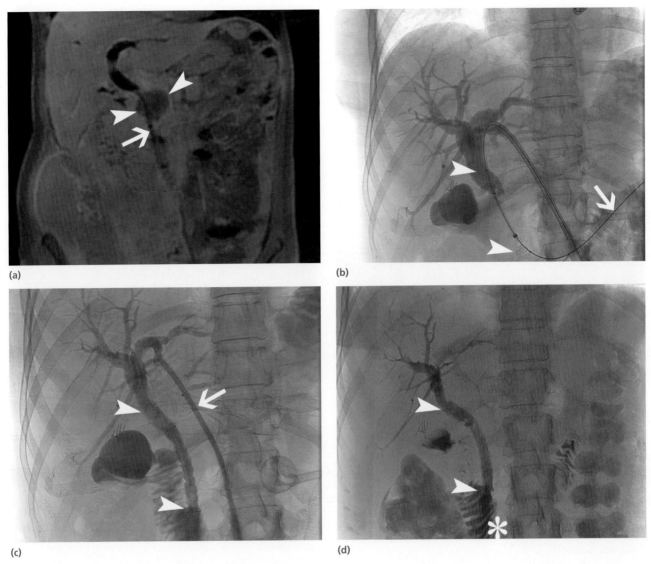

Figure 91.16 Pancreatic mass common bile duct stenting in a 49-year-old woman with pancreatic cancer. **(a)** Coronal T1-weighted fat-suppressed spoiled gradient-recalled echo image after injection of gadolinium showed a hypoenhancing mass in the pancreatic head encasing the distal common bile duct (arrowheads) and a left-sided 16 Fr locking biliary drainage catheter (arrow). **(b)** After removal of the existing tube over an 0.035 inch Amplatz Super Stiff guide wire (Boston Scientific) (arrow), a 10 mm × 8 cm self-expanding endoprosthesis (Gore Viabil) was deployed in the common bile duct (arrowheads). **(c)** Completed deployment of the stent (arrowheads) and placement of a foreshortened 18 Fr silastic biliary tube (Heyer-Schulte, Bentec, Sacramento, CA) to maintain access (arrow). **(d)** After 24 h, a tube cholangiogram showed a patent common bile duct stent (arrowheads) with no intrahepatic biliary duct dilatation and free passage of contrast into the bowel (*). The foreshortened tube was removed.

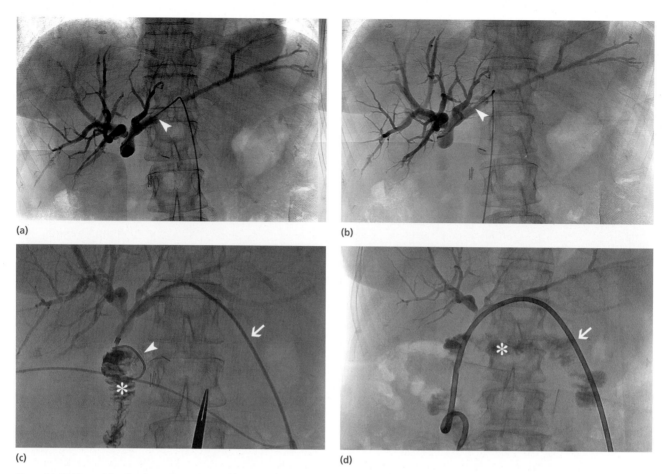

(a)

(b)

(c)

(d)

Figure 91.17 Hepatojejunal stricture in a 65-year-old woman following a Whipple procedure for pancreatic cancer with hepatojejunal anastomosis stricture and symptomatic jaundice. **(a)** Anteroposterior view: access site into the biliary tree is indicated by the arrowhead. **(b)** Lateral oblique view: after gaining access through the left-sided biliary system, contrast was injected through a micropuncture sheath (arrowhead) and the dilated biliary system was opacified. **(c)** A Brite Tip sheath (Cordis) was inserted over the wire and the tip was advanced just proximal to the stricture (arrow). A combination of glide wire (not shown) and 5 Fr catheter (arrowhead) were used to cross the stricture. Contrast injection confirmed good positioning into the small bowel (*). **(d)** Placement of a 10 Fr biliary drainage catheter (arrow) across the hepatojejunal stricture and opacification of the small bowel with contrast (*).

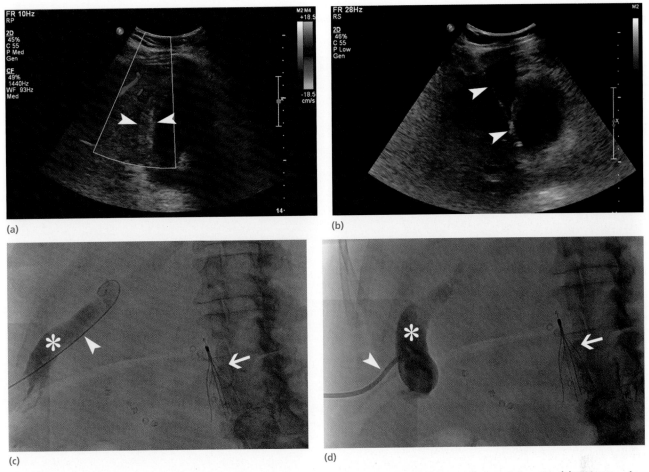

Figure 91.18 Cholecystostomy tube placement in a 66-year-old man with multiple comorbidities and acute acalculous cholecystitis. **(a)** Evaluation of the gallbladder with ultrasound demonstrated a thickened wall (arrowheads). **(b)** After choosing an intercostal transhepatic approach, the gallbladder was accessed under ultrasound using an 18-gauge trocar needle (arrowheads). **(c)** Contrast was injected through the needle into the gallbladder to confirm good positioning (*). A 0.035 inch Amplatz Super Stiff guide wire (Boston Scientific) was advanced through the needle and coiled in the gallbladder (arrowhead). Arrow indicates a Celect Vena Cava Filter (Cook Medical). **(d)** An 8 Fr locking all-purpose drainage catheter (arrowhead) was advanced over the wire in the gallbladder (*). Arrow indicates a Celect Vena Cava Filter (Cook Medical).

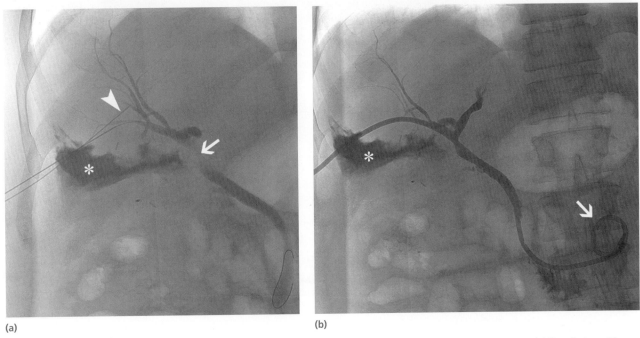

Figure 91.19 Biliary leak in a 65-year-old man with metastatic colon cancer to the liver following partial right hepatectomy with biliary leakage. The patient presented for biliary diversion. **(a)** Under fluoroscopic guidance, a 22-gauge Chiba needle was advanced into the liver parenchyma and into the biliary tree (arrowhead), and contrast was administered for a percutaneous cholangiogram. The biliary leakage is clearly identified (*). Triangulation and fluoroscopy were then used to target a posterior duct in the right hepatic lobe with a 21-gauge trocar needle, through which a 0.018-inch wire was advanced into the common bile duct (arrow). **(b)** Placement of a 10 Fr biliary drainage catheter (arrow) with extra side holes was carried out. Biliary leakage was seen (*).

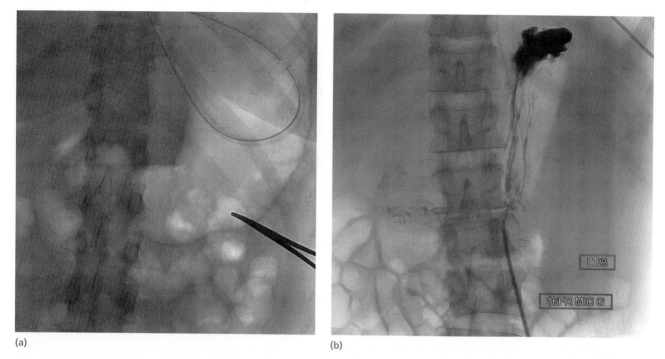

(a)   (b)

Figure 91.20 Gastric tube placement. **(a)** Scout abdominal X-ray showed a nasogastric tube terminating in the gastric fundus. The gastric lumen was distended with air. A clamp was positioned left of the left vertebral body and projecting over the gastric bubble. **(b)** The final anterior–posterior image showed contrast injection through the newly placed gastric feeding tube in a correct position. Contrast outlined the decompressed stomach. Two t-tacks can be seen surrounding the balloon of the feeding tube.

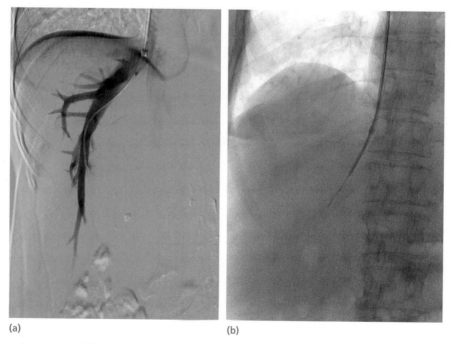

(a)   (b)

Figure 91.21 Transjugular liver biopsy. **(a)** Venogram of the right hepatic vein confirms catheter location prior to biopsy. **(b)** The inner metal cannula tip was located centrally and rotated anteriorly, and the biopsy needle was advanced into the liver tissue.

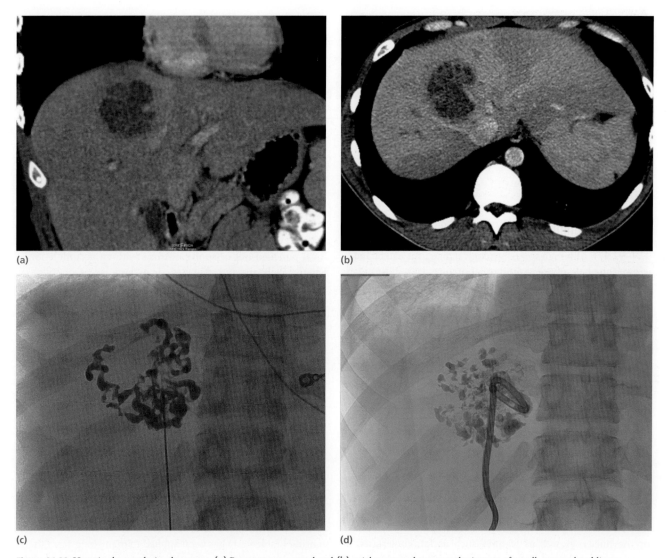

Figure 91.22 Hepatic abscess drain placement. (a) Postcontrast coronal and (b) axial computed tomography images of a well-encapsulated liver collection with multiple septations. (c) Needle contrast injection of the segment 8 multiloculated liver abscess showing the connections between the septations and no connection to normal hepatic structures. (d) Drainage catheter placement: contrast injection confirmed the position and purulent material was aspirated.

To access the videos for this chapter, please go to
www.yamadagastro.com/atlas

Video 91.1 Celiac arteriogram. Celiac trunk angiography shows classic three vessel branching pattern of the celiac trunk including the common hepatic, left gastric and splenic arteries. In this case of blunt splenic pseudoaneurysms, arteriovenous fistulas and petechial hemorrhage may be seen in the splenic parenchyma.

Video 91.2 Transjugular intrahepatic portosystemic shunt stent (TIPSS).

Video 91.2 (a) Hepatic venogram. A forward directing catheter is placed in an accessory hepatic vein and contrast is injected. Typically this vein is not used in TIPSS placement.

Video 91.2 (b) CO2 portovenogram. Here a balloon tipped catheter is wedged into a hepatic vein and CO2 as a contrast material is injected to show the portal venous system. The portal venous system shows a classic branching pattern.

Video 91.2 (c) Portal access. Fluoroscopic images obtained immediately after a needle was passed from the hepatic vein, through the liver parenchyma and into the portal vein. This venogram is confirming that the needle is in fact in the portal vein.

Video 91.2 (d) Portal and hepatic venograms. Simultaneous hepatic and portal venograms are performed outlining the intrahepatic course of the future TIPS stent.

Video 91.3 Cone beam roll movement. This movie show the fluoroscopic movement that is used to obtain imaging data is post processed into a Cone beam CT series. This is frequently performed in patients undergoing a liver embolization procedure.

CHAPTER 92

Liver biopsy and histopathological diagnosis

Sugantha Govindarajan
USC Keck School of Medicine, Downey, CA, USA

Evaluation of liver biopsy requires that the pathologist recognize the architecture and identify the pathological changes, and correlate the changes with clinical and laboratory data (Figures 92.1–92.97). Although some histological diagnosis can be made without the help of the clinical or laboratory data, most meaningful information is obtained with a proper clinical–pathological correlation.

Special stains, such as Masson trichrome, demonstrate fibrosis or cirrhosis of the liver, an indication of a chronic process. Other routine stains include stains for iron, reticulin, and diastase-resistant periodic acid Schiff-positive material. Granulomas of the liver require special stains for the etiological agent such as acid-fast organisms and fungi. Shikata or orcein stain identifies hepatitis B surface antigen as well as copper-binding protein, metallothionein. Immunoperoxidase stains detect viral and nonviral protein in the biopsy material using specific antibodies directed against the proteins.

Routine hematoxylin and eosin stained sections are the most valuable tools in the diagnosis. Well-embedded (3-μm) sections with good hematoxylin and eosin stain will provide great cellular details of hepatocytes, such as inclusions in the cytoplasm or the nuclei, as well as features such as fat, cholestasis, or dysplasia.

Initial assessment of the architecture is followed by a closer review of the portal tract or the fibrous septa if cirrhosis is present. Elements to be examined are the bile ducts, epithelial abnormalities or their absence or proliferation, cellular types of the inflammatory infiltrates, and the infiltrates' involvement of the bile ducts, the parenchymal limiting plate, or the vessels (vasculitis). The portal tracts or the fibrous septa should also be examined under polarized light for foreign material in the macrophages, which is usually seen in patients with a history of intravenous drug addiction.

The parenchyma is examined for cord sinusoidal pattern; normal one-cell thickness is altered in hepatocellular carcinoma to three to four or more cells that thicken the trabeculae. Parenchymal cytoplasmic inclusions such as Mallory bodies,

mega-mitochondria, α_1-antitrypsin, or of ground-glass cytoplasmic appearance are identified under higher magnifications in the review process. Areas of hepatocytolysis often appear as focal punched-out or spotty necrosis with an accumulation of Kupffer cells and lymphocytes, or as large areas of collapsed reticulin with loss of hepatocytes. Hepatocytolysis is often localized in the perivenular zones. Individual cell necrosis is seen as acidophil bodies or apoptotic cells.

Attention also should be paid to the sinusoidal lining cells, Ito cells, and the space of Disse. In alcoholic liver disease there is collagen deposition of the sinusoidal space, which stands out on Masson trichrome stain. Amyloid is also seen in this space, either as reticular or globular type, and is demonstrated by Congo red stain.

In addition to the histological diagnosis to confirm the clinical diagnosis, the liver biopsy has become a very important prognostic tool to assess the responses to treatment of chronic viral hepatitis B and C. The histological activity index (HAI) is measured using several standardized methods on pretreatment and 1- to 2-year follow-up biopsies. This quantitative measurement of necroinflammation and fibrosis either by Knodell or Ishak scoring (Table 92.1) has been applied to many long-term therapeutic protocols. Standardization of the scoring has been helpful in studies that compare different treatment modalities. Its application for individual cases also helps the clinician with patient follow-up and monitoring of other serological viral markers.

Liver biopsies are also extremely valuable in post-liver transplant settings. Standard protocols of liver biopsies help confirm the clinical diagnoses from rejection to opportunistic infections. Post-liver transplantation management of patients is largely dependent on the liver biopsy interpretations in conjunction with the other laboratory studies.

With proper indications and carefully chosen technique, a needle biopsy of the liver is an invaluable tool. Most often, the biopsy provides the final diagnosis when the pathology interpretation is made using the combined expertise of the pathologist and the hepatologist.

Yamada's Atlas of Gastroenterology, Fifth Edition. Edited by Daniel K. Podolsky, Michael Camilleri, J. Gregory Fitz, Anthony N. Kalloo, Fergus Shanahan, and Timothy C. Wang.
© 2016 John Wiley & Sons, Ltd. Published 2016 by John Wiley & Sons, Ltd.
Companion website: www.yamadagastro.com/atlas

Table 92.1 Histology Activity Index (HAI): Ishak score.

Modified HAI grading necroinflammatory scores	Score
A. Periportal piecemeal necrosis	
Absent	0
Mild (focal, few portal areas)	1
Mild/moderate (focal, most portal areas)	2
Moderate (continuous around <50% of tracts or septa)	3
Severe (continuous around >50% of tracts or septa)	4
B. Confluent necrosis	
Absent	0
Focal confluent necrosis	1
Zone 3 necrosis in some areas	2
Zone 3 necrosis in most areas	3
Zone 3 necrosis + occasional portal–central (P–C) bridging	4
Zone 3 necrosis + multiple P–C bridging	5
Panacinar or multiacinar necrosis	6
C. Focal necrosis and focal inflammation	
Absent	0
One focus or less per 10× objective	1
Two to four foci per 10× objective	2
Five to ten foci per 10× objective	3
More than ten foci per 10× objective	4
D. Portal inflammation	
None	0
Mild, some, or all portal areas	1
Moderate, some, or all portal areas	2
Moderate/marked, all portal areas	3
Marked, all portal areas	4
Modified staging: fibrosis and cirrhosis	
Change	
No fibrosis	0
Fibrous expansion of some portal areas	1
Fibrous expansion of most portal areas	2
Fibrous expansion with occasional portal to portal (P–P) bridging	3
Fibrous expansion with marked bridging	4
Marked bridging with occasional nodules, incomplete cirrhosis	5
Cirrhosis, probable or definite	6

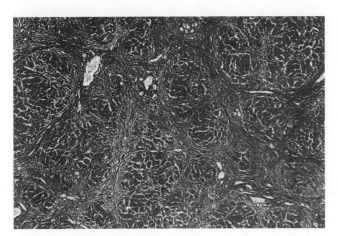

Figure 92.1 Cirrhosis of liver with fibrous septa and regenerative nodules. (Masson stain; original magnification ×40.)

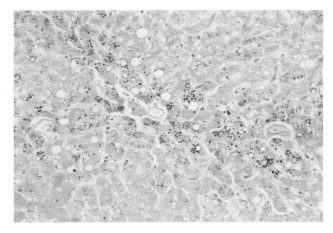

Figure 92.2 α_1-Antitrypsin globules in the periportal hepatocytes–diastase-resistant PAS-positive. (Di-PAS stain; original magnification ×200.)

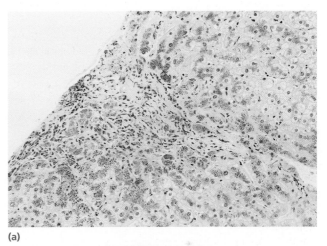

(a)

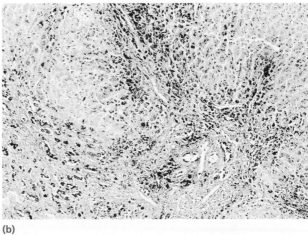

(b)

Figure 92.3 (a) H & E stain of hemochromatosis with iron deposits appearing as brown granules. **(b)** Perls' iron stain demonstrating bright blue granules in hepatocytes and duct epithelial cells in hemochromatosis. (Original magnification ×100.)

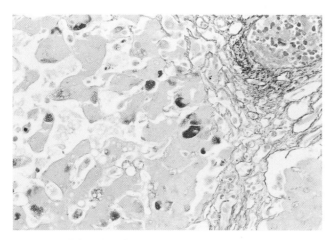

Figure 92.4 Shikata stain demonstrating the presence of HBsAg in the hepatocytes in chronic hepatitis B virus. (Original magnification ×200.)

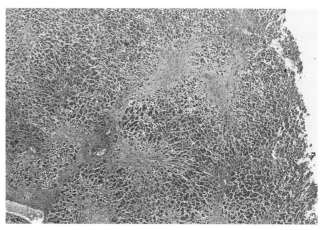

Figure 92.7 Submassive hepatic necrosis with collapsed perivenular reticulum network. (H & E stain; original magnification ×40.)

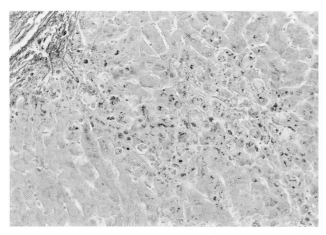

Figure 92.5 Shikata stain demonstrating dark black granules of copper binding protein in periseptal hepatocytes in Wilson disease. (Original magnification ×200.)

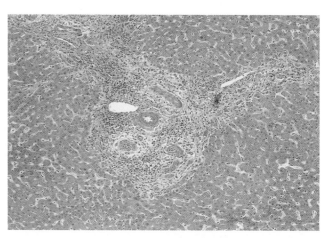

Figure 92.8 Portal area with prominent neutrophils in close proximity to the dilated interlobular bile duct in acute cholangitis. (H & E stain; original magnification ×100.)

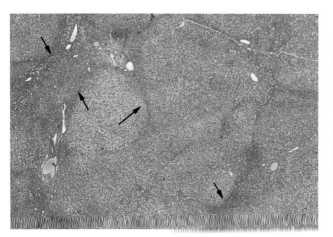

Figure 92.6 Nodular regenerative hyperplasia demonstrating regeneration of parenchyma compressing the surrounding parenchyma (arrows) without fibrous septa formation. (H & E stain; original magnification ×40.)

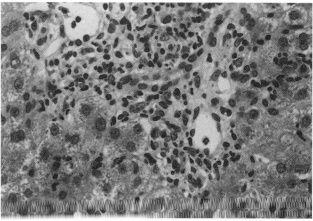

Figure 92.9 Portal area with prominent eosinophils among the inflammatory infiltrates in a case of Dilantin-induced hepatotoxicity. (H & E stain; original magnification ×200.)

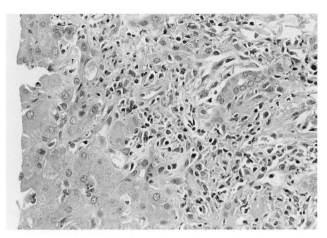

Figure 92.10 Portal area with increased number of eosinophils in a case of early rejection of orthotopic liver transplantation. (H & E stain; original magnification ×200.)

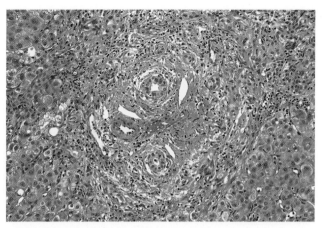

Figure 92.13 Lamellar periductal fibrosis in chronic bile duct obstruction. (H & E stain; original magnification ×100.)

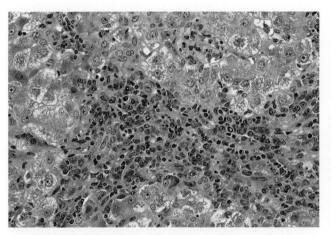

Figure 92.11 Prominent plasma cells among the infiltrates in the portal tract of autoimmune chronic hepatitis. (H & E stain; original magnification ×400.)

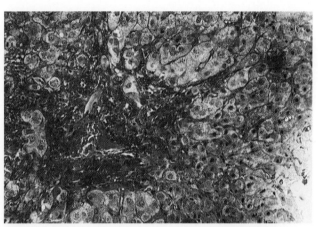

Figure 92.14 Arachnoid portal fibrosis with periportal extension of collagen in chronic alcoholic liver disease. (Masson trichrome stain; original magnification ×100.)

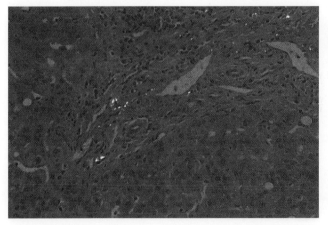

Figure 92.12 A portal area under polarizing light to demonstrate polarizable crystals in an intravenous drug user. (H & E stain; original magnification ×200.)

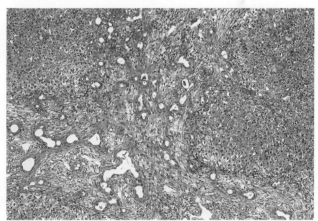

Figure 92.15 Portal area with marked cholangiolar proliferation in mechanical duct obstruction. (H & E stain; original magnification ×100.)

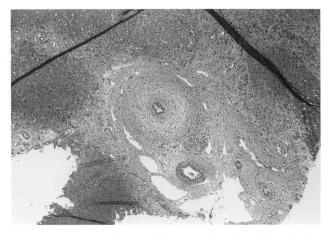

Figure 92.16 Primary sclerosing cholangitis with evidence of periductal fibrosis and chronic inflammatory infiltrate. (H & E stain; original magnification ×100.)

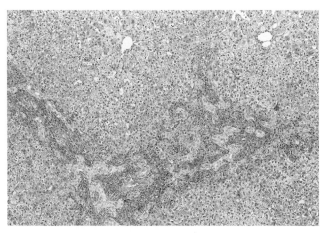

Figure 92.19 Biliary fibrosis and ductular proliferation in a 3-month-old infant with extrahepatic biliary atresia. (H & E stain; original magnification ×100.)

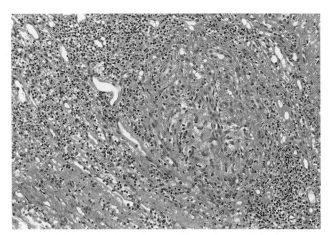

Figure 92.17 Primary biliary cirrhosis with granuloma. (Original magnification ×200.)

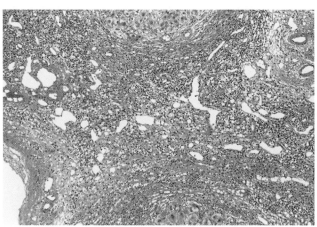

Figure 92.20 Increased number of thin-walled vascular structures representing portal venous radicles reflective of portal hypertension. (H & E stain; original magnification ×100.)

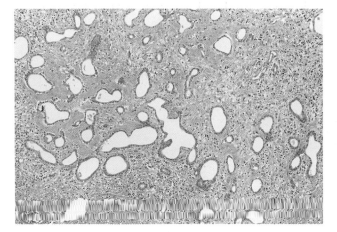

Figure 92.18 A few dilated duct structures with abnormal epithelium surrounded by loose collagen representing Meyenburg complex. (H & E stain; original magnification ×100.)

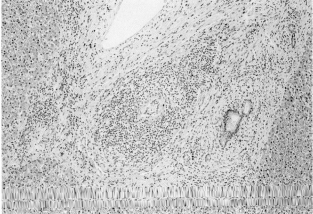

Figure 92.21 Severe necrotizing inflammatory reaction around hepatic arteriole in polyarteritis nodosa. (H & E stain; original magnification ×100.)

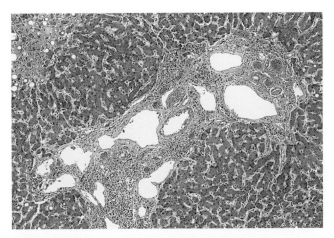

Figure 92.22 Increased number of abnormal vascular structures in a portal tract in Osler–Weber–Rendu syndrome. (H & E stain; original magnification ×100.)

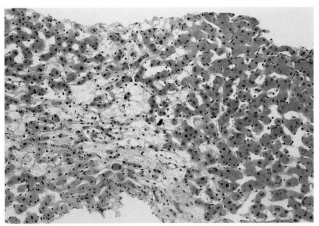

Figure 92.25 Budd–Chiari syndrome with perivenular hemorrhage, necrosis, and sinusoidal dilation. (H & E stain; original magnification ×200.)

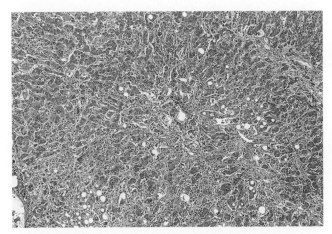

Figure 92.23 Marked perivenular fibrosis in alcoholic liver disease. (Masson trichrome stain; original magnification ×100.)

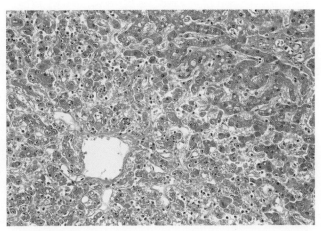

Figure 92.26 Confluent necrosis in the perivenular zone due to anoxia. (H & E stain; original magnification ×200.)

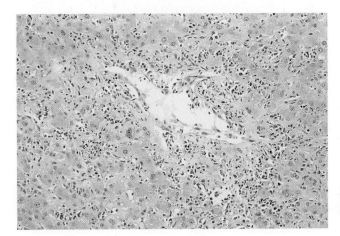

Figure 92.24 Endothelialitis showing inflammatory changes of a terminal hepatic venule in acute rejection of orthotopic liver transplantation. (H & E stain; original magnification ×200.)

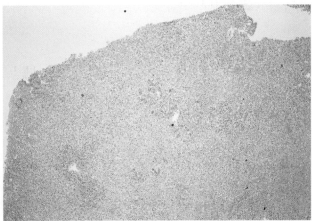

Figure 92.27 Massive hepatic necrosis involving the entire parenchyma with islands of portal tracts remaining. (H & E stain; original magnification ×40.)

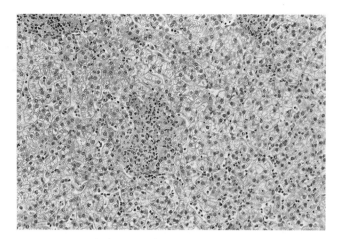

Figure 92.28 Punched-out granulomatous necrosis of the parenchyma in mononucleosis due to Epstein–Barr virus. (H & E stain; original magnification ×200.)

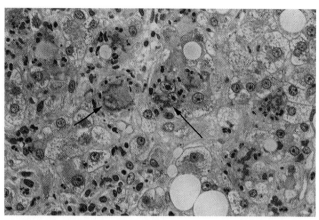

Figure 92.31 Perivenular hepatocytes containing Mallory hyaline (arrows) with neutrophilic reaction around them. (H & E stain; original magnification ×200.)

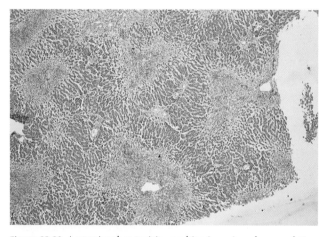

Figure 92.29 Acetaminophen toxicity resulting in perivenular coagulative necrosis without hepatocyte swelling. (H & E stain; original magnification ×100.)

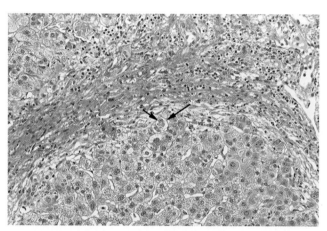

Figure 92.32 A periportal hepatocyte containing Mallory hyaline (arrows) in primary biliary cirrhosis. (H & E stain; original magnification ×200.)

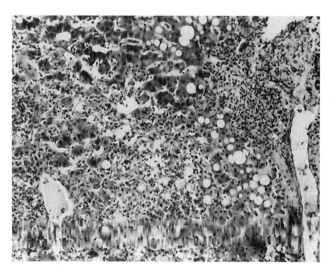

Figure 92.30 Halothane-induced perivenular and midzonal coagulative necrosis. (H & E stain; original magnification ×100.)

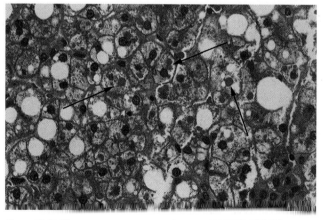

Figure 92.33 Hepatocytes containing spherical megamitochondria (arrows) in alcoholic liver disease. (H & E stain; original magnification ×200.)

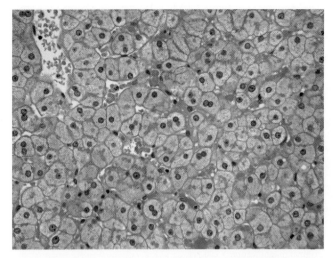

Figure 92.34 Focal regeneration with cobblestone arrangement of hepatocytes in chronic hepatitis. (H & E stain; original magnification ×200.)

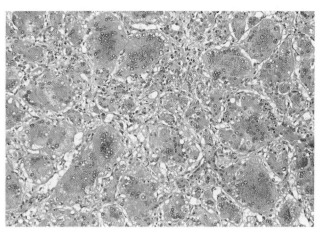

Figure 92.37 Syncytial hepatocytes in neonatal hepatitis. (H & E stain; original magnification ×200.)

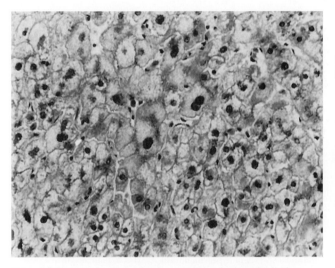

Figure 92.35 Focal dysplastic change consisting of enlarged cells, large nuclei in chronic hepatitis B. (H & E stain; original magnification ×200.)

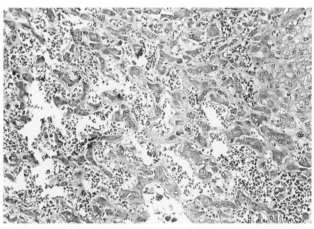

Figure 92.38 Chronic passive congestion causing perivenular sinusoidal dilation and atrophic hepatic cords. (Masson trichrome stain; original magnification ×400.)

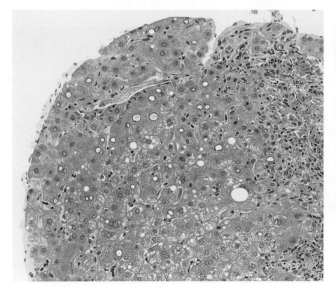

Figure 92.36 Hepatocytes with glycogen vacuolated nuclei. (H & E stain; original magnification ×200.)

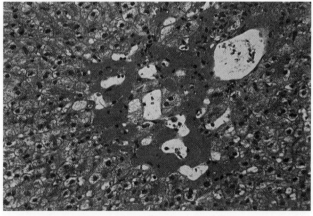

Figure 92.39 Perivenular hepatic parenchyma with dilated sinusoids and the presence of red blood cells within the hepatic cords in left-sided heart failure. (H & E stain; original magnification ×100.)

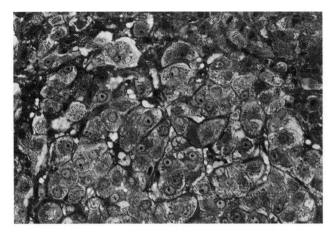

Figure 92.40 Collagen fibers along the sinusoids in the space of Disse in alcoholic liver disease. (Masson stain; original magnification ×200.)

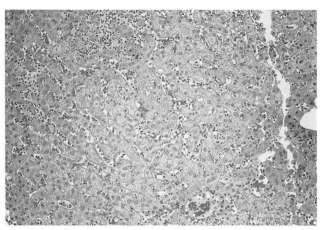

Figure 92.43 Hypertrophic Kupffer cells in salmonellosis. (H & E stain; original magnification ×200.)

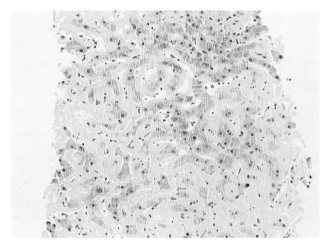

Figure 92.41 Reticular amyloid deposition in the space of Disse. (H & E stain; original magnification ×200.)

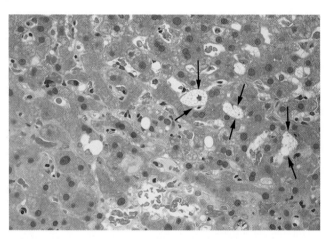

Figure 92.44 Ito cells with foamy fatty cytoplasm (arrows) along the sinusoidal surface in hypervitaminosis A. (H & E stain; original magnification ×400.)

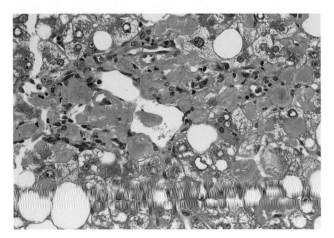

Figure 92.42 Globular amyloid deposition. (H & E stain; original magnification ×400.)

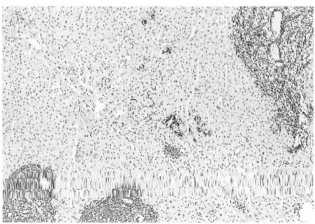

Figure 92.45 Leukemic cells in the sinusoidal blood space in a case of lymphocytic leukemia. (H & E stain; original magnification ×200.)

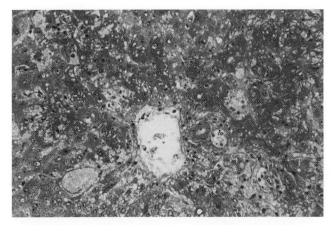

Figure 92.46 Periportal sinusoidal space filled with fibrin thrombi in toxemia of pregnancy. (H & E stain; original magnification ×100.)

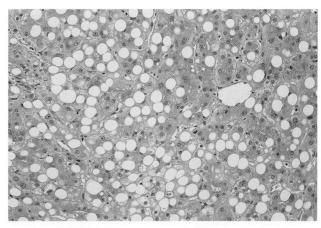

Figure 92.49 Macrovesicular fatty change of hepatocytes in alcoholic liver disease. (H & E stain; original magnification ×200.)

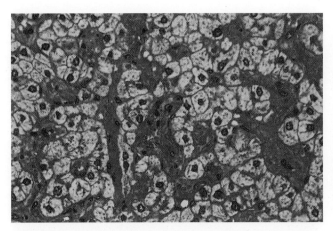

Figure 92.47 Clumps of sickled red blood cells packed in the sinusoidal spaces. (H & E stain; original magnification ×200.)

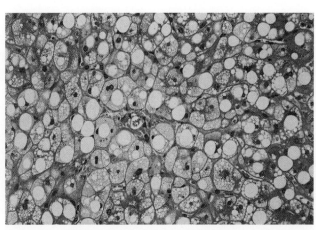

Figure 92.50 Diffusely enlarged hepatocytes with foamy fatty change in acute alcoholic liver disease. (H & E stain; original magnification ×100.)

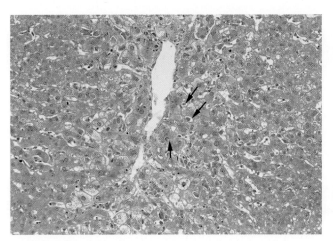

Figure 92.48 Cholestasis (arrows) in dilated canaliculi in zone 3 in chlorpromazine-induced liver disease. (H & E stain; original magnification ×200.)

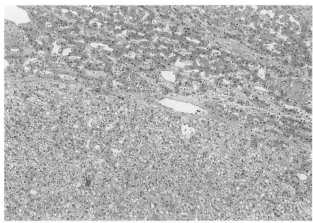

Figure 92.51 Liver cell adenoma with clear cells and the adjacent normal parenchyma. (H & E stain; original magnification ×100.)

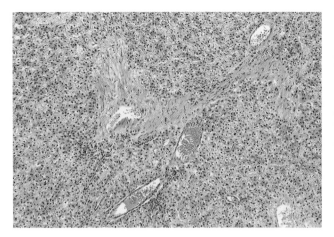

Figure 92.52 Liver cell adenoma with thick-walled vessels and lack of portal tracts. (H & E stain; original magnification ×100.)

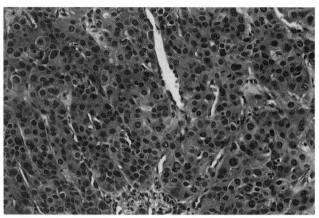

Figure 92.55 Well-differentiated trabecular hepatocellular carcinoma with endothelial lining. (H & E stain; original magnification ×100.)

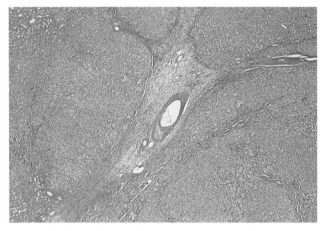

Figure 92.53 Focal nodular hyperplasia with central stellate scar. (H & E stain; original magnification ×40.)

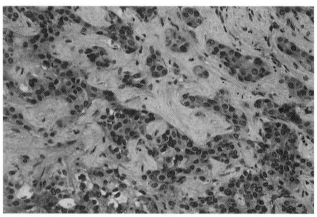

Figure 92.56 Sclerosing hepatic carcinoma with dense fibrous stroma. (H & E stain; original magnification ×100.)

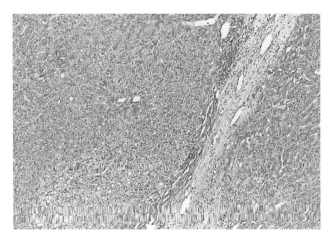

Figure 92.54 Focal nodular hyperplasia with the scar exhibiting lack of bile ducts and presence of vascular structures. Liver cells are uniform and regenerative in appearance. (H & E stain; original magnification ×100.)

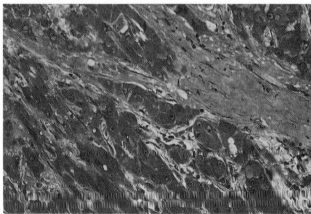

Figure 92.57 Eosinophilic neoplastic hepatocytes with lamellar fibrous stroma in fibrolamellar hepatocellular carcinoma. (H & E stain; original magnification ×100.)

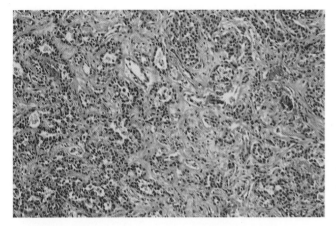

Figure 92.58 Neoplastic ductal structures with fibrous stroma in cholangiocarcinoma. (H & E stain; original magnification ×100.)

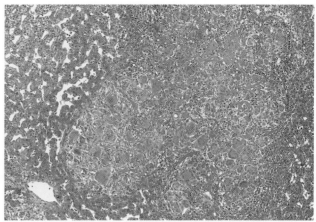

Figure 92.61 Partially segmented, exuberant epithelioid granuloma of sarcoidosis. (H & E stain; original magnification ×100.)

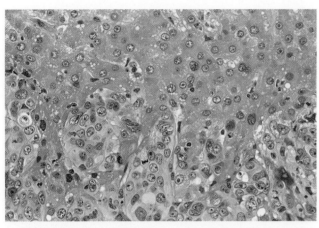

Figure 92.59 Metastatic, poorly differentiated adenocarcinoma infiltrating into the sinusoids. (H & E stain; original magnification ×200.)

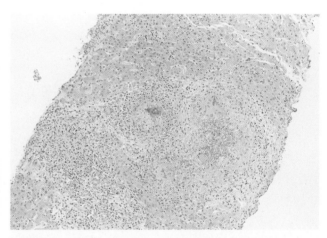

Figure 92.62 Epithelioid granuloma with Langhans giant cells in *Mycobacterium tuberculosis* infection of liver. (H & E stain; original magnification ×100.)

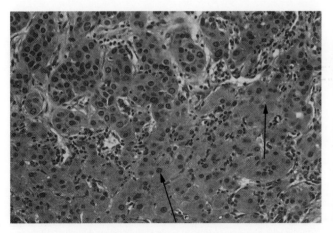

Figure 92.60 Junction of tumor and nontumor liver in hepatocellular carcinoma. The tumor cells grow into the hepatic cords (arrows). (H & E stain; original magnification ×100.)

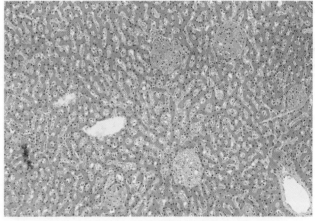

Figure 92.63 Well-circumscribed clusters of large foamy histiocytes in *Mycobacterium avium intracellulare* infection of the liver. These cells contain abundant acid-fast organisms on special stain (not shown). (H & E stain; original magnification ×100.)

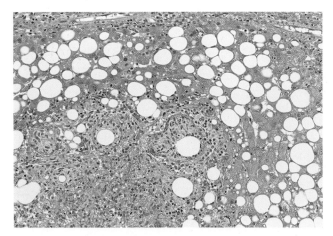

Figure 92.64 Granulomatous lesion with central vacuolization surrounded by a fibrin ring in Q fever. (H & E stain; original magnification ×200.)

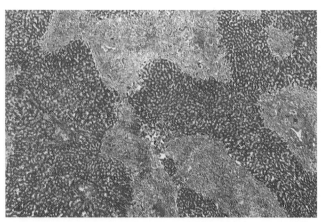

Figure 92.67 Jigsaw puzzle appearance of biliary cirrhosis. (Masson stain; original magnification ×40.)

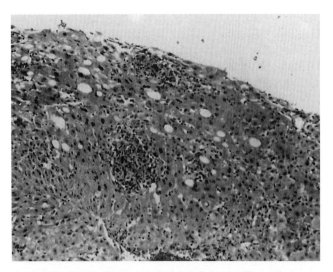

Figure 92.65 Small well-circumscribed granuloma in sulfonamide-induced hepatic necrosis. (H & E stain; original magnification ×100.)

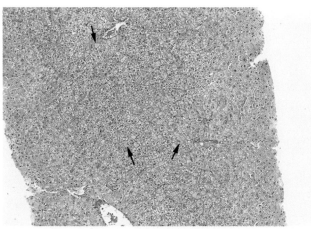

Figure 92.68 Scattered ground-glass cells (arrows) in chronic hepatitis, type B. (H & E stain; original magnification ×100.)

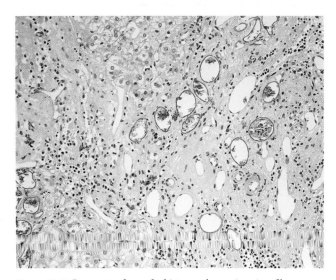

Figure 92.66 Remnants of ova of schistosomal organisms in a fibrous portal area. (H & E stain; original magnification ×200.)

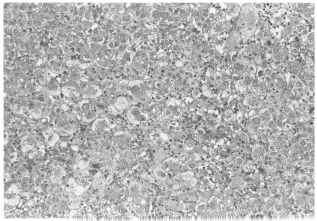

Figure 92.69 Perivenular zone in acute viral hepatitis demonstrating hydropic hepatocytes, hepatocytolysis, inflammatory exudate, and rare acidophilic bodies. (H & E stain; original magnification ×200.)

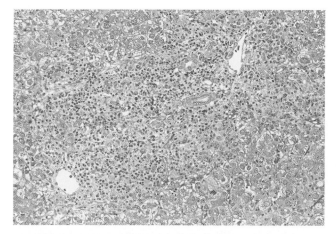

Figure 92.70 Portal area in acute viral hepatitis with mononuclear infiltration extending to the periportal regions. (H & E stain; original magnification ×200.)

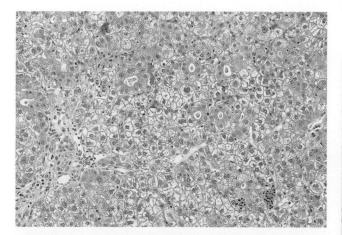

Figure 92.71 Prominent acinar transformation of hepatocytes in enterically transmitted acute hepatitis, type E. (H & E stain; original magnification ×200.)

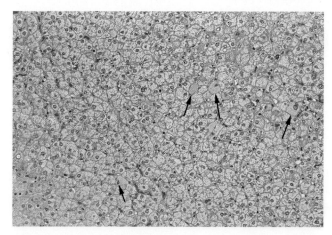

Figure 92.72 Uniform cobblestone appearance of parenchyma in chronic hepatitis, type B. A few ground-glass cells are seen (arrows). (H & E stain; original magnification ×200.)

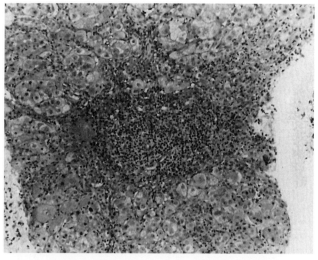

Figure 92.73 Portal areas with fibrosis and mononuclear inflammation extending to the parenchyma exhibiting piecemeal necrosis in chronic hepatitis. (H & E stain; original magnification ×100.)

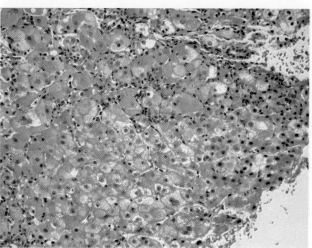

Figure 92.74 Inflammatory cells are seen cuffing around the hepatocytes in chronic hepatitis. (H & E stain; original magnification ×100.)

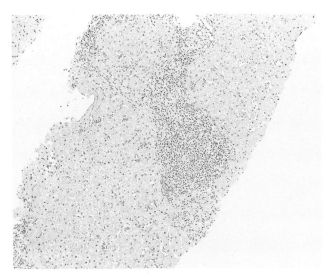

Figure 92.75 Chronic hepatitis C showing portal fibrosis and inflammation, macrovesicular fat, and inflammation in the adjacent parenchyma. (H & E stain; original magnification ×100.)

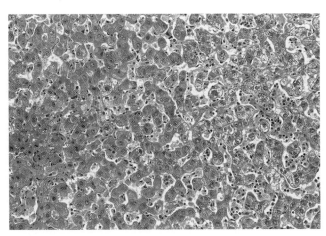

Figure 92.78 Striking sinusoidal lymphocytosis of atypical type in Epstein–Barr virus-induced mononucleosis. (H & E stain; original magnification ×200.)

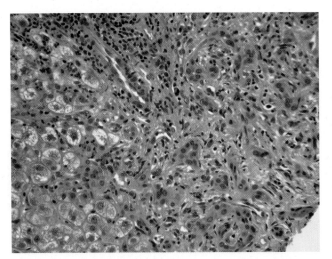

Figure 92.76 Atypical bile ducts in a portal tract of chronic hepatitis C. (H & E stain; original magnification ×200.)

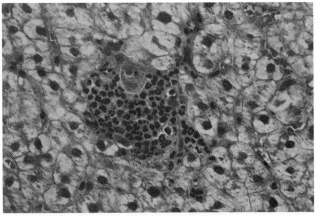

Figure 92.79 Intranuclear and cytoplasmic inclusions of cytomegalovirus (CMV) in a hepatocyte surrounded by polymorphonuclear leukocytes in an orthotopic liver transplant infected with CMV. (H & E stain; original magnification ×200.)

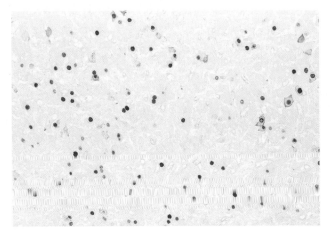

Figure 92.77 Immunoperoxidase stain demonstrating hepatitis D antigen in the nuclei of hepatocytes in chronic hepatitis D. (Original magnification ×100.)

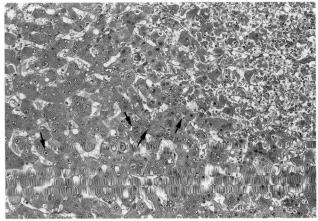

Figure 92.80 Intranuclear inclusions (arrows) of Cowdry type A of herpes simplex seen in hepatocytes. (H & E stain; original magnification ×200.)

Liver biopsy and histopathological diagnosis **CHAPTER 92**   **875**

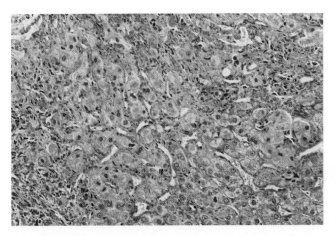

Figure 92.81 Diffuse interstitial fibrosis in chronic alcoholic liver disease. (Masson stain; original magnification ×100.)

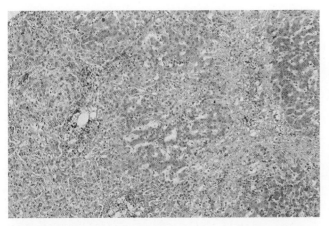

Figure 92.82 Marked perivenular fibrous scarring with mild portal fibrosis and lack of regenerative nodules in progressive perivenular fibrosis of alcoholic etiology. (Masson stain; original magnification ×100.)

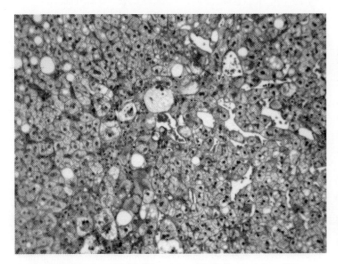

Figure 92.83 Perisinusoidal collagen in nonalcoholic steatohepatitis. (Masson trichrome stain; original magnification ×100.)

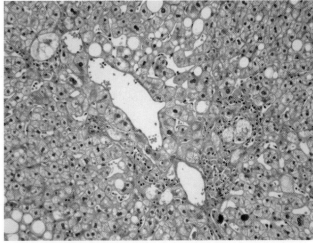

Figure 92.84 Hepatocytes with ballooning change and Mallory bodies in nonalcoholic steatohepatitis. (H & E stain; original magnification ×100.)

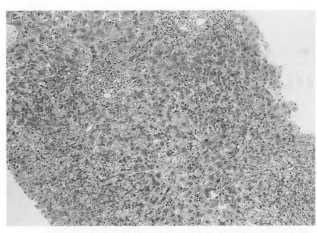

Figure 92.85 Hepatitis-like activity resembling acute viral hepatitis in Aldomet-induced hepatotoxicity. (H & E stain; original magnification ×200.)

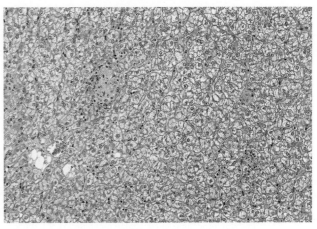

Figure 92.86 Dilantin-induced hepatic changes resembling mononucleosis. (H & E stain; original magnification ×100.)

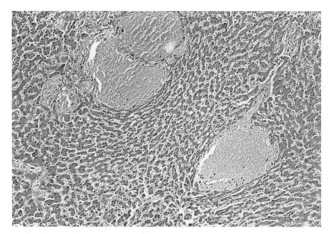

Figure 92.87 Peliosis hepatis with blood-filled spaces without endothelial lining. (H & E stain; original magnification ×100.)

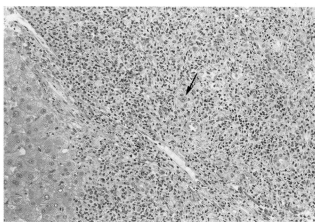

Figure 92.90 Portal infiltrate in Hodgkin lymphoma with an atypical Reed–Sternberg cell (arrow). (H & E stain; original magnification ×200.)

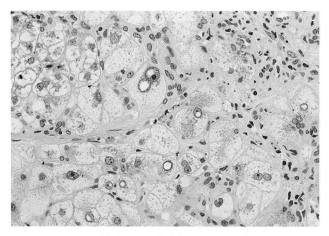

Figure 92.88 Sinusoidal fibrosis and nuclear dysplastic changes in methotrexate toxicity. (H & E stain; original magnification ×400.)

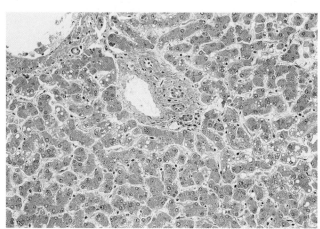

Figure 92.91 Portal area with lymphopenia in a patient with AIDS. (H & E stain; original magnification ×200.)

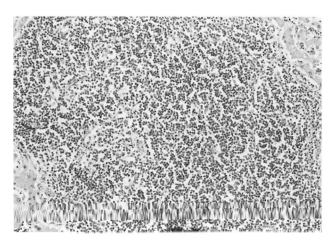

Figure 92.89 Portal infiltrate in non-Hodgkin lymphoma. (H & E stain; original magnification ×100.)

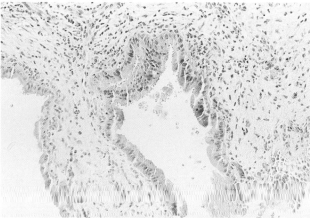

Figure 92.92 Bile duct epithelium along the luminal surface demonstrates the presence of cryptosporidiosis of 3- to 4-μm size. (H & E stain; original magnification ×400.)

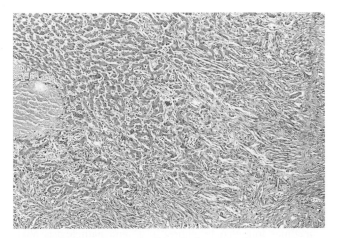

Figure 92.93 Kaposi sarcoma involving the liver. (H & E stain; original magnification ×100.)

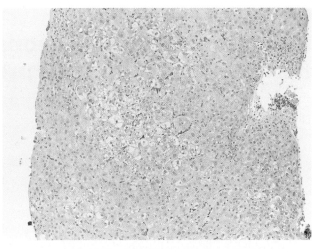

Figure 92.96 Marked ballooning of the hepatocytes in acinar zone 3 representing harvest injury. (H & E stain; original magnification ×100.)

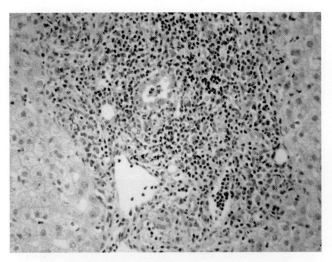

Figure 92.94 Portal inflammatory infiltrate, changes of interlobular bile ducts, and endothelialitis of portal vein radicles in acute rejection. (H & E stain; original magnification ×200.)

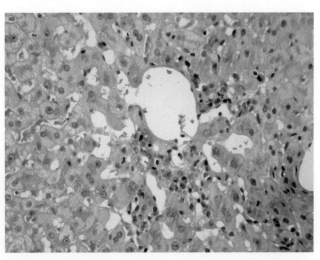

Figure 92.97 Perivenular zone with necroinflammatory changes in recurrent acute hepatitis B infection of allograft. (H & E stain; original magnification ×200.)

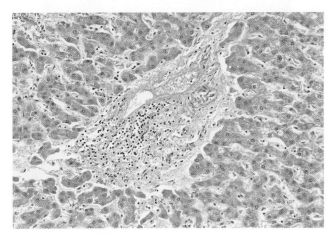

Figure 92.95 Portal inflammatory infiltrate with loss of bile ducts in chronic rejection. (H & E stain; original magnification ×200.)

CHAPTER 93

Endoscopic mucosal biopsy: histopathological interpretation

Elizabeth Montgomery and Anthony N. Kalloo

Johns Hopkins University, Baltimore, MD, USA

The key principle of biopsy interpretation of the gastrointestinal tract is that it has a limited repertoire of responses to a host of injuries, and diagnosing the type of injury in any given biopsy often requires correlation with clinical details. When dealing with mucosal biopsies of the gastrointestinal (GI) tract, it should also be noted that they only display the mucosa (and possibly a small amount of submucosa), a feature that is obvious but sometimes forgotten by endoscopists and pathologists alike. Correlating endoscopic imaging with histopathological findings may be critical in establishing correct clinical diagnosis. This chapter matches pathology with endoscopy for many common and uncommon gastrointestinal conditions (Figures 93.1–93.130).

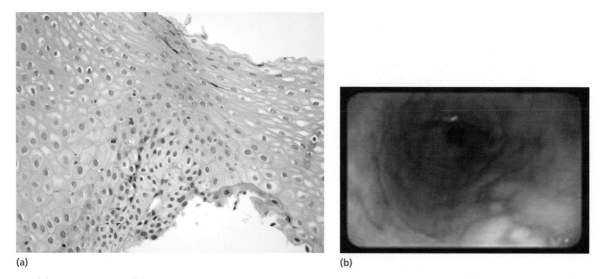

(a) (b)

Figure 93.1 (a) Reflux esophagitis. **(b)** Reflux esophagitis with erosions. Savary–Miller Grade III (circumferential lesion, erosive or exudative) reflux-type esophagitis and multiple erosions in the lower third of the esophagus can be seen in this image.

Yamada's Atlas of Gastroenterology, Fifth Edition. Edited by Daniel K. Podolsky, Michael Camilleri, J. Gregory Fitz, Anthony N. Kalloo, Fergus Shanahan, and Timothy C. Wang.
© 2016 John Wiley & Sons, Ltd. Published 2016 by John Wiley & Sons, Ltd.
Companion website: www.yamadagastro.com/atlas

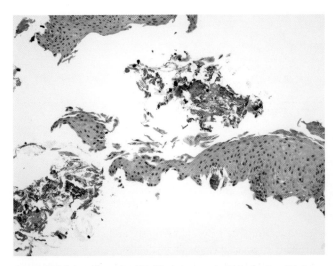

Figure 93.2 Iron pill esophagitis. The brown material in the image is iron pigment. The associated squamous epithelium shows reparative features.

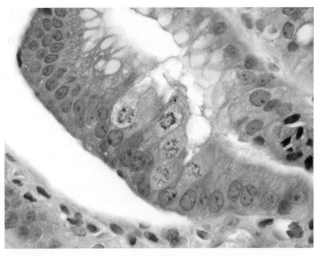

Figure 93.4 Taxol effect. This process involves metaplastic columnar mucosa in the esophagus. The ring mitoses are an indication of mitotic arrest.

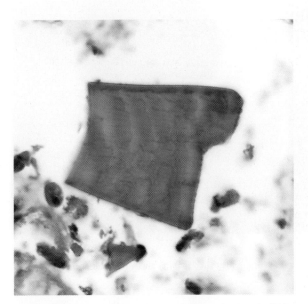

Figure 93.3 Kayexalate (sodium polystyrene sulfonate). Note the "fish scale"-like appearance of the crystalline material.

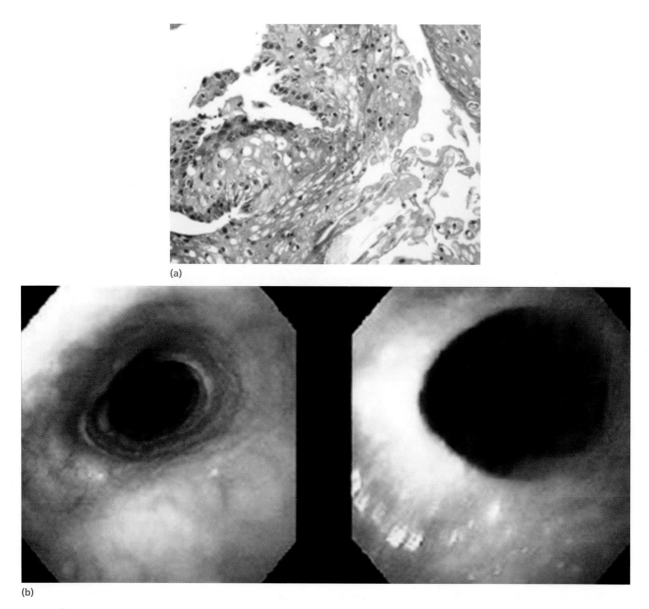

(a)

(b)

Figure 93.5 (a) Graft-versus-host disease (GVHD). There is extensive squamous epithelial apoptosis such that the nuclei resemble specks of dust. **(b)** GVHD of the esophagus with multiple fine mucosal webs present.

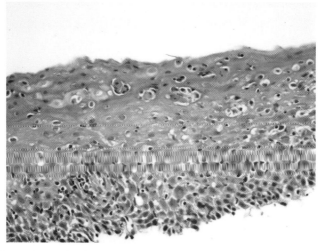

Figure 93.6 Lichen planus involving the esophagus. This field shows prominent intraepithelial lymphocytosis and necrotic squamous cells.

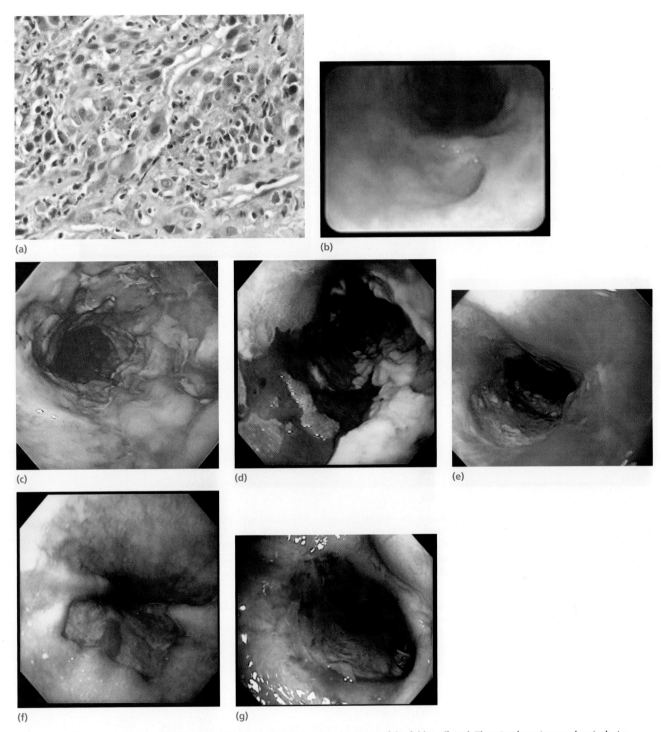

Figure 93.7 (a) Cytomegalovirus (CMV) esophagitis. An endothelial cell in the center of the field is affected. There is a large intranuclear inclusion. (b) Cytomegalovirus esophageal ulcer. Upper endoscopy in a patient with acquired immune deficiency syndrome (AIDS) and dysphagia revealed a distal esophageal ulceration. An immunohistochemical stain for CMV was positive. (c) Diffuse ulceration with a serpiginous appearance with overlying candidal debris. This patient with AIDS has CMV esophagitis and *Candida* coinfection. (d) Diffuse candidal plaque has been removed with the endoscope revealing a shallow serpiginous ulceration, which on biopsy confirmed CMV. (e) Large, deep ulceration in the proximal esophagus owing to CMV in a patient with AIDS. (f) Solitary, deep, well-circumscribed ulcer at the gastroesophageal junction caused by CMV. (g) Circumferential ulceration in the midesophagus as a result of CMV.

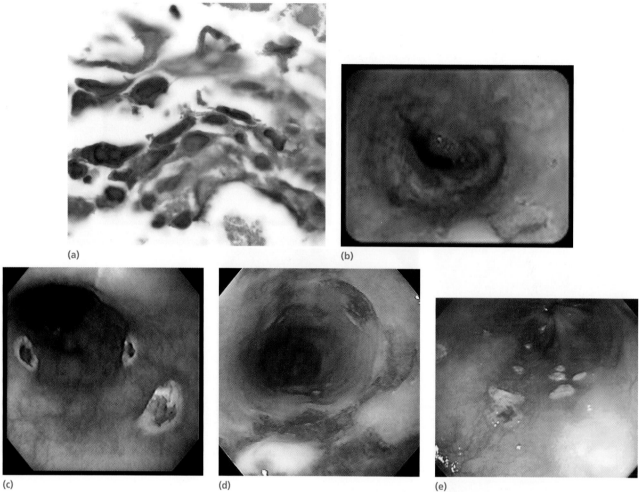

(a)

(b)

(c)

(d)

(e)

Figure 93.8 **(a)** Herpes simplex virus (HSV) esophagitis. The infected cells are multinucleated with "smudged" nuclei. **(b)** Herpetic esophageal ulcer. The earliest manifestation of herpes simplex esophagitis may be vesicular, though this is rarely seen. The herpetic lesions may coalesce. On endoscopy, a well-circumscribed, volcano-like appearance has been described. In this case, HSV-1 was cultured from esophageal biopsies. **(c)** Small volcano-like ulcers due to HSV. **(d)** Multiple well-circumscribed, shallow esophageal ulcers due to HSV esophagitis. **(e)** Small well-circumscribed areas of exudate resembling *Candida*. This is a classic appearance of mild HSV esophagitis. This patient had eutropenia.

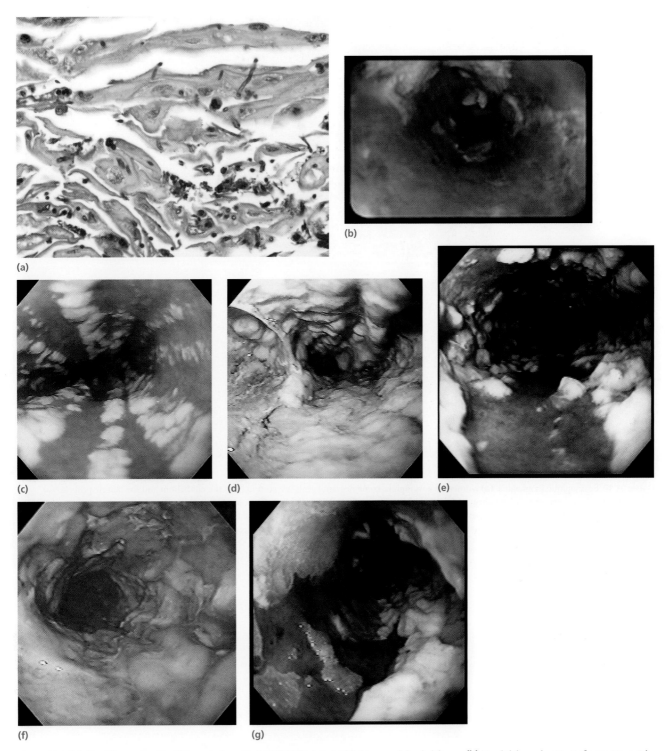

Figure 93.9 (a) *Candida* esophagitis. This periodic acid–Schiff (PAS) stain highlights pseudohyphal forms. **(b)** Candidal esophagitis. Inflammation with thick white adherent plaques in a patient with AIDS and candidal esophagitis. Fluconazole-sensitive *Candida albicans* was cultured from the esophageal brushing. **(c)** Multiple raised white plaques involving the esophagus with normal intervening mucosa. This would be classified as Grade II *Candida* esophagitis. **(d)** Exuberant yellow plaque material encroaching on the esophageal lumen typical for severe *Candida* esophagitis (Grade IV). **(e)** The plaque material has been removed with the endoscope revealing relatively normal underlying mucosa without ulceration. **(f)** Diffuse ulceration with a serpiginous appearance with overlying candidal debris. This AIDS patient has CMV esophagitis and *Candida* coinfection. **(g)** Diffuse candidal plaque has been removed with the endoscope revealing a shallow serpiginous ulceration, which on biopsy confirmed CMV.

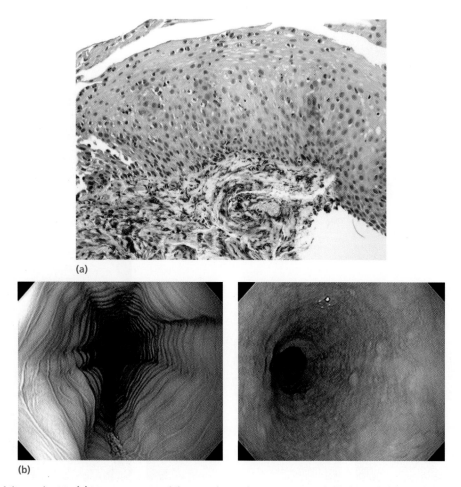

(a)

(b)

Figure 93.10 Eosinophilic esophagitis. **(a)** Numerous eosinophils, some degranulating, are seen in both the epithelium and the lamina propria. Far fewer eosinophils are seen in reflux esophagitis. Compare this image to Figure 93.1. **(b)** Feline esophagus demonstrating rippling or plications of the esophageal mucosa. This is a transient occurrence and disappears with continued observation, as shown in the right panel. Eosinophilic esophagitis can present with a similar appearance but the rings persist with air insufflation and are less tightly spaced apart (right panel).

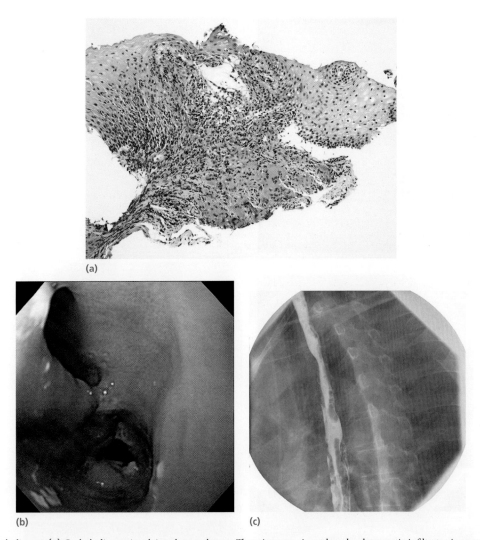

Figure 93.11 Crohn's disease. **(a)** Crohn's disease involving the esophagus. There is a prominent lymphoplasmacytic infiltrate. A granuloma is seen in the lower center portion of the field. **(b)** An endoscopic view of Crohn's disease of the esophagus with diffuse esophageal narrowing, a prominent sinus tract, and exudative plaques. **(c)** A barium swallow from the same patient shows esophageal narrowing, mucosal irregularity, ulceration, and nodularity, as well as sinus tracts parallel to the esophagus. **(d–i)** More examples of Crohn's esophagitis. Esophageal narrowing and deep sinus tracts again noted **(d)**, and on barium swallow, the barium tablet becomes lodged in the proximal esophagus **(e)**. Several fistulae with white exudate and possible *Candida* are seen opening from the esophagus **(f)**; barium swallow confirms a thin fistulous tract from the area of the gastroesophageal junction (GEJ) extending caudally to the right mainstem bronchus **(g)**. On CT scan, a thickened esophagus with multiple sinus tracts is readily apparent **(h)**, and just above the GEJ a fistulous tract is seen entering the lung **(i)**.

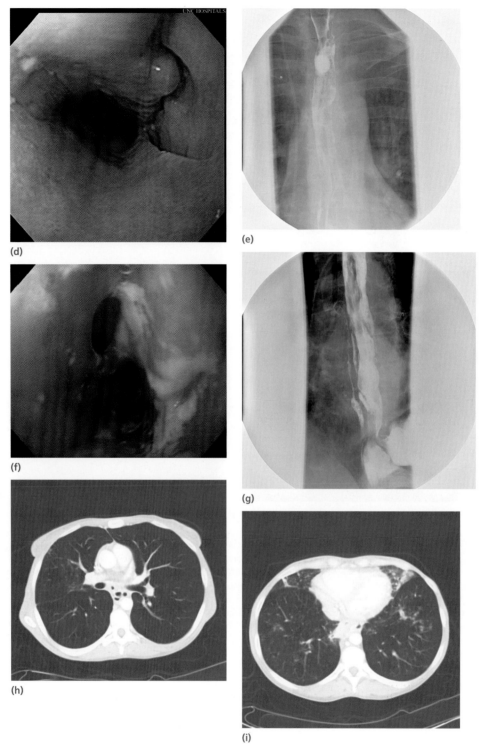

Figure 93.11 (*Continued*)

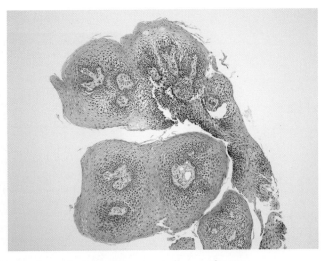

Figure 93.12 Squamous papilloma of the esophagus. Squamous mucosa coats fibrovascular cores.

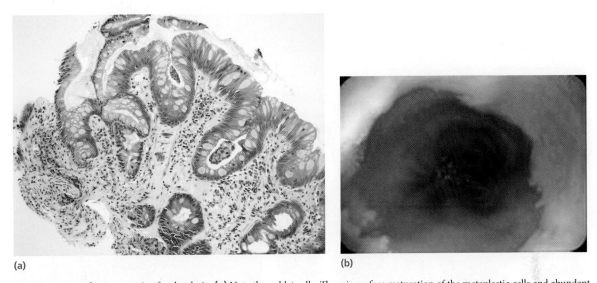

(a)   (b)

Figure 93.13 Barrett esophagus, negative for dysplasia. **(a)** Note the goblet cells. There is surface maturation of the metaplastic cells and abundant lamina propria. **(b)** This image demonstrates the characteristic salmon pink mucosa of Barrett esophagus extending proximally from the gastroesophageal junction. The normal esophageal squamous mucosa is pearly white and can be seen here in the proximal portion of the esophagus.

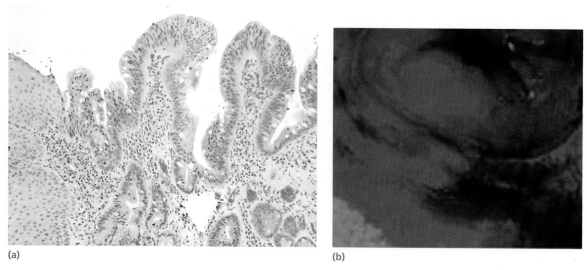

(a)

(b)

Figure 93.14 Low-grade dysplasia in Barrett esophagus. **(a)** The epithelial changes are seen both in deep glands and on the surface but the nuclei are aligned perpendicularly to the basement membrane (maintained nuclear polarity). **(b)** Chromoendoscopy. This involves staining the gastrointestinal mucosa for better endoscopic visualization, usually for the detection of malignant or premalignant lesions. In this image, Lugol solution has been used to stain the distal esophagus. Negative staining of nodular mucosa can be seen, and biopsy confirmed Barrett esophagus with mild dysplasia. Source: Courtesy of Dr. Moises Guelrud.

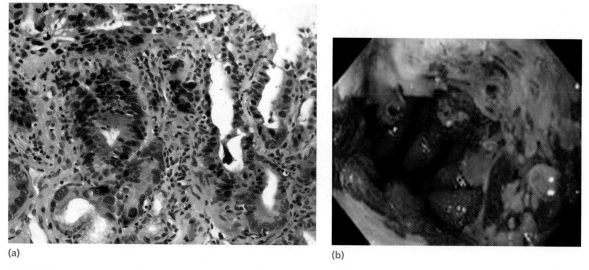

(a)

(b)

Figure 93.15 High-grade dysplasia and intramucosal carcinoma in Barrett esophagus. **(a)** Hyperchromatic nuclei have lost their polarity (relation to the basement membrane). **(b)** Narrow band imaging (NBI), Barrett esophagus with high-grade dysplasia. NBI is a high-resolution endoscopic technique that may enhance the visualization of the fine vasculature and mucosal morphology. In this patient with Barrett esophagus, high-grade dysplasia, and squamous overgrowth, NBI demonstrates dysmorphic glands and vasculature. Source: Courtesy of Drs Herbert C. Wolfsen and Michael B. Wallace.

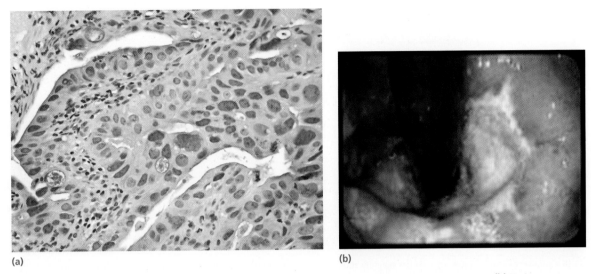

Figure 93.16 Esophageal adenocarcinoma. **(a)** In this field, the adenocarcinoma undermines adjoining squamous mucosa. **(b)** Endoscopic appearance of an ulcerated gastroesophageal junction mass, which revealed poorly differentiated esophageal adenocarcinoma on biopsy. In this image, the mass can be seen extending from the gastroesophageal junction in a retroflexed view.

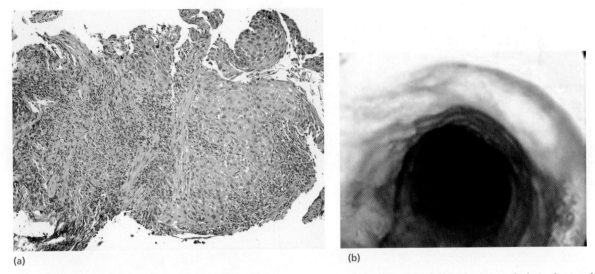

Figure 93.17 Esophageal squamous cell carcinoma. **(a)** There is a squamous pearl towards the right of the field. In this biopsy, the lesion has invaded the muscularis mucosae, seen as slender pink strips. **(b)** In the mid esophagus, an irregular nodular plaque was observed in a patient with a history of alcohol and tobacco use. Biopsies revealed moderately differentiated squamous cell cancer of the esophagus.

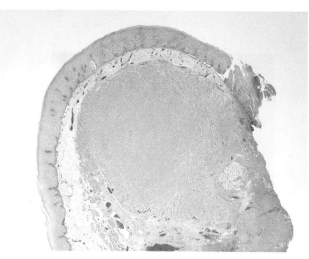

Figure 93.18 Granular cell tumor esophagus. At low magnification, a well-marginated nodule is seen in the lamina propria.

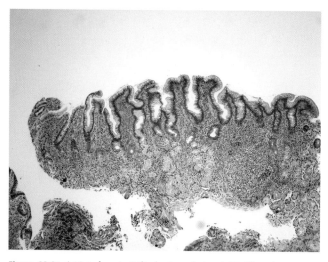

Figure 93.21 Active chronic *Helicobacter pylori* gastritis. Note the lymphoid follicles in this low-magnification field.

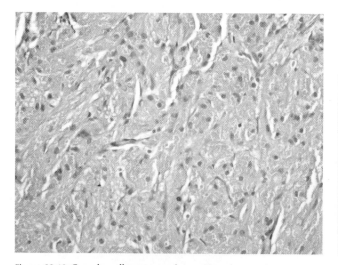

Figure 93.19 Granular cell tumor esophagus. Note the granular appearance of the eosinophilic proliferating cells.

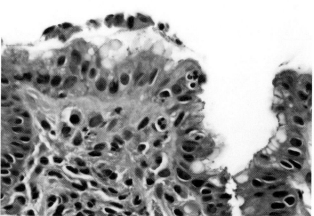

Figure 93.22 Active chronic *Helicobacter pylori* gastritis. At high magnification, neutrophils are seen in the epithelium. Organisms are easily identified on this hematoxylin and eosinstain but it is usually best to apply one of several other stains to detect them.

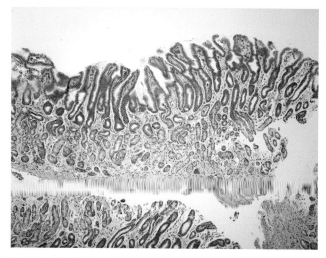

Figure 93.20 Chemical gastritis/reactive gastropathy. The antral mucosa has a villiform appearance and there is mucin loss in the epithelium. There is very little inflammation.

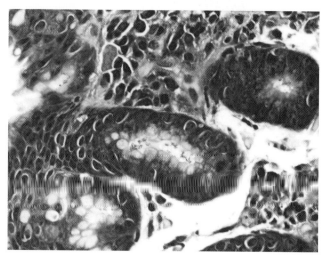

Figure 93.23 Active chronic *Helicobacter pylori* gastritis. A DiffQuik® stain highlights the organisms, seen as curved bacilli in the gland at the center of the field.

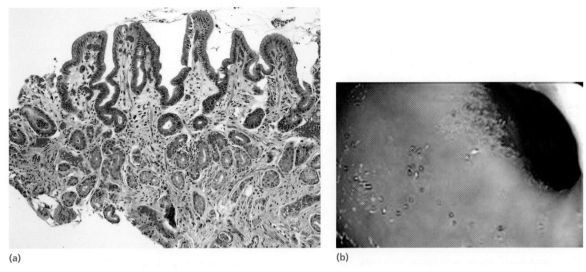

(a)   (b)

Figure 93.24 Autoimmune metaplastic atrophic gastritis. **(a)** The antrum from this patient shows chemical gastritis – there are few inflammatory cells. **(b)** This patient had diffuse atrophic gastritis. The image of the antrum reveals thin mucosa with visible submucosal vessels. Biopsy confirmed chronic antral gastritis with marked intestinal metaplasia consistent with atrophic gastritis.

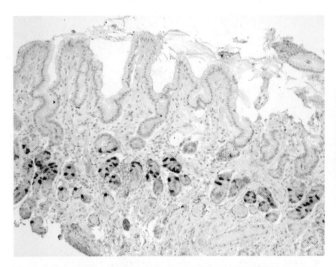

Figure 93.25 Autoimmune metaplastic atrophic gastritis. This is a gastrin stain from the field depicted in Figure 93.24. There are many gastrin-producing cells. The patient was probably hypergastrinemic.

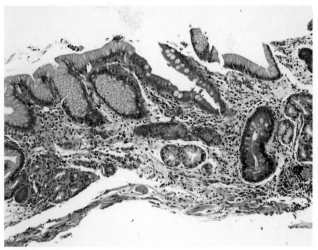

Figure 93.26 Autoimmune metaplastic atrophic gastritis. This biopsy is from the gastric body but there are no acid-producing cells. There is intestinal metaplasia in the center portion of the field (goblet cells).

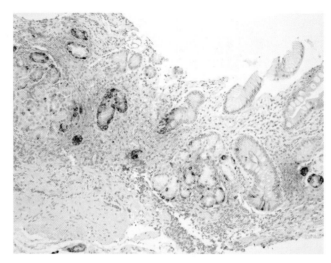

Figure 93.27 Autoimmune metaplastic atrophic gastritis. This chromogranin stain highlights endocrine cell hyperplasia in the area seen in Figure 93.26. Such proliferation can lead to Type 1 carcinoid tumors.

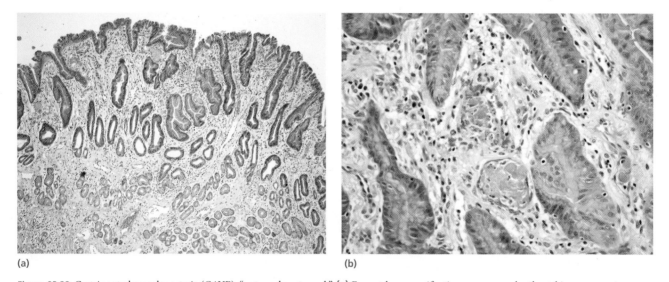

(a)

(b)

Figure 93.28 Gastric antral vascular ectasia (GAVE), "watermelon stomach". (a) Even at low magnification, many vascular thrombi are apparent. (b) High magnification of fibrin thrombi.

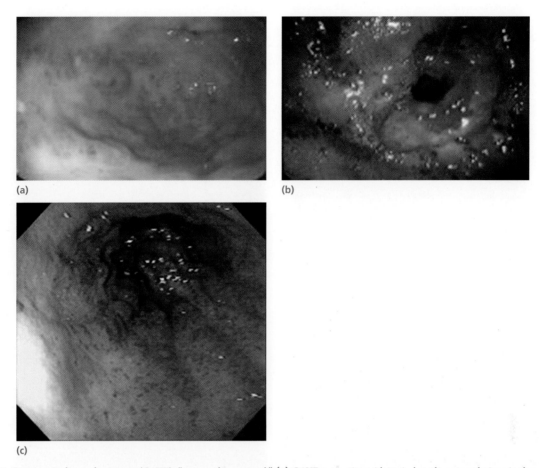

Figure 93.29 Gastric antral vascular ectasia (GAVE), "watermelon stomach". **(a)** GAVE presenting with typical erythematous lesions in the antrum of the stomach. These lesions may require repeated treatments with argon plasma coagulation or electrocautery to prevent recurrent GI bleeding. **(b)** Watermelon stomach. Another term for gastric antral vascular ectasia (GAVE), watermelon stomach refers to the watermelon-like appearance of the antrum in the presence of the striped lines of GAVE. In this patient, multiple bleeding angioectasias can be seen in the gastric antrum. These were treated with argon plasma coagulation with successful hemostasis. **(c)** Gastric antral vascular ectasia.

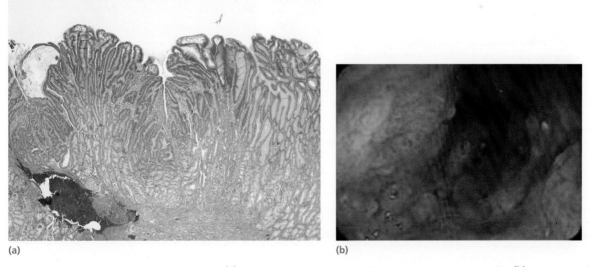

Figure 93.30 Hypertrophic gastropathy/Ménétrier disease. **(a)** There is striking hyperplasia of foveolar (mucin-producing cells). **(b)** Giant gastric folds/ Ménétrier disease. This patient with hypoalbuminemia presented with markedly enlarged gastric folds. Biopsies revealed edematous gastric mucosa with foveolar hyperplasia and no evidence of malignancy, confirming Ménétrier disease; however, years later he developed gastric leiomyosarcoma.

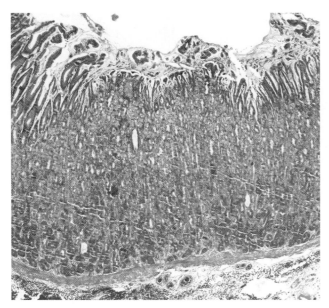

Figure 93.31 Gastric mucosa in Zollinger–Ellison syndrome. There is striking hyperplasia of parietal cells. Contrast this to Figure 93.30a.

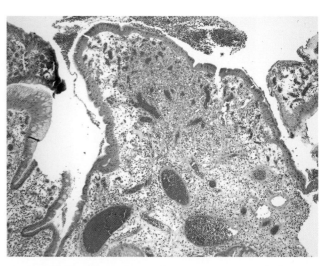

Figure 93.33 Gastric hyperplastic polyp: it is not uncommon for large hyperplastic polyps to display surface erosions or ulcers and reparative epithelial changes.

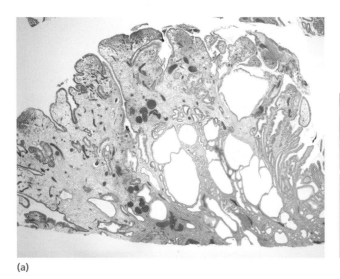

(a)

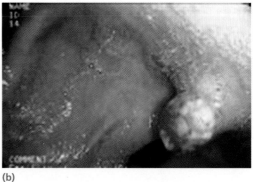

(b)

Figure 93.32 Gastric hyperplastic polyp. **(a)** There is prominence of mucin-producing epithelium and cystically dilated glands. This lesion has overlap with hypertrophic gastropathy and diagnosis of either condition requires correlation with the endoscopic appearance. **(b)** Gastric inflammatory polyp: hyperplastic polyp. An inflamed hyperplastic polyp is seen here in the antrum of the stomach. Hyperplastic polyps are the most common type of gastric polyp and, while they have a low malignant potential, should be removed at the time of endoscopy.

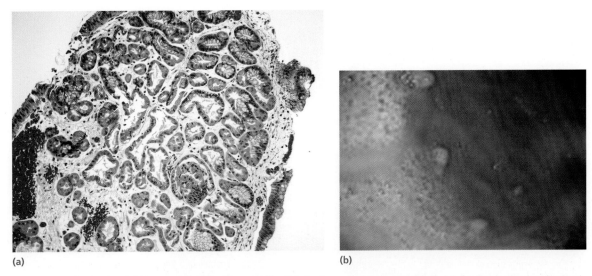

Figure 93.34 Fundic gland polyp. **(a)** The cystically dilated oxyntic (fundic) glands are the key feature. **(b)** Gastric fundic gland polyp: fundic gland polyps. These small sessile polyps that are distributed in the body and fundus in a patient with a history of proton pump inhibitor therapy are characteristic of fundic gland polyps.

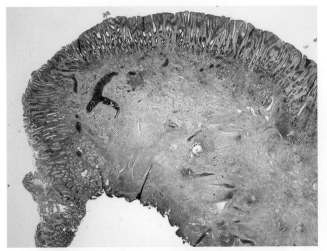

Figure 93.35 Inflammatory fibroid polyp. These tumors have their epicenters in the superficial submucosa.

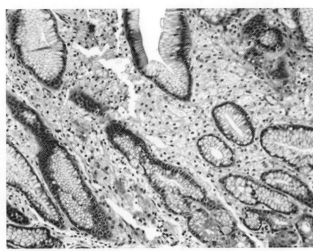

Figure 93.37 Gastric xanthoma. Numerous lipid-laden macrophages are seen in the lamina propria.

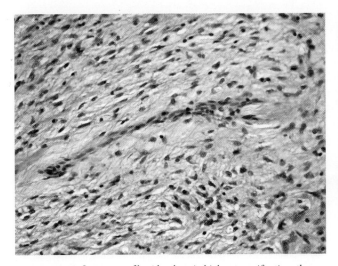

Figure 93.36 Inflammatory fibroid polyp. At higher magnification, there is a spindle cell lesion punctuated by many eosinophils.

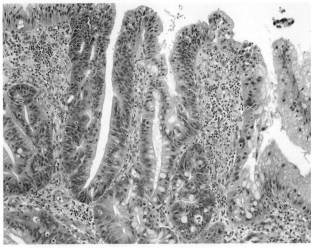

Figure 93.38 Gastric adenoma intestinal type. This example shows both intestinal metaplasia and high-grade dysplasia.

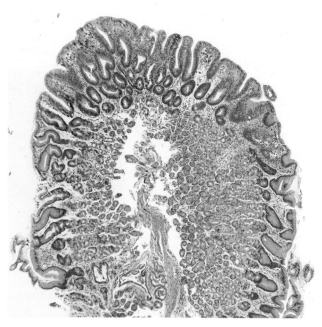

Figure 93.39 Gastric adenoma "gastric" type. Such a lesion, arising in normal background mucosa, is a "low-risk" lesion unlikely to be associated with either high-grade dysplasia or invasive carcinoma.

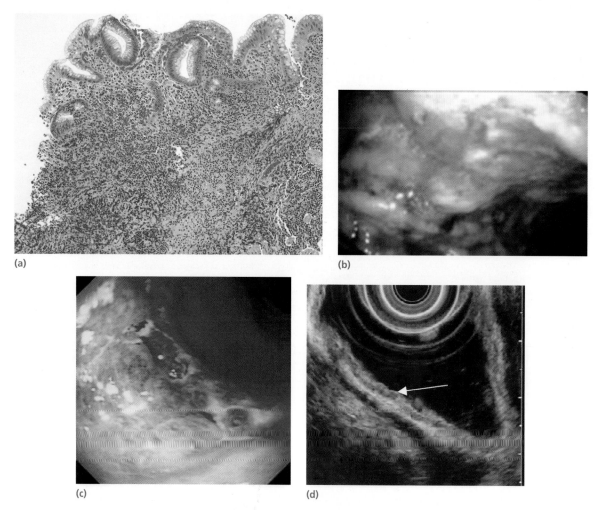

Figure 93.40 Mucosa-associated lymphoid tissue (MALT) lymphoma. **(a)** MALT lymphoma, also called extranodal marginal zone B-cell lymphoma. Note the "bottom-heavy" distribution of the lymphoid infiltrate. **(b)** Gastric MALT lymphoma. Friable ulcerated mucosa on the lesser curvature of the stomach. Biopsies revealed a dense lymphoid infiltrate with focal ulceration consistent with low-grade marginal zone MALT B-cell lymphoma. **(c)** MALT lymphoma: endoscopic appearance. **(d)** MALT lymphoma: thickened gastric mucosa without submucosa involvement (arrow) as shown by endoscopic ultrasonography (stage IE1).

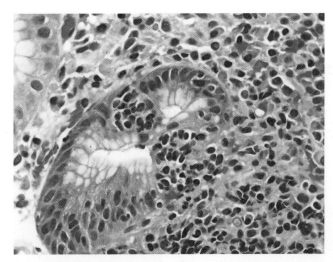

Figure 93.41 Mucosa-associated lymphoid tissue (MALT) lymphoma. This field shows a "lymphoepithelial lesion" in which lymphoid cells proliferate in the epithelium itself.

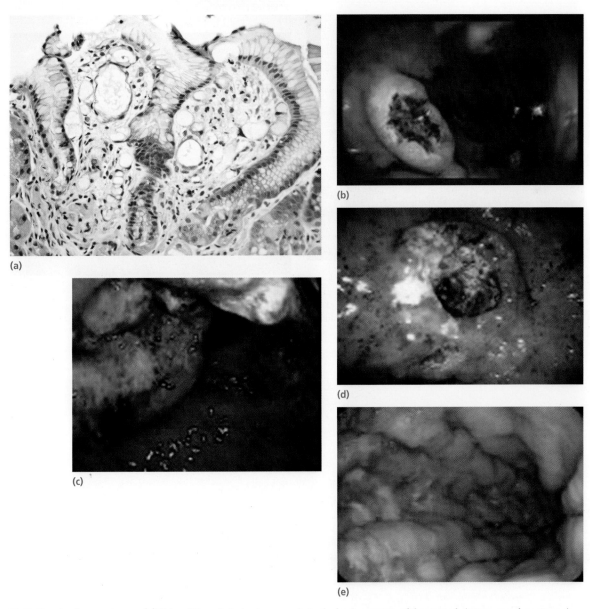

Figure 93.42 Gastric adenocarcinoma. **(a)** This subtle early lesion is seen only in the lamina propria of the stomach (intramucosal carcinoma). **(b)** Malignant gastric ulcer. This large cratered gastric ulcer had heaped margins and a chronic appearance. Biopsies from this ulcer revealed a signet ring cell adenocarcinoma with ulceration and candidal overgrowth. **(c)** Moderately differentiated invasive gastric adenocarcinoma. An ulcerated mass in the antrum of the stomach seen here in an 84-year-old woman from Korea with iron deficiency anemia. Stomach cancer is the most prevalent malignant neoplasm in Korea. **(d)** Advanced gastric carcinoma: irregular fungating ulcerated pyloric channel mass. The mass was an invasive, poorly differentiated adenocarcinoma on biopsy. **(e)** Linitis plastica. In this image, the rugal folds of the stomach are thickened diffusely. This patient was found to have poorly differentiated metastatic adenocarcinoma of the breast.

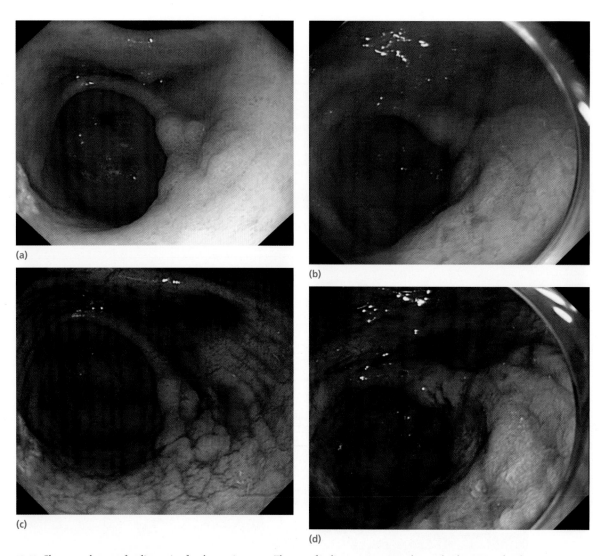

Figure 93.43 Chromoendoscopy for diagnosis of early gastric cancer. The use of indigocarmine can enhance the detection of early gastric cancer. **(a, b)** Type I protruded gastric cancer; **(c, d)** Type IIc depressed lesion.

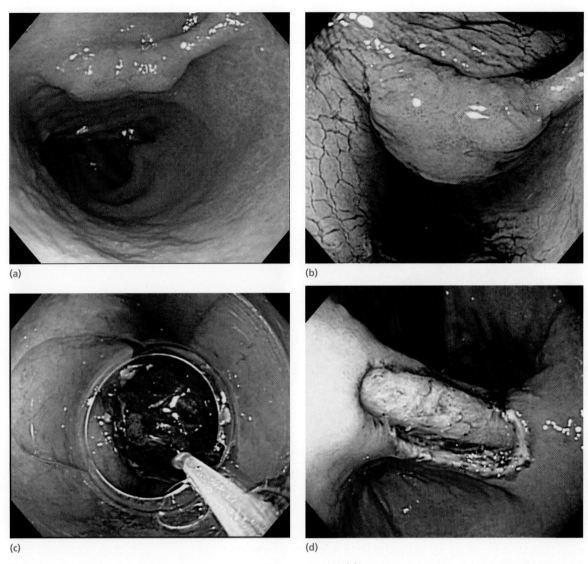

(a)

(b)

(c)

(d)

Figure 93.44 Endoscopic mucosal resection of early gastric cancer. Early gastric cancer (a) was first stained with indigocarmine and injected with normal saline to lift up the lesion (b). The lesion was then sucked into the suction cap (c) and removed by an endoscopic mucosal resection snare (d).

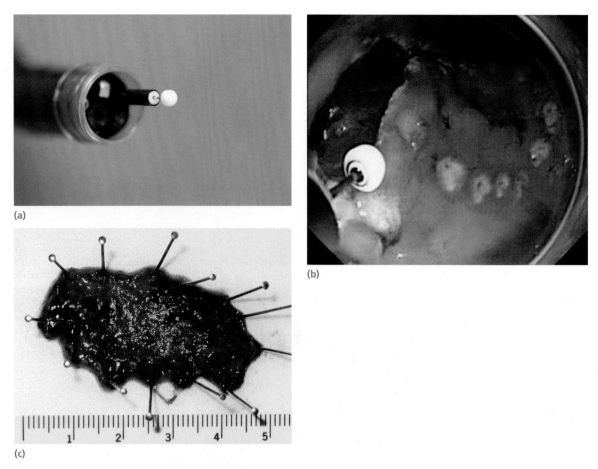

Figure 93.45 Endoscopic submucosal dissection of early gastric cancer. **(a)** The insulation-tipped needle knife consists of a conventional diathermic needle knife with a ceramic ball at the top to minimize the risk of perforation; **(b)** The knife can be used in submucosal dissection and complete en bloc resection of larger lesion; **(c)** One-piece removal of early gastric cancer.

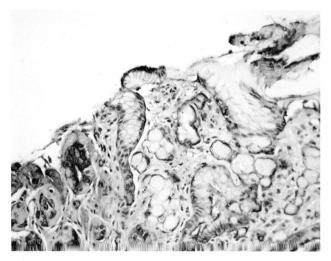

Figure 93.46 Gastric adenocarcinoma. A keratin stain highlights the cancer cells from the field seen in Figure 93.42a.

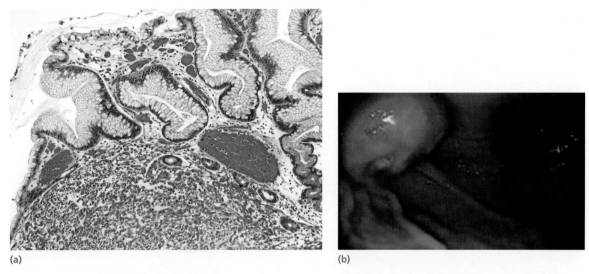

(a)

(b)

Figure 93.47 Gastrointestinal stromal tumor (GIST), spindle cell type. **(a)** This lesion displays mucosal invasion, a feature of malignant GIST. **(b)** Endoscopic appearance of a 3.4-cm GIST in the stomach. These submucosal tumors may have an overlying ulceration as seen here.

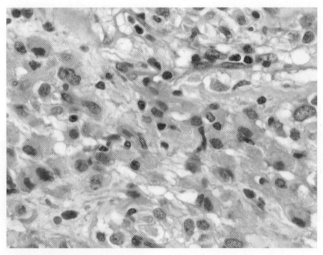

Figure 93.48 Gastrointestinal stromal tumor (GIST), epithelioid type. Note the eosinophilic appearance of the lesional cells. Such tumors were referred to as "leiomyoblastoma" in the past.

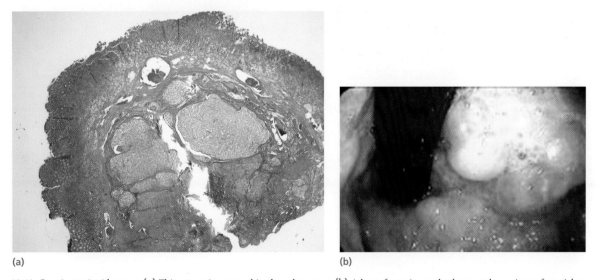

(a)

(b)

Figure 93.49 Gastric carcinoid tumor. **(a)** This tumor is centered in the submucosa. **(b)** A large fungating and submucosal noncircumferential mass was found in the cardia in this patient with multiple endocrine neoplasia type 1. Biopsies confirmed a low-grade carcinoid tumor.

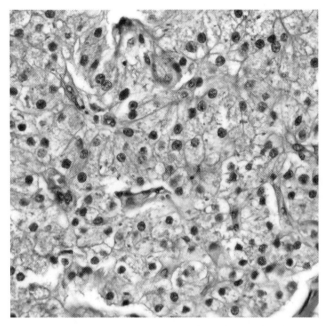

Figure 93.50 Gastric carcinoid tumor. Note the uniform nuclear features.

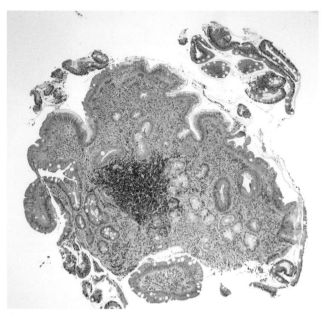

Figure 93.52 Chronic peptic duodenitis. At low magnification, normal duodenal mucosa is seen at the left (goblet cells are present) but the central portion shows gastric-type epithelium that is metaplastic.

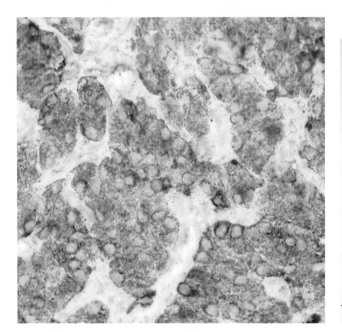

Figure 93.51 Gastric carcinoid tumor. The lesional cells are reactive with synaptophysin antibodies.

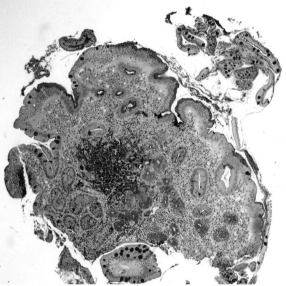

Figure 93.53 Chronic peptic duodenitis. A periodic acid Schiff stain with alcian blue shows the gastric metaplasia to advantage; it appears magenta.

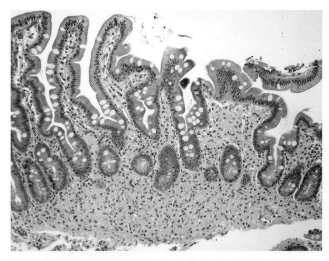

Figure 93.54 *Mycobacterium avium* intracellular duodenitis. The villi are expanded with macrophages.

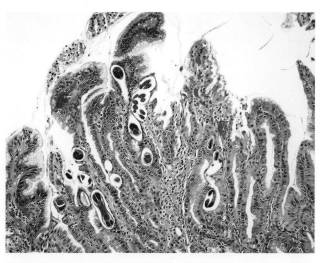

Figure 93.56 Strongyloidiasis. Multiple larval forms are seen in the small intestinal mucosa.

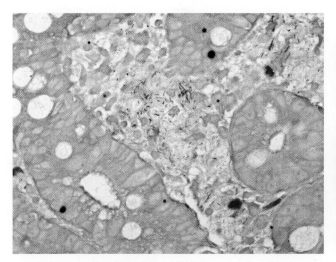

Figure 93.55 *Mycobacterium avium* intracellular duodenitis. This acid-fast stain highlights the organisms.

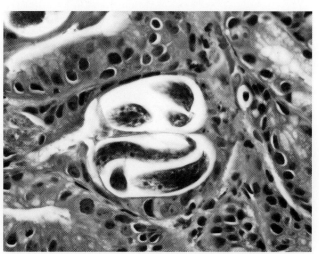

Figure 93.57 Strongyloidiasis. Higher magnification of image Figure 93.53.

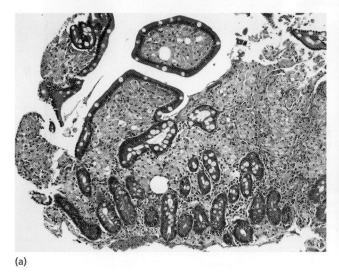

(a)

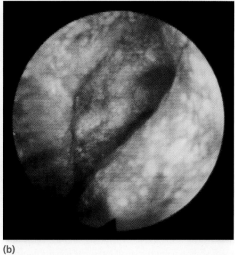

(b)

Figure 93.58 Whipple disease. **(a)** Like Figure 93.51, this image shows many foamy macrophages expanding the villi. In contrast, dilated lacteals are a feature of Whipple disease. **(b)** Characteristic duodenoscopic appearance of the duodenum of an untreated patient with Whipple disease. The folds are thickened and are covered with small yellowish-white plaques. This endoscopic appearance may be the first clue to the diagnosis.

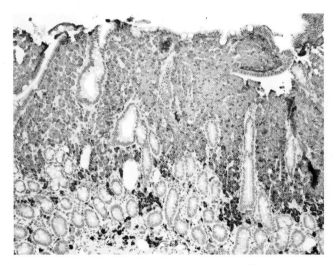

Figure 93.59 Whipple disease. This is an immunohistochemical preparation using an antibody directed against the organism.

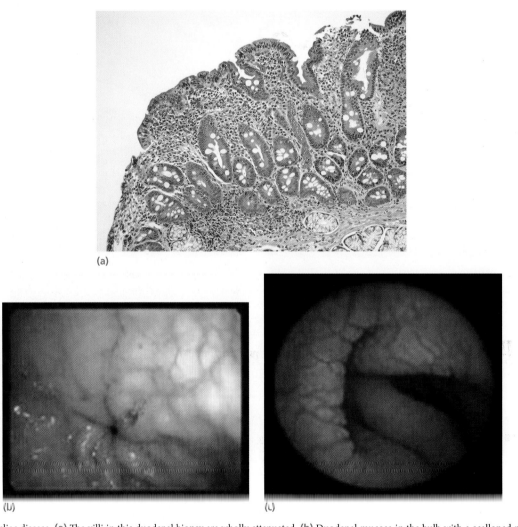

(a)

(b)

(c)

Figure 93.60 Celiac disease. (a) The villi in this duodenal biopsy are wholly attenuated. (b) Duodenal mucosa in the bulb with a scalloped mosaic appearance in a patient with celiac disease. This patient had a high titer of antiendomysial and tissue transglutaminase antibodies. Small bowel biopsies confirmed villous blunting, crypt hyperplasia, and markedly increased intraepithelial lymphocytes. (c) Capsule endoscopy in a patient with celiac disease reveals scalloping of the small intestinal mucosa. Source: Courtesy of Dr. Myles D. Keroack.

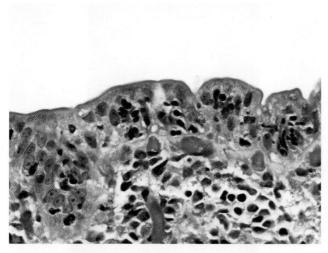

Figure 93.61 Celiac disease. Prominent intraepithelial lymphocytes are a key diagnostic feature.

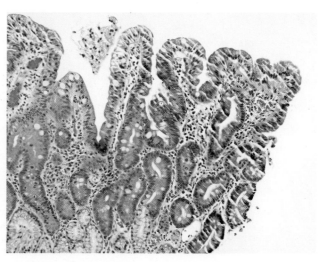

Figure 93.63 Colchicine toxicity. This patient's duodenal biopsy shows attenuated villi and an expanded proliferative compartment. Mitotic arrest is seen as ring mitoses.

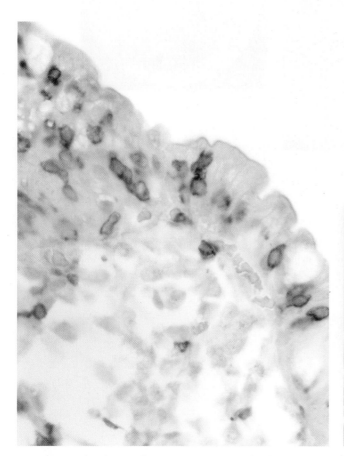

Figure 93.62 Celiac disease. This CD3 immunostain highlights the T cells in the epithelium.

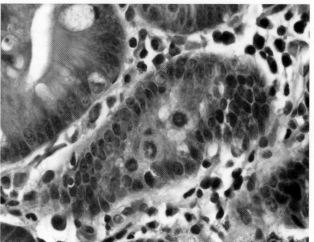

Figure 93.64 Colchicine toxicity. Higher magnification of arrested mitoses.

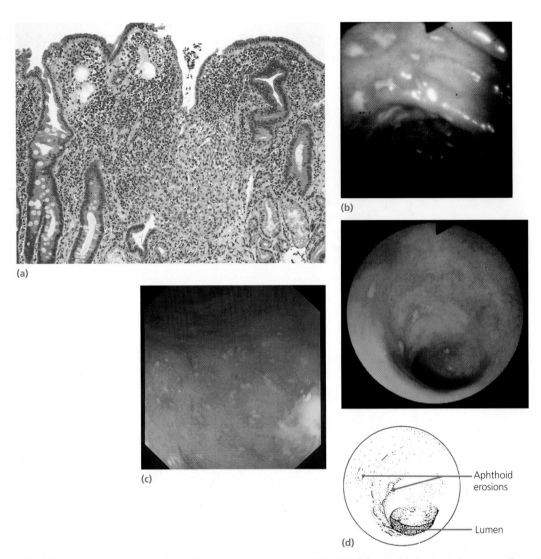

Figure 93.65 Crohn's disease. **(a)** Crohn's disease. A granuloma is seen in the center of the field. **(b)** Crohn's colitis with discrete small, round ulcers separated by normal mucosa. **(c)** Crohn's disease involving the transverse colon with multiple aphthous ulcers. A 26-year-old woman with Crohn's disease for 2 years has persistent symptoms despite prednisone 25 mg daily and sulfasalazine 3 g daily. Endoscopic image shows multiple aphthous ulcers; edematous and erythematous mucosa with a loss of normal vascular markings and mucous exudate. **(d)** Characteristic superficial aphthoid erosions in Crohn's disease have erythematous rings.

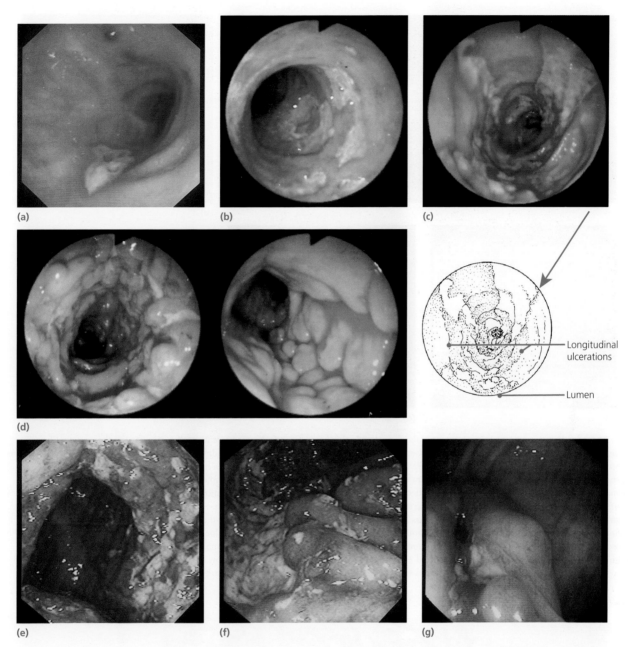

Figure 93.66 **(a)** Crohn's disease of the colon with focal ulcer. A 24-year-old man with Crohn's disease for 2 years currently has minimal symptoms while taking metronidazole 250 mg three times daily and mesalamine 2.4 g daily. There is a focal ulcer in the distal sigmoid colon, mild inflammatory changes of the surrounding mucosa, distortion of the vascular markings, mild granularity, and erythema. **(b)** Multiple large, deep, excavated ulcers in severe ulcerating Crohn's disease show distinct margins. This patient has concomitant sclerosing cholangitis. **(c)** Longitudinal alignment of ulceration causes a railroad-track appearance in Crohn's disease. **(d)** Active phase of Crohn's disease shows cobblestoning caused by interconnecting ulcerations (left). Area of cobblestoning after therapy (right). **(e)** Severely active Crohn's disease of the colon. A 22-year-old man with a 1-year history of Crohn's disease has severe diarrhea, a 19-pound weight loss, and continuing symptoms despite prednisone 60 mg daily. Colonoscopic image shows severe ulceration in the transverse colon with markedly edematous, granular, and friable mucosa. **(f)** Severely active Crohn's disease of the colon (same patient as in part [i]). Deep rake ulcer in middescending colon with surrounding mucosal edema, granularity, and friability. **(g)** Crohn's disease with ulceration at the ileocecal valve. A 26-year-old woman with a history of Crohn's disease for 4 years has involvement of the terminal ileum. The disease was previously controlled with mesalamine 4 g daily, with worsening cramping abdominal pain in recent weeks. Colonoscopy revealed ulceration at the ileocecal valve with stenosis of the valve, which could not be intubated with a colonoscope. The colon otherwise appeared normal.

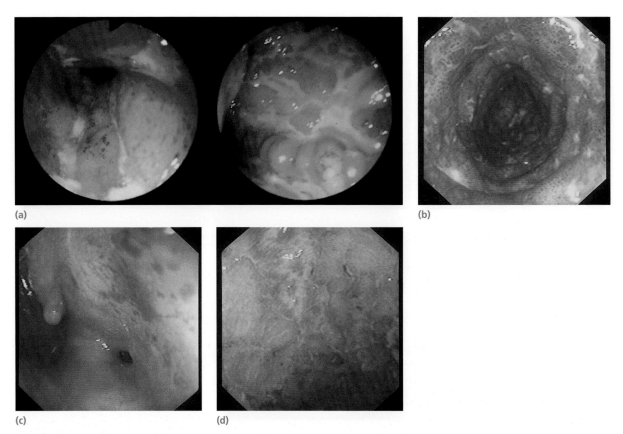

(a)

(b)

(c)

(d)

Figure 93.67 (a) Diffuse, concentric involvement of the distal terminal ileum in Crohn's disease presents itself as swelling, erythema, punctiform bleeding, and ulceration (left). Circumferential involvement of the distal terminal ileum with longitudinal ulcers and cobblestoning (right). **(b)** Crohn's disease involving the neoterminal ileum with multiple superficial ulcers. A 29-year-old woman with a history of Crohn's disease for 6 years had undergone resection of the terminal ileum and cecum with ileal-ascending colonic anastomosis. Symptoms of recurrent Crohn's disease (cramping abdominal pain and malaise) developed 4 months after resection. Colonoscopic image with visualization of the neoterminal ileum shows multiple focal superficial ulcers with edema, erythema, and granularity of the intervening mucosa. **(c)** Crohn's disease – view of the rectum with rectovaginal fistula and prominent anal papilla. A 40-year-old woman has a 10-year history of Crohn's disease involving the colon. A symptomatic rectovaginal fistula developed with gas and stool passed per vagina. Retroflexed view of the rectum shows a central fistulous opening communicating with the vagina. The endoscope is in the left field of the photo, and a prominent anal papilla is present. The mucosa is granular, edematous, and friable. **(d)** Mildly active Crohn's disease of the sigmoid colon in a 51-year-old man with a 4-year history of Crohn's colitis, now controlled with azathioprine 175 mg daily and metronidazole 250 mg twice daily. The mucosa shows superficial scarring, loss of normal vascular markings, and slight mucous exudate.

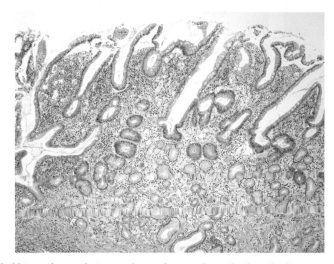

Figure 93.68 Crohn's disease. This ileal biopsy shows pyloric metaplasia – the metaplastic glands in the deep portion of the field lack goblet cells. (See also Fig. 93.67.)

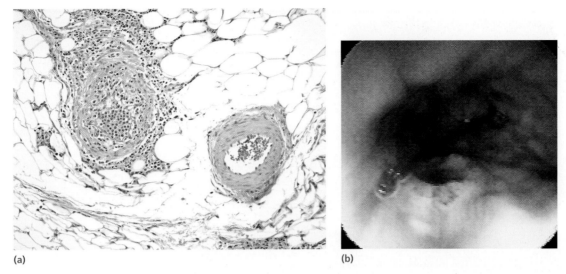

(a)   (b)

Figure 93.69 Behçet disease. **(a)** Vasculitis primarily affecting mesenteric veins is the hallmark. **(b)** An endoscopic view of esophageal ulceration in a patient with Behçet disease.

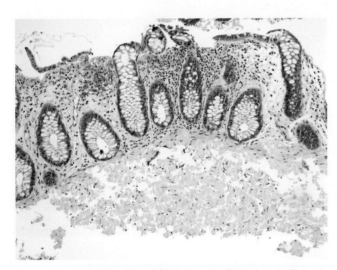

Figure 93.70 Amyloidosis. This field shows prominent submucosal deposits. This is from a colonic biopsy.

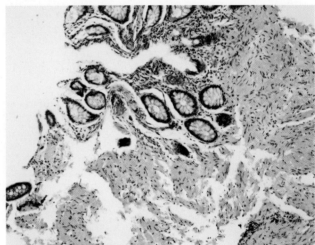

Figure 93.71 Amyloidosis. The Congo red preparation imparts an orange–brown color.

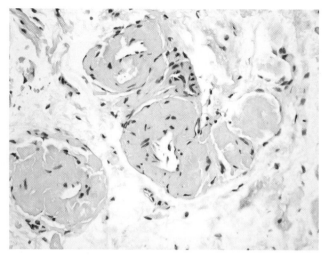

Figure 93.72 Amyloidosis. This vascular deposition was from a gastric biopsy.

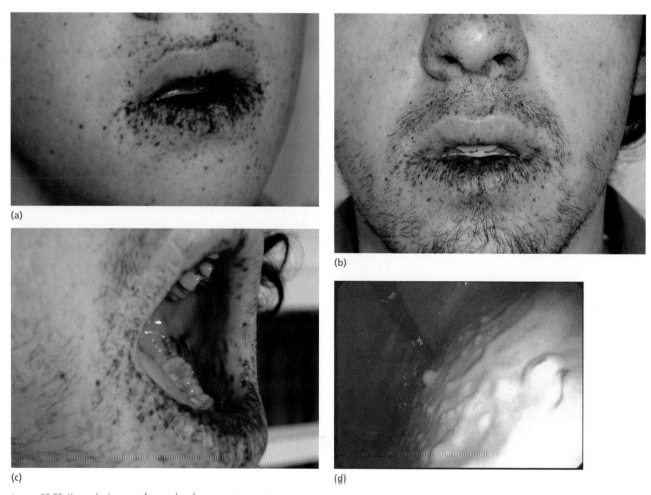

Figure 93.73 Peutz–Jeghers syndrome. (a–c) Perioral, lip, and buccal pigmentation. Courtesy of Dr. Abadur T. Tchekmedyian. (d) Gastric Peutz–Jeghers polyps.

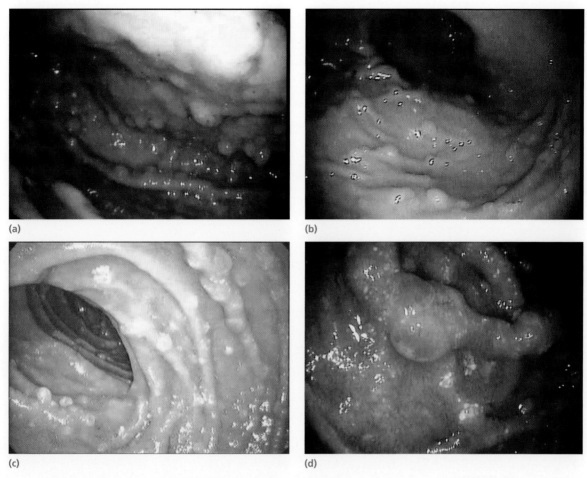

(a)

(b)

(c)

(d)

Figure 93.74 (a, b) Gastric Peutz–Jeghers polyps. **(c, d)** Duodenal Peutz–Jeghers polyps.

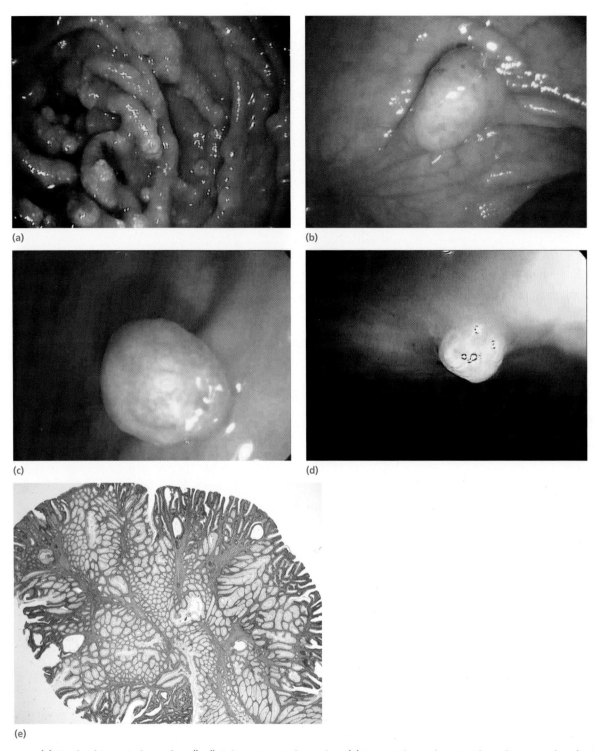

(a)

(b)

(c)

(d)

(e)

Figure 93.75 **(a)** Duodenal Peutz–Jeghers polyps. **(b–d)** Colonic Peutz–Jeghers polyps. **(e)** Peutz–Jeghers polyp. Note the striking muscular arborizing cores.

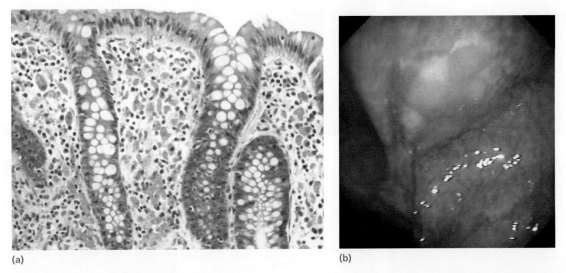

Figure 93.76 (a) Melanosis coli. The pigment in the lamina propria macrophages is lipofuscin rather than melanin. **(b)** Endoscopic photograph shows a 1-cm flat, multilobulated polyp adjacent to the cecal sling fold. The polyp is pale pink, whereas the surrounding mucosa is brown because of melanosis. Adenomas do not take up melanin and stand out in melanosis coli.

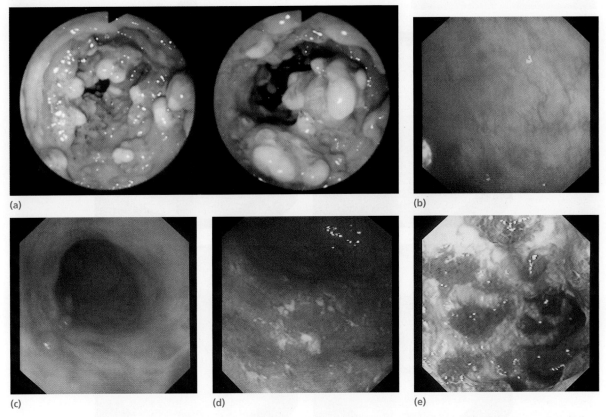

Figure 93.77 Ulcerative colitis. **(a)** Multiple pseudopolyps in ulcerative colitis. Their surface is smooth and glistening. Detailed view of exudate creating whitish caps. **(b)** Quiescent (inactive) ulcerative colitis in a 39-year-old woman with ulcerative pancolitis for 11 years, now asymptomatic. There is distortion of the vascular markings but no granularity, edema, friability, mucus exudate, or ulcerations. **(c)** Mildly active ulcerative colitis with pseudopolyps. Same patient as in part **(b)**, 1 year after the endoscopic examination in **(b)**, with a mild flare in symptoms. The disease now is responding to prednisone 20 mg daily and mesalamine 4 g daily. There are two small pseudopolyps; the mucosa is mildly granular and erythematous; and the vascular markings are distorted. **(d)** Moderately active ulcerative colitis in a 19-year-old woman with ulcerative pancolitis for 2 years. The patient has continuing symptoms despite oral mesalamine 4 g daily and prednisone 40 mg daily. Moderate granularity, edema, and mucus exudate is demonstrated. **(e)** Severely active ulcerative colitis in a 54-year-old woman with left-sided ulcerative colitis for 7 years. There is marked ulceration. At least half of the surface area depicted is denuded by ulcers, and there are intervening areas of edematous granular mucosa.

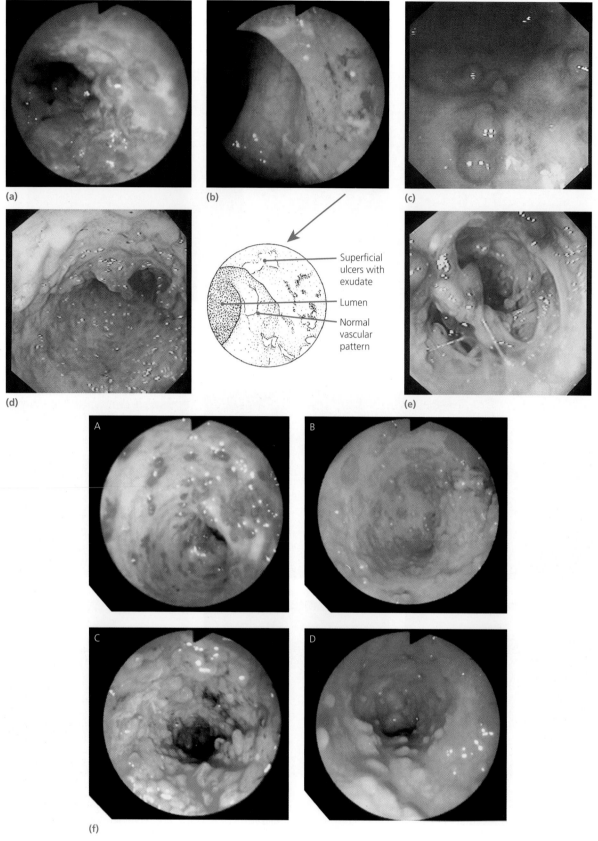

Figure 93.78 (a) Coarsely nodular deformity of mucosal contour in ulcerative colitis. Mucosa is intensely erythematous and friable. (b) Sharp transition from normal to inflamed bowel is discernible at the rectosigmoid junction. Erythema and superficial ulceration of diseased mucosa contrast to the normal vascular pattern. (c) Mildly active ulcerative colitis with multiple pseudopolyps. A 54-year-old woman (same patient as in Fig. 93.77d) about 1 year after a course of topical 5-ASA (mesalamine) and prednisone 60 mg daily tapered and discontinued 9 months previously. There is mild granularity and erythema; the vascular markings are distorted, and multiple small pseudopolyps are present. (d) Long-standing ulcerative colitis with scarring and pseudopolyps. A 25-year-old man had a 9-year history of ulcerative colitis. The patient is now asymptomatic with azathioprine 150 mg daily and mesalamine 2.4 g daily. There is scarring and loss of the normal vascular markings. Two small pseudopolyps are present. (e) Ulcerative colitis with bridging pseudopolyps. A 25-year-old man has had ulcerative colitis for 9 years (same patient as in part [d]) and the disease is asymptomatic with azathioprine 150 mg daily and mesalamine 2.4 g daily. Endoscopic picture shows bridging pseudopolyps in the transverse colon. (f) Sequential study of severe pancolitis. Massive ulceration of the colon was studied at intervals of 4–6 weeks after institution of medical therapy. A, view of the proximal sigmoid shows extensive ulceration before therapy. Some islands of remaining mucosa are visible; B, regression of inflammation and early reepithelialization; C, ulcers are regressing with pseudopolypoid elevation of nonulcerated mucosal islands; D, full reepithelialization and pseudopolypoid transformation characterize healing.

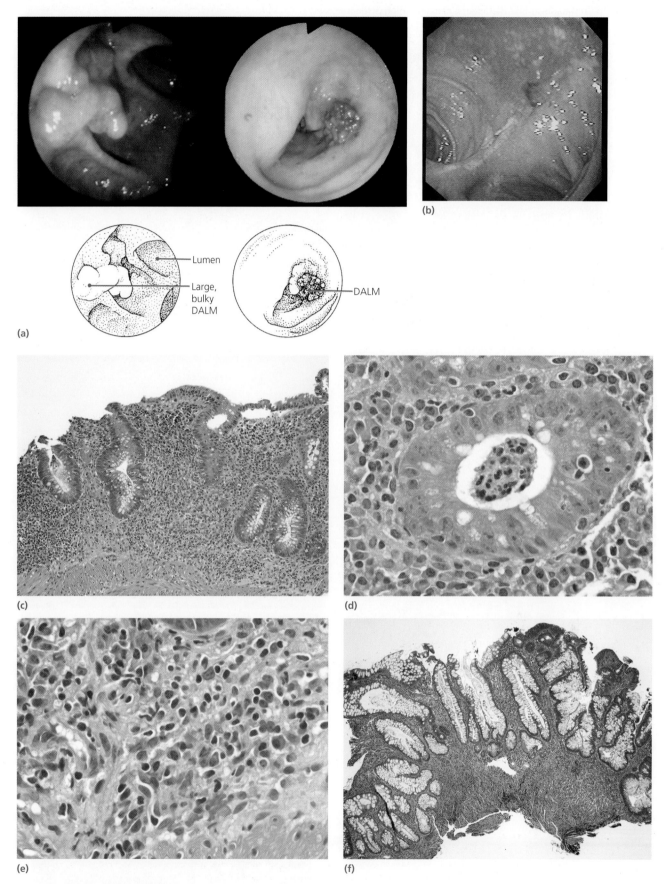

Figure 93.79 **(a)** Examples of dysplasia-associated lesions or masses in long-standing, inactive ulcerative colitis. **(b)** Mild to moderately active pouchitis. This 36-year-old woman has a history of ulcerative colitis for which she underwent colectomy with ileal J pouch-anal anastomosis 2 years previously. She had recurrent liquid stools and cramping discomfort relieved with bowel movements. Endoscopic image of the pouch, with views of the afferent limb of the neoterminal ileum in the left portion of the field and the blind end of the J pouch in the inferior aspect of the field, shows mucus exudate, superficial ulceration, and friability of the pouch mucosa but not of the mucosa in the neoterminal ileum. **(c–f)** Ulcerative colitis. In these fields, the crypts are distorted and do not reach the muscularis mucosae at the bottom of the fields.

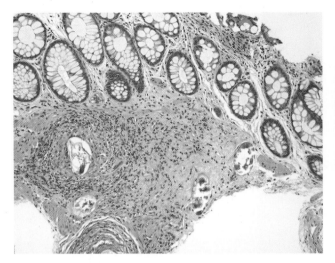

Figure 93.80 Schistosomiasis. Ova surrounded by eosinophils are seen in the submucosa.

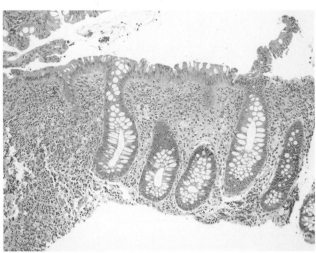

Figure 93.82 Spirochetosis. This biopsy was from an immunosuppressed person with diarrhea. The biopsy shows features of acute self-limiting colitis in that there is cryptitis without crypt distortion.

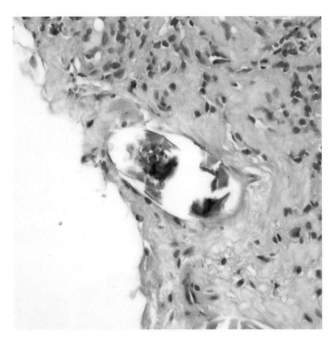

Figure 93.81 Schistosomiasis. The lateral spine of this ovum is in keeping with schistosomiasis mansoni.

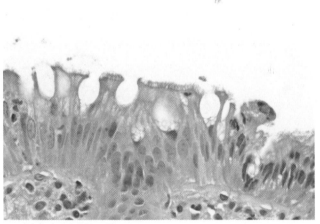

Figure 93.83 Spirochetosis. The hair-like structures emanating from the surface are the organisms.

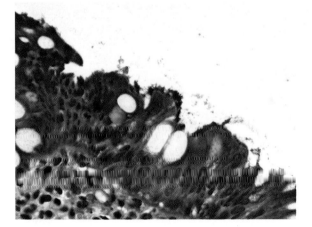

Figure 93.84 Spirochetosis. This Warthin-Starry silver stain highlights the organisms.

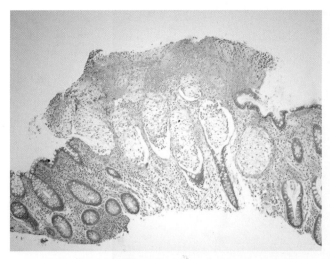

Figure 93.85 Pseudomembranous colitis. A pseudomembrane is seen at the center of the field.

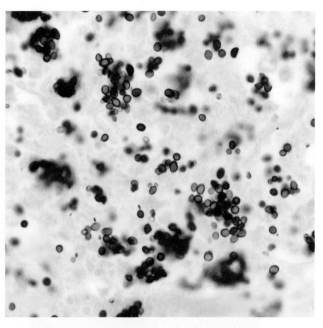

Figure 93.87 Histoplasmosis. A Gomori–methenamine silver stain from the image seen in Figure 93.80 shows budding yeast forms.

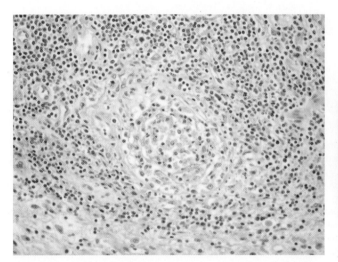

Figure 93.86 Histoplasmosis. This poorly-formed necrotizing granuloma was found in an immunosuppressed person and contained the organisms.

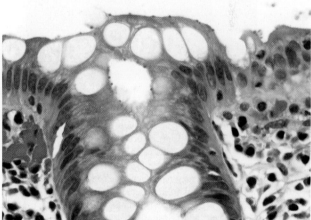

Figure 93.88 Cryptosporidiosis. Organisms appear as small beads at the epithelial surface.

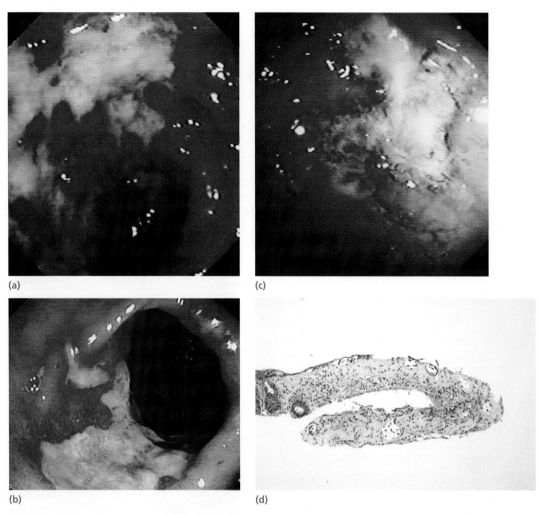

Figure 93.89 Ischemic colitis. **(a)** An 83-year-old female who presented with abdominal pain and bloody diarrhea. Colonoscopy revealed the presence of large ulcerations in the splenic flexure. Biopsies were compatible with the diagnosis of ischemic colitis. This region is commonly affected in colonic ischemia because of its relatively low perfusion (watershed area). Colonoscopy is the method of choice for the diagnosis of ischemic colitis, because it allows direct visualization of the mucosa and tissue sampling. **(b)** Large ulceration in the sigmoid region caused by ischemia. The sigmoid colon is another area that is particularly susceptible to ischemic lesions because of its relatively low perfusion. Although this lesion can be reached by a sigmoidoscopy, complete colonoscopy should be performed in patients suspected of having ischemic colitis because 50% of the ischemic lesions are proximal to the sigmoid colon. **(c)** Endoscopic findings in a 62-year-old female with ischemic colitis associated with a low-flow state (sepsis). The mucosa of the affected segment appears edematous, hemorrhagic, friable, and ulcerated. **(d)** Ischemic colitis. This example is from an individual who was receiving Kayexalate® but the features are similar regardless of etiology. This biopsy shows atrophic microcrypts and lamina propria hyalinization.

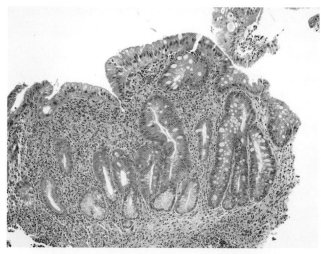

Figure 93.90 Common variable immunodeficiency. The features are similar to those of ulcerative colitis and it is easy for pathologists to make an incorrect diagnosis in such cases.

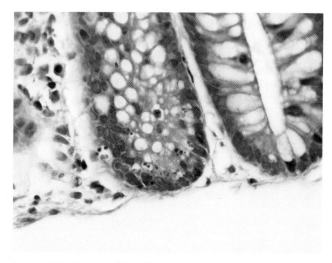

Figure 93.92 Graft-versus-host disease: note the crypt apoptosis. Crypt apoptosis may also result from phosphasoda bowel preparation so this method is not advised if assessing for graft-versus-host disease.

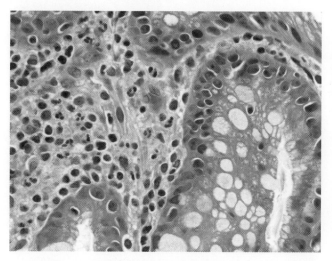

Figure 93.91 Common variable immunodeficiency. The key is the absence of plasma cells in the lamina propria; they would be a prominent constituent in the inflammatory backdrop of ulcerative colitis. The prominent lamina propria neutrophils in this biopsy are in keeping with an acute infection.

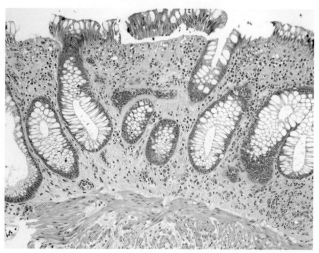

Figure 93.93 Radiation proctitis: note the prominent vessel parallel to the epithelial surface.

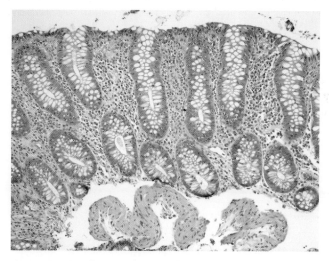

Figure 93.94 Lymphocytic colitis: note the intraepithelial lymphocytosis.

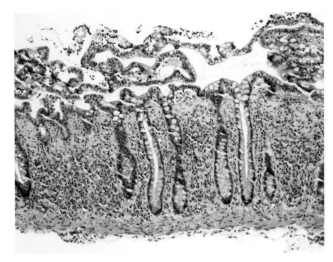

Figure 93.95 Collagenous colitis. Subepithelial collagen is the hallmark.

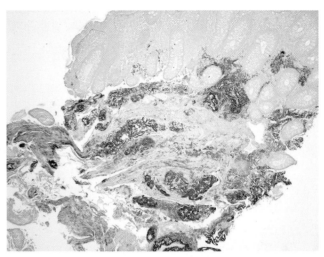

Figure 93.98 Elastosis. Elastic stain of the polyp seen in Figure 93.91.

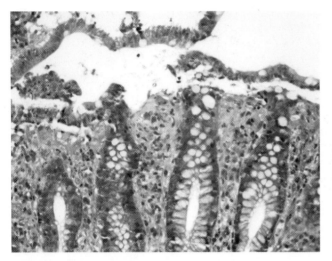

Figure 93.96 Collagenous colitis. This trichrome stain results in a blue color in the subepithelial collagen.

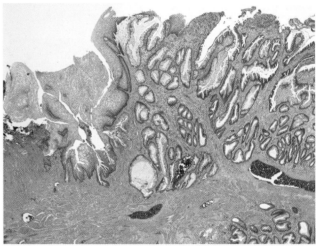

Figure 93.99 Inflammatory cloacogenic polyp. This prolapse lesion is found at the junction of anal squamous (left part of field) and rectal mucosa.

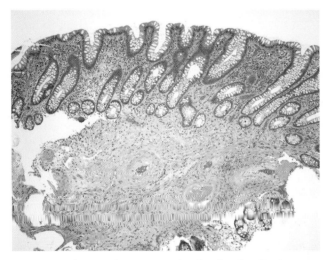

Figure 93.97 Elastosis. This process produced an "incidental" polyp.

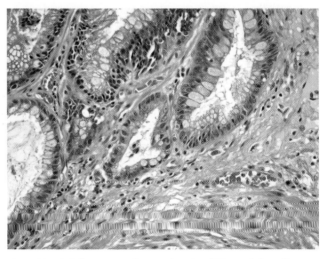

Figure 93.100 Inflammatory cloacogenic polyp. "Diamond-shaped" glands are a characteristic finding of colorectal prolapse lesions.

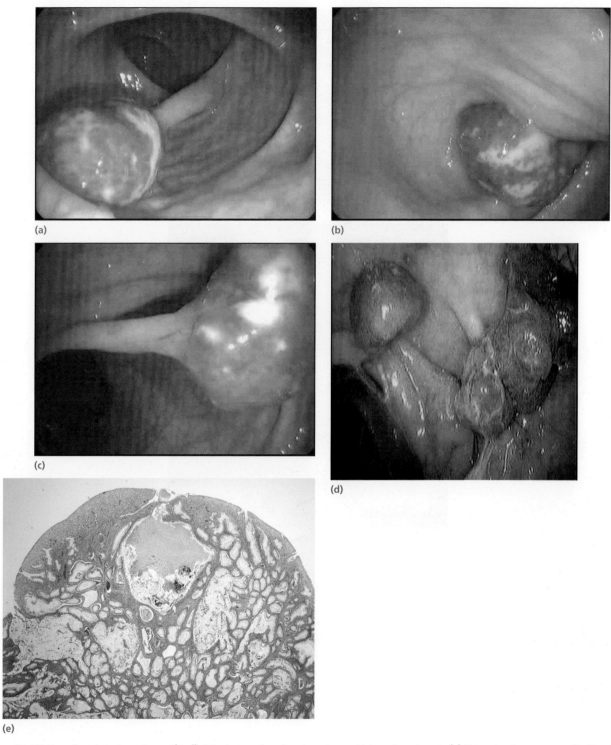

Figure 93.101 Juvenile polyposis syndrome. (a–d) Colonic juvenile polyps in patients with juvenile polyposis. (e) This polyp features cystically dilated glands, an expanded lamina propria and an eroded surface.

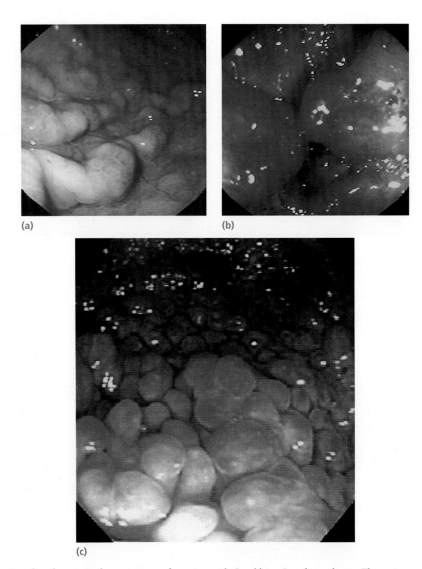

(a)

(b)

(c)

Figure 93.102 Cronkhite–Canada polyposis. Endoscopic views of a patient with Cronkhite–Canada syndrome. The patient presented with dysgeusia, alopecia, onychodystrophy, and diarrhea. **(a)** Stomach. **(b)** Colon: the largest polyp is a pedunculated adenomatous polyp; all other polyps shown exhibited histology typical of Cronkhite–Canada lesions. Source: Courtesy of Dr. Edward L. Krawitt. **(c)** Cronkhite–Canada polyposis. This endoscopic image is from the patient's cecum. He had polyps throughout his gastrointestinal tract, sparing only his esophagus.

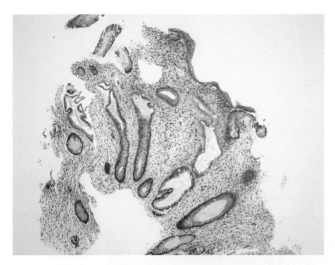

Figure 93.103 Cronkhite–Canada polyposis. This histological appearance of a colonic polyp is hardly specific – the polyp appears similar to a juvenile-type polyp. The distinction is made on clinicopathological grounds and by attention to the background flat mucosa, which is abnormal in Cronkhite–Canada polyposis but normal in juvenile polyposis.

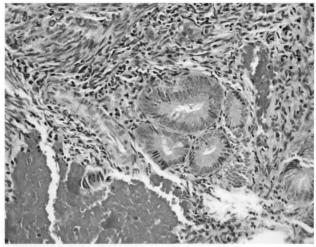

Figure 93.105 Colonic endometriosis. Higher magnification of the lesion seen in Figure 93.104.

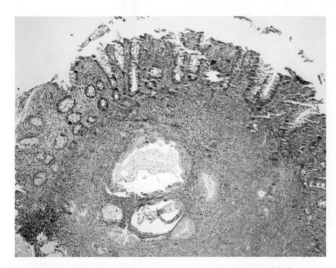

Figure 93.104 Colonic endometriosis. This is a diagnostic pitfall for endoscopists and pathologists alike. The key is for the pathologist to note the background stromal tissue accompanying the glands.

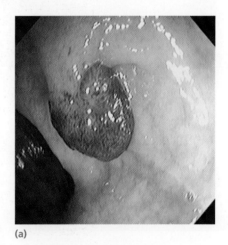

(a)

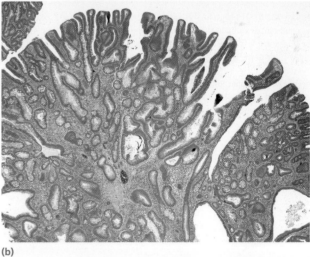

(b)

Figure 93.106 Tubular adenoma. **(a)** Colonoscopic photograph of an 8-mm tubular adenoma on a moderate sized stalk. **(b)** Histological appearance of a tubular adenoma. By definition, the epithelium is dysplastic (neoplastic) but not invasive carcinoma is evident.

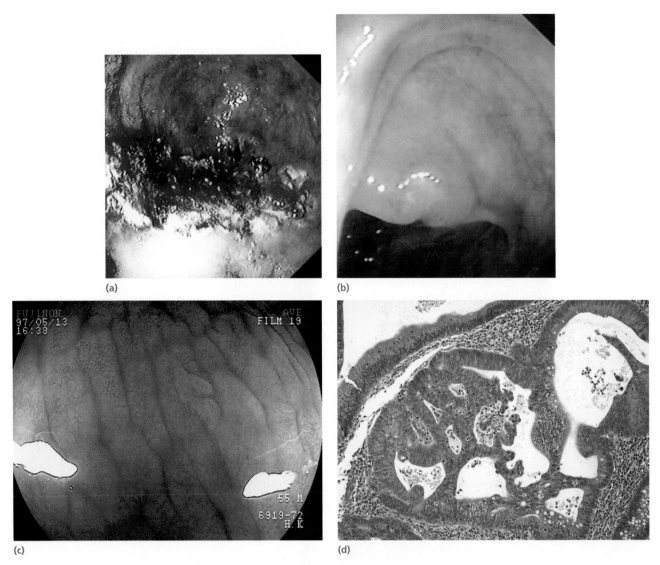

Figure 93.107 High-grade dysplasia in tubular adenoma. **(a)** Colonoscopic photograph of a villous adenoma after polypectomy followed by destruction of residual adenoma at the margins by argon plasma coagulation. Close follow-up is required to check for recurrence because total destruction cannot be guaranteed. **(b)** Colonoscopic photograph of a flat adenoma with slight central depression on the edge of a fold in sigmoid colon. These are likely to show high-grade dysplasia. Flat adenomas are recognized more commonly in Japan, and a recent study has shown that they may be as common in Western countries such as the United Kingdom. Source: Courtesy of Dr. Michael Bourke. **(c)** Magnifying colonoscopic view of a cluster of aberrant crypts with histopathological features of dysplasia. These are the earliest stage of adenoma formation. *APC* or *Ras* mutations (or both) may already be established in these lesions. **(d)** High-grade dysplasia in a tubular adenoma. The gland in the center is complex with a cribriform architecture. However, the basement membrane around it is intact.

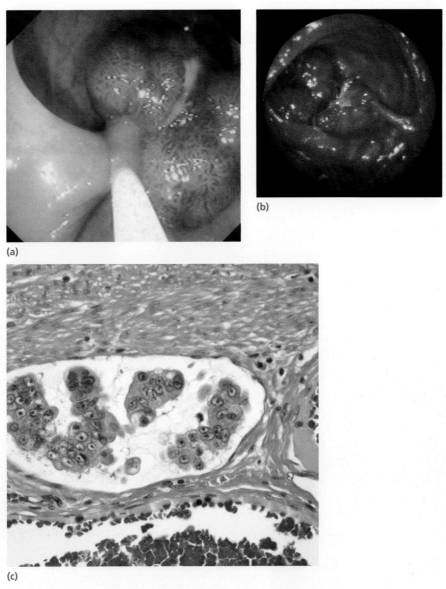

(a)

(b)

(c)

Figure 93.108 Carcinoma arising in adenoma. **(a)** Colonoscopic photograph of a large, multilobulated tubulovillous adenoma showing the diathermy loop secured to the stalk a good distance below the adenoma tissue. Histopathology confirmed total removal with a 4-mm margin. Such polyps have a chance of containing a focus of carcinoma and complete removal at the first attempt is desirable. Source: Courtesy of Dr. Michael Bourke. **(b)** Adenocarcinoma, sigmoid with synchronous (sentinel) adenoma. A cancer with an ulcerated mass appearance was found at the splenic flexure (in the distance at the 3 o'clock position). Just distal to this in the proximal descending colon, a pedunculated polyp is present as a sentinel neoplasm. The possibility that other adenomas or even cancers are present in this colon emphasizes the need to perform colonoscopy at the time of diagnosis to clear the colon of other lesions that could alter patient management. **(c)** Carcinoma arising in association with an adenoma; vascular space invasion. This is a feature that most authors believe should prompt resection following a diagnosis of "cancer in a polyp."

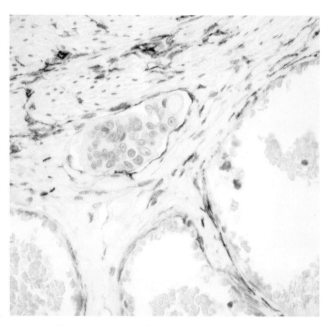

Figure 93.109 Carcinoma arising in association with an adenoma; vascular space invasion. This CD34 stain highlights endothelial cells lining the invaded vessel from the lesion seen in Figure 93.108.

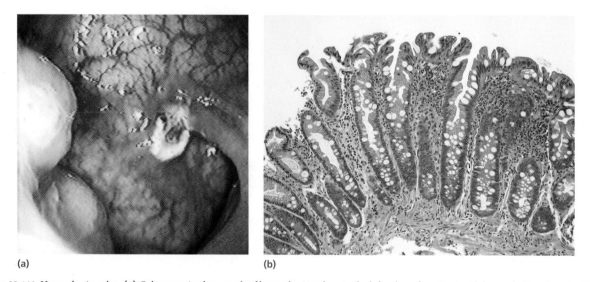

(a)   (b)

Figure 93.110 Hyperplastic polyp. **(a)** Colonoscopic photograph of hyperplastic polyps in the left colon of a patient with hyperplastic polyposis. These polyps are not distinguishable from adenomas without histological examination, preferably performed after polypectomy. **(b)** This serrated polyp shows cells with eosinophilic cytoplasm. Note that the bases of the glands are narrow.

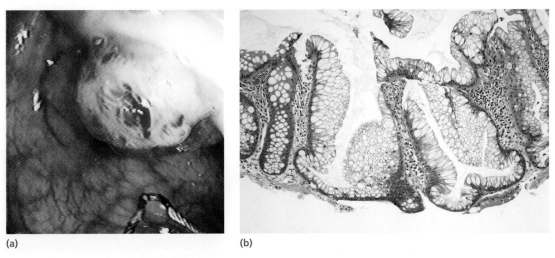

(a)   **(b)**

Figure 93.111 Sessile serrated adenoma. **(a)** Colonoscopic photograph of a large serrated adenoma about to be removed from a patient with hyperplastic polyposis. This lesion superficially resembles a hyperplastic polyp but differs **(b)** by having broad-based glands (compare to Figure 93.110). It lacks conventional dysplasia but is fully capable of progressing to invasive carcinoma.

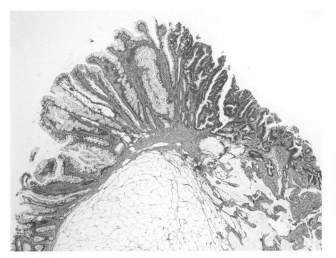

Figure 93.112 Sessile serrated adenoma with associated dysplasia and invasive carcinoma. The high-grade dysplasia and carcinoma component is at the right of the field.

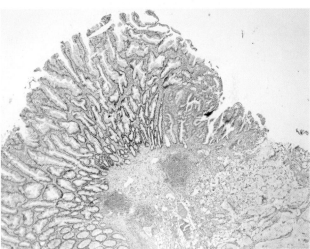

Figure 93.113 Sessile serrated adenoma with associated dysplasia and invasive carcinoma. In this immunohistochemical preparation for the mismatch repair protein MLH1, there is (nuclear) loss in the high-grade dysplasia and carcinoma component.

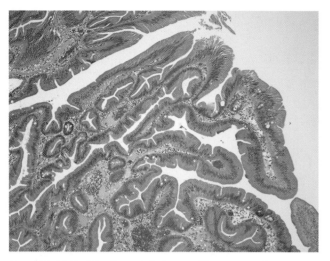

Figure 93.114 Traditional serrated adenoma. There is serrated architecture of the epithelial cells as well as traditional epithelial dysplasia like that of an ordinary adenoma.

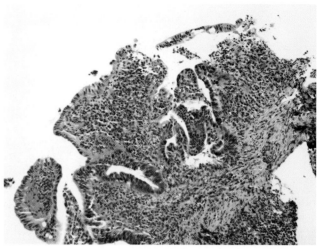

Figure 93.117 Dysplasia associated lesion or mass (DALM). This area shows high-grade dysplasia.

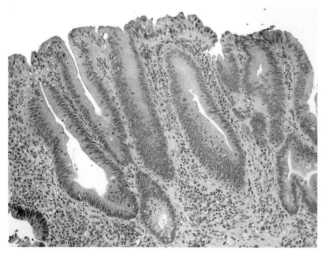

Figure 93.115 Dysplasia associated lesion or mass (DALM). This lesion has low-grade dysplasia and presented as an elevated visible lesion.

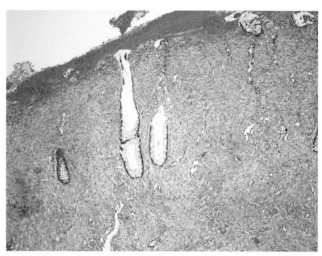

Figure 93.118 Benign fibroblastic polyp of the colon. The lamina propria is expanded by a benign spindle cell proliferation.

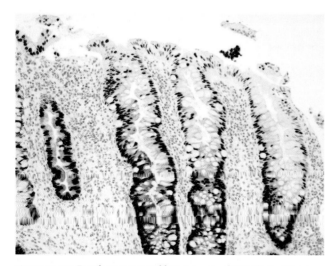

Figure 93.116 Dysplasia associated lesion or mass (DALM). A p52 stain can be useful in confirming an impression of DALM.

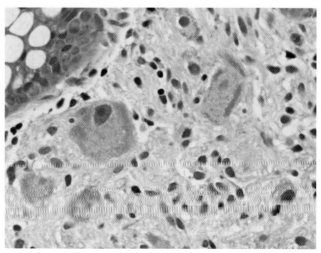

Figure 93.119 Ganglioneuroma. Aberrant ganglion cells and Schwann cells (bland spindled cells) proliferate in the colonic lamina propria. Most examples are isolated sporadic lesions.

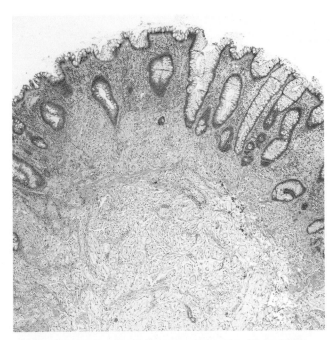

Figure 93.120 Benign epithelioid peripheral nerve sheath tumor. This lesion is centered around the lamina propria and superficial submucosa.

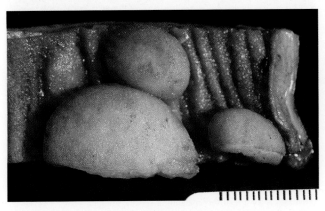

Figure 93.121 Colonic lipoma: surgical specimen.

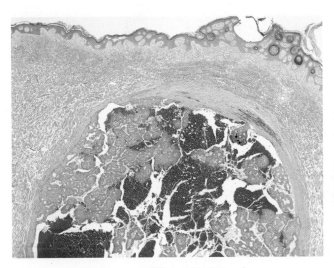

Figure 93.122 Hidradenoma papilliferum. This lesion shows differentiation along sweat gland lineage and is found in the perineum of females.

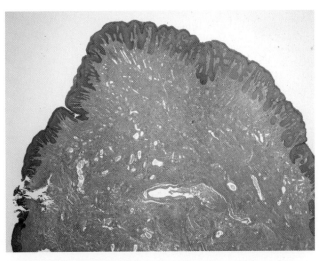

Figure 93.123 Anal fibroepithelial polyp. These appear similar to "skin tags" elsewhere.

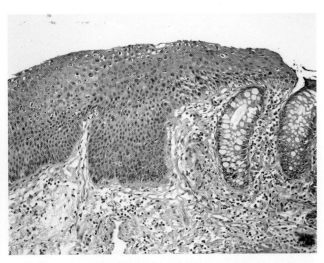

Figure 93.124 Anal intraepithelial neoplasia. This process often occurs at the anorectal transition.

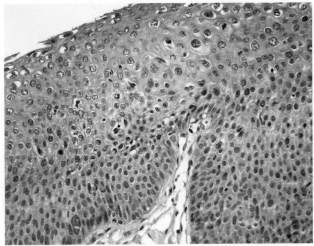

Figure 93.125 Anal intraepithelial neoplasia. The changes here are those of AIN 2 (moderate dysplasia) and would be subsumed under high-grade in situ lesions.

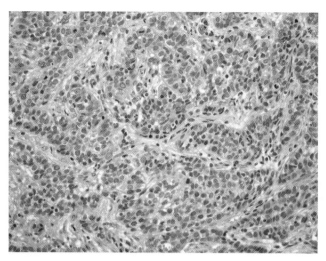

Figure 93.126 Anal squamous cell carcinoma. This example is basaloid (formerly "cloacogenic").

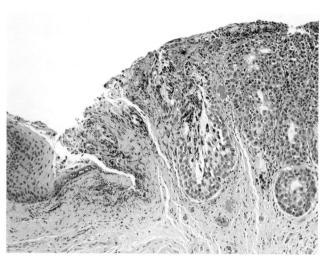

Figure 93.129 Anal melanoma: note the melanin pigment.

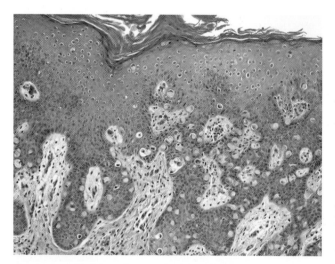

Figure 93.127 Anal Paget disease. Glandular cells proliferate in the squamous mucosa.

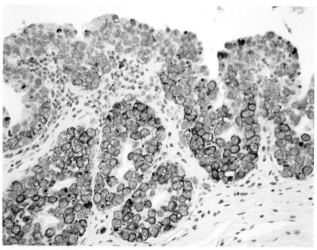

Figure 93.130 Anal melanoma. This immunohistochemical stain (HMB45) is for a relatively melanoma-specific antigen.

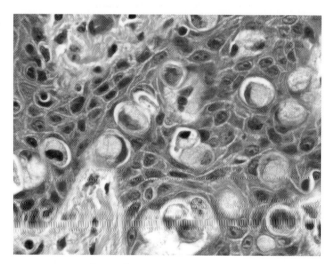

Figure 93.128 Anal Paget disease. At high magnification, intracellular mucin is apparent in these Paget cells.

Index

Page numbers in *italic* refer to figures.
Page numbers in **bold** refer to tables.
Page numbers suffixed with "b" refer to boxes.

abdominal cavity 36–42
  abscesses 477–483
  anatomy 36
abdominal compartment syndrome 296, 485
abdominal pain
  acute pancreatitis 295
  referred *342*
  see also acute abdomen
aberrant hepatic artery *823, 824*
abetalipoproteinemia 184–186, *187*
ABIC score, alcoholic hepatitis 426, 427
ablative therapies, liver tumors *842, 843*
abscesses
  abdominal cavity 477–483
  anorectal *275*
  liver 469–471, *481, 482, 515, 518*
    amebic 469–471, *515, 518*
    drainage *859*
    fistula from *481*
    MRI *469, 470, 482*
    PET *799*
  lung *652*
  retroperitoneal *484, 487*
  see also crypt abscesses
acanthosis nigricans *558*
acetaminophen
  CYS adducts *399*
  liver injury *397, 398,* **398,** *402–403, 866*
  metabolic pathways *399*
N-acetyl-p-benzoquinone imine 397
N-acetylcysteine *399*
achalasia, esophagus *67, 68, 69, 813*
achlorhydria 135
acidophil bodies
  acute viral hepatitis *386*
  nonalcoholic fatty liver disease *433*
acini, liver *52, 57*
acoustic shadowing *737*
acquired immunodeficiency syndrome
  complications 501–508
  esophagus 85–92
    Kaposi sarcoma *101*
    ulcers *85, 87, 88, 89, 90, 91, 92, 726*

liver histology *876*
  small intestine *see Mycobacterium avium* complex
acrodermatitis enteropathica *558*
Acta2 (actin isoform) 436, *440, 443*
actin, stellate cells 436, *440*
acute abdomen
  laparoscopy *698*
  see also abdominal pain
acute febrile neutrophilic dermatosis *562*
acute kidney injury, alcoholic hepatitis 427
acute mesenteric ischemia *582, 583*
acute necrotic collections, acute pancreatitis 297–300
acute peripancreatic fluid collections 297–300
acute renal failure, cirrhosis 448–449, *456, 457*
acute tubular necrosis 449
acute viral hepatitis 374–386, *872, 873*
  histology *386*
adenocarcinoma
  appendix *486*
    mucinous *789*
  biliary tract 370
  colon *630, 761, 925*
    Gardner syndrome *555*
    MSI-H *242*
  duodenum 202, *759*
  endometrium *785*
  esophagus 75, *93, 98, 99, 100, 609, 889*
    Barrett metaplasia and 75
    PET *783, 784*
  extramammary Paget disease *559*
  ischemic colitis *vs 594*
  Leser–Trelat sign *558*
  liver metastases, histology *871*
  lung, PET *800*
  microsatellite instability high colonic *242*
  pancreas *740, 750, 755, 765*
    MRI *768*
    PET *791*
  partial gastrectomy 147

rectum 238
  PET *786*
small intestine 202, *204*
stomach 149–152, *615, 616, 897*
  computed tomography *758*
  histology *900*
  PET *794*
ulcerative colitis 218
adenomas
  cancer screening 267, *268, 269*
  carcinoma from *925, 926*
  colorectal 234–237, *626, 923, 924*
  duodenal *619*
  liver
    histology *869, 870*
    rupture *836*
  serrated *see* serrated adenomas
  stomach
    gastric type *896*
    intestinal type *895*
  see also familial adenomatous polyposis; *specific types*
adherent clots, ulcers *614, 675, 676*
adhesions, laparotomy *699*
adjustable gastric band *495, 496*
  erosion *497, 499*
  leaks *498*
  prolapse *499*
adrenal gland, metastases, PET *783, 798*
adrenaline injection, peptic ulcers *129*
adult respiratory distress syndrome 298
aganglionosis, Hirschsprung disease 166
Agile Patency System *623*
AIDS *see* acquired immunodeficiency syndrome
air
  biliary tract *737*
  retroperitoneum *731*
  sonography *732, 733*
alanine aminotransferase
  acute viral hepatitis 376
  alcoholic liver disease 424, 425
albumin
  serum–ascites gradient 447, **449,** *451*
  for spontaneous bacterial peritonitis 448, 449, *455*

Yamada's Atlas of Gastroenterology, Fifth Edition. Edited by Daniel K. Podolsky, Michael Camilleri, J. Gregory Fitz, Anthony N. Kalloo, Fergus Shanahan, and Timothy C. Wang.
© 2016 John Wiley & Sons, Ltd. Published 2016 by John Wiley & Sons, Ltd.
Companion website: www.yamadagastro.com/atlas

alcohol abuse 423
alcoholic fatty liver 423
alcoholic hepatitis 425–427
alcoholic liver disease 423–427
  biopsy 860, 866, 875
    arachnoid portal fibrosis 863
    fatty infiltration 869
    mega-mitochondria 868
    perivenular fibrosis 865
  diagnosis and treatment 424–427
  prognostic assessment 426–427
  risk factors 423–424
alcoholic steatohepatitis (ASH) 425
Aldomet, hepatotoxicity 875
alkalis, esophagitis 102, *108*, 611
α-1-antitrypsin
  deficiency 419, *420*
  hepatocytes 861
α-fetoprotein 50, *51*
α-heavy-chain disease 214
amebiasis 469–470, 515, *517*, *518*
  see also Entamoeba histolytica
American dilator 644
ampulla of Vater *see* papilla of Vater
Amyand's hernia 37, *39*
amylase, acute pancreatitis 295, 296
amyloid, liver histology 868
amyloidosis
  colon 909
  esophagus 110, *112*
  macroglossia 581
  mesentery 484, *489*
  stomach 910
anal canal 24, *25, 26, 27*
  see also anorectal diseases; anus;
    sphincters
anal fissures 278
  Crohn's disease 230–231
anal retractors 272
anal transition zone 24
anal warts 170
anastomoses
  bariatric surgery 612
    ulcers 493, 495, 496, 497, 612
  Billroth II 613
  colon 731
  colorectal, rupture 787
  esophagogastric 611
    dilation (therapeutic) 645
  esophagojejunal 611
  gastrojejunostomy, NOTES 713
  ileal pouch–anal *see* ileal pouch–anal
    anastomosis
  Roux-en-Y hepaticojejunostomy
    642
Ancylostoma duodenalis 527, 528
aneurysms
  pancreas 826
  portal vein 822
  splenic artery 840
  see also under aorta

angiodysplasia
  colon *817*
  small intestine 209, *212*
angioectasia *614*
  colon 632–633
  small intestine *620, 623*
  see also gastric antral vascular ectasia;
    vascular ectasia
angiography 820–841
  gastrointestinal tract 820–833
  magnetic resonance angiography 768
  mesenteric 582, *586, 587*
    collaterals *587*
    inferior mesenteric artery *588*
    Leriche syndrome *589*
    treatment of thrombosis *585*
  portal vein 820, *831*
    with CO$_2$ *854*
  see also embolization; interventional
    radiology
angioplasty
  hepatic artery stenosis *848*
  inferior vena cava stenosis *853*
  superior mesenteric artery *586, 587, 851*
angular cheilitis 572, *580*
annular pancreas 15, *765*
anorectal diseases 270–286
  squamous cell carcinoma 245, *785*
  syphilis 170
  see also anus; *entries beginning* anal ...;
    rectum
anorectal examination
  fecal incontinence 279
  instruments 272
anoscopes 272
anoxia, liver histology 865
antibiotics
  liver abscesses 470–471
  pancreatic necrosis 304–306
  spontaneous bacterial peritonitis 448
anticoagulants
  intramural hematoma 544, *549*
  small intestinal ulcers 208, *211*
antidiarrheal therapies **190**
antigenome, hepatitis D virus 374
anti-HCV test 395, **395**
antinuclear antibodies, autoimmune
  hepatitis *406*
antiretroviral drugs, steatosis 508
antismooth muscle antibodies,
  autoimmune hepatitis *406*
anti-tumor necrosis factor, atypical
  psoriasis 230
antiviral therapy
  acute viral hepatitis 377
  hepatitis C virus **396**
    direct acting **396**
  antrum (stomach) 672
    dynamic contraction scintigraphy 116,
    119
    lipomas 616

anus 24
  anatomy *271*
  endoscopic microsurgery 720
  fibroepithelial polyp 929
  intraepithelial neoplasia 929
  melanoma 930
  Paget disease 930
  sonography *281*
  squamous cell carcinoma 285, 286, 930
    PET 796
  see also anorectal diseases; anorectal
    examination; *entries beginning*
    anal ...
aorta
  aneurysm, rupture 484, *486*
  dissection 586, *590*
  endoscopic ultrasonography *744*
aortic stenosis 544, *545*
aphthoid erosions, Crohn's disease *906*
aphthous stomatitis 560, *561*, 574, *581*
  Crohn's disease 230, *231*
  Sutton disease *562*
apoptosis, radiation injury 597, 598, 601
appendix 24–25, *27*
  abscess *479*
  adenocarcinoma 486
    mucinous *789*
  Amyand's hernia 37, *39*
  computed tomography *763*
  orifice, endoscopy *626*
  removal by NOTES *712*
  sonography *739*
apple peel atresia, small intestine 22
arc of Riolan 27, 582, *587*
arcuate line, pharynx *724*
argon plasma coagulation 629, 680, 687,
  689, 924
arteries
  colon and rectum 25–26, *28*
  gallbladder 43, *45*
  gastrointestinal tract 582
  liver 52
  pancreas 34
  radiation injury 597, 599, 600
  small intestine, atresia 22
  stomach 14
arterioportal fistula *826*
arteriovenous malformations 202, *829*
arthritis, ulcerative colitis 216
arthropathy, hemochromatosis 416
artifacts, PET 794
aryepiglottic folds *724*
  cyst *725*
arytenoid cartilage *724*
Ascaris (spp.) 542
Ascaris lumbricoides 525, 526
ascites 447–438
  fluid analysis 449
  nonalcoholic steatohepatitis 435
  tuberculosis 485
ascites total protein 447, **449**, *451*

aspartate aminotransferase
    acute viral hepatitis 376
    alcoholic liver disease 424, 425
aspergillosis, small intestine 180, *182*
aspiration, liver abscesses 469–470
aspirin, gastric erosions *146*
atresia
    biliary tract 43, 49, 807, 809, 864
    small intestine 21–22
atrophic gastritis 613, 891, 892
attenuated familial adenomatous
        polyposis **239**
attenuation correction, PET 794
atypia, cellular, radiation injury *601*
AUDIT-C (alcohol abuse screen) 423
autoimmune gastritis 140, *141*, 891, 892
    enterochromaffin-like cells *142*
autoimmune hepatitis 405–408
    histology *863*
    scoring systems **407**
    serology *406*
autoimmune pancreatitis 289–290
    biopsy 307
    histology *291*
    imaging *292*
    magnetic resonance imaging *293, 294*
autoinfection, *Strongyloides stercoralis* 530
Axios stent *303, 304*
azathioprine, autoimmune hepatitis **408**

baclofen 425
Balantidium coli **516**, 518–520
balloon dilation
    colon *647*
    duodenum *646*
    esophagus *654*
    ileum *648*
ballooning of cells, steatosis *429*
balloons, intragastric *494*
banded gastroplasty 495, *499*
banding *see* ligation; rubber-band ligation
bariatric surgery 491, 495–500
    anastomotic ulcers 493, 495, 496, 497,
        612
    endoscopic *494*
barium studies 722
    esophagus, squamous cell carcinoma *94*
    extravasation at *731*
    small bowel follow-through, Crohn's
        disease 225–226, *228*
Barrett esophagus 93, 98, 887, 888
    chromoendoscopy *609*, 888
    endoscopic mucosal resection *608*
    histology *99*
    after photodynamic therapy *607*
    Prague convention *75*
Bartonella infection 473
basal acid secretion, Zollinger–Ellison
        syndrome *136*
basaloid squamous cell carcinoma *930*
basket retrieval, polypectomy *629*

B cell lymphomas
    Burkitt lymphoma *801*
    diffuse large, PET *802*
    posttransplant lymphoproliferative
        disorder *793*
    small intestine 203–204, *207*
    stomach *507*
Behavioral Risk Factor Surveillance
        System *492*
Behçet syndrome
    esophagus 110, *112, 909*
    scrotal ulcers *561*
    small intestinal ulcers 208
belching
    esophageal manometry *78*
    pH-impedance testing *77*
    supragastric *71, 77*
benign intrinsic esophageal stenosis *607*
benign misplaced epithelium, Peutz–
        Jeghers syndrome *256*
benign mucous membrane
        pemphigoid 110, *113*
benign tumors, gallbladder 368b
bezoars
    esophageal diverticula *12*
    stomach *156*
bile 335, *338*
    phospholipids *338, 339*
bile crystals, Maltese-cross
        birefringence *340*
bile-reflux gastropathy 145–147
biliary atresia 43, *49*, 807, 809, 864
biliary cirrhosis, liver histology *872*
biliary colic *see* Charcot's triad;
        hepatobiliary pain;
        postcholecystectomy syndrome
biliary leak 807, *810, 857*
biliary pancreatitis
    algorithm *297*
    biochemistry *296*
    gallbladder sludge *344*
    hemorrhage *301*
    pain 295
biliary tract 43–49, 354–360
    anatomy 43, *44, 53, 54*
    anomalies 43, *45*
    canaliculi *52, 56*
    cysts 361–366
    drainage 752, *753, 857*
    embryology 43, *48, 50*
    hemorrhage into *837*
    infections 351, 354, *360*
    interventional radiology *842*
    intrahepatic 50, *52*
    obstruction
        common bile duct *765*
        histology *863*
        magnetic resonance imaging *777*
        radionuclide imaging 804–806, *807*
    portal cholangiopathy *472*
    radionuclide imaging *807*

sonography 737–738
stents *637, 752, 753*
    PET *791*
stones *see* choledocholithiasis;
        cholelithiasis
    tumors 368–373
    see also cholangiocarcinoma
biliopancreatic diversion, with duodenal
        switch 495, *500*
Billroth I anastomosis *612*
Billroth II anastomosis *613*
biopsy
    autoimmune pancreatitis 307
    colorectal polyps 627
    Cryptosporidium infection **516**
    endoscopic mucosal 878–930
    eosinophilic esophagitis 84
    esophagus 3
    Hirschsprung disease 166–167
    liver 860–877
        alcoholic liver disease *see under*
            alcoholic liver disease
        chronic hepatitis B *387*
        hemochromatosis 418b, *861*
        peroral transgastric *703, 706*
        primary sclerosing cholangitis 354,
            358, 360
        transjugular *839, 858*
    ulcerative colitis 221
    vertebra *708*
    Whipple disease *177*
bird beak pattern, gastroesophageal
        junction *67*
bladder
    schistosomiasis *531, 533*
    visceral myopathy *162*
bladder protocol, PET 782, *785*
Blastocystis hominis 515, **516**, *518*
blood investigations, total parenteral
        nutrition 193b
blue rubber bleb nevus syndrome *557,
        574, 579*
Bochdalek hernia 36, *38*
body mass index 491
body packer syndrome 208, *211*
Boerhaave syndrome 102, *104*
Bogota bag *485*
bone
    metastases, PET *786*
    primary sclerosing cholangitis 354,
        357
    sarcoidosis *790*
    see also osteoporosis
bone marrow transplantation 512–513
    neutropenic enterocolitis 548, *551, 552*
bougienage, esophagus *643*
Bowen disease 270, *286*
breath tests
    carbon-13, gastroparesis 116
    lactose malabsorption 184, *185*
    sucrase–isomaltase deficiency 186, *188*

bridging fibrosis, nonalcoholic fatty liver
   disease *432*
bronchoesophageal fistula *652*
Brunner's gland hyperplasia *17, 619*
Budd–Chiari syndrome *472, 473*
   angiography *836, 838*
   liver histology *865*
   portosystemic shunts *842*
   sonography *737*
budesonide, autoimmune hepatitis **408**
bullous pemphigoid
   esophagus *110, 113*
   IgG deposits *566*
   skin lesions *565*
Burkitt lymphoma *801*
N-butyl-2-cyanoacrylate *664*

C282Y test, hemochromatosis *415, 417b*
café-au-lait macules *556*
calcification
   chronic pancreatitis *308, 309*
   gallbladder *737, 738*
   serous cystadenoma *324*
calcium infusion test *135, 136*
Campylobacter jejuni infection *170, 171,
   506*
canaliculi, biliary *52, 56*
candidiasis
   esophagus *85, 86, 87, 546, 611, 725,
      881, 883*
   pharynx *725*
   small intestine *180, 183*
   spleen *552*
capsule endoscopy *208, 619, 620, 621–625*
   Crohn's disease *225*
   retention of capsule *648*
   see also wireless motility capsule
carbohydrate-deficient transferrin *423*
carbon-13 breath tests, gastroparesis *116*
carbon dioxide (as contrast agent) *820*
   splenoportography *840*
carcinoids
   mesentery *759*
   PET *802*
      metastases *803*
   rectum *244*
   single photon emission tomography *818*
   small intestine *202, 205, 729*
      angiography *832*
   somatostatin receptor imaging *811*
   stomach *615, 901, 902*
   Zollinger–Ellison syndrome *136*
carcinoma
   from adenomas *925, 926*
   biliary tract *368 373*
      see also cholangiocarcinoma
   chronic pancreatitis *323*
   colorectal *see* colorectal carcinoma
   esophageal invasion *608*
   esophagus *727, 746, 747*
   gallbladder *353, 372, 831*

Leser–Trelat sign *558*
pancreas *766*
   common bile duct compression *855*
   gastrojejunostomy *657–658*
   magnetic resonance imaging *780*
   PET *799*
PET *814*
in polyps *925, 926*
   screening *267, 268, 269*
rectum *630*
sebaceous *555*
stomach *728, 749*
   chromoendoscopy *898*
   endoscopic mucosal resection *899,
      900*
see also specific types
carcinomatosis
   peritoneum *484, 486, 784*
cardia, stomach *611*
cardiac glands, esophagus *4f*
Caroli disease *361, 364*
catheters
   angiography *820, 821*
   pancreatic drainage *303, 304*
cationic trypsinogen, hereditary
   pancreatitis *317, 322*
causality assessment methods, drug-
   induced liver injury *403b*
caustic esophagitis *102, 108, 109, 611*
cautery
   polyps *627*
   see also electrocoagulation
cavernoma, portal *474*
cavernous hemangioma of liver
   angiography *835*
   scintigraphy *809*
   SPECT/CT *812*
cavernous transformation, portal vein
   735
cecum
   dilation *28, 29*
   hemorrhage, interventional
      radiology *850*
   lipomas *243*
   neutropenic enterocolitis *551*
   vascular ectasia *830*
celiac axis *582, 823*
   dissection *544, 545*
   endoscopic ultrasonography *744, 755*
   median arcuate ligament
      compression *822*
   occlusion *826*
   stenosis *587, 851*
   variations *824*
celiac disease *618, 620, 624, 904, 905*
celiac plexus neurolysis *755*
cell-mediated immunity, acute viral
   hepatitis *375*
centroacinar cells, pancreas *30*
cestodes *524*
   see also specific species

CF transmembrane conductance
   regulator *317, 318, 319, 320*
Charcot's triad *346*
charge-coupled devices *605–606*
chemical gastropathy (reactive
   gastropathy) *143–145, 146, 147,
   890, 891*
chemoembolization *842*
   hepatocellular carcinoma *843, 844, 847*
   survival trial results *468*
cherry red spots, esophageal varices *668*
chest radiographs
   Ascaris lumbricoides infection *525*
   liver abscesses *469, 515, 518*
   pneumoperitoneum *723*
childhood visceral myopathies *158–159,
   161*, **161**
children, total parenteral nutrition, **195**
Child–Turcotte–Pugh score *459*, **461**
Chlamydia trachomatis *506*
cholangiocarcinoma *359, 368*
   algorithms *372, 373*
   choledochal cyst with *362*
   histology *871*
   magnetic resonance imaging *777*
   perihilar *370, 373*
   primary sclerosing cholangitis *354–355,
      358*
   tumor embolus *369*
cholangiopathy
   AIDS *508*
   portal *472, 474*
cholangitis
   acute *352, 862*
   bacterial *354, 360*
   see also pericholangitis; primary
      sclerosing cholangitis; sclerosing
      cholangitis
cholecystectomy *346*
   hemorrhage after *837*
   hybrid transgastric *713*
   prophylactic, indications **348**
   transvaginal NOTES *719*
cholecystitis *350*
   algorithms *349, 350, 351*
   computed tomography *344*
   fistula *481*
   gangrenous *351, 739*
   interventional radiology *857*
   radionuclide imaging *804, 806*
   sonography *737, 739*
cholecystokinin cholescintigraphy *804,
   806*
cholecystostomy *857*
choledochal cysts *43, 49, 361–366*
choledochoceles *361, 365*
choledochoduodenostomy *753*
choledocholithiasis *333*
   computed tomography *767*
   ERCP *346, 634, 636, 637*
   magnetic resonance imaging *776*

cholelithiasis *191, 298, 299, 335–353*
  acute pancreatitis *296–297*
  chronic calculous cholecystitis *804*
  ERCP *634*
  fistula *481*
  sonography *737, 738*
cholera *171*
cholestasis, liver histology *869*
cholesterol emboli *595*
cholesterol gallstones *335, 336, 348*
  crystals *340, 341*
  etiology *338, 339*
cholestyramine resin **190**
chromoendoscopy *609, 631*
  Barrett esophagus *609, 888*
  stomach, carcinoma *898*
chronic gallbladder disease *804, 806*
chronic hepatitis
  histology *867, 872, 873, 874*
    hepatitis B virus *389, 390, 391, 862, 867*
  viral *376, 377*
    biopsy *860,* **861,** *874*
chronic intestinal ischemia *589*
chronic mesenteric ischemia *582*
chronic ulcerative jejunoileitis *209–212*
cimetidine, Meckel scan *810*
cirrhosis *432, 435, 442, 446*
  acute renal failure *448–449, 456, 457*
  ascites *447–448, 452, 453, 454*
  biliary, liver histology *872*
  computed tomography *763*
  hemochromatosis *416*
  histology *861*
  magnetic resonance imaging *768, 775*
  portal hypertension *664, 666*
  sonography *732*
  transjugular portography *831*
  Wilson disease *420*
c-KIT, visceral neuropathies *159, 165*
clear cell carcinoma, kidney *788*
ClinOleic™ *191, 201*
clips
  hemostatic
    hemoclips *689*
    peptic ulcer disease *678, 679*
  over-the-scope *697, 714–715*
  polypectomy *690*
    for perforation *695–696*
  see also endoclips
cloaca *25, 28*
cloacogenic inflammatory polyps *920*
clonidine **190**
Clonorchis sinensis *535, 536*
Clostridium difficile *170, 174, 175*
  see also pseudomembranous colitis
closures, NOTES *716, 717*
  transcolonic *721*
Clouse plots *62*
coagulation defects *544*
coaxial catheterization *820, 821*

cobblestone appearance
  chronic hepatitis *873*
  Crohn's disease *907*
cocaine toxicity *544, 545*
coccygodynia *284*
codeine **190**
coins, esophagus *102, 107*
colchicine, duodenal toxicity *905*
colitis *628–629*
  Campylobacter *170, 171*
  collagenous *920*
  cytomegalovirus infection *504, 514*
  diverticular *626*
  enteroinvasive *170, 174*
  Escherichia coli *170, 171, 172, 173, 174*
  ischemic *see* ischemic colitis
  lymphocytic *919*
  pseudomembranous *170, 174, 175, 553, 631*
    computed tomography *763*
    histology *917*
  Shigella *170*
  spirochetes *916*
collagen, liver *51*
collagenous colitis *920*
collagen vascular diseases, small intestinal ulcers *208–209*
collar-button ulcers *220*
collaterals
  intestinal blood supply *582, 587, 826*
  portosystemic *665*
colon
  adenocarcinoma *630, 761, 925*
    Gardner syndrome *555*
  amyloidosis *909*
  anatomy *24–28*
  angiodysplasia *817*
  angioectasia *632–633*
  carcinoma *see* colorectal carcinoma; colon *under* adenocarcinoma
  Crohn's disease *906, 907*
  crypt apoptosis *919*
  dilation *28*
  dilation (therapeutic) *647, 656*
  double-contrast radiography *722, 730, 731*
  endometriosis *923*
  fibroblastic polyps *928*
  graft-versus-host disease *552, 919*
  infections *170–176*
  lymphoid hyperplasia *265*
  malignant tumors *238–245*
    fistula *480*
    see also colorectal carcinoma
  motility disorders *157–169*
  NOTES via *702, 721*
  pneumatosis *723*
  polypectomy *686*
  polyps *234–237*
  radiation injury *600*
  schistosomiasis *531, 532*

tubular adenoma *923, 924*
  see also magnetic resonance colonography; *specific parts e.g.* sigmoid colon
colonoscopy *626–633*
  virtual *762*
color CCDs *605*
colorectal carcinoma *238–245, 628, 629–631, 730, 925*
  adenocarcinoma *555, 630, 761, 925*
  ischemic colitis with *594*
  metastases *786*
  PET *786, 787, 819*
  polyps *234, 236*
    see also specific hereditary syndromes
  rectum *630*
  risk in polyposis syndromes **247**
  screening *266–269*
  ulcerative colitis *216*
  see also dysplasia
colorectal hamartoma *234, 237*
  see also PTEN hamartoma
colorectal lipomas *628, 929*
colorectal polyps *234–237, 626–627, 628, 629, 730, 913, 924, 926*
  argon plasma coagulation *629, 924*
  malignant *234, 236, 630, 730*
  melanosis and *913*
colorectal prolapse *920*
colostomy
  double-contrast radiography via *731*
  peristomal varices, ulcerative colitis *354, 357*
comb sign, Crohn's disease *227, 229, 760*
common bile duct *43, 48*
  anomalies *361, 363*
  choledochal cysts *362*
  chronic pancreatitis *310, 311, 312*
  drainage *752*
  obstruction *765*
  stents *759, 855*
  stones *see* choledocholithiasis
  strictures *357*
  time–activity curve *808*
  tumor invasion *831*
common variable immunodeficiency (CVID) *509–511, 512, 919*
compartment syndrome, abdominal *296, 485*
compensatory antiinflammatory response syndrome *287*
computed tomography *756–767*
  abdominal abscesses *478*
  enterography *756*
    Crohn's disease *227–228, 229*
  gastrointestinal fistulae *477*
  ischemic colitis *590, 592*
  liver abscesses *469, 470*
  neuroendocrine tumor of pancreas *795*
  pancreatic pseudocyst *14, 302*

computed tomography (*cont'd*)
pancreatitis 297, *299, 300*
severity index **296**
PET with 811–814
inflammation *796*
mesenteric metastases *784*
pancreatic neuroendocrine
tumors *795*
posterior renal fascia *787*
pseudomyxoma peritonei *789*
sarcoidosis *790*
small intestinal metastases *787*
computed tomography severity index
acute pancreatitis **296**
condylomata acuminata 170
condylomata lata 170, *176*
confocal laser endomicroscopy *609*
congenital hepatic fibrosis 361–366, *367*
congenital hypertrophy, retinal pigment
epithelium *253*
congenital lactase deficiency 184
congenital venous malformations,
esophagus 3, 6f
congestion, chronic passive, liver *867*
conjunctivitis, Sweet syndrome *562*
constipation, slow-transit 162, *164, 165,*
167b, 168
constitutional mismatch repair deficiency
syndrome **249**
contractile deceleration point,
esophagus *67*
contractile front velocity, esophagus *67*
contractile stellate cells 436
contrast agents
angiography *820*
computed tomography 756–757
see also carbon dioxide
copper
primary biliary cirrhosis *413*
Wilson disease 419
core antigen immunoassay, hepatitis C
virus **395**
corkscrew esophagus *67*
corkscrew hepatic artery *735*
coronary ligament *52*
corrosive substances, esophagitis 102, *108,*
611
Cowden syndrome *see* PTEN hamartoma
Cowdry type A intranuclear
inclusions *874*
CREST syndrome
telangiectasia *410*
cricoid cartilage *724*
cricopharyngeal bar 3, *10,* 63, *64*
critical micellar concentration, bile
acids *338*
Crohn's disease 225–233, *624, 906, 907*
algorithm 622
computed tomography *760, 761*
dilation (therapeutic) 643
esophagus 110, *111,* 885–886

fistula *480, 483*
anal *231*
oral lesions *574, 576*
perianal 230–231, *559*
positron emission tomography *811*
postoperative recurrence 232–233
terminal ileum *630, 633, 907, 908*
see also inflammatory bowel disease
Crohn's Disease Activity Index 225, **226**
Crohn's Disease Endoscopic Index of
Severity 225
Cronkhite–Canada syndrome **249,** *264,*
265, 922, 923
crypt abscesses 216, *217*
crypt apoptosis, colon *919*
crypt branching 216, *217*
Cryptosporidium infection *502,* 520, 522
ampulla of Vater *508*
life cycle *521*
liver histology *876*
mucosal histology *917*
stool *519*
stool and biopsy **516**
CTP score 459, **461**
Cullen's sign 295–296
Cushing syndrome, ectopic, Zollinger–
Ellison syndrome *138*
cutaneous larva migrans *541, 542*
cyanoacrylate 664
Cyclospora cayetanensis **516,** 520, *522*
cystic artery, variations *46*
cystic duct 43
anomalies *45*
cysticerci *539*
cystic fibrosis 184, *185, 186, 187,* 317–323
cystocele *282*
cysts
abdomen 36
aryepiglottic folds *725*
biliary tract 361–366
choledochal 43, *49,* 361–366
endoscopic ultrasonography *751*
epidermal inclusion cysts *555, 556*
esophagus 8f
hydatid disease *540, 541*
liver *361, 366, 769*
mucus retention cysts *258*
pancreas 324–328
PET *791*
see also pseudocyst
cytochrome P450 enzymes,
polymorphisms *399*
cytomegalovirus infection *505,* 513
colitis *504, 514*
esophagus *85, 881*
cytopathy *90*
ulcers *87, 88, 89, 610, 881, 883*
inflammatory bowel disease *228*
liver histology *874*
cytotoxic T lymphocytes
acute viral hepatitis 375–376

Dane particle 374
danger hypothesis, idiosyncratic drug-
induced liver injury *397, 400*
deep enteroscopy 621
defecation *278, 279*
Degos disease *567*
dehiscence, vertical sleeve
gastrectomy 660–661
delta antigen 374–375
dentate line, rectum 24
dermatitis herpetiformis *562, 563*
dermatomyositis *573*
desmoid, mesentery 484, *489*
diabetes mellitus 544, *547*
chronic pancreatitis 323
gastroparesis 115, 117, *165,* 546
intestinal dysmotility 168
diaphragm, hernias 36, 37, *38*
hiatus hernia 72, *79,* 153–155, *156,*
612
diarrhea
infections 170–176
short bowel syndrome 189
Dientamoeba fragilis **516,** 518, *519*
diet
colorectal cancer 239
for PET *782*
Dieulafoy lesion *613*
diffuse idiopathic skeletal hyperostosis
(DISH) 4, *12*
diffuse type gastric adenocarcinoma 149
digital examination, anorectal *279, 284*
Dilantin, hepatotoxicity *862, 875*
dilation (therapeutic)
esophageal strictures *74, 114,* 643, *645*
perforation 102, *104*
gastrointestinal tract 643–663
gastrojejunostomy strictures *497,*
657–658
instruments *644*
mesenteric angiography *587*
pyloric stenosis *17, 130*
Roux-en-Y hepaticojejunostomy *642*
see also stents
diphenoxylate atropine sulfate **190**
Diphyllobothrium latum 537
direct-acting antiviral therapies, hepatitis
C virus **396**
direct vision endoscopy technique 606
discriminant function (Maddrey),
alcoholic liver disease 426
dissection
aorta *586, 590*
celiac axis 544, *545*
distal contractile integral 65, *66*
distal esophageal spasm *67*
distal intestinal obstruction
syndrome 104, *105, 186,* 317, *321*
distal latency, esophagus *67*
disulfiram 425
diuretics, ascites 447–448, *453*

diverticula
    duodenum *18, 617*
    esophagus *3–4, 10–12, 607*
diverticular colitis 626
diverticulitis
    abscess *479*
    computed tomography *762*
    ischemic colitis with *591*
diverticulosis 626, *627*
    small intestine *215*
DOPA (⁶⁸Ga), PET radiotracer *782, 802*
Doppler ultrasonography 732–735
    ascites *447*
    biliary tract tumors *371*
    Budd–Chiari syndrome *473*
    hepatic artery *734, 735*
        liver transplantation *736*
DOTA-TOC (⁶⁸Ga), PET radiotracer *782,
        803*
double-contrast radiography 722
    colon *722, 730, 731*
    pharynx *722, 724*
double pigtail stents *647*
drainage
    abdominal abscesses *478, 483*
    acute pancreatitis *300–304*
    biliary tract *752, 753, 857*
    chronic pancreatitis 308, *315*
    after laparotomy *699*
    liver abscesses *859*
    pancreatic necrosis *704, 754*
drug-eluting beads 843, *845, 847*
drugs
    Crohn's disease, adverse reactions
        229–230
    liver disease from 397–404
        acetaminophen *866*
        chlorpromazine *869*
        Dilantin *862*
        histology *401, 402–403*
        illicit drugs *863*
        methotrexate *876*
        methyldopa *875*
        sulfonamides *872*
    small intestinal injury 208, 209, **210,**
        211
dual-source MDCT *756*
ductal plate, liver 50, *51*
ductopenia, primary biliary cirrhosis *412*
ducts of Hering *52*
duodenal switch, biliopancreatic diversion
        with 495, *500*
duodenitis, peptic *902*
duodenojejunal bypass sleeve *494*
duodenum 18, *617, 618, 619,* 621
    adenocarcinoma 202, *759*
    anatomy 13, *621*
    annular pancreas *15*
    arteriovenous malformations *829*
    Brunner's gland hyperplasia *17*
    carcinoids *205*

colchicine toxicity *905*
dilation (therapeutic) 646, *655*
diverticulum 18, *617*
epithelioid angiosarcoma
        PET *798*
familial adenomatous polyposis 252
gastrinoma 135–136, *137, 138*
gastrointestinal stromal tumors 206
hamartoma *203*
juvenile polyposis *259*
malrotation *37*
Mycobacterium avium complex
        infection 506, *548*
Mycobacterium avium intracellulare
        903
necrotizing pancreatitis *314*
peptic ulcer disease 131, 132, *133,* 676
        hemorrhage *828*
Peutz–Jeghers syndrome 257, *911, 912*
polypectomy *685*
PTEN hamartoma *263*
superior mesenteric artery syndrome
        15
ulcer 617, *728*
Whipple disease 178, *179, 180*
duplication
    esophagus 3, *7f*
    small intestine 21
    stomach *14*
Dupuytren contracture *573*
dynamic antral contraction
        scintigraphy 116, *119*
dyspepsia, functional 117, *118*
dysphagia, Schatzki ring 3
dysphagia lusoria 3, *6f*
dysplasia
    colorectal 234, *236,* 629–631, *730*
        juvenile polyposis *258*
        ulcerative colitis 216, *218, 222–224*
    stomach *152*
        familial adenomatous polyposis *251*
        intestinal type adenomas *895*
    tubular adenoma *924*
dysplasia-associated lesion or mass
        (DALM) 222–224, *928*
dysplasia-associated lesions
    ulcerative colitis 222–223, *915*
dysplastic polyps 626

Echinococcus spp. *541*
ectopic Cushing syndrome, Zollinger–
        Ellison syndrome *138*
ectopic gastric mucosa, esophagus 3, *8f,
        13, 16, 610*
ectopic pancreatic tissue *614*
Ehlers–Danlos syndrome *557*
elastography
    magnetic resonance elastography 442,
        445
    transient elastography 425, 442, *444*
elastosis *920*

electrical stimulation, gastric 119
electrocoagulation
    peptic ulcer disease *677*
    polyps *681*
    see also cautery
electrocoagulation catheter 677, *678*
electrogastrography 116–117, *122, 123*
embolism, mesenteric arteries 582, *583*
embolization (therapeutic)
    acute pancreatitis *300*
    cecal hemorrhage *850*
    hepatocellular carcinoma, trials *468*
    for peptic ulcer disease *134*
    pseudoaneurysm *822*
        superior mesenteric artery *849, 852*
    radioembolization 842, *846*
    splenic artery 830, *839–840, 841*
    see also chemoembolization
embryology
    biliary tract 43, *48, 50*
    gastrointestinal tract 19, *20*
    liver 48, *50, 51*
    pancreas 30, *31, 43, 48*
emphysematous cholecystitis *739*
enamel erosion, gastroesophageal reflux
        disease 574, *575*
endoclips 680, *716*
    see also clips; hemoclips
endocrine cell hyperplasia, stomach *892*
endocrine tumors
    pancreas 325
    see also neuroendocrine tumors
endometriosis 544, *547, 923*
endometrium, adenocarcinoma *785*
endoplasmic reticulum, hepatocytes 51
EndoSAMURAI *709*
endoscopic mucosal biopsy 878–930
endoscopic mucosal resection
    Barrett esophagus *608*
    instruments *900*
    polyps 627
    stomach cancer *899, 900*
endoscopic retrograde
        cholangiopancreatography
        294–295, 634–642
    chronic pancreatitis 307, *308*
    common bile duct, stones *346*
endoscopic submucosal dissection 680,
        683–684, 692, 693–694
    perforation *695–696*
endoscopic ultrasonography 741–755
    biliary drainage *752, 753*
    colorectal 238, *244*
    gastric varices 664, *671*
    instruments 741, *742*
    intrauterine *719*
    islet cell tumor *833*
    mediastinal leiomyoma *707*
    pancreas 744, *750*
        drainage *300–304*
    polyps *685*

endoscopic ultrasonography (*cont'd*)
  stomach 13, *16, 743, 748, 749*
    NOTES via *710*
endoscopy
  colon *see* colonoscopy
  dilation (therapeutic) 643
  lower intestinal 626–633
  procedures
    bariatric 491, *494*
    polyps 680–697
    see also entries beginning
      endoscopic …
  small intestine 208, 621
  upper gastrointestinal 605–620
    hemorrhage 675–679
    techniques 606
  see also capsule endoscopy
endothelialitis
  liver histology 865
endothelin B system
  visceral neuropathies 159
Entamoeba histolytica 515, **516**, *517*
  see also amebiasis
enteral nutrition
  acute pancreatitis 306
enteric nervous system 157, *158*, 159
enteritis, radiation injury *602*
Enterobius vermicularis 529
enterochromaffin-like cells
  autoimmune gastritis *142*
enteroclysis *see* small bowel enema
enterocutaneous fistula *483*, 500
enterography
  computed tomography 756
    Crohn's disease 227–228, *229*
  Crohn's disease 227–228
  magnetic resonance 227–229
enterohemorrhagic *E. coli* 170
enteroinvasive colitis 170, *174*
enteroscopy 208
  deep 621
  ERCP 635
  Roux-en-Y hepaticojejunostomy *642*
eosinophilic esophagitis 3, 5f, 82–84, *607*,
  884
  strictures *74*
eosinophilic gastritis *549*
eosinophilic myocarditis *549*
epidermal inclusion cysts *555, 556*
epidermolysis bullosa acquisita *563, 564*
epidermolysis bullosa dystrophica,
  esophagus 110, *114*
epiglottic tip *724, 726*
epiphrenic diverticula 3, *11*
episcleritis, Crohn's disease *229*
epithelioid angiosarcoma, duodenum,
  PET *798*
epithelioid granulomas, liver *871*
epithelioid peripheral nerve sheath
  tumor *929*
epithelioid-type GIST *901*

epithelium, radiation injury 597, *598, 601*
Epstein–Barr virus
  liver histology *866, 874*
  posttransplant lymphoproliferative
    disorder *793*
Erlenmeyer flask deformity, femur *545*
erosion of teeth, gastroesophageal reflux
  disease *574, 575*
erosions
  Crohn's disease *906*
  duodenum *618*
  reflux esophagitis *878*
  stomach, aspirin *146*
erosive gastritis *126, 128, 147*
  NSAIDs 144–145, *146*
erythema nodosum 216, 229, *560*
Escherichia coli, colitis 170, *171, 172, 173,*
  174
esophagitis
  caustic 102, 108, *109, 611*
  cytomegalovirus infection *881*
  eosinophilic 3, 5f, 82–84, *607*, 884
    strictures *74*
  herpes simplex virus infection 85, *87,*
    88, 89, 505, 610, 882
  iron pill *879*
  lymphocytic 109, *110*
  reflux 73, *607, 878*
  from tablets 102, *108*
esophagogastric anastomosis *611*
  dilation (therapeutic) *645*
esophagojejunal anastomosis *611*
esophagus 102–114
  acquired immunodeficiency
    syndrome 85–92
    Kaposi sarcoma *101*
    ulcers 85, *87, 88, 89, 90, 91, 92, 726*
  adenocarcinoma 75, 93, *98, 99, 100,*
    609, 889
    Barrett metaplasia and 75
    PET *783, 784*
  anatomy 3–4
  anomalies 3–12
  Behçet syndrome 110, *112, 909*
  candidiasis 85, *86, 87, 546, 611, 725,*
    881, 883
  carcinoma *727, 746, 747*
    see also specific types
  computed tomography *758*
  Crohn's disease 110, *111, 885–886*
  dilation (therapeutic) 643, *649, 650, 659*
  endoscopic ultrasonography *746, 747*
  endoscopy *606*
  fistula *see* fistulae, esophagus
  glycogenic acanthosis *262, 607*
  graft-versus-host disease 110, *112, 880*
  granular cell tumor *929*
  herpes simplex virus infection 85, *87,*
    88, 89, 505, 610, 882
  heterotopic gastric mucosa 3, 8f, 13, *16,*
    610

intramural hematoma 102, *105, 549*
lichen planus *880*
motility disorders 61–71, *78, 81, 813*
  see also gastroesophageal reflux
    disease
neoplasms 93–101
  see also specific types
  NOTES via *702, 705, 706, 707, 708*
peptic stricture 74, *105, 654*
peroral endoscopic myotomy *706*
radionuclide imaging *809*
rupture (Boerhaave syndrome) 102, *104*
squamous cell carcinoma *see under*
  squamous cell carcinoma
squamous papilloma *887*
stents *see* stents, esophagus
strictures *see* stents, esophagus;
  strictures, esophagus
taxol on *879*
ulcers *see under* ulcers
varices 608, 664–674
  grading 664, *667*
  see also Barrett esophagus; esophagitis
ethnicity, gallstones *337*
exomphalos (omphalocele) 22, *23, 36*
extended-criteria donor organs 459, *461b*
extracorporeal albumin dialysis *457*
extraintestinal manifestations
  Crohn's disease 229–231
  familial adenomatous polyposis *253*
  ulcerative colitis 216–218
extramammary Paget disease *559*
extravasation, at barium studies *731*
eye
  Crohn's disease 229
  retinal pigment epithelium, congenital
    hypertrophy *253*
  ulcerative colitis 216, *219*

falciform ligament *52*
fallopian tube, ligation by NOTES *718*
familial adenomatous polyposis **239**, **247**,
  250, 251, 252
  endoscopy 240, *626, 628*
  extraintestinal manifestations *253*
familial visceral myopathies 157–158, *159,*
  160, 161, **167**
Fasciola hepatica *534*
fasting, for PET *782*
fasting gastrin level *135*
fat necrosis, acute pancreatitis *288*
fatty infiltration
  liver
    alcoholic fatty liver 423
    see also steatosis
  pancreas *740*
focal nodular hyperplasia, liver *761*
fecal impaction *280*
fecal incontinence
  anorectal examination *279*
  functional *280*

magnetic resonance imaging *282*
manometry **270**
   squeeze pressures *283*
sonography *281*
fecal occult blood tests *267*
feeding tube placement *858*
feline esophagus *3, 5f, 607, 884*
female sex, alcoholic liver disease *423–424*
femoral hernia *37, 39, 40*
femur, Erlenmeyer flask deformity *545*
ferritin, hemochromatosis *415, 418b*
fetus, NOTES *719*
fiber, colorectal cancer and *239*
fibroblastic polyps, colon *928*
fibroblasts
   portal *436*
   radiation injury *601*
fibrocytes, liver *436, 438*
fibroepithelial polyp, anus *929*
fibroid inflammatory polyps *237, 895*
fibrolamellar hepatocellular
     carcinoma *467, 870*
fibromas (skin), familial adenomatous
     polyposis *253*
fibromatous proliferation, mesentery *484,
     489*
Fibroscan (transient elastography) *425,
     442, 444*
fibrosis
   mesentery *487*
   radiation injury *597, 600*
fibrosis (liver) *436–446*
   alcoholic liver disease *424–425, 863,
     865*
   measurement *441–442*
     magnetic resonance
       elastography *442, 445*
     transient elastography *425, 442, 444*
   nonalcoholic fatty liver disease *428,
     431, 432*
   perisinusoidal *476*
   reversion *441, 444*
fiducials, endoscopic ultrasonography
     755
fistulae
   abdominal cavity *477, 480, 481*
   anorectal *276*
   arterioportal *826*
   bronchoesophageal *652*
   chronic pancreatitis *307, 312*
   Crohn's disease *480, 483*
     anal *231*
   enterocutaneous *483, 500*
   esophagus
     AIDS *90, 91*
     carcinoma *608*
     Crohn's disease *110, 111, 885–886*
     Nissen fundoplication *81*
     stenting *100*
   gastrogastric *499*
   rectovaginal *908*

flap, mucosal, transcolonic NOTES *721*
flap valve, gastroesophageal junction *79*
flat adenomas, colon *924*
fluid analysis, ascites **449**
fluid collections
   acute pancreatitis **302**
   acute peripancreatic *297–300*
flukes *see* trematodes; *specific species*
fluorescent in situ hybridization (FISH),
     cholangiocarcinoma *359*
[18]F-fluorodeoxyglucose *782*
   gastrointestinal malignancies *811–814*
foam cells, radiation injury *599*
foamy histiocytes, liver infection *871*
focal nodular hyperplasia
   angiography *835*
   computed tomography *764*
   histology *870*
   magnetic resonance imaging *770*
   sonography *732, 734*
folds of rectum *626*
follicular gastritis *143, 145*
follicular lymphoma, small intestine *204,
     207*
food impaction, esophageal strictures *102,
     609*
foods
   colorectal cancer *239*
   high in oxalate *191b*
foreign bodies
   esophagus *102, 105, 106, 107*
   gossypiboma *484, 485*
   stomach *155*
     perforation *697*
   see also bezoars
foveolar dysplasia *251*
foveolar hyperplasia *146, 147, 148*
free fatty acids, PET and *782*
functional dyspepsia *117, 118*
functional fecal incontinence *280*
fundic gland polyps *251, 615, 895*
fundoplication *81*
fungal infections
   esophagus *85, 86, 87*
   pancreatic necrosis *304–306*
   skin, Crohn's disease *230*
furosemide, ascites *448, 453*
furrowing, eosinophilic esophagitis *83*

gallbladder *43–49*
   anatomy *43, 44*
   benign tumors *368b*
   cholelithiasis *191*
   endoscopic ultrasonography *745*
   malignant tumors *369b, 372, 831*
     carcinoma *353*
   polyps *343*
   puncture at NOTES *710*
   radionuclide imaging *804, 805, 806*
   sludge *344, 738, 739*
   sonography *737–738, 738, 739*

   stasis *341*
   variations *48*
gallbladder ejection fraction *804, 806*
^{68}Ga-DOTA-TOC, PET radiotracer *782,
     803*
gallstone ileus *352*
gallstones *see* cholelithiasis
gamma-glutamyltransferase *423*
ganglioneuroma *928*
ganglioneuromatosis, transmural
     intestinal *163*
gangrene, ischemic colitis *595*
gangrenous cholecystitis *351, 739*
Gardner syndrome *555*
   osteomas *574, 580*
gas
   contrast media *756*
     see also carbon dioxide
   portal vein *723*
   see also air
gastrectomy
   bile-reflux gastropathy *145–147*
   partial *147*
   vertical sleeve gastrectomy,
     dehiscence *660–661*
gastric antral vascular ectasia *548, 613,
     674, 892, 893*
   watermelon stomach *147–148, 893*
gastric band *495, 496, 497, 499*
   leaks *498*
gastric bypass *495, 496, 498, 500*
   anastomoses *612*
   ERCP *635, 641*
gastric electrical stimulation *119*
gastric feeding tube placement *858*
gastric outlet obstruction *655, 657*
   pancreatic pseudocyst *311*
   see also pyloric stenosis
gastric sleeve *495*
gastrin *135, 136*
gastrinoma *135–136*
   angiography *833*
   duodenum *135–136, 137, 138*
gastritis *125, 126, 140–148*
   atrophic *613, 891, 892*
   eosinophilic *549*
   erosive *126, 128, 147*
     NSAIDs *144–145, 146*
   H. pylori 125, 126, 141–143, 144, 145, 890
gastritis cystica polyposa *147*
gastroduodenal artery,
     pseudoaneurysm *833*
gastroesophageal junction
   flap valve *79*
   incompetence *72*
   motility disorders *67, 68, 70*
   transient relaxation *78*
   see also lower esophageal sphincter
gastroesophageal reflux disease *72–81*
   gastroparesis *116, 118*
   oral lesions *574, 575*

gastroesophageal reflux disease (cont'd)
  radionuclide imaging 809, *814*
  see also reflux
gastrogastric fistula *499*
gastrohepatic ligament, tumor
      involvement *758*
gastrointestinal stromal tumors (GIST)
  PET *788*
    small intestine 202–203, *206*
    stomach *16*, *616*, *759*, *901*
      resection *700*
gastrojejunostomy
    self-assembling magnets *713*
    stricture dilation *497*, 657–658
gastroparesis 115–119
    diabetes mellitus 115, 117, *165*, *546*
    radionuclide imaging 116–117, *118*,
      120, 809–810, *816*
Gastroparesis Cardinal Symptom
      Index 115, **116**
gastropathy
    bile reflux 145–147
      portal hypertension *614*, *664*, *673*
      reactive 143–145, *146*, *147*, *890*, *891*
gastroplasty, vertical banded *495*, *499*
gastroschisis 22, *23*, *36*
gastrotomy *see* NOTES *under* stomach
Gaucher disease, type 1 *544*, *545*
gel submucosal dissection *692*
genomes, hepatitis viruses 375, 379, 381,
      383, *393*
genome-wide association studies,
      idiosyncratic drug-induced liver
      injury 397–398, *400*
genotyping, hepatitis C virus **395**
germ cell tumor, retroperitoneal
      metastases *487*
GGT-CDT (alcohol abuse test) 423
giardiasis *510*, 515–518, *519*
GIST *see* gastrointestinal stromal tumors
glomus tumor, stomach *616*
glucagonoma 331
    angiography *834*
    necrolytic migratory erythema *330*,
      559
glucose levels, PET and 782
glutathionine 399
gluten-sensitive enteropathy 209–212
glycogen
    embryonic liver *50*
    liver histology *867*
    nonalcoholic fatty liver disease *433*
glycogenic acanthosis, esophagus *262*,
      607
glycogen storage diseases 419–420, *421*,
      422
goblet cells, colon *24*
gold enterocolitis *709*
Golgi apparatus *51*
Gorlin syndrome **249**
gossypiboma *484*, *485*

graft-versus-host disease 501, *508*,
      512–513
    colon *552*, *919*
    esophagus 110, *112*, *880*
    oral lesions *574*, *578*
    PET *796*
granular cell tumor, esophagus *890*
granulomas *544*
    Crohn's disease *225*, *228*
    liver *511*, *512*
      epithelioid *871*
      histology *864*
      schistosomiasis *532*
    primary biliary cirrhosis *413*
    spleen *548*
Griffiths' critical point *27*
ground glass cells, liver *872*
guaiac-based fecal occult blood tests 267
guidewires
    biliary drainage *752*, *753*
    esophageal dilation *649*
    Seldinger technique *821*
gynecomastia, PET *792*

H63D mutation, hemochromatosis 417b
halothane hepatotoxicity *866*
hamartoma
    colorectal *234*, *237*
      see also PTEN hamartoma
    Peutz–Jeghers syndrome *256*, *257*
    small intestine 202, *203*, *624*
harmless acute pancreatitis score 288b
harvest injury, liver histology *877*
HBeAg *384*
HBsAg *384*
heart, PET *797*, *802*
heart failure, liver histology *867*
Helicobacter pylori 124, *125*, *126*
    detection 142–143
    gastric cancer 149
    gastritis *125*, *126*, 141–143, *144*, 145,
      890
    intestinal metaplasia 140
helminths 524–543
helper T lymphocytes, acute viral
      hepatitis 375
hemangioma
    liver *763*, 768, *770*
    small intestine *625*
    see also cavernous hemangioma of liver
hematoma, intramural 102, *105*, *544*, *549*
hematopoiesis, in liver *50*, *51*
hemochromatosis 415–418, *861*
hemoclips *689*
hemolytic–uremic syndrome *173*
hemorrhage
    into biliary tract *837*
    gastrointestinal *544*, *545*
      algorithm *622*
      angiography 820, *822*, *827*, *828*
      diverticulosis *626*

    interventional radiology *849*, *850*
    radionuclide imaging 810, *817*
    see also upper gastrointestinal
      hemorrhage
    intraabdominal, acute pancreatitis *301*
    liver adenoma *836*
    polypectomy 680, *681*, *690*, *691*
hemorrhoids 24, 270, *273*, *274*
    rubber-band ligation *274*
      instruments *272*
hemosiderin, embryonic liver *50*
hemosiderosis, liver, MRI *774*
Hemospray *130*
hemostatic clips
    hemoclips *689*
    peptic ulcer disease 678, *679*
Henoch–Schönlein purpura *570*, *571*
hepatic artery *50*, *52*, *53*, *54*
    aberrant *823*, *824*
    Doppler ultrasonography *734*, *735*
      liver transplantation *736*
    fistula from *826*
    injury *837*
    pseudoaneurysm *837*
    stenosis
      angioplasty *848*
hepatic flexure, endoscopy *626*
hepatic hydrothorax *448*
hepatic vein *50*
hepatic venography 836–839
hepatic venoocclusive disease
    radiation injury *599*
    see also sinusoidal obstruction
      syndrome
hepatic venous pressure gradient **449**
hepatic venous pressure measurement *666*
hepatitis
    alcoholic 425–427
    chronic, histology 390, *391*, *862*, *867*,
      872, *873*, *874*
    sonography *732*, *733*
    see also autoimmune hepatitis; viral
      hepatitis
hepatitis A virus 374, 377
    serology *383*
    structure *379*
    world prevalence *375*
      liver failure 398, **398**
hepatitis B virus 374, 377
    acute hepatitis, allograft *877*
    chronic hepatitis 387–391
      histology 389, *390*, *391*, *862*, *867*
      management **390**
      monitoring 387
      prevention 390
      progression 388
      world prevalence 388
      genome 379
    hepatitis D virus with 385
    immune response 383
    replication 380

serology *384*
world prevalence *376, 378*
liver failure *398*, **398**
hepatitis C virus 374, 377, 392–396
diagnostic testing 392, **394**, **395**
genome *381, 393*
histology *394*
liver histology *874*
progression *394*
replication *382*
serology *384*
world prevalence *377*
hepatitis D virus 374, 377
genome *383*
liver histology *874*
ribonucleoprotein complex 374–375
serology *385*
superinfection *385*
world prevalence *378*
hepatitis E virus 374, 377
genome *375, 383*
serology *385*
world prevalence *378*
liver failure *398*
hepatobiliary pain *342, 349*
hepatocellular carcinoma 465–468
chronic hepatitis B 389–390, *391*
computed tomography *764*
cTACE *844, 845*
DEB-TACE *843, 845, 847*
histology *870, 871*
MRI *465, 771, 775*
PET *792*
portal vein invasion *836*
radiofrequency ablation *843*
sonography *732*
hepatocytes *51, 55, 56*
α-1-antitrypsin *861*
glycogen accumulation *433*
hepatocytolysis *860*
hepatojejunal stricture *856*
hepatoma *see* hepatocellular carcinoma
hepatorenal syndrome *447, 448–449, 453, 457*
hepatosplenomegaly, schistosomiasis *531*
herbal medications, liver injury *399, 404*
hereditary colorectal cancer
syndromes 238, **239**
see also polyposis syndromes; *specific syndromes*
hereditary hemorrhagic telangiectasia *556, 579*
hereditary mixed polyposis syndrome **249**
hereditary pancreatitis *317, 322*
hernias 36–42
hiatus hernia *72, 79, 153–155, 156, 612*
inguinal *36, 38, 39, 40, 458, 767*
laparotomy *699*
parastomal *see* incisional hernia
umbilical *37, 40, 458*
see also paraesophageal hernia

herpes simplex virus infection
esophagus *85, 87, 88, 89, 505, 610, 882*
liver histology *874*
perianal *505*
heterotopic gastric mucosa, esophagus *3, 8f, 13, 16, 610*
heterotopic mucosa, Meckel
diverticulum *19*
HFE gene *415*
hiatus hernia *72, 79, 153–155, 156, 612*
hidebound appearance, scleroderma *546*
hidradenoma papilliferum *929*
high-resolution manometry,
esophagus *61, 62, 63*
Hill grades, gastroesophageal junction flap
valve *79*
Hirschsprung disease 162–167
histological activity index, chronic viral
hepatitis *860*, **861**
histological score (AHHS), alcoholic
hepatitis *426, 427*
histoplasmosis
histology *917*
small intestine *180, 182*
Whipple disease *vs* *177*
historical aspects, endoscopy *605*
HIV-associated idiopathic ulcers,
esophagus *90, 91, 92*
HIV infection *see* acquired
immunodeficiency syndrome
HLA haplotypes, idiosyncratic drug-
induced liver injury 397–398, *400*
Hodgkin lymphoma, liver histology *876*
hookworms *527, 528, 542*
Houston's valves *626*
human immunodeficiency virus *see*
acquired immunodeficiency
syndrome
hybrid NOTES *702, 711, 713, 719*
hydatid disease *540, 541*
hydramnios, small intestinal atresia *22*
hydrogen breath test
lactose malabsorption *184, 185*
sucrase–isomaltase deficiency *186, 188*
hydronephrosis, schistosomiasis *531*
hydrothorax, hepatic *448*
hypereosinophilic syndrome *544, 549*
hyperglycemia, gastroparesis *117*
hyperpigmentation
hemochromatosis *416*
primary biliary cirrhosis *410*
hyperplastic polyp
colorectal *626, 627, 926*
stomach *615, 894*
hypertensive peristalsis, esophagus *65, 78*
hypertrophic lichen planus *569*
hypochlorhydria *135*
hypogammaglobulinemia *510*
hyponatremia, ascites *447, 453*
hypopharynx, squamous cell
carcinoma *726*

hypopyon *219*
Hy's Law *399, 404*

idiopathic HIV-associated ulcers,
esophagus *90, 91, 92*
idiopathic noncirrhotic portal
hypertension *473*
idiopathic nonfamilial visceral
neuropathies 167–168
idiosyncratic drug reactions, liver
injury 397–398
danger hypothesis *400*
genome-wide association studies *400*
HLA haplotypes *400*
regulatory actions **403**
IgA deficiency *510*
IgG4 sclerosing cholangitis *290*
ileal ischemia, acute *583*
ileal pouch–anal anastomosis *233, 915*
familial adenomatous polyposis *252*
see also pouchitis
ileocecal valve
Crohn's disease *907*
endoscopy *626, 627*
ulcerative colitis *218*
ileocolic intussusception *740*
ileus
paralytic *298*
see also gallstone ileus
imatinib mesylate, PET, treatment
monitoring *788*
immune response
acute viral hepatitis 375–376
hepatitis B virus *383*
idiosyncratic drug-induced liver
injury *397*
immunochemical tests, fecal *267*
immunodeficiency 501–508, 509–514, *548*
see also acquired immunodeficiency
syndrome; common variable
immunodeficiency
immunoperoxidase stains *860*
immunoproliferative small intestinal
disease **248**
immunosuppressive therapy, for
autoimmune hepatitis *405*, **408**
Imodium (loperamide) **190**
impaction
at esophageal strictures *106, 609*
fecal *280*
impedance, intraluminal, esophagus *61, 62*
incisional hernia *37, 41*
incisions, laparotomy *699*
inclusion cysts, epidermal *555, 556*
indigocarmine, chromoendoscopy *898*
indium-111 pentreotide *811*
indium-111 radiolabeled solid meal *116, 120*
infarction
intestinal *723*
omental *484, 490, 547*

infections
  biliary tract *351*, *354*, *360*
  colon 170–176
  Crohn's disease *vs* 232
  esophagus, viral 85, *87*, *88*, *89*, *90*
  fungal *see* fungal infections
  liver
    foamy histiocytes *871*
    see also viral hepatitis
  opportunistic 501–508, 512
  pancreatic necrosis 304–306
  retroperitoneal 484
  small intestine 177–183
  see also specific organisms
inferior mesenteric artery 26–27, 582
  collaterals from *826*
  stenosis *588*
inferior vena cava
  liver transplantation *736*
  stenosis *853*
inflammatory bowel disease
  cytomegalovirus infection 228
  positron emission tomography *800*,
    807, *811*
  see also Crohn's disease; ulcerative
    colitis
inflammatory polyps 258
  cloacogenic *920*
  Crohn's disease 225, *227*
  fibroid *237*, *895*
  polyposis syndromes with **248**
  ulcerative colitis 216, *217*
inguinal hernias 36, *38*, *39*, *40*, *458*, *767*
injection therapy
  needle *678*
  peptic ulcer disease *129*, 677
inlet patches, esophagus 8f, 13, *16*, *610*
innate immunity, acute viral hepatitis 375
instrument channels, endoscopes 606
insulin, PET and 782
insulinoma 742, *766*
  angiography *833*
integrated relaxation pressure,
    gastroesophageal junction 68
intensive care units, laparoscopy in 698
interleukin-6, severe acute
    pancreatitis 287
internal hernias, abdominal cavity 37, *42*
interstitial cells of Cajal (ICCs) 162, *164*,
    165
interventional radiology 842–859
  liver abscesses 471
  mesenteric 582, *585*, *586*, *587*, *588*
  see also embolization
interventional sonography 735
intestinal dysmotility **159**, **161**, **162**,
    167–169
  distal intestinal obstruction
    syndrome 184, *185*, *186*, 317, *321*
intestinal failure 189
  algorithm *199*

intestinal malrotation *18*, 36, *37*
intestinal metaplasia
  stomach 140–141, *142*, *144*
  see also Barrett esophagus
intestinal transplantation 189–191, *200*
intestinal type adenomas, stomach *895*
intestinal type gastric
    adenocarcinoma 149, *151*
intraductal mucinous neoplasm,
    pancreas 766
intraductal papillary mucinous neoplasm,
    pancreas *326*, *327*, *328*
intraepithelial lymphocytosis *919*
intraepithelial neoplasia, anus *929*
intragastric balloons *494*
intragastric resection, GISTs *700*
intrahepatic cholangiocarcinoma *372*
Intralipid *201*
intraluminal impedance, esophagus 61, *62*
intramucosal carcinoma 234, *236*, *897*
intramural hematoma 102, *105*, 544, *549*
intramural pseudodiverticulosis 3–4, *65*
intraoperative ultrasonography 740
intravenous contrast agents 757
intussusception
  ileocolic *740*
  rectum *282*
iritis 216
iron
  liver cirrhosis *416*
  overload 417b, **417**
    nonalcoholic fatty liver disease *434*
  small intestinal injury *210*
iron pill esophagitis *879*
ischemia, intestinal 582–596
ischemic colitis 582, *590*, *591*, *593*, 632,
    918
  carcinoma and *594*
  computed tomography *590*, *592*
  fulminant *595*
  histology *596*
ischiorectal abscess *275*
Ishak score, chronic viral hepatitis **861**
islet cell tumor
  endoscopic ultrasonography *833*
  somatostatin receptor imaging *817*
  see also insulinoma
islets of Langerhans 30, *35*
Isospora belli *503*, **516**, 520, *522*, *523*
Ito cells *868*

jackhammer contraction, esophagus 66, 68
Jass and Filipe classification, intestinal
    metaplasia 140
jigsaw puzzle appearance, biliary
    cirrhosis *872*
juvenile polyposis **239**, **247**, *258*, *259*, *921*

Kaposi sarcoma *507*, *550*, 573
  esophagus *101*
  liver histology *877*

Kartagener's syndrome 3, 5f
kayexalate *879*
Kayser–Fleischer ring 419, *421*
keratoacanthoma *555*
kidney
  acute renal failure, cirrhosis 448–449,
    456, *457*
  alcoholic hepatitis 427
  chronic disease 544
  clear cell carcinoma *788*
  see also renal cell carcinoma
koilonychia 568
Kupffer cells 51

lacrimal glands, lymphoma *801*
lactase nonpersistence 184
lactose malabsorption 184, *185*
Langhans giant cells, liver *871*
laparoscopy 698–700
  complications 699
  technique 698–699
  see also adjustable gastric band
laparotomy 698
  complications 699
  technique 699
large-volume paracentesis 448, *454*
larva migrans, cutaneous *541*, *542*
larynx, double-contrast radiography *724*
leaks
  adjustable gastric band *498*
  biliary 807, *810*, *857*
  pancreatic duct *640*
  Roux-en-Y gastric bypass *500*
leiomyoma
  esophagus *101*, *608*
  submucosal tunneling endoscopic
    resection 707
leiomyomatosis, gastrointestinal **249**
leiomyosarcoma *829*
lepidic growth pattern, adenocarcinoma of
    lung *800*
Leriche syndrome *589*
Leser–Trelat sign *558*
leukemia, lymphocytic, liver histology
    868
leukocytoclastic vasculitis *571*
levator ani 24
lichen planus *569*, *570*, *880*
ligamentum teres 52
ligation
  bleeding polyps *691*
  esophageal varices *664*, *670*
  fallopian tube, NOTES *718*
  see also rubber-band ligation
Lille Model, alcoholic hepatitis 427
linear echoendoscopes *741*, *742*
linitis plastica *616*, *897*
lipase, acute pancreatitis *273*, *290*
lipid emulsions 191, **201**
lipogranuloma, nonalcoholic
    steatohepatitis *433*

lipomas
  cecum *243*
  colorectal *628, 929*
  duodenum *619*
  gastric antrum *616*
  skin *556*
lipomatous polyposis **249**
lipophages, radiation injury *599*
Liposyn II *201*
litholysis, oral *346, 347*
lithotripsy, biliary tract *637*
Littre's hernia *37*
liver *50–57*
  ablative therapies *843*
  abscesses *469–471, 481, 482, 515, 518*
    amebic *469–471, 515, 518*
    drainage *859*
    fistula from *481*
    MRI *469, 470, 482*
    PET *799*
  alcoholic disease *see* alcoholic liver
    disease
  anatomy *50, 52, 53*
  angiography *834–839*
  biopsy *see under* biopsy
  cavernous hemangioma
    angiography *835*
    scintigraphy *809*
    SPECT/CT *812*
  cirrhosis *see* cirrhosis
  cystic fibrosis *317, 321*
  cysts *361, 366, 769*
  drug-induced injury *397–404*
  embryology *48, 50, 51*
  fibrosis *see* fibrosis (liver)
  focal nodular hyperplasia *see* focal
    nodular hyperplasia
  granulomas *511, 512*
    epithelioid *871*
    histology *864*
    schistosomiasis *532*
  hemangioma *763, 768, 770*
  hemosiderosis *774*
  interventional radiology *842*
  magnetic resonance imaging *768*
  metabolic diseases *419–422*
  metastases
    angiography *824*
    carcinoids *818*
    histology *871*
    magnetic resonance imaging *772, 773*
    radioembolization *846*
    renal cell carcinoma *832*
    Zollinger–Ellison syndrome *138*
  microanatomy *51–52*
  nonalcoholic fatty liver disease *428–435*
  pseudoaneurysms *852*
  radiation injury *597, 599*
  radionuclide imaging *809*
  sarcoidosis *790*
  sonography *732–735*

  steatosis *see* steatosis
  stellate cells *51, 436, 438, 439–440, 442,
    443*
  submassive necrosis *386, 862*
  transplantation *see* liver transplantation
  vascular diseases *472–476*
liver cytosol autoantibodies *406*
liver failure, world etiologies *398,* **398**
liver kidney microsome
    autoantibodies *406*
liver transplantation *355, 459–464*
  acetaminophen injury *397*
  α-1-antitrypsin deficiency *419*
  biopsy *860*
  harvest injury *877*
  hepatocellular carcinoma *465, 468*
  PET *793*
  rejection *863, 865, 877*
  sonography *735, 736*
living donor liver transplantation *459, 461*
local anesthesia, laparoscopy *699*
Loeffler's syndrome *525*
Lomotil **190**
loops, detachable (PolyLoop®) *688, 691*
loperamide **190**
Los Angeles convention, reflux
    esophagitis *73*
lower esophageal sphincter, dilation
    (therapeutic), perforation *102, 104*
  endoscopy *606*
  see also gastroesophageal junction
lower gastrointestinal tract, definition *621*
lumbar hernia *37, 41*
lumiracoxib, liver injury *400*
lung
  abscesses *652*
  adenocarcinoma, PET *800*
  sarcoidosis *790*
lymphadenopathy
  endoscopic ultrasonography *746*
  mediastinum, CT *758*
  mesentery *489, 802*
  PET *783, 802*
  sarcoidosis *548, 790*
lymphangiectasia *215, 510, 618, 729*
lymphangioma *37*
lymphatics, rectum *28, 29*
lymphocytic colitis *919*
lymphocytic esophagitis *109, 110*
lymphocytic leukemia, liver histology *868*
lymphoepithelial lesions, MALT
    lymphoma *897*
lymphogranuloma venereum *506*
lymphoid hyperplasia *509*
  colon *265*
  multiple **248**
  nodular **248,** *509, 511*
lymphoma
  Burkitt lymphoma *801*
  duodenum *619*
  Leser–Trelat sign *558*

  mucosa-associated lymphoid tissue *617,
    797, 896, 897*
  posttransplant *793*
  small intestine *203–204, 207, 214*
  spleen *545*
  see also B cell lymphomas; non-
    Hodgkin lymphoma
Lynch syndrome *238, 239, 269*
lysosomes, hepatocytes *51*

macroamylasemia *296*
macroglobulinemia, Whipple disease
    vs 177
macroglossia, amyloidosis *581*
macronodular cirrhosis *442, 446*
Maddrey's discriminant function, alcoholic
    liver disease *426*
magnetic resonance angiography *768*
magnetic resonance cholangiography *768*
magnetic resonance
    cholangiopancreatography *345,
    768*
  choledocholithiasis *776*
  chronic pancreatitis *307, 310, 779*
  liver cyst *769*
  normal appearances *345, 778*
  stones *345*
magnetic resonance colonography *781*
magnetic resonance elastography *442, 445*
magnetic resonance enterography *227–229*
magnetic resonance imaging *768–781*
  autoimmune pancreatitis *293, 294*
  fecal incontinence *282*
  gastrointestinal fistulae *477*
  liver abscesses *469, 470, 482*
magnets (self-assembling),
    gastrojejunostomy *713*
major papilla, duodenum *18*
malignant atrophic papulosis *567*
malignant melanoma metastases
  duodenal *618*
  MRI *773*
  PET *787*
malignant polyps *234, 236, 630*
malignant ulcers, gastric *615, 897*
Mallory bodies *413, 875*
Mallory hyaline *430, 866*
Mallory–Weiss tears *102, 103, 613, 676,
    677*
malrotation, intestinal *18, 36, 37*
Maltese-cross birefringence, bile
    crystals *340*
MALT lymphoma *617, 797, 896, 897*
manometry
  esophagus *61, 62, 63*
  fecal incontinence **270**
    squeeze pressures *283*
  pancreatic sphincter *640*
marginal artery of Drummond *27, 582*
marginal ulcers, bariatric surgery *493,
    495, 496, 497, 612*

massive necrosis, liver *865*
Masson trichrome *860*
maximal acid secretion, Zollinger–Ellison syndrome *136*
maximum intensity projection, computed tomography *757*
Maydl hernia *37*
McCune–Albright syndrome **249**
meal test, Zollinger-Ellison syndrome *135, 136*
Meckel diverticulum *19–21*
  hemorrhage *828*
  histology *16*
  radionuclide imaging *19, 810*
meconium ileus *184, 317*
median arcuate ligament compression, celiac axis *822*
median glossoepiglottic fold *724*
mediastinum
  access by NOTES *705, 707*
  endoscopic ultrasonography *745*
  lymphadenopathy *758*
megacolon, toxic *218, 219*
megacystis-microcolon-intestinal hypoperistalsis **161**
megaesophagus *499*
mega-mitochondria *430, 866, 868*
melanoma
  anus *930*
  see also malignant melanoma metastases
melanosis coli *913*
MELD score *459–460, 462b, 462*
Menetrier disease *613*
mesenteric arteries *582*
  diseases affecting *208–209, 210*
  embolism *582, 583*
  radiation injury *599, 600*
mesenteric ischemia
  acute *582, 583*
  subacute *584*
mesenteric veins
  thrombosis *209, 211, 544, 549*
  see also superior mesenteric vein
mesentery *484*
  carcinoids *759*
  desmoid tumor *489*
  disease classification *489b*
  fibrosis *487*
  lymphadenopathy *489, 802*
  metastases *787, 832*
    angiography *832*
    PET/CT *784*
  see also infarction
metabolic bone disease, primary sclerosing cholangitis *354, 357*
metabolic diseases, liver *419–422*
metabolic syndrome *401*
metaplasia
  intestinal type adenomas *895*
  peptic duodenitis *902*
  see also Barrett esophagus; intestinal metaplasia

metaplastic atrophic gastritis *891, 892*
metastases *548, 550*
  carcinoids, PET *803*
  colon *243*
  duodenum *618*
  epithelioid angiosarcoma *798*
  esophageal cancer *783*
  linitis plastica *897*
  liver *see under* liver
  mesentery *787, 832*
    angiography *832*
    PET/CT *784*
  pancreas *832*
  PET *783, 784, 786, 814, 819*
  retroperitoneal, germ cell tumor *487*
  small intestine *550, 728, 787*
  SPECT/CT *817*
  Zollinger–Ellison syndrome *138*
methotrexate, hepatotoxicity *876*
methyldopa, hepatotoxicity *875*
Meyenburg complexes *864*
MHC haplotypes, idiosyncratic drug-induced liver injury *397–398, 400*
micelles *338*
micronodular cirrhosis *442, 446*
microparticles, TACE *845*
microsatellite instability high colonic adenocarcinoma *242*
Microsporidia infection *503*
midgut, definition *621*
midodrine *449*
migration, esophageal stent *662–663*
Milan criteria, hepatocellular carcinoma *465, 468*
minilaparoscopy *700*
minor papilla *18, 641*
mitochondria
  mega-mitochondria *430, 866, 868*
  Reye syndrome *421*
mitochondrial neurogastrointestinal encephalomyopathy syndrome *158,* **159**
mixed cholesterol gallstones *336*
Model for End-stage Liver Disease score *459–460, 462b, 462*
monitoring, hepatitis B virus infection *387*
mononuclear cells, *H. pylori* gastritis *142*
mononucleosis *see* Epstein–Barr virus
Montreal definition, gastroesophageal reflux disease *73*
Morgagni hernia *36, 37*
morphine, radionuclide imaging of gallbladder *804, 805*
motility disorders
  esophagus *61–71, 78, 81, 813*
    see also gastroesophageal reflux disease
  intestines *157–169*
  stomach *115–123*
    radionuclide imaging *809–810, 815, 816*

mucinous adenocarcinoma
  appendix *789*
  pancreas *791*
mucinous cystadenoma, pancreas *328*
mucinous neoplasm, intraductal papillary, pancreas *326, 327, 328*
mucin typing, intestinal metaplasia *140–141*
mucosa-associated lymphoid tissue lymphoma *617, 797, 896, 897*
mucosal biopsy, endoscopic *878–930*
mucosal breaks, reflux esophagitis *73*
mucosal flap, transcolonic NOTES *721*
mucosal prolapse syndrome *248, 265*
mucosal resection, esophagus *608*
  see also endoscopic mucosal resection
mucous membranes, pemphigoid *565*
mucus, cystic fibrosis *185*
mucus retention cysts *258*
Muir–Torre syndrome, skin lesions *555*
multichannel electrogastrography *116, 123*
multidetector CT *756*
multiplanar reconstructions, CT *757*
multiple endocrine neoplasia syndromes
  type 1 *135, 137–139*
  type 2b *163,* **248**
multiple lymphoid hyperplasia **248**
multiple organ failure, severe acute pancreatitis *287*
multipolar electrocoagulation catheter *677, 678*
Murphy sign, sonographic *737*
MUTYH-associated polyposis **239, 247**
Mycobacterium avium complex
  duodenum *506, 548*
  small intestine *177, 179*
Mycobacterium avium intracellulare
  duodenum *903*
  liver histology *871*
myocarditis, eosinophilic *549*
myofibroblasts, liver *437, 438*
myotomy, peroral endoscopic *706*

N-acetyl-*p*-benzoquinone imine *397, 399*
N-acetylcysteine *399*
naltrexone *425*
narrow band imaging
  Barrett esophagus *888*
  gastric cancer *150*
nasogastric tube placement *858*
natural orifice transluminal endoscopic surgery *702–721*
N-butyl-2-cyanoacrylate *664*
Necator americanus *527, 528*
necrolytic migratory erythema *330, 559*
necrosis
  periportal *199*
  liver *800, 803, 872, 873*
    piecemeal *413*
    submassive *386, 862*
  pancreas *see* walled-off necrosis
necrotizing enterocolitis *212–213, 214*

necrotizing pancreatitis 300, 302–306, 307, *309*, *314*, *316*
nematodes 524
  see also specific species
neonatal hepatitis, histology *867*
neonatal necrotizing enterocolitis 213
nephrectomy, abscess *479*
nerve supply
  anal sphincters *26*, 283
  biliary tract *47*
  enteric nervous system 157, *158*, 159
  levator ani 24
neuroendocrine tumors 135, 137–139
  colorectal 238
  pancreas 135, 137–139, 329–334
    angiography *833*
    PET *334*, *795*
    somatostatin receptor imaging 810–811
neurofibromatosis **248**
neurofibromatosis type 1 *556*, *557*
neuromodulation, gastric 119
neurotransmitters, visceral neuropathies **167**, 168
neutral contrast agents *756*
neutropenic enterocolitis 548, *551*, *552*
neutrophils, *H. pylori* gastritis 141–142
Nissen fundoplication *81*
nodular hepatocellular carcinoma *468*
nodular lymphoid hyperplasia **248**, 509, *511*
nodular regenerative hyperplasia 472–473, *475*, *476*, *862*
nodule-in-nodule hepatocellular carcinoma *468*
nonalcoholic fatty liver disease 428–435
nonalcoholic steatohepatitis 428, *432*, *433*, *435*, *875*
noncirrhotic idiopathic portal hypertension *473*
nonfunctional pancreatic neuroendocrine tumors 137–139
non-Hodgkin lymphoma 548
  liver histology *876*
  small intestine *729*
  stomach *507*, *551*
nonlifting sign *630*
nonocclusive mesenteric ischemia *582*
nonsteroidal anti-inflammatory drugs
  gastropathy 144–145, *146*
  peptic ulcer disease 124, *125*, *127*, *128*, *133*, *614*
  small intestinal ulcers 208
NOTES (natural orifice transluminal endoscopic surgery) 701–721
nucleoside analog reverse transcriptase inhibitors, steatosis *508*
nutrition
  cystic fibrosis 317, *322*
  enteral, acute pancreatitis 306
  primary biliary cirrhosis *414*
  see also total parenteral nutrition

obesity 491–494
  alcoholic liver disease 424
  see also bariatric surgery
obstruction
  biliary tract
    common bile duct *765*
    histology *863*
    magnetic resonance imaging *777*
    radionuclide imaging 804–806, *807*
  distal intestinal obstruction syndrome 184, *185*, *186*, 317, *321*
  gastric outlet *see* gastric outlet obstruction
  small intestine *761*, *767*
  see also pseudoobstruction
obturator hernia 37, *42*
OctreoScan® (indium-111 pentreotide) *811*
octreotide **190**, 449
octreotide analog, PET radiotracer *782*, *803*
ocular manifestations *see* eye
odontomes *574*, *580*
oil red O, stellate cells *436*, *439*
Omegaven 191, *201*
omentum *see* mesentery
omphalocele 22, *23*, 36
onychodystrophy, Cronkhite–Canada syndrome *264*
ophthalmic manifestations *see* eye
opioids, antidiarrheal **190**
Opisthorchis spp. 535, *536*
opportunistic infections 501–508, 512
Optical dilator *644*
oral contrast agents, computed tomography *756*
oral lesions 574–581
  Peutz–Jeghers syndrome 241, *255*, *910*
oral litholysis 346, *347*
orcein stain (Shikata stain) *860*, *862*
Osler–Weber–Rendu syndrome, liver histology *865*
osteomas
  familial adenomatous polyposis 253
  Gardner syndrome *574*, *580*
osteoporosis
  primary biliary cirrhosis, management *414*
  primary sclerosing cholangitis 354, *357*
Overstitch device *717*
over-the-scope clips *697*, 714–715
oxalate, foods high in *191b*
oxaluria *191*
oxyntic gland polyps *251*, 615, *895*

pacing, gastric 119
Paget disease
  anus *930*
  extramammary *559*
pain *see* abdominal pain
pancolitis, ulcerative colitis *914*

pancreas 30–35
  adenocarcinoma *740*, *750*, *755*, *765*
    MRI *768*
    PET *791*
  anatomy 30–35
  aneurysm *826*
  angiography 833–834
  annular 15, *765*
  arteriovenous malformations *829*
  carcinoma 766
    common bile duct compression *855*
    gastrojejunostomy *657–658*
    magnetic resonance imaging *780*
    PET *799*
  cystic fibrosis 184, *185*, *186*, *187*, 317–323
  cysts 324–328
    PET *791*
  embryology 30, *31*, 43, 48
  ERCP 634–635, 639
  insulinoma *742*, 766
    angiography *833*
  islet cell tumor *see* islet cell tumor
  magnetic resonance imaging 768, *778*
  metastases *832*
  neuroendocrine tumors 135, 137–139, 329–334
    angiography *833*
    PET *334*, *795*
  pseudocyst *see* pseudocyst
  Shwachman–Diamond syndrome 318
  stones, ERCP 634–635, 639
  transgastric necrosectomy 304, *316*
  ultrasonography 738, *740*
    endoscopic *744*, *750*
    pseudocyst *308*
pancreas divisum 32, 290–292, *294*, 641
pancreatic duct 48
  anomalous union with common bile duct 361, *363*
  leaks *640*
  sphincterotomy *640*
  stents *314*, 635, *636*, 639
  strictures *639*
pancreatic rest *614*
pancreatic secretory trypsin inhibitor *322*
pancreatitis
  acute 287–306
    classification *301b*
    see also walled-off necrosis
  chronic 307–316
    carcinoma 323
    diabetes mellitus 323
    endoscopic ultrasonography *750*
    magnetic resonance imaging 768, *779*
    pseudoaneurysm 308, *313*, *833*
    steatorrhea 323
  ERCP
    prevention 634
    recurrent acute 635, *640*, 641
  gallbladder sludge 344
  hereditary 317, *322*
  sonography 738

panhepatic angiography 836
pantaloon hernia 37
papilla of Vater 43, 48, 617
  AIDS 508
  associated mass 618
  chronic pancreatitis 311
  ERCP 634, 636, 637, 638, 641
  major papilla 18
  minor papilla 18, 641
papillary mucinous neoplasm, intraductal,
  pancreas 326, 327, 328
paracentesis (large-volume) 448, 454
paraduodenal hernia 37
paraesophageal hernia 153–155
  after Nissen fundoplication 81
paralytic ileus 298
parasitic diseases
  helminths 524–543
  protozoa 515
parastomal hernia (incisional hernia) 37,
  41
parenteral nutrition see total parenteral
  nutrition
patatin-like phospholipase domain-
  containing protein 3 424
patency capsule 621, 623
pedunculated polyps 626, 628
  resection 681, 688
peginterferon, HCV, contraindications
  396
peliosis 473, 476, 876
pellagra 572
pelvis
  abscesses 482
  hernias 37
pemphigoid 565
  benign mucous membrane
    pemphigoid 110, 113
  see also bullous pemphigoid
pemphigus vulgaris 566
  esophagus 110, 113
pentreotide, indium-111-labeled 811, 818
peptic duodenitis 902
peptic stricture, esophagus 74, 105, 654
peptic ulcer disease 124–134, 614
  endoscopic treatment 677, 678, 679
  hemorrhage 675, 676, 679, 827, 828
  strictures 130, 654
  Zollinger–Ellison syndrome 135–139,
    894
percutaneous ports, ERCP, Roux-en-Y
  gastric bypass 641
percutaneous splenoportography 840
percutaneous transluminal angioplasty see
  angioplasty
perforation
  colorectal polypectomy 681, 688, 695, 696
  endoscopic submucosal dissection
    695–696
  esophagus 102, 104, 608
  foreign bodies 697

pneumoperitoneum 723
  polypectomy 680
periadenitis mucosa necrotica
  recurrens 562
periampullary masses 618
perianal Crohn's disease 230–231, 559
perianal herpes simplex virus
  infection 505
pericellular fibrosis, nonalcoholic fatty
  liver disease 431
pericholangitis 218
perihilar cholangiocarcinoma 370, 373
perinuclear antineutrophil cytoplasmic
  antibodies (pANCA), autoimmune
  hepatitis 406
periodic acid–Schiff staining, small
  intestine 177, 178, 179
peripheral nerve sheath tumor,
  epithelioid 929
perisinusoidal fibrosis 476
peristalsis, esophagus 62
  abnormalities 65, 66, 78
peristomal varices, ulcerative colitis 354,
  357
peritoneoscopy, transgastric 703, 711
peritoneum 484, 485, 486
  abscesses 477–483
  anatomy 36
  carcinomatosis 484, 486, 784
  lymphoma 802
  sonography 740
  see also pseudomyxoma peritonei
peritonitis 484
  PET 787
  see also spontaneous bacterial
    peritonitis
pernicious anemia see autoimmune
  gastritis
peroral endoscopic myotomy 706
peroral transgastric biopsy, liver 703, 706
petechial hemorrhages, stomach 126, 128
Peutz–Jeghers syndrome **239, 247**
  mouth 241, 255, 580, 910
  polyps 256, 257, 910, 911, 912
  small intestinal hamartoma 624
pH, stomach 135
pharynx
  anatomy 724
  candidiasis 725
  double-contrast radiography 722, 724
pH-impedance testing
  belching 77
  gastroesophageal reflux 76
phonation, double-contrast
  radiography 724
phospholipids, bile 338, 339
photodynamic therapy, cholangiocarcinoma 377, 611
piecemeal necrosis, primary biliary
  cirrhosis 413
pigmentation see hyperpigmentation
pigment gallstones 335, 336

pigment-laden macrophages, nonalcoholic
  fatty liver disease 432
pill esophagitis 102, 108
  iron pill esophagitis 879
Pima Indians, gallstones 337
pinworms 529
plasma cells, liver histology 863
plicae circulares 621
pneumatosis
  acute mesenteric ischemia 583
  colon 723
  small intestine 760
pneumatosis cystoides intestinalis **249,
  265, 632**
pneumobilia 737
pneumoperitoneum 723
PNPLA3 (patatin-like phospholipase
  domain-containing protein 3) 424
POEM (peroral endoscopic myotomy)
  706
polarized light, liver histology 860, 863
polyarteritis nodosa 212
  liver histology 864
polycystic liver disease 366, 367, 733
polyhydramnios, small intestinal
  atresia 22
PolyLoop® 688, 691
polypectomy
  argon plasma coagulation 687
  clips 690
    for perforation 695–696
  colorectal 627–628, 629, 686
  duodenum 685
  hemorrhage 680, 681, 690, 691
  saline-assisted 680, 682, 683–684
  snare polypectomy 629, 681, 682,
    683–684, 685, 688
polyposis syndromes 246–265
  juvenile polyposis **239, 247**, 258, 259,
    921
  serrated polyposis syndrome 240, **247**,
    254, 927, 928
  see also familial adenomatous polyposis;
    hereditary colorectal cancer
    syndromes
polyps
  anus, fibroepithelial 929
  carcinoma 925, 926
    screening 267, 268, 269
  colorectal see carcinoma; colorectal
    polyps
  Crohn's disease 225, 227
  Cronkhite–Canada syndrome 922, 923
  elastosis 920
  endoscopic therapy 680–697
  fibroblastic, colon 928
  fundic gland polyps 161, 916, 919
  gallbladder 343
  hyperplastic see hyperplastic polyp
  inflammatory see inflammatory polyps
  juvenile polyposis 921

Peutz–Jeghers syndrome *256, 257, 910, 911, 912*
schistosomiasis *531, 532*
sessile *see* sessile polyps
small intestine *624, 625*
stomach *615*
virtual colonoscopy *762*
see also pseudopolyps
porcelain gallbladder *737, 738*
porphyria cutanea tarda *568*
portal fibroblasts *436*
portal fibrosis *431*
portal hypertension 436–446
gastropathy *614, 664, 673*
liver histology *864*
noncirrhotic idiopathic *473*
transjugular portography *831*
upper gastrointestinal hemorrhage 664–674
portal tracts 51, *54, 55*
portal vein 50, *52, 53, 54, 665*
aneurysm *827*
angiography *820, 831*
with CO_2 *854*
cavernous transformation *735*
fistula into *826*
gas *723*
interventional radiology *842*
invasion *836*
occlusion *839*
relations with pancreas *33*
schistosomiasis *531*
thrombosis *472, 473, 474, 763*
portosystemic collateral circulation *665*
portosystemic shunts *842*
see also transjugular intrahepatic portosystemic shunt
positive contrast agents 756–757
positron emission tomography (PET) 782–803
cholangiocarcinoma *358*
gastrointestinal malignancies 811–814
inflammatory bowel disease *800, 807, 811*
pancreatic neuroendocrine tumors *334, 795*
postcholecystectomy syndrome, radionuclide imaging *806, 808*
post-ERCP pancreatitis 294–295
posterior renal fascia, peritonitis, PET *787*
postprocessing, computed tomography *757*
posttransplant complications, liver transplantation *460, 464*
posttransplant lymphoproliferative disorder *793*
pouchitis 224, 354, 357, *915*
see also ileal pouch–anal anastomosis
Prague convention, Barrett metaplasia *75*
prednisolone, alcoholic hepatitis response *427*

prednisone, autoimmune hepatitis **408**
pregnancy, toxemia, liver histology *869*
prenatal diagnosis, omphalocele *22*
primary biliary cirrhosis 409–414
course and management *414*
histology *411, 412, 413, 864, 866*
primary peritoneal cancer *484*
primary sclerosing cholangitis 216–218, 354–360, *864*
PRKCSH gene *366*
proctalgia fugax *284*
proctosigmoidoscopy, instruments *272*
prokinetic agents *119*
prolapse
colorectal *920*
rectum *277*
prosthesis, esophagus *650*
protein C deficiency *549*
protein-losing gastroenteropathy 213, 214b
proton pump inhibitors
gastroesophageal reflux disease *72, 80*
Helicobacter pylori detection and *143*
nonresponder algorithm *80*
on oxyntic glands *144*
protozoa *515*
PRSS1 gene *317*
prurigo *567*
pseudoaneurysms
celiac axis *822*
chronic pancreatitis 308, *313, 833*
hepatic artery *837*
interventional radiology *852*
splenic artery *841*
superior mesenteric artery *849, 852*
pseudocyst (pancreatic) *307*
angiography *834*
computed tomography *14, 302*
gastric outlet obstruction *311*
treatment 308, *315*
ultrasonography *308*
pseudodiverticulosis, intramural, esophagus 3–4, *65*
pseudomembranous colitis 170, *174, 175, 553,* 631
computed tomography *763*
histology *917*
pseudomyxoma peritonei 484, *486, 767*
PET *789*
pseudoobstruction, chronic intestinal **159, 161, 162, 167,** *169*
idiopathic nonfamilial 167–168
pseudopapillary neoplasm, pancreas *325*
pseudopolyps
colorectal 234, *237, 243, 629, 631*
Crohn's disease *227*
ischemic colitis *593*
ulcerative colitis 217, 221, *222, 223, 913, 914*
pseudovein sign *827*
pseudoxanthoma elasticum *556*

psoriasis, atypical, Crohn's disease *230*
psyllium **190**
PTEN hamartoma **239, 247**
endoscopy *241, 260, 261, 262, 263*
glycogenic acanthosis *607*
histology *262*
puborectalis muscle *278, 279*
pyloric stenosis *17*
peptic ulcer disease *130*
see also gastric outlet obstruction
pylorus, stomach *612*
pyoderma gangrenosum 216, 218, 229, *559, 560*
facial lesion *230*
vegetating *577*
pyostomatitis vegetans 230, 574, *577*
pyriform sinuses, pharynx *724*

Q fever, liver histology *872*
quality of life, total parenteral nutrition **198**

radial echoendoscopes *741, 742*
radiation injury 597–602
esophagus *610, 649, 659*
proctitis 553, 632, *919*
small intestine 209, *213*
radioembolization *842, 846*
radiofrequency ablation, hepatocellular carcinoma *843*
radiology 722–731
small bowel follow-through, Crohn's disease 225–226, *228*
see also barium studies; chest radiographs; interventional radiology
radionuclide imaging 804–819
gastroparesis 116–117, *118, 120, 809–810, 816*
Meckel diverticulum 19, *810*
ragged red fibers *160*
railroad-track appearance, Crohn's disease *907*
reactive gastropathy 143–145, *146, 147, 890, 891*
rebleeding risk, peptic ulcer disease 675, *676, 679*
recombinant immunoblot assay (RIBA), HCV **395**
rectovaginal fistula *908*
rectum 24, *25, 271*
adenocarcinoma *238*
PET *786*
blood supply 25–26, *28*
carcinoids *244*
carcinoma *630*
Crohn's disease *908*
distention test *167*
endoscopy *626*
folds of *626*
hemorrhage *828*

rectum (*cont'd*)
   intussusception *282*
   lymphatics 28, *29*
   NOTES via 702, *720*
   PET *785*
   polyps 234–237
   prolapse *277*
   radiation injury 553, 600, 602, 632
   transanal endoscopic microsurgery
      720
   ulcers *277*
   Whipple disease, biopsy *177*
   see also anorectal diseases; anorectal
      examination
recurrent acute pancreatitis, ERCP 635,
   640, 641
red blood cells, Tc-99m-labeled 809, 810,
   812
red meat, colorectal cancer *239*
red signs, esophageal varices *668*
Reed–Sternberg cells *876*
reflux, gastroesophageal *63*
   esophagitis 73, 607, 878
   pH-impedance testing *76*
   radionuclide imaging *809*
   see also gastroesophageal reflux disease
refractory ascites 447, 448, 454, 455
regurgitation *71*
renal cell carcinoma
   metastases *832*
   PET *788*
renal failure, cirrhosis 448–449, 456, 457
rendezvous technique, biliary
      drainage *752*
resection
   gastrointestinal stromal tumors
      (GIST) *700*
   mucosal, esophagus *608*
      see also endoscopic mucosal
         resection
   pedunculated polyps 681, 688
   sessile polyps 682, 683–684, 685, 686,
      689, 693–694
   submucosal tunneling endoscopic
      resection, leiomyoma *707*
   see also endoscopic mucosal resection
resolution, CCDs 605–606
retained foreign objects *see* foreign bodies;
   gossypiboma
RET gene, visceral neuropathies *159*
retinal pigment epithelium, congenital
      hypertrophy *253*
retractors, anal *272*
retroflexion, endoscopy 627, 693–694
retroperitoneum 484, 487, 488
   air *731*
Reye syndrome 120, 121, 122
Rezulin, withdrawal *403*
RIBA (recombinant immunoblot assay),
      HCV **395**
ribavirin, HCV, contraindications **396**

ribonucleoprotein complex, hepatitis D
      virus 374–375
Richter hernia *37*
rigid proctosigmoidoscopy,
      instruments *272*
rim sign, acute cholecystitis 804, *806*
RNA tests, hepatitis C virus **395**
Roth Net® 686, *694*
Roussel Uclaf causality assessment
      method 403b
Roux-en-Y gastric bypass 496, 498, 500
   ERCP 635, *641*
Roux-en-Y hepaticojejunostomy,
      enteroscopy *642*
rubber-band ligation
   esophageal varices *670*
   hemorrhoids *274*
      instruments *272*
rugae, stomach 15, *125*
rumination syndrome *71*
rupture of esophagus 102, *104*
Rutgeerts score 232–233

sacral nerve stimulators *283*
saline-assisted polypectomy 680, 682,
      683–684
saline injection, peptic ulcer disease *678*
Salmonella infection *506*
   liver histology *868*
Sandostatin **190**
Santorini's duct *31*
sarcoidosis *548*
   esophagus 109, *110*
   liver histology *871*
   PET *790*
   skin lesions *572*
Sarin's classification, gastric varices *668*
Savary–Gilliard dilator *644*
Schatzki ring 3, 9f, 74, *607*
schistosomiasis 531, *532*
   histology *916*
   life cycle *533*
   liver *872*
Schwann cells *928*
schwannoma, retroperitoneal *488*
scintigraphy *see* radionuclide imaging
scleritis, Crohn's disease *229*
scleroderma *546*
   esophagus *70*
   intestinal dysmotility 168, *169*
sclerosing cholangitis *355*
   IgG4 *290*
   primary 216–218, 354–360, *864*
sclerosing hepatic carcinoma,
      histology *870*
screening
   alcohol abuse *100*
   colorectal cancer 266–269
scrotum, Behçet syndrome *561*
scurvy *572*
sebaceous carcinoma *555*

seborrheic keratoses 558, *559*
SEC63 gene *366*
secretin stimulation 135, *136*
   MRCP *310*
Seldinger technique *821*
self-assembling magnets,
      gastrojejunostomy *713*
self-expandable plastic stent,
      esophagus *659*
sentinel adenoma *925*
sentinel piles, anal fissures *278*
sequential circumferential direct muscle
      stimulation, gastric *119*
serous cystadenoma, pancreas *324*
serrated adenomas 626, *627*
   cancer screening *269*
serrated polyposis syndrome 240, **247**,
      254, 927, 928
serum–ascites albumin gradient 447, **449**,
      451
sessile polyps 626, 627, 629, 630, *927*
   cancer screening *269*
   chromoendoscopy *631*
   resection 682, 683–684, 685, 686, 689,
      693–694
sessile serrated adenomas 254, *927*
Shigella infection 170, *506*
Shikata stain 860, *862*
short bowel syndrome 189–201
shunts, portal hypertension 673, *842*
   see also transjugular intrahepatic
      portosystemic shunt
Shwachman–Diamond syndrome 318,
      323
sickle cells, liver histology *869*
sigmoid colon
   ischemic colitis *918*
   volvulus 28, *29*
signal intensity, MRI *768*
signet-ring cells, gastric cancer *149*
Simple Endoscopic Score, Crohn's
      disease *225*
sincalide, cholescintigraphy 804, *806*
single photon emission tomography
      (SPECT)
   carcinoids *818*
   gastroparesis 116, *120*
   islet cell tumor *817*
   liver *809*
   metastases *819*
single-port laparoscopic surgery 699–700
sinusoidal obstruction syndrome 472, 474,
      475
   radiation injury *599*
sinus tracts, Crohn's disease,
      esophagus 885–886
skin lesions 551–573
   Crohn's disease 229, *230*
   esophageal involvement *110*
   fibromas, familial adenomatous
      polyposis *253*

necrolytic migratory erythema *330, 559*
ulcerative colitis 216
see also enterocutaneous fistula
skin tags, anal, Crohn's disease 231
slow-transit constipation 162, *164, 165,*
167b, 168
slow waves, gastrointestinal 162
sludge, gallbladder *344, 738, 739*
small bowel enema 722
non-Hodgkin lymphoma *729*
small bowel follow-through, Crohn's
disease 225–226, *228*
small intestine 19–23, 208–215, 62
AIDS *see Mycobacterium avium*
complex
anomalies 19–23
capsule endoscopy *619, 620*
carcinoids 202, *205,* 729
angiography *832*
chronic infections 177–183
cystic fibrosis 317, *321, 322*
dilation (therapeutic) 648
function disorders 184–188
immunoproliferative disease **248**
metastases *550, 728, 787*
motility disorders 157–169
non-Hodgkin lymphoma *729*
obstruction *761, 767*
Peutz–Jeghers syndrome *624*
pneumatosis *760*
tumors 202–207
algorithm *623*
capsule endoscopy *625*
SmartPill (wireless motility capsule) 116,
121
SMOF lipids (lipid emulsion) 191, *201*
smooth muscle actin, stellate cells 436,
440, 443
snare polypectomy *629, 681, 682,*
683–684, 685, 688
snares, detachable *680, 688*
sodium polystyrene sulfonate *879*
sodium taurocholate cotransporter
polypeptide *380*
solid meal, indium-111 radiolabeled 116,
120
solid pseudopapillary epithelial neoplasm,
pancreas *325*
somatostatin receptor analog, PET
radiotracer *782, 803*
somatostatin receptor imaging 810–811
islet cell tumor *817*
SOX-10 (transcription factor), visceral
neuropathies 159
space of Disse 51
stellate cells 439
sphincter of Oddi 43, *48*
dysfunction 292–294, *806, 808*
sphincterotomy
ERCP 634
pancreatic duct *640*

sphincters
anal 24, *26*
dysfunction **270,** *280*
sonography *281*
squeeze pressures **270,** *283*
see also lower esophageal sphincter
spider angioma *567*
Spigelian hernia 37, *41*
spindle cell sarcoma, retroperitoneal *488*
spine, access by NOTES *708*
spirochetes
anorectal 170
colitis *916*
spironolactone, ascites 448, 453
spleen
candidiasis *552*
lymphoma *545*
radionuclide imaging *809*
sarcoidosis *548*
splenectomy, laparoscopic *700*
splenic artery
angiography 839–840
embolization *830,* 839–840, *841*
pseudoaneurysm *841*
splenic flexure, watershed areas *918*
splenomegaly
angiography *841*
computed tomography *763*
schistosomiasis *531*
splenoportography, percutaneous 840
splenosis, SPECT/CT *812*
spontaneous bacterial peritonitis 447, 448,
449, 456
albumin for 448, 449, *455*
sprue
CVID 510
see also celiac disease
squamous cell carcinoma
anorectal 245, *785*
anus 285, *286, 930*
PET *796*
esophagus 93, *889*
barium studies *94*
endoscopy *95, 610*
fistula *652*
histology *96*
PET *792*
prosthesis *650*
hypopharynx *726*
squamous papilloma, esophagus *887*
squeeze pressures, anal sphincters **270,**
283
staging laparoscopy 698
stains
Helicobacter pylori 142–143, *144*
intestinal metaplasia 140
liver biopsy *860*
oil red O, stellate cells *436, 439*
periodic acid–Schiff staining, small
intestine 177, *178, 179*
starry sky pattern, sonography *732, 733*

steatorrhea
chronic pancreatitis *323*
primary sclerosing cholangitis 354
steatosis 428, *429, 434*
AIDS *508*
magnetic resonance imaging *774*
sonography *732, 733*
stellate calcification, serous
cystadenoma *324*
stellate cells, liver 51, 436, *438, 439–440,*
442, 443
stent-in-stent removal 660–661
stents
Axios stent *303, 304*
biliary tract *637, 752, 753*
PET *791*
colon *656*
common bile duct *759, 855*
double pigtail *647*
duodenum *655*
esophagus *609, 651, 653, 654*
computed tomography *758*
fistula *100*
migration 662–663
self-expandable plastic *659*
gastrointestinal *643*
gastrojejunostomy 657–658
inferior vena cava stenosis *853*
mesenteric *582, 586, 587, 588*
pancreatic duct *314, 635, 636, 639*
superior mesenteric artery stenosis *851*
transjugular intrahepatic portosystemic
shunt 448, *854*
vertical sleeve gastrectomy
dehiscence 660–661
stiffness, liver 425, 442, *444*
stomach 13, 153–156, *743*
adenocarcinoma 149–152, *615, 616, 897*
computed tomography *758*
histology *900*
PET *794*
adenomas
gastric type *896*
intestinal type *895*
amyloidosis *910*
arteries to *14*
balloons *494*
carcinoids *615, 901, 902*
carcinoma *728, 749*
chromoendoscopy *898*
endoscopic mucosal resection *899,*
900
cytomegalovirus infection *505*
duplication *14*
endoclips *716*
endoscopic ultrasonography 13, *16,*
743, 748, 749
NOTES via *710*
endoscopy *611*
familial adenomatous polyposis *240,*
251

stomach (*cont'd*)
  foreign bodies *155*
    perforation *697*
  gastrointestinal stromal tumor *16, 616, 759, 901*
    resection *700*
  hyperplastic polyp *615, 894*
  liver biopsy via *706*
  minimally invasive surgery via *see entries beginning* transgastric …
  motility disorders *115–123*
    radionuclide imaging *809–810, 815, 816*
  non-Hodgkin lymphoma *507, 551*
  NOTES via *702, 703*
    appendectomy *712*
    endoscopic ultrasonography *710*
    fallopian tube ligation *718*
    hybrid technique *711*
    walled-off pancreatic necrosis *704*
  pancreatic necrosectomy via *304, 316*
  Peutz–Jeghers syndrome *257, 910, 911*
  PTEN hamartoma *263*
  rugae *15, 125*
  surgery
    vertical banded gastroplasty *495, 499*
    see also gastrectomy; gastrojejunostomy
  ulcers *727*
    malignant *615, 897*
  varices *664–674, 830*
    chronic pancreatitis *307, 312*
  Whipple disease, biopsy *177*
  xanthomas *895*
  see also entries beginning gastric … or gastro …; gastritis
stomal ulcers, bariatric surgery *493, 495, 496, 497, 612*
stones
  kidney, ulcerative colitis *218*
  pancreas, ERCP *634–635, 639*
  see also choledocholithiasis; cholelithiasis; oxalate
straight-line sign, peritoneal carcinomatosis *784*
strictures
  anorectal *751*
  bariatric surgery *495, 497, 498, 500*
  biliary tract, ERCP *634*
  colon *647*
  Crohn's disease *225, 227*
  dilation *see* dilation (therapeutic)
  duodenum *18*
  esophagus *74, 102, 108, 746*
    caustic *102, 108*
    food impaction *102, 609*
    foreign body impaction *106, 108*
    malignant *746*
    peptic *74, 105, 654*
    see also stents, esophagus

hepatojejunal *856*
pancreatic duct *639*
peptic ulcer disease *130, 654*
primary sclerosing cholangitis *354, 357, 358*
radiation injury *597, 600, 602*
see also stents
Strongyloides stercoralis *529, 530, 903*
subacute mesenteric ischemia *584*
submassive necrosis, liver *386, 862*
submucosal tunneling, NOTES *705, 706, 721*
submucosal tunneling endoscopic resection, leiomyoma *707*
subphrenic abscess *478*
subxiphoid hernia *40*
sucrase–isomaltase deficiency *186, 188,* **188**
Sudeck's point *27*
sulfonamides, hepatotoxicity *872*
sulfur colloid scintigraphy *809*
superior mesenteric artery *26, 582*
  aberrant hepatic artery from *823*
  endoscopic ultrasonography *744*
  occlusion *825*
  pseudoaneurysm *849, 852*
  stenosis *587*
    interventional radiology *851*
  thrombosis *582, 760*
  tumor encasement *759*
  variations *824*
superior mesenteric artery syndrome *15*
superior mesenteric vein
  schistosomiasis *533*
  thrombosis *211, 549, 582, 584, 585*
  tumor encasement *765*
  see also mesenteric veins
supragastric belching *71, 77*
Sutton disease *562*
sutures
  after laparotomy *699*
  NOTES *717*
swallowing, cricopharyngeal bar *63*
Sweet syndrome *562*
syphilis, anorectal *170*
systemic inflammatory response syndrome *287, 288b, 289*
  alcoholic hepatitis *427*
systemic lupus erythematosus, small intestinal ulcers *208*

tablets *see* pill esophagitis
TACE *see* chemoembolization
Taenia spp. *538, 539*
Takayasu arteritis *550*
tapeworms *see* cestodes; *specific species*
target sign, Crohn's disease *227, 228*
tattooing of polyps *682, 683, 684, 688*
taxol, on esophagus *879*
T-cell lymphoma, enteropathy-associated *214*

technetium-99m radionuclide imaging
  gastroparesis *116–117, 118, 120*
  Meckel diverticulum *19*
teduglutide *191*
teeth, gastroesophageal reflux disease *574, 575*
telangiectasia
  colon *632*
  hereditary hemorrhagic *556, 579*
  primary biliary cirrhosis *410*
  radiation injury *597, 601, 602*
terlipressin *449*
terminal ductules *52*
terminal ileum
  carcinoids, PET *803*
  Crohn's disease *630, 633, 907, 908*
  cystic fibrosis *317, 321*
  endoscopy *626, 633*
  ulcerative colitis *218, 633*
Terry nails *568*
thermal therapy
  peptic ulcer disease *678*
  see also electrocoagulation
threads and streaks sign *836*
three-dimensional computed tomography *757*
thrombi, watermelon stomach *148*
thrombosis
  mesenteric veins *209, 211, 544, 549*
  portal vein *472, 473, 474, 763*
  superior mesenteric artery *582, 760*
  superior mesenteric vein *211, 549, 582, 584, 585*
thumbprinting, ischemic colitis *590, 591, 594*
total parenteral nutrition *189, 190, 191,* **192**, *193b*
  children **195**
  complications **197**
  quality of life **198**
  survival rates **199**
toxemia of pregnancy, liver histology *869*
toxic megacolon *218, 219*
trace elements, for short bowel syndrome **193, 195**
trachealization, eosinophilic esophagitis *83*
transanal endoscopic microsurgery *720*
transferrin
  carbohydrate-deficient *423*
  saturation *418b, 418*
transgastric biopsy, liver *706*
transgastric necrosectomy, pancreas *304, 316*
transgastric NOTES
  endoscopic ultrasonography *710*
  hybrid *711, 718*
  transgastric peritoneoscopy *703, 711*
transient elastography *423, 442, 444*
transient relaxation, gastroesophageal junction *78*

transjugular intrahepatic portosystemic shunt (TIPS) *454*, *672*, *831*, *842*, *854*
  Doppler ultrasonography *735*
  refractory ascites *448*
transjugular liver biopsy *839*, *858*
transjugular portography *831*
transmural intestinal ganglioneuromatosis *163*
transplantation
  bone marrow *512–513*
    neutropenic enterocolitis *548*, *551*, *552*
  intestinal *189–191*, *200*
  liver *see* liver transplantation
transverse colon, endoscopy *626*
trauma, laparoscopy for *698*
trematodes *524*
  see also specific species
Trichinella spp. *543*
Trichuris trichuria *527*
trimethoprim-sulfamethoxazole, liver injury *402–403*
tuberculosis
  esophagus *90*, *91*
  liver histology *871*
  peritonitis *484*, *485*
  small intestine *180*, *181*
tuboovarian abscess *483*
tubular adenoma
  colon *923*, *924*
  duodenum *618*
tubulovillous adenoma *925*
  rectum *235*
  small intestine *202*, *203*
tumefactive sludge, gallbladder *739*
tunneling *see* submucosal tunneling
Turner's sign *296*
tyrosine kinase receptor *159*, *163*

ulcerative colitis *216–224*, *630*, *631*, *913*, *914*
  carcinoma *see* dysplasia
  double-contrast radiography *216*, *220*, *730*
  dysplasia-associated lesions *222–223*, *915*
  oral lesions *574*
  peristomal varices *354*, *357*
  PET *800*
  primary sclerosing cholangitis *216–218*, *354*
  terminal ileum *218*, *633*
  see also inflammatory bowel disease
ulcers
  adrenaline injection *129*
  anastomotic, bariatric surgery *493*, *495*, *496*, *497*, *612*
  aphthous *see* aphthous stomatitis
  colitis *629*
  colorectal cancer *628*

Crohn's disease *225*, *226*, *227*, *630*, *907*
  duodenum *617*, *728*
  esophagus *726*
    AIDS *85*, *87*, *88*, *89*, *90*, *91*, *92*, *726*
    Behçet syndrome *909*
    candidiasis *883*
    cytomegalovirus infection *87*, *88*, *89*, *610*, *881*, *883*
    herpes simplex virus infection *610*, *882*
  ileum *624*
  ischemic colitis *918*
  malignant, gastric *615*, *897*
  peptic ulcer disease *124*
    bleeding *132*, *133*, *675*, *676*
    endoscopy *125*, *126*, *127*, *128*, *131*
  radiation injury *600*
  rectum *277*
  scrotum
    Behçet syndrome *561*
  small intestine *208–212*
  stomach *727*
    malignant *615*, *897*
  ulcerative colitis *219*, *220*, *913*
ultrasonography *732–740*
  abdominal abscesses *483*
  anal *281*
  ascites *447*, *450*, *737*
  chronic hepatitis B *387*
  Doppler *see* Doppler ultrasonography
  endoscopic *see* endoscopic ultrasonography
  gastrointestinal tract *738–740*
  hepatitis *732*, *733*
  liver abscesses *469*, *470*
  pancreas *738*, *740*, *744*, *750*
    pseudocyst *308*
umbilical hernia *37*, *40*, *458*
umbilical vein, injection into *719*
unilamellar vesicles, bile *338*
upper gastrointestinal endoscopy *605–620*
  hemorrhage *675–679*
  techniques *606*
upper gastrointestinal hemorrhage
  chronic pancreatitis *307–308*
  endoscopy *675–679*
  management *124–128*, *129*, *130*
  portal hypertension *664–674*
upper gastrointestinal tract, definition *621*
  urethra, NOTES via *702*
urinary tract, PET and *782*
ursodeoxycholic acid, for primary biliary cirrhosis *414*
uterus, NOTES in *719*

vaccination, acute viral hepatitis *377*
vagina, NOTES via *702*, *702*, *719*
valleculae, pharynx *724*
varices
  esophageal *608*, *664–674*
    grading *664*, *667*

gastric *612*, *614*, *664–674*, *830*
  chronic pancreatitis *307*, *312*
  peristomal, ulcerative colitis *354*, *357*
vascular anomalies, esophagus *3*, *6f*
vascular ectasia *544*, *545*, *548*
  cecum *830*
  see also angioectasia; gastric antral vascular ectasia
vasculitis *582–596*
  leukocytoclastic *571*
vegetating pyoderma gangrenosum *577*
venesection *415*
venoocclusive disease, hepatic
  radiation injury *599*
  see also sinusoidal obstruction syndrome
venous drainage, liver *53*
venous malformations
  esophageal *3*, *6f*
  oral *574*, *579*
vertebra, biopsy *708*
vertical banded gastroplasty *495*, *499*
vertical sleeve gastrectomy, dehiscence *660–661*
videoendoscopes *605–606*
villi, radiation injury *598*
vimentin, stellate cells *440*
VIPoma *331*
viral hepatitis
  acute *374–386*, *872*, *873*
    histology *386*
  chronic *376*, *377*
    biopsy *860*, **861**, *874*
    see also under hepatitis B virus
  Epstein–Barr virus *866*, *874*
viral infections, esophagus *85*, *87*, *88*, *89*, *90*
virtual colonoscopy, polyps *762*
visceral myopathies *157–159*, **159**, *160*, *161*, **161**
visceral neuropathies *159*, *162*, *166–168*
  c-KIT *159*, *165*
  idiopathic nonfamilial *167–168*
vitamin(s)
  pellagra *572*
  primary biliary cirrhosis *414*
  for short bowel syndrome **193**, **195**
vitamin A excess, liver histology *868*
vitamin B-12 deficiency, tongue *581*
vitamin C deficiency *572*
vitamin D, supplementation algorithm *196*
vocal cords *724*
Volumen *756–757*
volume rendering, computed tomography *757*
volvulus
  sigmoid colon *28*, *29*
  small intestine *22*, *23*
  stomach *156*

Waardenburg syndrome *159*
waist circumference *492*

wall-echo-shadow sign 737, *738*
walled-off necrosis, acute pancreatitis 300, *303*, *304*
   endoscopic drainage *704*, *754*
WallFlex stents *657–658*
   Colonic *656*
warfarin, intramural hematoma 544, *549*
watermelon stomach 147–148, *893*
watershed areas
   colorectal blood supply 27
   splenic flexure *918*
weak peristalsis, esophagus *66*, *78*

webs, esophagus 8f, 9f, *610*
wedged hepatic venography *836–839*
Wegener granulomatosis *212*
Whipple disease 177–180, *903*, *904*
Whipple procedure, hepatojejunal stricture *856*
Wilson disease 419, *420*, *421*, *862*
wireless capsule endoscopy *see* capsule endoscopy
wireless motility capsule 116, *121*
Wirsung's duct *31*
withdrawal of drugs, for hepatotoxicity 398–399, *403*

xanthomas *410*
   stomach *895*

Yersinia spp., small intestinal infections 180, *181*
yttrium-90 radioembolization *846*

Zenker diverticulum 3, *10*, *64*
Zimmerman, Hyman *404*
zinc deficiency *190*
Zollinger–Ellison syndrome 135–139, *894*
zones of Rappaport 52